ESSENTIALS OF CLINICAL PSYCHIATRY

Second Edition

ESSENTIALS OF CLINICAL PSYCHIATRY

Second Edition

Edited by

Robert E. Hales, M.D., M.B.A.

Joe P. Tupin Professor and Chair,
Department of Psychiatry and Behavioral Sciences,
University of California, Davis School of Medicine
Medical Director, Sacramento County Mental Health Services,
Sacramento, California

Stuart C. Yudofsky, M.D.

D.C. and Irene Ellwood Professor and Chairman,
Menninger Department of Psychiatry and Behavioral Sciences,
Baylor College of Medicine
Chief, Psychiatry Service, The Methodist Hospital,
Houston, Texas

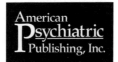

American Psychiatric Publishing, Inc.

Washington, DC
London, England

Typeset in Adobe's Revival, Caecilia, and Formata

Manufactured in the United States of America on acid-free paper
07   06   05   5   4   3   2

American Psychiatric Publishing, Inc.
1000 Wilson Boulevard
Arlington, VA 22209-3901
www.appi.org

Library of Congress Cataloging-in-Publication Data
Essentials of clinical psychiatry, second edition / edited by Robert E. Hales, Stuart C. Yudofsky.
    p. ; cm.
  Includes bibliographical references and index.
  ISBN 1-58562-033-5 (alk. paper)
   1. Psychiatry. I. Hales, Robert E. II. Yudofsky, Stuart C. III. American Psychiatric Publishing textbook of clinical psychiatry. 4th ed.
   [DNLM: 1. Mental Disorders. 2. Psychiatry. WM 140 E778 2004]
RC454.E823 2004
616.89—dc21

                                                                        2002043673

British Library Cataloguing in Publication Data
A CIP record is available from the British Library.

Essentials of Clinical Psychiatry,
Second Edition,
is dedicated to

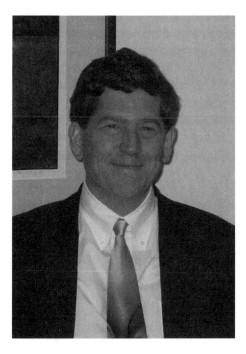 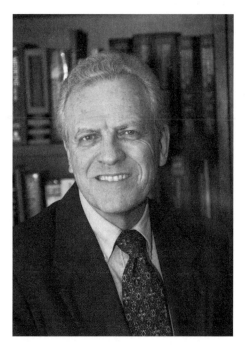

Mark E. Servis, M.D.
Roy Brophy Professor of Psychiatry and
Behavioral Sciences and Vice Chair for
Education, Department of Psychiatry and
Behavioral Sciences, University of
California, Davis School of Medicine,
Sacramento, California

James A. Lomax, M.D.
Associate Chairman for Education,
Menninger Department of Psychiatry and
Behavioral Sciences, Baylor College of
Medicine, Houston, Texas

We thank you for being inspiring educators,
devoted mentors, and perennial friends
for a generation of medical students and residents in psychiatry.

Contents

Contributors

Nancy C. Andreasen, M.D., Ph.D.
Andrew H. Woods Professor of Psychiatry and Director, Iowa Schizophrenia Clinical Research Center, Department of Psychiatry, University of Iowa Roy J. and Lucille A. Carver College of Medicine, Iowa City, Iowa; Director, The MIND Institute, University of New Mexico, Albuquerque, New Mexico

Charles E. Bailey, M.D.
Medical Director, CNS Healthcare, Orlando, Florida

Judith V. Becker, Ph.D.
Professor of Psychology and Psychiatry, Department of Psychology, University of Arizona College of Medicine, Tucson, Arizona

Donald W. Black, M.D.
Professor of Psychiatry, Department of Psychiatry, University of Iowa Roy J. and Lucille A. Carver College of Medicine, Iowa City, Iowa

James A. Bourgeois, O.D., M.D.
Associate Professor of Clinical Psychiatry and Behavioral Sciences and Director of the Psychiatry Consultation-Liaison Service, University of California, Davis School of Medicine, Sacramento, California

Michael Brook, B.S.
Postgraduate Researcher, Department of Psychiatry and Behavioral Sciences, University of California, Davis School of Medicine, Sacramento, California

Stephen J. Cozza, M.D.
Associate Professor of Psychiatry and Vice Chairman of the Department of Psychiatry, F. Edward Hébert School of Medicine, Uniformed Services University of the Health Sciences, Bethesda, Maryland; and Chief, Department of Psychiatry, Walter Reed Army Medical Center, Washington, D.C.

Glen C. Crawford, M.D.
Assistant Professor of Psychiatry, F. Edward Hébert School of Medicine, Uniformed Services University of the Health Sciences; and Staff Child and Adolescent Psychiatrist, Department of Psychiatry, National Naval Medical Center, Bethesda, Maryland

Robert Davies, M.D.
Assistant Professor of Psychiatry, University of Colorado School of Medicine, Denver, Colorado

Amelia N. Dubovsky, B.A.
Graduate Student, Premedical Studies, Columbia University, New York, New York

Steven L. Dubovsky, M.D.
Professor of Psychiatry and Medicine and Vice Chair of the Department of Psychiatry, University of Colorado School of Medicine, Denver, Colorado

Mina K. Dulcan, M.D.
Professor of Psychiatry and Pediatrics, Head of the Department of Child and Adolescent Psychiatry, and Margaret C. Osterman Professor of Child Psychiatry, Children's Memorial Hospital; and Professor of Psychiatry and Behavioral Sciences, Northwestern University Medical School, Chicago, Illinois

Marc D. Feldman, M.D.
Professor, Department of Psychiatry and
Behavioral Neurobiology, and Vice Chair
of Clinical Services, University of Alabama
at Birmingham, Birmingham, Alabama

Richard J. Frances, M.D.
Clinical Professor of Psychiatry, New York
University School of Medicine, New York,
New York; Adjunct Professor of Psychia-
try, University of Medicine and Dentistry
of New Jersey, Newark, New Jersey; and
President and Medical Director, Silver Hill
Hospital, New Canaan, Connecticut

John E. Franklin Jr., M.D., M.Sc.
Associate Professor of Psychiatry and Director of Addiction Psychiatry, Northwestern University Medical School, Evanston,
Illinois

G. Davis Gammon, M.D.
Assistant Clinical Professor, Child Study
Center, Yale University School of Medi-
cine, New Haven, Connecticut

Donald C. Goff, M.D.
Associate Professor of Psychiatry, Harvard
Medical School; and Director, Schizophrenia Program, Massachusetts General Hospital, Boston, Massachusetts

John G. Gunderson, M.D.
Professor of Psychiatry, Harvard Medical
School, Boston; and Director, Psychosocial
Research Program, McLean Hospital, Bel-
mont, Massachusetts

Robert E. Hales, M.D., M.B.A.
Joe P. Tupin Professor and Chair, Depart-
ment of Psychiatry and Behavioral Sciences,
University of California, Davis School of
Medicine; and Medical Director, Sacra-
mento County Mental Health Services,
Sacramento, California

Katherine A. Halmi, M.D.
Professor of Psychiatry, Weill Medical Col-
lege of Cornell University, White Plains,
New York

Margaret E. Hertzig, M.D.
Professor of Psychiatry, Payne Whitney
Clinic, Department of Psychiatry, Weill
Medical College of Cornell University,
New York, New York

Donald M. Hilty, M.D.
Associate Professor of Clinical Psychiatry
and Behavioral Sciences, University of California, Davis School of Medicine, Sacramento, California

Beng-Choon Ho, M.R.C.Psych.
Assistant Professor of Psychiatry and Clin-
ical Director, Iowa Schizophrenia Clinical
Research Center, Department of Psychia-
try, University of Iowa Roy J. and Lucille
A. Carver College of Medicine, Iowa City,
Iowa

Eric Hollander, M.D.
Professor of Psychiatry and Director of
Clinical Psychopharmacology, Department
of Psychiatry, Mount Sinai School of Medicine, New York, New York

Bradley R. Johnson, M.D.
Assistant Professor of Psychiatry, University
of Arizona College of Medicine, Tucson;
and Chief of Psychiatry, Arizona Community Protection and Treatment Center,
Phoenix, Arizona

David J. Kupfer, M.D.
Thomas Detre Professor and Chairman,
Department of Psychiatry, University of
Pittsburgh School of Medicine, Pittsburgh,
Pennsylvania

Martin H. Leamon, M.D.
Assistant Professor of Clinical Psychiatry
and Behavioral Sciences, University of California, Davis School of Medicine, Sacramento, California

Avram H. Mack, M.D.
Fellow, Columbia University College of
Physicians and Surgeons; and Resident Psychiatrist, New York State Psychiatric Institute, New York, New York

José R. Maldonado, M.D.
Assistant Professor and Chief, Medical Psychiatry Section, and Director, Medical Psychotherapy Clinic, Department of Psychiatry and Behavioral Sciences, Stanford University School of Medicine; and Medical Director, Consultation/Liaison Service, Stanford University Medical Center, Stanford, California

Lauren B. Marangell, M.D.
Brown Foundation Professor of Psychopharmacology of Mood Disorders, Menninger Department of Psychiatry and Behavioral Sciences, Baylor College of Medicine, Houston, Texas

Jeffrey Newcorn, M.D.
Associate Professor of Psychiatry and Director of the Child Psychiatry Division, Division of Child and Adolescent Psychiatry, Department of Psychiatry, Mount Sinai School of Medicine, New York, New York

Thomas C. Neylan, M.D.
Assistant Professor in Residence, University of California, San Francisco School of Medicine and Veterans' Affairs Medical Center, San Francisco, California

Katharine A. Phillips, M.D.
Professor of Psychiatry, Brown Medical School; and Director, Body Dysmorphic Disorder Program, Butler Hospital, Providence, Rhode Island

Charles W. Popper, M.D.
Clinical Instructor in Psychiatry, Harvard Medical School, Boston; and Attending Psychiatrist, McLean Hospital, Belmont, Massachusetts

Charles F. Reynolds III, M.D.
Professor of Psychiatry and Neurology and Director of the Mental Health Clinical Research Center for Late-Life Mood Disorders, University of Pittsburgh School of Medicine, Pittsburgh, Pennsylvania

Stephen C. Scheiber, M.D.
Adjunct Professor of Psychiatry, Northwestern University Feinberg School of Medicine, Chicago, Illinois; Adjunct Professor of Psychiatry, Medical College of Wisconsin, Milwaukee, Wisconsin; and Executive Vice President, American Board of Psychiatry and Neurology, Deerfield, Illinois

Charles L. Scott, M.D.
Assistant Professor of Clinical Psychiatry and Behavioral Sciences and Chief of Forensic Psychiatry, University of California, Davis School of Medicine, Sacramento, California

Jeffrey S. Seaman, M.S., M.D.
Clinical Assistant Professor in Psychiatry, University of Texas Health Sciences Center at San Antonio; and Director, Consultation-Liaison Service, Department of Psychiatry, Wilford Hall Medical Center, Lackland Air Force Base, San Antonio, Texas

Mark E. Servis, M.D.
Roy Brophy Professor of Psychiatry and Behavioral Sciences, Associate Professor of Clinical Psychiatry and Behavioral Sciences, and Vice Chair for Education, Department of Psychiatry and Behavioral Sciences, University of California, Davis School of Medicine, Sacramento, California

Theodore Shapiro, M.D.
Professor of Psychiatry and Professor of Psychiatry in Pediatrics, Payne Whitney Clinic, Department of Psychiatry, Weill Medical College of Cornell University, New York, New York

Edward K. Silberman, M.D.
Clinical Professor of Psychiatry and Human Behavior and Director of Residency Education, Department of Psychiatry and Human Behavior, Jefferson Medical College of Thomas Jefferson University Hospital, Philadelphia, Pennsylvania

Jonathan M. Silver, M.D.
Clinical Professor of Psychiatry, New York University School of Medicine; and Assistant Director for Clinical Services and Research, Department of Psychiatry, Lenox Hill Hospital, New York, New York

Daphne Simeon, M.D.
Associate Professor of Psychiatry, Mount Sinai School of Medicine, New York, New York

David Spiegel, M.D.
Willson Professor and Associate Chair of Psychiatry and Behavioral Sciences, Department of Psychiatry and Behavioral Sciences, Stanford University School of Medicine, Stanford, California

James J. Strain, M.D.
Professor of Psychiatry, Mount Sinai School of Medicine/New York University Medical Center Health Service, New York, New York

Robert J. Ursano, M.D.
Professor of Psychiatry and Neuroscience and Chairman of the Department of Psychiatry, F. Edward Hébert School of Medicine, Uniformed Services University of the Health Sciences, Bethesda, Maryland

Scott A. West, M.D.
President and Chief Executive Officer, CNS Healthcare, Orlando, Florida

Shirley Yen, Ph.D.
Assistant Professor, Department of Psychiatry and Human Behavior, Brown Medical School, Providence, Rhode Island

Stuart C. Yudofsky, M.D.
D.C. and Irene Ellwood Professor and Chairman, Menninger Department of Psychiatry and Behavioral Sciences, Baylor College of Medicine; and Chief, Psychiatry Service, The Methodist Hospital, Houston, Texas

Sean H. Yutzy, M.D.
Associate Professor of Psychiatry and Director of Forensic Services, Department of Psychiatry, University of New Mexico, Albuquerque, New Mexico

Preface

The *Essentials of Clinical Psychiatry* provides a synopsis of the most important material included within the fourth edition of *The American Psychiatric Publishing Textbook of Clinical Psychiatry* and was developed specifically for those needing a concise reference of clinical psychiatry. Although this work will provide psychiatry residents, fourth-year medical students on psychiatry electives, and practicing psychiatrists a complete, yet abridged, overview of clinical psychiatry, it will also serve anyone seeking a clear and direct reference on this subject. As such it will prove useful to both physicians in other fields as well as lay persons who are interested in clinical psychiatry.

With its more concise structure, this book intends to provide core knowledge to the busy trainee or practitioner on psychiatric assessment and treatment of children, adolescents, adults, and seniors. It takes a biopsychosocial approach to patient treatment, including both psychotherapy and psychopharmacology.

In recognition of the importance of the clinical treatment of children and adolescents, a quarter of this work is dedicated to this subject: three of its chapters are titled "Normal Child and Adolescent Development," "Disorders Usually First Diagnosed in Infancy, Childhood, or Adolescence," and "Treatment of Children and Adolescents."

To develop the subject matter of this work, we carefully reviewed the 40 chapters contained within *The American Psychiatric Publishing Textbook of Clinical Psychiatry* and selected the 20 that we felt were most important and relevant for clinical practice in a variety of settings: inpatient, partial hospitalization, outpatient, and rehabilitation programs. Our goal was create an economical paperback version of the *Textbook* that remained focused on key clinical information concerning selected psychiatric disorders. At the same time, we endeavored to present this essential knowledge base and the methods of psychiatric treatment in a manner that was both exciting and accessible.

One important feature that gives *Essentials of Clinical Psychiatry* its particular effectiveness is the combined effort of senior and junior authors in certain chapters. The addition of junior authors has infused the chapters with new research insights and fresh and expanded perspectives on the subject matter. The senior authors have complemented these new ideas with their considerable wisdom and vast research and clinical experience. We believe that these collaborations both increase the appeal of the chapters to readers at all levels of educational and clinical experience and enrich the diversity and quality of the material presented.

The challenging task of condensing the 1,758-page *Textbook* into an abbreviated volume required outstanding editorial skills from the APPI team. We are fortunate that Jennifer Wood assumed the role of Project Editor and performed in her usual outstanding fashion. A number of other people at American Psychiatric Publishing, Inc. (APPI) also helped us a great deal with this project. First, we would like to thank CEO Ron McMillen for his support and encouragement in developing the work. In addition, John McDuffie, Editorial Director, and Pam Harley, Managing Editor, Books Department, provided a number of helpful suggestions concerning its structure and formatting. Bob Pursell, Director of Marketing, designed an effective marketing strategy to "spread the word" on the book and its approach to its subjects. Anne Barnes, Graphic Design Manager, and Judy Castagna, Manufacturing Manager, are to be congratulated for producing this book in a very short period of time. We also would like to thank Robin Simpson, who coordinated the contractual paperwork between APPI and the authors.

The editorial headquarters for this work was located at the University of California, Davis. Tina Coltri-Marshall handled all of the complex interactions with our 49 authors and APPI editorial staff with her usual efficiency, skill, and good humor. The project would not have been accomplished on time without her invaluable help.

Last and most importantly, we would like to thank our outstanding authors for carefully reviewing their chapters and skillfully sculpting them into well-edited summaries of their topics. Because of their efforts, readers of this work will find the information it contains is easily accessible, concise, and clinically relevant to psychiatric practice. As a result, we believe that *Essentials of Clinical Psychiatry* will prove to be a useful companion volume to the fourth edition of *The American Psychiatric Publishing Textbook of Clinical Psychiatry* and will establish itself as a vital source for clinical information.

Robert E. Hales, M.D., M.B.A.
Sacramento, California

Stuart C. Yudofsky, M.D.
Houston, Texas

Normal Child and Adolescent Development

Theodore Shapiro, M.D.

Margaret E. Hertzig, M.D.

The current focus in modern psychiatry on descriptive nomenclatures, diagnosis, and treatment does not necessarily include a developmental point of view. On the other hand, there are strong historical and clinical reasons why any student of personality and pathology within a medical framework should be interested in what is known about the normal developmental process.

Historical Background

The understanding of psychiatrists such as Pinel, who recorded longitudinal histories from patients in the French asylums, that psychopathology in adulthood may have something to do with life history is deeply ingrained in the notion of "humane treatment." In the United States, Adolf Meyer, founder of the concept of psychobiology, emphasized the life event chart as a mainstay of clinical knowledge. Freud, at the beginning of the twentieth century, elaborated the idea that the first 5 years of life had a determining effect on later psychopathology and development.

From a more general medical vantage point, pediatrics was split off from general medicine. Most pediatricians consider themselves practitioners of developmental medicine. Thus, the notions of developmental medicine and developmental psychiatry are the historical roots from which specific areas of knowledge and skill have grown. Such increased awareness has compelled us to look at normal growth and development as a key component of our work as well as an essential basis for etiological thought.

Outside of medicine, the language of developmental psychology derives from Darwin's linking of variation in forms of life to their survival value in evolution. Darwin's formulations then led to Ernst Haeckel's biogenetic law that "ontogeny recapitulates phylogeny." Concepts such as maturation, development, differentiation, pleiomorphism, and organizers all have been borrowed from embryology and have enriched our understanding of how children start to be, beginning with gametization, embryogenesis, and then birth and progressing to later developmental stages that can be observed and staged.

Developmental Principles

The terms *growth*, *maturation*, and *development*, although used imprecisely in common parlance, connote a direction from more global reactiveness to more specified reactiveness and from a less complex organization to a more complex state of organization. *Growth* usually refers to the simple accretion of tissue (i.e., an increase in size or in the number of cells). Changes in height and weight are examples of growth. *Maturation* is a convenient fiction that has a somewhat teleological implication of a direction toward which the individual is headed in accord with his or her functions, abilities, structures, and competencies. In its most narrow meaning, the term suggests that there is a natural unfolding of genetic potential toward an end that is known as "maturity." This end can come about in average, expectable environments given the premise that the organism has average species-specific biological equipment. The concept does not invoke the variation that may occur in certain special ecologies. *Development*, on the other hand, includes whatever the maturational potential provides plus the variations in social and environmental influence. This concept refers to the changing structure of behavior and thought over time.

Normative studies suggest a cephalocaudal developmental sequence, with the head end of the organism at the beginning of life presenting as a more highly differentiated functional entity than the tail end. Biological forces such as myelinization of the central long tracts progressing from head to toe help us to understand that regardless of the cultural variation in the early months, most human children begin to walk between the ages of 10 and 18 months (Gesell and Amatruda 1947). Similarly, along with the achievement of that motor landmark, the landmarks of language development occur in a lockstep sequence.

No matter what language is spoken by the parent, by the time the child is 2 years old, he or she usually can string together two- and sometimes three-word utterances with some competence in grammatical formatting. Any errors that are made derive from overgeneralization of grammatical rules and are not random. However, to add complexity, each line of development may mature independently, such as in a limited cerebral palsy affecting only the small section of the cortex that controls limb motor pathways.

From the developmental vantage, these maturational regularities are acted on by social nurturing influences; the achievements are not entirely innate. For example, if a child is tied down or forced to remain recumbent, the maturational event of walking surely will be delayed because of muscular disuse. Similarly, although the capacity for language and grammar may be built in, children will not achieve speech and language in the usual manner if they are deaf or if they are not spoken to.

Differentiation and Integration

Maturation within individual systems also requires that we consider another central theme in development, *differentiation*. Just as the blastosphere differentiates into endoderm, ectoderm, and mesoderm, and these further mature into more highly differentiated tissues, so, too, do psychological and social systems differentiate. In a psychological sense, the general arousal of infants differentiates selectively into responses signifying that the child distinguishes between human and nonhuman, mother and nonmother, friend and foe.

Integration also emerges between and among the varying senses. In the beginning the eye sees what impinges on it; the hand grasps that which is put into it. At 3 or 4 months, if the child sees the hand and the thing to be grasped in the same visual field, he or she will grasp. It is not until some time later that the child reaches for that which he or she sees even if the hand is not in the visual field. At a psychological level, the capacity to put together good and bad experiences with a person and also to change set in relation to varying exposures requires integration. As the infant, showing more differentiated and integrated functioning, moves from the more global apprehension of the world, he or she may also lose some functions that were natively available.

Hierarchic Reorganization and Critical Periods

As each stage unfolds, the question arises as to whether it could unfold without the child having had to pass through the prior stage. *Epigenesis* is the concept of sequential steps influencing subsequent steps. Each stage in that model is highly dependent on resolution of the experiences of the prior stage. The epigenetic vantage point permits, but it does not necessarily include, another model that is known as *hierarchic reorganization.* According to this concept, each new integration of biological and neuronal function meshes with psychocognitive capacities that are more than the sum of their parts. Each stage is truly a new structure permitting functions and adaptations that are not easily predicted from their precursors. These reorganizations permit the next level of behavior and competence as the child pulls himself or herself along the chronological ladder.

Invoking a hierarchically reorganized

sequence permits consideration of a concept known as *critical periods*, which require that an environmental releaser stimulate the emergence of a developmental capacity that is inborn and ready for use only within a limited time period. If no release occurs, the function is said to *involute*. However, such releasers may not adequately describe the way in which human biological development takes place, because the time lines are not as critically limited as in other mammals.

Developmental Psychologies

Most psychiatrists are well versed in the retrospective reconstructive attitude of the Freudian developmental system. The *genetic point of view* was Freud's attempt to retrospectively divine the infantile roots of adult behavior and pathology. His assumptions of polymorphously perverse infantile sexuality and the maturational sequences described in libido theory were based on retrospective reconstructions of how men and women seem to organize their fantasy lives. Later psychoanalytic thinkers (e.g., Mahler et al. 1975; Spitz 1965) created their own developmental systems that elaborated Freud's system.

The behavioral vantage point, which was well outlined in the initial work of Watson (1919) and then B.F. Skinner (1953), is based on learning theory and takes a Lockean philosophical position in which experience is said to be inscribed on a blank slate of mind, thereby transforming it. No competence becomes possible that is not learned. Furthermore, nothing can be learned that is not within the capacity of the species, which in turn determines the limits of responsiveness. The virtue of a learning model for development is that such a model can be empirically apprehended and there is little inferred substructure and very few intervening variables.

Jean Piaget set out to determine how intelligent behavior evolves. Calling himself a "genetic epistemologist," he addressed the issue of how children strategically arrive at right or wrong answers by means of their native capacities and regularized sequence of stages. The normative developmental theory of Arnold Gesell (Gesell and Amatruda 1947) is more closely related to those of the learning theorists, but within the medical framework. Gesell attempted to unify the biological and neurodevelopmental principles that were available at that time from embryogenesis and the normative sequences of observed behaviors. Gesell's studies inspired others to examine large numbers of children "cross-sectionally" in order to find out what they do at each chronological age. Normative, cross-sectional studies, however, do not tell how one progresses (i.e., the process) throughout the longitudinal cycle from one stage to another. *Longitudinal studies* more easily address such issues. Although longitudinal studies are not generally reported in terms of how child A responds at point X and then at point Y, investigators in such studies do have the potential to do just that: to track developmental facts in individual subjects at varying stages, looking for outcomes from past behaviors and checking on retrospective suggestions.

Psychoanalytic Developmental Viewpoint

The psychoanalytic view of childhood derives from two sources. The first source (i.e., *genetic*) uses retrospective and reconstructive inferences about the patient's past to construct a coherent and plausible sequenced history. The other source (i.e., *developmental*), based on the prospective studies by psychoanalytically oriented observers, attempts to observationally flesh out the models of development derived from the genetic point of view.

The Freudian Perspective

Freud's initial view of childhood as a period of polymorphously perverse infantile sexuality grew out of his observation that adult disorder reveals certain constant, compelling features. Adult sexuality consists not only of coitus and gametization, but of erotic arousal that depends on stimulation of various bodily zones. Perverse activity and normal foreplay both led to arousal and orgasmic behavior. In Freud's view, neurotic individuals did not dare think about the things that perverse individuals perpetrated. On these grounds, Freud suggested that repression was the prime mechanism that both hid and modified early sexual thoughts from the conscious minds of neurotic individuals. Libido theory was introduced to describe the maturational sequence that children were expected to traverse en route to adulthood. The theory included the active and passive aims of children seen retrospectively in relation to their primary objects, mother and father. These aims became what Erikson (1963) called the enactments and fantasies of the tragedies and comedies that occur around the orifices of the body.

Psychopathology was viewed by Freud as the result of either a fixation at (i.e., an arrest in the progress of psychosexual maturation) or a regression to (i.e., a symbolic or functional return to earlier ways of acting or thinking) one or another of these stages. As Erikson (1963) noted, the body zones and modes of function are analogous to other behaviors in life. For example, ingesting and spitting out as bodily acts were thought to become introjection and projection as mental defenses, and so forth.

Freud took up a strongly developmental position in response to the challenge thrown before him by Otto Rank, who wrote that birth anxiety was at the center of symptom formation. Freud (1926/1959b) suggested that anxiety only breaks through to consciousness when successful repression does not take place and that anxiety functions as a signal that a dangerous situation is at hand in response to the emergence of specific thoughts as they threaten to break into consciousness. Freud posited a hierarchy of threats that humans have to evaluate and cope with during early childhood. Helplessness is the first signal of danger. Separation, occurring somewhere between 7 and 24 months, follows, and then castration anxiety (or body integrity anxiety) takes over from the third to the sixth years. Finally, danger of punishment by guilt ensues from an internalized value system embodied in the superego, which is an agency of the tripartite mind of the new structural model. The progression moves, as Freud (1926/1959b) suggests, from fear of loss of the object to fear of loss of the love of the object, with, in this instance, the mental object being a representation of the mother.

The Perspective of Ego Psychology

Freud's work was followed by empirical observations by others who moved away from depth psychology toward what was called *ego psychology*.

Spitz's genetic field theory. Rene Spitz's (1965) genetic field theory was derived from direct observation of infants. He invoked the concept of the "organizer" in the development of human behavior, and there are three organizers that have significance for the differentiation process.

Spitz's first organizer, the *smiling response*, includes a consistent and repeatable social smile in response to a full face or a moving oval with darkened areas representing eyes. The format of the human face entailed here suggests that this is the first "not-me" object to be appreciated by an infant. This maturational landmark links outside experience and autonomous function, supporting the notion of a regularly responsive internalization en route to what psychoanalysts call *object constancy*.

The next organizer, the *stranger response*, occurs at about 7 months. The child now turns away from the stranger with apprehension, terminating what Anna Freud (1965) has called the period of *need satisfying object*. This second organizer marks the attachment to a specific other.

The third organizer, the *development of the signal for no*, then signifies a fully internalized and individuated human toddler who now can undo with a verbal signal.

Mahler's separation-individuation theory. Mahler's (Mahler et al. 1975) separation-individuation theory continues the process of development into the postuterine period, involving the "hatching" of human consciousness, with the toddler as a separate, discrete autonomous agency. In Mahlerian terms the child moves from an autistic to a symbiotic stage in which he or she is initially enmeshed psychologically with the mother as though he or she were not separate from the mother.

During the *differentiation* subphase, psychological birth occurs under the rubric of hatching, which is characterized by a permanently alert sensorium in which visual and manual examination of the external world become central. Next emerges the *practicing subphase*, which is characterized by increased curiosity. The child now appears as if he or she were omnipotent and as if an internal agency were not dissociated from an external agency. Only with the understanding that the mother is separate, during the next subphase, does the child arrive at what is called *object constancy*, which ensues at about 25 months to 3 years. Relative independence can occur when a child is able to maintain a stable mental image of an important caretaker.

Anna Freud's multilinear theory. Anna Freud (1974) described a series of developmental lines according to which the child moves 1) from being nursed to rational eating, 2) from wetting and soiling to bowel and bladder control, 3) from egocentricity toward companionship with peers, 4) from play to the capacity to work, 5) from physical to mental pathways of discharge of drives, 6) from animate to inanimate objects, and 7) from irresponsibility to guilt. One can infer from these observations and their variations that a central theme evolves concerning how the child organizes behavior in an affective climate and in relation to others. This has become the observational groundwork of what now is called *object relations theory* in psychoanalysis, in which the object referred to is the child's mental representation of significant adults such as parents.

In recent years psychoanalytic theory has turned toward self psychology. Daniel Stern (1985) offered developmental empirical data delineating the emergence from a core sense of self to a verbal self within the evolving matrix of mother–infant communication.

Normative Cross-Sectional Development

Cross-sectional developmental observers determine what children can do at varying ages and seek to construct sequential maps consisting of stages (Table 1–1). Gesell divided behavior into four sectors: motor, adaptive, language, and personal-social (Gesell and Amatruda 1947). He tracked these behavioral observations over the long period of infancy and described a

normative timetable. The essential question asked is, Does the child at age X achieve behavior in accord with what most children at age X can do? Gesell's organizing principle was neurodevelopmental integrity. He watched the child in the supine and prone positions give way to the sitting position and then to the standing and walking position. Nonetheless, Gesell matched Freud when he stated that the developmental span that lies between birth and 5 years is formative and of major significance for the entire life of the human organism. The developmental quotient (i.e., maturational age divided by chronological age and then multiplied by 100 [$(MA/CA) \times 100$]) gives a rough index of what the child tested can do at each stage.

Other cross-sectional schemes of childhood pertain largely to the development of intelligence. Binet (1905) invented the IQ measure for that purpose. His test was revised in the United States as the Stanford-Binet Intelligence Test, which has been in continuous use as the IQ standard ever since. It has become, with revisions, a normative outline of what children are, on the average, capable of at each age.

Most studies of development rest on cross-sectional visions similar to the IQ and Gesell's developmental quotient. The most recent studies of cross-sectional behavior have tried to include a large sector of behaviors other than verbal behavior. Thus, the Wechsler Intelligence Scale for Children (WISC; Wechsler 1949) was designed to include both verbal and performance scales.

Piagetian Cognitive Development

Piaget took a unique stance when he noted that getting the right answer is only one aspect of intelligence. He wished to understand *how it is that children come to*

TABLE 1–1. Landmarks of normal behavioral development—the revised Gesell developmental schedules

Age	Motor (gross/fine)	Adaptive	Language	Personal/social
4 weeks	Tonic neck reflex position; rotates head when prone; makes alternating crawling movements	Responds to sound; follows moving objects to midline	Small throaty noises	Regards face; reduces activity
8 weeks	Symmetric posture seen; head bobbingly erect	Follows moving objects past midline	Vocalizes in response to social stimulation; sustained "cooing"	Follows moving person; smiles responsively
16 weeks	Symmetric posture predominates; holds head balanced; hands engage in midline; rolls to prone	Looks at object in hand	Laughs and squeals; "talks" to people/toys spontaneously	Initiates social smile; smiles and vocalizes at mirror; discriminates strangers (20 weeks)
28 weeks	Sits unsupported with hands up (1 minute); gets to hands and knees	One hand reach and grasp of toy; transfers toy	Vocalizes "m-m-m" when crying; understands name (32 weeks)	Gets feet to mouth; tries to obtain toys out of reach
40 weeks	Sits indefinitely with hands free (36 weeks); pulls to stand (36 weeks); cruises; lets self down; inferior pincer grasp	Matches two objects in midline; uncovers toy (44 weeks)	"Mama" or "Dada" and two "words" with meaning; responds to "no-no"	Initiates "pat-a-cake" and "peek-a-boo"; holds own bottle (36 weeks); helps in dressing; gives toy on request (44 weeks)
52 weeks	Picks up object from floor from standing position; walks several steps; helps turn pages (56 weeks)	Releases toy; imitates scribble; puts round block in formboard spontaneously	Six "words"; uses jargon	Points for wants; hugs doll; offers toy to image in mirror
15 months	Walks alone, seldom falls; walks up stairs, one hand held; creeps down; hurls ball; builds tower of three blocks	Spontaneous scribble; gets toy with stick after demonstration	10–19 words; knows one body part	Feeds self with spoon (spills); says "Thank you"; seeks help; pulls adult's hand to show
18 months	Walks down stairs, one hand held; builds tower of four blocks	Imitates stroke of crayon; places three blocks in formboard after demonstration	20–29 words including names of siblings, friends, relatives; combines two to three words ("daddy go"); asks for more food and drink	Gets spoon to mouth right side up; passes empty dish; echoes two or more last words; imitates mother/father sweeping, hammering, etc.

TABLE 1–1. Landmarks of normal behavioral development—the revised Gesell developmental schedules (*continued*)

Age	Motor (gross/fine)	Adaptive	Language	Personal/social
24 months	Jumps, both feet off floor; kicks large ball on request; builds tower of seven blocks	Imitates vertical stroke; imitates circular scribble; inserts circle, square, triangle in formboard spontaneously	50+ words; uses *I* and *you*; three- to four-word sentences; uses plurals	Occasionally indicates toilet needs; calls self *me*; helps put things away
30 months	Alternates feet going up stairs; rides tricycle using pedals; turns pages singly; builds tower of nine blocks	Names own drawing; imitates horizontal stroke, circle; adapts to rotation of formboard; repeats two digits (1–3 trials)	Eight- to nine-word sentences; carries tune; uses *he* and *she* correctly; relates events of 2–3 days ago	Pours from glass to glass; keeps time to music; pulls up pants; puts shoes on; names self in mirror
36 months	Alternates feet going down stairs; throws ball overhand; builds tower of 10 blocks	Copies vertical and horizontal stroke; copies circle; imitates cross, repeats three digits (1–3 trials); imitates bridge	Uses *and* or *but*; recites all of a song; knows up and down; follows three commands (three of the following: on, under, in back of, in front of, beside); knows two colors	Fully toilet trained; understands taking turns; plays with other children; washes and dries hands; knows front from back
48 months	Stands on one foot (4–8 seconds); skips on one foot only	Draws person with two parts; adds three parts to incomplete man	Follows four commands	Laces shoes; cooperates with children; goes on errands
60 months	Skips using feet alternately; walks on tiptoe	Adds eight parts to incomplete man; copies square (54 months) and triangle; counts 10 objects pointing; prints first name	Names penny, nickel, dime; describes pictures; asks meanings of words; gives first and last name	Dresses and undresses with little assistance; dresses up in adult clothes; ties a bow

know what they seem to know. Piaget found the regularities in sequence that permit abstract intelligent behavior.

Piaget proposed that the infant is born with two kinds of reflexes: those that remain fixed through life and those that are plastic in response to experience. The experiential world impinges on the child reflexively, and gradually a mental organization, called a *schema*, develops around repeated interactions. The *process* of development remains the same throughout life, but the *structures* change. The repeated process involves a reexperiencing in *assimilation*, but the assimilative schemas can change as they *accommodate*, leading to *adaptation*. For Piaget, assimilation is the incorporation into existing schemas of a structure of action that the subject judges to be equivalent. Accommodation, in turn, occurs when the schema must change to appreciate new objects and differentiate them from old assimilatory forms. Around this universal complementary functional format, the child then passes through four stages: sensorimotor, preoperational, concrete operational, and formal operational.

During the *sensorimotor stage*, no behavior and its schema are separated into sensory and motor components. A thing to be acted on is appreciated as the thing acted on. It does not exist as a sensorily discrete entity without action. It is as though the infant were constantly embedded in a trial-and-error world.

As the infant strips away the motor component, he or she can, between the ages of 18 months and 2 years, maintain a stable mental representation and create a representational world. This inaugurates the *preoperational period*, during which things are worked on in accord with how effective the child is.

The *concrete operational stage*, from 7 to 14 years, introduces a series of functional components suggesting that behav-

ior becomes more rule-governed and that the rules permit decentering. When the child decenters, he or she loses his or her literal egocentricity—that is, he or she can generalize. However, he or she cannot yet generalize from data. Conservation becomes possible, and change in surface appearance does not necessarily signify basic change as in the concepts of volume or weight. Reversal operations may become possible, and trial and error are superseded by mental work employed to solve problems in one's mind, as in equation reversibility.

The later stage, that of *formal operations*, involves reasoning from empirical observations that then can be abstracted as general rules that can be used to dictate future actions. The child is now sufficiently decentered to take on another's vantage point, and reversibility is well established. The rules of logic of language are established. Piaget wrote also about imagination and dreams and about language itself. He looked at these functions as having various logical structures.

Ethological Development

Bowlby recognized the nature of human ties as an organizing precursor to later mature development. He reviewed the nature of the maternal tie and established what he called a component instinctual response system that bore some similarity to Freud's 1905 theory. The infant is described as having five components that make up attachment behavior. Experiences are integrated to create a unified mental representation. The activated reflexes of *sucking*, *clinging*, and *following* have representation in other species, but are also present in the human. *Crying* and *smiling* achieve their ends by reciprocal maternal behavior: they bring the mother to the child. Each of these component instincts is considered to be an inborn response activated by an external caregiver (e.g., the mother). The evolutionary basis for this attachment is accounted for in the survival value and the natural selection for these responses.

Protest, despair, and *grief* were repeatedly observed on separation, and then, if these responses were carried on too long, *denial of need* ensued. These behaviors serve as negative indicators that the normal process of the attached state has been interrupted. This work has been seminal in producing further empirical study of time of attachment, bonding and separation, and strange situation paradigms by which investigators explore attachment (see the "Affective-Interactive Organization" subsection later in this chapter).

Normal Growth and Development: Birth to Prepuberty

Neurodevelopmental and Cognitive Organization

Biodevelopmental Reorganizations in the First 2 Years of Life

The human infant is born with a largely prewired nervous system, with many capacities designed for survival already built into the organism (Stern 1985). Variations in the environment seem to influence the CNS and neuronal networks largely through increases and decreases in the proliferation of synaptic connections and dendritic growth. There is a general proliferation of neural connections through the sixth and seventh year of life, followed by a decline, so that at puberty the network appears less dense (but not, however, as sparse as the network found in the human brain at birth) (Huttenlocher 1979).

Changes on the electroencephalogram (EEG), clinical neurological status, and cognitive levels can be cited to document periods of radical change. These observations have led to formulations on the psychobehavioral level known as *discontinuities in development*, or as *biodevelopmental shifts* by other developmentalists intent on bringing the behavioral level into relation with the substrate (Emde et al. 1976).

Neurological organization.   The first suggestion of a biodevelopmental shift occurs at the time of the first social organizer, the social smile, described by Spitz as signaling the recognition of an external stimulus of the human face as a releaser. The EEG becomes reorganized at a physiological level. Moreover, the rapid heartbeat of early infancy during disposition of attention gives way to slowing of the heartbeat with attentive staring after 2 months.

The six or seven regularly recurring REM periods during adult sleep only gradually emerge, evolving from early infancy (less than 3 months), when light sleep (Stages 1 and 2) dominates the EEG (Roffwarg et al. 1966). Moreover, sleep EEGs of premature infants show that up to 70% of sleep time is spent in a Stage 1 REM pattern. Sleep spindles appear only at 3–4 months, and by 3 months the infantile form of going to sleep that is characterized by rapid shifts from Stage 1 to Stage 4 recedes. These changes parallel the behavioral characteristics known as *settling*, when 70% of babies become night sleepers, rescinding their former pattern of waking at 3- to 4-hour intervals. By the end of the first year of life, the adult pattern of sleep is established on a physiological level.

Motoric behavior.   Gesell emphasized the capacity to turn over, sit upright, and, finally, use bipedal locomotion as developmental markers of maturation. These achievements are signs of the integration of CNS structures. Not only do they sub-

sume the progression from cephalic dominance to the importance of manual dexterity and locomotion in human children, but they also mark the growing capacity of the child to become separate from the caretaking parent on the grounds of motor competence.

Behaviorally, the infant at birth lies in a "fencer" position (tonic neck reflex) and during alert wakeful times can be stimulated to focus, grasp, and respond reflexively to rooting and sucking, all of which are adaptive for survival. These behaviors later give way to lying in a supine position and beginning to use both hands for grasping and mouthing objects as hand–mouth integrations become possible. Only by 10 months does the infant grasp objects in both hands and bring them to the midline. Symmetrical use of limbs and axial support become essential to the child's being able to turn over at 4 months and, ultimately, to achievement of the sitting position at 6 months.

Linguistic behavior. The vocal apparatus is used to produce protolinguistic expressions attracting the environment to the child while the child is incorporating the vocalizations of the surround. Even at this stage, infants seem to be prepared to selectively attend to congruent visual and acoustic signals (MacKain et al. 1983). Infants' babbling begins to take on meaning and significance as it differentiates into the speech of their mothers. Sapir (1921) suggested that in the beginning the child is overheard. Overheard expressive vocalizations in infancy, usually beginning with vowel sounds and gutturals, have been operationally divided into comfort and discomfort series based on the assumption that they have social significance (Lewis 1936). Infants move from expression to appeal to propositioning.

We now understand that the child is well prepared for phonetic distinctions in

that he or she can discriminate phonetic contrasts during the first 4 months (Eimas et al. 1971). This refinement may undergo both specialization and involution as development proceeds so that distinctions that are selectively important in one's language flourish, whereas others disappear (Kuhl 1992).

Cognitive behavior. The cognitive substructures that subsume representational reality and thus constancy are dependent on the achievement of the passage through the sensorimotor period to the preoperational and early concrete operational stages. During this first year of development, the child is undergoing major cognitive shifts in his or her capacity to apprehend the external environment in a manner consonant with commonsense cultural reality. The period from birth to 18 months, from the standpoint of the development of intelligent action, concerns the development of a representational reality that spans the six stages of sensorimotor intelligence, as described by Piaget.

The first and second stages refer to *heterologous and practical groups* in which no behavior pattern relative to vanished objects is observed and each event in time and space does not seem to be connected to its contiguous event. It is as if the experience is fragmented, or cut into frames. As noted, sensory impressions are intimately entwined with motor activity— hence the term *sensorimotor intelligence*. In fact, paradoxically, our adult concept of a distinctive perceptual sensory experience apart from motor activity should be viewed as an achievement of development. Recent work indicates that earliest memories are stored as procedural sequences, only later to be translated into nominal and verbal propositions. The latter changes are related to hippocampal development (Cohen et al. 1985).

The third stage of cognitive development is presumed when the child *extends movements already started*, which indicates that there is some sense of "thing permanence" so that, for example, the child follows the trajectory of the dropped ball to a vanishing point.

The fourth stage is characterized by *reversible operations* of seeking and finding with an active search for the vanished object. However, the child is not yet able to take into account the *sequential displacements* that go on out of sight.

By the fifth stage, *objective groups* are established and there is some sense of the permanence of the object that is extended into the sixth and final stage, that of *representative groups*. Only then can the child imagine invisible displacements. The "thing" finally exists as a mental property, naively but practically assumed to be in the world. From age 16 to 18 months, "things" are freed of their motor components. The child can begin to mentally retrace movements. The possibility of a mental world has become established on purely cognitive grounds.

The establishment of a representational world has some bearing on other matters of representations that touch on emotions. For example, how does the child represent the mother? How does the child keep an image alive as a mental property even in the absence of a stimulus? What are the precursors to fantasying, imagining, and, finally, projecting the future? These features are abstracted in Piaget's model into the minimum set of achievements that are required in the mental schemata that lead to the accession of well-established representations of the external world.

Toddler and Preschool Years: Language and Cognition

From 3 years of age on, the toddler can begin to copy geometric forms, name them, and progressively begin to represent the human figure. The 3-year-old, full of exuberance, is also a language user. He or she can participate at table and can behave in limited social situations. Attendance at nursery school, with its routinized group demands of sharing and taking turns, becomes possible. Fantasy pretend play emerges in the early socialization process as well.

During the preoperational period, the child is still not able to decenter or imagine the vantage point from different positions in a room. There is no conservation of weight or volume and no cardinality of number or reversibility.

Qualitative differences between stages may not be as clear-cut as was formerly thought. An uncanny experiment suggests that some abilities are present early but must reemerge later during the age period of 2–6 years with new cognitive underpinnings. If one puts a cube in an infant's mouth and then presents different shaped objects visually, the child focuses on the cube. Certain children at 3 or 4 years of age can solve some conservation problems, but these problems must be presented in language that is appropriate to the age. This indicates that perhaps some of the failures and difficulties of younger children are due to the kind of language that was used in the initial experiments.

Social referencing is one area in which an early relationship influences cognitive performance. A young child who is capable of crawling (i.e., age 8 months and older) can recognize a "visual cliff" (i.e., an illusion that there is a drop-off, although a transparent Plexiglas plate covers the drop). The child stops crawling at the cliff margin. However, if the mother is at the other end encouraging him or her, the child will proceed in accord with the afforded confidence.

As the child moves into the toddler years, much of what takes place in the cognitive sphere well into the beginnings of school rests on the acquisition of language and communicative ability. The emotional and social climate of learning also becomes very important, and we tend to take the neurodevelopmental aspects and cognitive aspects more for granted until the changes that occur at ages 6 and 7 years. Language competence and performance develop at a rapid pace. The 2-year-old rapidly achieves telegraphic speech of two words, which indicates his or her understanding that some words are more important than others when a message is to be conveyed. The child then adds grammatical morphemes (i.e., small endings on words that signify tense, person, etc.). These rapid shifts occur sequentially, in an orderly manner, in accord with the language that is spoken. By 3 years of age, the child is a fairly competent speaker, with a three- to six-word mean length of utterance (MLU).

It was formerly thought that the first 50-word corpus consisted of only nouns. However, some children have a higher concentration of prepositions and verbs that refer to rather complicated concepts (Nelson 1981). There is general agreement that the child may imitate before he or she comprehends, and that production follows. Thus, there is a greater constraint developmentally on expression production than on understanding. A most remarkable finding that undoes some of the mechanical presuppositions about language development concerns the early detection of narrative lines in children's learning, even with children at age 2 or 3 years (Bretherton 1989; Nelson 1986).

The remarkable achievement of deixis suggests a very early capacity to distinguish a "this" from a "that," or "I" from "you" from "me." These distinctions are regularly achieved by age 2 years. Similarly, concreteness begs for explanation. The child of limited vocabulary who designates his or her dog "Rex" may then see a horse or a sheep and call either "Rex."

The child may exhibit concreteness in other ways because of a limited understanding of the nuances of language. This is most apparent in the adult concept of the *joke*. Jokes told by 5- to 10-year-olds tend to be puns or restatements of naughty words and are not very funny to adults. The child practices with the laughter that goes with the presumed joke. He or she also seems to thrive on repetition.

Although the cognitive and neurodevelopmental capacities necessary for independence may be present before 7 years of age, the maturity of the mental apparatus and judgments about the world are not sufficient for the child to take his or her place in the larger social world. We have instituted nursery schools for day care and kindergartens since the late nineteenth century, but these are generally places where socialization occurs and manipulative skills are stressed. Although variation is apparent early in life and may persist, most cultures have decided that formal schooling should take place somewhere between 6 and 7 years.

The Second Biodevelopmental Shift

Every level of study, from the neurodevelopmental to the cognitive and social, suggests that there is a hierarchic reorganization at age 7 years that would correspond to a second biodevelopmental shift. The brain attains its adult format and reaches the asymptote of its maximum weight at 7 years. Neuronal dendrites are most dense at this age. Moreover, it is after age 7 that children begin to understand that their feelings, intuitions, and thoughts may be of interest to others and, more important, may be thought about by others. Children of age 7 have had the experience of viewing the actions of others in terms of separate motivation, and they can infer feelings. They also seem to begin to understand cause-and-effect relationships between objects, events, and situations, and they can begin to understand concepts such as ambivalence. They can grasp the concept of conservation of weight (despite how much a piece of clay is distorted in shape), of volume (despite container shape), or of number (despite, for example, the length of a line of coins).

Children ages 7 years and older may also develop rigidities. They become rule-bound and even moralistic about rules, outreasoning their parents in accord with the rules they have been taught. They chastise parents for smoking or for minor infractions of the law. Although they expect devotion and rigor from their parents, children this age sometimes break rules too. They are exceedingly fickle in friendships, but at the same time demand absolute allegiance. "Best friends" may turn out to be different individuals each day. Children during this period tend to set up clubs with complicated rule structures. Rituals are also rampant.

The period that Freud called *latency* and that is now more neutrally named *middle childhood* becomes a time of mastering a great number of facts and skills. The period through fourth grade is considered a time of skill development. Self-righteousness and preoccupation with being admired and cared for, and acceptance of the ministrations of parents, are the hallmark of this stage. This is a period when games are paramount and when persistence at games and collecting are central concerns.

Affective-Interactive Organization

The Newborn Infant

From the very first moments of life, the infant's physical characteristics and behavioral patterns attract the caring attention of the people in its environment.

Bowlby (1969) proposed that attachment originates in inherited species-characteristic behavior called *inborn response systems*. By clinging, sucking, vocalizing, crying, smiling, and following, the infant brings or keeps the caregiver close. Human babies initially follow with their eyes, cling as part of a grasp reflex, and suck to obtain nutrition needed for survival. The behavioral patterns of the newborn ensure the proximity of the caretaker that is necessary for sheer physical survival.

Among these inborn response systems, *affectivity* is essential. For the first 2 months of life, the care of the infant is primarily concerned with the regulation and stabilization of sleep–wake and hunger-satiation cycles. The parents of newborns are focused on the tasks of responding to signals of distress: of feeding, changing, and getting the infant to sleep.

The newborn infant seeks sensory stimulation in periods of quiet alertness. The world of the newborn is not the blooming, buzzing confusion postulated by William James. Between birth and 2 months of age, infants select out the movement and size attributes of visual stimuli. These very young infants are capable of recognizing similarities and differences not only within sense systems but across sensory modalities as well. By 6 weeks of age, babies tend to look more closely at faces that speak, and in experimental situations they focus longer on faces that move in ways consistent with, rather than discrepant from, a simultaneously presented auditory stimulus.

Infants can perceive persons as unique forms from the very beginning. Newborns act differently when scanning live faces than when scanning inanimate patterns; they vocalize more and their movement patterns are smoother and more coordinated (Brazelton et al. 1974). Infants as young as 2 days have been found to be able to reliably imitate an adult model who either smiled, frowned, or showed a surprise face (Field et al. 1982), and by 6 weeks of age infants display evidence of delayed imitation. Infants presented with a person who pulled his tongue in and out repeatedly, pushed out their tongues when viewing the same person, this time with lips closed, after an interval of 24 hours. Such behaviors were not generated in response to new faces seen for the first time (Meltzoff and Moore 1994). Babies are particularly receptive to the ways in which people interact with them. Mothers have little difficulty in deciding whether their babies are content or distressed, and only somewhat more difficulty in attaching specific affective labels to facial expressions.

Emergence of Emotional Experience

Emotional experiences require a sense of self—an "I" to evaluate changes in "me"—as well as the cognitive capacity to perceive, discriminate, recall, associate, and compare. From this perspective, the very young baby's emotional expressions tell us little of his or her emotional experience.

In Stern's (1985) view, an emergent sense of self—in relation to others—is present from birth. The affects, perceptions, sensorimotor events, memories, and other cognitions that accompany social interactions become increasingly integrated over time, providing a framework for the further elaboration of both a sense of self and an awareness of and attachment to others.

Even though newborn infants have the capacity to deal with the stimulation afforded by the external world and can become deeply engaged in and related to social stimuli, their tolerance is limited. Gesell and Amatruda (1947) noted that the 4-week-old child sleeps for as many as 20 hours each day. Often it is only in the late afternoon (typically between 4 and 6 o'clock) that there is a more sustained opportunity for social interaction. By 2 months of age, biobehavioral transformations affecting the nature and quality of social interactions are well underway (Emde et al. 1976; Spitz 1965). Sleep and activity cycles have stabilized, motor patterns are more mature, and altered visual scanning patterns permit new strategies for attachment to the world. Symmetry, complexity, and novelty are becoming salient attributes of visual stimuli. Learning occurs more rapidly and more inclusively. The perceptual preferences for the human face and voice, present at birth, are fully operative. The social smile is well established, vocalizations directed at persons entering the infant's range of vision have begun, and mutual gaze is actively sought.

The period between 2 and 7 months is perhaps the most exclusively social period of life. Typically, caregivers repeat their exaggerated facial expressions, gestures, and vocalizations with minor variations, which serve to regulate the infant's level of arousal and excitation within a tolerable range. Infants, too, are able to regulate their level of social engagement, using gaze aversion to cut out stimulation that has risen above an optimal range, and vocalizations and alterations of facial expression to invite new levels of stimulation when excitation has fallen too low. Infants draw on these daily life experiences to consolidate a sense of a core self as a separate, cohesive, bounded physical unit. During this period, they are increasingly able to recognize relations between actions and reactions, to engage in voluntary activities, and to anticipate the consequences of such activities.

Emergence of Seventh-Month Wariness (Stranger Anxiety)

The development of a core sense of self is paralleled by an increasing ability to engage in social discriminations. At about this time a wariness of strangers first becomes apparent (Schaffer and Emerson 1964). The baby appears cautious and watchful in the presence of strangers. Although facial expressions of fear begin to be noted at 6 months of age (Cicchetti and Sroufe 1978), outright fear in the presence of a stranger is not regularly observed until somewhat later (8–12 months), and even then it is dependent on the situation. Fear is most likely when strangers intrude rapidly and seek to pick up the infant (Horner 1980).

Affective Attunement

Infants of 9 months appear to be capable of joint attention. Not only will they visually follow the direction of the mother's pointing finger beyond her hand to the target, but after their gaze reaches the target they will look back at the mother and appear to use the feedback from her face to confirm that they have arrived at the intended goal. Similarly, babies at this time are increasingly capable of communicating intention and of sharing affective experiences.

Stern (1985) provided rich behavioral descriptions of the process of affective sharing that characterizes attunement. *Attunement* refers to that dimension of the caregiver's behavior that matches not behavior per se, but rather some aspect of the behavior that appears to underscore the baby's feeling state. In attunements, the matching is largely cross-modal—that is, the modality of expression used by the mother to match the infant's behavior is different from that used by the infant. These experiences play a role in the infant coming to recognize that internal feeling states are forms of human experience that are shareable with others. The baby's behavior is also beginning to be influenced by the emotional expressions of others—a phenomenon called *social referencing*.

Taken together, Stern's sense of a core self and his sense of intersubjective self correspond to what self psychologists term the *subjective* or *existential self*—the "me" (Harter 1983).

Selective Attachment

By 10 months of age most infants not only exhibit wariness of strangers but also have developed selective attachments to a small number (usually three or four) of specific persons. There is usually a marked hierarchy among various attachments, with the mother at the top. Once attachment has developed, babies actively seek proximity and contact with the mother, particularly when faced with an unfamiliar or frightening situation. When they are with their mother, they tend to comfortably play and explore the environment, but when mother is out of sight, the infants will very likely follow or protest, either immediately or after a short while. The term *separation anxiety* has been used to describe the distress exhibited by the baby when mother is unavailable.

The Strange Situation

Ainsworth et al. (1978) developed a research method for assessing the quality of attachment in 12- to 18-month-old children. The *strange situation procedure* involves a set series of 3-minute separations and reunions with a caregiver and with a stranger in an unfamiliar room. Children who show mild protest following the departure, who seek the mother when she returns, and who are easily placated by her (about two-thirds of a sample of middle-class 1-year-old American children) are considered as the most *securely attached*. Infants who do not protest maternal departure and who do not approach the mother when she returns (about one-quarter of the sample) are characterized as *avoidant*. Children who become markedly upset by departure and who resist the mother's efforts to comfort them when she returns (about a tenth of the sample) are described as *resistant* or *anxiously attached.*

Changes in attachment status occur in one-quarter to one-third of subjects followed from infancy through early adulthood (Hamilton 2000; Waters et al. 2000), suggesting that experiences beyond infancy influence adult security. Babies designated as showing "secure" attachments tend later to exhibit greater social competence and better peer relationships and to experience fewer negative life events (Sroufe and Fleeson 1984). However, an "insecure" attachment early in life does not inevitably predict the later emergence of psychopathology. Rather, varying patterns of attachment in infancy are initiating conditions that frame the ways in which relationships develop over time.

Separation-Individuation

In the period between approximately 10 and 16 months, the child devotes considerable energy to practicing locomotor skills and exploring the environment. Early in this period, the infant will search for the absent mother or repeat "Mama." Later the child shows a greater tolerance for separation and may seem unconcerned with the mother's whereabouts.

Between 16 and 24 months, ambivalence is often intense. The child seems to want to be united with but at the same time be separate from the mother. Temper tantrums, whining, sad moods, and intense separation reactions are at their peak. Mahler suggests that during this *rapprochement subphase* the mental image of mother is considered to be insufficiently strong to provide comfort in periods of upset.

Between 18 months and 3 years, the development of language contributes to the further organization of the sense of self and the sense of others. Language provides the self and others with a new medium for exchange with which to create shared meanings. With the advent of what Stern (1985) refers to as the "verbal self," children begin to see themselves objectively. By 18 months of age they are able to recognize themselves in mirrors, still pictures, and videotapes. By 2 years they begin to use "I" to refer to themselves, and shortly thereafter to call other people "you." Genetic, prenatal-hormonal, pubertal-hormonal, and socialization factors all contribute to the determination of subsequent sexual status and orientation (Money 1987), but for most children, core gender identity becomes established as well.

Emotions in Toddlers and Middle Childhood

The recognition and labeling of the basic emotions of joy, sadness, anger, and fear develop earlier than those of emotions such as contempt and shame. By 2 years of age, children can dissimulate emotions and pretend to assume emotional states. Between 2 and 4 years of age, children produce increasingly appropriate facial expressions when provided with a verbal label, and between 3 and 4 years they begin to be able to designate what emotions are appropriate to particular situations. Emotional experiences become increasingly clearly defined through the interaction of children with their social environment.

By 3 years of age, children have developed a well-articulated sense of both the subjective self and the objective self. The advent of language facilitates the capacity for symbolic play reflective of daily life experiences, as well as the identification and sharing of affective states. Children come to know the names of their feelings and when to display what affects and increasingly to experience empathy.

Between 3 and 5 years of age, the concept of a private self that is not observable by others begins to be elaborated. Expressed emotions, which encompass a full range of affects, fluctuate easily at age 4 but have become more stable by age 5. The ability to use language to distinguish among affects expands, as does the capacity to identify situation-appropriate emotions. Children begin to elaborate a "theory of mind" as they become increasingly adept at inferring what it is that others know and feel (Baron-Cohen 1989). Relationship patterns become more complicated, and rivalries, jealousies, secrets, and envy begin to emerge. Fantasies become increasingly complex. Behavioral differentiation of the sexes is minimal when children are observed or tested individually. Sex differences emerge primarily in social situations, and their nature varies with the gender composition of dyads and groups.

The period of middle childhood is marked by changes in the ability to regulate and modulate affects. Six-year-olds can be highly emotional, and angry outbursts are frequent. By age 7, children may appear to be moody and sulky and complain that no one likes them and that people are mean and unfair. By age 8, children are described as impatient and demanding, frequently bursting into tears or laughing uproariously. Humor begins to play a role in the modulation of affects. A sense of right and wrong emerges, and children may feel guilty and inwardly unhappy and frankly sad if they have failed to live up to a standard. First-graders have come to appreciate that they cannot change—say, become an animal or a child of the opposite sex—and that the self is continuous from past to future (Guardo and Bohan 1971).

During this period children are also interested in defining their place in the family and in relation to other family members. Children fluctuate between love for family and worries about not belonging. Fantasies of having been adopted and of having rich and powerful natural parents are frequent. Studies of siblings throughout childhood and adolescence report a marked range of individual differences between sibling pairs in measures of friendliness, conflict, rivalry, and dominance.

During middle childhood, interests in relationships with peers and teachers expand. Childhood games with rules emerge, as does a capacity for intimacy with a "best friend." However, the two sexes engage in fairly different kinds of activities and games. Boys play in somewhat larger groups, on the average, and their play is rougher and more expansive. Girls tend to form close, intimate friendships with one or two other girls, and these friendships are marked by the sharing of confidences. Boys' friendships are more oriented around mutual interests in activities.

Boys in groups are more likely than girls in all-girl groups to interrupt one another, refuse to comply with another child's demand, heckle a speaker, or call another child names. Girls in all-girl groups are more likely than boys to express agreement with what another speaker has just said, pause to give another girl a chance to speak, and acknowledge a point made by another speaker.

Between 9 and 10 years of age, children still define themselves in terms of concrete objective categories such as address, physical appearance, possessions, and play activities. Self-criticism is prominent, but children are also beginning to be able to accept jokes by others about themselves. The concept of family continues to be important to most children, although they often prefer to be either on their own, with friends, or with other adults who, like the parents, may serve as role models. There are well-developed capacities for empathy, love, compassion, and sharing, as well as outbursts of person-directed anger, self-evaluative depression, and self-centered righteousness.

Adolescence

What Is Adolescence?

Adolescence has come to represent the developmental bridge between middle childhood or latency and adulthood. It also marks a discontinuity in development based on biological, psychological, and social factors that set this period apart from both childhood and adulthood. Modern theorists suggest that developmental processes continue throughout the life cycle and that each phase or period may be subjected to a developmental analysis. In that sense this chapter on development is incomplete. Adolescence stands out because of the disruptions in behavior, the moodiness, and the difficulties in living, as well as the conflicts and strife with families that have been considered normative.

These popular opinions are striking in view of the fact that adolescence is relatively new on the developmental scene, partly so because there remains some uncertainty as to how to define adolescence and whether adolescence existed in preindustrial society or exists in non-Western communities (Esman 1990). From a sociological vantage point, the rites of passage that mark the terminus of childhood mark entry into adulthood rather than into an intermediate phase. More recent work seeks to define adolescence as a distinct subculture with its own lore and rules.

Puberty

Biologically, *puberty* refers to attaining the capacity to procreate as a mature member of a species. The notion of puberty as a phase in the biological life cycle is more important from a psychosocial vantage point because the external characteristics (i.e., secondary sexual characteristics) of both sexes become prominent social signs. In females puberty occurs 2 years earlier than in males, and the first signs are breast buds, followed by the growth of pubic and axillary hair and the attainment of a feminine body habitus with broadening of the hips (Tanner 1968). In the United States, girls achieve menarche at a mean age of 12.7 years (Zacharias et al. 1970), with 5% beginning at 11–11.5 years, 25% at 12–12.5 years, and 60% by age 13. Nine percent of normal females experience menarche up to 5 years after the beginning of breast development. A height spurt also begins to take place at age 11 that peaks at 12 and then falls off at 14 or 15. Menarche is frequently followed by irregular anovulatory periods for 12–18 months before a more regular menstrual cycle ensues (Tanner 1968).

In boys, the height spurt begins somewhat later, at age 12, peaking at around 14 years, and begins to fall by age 16 or 17. Correspondingly, the penis and the testes are already on their way to achieving adult size and form. The pubic escutcheon and axillary hair likewise begin to be prominent, as does the masculine habitus, and there is deepening of the voice.

In both sexes these primary and secondary sexual changes correspond to activation of hypothalamic functions that in turn stimulate the gonadotropic hormones of the pituitary. These hormones stimulate both estrogen and luteinizing hormone at the periphery as well as testosterone, especially in boys. The changes are thought to be coordinated with maturation of the hypothalamic cells. They become less sensitive to the feedback-dampening effect of circulating sex hormones. In males, nocturnal emissions are observed to occur about a year after the secondary sexual characteristics develop and mark the beginning of the capacity to procreate.

The regular trend toward earlier puberty, especially in girls, in European and American populations has been attributed to better diet. There is also some suggestion that menarche and physical maturity may have long historical cycles so that the early onset of puberty in our time may be a temporary event.

Cognitive Organization in Adolescence

Piaget (1952) suggested that operational intelligence gained at age 7 years is advanced to *abstract* intelligence in adolescence. Achievement of the landmark of abstract intelligence, however, does not occur as uniformly at the age of 14 as previously thought. There are data to suggest that only 10% of 14-year-olds, and 35% of 16- to 17-year-olds, achieve formal operations. Sixty percent of those classified as gifted adolescents attain formal operations.

Social Determinants of Adolescence

The social significance of adolescence did not take hold until economic gain became attached to long periods of education and continuation of economic dependency. One of the by-products of adolescence is the conflict experienced by biologically mature organisms who are still dependent on family support both socially and psychologically.

At the same time, changing social patterns affect youngsters from ages 12 to 18 years. For example, there are more than 8 million one-parent families in the United States. In addition, divorce rates peak early in the first 2 years of marriage but then again just when families are rearing young teenagers. Other social forces involving the women's movement have changed family patterns, with both parents going out to work and women beginning or finishing their education just as their children can begin to be physically, but not psychologically, able to care for themselves. Poverty continues to have a major effect as well. Sociopathy, drug use, and legal entanglements associated with psychiatric disorder have much higher representation in the lower-socioeconomic-status classes.

Psychology of Adolescence: Normative Studies

Adolescence was largely ignored by analysts until Anna Freud (1946) described a rapid oscillation between excess and asceticism during adolescence. She viewed the rapid swings of behavior and mood as secondary to the surgent effect on behavior of the drives stimulated by sexual maturity and the hormones of puberty. The instability of the newly stressed defenses against impulse was seen as the ego's contribution to the erratic behaviors being manifested.

Erikson's (1959) concept of *adolescent turmoil* and his concomitant notion of *identity diffusion* became the hallmarks of our view of normal adolescence. Although Erikson cautioned that diffusion was a maladaptive, temporary state, he implied that we all traverse the stage more or less. Only now do we generally accept the formulations of Offer and Offer (1975), who showed that, by and large, adolescence is more quiescent than was formerly thought. Offer and Offer studied two Midwestern middle- and upper-middle-class community high schools. Their findings, although based on only adolescent males, were later extended and verified by others (see Emde 1985; Hauser et al. 1991). The young men in Offer and Offer's sample were 14 years old and entering high school in 1962.

Those individuals who were within at least one standard deviation from the mean in 9 of 10 scales of personal and social adjustment were the subjects of the study. Sixty-one adolescents were then studied more intensively by a questionnaire technique and were followed well into later life to determine outcome. To convey the advantaged status of the sample, it is worth noting that 74% went to college during the first year after high school graduation. The adolescents came largely from intact families, and through the 8 years of study, from 1962 to 1970, there were no serious drug problems or any major delinquent activity, and no one was arrested for political sit-ins. The group showed no visible generational gap or difference in basic values from their parents.

Varieties of Adolescent Psychological Development

The Offers found three developmental routes, which they designated as *continuous growth* (23% of the sample), *surgent growth* (35%), and *tumultuous growth* (21%). The remaining 21% were not easily classified but were closer to the first two categories than the third. In the *continuous growth* group, major separation, death, and severe illness were less frequent. Parents were described as encouraging independence, and the adolescents showed a capacity for what were described as good human relationships. They were able to achieve Eriksonian intimacy and to display shame and guilt and had few problems of major intrapsychic complexity as far as the methods of investigation could provide. The *surgent* group were "late bloomers," as the term implies. They were not as action-oriented as the first group and were given to more frequent depressive and anxious moments. They were often successful but tended to

be less introspective and reported more areas of disagreement between parents about child raising. Finally, the *tumultuous* group reported recurrent self-doubt and conflict with their families and came from less stable backgrounds. Academically this group preferred the arts, humanities, and social sciences to professional and business careers.

The results of studies such as those by the Offers (Offer 1969; Offer and Offer 1975; Offer and Sabshin 1974) and those by Block and Haan (1971) and Vaillant (1977) tend to negate the notion that turmoil is necessary for adolescent development.

Block and Haan (1971) showed a persistence of character style as individuals develop. The 84 males and 86 females in their study were divided into five and six types, respectively. Among the males the following groups were isolated:

1. Ego-resilient adolescents
2. Belated adjusters (who seem very similar to Offer's surgent group)
3. Vulnerable overcontrollers
4. Anomic extroverts (who seem to have less inner life and relatively uncertain values)
5. Unsettled undercontrollers (who are given to impulsivity)

The categories represented by these individuals are not meant to refer to pathological entities but rather to styles of adaptation.

They divided the cohort of females into the following:

1. Female prototypes (exemplifying stereotyped descriptions of what the authors thought of as feminine in the 1980s)
2. Cognitive types (who tend to be intellectualized in the way in which they negotiate problems)

3. Hyperfemine repressors (who are close in description to persons with hysterical personality disorders)
4. Dominating narcissists
5. Vulnerable undercontrollers
6. Lonely independents

Hauser et al. (1991) studied a sample of 133 14-year-olds longitudinally. Almost half the sample had been inpatients in a psychiatric hospital. However, these authors' mode of study did not show crucial differences in the outcome of this largely middle-class group through their teen years. An ego scale was used that describes stages in maturation with designations such as preconformist, conformist, and postconformist. The authors found three paths of progression from the steady conformist group: early, advanced, and dramatic. This central group of progressive development represents the "team players" of adolescence and constitutes one-third of the group. Only six teenagers attained the level designated as a stage of integrity and conscience, the highest level on the scale. Their parental environment was of a model sort, but as a group they did not differ significantly from the steady conformists in the measures taken.

Developmental Themes of Adolescence

Dependence Versus Independence

The *dependence/independence* interaction refers to the intrapsychic struggle for a sense of emancipation from the nuclear family that permits goals to be formed as a personal claim. Adolescents feel that they must extricate themselves from the caretaking hold of their parents. They see their elders as either exacting gratitude or inducing guilt and shame as internal controls over individual action. On the other hand, these actions may

strike families as egocentric and selfish.

In contrast to nuclear families, children growing up in collectivist societies, where the group rather than the parents is the controlling social force, find it very difficult to move into the larger society where independent individualized action seems to be required (Ainsworth 1962). The notion of an individual achiever and self-starter seems to be related to social values, and these values then become the prominent dynamism in regard to what Blos (1985) called a *second separation-individuation phase*, in which biological, motor, and social equipment are developed to the point that a youth can take his or her place in society and begin to move away from the dependent relationships with parents. This is achieved only with ambivalence and conflict in many families.

License Versus Intellectualized Control

The conflict between *license* and *intellectualized control* is probably best exemplified by Anna Freud's descriptions. Adolescence may be a period of experimentation regarding sexuality, drug use, general disobedience, and other opportunities seen as temptations. Newly formed cognitive skills also permit intellectuality to be used as a controlling mechanism both on a defensive basis and as an interpersonal tool to resist indulgence of wishes and to help define one's goals during adolescence.

Family Versus Peer Group

The third theme, *group formation* in adolescence, is intimately related to the first two themes. Large or small peer group formation brings the adolescent's attempt at removal from family life into sharp focus. Whether this removal is used as a substitution for or regression from family life depends on how the group is used and how the adolescent determines his or her role in that group. During the juvenile period just prior to adolescence, or in early adolescence, Sullivan (1953) described the "chumship" as a time of same-sex social companionship and interest in which sharing and comparing of personal secrets take place. During this initial small-group formation, the adolescent is gradually made aware that companionship, companionableness, and the inner life can somehow now be translated into intimate relations with same-age, same-sex peers for developmental advantage. These small groups of two then gradually develop into larger groups during the early adolescent phase.

Phenomenologically, young women begin to wear the same clothes and share the same style, and young men belong to a team and exhibit the common expressions of individuality in pairs, bringing to light a kind of twinning effect that then proceeds into larger group formation.

If these new social groups take on an antifamily stance or become indifferent to the values of the community, they may become degenerated groups or gangs. A study of 221 African American adolescents in ninth through twelfth grades demonstrated the important positive effect of peer support when stress was high (McCreary et al. 1996). The issue of license for groups or gangs becomes a public concern when illicit drugs, drag racing, public sexual display, or harassment of "grownups" or elderly people are at the forefront.

During the 1990s and into the new millennium, we have witnessed the effect of the new technology and the media on adolescents. Chat rooms and films have brought adolescents together in a new way, exploiting their sexual interests and curiosities and gratifying their need for contact and community while ignoring intimacy. The adolescent culture is newly abuzz with the search for immediate gratification, with many validations for their actions in film and television. We do not know the long-term effects of such reinforcement on institutions such as marriage and family and on social responsibility.

Normalization Versus Privacy

The normalizing function of adolescent community must be contrasted with the need for privacy. These two issues are sometimes, but not always, in opposition to each other. The normalizing function addresses issues of what the adolescent can tell a peer, what is private, and what the adolescent must feel is either sacred to the family or sacred to himself or herself. The tempting possibility of sharing a special or "weird" fantasy with somebody involves risk taking for the adolescent and is an essential part of learning where he or she fits into the expanding world.

Even as the adolescent clings to groups, he or she also craves privacy. The closed door, secret telephone conversations, chat rooms, instant messaging, diaries, and music blasting through earphones are but a few examples of how the adolescent counteracts the urge to tell with the need to hide.

We have ample recent examples from the gay rights movement to suggest that some young men and women understand early—in their eleventh to fifteenth year—that their homosexual impulses are dominant, and yet their ability to "come out" continues to be under social and familial constraints. It is perhaps more the case than not that, whatever one's sexual preference, adolescence is a time for seeing how others feel about the same ideas or of becoming ashamed with the conviction that one's thoughts are unnatural.

Idealization Versus Devaluation

While attempting to normalize his or her experience, the adolescent often spends a great deal of time in *idealizing and devaluing adults or peers*. Crushes, pinups, and hero worship are the hallmark of the adolescent. Indeed, sometimes one's parent or parents may be temporarily idealized. The usual, expected adolescent sequence involves devaluing one's parents while idealizing a public figure or special teacher. Such idealization and devaluation, however, are fragile and frequently lose their power as rapidly as they are constructed. As these processes are taking hold, the adolescent is beginning to establish his or her own character or identity.

Identity, Role, and Character

Identity, role, and *character* have been associated in the developmental literature with the name of Erik Erikson (1963), who contended that "the sense of ego identity… is the accrued confidence that the inner sameness and continuity prepared in the past are matched by the sameness and continuity of one's meaning for others, as evidenced in the tangible promise of a 'career'" (pp. 261–262). The adolescent seeks to establish continuity with the past and to mentally work over the various and sometimes fragmentary idealizations and identifications to ultimately form a coherent unity in character. Thus, identity not only extends backward but is projected forward in the form of establishment of goals, aims, and anticipated career and lifestyle.

Identity contains many of the elements that might be addressed under concepts such as character and personality. Adolescence is a period involving the rapid establishment of these presumed structures. If a failure occurs, there may be a functional breakdown akin to what Erikson called identity diffusion, a condition that is marked by doubt, confusion, insecurity, and aimlessness.

Sexuality: Identity, Role, and Partner

Sexuality may be seen as a substructure of identity, but it is important during the adolescent period not only in terms of role establishment but in terms of matching one's core sexual identity with sexual role and sexual object choice. The early phases of sexual functioning are characterized by a recrudescence of masturbation, especially in males. It is only as the teenager moves into the second part of adolescence (ages 15–20) that this overuse of masturbation as a discharge channel gives way to more differentiated sexual activity guided by fantasies about others with a clearer determination of mental partners in pleasure. Whether this object is heterosexual or homosexual, the maturational thrust is in the direction of permitting one's sexuality to be expressed as a bid for an affiliation that ultimately will bind affection and bodily pleasure. One of the important aspects of masturbatory activity in adolescence concerns the idiosyncratic establishment of the masturbation fantasy created to satisfy many features of past problems and current understanding. In short, the adolescent can in fantasy be active and passive, sadistic and compliant, tender and vigorous, male and female, observer or exhibitor.

As adolescents move into the world and attempt to express their sexuality, they seek a person who more or less matches their mental object. Adolescents then attempt to work out the varying aspects of what is arousing and what creates a human interaction and brings the elements of satisfaction and security together. Sexual experimentation may take place. Adolescence is a time of dating, going together, and experimentation with others. Even if sexual intercourse or its arousing foreplay is not accomplished, it is on the mind of the adolescent. If there is sexual enactment during the periods of turmoil and rebellion, developmental conflicts concerning dependence and independence, license and intellectualization, and removal from family groups in favor of the sexual alliance are the themes of the enactment. Choosing someone who is the opposite of one's mother or father in appearance or removed from one's ethnic group may be an example of reaction formation in the face of threatened oedipal impulses. On the other hand, choices too close to home may have the same meaning of oedipal patterning and dependency.

Young men, accustomed to counterdominance and competitive reactions to their own power assertions, may find themselves relating to women who agree with them and otherwise offer enabling responses. Young women, in interactions with men, are less likely to receive the reciprocal agreement and opportunities to talk that they have learned to expect from other women. Whereas the behavior of men in mixed-sex and same-sex groups tends to be similar, women's behavior in mixed groups is more complex. Some women become more like men as tradition would describe them—raising their voices, interrupting, and otherwise becoming more assertive than they would be when interacting with women only. Others appear to behave as they do in same-sex groups, sometimes in exaggerated form, and may end up speaking less and smiling more than they would in a women's group.

Although patterns of mutual influence can become more symmetrical in intimate male–female dyads, the distinctive styles of the two sexes still persist. On balance, the interactive styles of girls and women appear to put them at a disadvantage in cross-sex encounters, a factor of increasing importance as more and more women enter the workplace in traditionally male

occupations. Moreover, the centrality of interdependence and caring relationships in the lives of girls and women tends to be viewed pejoratively by those persons, including many women themselves, who stress the importance of self-actualization through competitive success (Gilligan 1982).

Reshuffling of Defenses (Style)

In the beginning of adolescence there is a tendency to project outward and to make adaptations that are alloplastic (i.e., externalized). The world, not the adolescent's inner wishes or aims, becomes the reason why the adolescent acts the way he or she does. Blame is placed outside of the individual; responsibility for actions are seen as exterior to the self. This tendency toward denial and projection has led some investigators to suggest that the adolescent acts in a way that may be dystonic to consensual reality. In other adolescents identifications take hold early in a firmer way, and reaction formations and repression begin to help the individual to cut loose from earlier oedipal ties. We begin to see in adolescents a clear establishment of defensive operations in line with productive work and adaptation using their idealized images as guides to planning future aims.

References

Ainsworth MDS: The effects of maternal deprivation: a review of findings and controversy in the context of research strategy, in Deprivation of Maternal Care: A Reassessment of Its Effects. Public Health Papers No 14. Geneva, World Health Organization, 1962

Ainsworth MDS, Blehar MD, Waters E, et al: Patterns of Attachment: A Psychological Study of the Strange Situation. Hillsdale, NJ, Lawrence Erlbaum, 1978

Baron-Cohen S: The autistic child's theory of mind: a case of specific developmental delay. J Child Psychol Psychiatry 30:285–298, 1989

Binet A: New methods for the diagnosis of the intellectual level of the subnormals. L'Annee Psychologique 12:191–244, 1905

Block J, Haan N: Lives Through Time. Berkeley, CA, Bancroft Books, 1971

Blos P: Son and Father: Before and Beyond the Oedipus Complex. New York, Free Press, 1985

Bowlby J: Attachment and Loss, Vol 1: Attachment. New York, Basic Books, 1969

Brazelton TB, Koslowski B, Main N: The origins of reciprocity: the early mother-infant interaction, in The Effect of the Infant on Its Caregiver. Edited by Lewis M, Rosenblum L. New York, Wiley, 1974, pp 49–76

Bretherton I: Pretense: the form and function of make-believe play. Developmental Review 9:383–401, 1989

Cicchetti D, Sroufe LA: An organizational view of affect: illustration from the study of Down's syndrome infants, in The Development of Affect. Edited by Lewis M, Rosenblum LA. New York, Plenum, 1978, pp 309–335

Cohen NJ, Eichenbaum H, Deacedo BS, et al: Different memory systems underlying acquisition of procedural and declarative knowledge. Ann N Y Acad Sci 444:54–71, 1985

Eimas PD, Squeland ER, Josczyk P, et al: Speech perception in infants. Science 171:303–306, 1971

Emde RN: From adolescence to midlife: remodeling the structure of adult development. J Am Psychoanal Assoc 33 (suppl):59–112, 1985

Emde RN, Gaensbauer T, Harmon R: Emotional Expression in Infancy: A Bio-Behavioral Study. New York, International Universities Press, 1976

Erikson E: Growth and Crises of the Healthy Personality. New York, International Universities Press, 1959

Erikson E: Childhood and Society, 2nd Edition, Revised and Expanded. New York, WW Norton, 1963

Esman A: Adolescence and Culture. New York, Columbia University Press, 1990

Field M, Woodson R, Greenberg R, et al: Discrimination and imitation of facial expressions by neonates. Science 218:179–181, 1982

Freud A: The Ego and the Mechanisms of Defense. New York, International Universities Press, 1946

Freud A: The Assessment of Normality in Childhood. New York, International Universities Press, 1965

Freud A: A psychoanalytic view of developmental psychopathology. Journal of the Philadelphia Association for Psychoanalysis 1:7–17, 1974

Freud S: Inhibitions, symptoms and anxiety (1926), in The Standard Edition of the Complete Psychological Works of Sigmund Freud, Vol 20. Translated and edited by Strachey J. London, England, Hogarth Press, 1959, pp 75–175

Gesell AL, Amatruda CS: Developmental diagnosis, in Normal and Abnormal Child Development: Clinical Methods and Psychiatric Applications, 2nd Edition. New York, Hoeber, 1947, pp 3–14

Gilligan C: In a Different Voice: Psychological Theory and Women's Development. Cambridge, MA, Harvard University Press, 1982

Guardo CJ, Bohan JB: Development of a sense of self-identity in children. Child Dev 42:1909–1921, 1971

Hamilton CE: Continuity and discontinuity of attachment from infancy through adolescence. Child Dev 71:690–694, 2000

Harter S: Developmental perspectives on the self-system, in Handbook of Child Psychology, Vol 4: Socialization, Personality, and Social Development. Edited by Hetherington EM. New York, Wiley, 1983, pp 275–385

Hauser ST, Powers S, Noam GG: Adolescents and Their Families. New York, Free Press, 1991

Horner TM: Two methods of studying stranger reactivity in infancy: a review. J Child Psychol Psychiatry 21:203–219, 1980

Huttenlocher PR: Synaptic density in human frontal cortex: developmental changes and effects of aging. Brain Res 163:195–205, 1979

Kuhl P: Linguistic experience alters phonetic perception in infants by six months. Science 255:606–608, 1992

Lewis MM: Infant Speech. New York, Harcourt Brace, 1936

MacKain K, Studdert-Kennedy M, Spieker S, et al: Infant intermodal speech perception is a left-hemisphere function. Science 219:1347–1349, 1983

Mahler MS, Pine F, Bergman A: The Psychological Birth of the Human Infant: Symbiosis and Individuation. New York, Basic Books, 1975

McCreary ML, Slavin LA, Berry EJ: Predicting problem behavior and self-esteem among African American adolescents. Journal of Adolescent Research 11:216–234, 1996

Meltzoff AN, Moore MK: Imitation, memory and the representation of persons. Infant Behavior and Development 17:83–99, 1994

Money J: Sin, sickness, or status? Homosexual gender identity and psychoneuroendocrinology. Am Psychol 42:384–399, 1987

Nelson K: Individual differences in language development. Developmental Psychology 17:170–187, 1981

Nelson K: Event Knowledge: Structure and Function in Development. Hillsdale, NJ, Lawrence Erlbaum, 1986

Offer B, Offer JB: From Teenage to Young Manhood: A Psychological Study. New York, Basic Books, 1975

Offer D: The Psychological World of the Teenager: A Study of Normal Adolescent Boys. New York, Basic Books, 1969

Offer D, Sabshin M: Normality: Theoretical and Clinical Concepts of Mental Health, Revised Edition. New York, Basic Books, 1974

Piaget J: The Origins of Intelligence in Children. Translated by Cook M. New York, International Universities Press, 1952

Roffwarg H, Muzio J, Dement W: Ontogenetic development of the human sleep-dream cycle. Science 152:604–619, 1966

Sapir E: Language: An Introduction to the Study of Speech. New York, Harcourt, Brace & World, 1921

Schaffer HR, Emerson PE: The development of social attachments in infancy. Monogr Soc Res Child Dev 29(Ser No 94), 1964

Skinner BF: Science and Human Behavior. New York, Macmillan, 1953

Spitz RA: The First Year of Life: A Psychoanalytic Study of Normal and Deviant Development of Object Relations. New York, International Universities Press, 1965

Sroufe LA, Fleeson J: Attachment and the construction of relationships, in Relationships and Development. Edited by Hartup W, Rubin Z. New York, Cambridge University Press, 1984, pp 51–71

Stern DN: The Interpersonal World of the Infant: A View From Psychoanalysis and Developmental Psychology. New York, Basic Books, 1985

Sullivan HS: Interpersonal Theory of Psychiatry. Edited by Perry HS, Gawel ML. New York, WW Norton, 1953

Tanner JM: Growth of bone, muscle and fat during childhood and adolescence, in Growth and Development of Mammals. Edited by Lodge ME. London, England, Butterworths, 1968

Vaillant GE: Adaptation to Life. Boston, MA, Little, Brown, 1977

Waters E, Merrick S, Treboux D, et al: Attachment security in infancy and early adulthood: a twenty-year longitudinal study. Child Dev 71:684–689, 2000

Watson J: Psychology From the Standpoint of a Behaviorist. Philadelphia, PA, JB Lippincott, 1919

Wechsler D: Wechsler Intelligence Scale for Children. New York, The Psychological Corporation, 1949

Zacharias L, Wurtman RJ, Shatzoff M: Sexual maturation in contemporary American girls. Am J Obstet Gynecol 108:833–846, 1970

Glossary

Accommodation   A functional aspect of Piaget's model of cognitive development. Accommodation occurs when existing schemas (mental organization) differentiate into new structures ready for new psychic elements.

Assimilation   A functional aspect of Piaget's model of cognitive development that refers to the incorporation of a sensorimotor schema that is repeated with new experiences judged to be equivalent to existing mental organizations.

Adolescence   The developmental period between middle childhood (i.e., latency) and adulthood, characterized by puberty and psychological and social discontinuities in development.

Biosocial organization   Social behavior determined by biological determinants, such as pheromones emanating from a queen ant or bee. The biological agent is active throughout life.

Core self   The self as a cohesive and bounded psycho-physical unit, a dawning sense of which begins to emerge by 2 months of age and becomes consolidated by 30 months.

Critical period   Time frame during which an environmental releaser stimulates the emergence of a developmental capacity that is inborn. If no release occurs, that function is said to *involute*. Concept derives from ethological study of nonmammalian species. Among mammals, however, time lines are not as critically limited; therefore, caution must be exercised in applying data across species.

Development   The changing structure of behavior and thought over time. Development includes whatever is provided by maturational potential plus variations in social and environmental influences.

Differentiation   The move from more global reactions to increasingly individuated processes within systems that occurs in the course of maturation and development.

Ego psychology   A psychoanalytic model and movement that superseded depth Id psychology in the late 30s and has persisted. It is to be distinguished from self psychology, intersubjectivity, and object relations theory. Anna Freud may be said to have begun the idea with *The Ego and the Mechanisms of Defense* (A. Freud 1946), and Hartmann, Kris, and Lowenstein were major exponents of the model in the 1950s and 1960s. Its focus is on the ego as an organizing mediator between drive and reality.

Epigenesis   A description of how early sequential steps influence subsequent steps in development. In this linear model of development, each stage is dependent on the resolution of the experiences of the prior stage.

Gender identity   An individual's belief and self-awareness of being male or female. Gender identity is generally established by age 3 years and is usually determined by the sex in which an individual is reared independent of biological factors.

Growth   Biologically, simple accretion of tissue or increase in size or in the number of cells. Change over time in height and weight is an example of growth. Metaphorically, used for describing development.

Hierarchic reorganization   Changes in organization that are not the logical or necessary outcome of prior stages. In this nonlinear model of development, each new integration of biological and neuronal function meshes with psycho-cognitive capacities so that the result is more than the sum of the parts. Each new stage is a new structure that permits qualitatively different functions and adaptations.

Integration   The increasing complexity of relations between and among the senses and the motor apparatus that occurs in the course of maturation and development. Can be applied to psychological functions as well.

Latency   In psychoanalytic theory, the period between the resolution of the Oedipus complex and the onset of puberty during which the drives are relatively quiescent. More neutrally described as middle childhood, this is a period of skill and social development and increasing ability to regulate and modulate affects.

Lines of development   Anna Freud's proposal that in the course of development the child moves 1) from being nursed to rational eating; 2) from incontinence to bowel and bladder control; 3) from egocentricity toward companionship with peers; 4) from play to a capacity for work; 5) from physical to mental pathways of discharge of drives; 6) from animate to inanimate objects; and 7) from irresponsibility to guilt. Symptoms are viewed as regressions or arrests in these lines.

Maturation   The natural unfolding of genetic potential toward an end characterized by full functioning.

Object constancy   The capacity of the developing child (2–3 years) to maintain a stable mental image of the important caregiver in his or her absence.

Organizer   A behavior identified by Spitz as being analogous to an embryonic organizer in general biology. Examples of these behaviors are the smiling response (2 months), the stranger response (7 months), and the signal for "No" (around 2 years).

Practicing   Subphase of Mahler's theory of the process of separation-individuation (10–16 months) during which the child "practices" newly found locomotor and psychological skills and actively explores his or her environment with exuberance.

Psychosocial organization   Social behavior is primarily determined by early experience and its organizational effect in memory rather than by ongoing biological processes.

Puberty   Attainment of the capacity to procreate as a mature member of a species (see Tanner 1968).

Rapprochement   Subphase of Mahler's theory of the process of separation-individuation (16–24 months) during which temper tantrums, whining behavior, moodiness, and intense separation reactions are at their peak.

Separation-individuation   Mahler's descriptive theory of the process by which the baby becomes a separate, discrete, and autonomous toddler.

Social referencing   The ability of the baby, established during the final quarter of the first year of life, to respond behaviorally to the emotional expressions of others. Crawling babies can be induced to cross a "visual cliff" (i.e., an illusion that there is a drop-off, although a transparent Plexiglas plate covers the drop) if their mother smiles in encouragement and will turn away if the mother assumes a fearful facial expression. Eye gaze for permission is a later behavioral organizer.

Sensorimotor   The first stage of Piaget's model of cognitive development, in which the ability to maintain a stable mental representation and to create a representative world matures. During this stage, sensory and motor behaviors are fused.

Appendix: Major Names in Developmental Psychiatry

Ainsworth, Mary   Canadian-educated American psychologist, collaborator and student of John Bowlby, who developed the strange situation procedure, a laboratory method for assessing the quality of attachment in 12- to 18-month-old children, and fostered further empirical study of attachment research paradigms.

Bowlby, John   British psychiatrist and psychoanalyst, known as the "father of attachment," who was the first to build a human developmental psychology that melded the psychoanalytic and ethological literature. Bowlby recognized the nature of human ties as an organizing precursor to later mature development. His work stimulated further empirical study of attachment, bonding, and separation.

Erikson, Erik Homburger   German-born American psychoanalyst who proposed that personality development takes place through a series of crises that must be overcome and internalized by the individual as he or she passes through eight stages of development from infancy to old age. Additional interests included social psychology and the interactions of psychology with history, politics, and culture. Erikson is best known for his work on identity in adolescents.

Freud, Anna   Psychoanalyst of children, daughter of Sigmund. She introduced play therapy, ego defenses, and developmental lines as significant ideas in child development.

Freud, Sigmund   Viennese founder of psychoanalysis, a treatment and theoretic system that has influenced a century of thought. Freud introduced the idea of polymorphous perverse infantile sexuality and created interest in childhood experience as the basis for adult neurosis.

Gesell, Arnold   American psychologist and pediatrician whose pioneering studies of normal physical and mental development resulted in the establishment of a schedule describing the motor, adaptive, language, and personal/social achievements of infants and young children from birth through 5 years of age. Gesell's normative schedule has been adapted as the Denver Developmental Screen, which is widely used by pediatricians.

Mahler, Margaret   Originally a Hungarian pediatrician, she became an American psychoanalyst and was responsible for the introduction of separation-individuation theory, which was based on direct observation of children in a systematic manner.

Main, Mary   Berkeley University of California Professor of Psychology who introduced the Adult Attachment Interview, an instrument that uses narrative analysis based on Gricean constructs to determine an adult's attachment status.

Piaget, Jean   Swiss psychologist who was one of the first to make a systematic study of the acquisition of understanding in children. Piaget described four stages of development: sensorimotor stage, preoperational stage, concrete operational stage, and formal operational stage. Self-designated as a "genetic epistemologist," he fathered development of cognitive psychology known as the Geneva School.

Skinner, Burrhus Frederic   American psychologist whose work profoundly influenced psychology during the second half of the twentieth century. Skinner's principles of operant conditioning provide the basis for much of modern-day behavior therapy.

Spitz, Rene   A European psychoanalyst who spent most of his professional life in the United States, Spitz studied infants in institutions and mother–infant interaction empirically. He was responsible for the term *anaclitic depression* and the earliest theories of infant ego development. Spitz spent his last years at the University of Colorado, where he influenced Robert Emde.

Stern, Daniel   American psychoanalyst and developmental investigator of mother–infant interaction using microanalytic observational techniques. Stern introduced the terms *motherhood constellation* and *attunement* and has had a significant impact on late-twentieth-century infant research and theory.

Watson, John Broadus   American psychologist whose work in the early years of the twentieth century earned him the title "Founder of Behaviorism." Watson defined psychology as the "science of behavior" and sought to develop a behavioral theory of emotions. His studies of "Little Albert" demonstrated the artificial conditioning of emotional responses in children.

CHAPTER 2

The Psychiatric Interview, Psychiatric History, and Mental Status Examination

Stephen C. Scheiber, M.D.

The *psychiatric interview* remains the essential vehicle for the assessment of the psychiatric patient. The psychiatrist is the medical specialist in psychiatric diagnosis, psychiatric treatment, and understanding interpersonal relationships. The patient reveals what is troubling him or her in the context of a confidential doctor–patient relationship. The psychiatrist listens and responds, attempting to obtain as clear an understanding as possible of the patient's problems in the context of the patient's culture and environment. The psychiatrist encourages a free-flowing exchange with the patient and then, at the conclusion of the interview, arrives at a diagnostic formulation of the patient's problems. The more accurate the diagnostic assessment, the more appropriate the treatment planning (Halleck 1991).

The *psychiatric history* includes information about the patient as a person, the chief complaint, the present illness, premorbid adjustment, pertinent past history, history of medical illnesses, family history of psychiatric and medical disorders, and a developmental history of the patient. The psychiatrist obtains as much history as needed to arrive at a differential diagnosis. With subsequent interviews, the psychiatrist refines his or her working diagnosis and examines the influences of biological, psychological, cultural, familial, and social factors on the patient's life. During the course of a psychiatric history, the psychiatrist evaluates the patient's perceptions of himself or herself and his or her experiences, the patient's perspectives on his or her problems, the goals of treatment, and the desired treatment relationship.

The *mental status examination* is a cross-sectional summary of the patient's behavior, sensorium, and cognitive functioning. Information pertaining to the mental status of the patient is obtained informally during a psychiatric interview as well as through formal testing. Informal information is based on the psychiatrist's observations of the patient and his or her listening to what the patient says. Categories of such information include appearance and behavior, motor activity, eye contact, mode of relating, mood, affect, quality and quantity of speech, thought content, thought processes, and use of vocabulary.

Formal testing considers orientation, attention and concentration, recent and remote memory, fund of information, vocabulary, abilities to abstract, judgment and insight, and perception and coordination. The need for and specificity of formal testing are based on information and clues derived from the psychiatric interview (Othmer and Othmer 1994).

The Psychiatric Interview

Psychiatric Diagnosis

The single most important method of arriving at an understanding of the patient who exhibits the signs and symptoms of a psychiatric disorder is by the psychiatric interview. Although having many features in common with a medical interview, the psychiatric interview has significant elaborations and departures from the medical interview. In addition to the descriptive features of psychiatric diagnoses, which are detailed in DSM-IV-TR (American Psychiatric Association 2000), the psychiatric interview serves as an entrée into a multidimensional understanding of the patient as a person. The psychiatric interview focuses on multiple areas (Table 2–1).

Distinctive features of the psychiatric interview include examining feelings about significant events in the individual's life, identifying significant persons and their relationship to the patient in the course of his or her life, and identifying and tracing the major influences on the biological, social, and psychological development of the individual. The interviewer gathers cross-sectional data related to the signs and symptoms of primary psychiatric disorders, such as anxiety disorders, mood disorders, schizophrenic disorders,

TABLE 2–1.   Areas of focus in the psychiatric interview

1. Patient's psychological makeup
2. How the patient relates to his or her environment
3. Significant social, religious, and cultural influences on the patient's life
4. Conscious and unconscious motivations for the patient's behavior
5. Patient's ego strengths and weaknesses
6. Coping strategies used by the patient
7. Defense mechanisms that are predominant and under what conditions
8. Available support systems and networks for the patient
9. Patient's points of vulnerability
10. Patient's aptitude and achievement

substance-related disorders and cognitive disorders—that is, those categorized under Axis I of the five axes of DSM-IV-TR. The interviewer simultaneously looks for lifetime patterns of the individual's adaptation and relation to the environment in the form of character traits and, at times, character disorders that are described formally under Axis II of DSM-IV-TR.

The psychiatrist in the course of the interview assesses whether the patient exhibits psychotic thinking and/or behavior and whether the patient is harboring suicidal or homicidal thoughts or plans. Safety issues are always foremost in the psychiatrist's evaluation of patients. The patient's capacity to control impulses is also assessed. If in the course of an interview it is determined by the psychiatrist that a patient may be a danger to himself or herself or to others by virtue of a major mental disorder, the psychiatrist is obligated to consider psychiatric hospitalization to protect the patient and/or society. Some states mandate that a psychiatrist notify potential victims of threatened harm revealed during the course of an interview (Halleck 1991).

General Considerations

Initiation

Most calls are not emergencies. The psychiatrist, when returning a call, requires sufficient time to assess several critical subjects (Table 2–2).

TABLE 2–2. Critical subjects to assess when returning patient phone calls

1. What are the circumstances that led to the patient's calling?
2. What are the presenting complaints?
3. Who referred the patient?
4. Is (or was) the patient in treatment with another psychiatrist?
5. What does the patient hope to gain by seeing a psychiatrist?
6. Does the identified problem require the expertise of a psychiatrist?
7. Does the caller need to be referred elsewhere?

The psychiatrist elicits enough information to determine whether the patient is in need of an immediate assessment and examination for a psychiatric hospitalization. If the psychiatrist judges that the patient may need hospitalization, the psychiatrist tells the patient to go to the emergency department. The psychiatrist then either goes to the emergency department or arranges for someone at the emergency department to evaluate (not admit) the caller (Morrison 1993).

Coordinating care with a referring physician is important, particularly when there are overlapping medical/psychiatric problems and when medications are prescribed. This coordination is critical in working with primary care physicians. The psychiatrist should welcome as much data as the primary physician can offer regarding the patient's history and mental status.

Initial telephone contacts set the stage for subsequent psychiatric interviews. The psychiatrist exhibits the capacity to be an expert listener who will work to understand the patient and his or her problem. Rapport with a patient begins with the initial contact. In addition to listening to the patient's problems, the psychiatrist advises the patient about what to expect when coming for an evaluation. The patient is told the minimum amount of time that the psychiatrist expects will be needed to do a complete assessment, how much time will be allowed per visit, over what period of time the assessment will be conducted, what the hourly cost will be, the charge for missed appointments, and whether the psychiatrist anticipates being available to treat the patient when the assessment is completed. The psychiatrist inquires about when the patient would be available to come for an evaluation and sets up a time that is mutually agreeable (Table 2–3).

TABLE 2–3. Initial steps of the psychiatric interview

Background information
  Reason for call
  Location of patient
  How caller can be reached
  Presenting complaints
  Referral source's name and telephone number
  Treatment history
  Concurrent medical conditions
  What patient hopes to gain
  Determination of urgency
  Primary physician's name and phone number
Expectations
  Time for assessment
  Cost of evaluation
  Purpose of assessment
  Psychiatrist's availability for treatment

Requests for appointments with a psychiatrist can also be initiated by third parties, who can include relatives, treating physicians, judges, lawyers, staff of employee health services or student health services, staff of disability evaluation organizations, military superiors, and others. In every instance, it is essential for the psychiatrist to learn what the patient has been told about requests for a psychiatric consultation or evaluation and to find out what the patient expects from seeing a psychiatrist. The purpose of the examination should be explicit. If the purpose is to advise an employer about the patient's psychiatric fitness to continue employment, the psychiatrist advises the employer to inform the patient that this is the purpose and to make sure the patient knows that the psychiatrist's conclusions will be shared with the employer.

If a relative is calling, it is important not only to ascertain what the patient knows of the call but to find out the reasons why the patient is not calling directly. The psychiatrist does everything possible to dissuade a family member from using deception in getting the patient to agree to an appointment.

Third-party callers should also be advised of what information they can expect following a psychiatric examination. In most instances, no information will be shared without the patient's consent. In the case of a minor, the information may be shared with the parent. If the purpose of an examination is to collect information as an expert witness in a court of law, the patient is advised at the onset of the interview that everything he or she says may be used as part of the psychiatrist's expert testimony in court. In this instance, the usual doctor–patient confidentiality is not in force.

Time

The amount of time set aside for an initial psychiatric outpatient evaluation varies, ranging from 45 minutes for some evaluations to 90 minutes for others. If the evaluation is conducted at the bedside on a medical service, the length of the interview is often shorter because of the patient's medical condition, and more frequent, brief visits may be necessary. In emergency department settings, the evaluation may be prolonged, particularly if hospitalization is in question and supporting data are needed from resources not immediately available, such as from relatives and treating physicians who have to be reached by telephone. If a patient is exhibiting psychotic behaviors during an outpatient appointment, the interview may be abbreviated if, in the judgment of the psychiatrist, prolonging the interview will aggravate the patient's condition. When possible, the psychiatrist should have some flexibility in his or her schedule at the time of an initial interview. In most instances, evaluations for treatment require scheduling additional meetings beyond the initial hour.

Setting

The most important space consideration for a psychiatric interview is establishing privacy so that the interview proceeds in a setting where confidentiality can be ensured. In academic settings, where audiovisual equipment and one-way viewing mirrors are used for teaching, the patient is owed an explanation by the resident about the purposes for which recording devices are being used. The patient has the right of refusal regarding the use of such devices. Most patients attending a clinic in a teaching institution expect that part of going to such an institution for help will involve using them as teaching aids for residents. The resident's dealing directly and honestly with a patient's questions and concerns is essential and also will enhance the doctor–patient relationship. The resident learns the importance of being sensitive to the patient's reactions to the use of such equipment. For instance, adolescent patients may be reluctant to discuss negative feelings toward their parents or other authority figures in the face of a camera or recording device until they are ensured that such data will not be shared with the parents.

The psychiatrist does everything possible to put the patient at ease during the interview. The setting should be one that promotes comfort for both patient and psychiatrist.

Special populations and settings require variations from an office setting with comfortable chairs. Hospital bedside consultations are difficult to conduct while ensuring privacy. The psychiatrist should check with the nursing staff to see whether the patient's medical condition will permit his or her being moved to a quiet room to avoid multiple interruptions at the bedside by hospital personnel, visitors, shared bedside telephones, and roommates in semiprivate rooms and ward settings.

For young children, a playroom setup, with toys that children can express themselves with, is preferable for diagnostic interviewing. Much formal training, skill, and experience are needed to appropriately evaluate a child in a playroom setting (Greenspan and Greenspan 1991; Kestenbaum 1997; Robson 1986; Rutter et al. 1988).

In hospital emergency department settings, a quiet room should be available with a mattress and no removable (and potentially dangerous) objects. Such a room will prove to be the safest setting in which to interview a psychotic patient who has exhibited out-of-control behaviors. In addition to privacy and comfort, safety is an important consideration. With a potentially agitated paranoid patient, it is important for the psychiatrist to have unimpeded access to an exit door.

Note Taking

The purpose of taking written notes during a psychiatric interview is so that the psychiatrist has accurate information for preparing the report of the interview. Newly trained psychiatrists, when interviewing, tend to take extensive notes, because they are lacking in knowledge and experience about what is relevant and what is not. For the newly trained psychiatrist who often uses audiovisual aids such as audio- or videotape recorders for supervisory review, these same devices can be used for reviewing databases and can substitute for note taking. Any recording devices need to be in clear view of the patient, and an explanation is to be given to the patient about its use. The patient should be assured that the tapes will be erased after they are reviewed.

The greatest limitation in excessive note taking is that it can inhibit the free flow of exchange between patient and physician. If the interviewer is preoccupied with note taking, he or she will miss important nonverbal messages and will not pursue important leads in the interview.

If a patient requests that the psychiatrist not take notes, this request should be respected. Patients may react to the relative absence of note taking as well. They may comment, "How can you remember everything I have to say?"

Notes help psychiatrists remember information accurately. The psychiatrist should record his or her notes, observations, and conclusions as soon after the interview as possible. Prompt recording of data and information while still fresh in the psychiatrist's mind maximizes the accuracy of the information and minimizes distortions and gaps in the database that will result when the psychiatrist delays his or her recording. The psychiatrist should set aside time at the conclusion of the interview to accomplish this task. For the experienced psychiatrist, 5–10 minutes at the conclusion of a 45- to 50-minute interview usually suffices. The newly trained psychiatrist will require additional time.

The notes that are incorporated in the patient's record are necessarily more comprehensive following initial interviews than subsequent ones, because all the data constitute new information. With subsequent interviews, only new, pertinent information needs to be recorded. Psychiatrists need to be particularly sensitive to what information is incorporated into a general hospital chart that is available to multiple caretakers and to third-party reviewers. Only essential information for the overall care of the patient should be included in a general medical chart.

Interruptions

The time set aside and agreed upon for a patient interview is viewed as sacred and protected time for the patient. Calculated measures are taken to discourage interruptions. If the door to the interview room is in an area where others may knock, a sign should be hung on the door with an instruction such as "Do not disturb" or "Interview in progress" or "In session."

Relatives or Friends Accompanying the Patient

When relatives arrive with the patient, the psychiatrist always interviews the patient first and tells relatives that he or she may want to talk with them later. (An exception would be a couple coming for couple evaluation and possible couple therapy.) In the course of the patient's interviews, the psychiatrist can indicate his or her desire to speak with the relatives and can explore the patient's feelings about the psychiatrist's doing so. The patient must grant permission before relatives are interviewed.

An exception to this rule occurs when the psychiatrist judges the patient to be in imminent danger of hurting himself or herself or others and when the patient refuses voluntary hospitalization. In such an instance, the patient must be told why the psychiatrist is obliged to talk to a third party without the patient's permission.

If the psychiatrist wants to meet with the patient's relatives, he or she must advise the patient whether the meeting will take place with or without the patient present. If in doubt, the psychiatrist chooses to have the patient present. This signals to the patient that the psychiatrist does not want to jeopardize the doctor–patient relationship. This relationship is more important than obtaining additional information that relatives may not want to reveal in the patient's presence.

If the psychiatrist chooses to see relatives without the patient present, the ground rule needs to be established with relatives that the psychiatrist is not at liberty to share, without the patient's permission, any information obtained from the patient in confidence but is at liberty to share with the patient any information that relatives reveal.

Sequence

The psychiatrist's first impressions of the patient begin with the initial telephone contact. The formal assessment of the patient begins with the psychiatrist's initial observations of the patient. The psychiatrist observes the patient's appearance and behavior in the waiting area, who is with the patient, how the patient responds when the psychiatrist greets him or her by name, and how the patient responds to a handshake. It is preferable with adult patients to refer to them by their last names during the initial encounter, and then, when they are in the interview room, to inquire what the patient's preference is regarding first- or last-name usage. Referring to geriatric patients by first names without the patients' permission is particularly demeaning and infantilizing.

The psychiatrist then walks with the patient to the interview room and indicates interest in the patient by being friendly but does not make any clinical inquiries or comments until the interviewing room door is closed. The psychiatrist indicates which seat he or she will sit in while offering the patient a choice if there is more than one seat available.

At the beginning of the interview, the psychiatrist encourages the patient to speak as spontaneously and openly as possible about the reasons for his or her coming at this time (Table 2–4). The psychiatrist can facilitate this process by briefly summarizing what he or she has learned about the patient and the patient's problems and then saying that he or she would like to hear in the patient's own words what is troubling the patient. An opening inquiry such as "Tell me what brings you here today" encourages the patient to express what currently is troubling him or her. The psychiatrist establishes a primary posture of listening, allowing the patient to tell his or her story with minimal interruptions or direction. In the early part of the interview, if the patient stops talking, the psychiatrist encourages him or her to continue, using comments such as "Tell me more about [a particular incident]." If the patient describes a significant event in his or her life and expresses no emotion, the psychiatrist inquires, "How do you feel about this?" If the patient describes a disturbing event and starts clenching his or her fists and exhibiting flushing, the psychiatrist inquires about the patient's feelings at the moment. If the patient denies any feelings, the psychiatrist advises him or her that most people would react to similar circumstances with anger. Thus, in the initial part of the interview, the psychiatrist establishes that he or she is interested in not only the chronology of

events that led to the patient's coming but also the feelings that accompany such events and encourages the patient's expression of these feelings. At times, when the expression of feelings is too overwhelming for the patient, the psychiatrist must not push the patient beyond his or her tolerance for expressing them. If the patient has had one or more psychiatric hospitalizations, the psychiatrist should learn details about each hospitalization and most particularly the events leading up to the initial hospitalization. It is also key to inquire what was most helpful during a patient's hospitalization as well as what follow-up care was most beneficial.

TABLE 2–4. Phases of the psychiatric interview

Initial
  Chief complaint
  Present illness
  Feelings about significant events
Middle
  Patient as a person
  Multigenerational family history
  Current living situation
  Occupation
  Avocations
  Education
  Value systems
  Religions and cultural background
  Military history
  Social history
  Medical history
  Developmental history
  Sexual history
  Typical day
  Strengths and weaknesses
Concluding
  Time remaining
  Important areas not covered
  Patient's questions
  Sharing clinical impressions
  Permission to obtain records
  Permission to speak with others
  Treatment plan and patient's reaction

Throughout the interview the psychiatrist tries to learn how the patient experiences life events and to understand the patient's perceptions of how such events evolve. Once the psychiatrist has a grasp of the essentials of the present illness and accompanying feelings, he or she then shifts the focus to other subjects.

In the middle portion of the interview, the psychiatrist tries to learn about the patient as a person. There are numerous areas of the patient's life to explore: significant relationships, multigenerational family history, current living situation, occupation, avocations, education, value systems, religious and cultural background, military history, social history, medical history, developmental history, sexual history, and legal history, to name a few. The breadth of material requires several interview sessions for the psychiatrist to gather the pertinent data.

The patient will frequently be asked to describe a typical day in his or her life. The psychiatrist tries to establish the patient's highest level of functioning and assesses when current symptoms began to interfere with the patient's functioning. The decision regarding the order in which the psychiatrist inquires about these data is a matter of clinical judgment. The patient usually signifies his or her comfort with particular subjects by raising them in the interview, and the psychiatrist then follows up with questions to get more in-depth information.

As a rule, the psychiatrist moves from areas assumed to be of positive value to those of neutral interest and, finally, to those that the psychiatrist anticipates will be more emotionally charged for the patient.

Throughout these initial inquiries, the psychiatrist is ascertaining the patient's strengths and weaknesses and is monitoring the responses to ascertain potential areas of conflict for the patient. Again, the psychiatrist is guided by the patient's responses in terms of inquiring about areas in which the patient may be reluctant to respond. When inquiring about the sexual history of a boy or man, the psychiatrist begins with, "Do you have a girlfriend?" If yes, the psychiatrist follows with "Tell me about her" and can then inquire about the nature of the relationship. The psychiatrist follows up by asking about specific areas of sexual conduct. Beginning with questions regarding kissing and then petting and then sexual intercourse, the psychiatrist then asks about the patient's feelings in regard to various sexual activities, inquiring about both heterosexual and homosexual interests and relationships. Histories of sexual abuse should be elicited (Morrison 1993). Inquires should also be made about sexually transmitted diseases such as AIDS.

In the concluding portion of the interview, the psychiatrist notes for the patient the remaining time left. The patient is asked whether there are any important areas that he or she has not talked about. The psychiatrist asks whether the patient has any questions, then answers each of the patient's questions. If the psychiatrist has insufficient information to answer a question, he or she tells the patient just that.

At this time the psychiatrist shares with the patient his or her clinical impressions in words that the patient understands, avoiding psychiatric jargon. The psychiatrist then presents a treatment plan to the patient. It is important to ascertain the patient's fiscal status as well as to determine the third-party insurance that will cover the patient's care. It may be that, under the limitations of a managed-care situation, the psychiatrist will have to advise the patient that the tried and true treatment modalities may not be available to him or her because of the limitations of his or her reimbursement system. Psychiatrists have the ethical responsibility to try to assist patients to receive optimal care. On the other hand, patients must decide within the limitations of their fiscal abilities what is feasible for themselves and their families.

If records and information are available from other sources, the psychiatrist requests written permission from the patient to obtain medical records from hospitals or other physicians. If the psychiatrist wishes to contact others by telephone, he or she obtains permission from the patient before doing so. If the patient is receiving medical care from other physicians, the psychiatrist obtains consent to contact them.

It is important to solicit patients' reactions to as well as agreement with a given treatment plan. Patients are entitled to know the various treatments available for their disorder. The psychiatrist shares with the patient his or her specific recommendations for treatment and responds to the patient's questions about why the psychiatrist believes these suggestions are best for the patient. If the patient wants an alternative plan, it is best for the psychiatrist to postpone implementation of specific treatment until there is mutual agreement. There is a better likelihood for patient compliance when the patient understands a treatment plan and agrees to it (Garrett 1942; Gill et al. 1954; Group for the Advancement of Psychiatry 1961; Leon 1982; Nurcombe and Fitzhenry-Coor 1982; Rutter and Cox 1981; Strupp and Binder 1984; Sullivan 1954; Whitehorn 1944).

The Physician–Patient Relationship

Transference

Transference is a process whereby the patient unconsciously projects his or her emotions, thoughts, and wishes related to significant persons in his or her past onto people in his or her current life and, in the context of the psychiatrist–patient relationship, onto the psychiatrist. The patient is reacting to the psychiatrist as if the psychiatrist were part of the patient's past. Whereas the reaction patterns may have been appropriate in an earlier situation, they are inappropriate when applied to figures in the present, including the psychiatrist. This theoretical construct is borrowed from the psychoanalytic literature.

For example, a 24-year-old male patient notices the long braided hair and blue eyes of the psychiatrist. He starts making several demands of the psychiatrist using a whining voice, without being consciously aware that he is doing so. Such demanding behavior replicates how he behaved in the presence of a significant aunt in his youth with similar physical features, with whom he had a highly dependent relationship and in whose presence he had exhibited similar whining voice intonations.

It is important for the psychiatrist to recognize these patterns and to treat them as distortions, not to respond in kind. An ultimate understanding of such unconscious behaviors is one of the goals of insight-oriented psychotherapy. In the early training of a psychiatrist, the psychiatric supervisor devotes considerable time to the resident's understanding of the process of transference so that the resident will not treat these reaction patterns as personal assaults.

Countertransference

Countertransference is a process whereby the psychiatrist unconsciously projects emotions, thoughts, and wishes from his or her past onto the patient's personality or onto the material that the patient is presenting, thus expressing unresolved conflicts and/or gratifying the psychiatrist's own personal needs. These reactions are inappropriate in the physician–patient relationship. In this instance, the patient assumes the role of an important person from the psychiatrist's earlier life. This construct is also gleaned from the psychoanalytic literature. In such instances, the psychiatrist mistakenly attributes to the patient feelings and thoughts that are based on the psychiatrist's own life experiences, which can interfere with his or her understanding of the patient.

For example, a male psychiatrist responds inappropriately to an internist's consultation request on a 76-year-old, dying, hospitalized female patient. The psychiatrist has been making twice-daily hour-long bedside visits followed by frequent calls to the patient's internist. The psychiatrist questions the internist's medical care of the patient and recommends antianxiety agents to treat the patient's presumed anxiety. As a child, the psychiatrist had experienced strong attachment to his grandmother, who had died in his childhood home. He unconsciously retained guilt feelings for not doing something to prevent her death. The psychiatrist's handling of the consultation is in essence an attempt to cope with his own anxieties and guilt about his grandmother's death without consciously realizing that he is doing this or being cognizant of the inappropriateness of his behavior.

The psychiatrist in this case would benefit from consultation with a colleague, who could help clarify the psychiatrist's reaction patterns and guide him toward more appropriate professional behavior.

One of the values of personal psychoanalysis for psychiatrists is to enhance their awareness of their unconsciously motivated behaviors so that they can better use their countertransference reactions to understand their patients. In their training, residents will be helped by a supervisor to examine their countertransference reactions so that these reactions will not interfere with patients' treatment but will aid the residents in understanding their patients.

Therapeutic Alliance

The therapeutic alliance, a third theoretical construct from the psychoanalytic literature, is a process whereby the patient's mature, rational observing ego is used in combination with the psychiatrist's analytic abilities to advance the psychiatrist's understanding of the patient. The basis for such an alliance is the trusting relationship established in early life between the child and the mother, as well as other significant trusting relationships from the patient's past. The psychiatrist encourages the development of this alliance, and both persons must invest in cultivating the alliance so that the patient can benefit. The psychiatrist enhances this alliance by his or her professional conduct and attitudes of caring, concern, and respect.

Psychiatrists accept and respect patients' value systems and their integrity as persons. Without a therapeutic alliance, patients cannot reveal their innermost thoughts and feelings. It is unethical for psychiatrists to exploit patients sexually or to exploit them for personal financial gain by inquiring about investment opportunities from patients knowledgeable about such matters. These are violations of the physician–patient relationship. Psychiatrists must never victimize patients by exploiting their roles as physician-healers (American Psychiatric Association 2001).

Resistance

Resistance is a theoretical construct that reflects any attitudes or behaviors that run counter to the therapeutic objectives of the treatment. Understanding resistance is critical to the conduct of dynamic psychotherapy. Freud described several types of resistance, including conscious resistance, ego resistance, id resistance, and superego resistance.

Conscious resistance by patients occurs for a variety of reasons, such as lack of trust of psychiatrists, shame on the part of patients in revealing certain events and aspects of themselves or feelings that they are experiencing, and fear of displeasing or risking rejection by psychiatrists. One form of conscious resistance by patients is silence. The psychiatrist must acknowledge the difficulties the patient is experiencing and encourage the patient to verbalize material that is difficult to express. This should be done in a tactful, sensitive manner.

There are three forms of *ego resistance*: repression resistance, transference resistance and secondary-gain resistance. The first form is *repression resistance*, whereby, for mostly unconscious reasons, the same forces that led to the patient's symptoms keep him or her from developing an awareness of the underlying conflicts. A second type of ego resistance, *transference resistance*, can take many forms. Such resistance may occur when the patient projects undesirable feelings onto the psychiatrist and ascribes these feelings to the psychiatrist. This, in turn, can lead to the patient's attacking the psychiatrist, and a negative transference can result. It is critical that the psychiatrist understand the underpinnings of such a transaction and, rather than retaliate, treat the patient's expressions as a resistance. A third type of ego resistance is *secondary-gain resistance*. In this form, a patient's symptoms serve to elicit nurturing responses from significant figures and thus allow the patient to gratify his or her dependency needs.

Id resistance occurs in psychoanalytic practice when a patient repeatedly brings up the same material in the face of repeated interpretations of the behavior.

Superego resistance occurs most frequently with obsessional, depressed patients who, by virtue of their guilt feelings and self-defeating behaviors, exhibit a need for punishment. Thus, patients continue to exhibit symptoms that serve as punishment, and they are resistant to relinquishing them (Luborsky 1984).

Resistance takes many forms. These include patients' censoring of what they are thinking, intellectualization, generalization, preoccupation with one phase of life, concentration on trivial details while avoiding important topics, affective displays, frequent requests to change appointment times, using minor physical symptoms as an excuse to avoid sessions, arriving late or forgetting appointments, forgetting to pay bills, competitive behaviors with the psychiatrist, seductive behaviors, asking for favors, and acting out (MacKinnon and Michels 1971).

Confidentiality

Psychiatrists are bound by medical ethical principles to not divulge any information revealed to them unless they have patients' consent. They must protect patients and assume responsibility for seeing that no harm will come to patients by virtue of the patients' revealing information about themselves. If patients refuse to give permission to psychiatrists to reveal information, whether it be to a referring physician or for filling out an insurance form, psychiatrists must respect the patients' wishes.

In hospital or clinic settings, the patient is told about the types of information that will be recorded and who may have access to the information. When psychiatrists record information in the general hospital record, they record only data pertinent to the overall care of the patient, such as medications prescribed, and minimize recording personal information that has no relevance to the general medical care of the patient. In general hospital settings, it is preferable to have separate psychiatric records that can be housed and locked in an area separate from the general hospital records, to which only trained psychiatric personnel will have access.

Only when patients are in danger of hurting themselves or others by virtue of their mental illness is the psychiatrist obliged to reveal such information in order to institute involuntary hospitalization.

When third-party carriers are seeking psychiatric information, psychiatrists review with patients the information that has been prepared for the carrier and obtain patients' permission to submit reports.

Interview Technique

Facilitative Messages

The most important component in the psychiatrist–patient relationship is the interest psychiatrists show in their patients. The most important element in the psychiatric interview of patients is for psychiatrists to allow patients to tell their stories in an uninterrupted fashion. Psychiatrists assume an attentive listening posture; they do not ask excessive questions that would interrupt the flow of the interview. Throughout the interview, patients will experience resistance to revealing themselves that is based on the realities of the interview situation as well as on transference issues.

Newly trained psychiatrists often mistakenly believe that sitting in an unresponsive, silent posture emulates a psychoanalyst's approach to a patient and that this is the optimal way to interview a psychiatric

patient. On the contrary, residents need to learn a repertoire of interviewing techniques that will facilitate communication as much as possible (Table 2–5). Some of these techniques are described here.

Open-ended questions. An open-ended question reflects a topic that the psychiatrist is interested in exploring but leaves it to the patient to choose the areas he or she believes are relevant and important to share.

Reflections. The psychiatrist often wishes to draw patients' attention to the affective concomitants of their verbal productions. One way of doing this is by rephrasing what the patient has stated and stressing the feelings that accompany a reported event. By restating the patient's verbalizations, the psychiatrist provides the patient with an opportunity to correct any misconceptions that the psychiatrist may have about the patient's condition. This technique is referred to as *reflections*.

Facilitation. In this technique, the psychiatrist uses body language and minimal verbal cues to encourage and reinforce the patient's continuing along a particular line of thought with minimal interruptions in the patient's flow of verbalizations. Examples of these cues include attributes that are frequently ascribed to psychiatrists, such as the nodding of their heads or comments such as "Uh-huh." Other examples include raising of eyebrows, cocking of head, leaning toward patients, and verbalizations from the psychiatrist such as "I see," "Go on," "What else?" "Anything more?" and "Proceed." Facilitations indicate to the patient that the psychiatrist is interested in the patient's particular train of thought and that he or she is attentive to what the patient is saying. Excessive reliance on a single facilitation will, how-

TABLE 2–5.   Facilitative messages

Type	Example
Open-ended questions	"Tell me about…"
Reflections	"You're anxious about succeeding."
Facilitation	"Uh-huh."
Positive reinforcement	"Good. That helps me understand you."
Silence	Long pause allowing patient to take distance from verbal material.
Interpretation	"When you can't perform the way you think you should, you try to do something to please."
Checklist questions	"When you feel nervous, do you develop sweaty palms? heart palpitations? rapid breathing? butterflies in your stomach?"
"I want" messages	"We should explore other topics besides your depression. Tell me about your family."
Transitions	"Now that you've told me about your job, tell me what a typical day is like."
Self-disclosure	"When I've been in similar situations, I've felt terrified."

ever, approach the parody of a psychiatrist and become counterproductive.

Positive reinforcement.   The subjects that the psychiatrist explores with the patient are frequently ones that the patient is unaccustomed to talking about and finds difficult to explain. When the patient has struggled with a particular topic and is then able to communicate clearly, the psychiatrist signals his or her approval by using positive reinforcement.

Silence.   The judicious use of silence when interviewing a patient is an important component of the psychiatrist's repertoire of interviewing techniques. Silences allow patients to create some distance from what they have been saying and can help them put their thoughts in order or enable them to understand better the psychological meaning and context of what has happened in the interview.

Interpretation.   The psychiatrist works with patients to try to help them understand their motivations and the meanings of their thoughts, feelings, and actions.

The psychiatrist examines repeated patterns of behaviors and draws inferences regarding these patterns. Such inferences are called *interpretations*. Several interpretation techniques may be used to help patients.

Checklist questions.   The psychiatrist spells out a list of potential responses for a patient when the patient is unable to describe or quantify to the degree of specificity that the psychiatrist believes is important to know in particular situations. The psychiatrist uses a checklist of questions when open-ended questions do not yield the necessary information and when more specific information than what has been obtained with the open-ended questions is needed. The checklist format is often helpful for elucidating medical problems.

"I want" messages.   When the psychiatrist senses that an interview has failed to progress because of the patient's need to focus on a single theme, the psychiatrist asserts that they need to move on to other areas of inquiry. The psychiatrist is firm with the patient that sufficient information has been obtained about the single theme and that he or she understands the patient's concerns and feelings about that particular topic.

Transitions. Once sufficient information regarding a particular part of a patient's history is obtained, the psychiatrist then signals to the patient his or her satisfaction with the understanding of that portion of the interview and invites the patient to move on to another area. This technique is referred to as *transitions*. Transitions allow the psychiatrist to guide the patient from one significant topic to another while signaling to the patient the areas that are important for the psychiatrist to learn about. Once the patient has given clues that he or she is prepared to talk about a particular area, the choice of ordering of topics is best dictated by the patient. The psychiatrist, by keeping attuned to the patient's readiness to discuss a topic, will orchestrate a smooth transition from one topic to another.

Self-disclosure. The psychiatrist, at times, will judge that it is in the patient's best interest for the psychiatrist to disclose certain thoughts, feelings, or actions about himself or herself. This self-disclosure may be in response to the patient's questions, or it may occur when the psychiatrist believes that sharing his or her own experiences will benefit the patient.

Obstructive Messages

Obstructive messages tend to interfere with the uninterrupted flow of the patient's verbalizations and stand in the way of the establishment of a trusting relationship between psychiatrist and patient (Table 2–6). These communications are interview techniques that should

be avoided. Some were learned in medical school, and psychiatric residents need to be coached in how to avoid using them.

Excessive direct questions. Excessive direct questions represent the antithesis of open-ended questions. They occur when the psychiatrist directs the patient to a single response. This technique does not allow the patient to choose those areas that are of greatest concern to him or her. The excessive use of direct questions lends itself to the patient's answering only what is on the psychiatrist's list of questions. It presupposes that the psychiatrist alone knows the issues, priorities, and relevant information. The patient thus becomes a passive recipient of the psychiatrist's inquiries and fails to become an equal partner with the psychiatrist.

Run-on questioning. Rather than giving the patient a chance to respond to a single question, the psychiatrist asks several questions at one time. The patient may not know which question to answer or attempt to condense all the questions into one and respond with a yes or no response.

Preemptive topic shifts. Rather than responding to the patient's cues about meaningful events, the psychiatrist moves from one topic to another, seemingly insensitive to what is important to the patient. Instead of focusing on the patient's shaky feelings and exploring this area in depth, the psychiatrist shifts to other areas that he or she wants to cover and fails to investigate issues that are of immediate concern to the patient. The patient is left feeling that the psychiatrist is unconcerned about the patient's troubles. Preemptive topic shifts may be a conscious or unconscious defense by the psychiatrist when he or she is threatened or unhappy with the topic.

TABLE 2–6.   Obstructive messages

Type	Example
Excessive direct questions	Psychiatrist: What's making you sad? Patient: I've lost a girlfriend. Psychiatrist: Do you cry a lot? Patient: Probably not. Psychiatrist: Did you grieve inadequately? Patient: I'm not sure.
Run-on questioning	Psychiatrist: Is there a family history of mental illness such as anxiety disorders, depressive disorders, major psychotic disorders, dementia, drug or alcohol problems, suicide, and/or personality disorders? Patient: Yes.
Preemptive topic shifts	Patient: I feel suicidal. Psychiatrist: Are you feeling despondent? Patient: I'm terribly depressed. Psychiatrist: Are you having trouble with your marriage? Patient: I can't say.
Premature advice	Patient: I have an upset stomach. Psychiatrist: You may want to try antacids and warm milk at bedtime and six meals a day.
False reassurance	Psychiatrist: You need not worry about your phantom pains—lots of persons with amputations experience the same problem.
Doing without explanation	Psychiatrist: I know what your problem is. You're suffering anxiety from too much stress. Cut back your hours of study. Take these pills three times a day. Start eating three meals a day.
Put-down questions	Psychiatrist: How can you continue to complain about your academic inadequacies when you have all A's and just made Phi Beta Kappa?
"You are bad" statements	Psychiatrist: You keep crying when you mention your mother—hysterics are known to do that.
Trapping patients with their own words	Psychiatrist: You just said you were pleased with your progress; now you're complaining that you're still depressed.
Nonverbal messages of resentment	Psychiatrist turns away from patient, shuffles papers on desk, and closes eyes when patient repeats same verbalization.

Premature advice.   The psychiatrist may assert his or her authority by telling the patient what to do without sufficient information and without engaging the patient in seeking solutions to his or her own problems. Rather than pursuing what may be the etiology of the patient's complaint and getting details of what may be going on in the patient's life, the psychiatrist advances a series of solutions that may be totally inappropriate for the patient. Such premature advice leads the patient to react with resentment and hinders his or her relationship with the psychiatrist (Balint 1972).

False reassurance.   When the psychiatrist tells the patient that something will or will not occur, and either he or she has insufficient information to draw that conclusion or the clinical situation suggests that just the opposite may happen, the psychiatrist is giving the patient false reassurance.

Doing without explanations. When psychiatrists do something to or for patients without reviewing their rationale and without getting the patients' consent, they falsely assume that patients accept their authority without question and are passive recipients of their ministrations.

Put-down questions. Although the psychiatrist may pose a question, the underlying message is one of criticism, derision, or annoyance with the patient.

"You are bad" statements. In another form of derision of a patient, the psychiatrist, falsely believing that he or she is making an interpretation, makes a statement critical of the patient.

Trapping patients with their own words. The psychiatrist may focus on contradictions in the patient's verbalizations to the point of trapping the patient. An example would be a patient who protests that he is very fond of a teacher whom he describes as not treating him fairly in the classroom. Confronting the patient with a contradiction in his verbalizations is counterproductive.

Nonverbal messages of resentment. A psychiatrist may be annoyed at or disapprove of a patient's behaviors. Rather than dealing directly with the patient, he or she uses body language to signal disapproval. For example, a patient walks into the psychiatrist's office and ignores "No Smoking" signs. The patient lights up a cigarette. Instead of confronting the patient's behavior, the psychiatrist begins coughing frequently and frowning at the patient. The patient picks up from these nonverbal cues that the psychiatrist is signaling disapproval. The patient believes that the psychiatrist disapproves of her as a patient. Because of the psychiatrist's behavior, the patient experiences diminished self-esteem and feels demeaned (Platt and McMath 1979; Strayhorn 1977).

Specific Interviewing Situations

Psychiatrists learn to adapt their interviewing methods and styles on the basis of multiple variables that any individual patient presents, including particular psychiatric problems.

Interviewing the Delusional Patient

A delusion is a fixed, false belief that the patient holds to even though it has no basis in reality. There are several types of delusions: delusions of persecution, delusions of grandiosity, erotomania, delusions of jealousy, delusions of reference, and somatic delusions. The psychiatrist inquires whether the patient has ever acted on a delusional belief or has plans to do so.

The psychiatrist's examination of the patient's delusional beliefs will yield significant information regarding the patient's underlying psychodynamic conflicts. The psychiatrist can also observe how the patient defends against painful realities in his or her life and uses his or her delusional system as a form of protection. The psychiatrist looks for the precipitating stresses in the patient's life that led to the formation of these delusions.

The delusional patient is most often brought to treatment by third parties against his or her will. It is important for the psychiatrist to empathically acknowledge the patient's wishes not to be a patient, but also to point out how the psychiatrist may be helpful to the patient and to encourage the patient to communicate with him or her.

The most common error for the newly trained psychiatrist is to try to convince the patient with delusions that his or her false beliefs make no logical sense. Such an approach is counterproductive. Instead, the psychiatrist takes a neutral stance with the patient and neither agrees with a delusional belief nor openly challenges its verity. Only at such a point that the patient expresses doubt about a delusion should the psychiatrist support this doubt. Patients usually do not consider their delusions to be a clinical problem. It is preferable for the psychiatrist to focus on other signs and symptoms for which the patient may want help.

Very often, as the patient's overall clinical condition improves, he or she stops talking about his or her delusional beliefs. It is not necessary for the psychiatrist to raise questions about the delusions, even though he or she may be curious about how steadfast the patient is in retaining the delusions.

Interviewing the Depressed and Potentially Suicidal Patient

Depression, one of the most common problems that psychiatrists evaluate and treat in their practice, can be either a primary psychiatric disorder or secondary to medical disorders or other psychiatric disorders. It is frequently part of a dual diagnosis. For every depressed patient, it is imperative that psychiatrists explore the risk of suicide.

The assessment of depression begins with the patient's appearance and behavior. The psychiatrist observes the patient's general demeanor and posture. The patient walks slowly, holding his or her head down, and lacks spontaneity. Some patients present with an anxious or an agitated depression, with the wringing of hands and pacing. Others exhibit a retarded depression, with a paucity of spontaneous movements. The pace of the interview itself is usually slow, with the patient responding to questions with long pauses and short answers. Very often there is a blunted range of facial expres-

sions, and, at other times, the patient may cry or fight back tears. Not all patients will verbalize feeling depressed. They will often give clues through their verbalizations that indicate a sense of giving up and of not wanting to go on. A depressed patient's thinking and verbalizations are also slowed. Voice intonation patterns are often monotonal. Thinking often reveals excessive guilt, feelings of loss of self-esteem and self-confidence, and a general lack of interest in activities that the patient had previously participated in. These patients exhibit low energy, and their social contacts are diminished as well.

Because the patient often has a number of physical manifestations that are part of the depression, the psychiatrist explores problems with sleep, appetite, bowel habits, sexual functioning, and pain syndromes, among others. The psychiatrist explores the nature of these disturbances and how they have interfered with the patient's functioning. The patient is helped to understand that these physical changes are part of the depression. Because the patient often does not associate the physical complaints with depression, this new knowledge can be a relief.

In exploring the origins of a depression, the psychiatrist looks for significant losses and separations in the patient's life. Death or separation from a loved one often leads to depression. The onset of the syndrome of depression is often delayed following a significant loss. The psychiatrist should also explore anniversary phenomena—depression that occurs on the anniversary of a significant loss.

The psychiatrist takes an active role when interviewing the depressed patient. The patient is encouraged to verbalize what he or she is experiencing. The psychiatrist empathizes with the patient's pain and mental anguish. Prolonged silences on the part of the psychiatrist are rarely helpful with these patients and should be discouraged.

The newly trained psychiatrist is often reluctant to inquire about suicide with a depressed patient, fearing that he or she may be planting an idea that the patient may not have had or fearing that the patient will take offense. Psychiatrists' inquiries about suicide are, on the contrary, a relief to patients. It is essential that the psychiatrist find out what kinds of thoughts the patient has had regarding suicide and whether the patient has ever acted on these thoughts, what plans he or she currently has, and what has kept him or her from acting on these plans.

The subject of suicide is introduced with such questions as "Have things ever gotten so bad that you've had thoughts of ending your life?" If the patient answers in the affirmative, the psychiatrist follows with "Tell me about them." In inquiring about past suicidal behavior, the psychiatrist asks, "Have you ever done anything to hurt yourself?" Again, the psychiatrist pursues details. If all the responses are about the past, the psychiatrist inquires about the present with "Have you had any thoughts of ending your life lately?" The interest here is not only in thoughts or actions but also in the patient's ability to control these impulses. To assess this, the psychiatrist inquires, "What is it that has kept you from carrying out your plans?"

By pursuing the topic of suicide, the psychiatrist arrives at a clinical judgment about the imminent danger of suicide in the patient's life. He or she also learns about what suicide means to an individual patient.

Interviewing the Psychosomatic Patient

Patients with psychosomatic illnesses are usually referred by their primary care physician and rarely seek psychiatric consultation on their own. Their greatest fear is that psychiatric consultation is being sought because they are "crazy" or because the primary physician does not believe that they have a legitimate reason for their complaints. Psychosomatic patients may interpret psychiatric consultation as a signal that their primary physician has given up on them. It is important for the psychiatrist to discuss with the referring physician what the patient has been told about the consultation and to ascertain what clinical questions the referring physician wants the psychiatrist to address in the consultation. Before seeing the patient, the psychiatrist reviews the patient's medical history, including medications and medical procedures and the results of any tests given.

After introducing and identifying himself or herself as a psychiatrist, the consultant psychiatrist reviews with the patient the complaints that led to the patient's seeking care. The psychiatrist then explores with the patient his or her understanding of the reasons for the primary physician's wanting a psychiatric consultation. The psychiatrist establishes his or her interest in the patient's physical complaints as well as any emotional concomitants and also follows up with the patient in clarifying any misunderstandings about the psychiatrist's role as a consultant.

While reviewing the patient's medical history with the patient, the psychiatrist looks for clues to any psychological stresses that may be accompanying the patient's physical symptoms. The psychiatrist checks for autonomic signs of distress during the interview and inquires about the patient's feelings at these points. As the interview progresses, the psychiatrist reviews the specific circumstances that were occurring in the patient's life when he or she first became symptomatic, any significant antecedent events, and the range of feelings that the patient experienced with the onset of the illness.

The psychiatrist inquires about how the patient's symptoms may be interfering with the patient's level of functioning and looks for both the primary and the secondary gains of the symptoms. The psychiatrist explores what the patient feels is wrong with himself or herself, what he or she fears will happen as a result of the illness, and in what ways the symptoms will interfere with the patient's future life.

Because the patient's presenting complaints are physical, the psychiatrist establishes that he or she is interested in these complaints and that in no way is his or her intention to minimize the significance of the complaints. The psychiatrist acknowledges that subjective complaints are real and that his or her inquiries about emotional concomitants are necessary to gain a better understanding of the patient.

The psychiatrist leaves time at the end of the psychiatric consultation visit to answer specific questions that the patient may have or to clarify any misunderstandings. The psychiatrist also summarizes his or her findings and shares any specific recommendations, including return visits to further explore areas not covered in the initial visit. Usually several visits are needed before patients are ready to accept the importance of the impact of emotional reactions on their physical complaints.

Interviewing the Elderly Patient

Elderly patients often need special attention during a psychiatric interview. Psychiatrists usually need to slow the pace of the interview and may need several short interviews instead of one prolonged interview. They need to pay special attention to any physical limitations, whether sensory, motor, coordination, extrapyramidal, or other. For example, hearing-impaired

individuals might need to be seated closer to the psychiatrist. The psychiatrist must speak in clear, loud tones for a hearing-impaired elderly patient to be able to understand him or her. Visual impairments such as cataracts and macular degeneration may lead to elderly patients' not being able to clearly see those interviewing them. Unlike younger patients, with whom an initial handshake may and should be the only physical contact, elderly patients may need to have psychiatrists assist with the patients' safely walking into and out of the room, and a gentle pat on the shoulder or a grasping of elderly patients' hands as a signal of reassurance is often indicated.

The physical status of elderly patients needs special attention so that those with cardiac or respiratory limitations are not overly stressed in an individual interview session. The psychiatrist needs to review medications prescribed and those taken over the counter so that he or she is especially attuned to any drug interactions and aware of the influences of these medications on the elderly patient's mental status and behavior.

Interviewing the Violent Patient

Patients exhibiting violent behavior are most frequently seen in a hospital emergency department setting. The police often bring violent patients to the hospital. One of the first judgments that a psychiatrist must make is the safety of removing physical restraints from patients. Before the police remove handcuffs, the psychiatrist makes contact with the patient to assess his or her reality testing and ability to verbalize. If the patient is judged to be unable to communicate verbally or to be out of touch with reality, the psychiatrist, before proceeding with the interview, requests that the patient be placed in a quiet room where he or she may be restrained. Restraints can be physical or chemical. The psychiatrist first talks with a patient who can communicate verbally about whether to remove restraints. If the patient exhibits any hostile or belligerent behavior when the restraints are being removed, the psychiatrist requests that the restraints remain in place until the patient is calmer. The interview is often conducted with a security officer present, as the officer's uniform is often a deterrent to patients' acting out their impulses. The psychiatrist emphasizes to the patient that the restraints are needed both for the patient's safety and for the safety of other persons in the immediate area.

The psychiatrist never confronts or challenges a violent patient. The psychiatrist lets the patient know when the psychiatrist is frightened by the patient's behavior, and he or she seeks assistance in placing a potentially violent patient in a safe setting. On inpatient units, a seclusion room is used as a temporary placement for violent patients until their behavior is judged not to be dangerous to themselves or others.

The key factor in the approach to violent patients is safety. The psychiatrist works with available staff to maintain the safety of the patient, the staff, and other patients. At no time should the psychiatrist resort to individual heroics in trying to subdue a violent patient. Each hospital is advised to have an emergency plan of action for the management of violent patients, with nursing personnel trained to respond to help control violent patients' behavior. This plan should be rehearsed at staff meetings from month to month, because personnel may change or may forget procedures (Slaby et al. 1981).

Interviewing Relatives

The importance of obtaining consent from the patient before interviewing relatives was addressed earlier in this chapter.

Interviewing relatives can serve several useful functions. The relatives' observations of the patient's presenting problems, their impressions of his or her current living situation, their understanding of the family, their knowledge of the patient's past history, and their recital of developmental milestones can aid in the diagnosis and add to the psychiatrist's understanding of the patient. Relatives can also serve as valuable allies in the treatment process. They can learn to recognize early signs of decompensation and to seek help to prevent further decompensation. They can participate in treatment and aid with compliance, such as with medications, and they can work with the patient and psychiatrist in noting significant changes in the patient's condition. Such changes can include the onset of manic symptoms, suicidal thoughts or behaviors, and psychotic behaviors. The psychiatrist can assess whether couples or family therapy may benefit the patient. The more serious the psychiatric condition, the more likely that the patient will benefit from a relative's participation in assessment and/or treatment. The relative's participation is contingent on the knowledge and agreement that the psychiatrist cannot, without obtaining consent, divulge to a relative any material that the patient presented in confidence to the psychiatrist. On the other hand, the psychiatrist can share any material with the patient that a relative presents. It is of vital importance to consider involving family members and other significant persons in the treatment of most (although not all) patients.

Past History

The previous section on interviewing emphasized the importance of the psychiatrist's pursuing a patient's history according to the leads that the patient presents. However, when recording the material, a specific format is used. This section provides an outline of such a format for the patient's record.

Identification of the Patient

The psychiatrist begins with a brief report of who the patient is, including the following:

- Full name
- Age
- Race
- National/ethnic origin
- Religious affiliation
- Marital status and number of children
- Current employment (past employment, if the patient is unemployed)
- Living situation
- Total number of hospitalizations (and in each case the name of the hospital), including nonpsychiatric hospitalizations
- Total number of hospitalizations for the presenting problem (if the patient has been hospitalized)
- Names and phone numbers of the patient's primary physicians
- Name and phone number of the nearest living relative

Circumstances of Referral

The psychiatrist describes how the patient came to see him or her, who referred the patient, and how the patient was transported. If a patient is referred by a professional, the name and phone number of the referring agent are recorded. If a third party brought the patient, the psychiatrist notes the third party's name and relationship to the patient. The psychiatrist records his or her judgment of the reliability of the third-party informant.

Chief Complaint

The psychiatrist records verbatim the patient's reasons for seeking help at the time of the initial interview. If the patient is too disturbed to verbalize his or her reasons for being seen, a statement from a third party is recorded and the informant is identified. The chief complaint is not always evident in the first interview, particularly in patients with long, complex histories.

History of Present Illness

The psychiatrist records the chronology of events from the onset of symptoms up to the present. With patients who can give a coherent account of their problems, the psychiatrist inquires when the symptoms began. The patient's highest level of functioning is established, and a description is made of how the patient's problems are interfering with his or her optimal functioning. The psychiatrist examines the patient's functioning in the biological, psychological, and social spheres. The psychiatrist documents all the relevant symptoms with which the patient presents. For psychotic patients, psychiatrists need to structure the interview in a way that will obtain the necessary data and to record the data in an organized fashion. The psychiatrist also notes the precipitating stressors at the time the patient became symptomatic and assesses the secondary gains of the patient's symptoms but, again, does not confront the patient with his or her findings.

Psychiatric History

The psychiatrist inquires about the first time the patient was aware of any psychiatric problems. The psychiatrist asks whether any help was sought at that time, and, if help was sought, he or she notes the following:

- Who saw the patient and for how long
- The nature of the treatment
- Medications, if any, that were prescribed

- Modality that was helpful (i.e., individual therapy, group therapy, psychopharmacological interventions)
- Length of treatment
- Reason for discontinuing treatment

Significant events such as hospitalizations, as well as information on where they took place, which treatment modalities were used in these settings, and the length of stay and outcomes should also be noted. Contact with previous treating psychiatrists is most helpful in assisting with understanding past evaluations and treatments.

Alcohol and Drug History

The psychiatrist obtains a history from the patient on the consumption of alcohol and drugs. Inquiries are made about the precise amounts that are consumed and the method of administration, whether it be oral (alcohol), by sniffing (cocaine), or by injections (heroin). The frequency of use is noted. The social setting in which the substances are used is recorded. The psychiatrist learns about the patient's reasons for using drugs—that is, for recreational purposes, to treat or mask one's symptoms (e.g., hallucinations or depression), to succumb to peer pressure, or as part of an addiction pattern. Tolerance for drugs such as sedatives or narcotics is ascertained. The psychiatrist asks whether the patient has ever considered drug taking or alcohol consumption a problem. If so, the psychiatrist learns whether the patient has 1) overdosed on drugs, 2) lost consciousness in the past, and 3) ever suffered from withdrawal effects from drugs. Medical, orthopedic, and surgical complications (including head trauma) as a result of drug consumption are recorded. Any previous efforts toward withdrawal from addicting substances are noted, including problems such as delirium tremens with alcohol withdrawal. The psychiatrist also notes

whether the patient has been in psychiatric treatment or has been treated in separate chemical dependency programs, including self-help groups.

The effects of alcohol consumption and drug taking on the patient's life are also evaluated. These effects include the patient's ability to maintain employment, his or her ability to maintain social relationships, and whether the patient has had any trouble with the law, such as charges of driving while intoxicated.

The effectiveness of previous therapeutic interventions is assessed. The consideration of dual diagnoses with other DSM-IV-TR Axis I diagnoses is reviewed, along with Axis II considerations.

Collateral histories are often vital, because drug- and alcohol-consuming populations are notorious for historical distortions, particularly about the amounts consumed.

Family History

The psychiatrist reviews and records a family tree and lists names and ages of living relatives and names, ages, and time of death of deceased relatives. Any emotional problems as well as organic diseases in family members are indicated (Table 2–7).

Family histories are particularly useful in families who seem to have a genetic vulnerability for psychiatric or organic diseases, including schizophrenia, major affective disorders, Huntington's chorea, and epilepsy.

The family history also describes who the significant relatives in the patient's life have been, what they were like as persons, how the patient related to them, and what roles they played in the patient's upbringing, as well as a description of current significant relationships. When obtaining information about the family from relatives, the psychiatrist notes the sources and reliability of each of the historians. The psychiatrist is also interested in assessing who

TABLE 2–7. Pertinent family psychiatric history

Who had sought psychiatric help and their diagnosis, if known

Psychiatric hospitalizations, if any

What treatment modalities were administered

The names of specific drugs taken, if known

The outcome of treatment

Suicidal behaviors or death by suicide

the supportive figures currently are in the patient's life.

Personal History

The psychiatrist obtains information on the patient's personal history in order to help determine a psychodynamic formulation of the patient's problems. The psychiatrist seeks to understand the critical past events that have led the patient to be the way he or she is today as a person. The clues regarding relevant areas to explore are gleaned from the patient's presentations of the present illness.

A patient's history is never complete. The organization of the data follows a chronology of life events.

Prenatal Period

The psychiatrist records information on the patient from conception to birth. The principal family members are described, and the environment and the household before the patient was born are noted. Significant data include whether a pregnancy was "planned," whether the baby was "wanted," what the toxicological and nutritional status of the mother was during pregnancy, whether the mother had any medical problems such as infections or obstetrical complications, and what type of prenatal care she received. Particular prenatal wishes are noted, such as whether the parents wanted a boy or a girl, what the parental expectations were

for the child when he or she was growing up (e.g., to be an astronaut), whether the child was replacing one lost through a miscarriage or childhood death, and any other special characteristics that were expected of the child. Learning how names were selected and whom the child was named after (if anyone) can give important clues as to parental expectations. The recording of the father's role during the pregnancy and delivery can also yield helpful information. Data about any problems with the delivery, such as a cesarean section and the reasons for it, and any defects at birth are also important to record. Drugs taken by the mother, whether prescribed, over the counter, or illicit, are important to know.

Infancy and Early Childhood Development

The psychiatrist describes the early infant–mother relationship, noting any problems in feeding and sleep patterns, as well as development milestones such as smiling, sitting, standing, and walking. Infantile illnesses or illnesses of the infant's caregivers are noted, as well as how such illnesses may have affected the development of the baby. The psychiatrist also ascertains who the significant people were in the caregiving of the baby and what particular influences each individual had on the child's development.

Symptoms of unusual rocking behaviors, head banging, screaming, thumb sucking, temper tantrums, bed wetting, and nail biting are explored and recorded in detail. Delays of motor activities, speech development, and socialization are noted as well.

A description is given of each of the siblings at home and of how the early sibling relationships developed. The psychiatrist looks for the caregiving roles of siblings as well as roles in which rivalries, if any, developed.

To assess social development, the psychiatrist examines the child's play activities. Independent behaviors and the capacity to concentrate and to look for social interactions are assessed. The patient's earliest memories and the events and feelings associated are important to record. The psychiatrist also explores favorite childhood stories and the patient's associations with them, as well as favorite activities and favorite people.

Middle Childhood (Ages 3–11)

The psychiatrist, who is interested in the intellectual development of the child, inquires about nursery school experiences and how the child adapted to social situations. The child's reactions to first going off to school and leaving home are noted. The psychiatrist inquires about important figures in the patient's life: schoolteachers, ministers, camp counselors, and childhood friends. The child's recreational, athletic, and cultural activities are explored, as well as how the child would spend a typical day. Explorations regarding academic development include the child's favorite subjects, subjects in which he or she excelled, and those that he or she found difficult. If the child repeated any grades, the reasons for having done so are noted.

The psychiatrist also records any prolonged illnesses, surgeries, and accidents with injuries and the influence of these medical/surgical events on the patient's life. In children who were "accident prone" or had multiple soft-tissue injuries and multiple fractures, the psychiatrist is alerted to the possibility of child abuse. Patterns of neglect are also explored.

Areas that relate to discipline and the types of punishment that were used are also explored. The psychiatrist learns who the figures were who meted out punishment and assesses the effects that these behaviors had on the child's development. The psychiatrist also explores any signifi-

cant personal losses or separations during this period, such as the death of significant figures and whether there were any parental separations or divorces and remarriages. The emotional impact of these events is also recorded.

Symptoms reflecting emotional distress are noted. These would include enuresis, nail biting, night terrors, and excessive masturbation.

Late Childhood and Adolescence

The teenage years are important transitional years in the development of the individual from a dependent child to an independent adult. The psychiatrist traces biological development in terms of major body changes and their influence on the individual, as well as the child's psychological development and social development. The psychiatrist inquires about the child's interests and activities, participation in organized sports, hobbies, church activities, introduction to civic responsibilities, work history (often beginning with baby-sitting and newspaper delivery routes), social network, and the influence of religious instruction and the commonalities and differences of the child's belief systems with those of his or her family. In addition to noting the grades and achievements in academic work, the psychiatrist further studies the child's academic potential and his or her areas of special interest and the child's relationship with his or her peer group and with people whom the child likes and wants to emulate, such as teachers, coaches, or public figures.

The psychiatrist examines areas that have led to psychological stress, such as problems in relationships with authority figures, with peers, and with siblings. The psychiatrist also inquires about eating disorders, sleep disturbances, periods of depression, self-mutilation, suicidal ideation, alcohol and drug intake, and problems that relate to the personal identity of the teenager.

Adulthood

The psychiatrist explores the patient's capacities for intimacy, development of friendships, social networks, adult educational history, employment record, intellectual pursuits, recreational activities, and avocational interests. The patient's military history, civic responsibilities, religious affiliations, value systems, political involvements, fiscal security, vacation habits, and relationship with his or her family are also reviewed. The psychiatrist documents what the patient's plans are for the future, whether such plans are achievable, and how the patient intends to implement them. The psychiatrist then records the impact of illnesses, both the patient's own and those affecting close relationships and affecting the patient's life.

Sexual History

The psychiatrist inquires about the patient's early life experiences related to sexual development. The patient's childhood sexual playing experiences, such as playing "doctor" and "nurse," observing the genitalia of other children, and fantasies about sexuality as a child, are explored. The psychiatrist notes not only the child's reactions to these fantasies and play activities but also how family members reacted when the child revealed them or was found engaged in them.

The psychiatrist inquires about what and how the patient learned about sexual activities, conception, and pregnancy and who was responsible for the learning. The reactions of the patient's parents to the patient's inquiries about how babies are born are elicited. The psychiatrist also inquires about a history of sexual abuse.

The psychiatrist asks both male and female patients about their experiences in puberty. With female patients, the inquiries begin with menarche. The female patient is asked about who prepared her for menses, what she was told about what to expect, what the meaning of menses was to the patient, and what the parents' reactions to the menarche were. For both male and female patients, a masturbatory history is obtained with explorations about fantasies that accompanied masturbation. Descriptions of sexual experiences, both heterosexual and homosexual, are elicited, including activities such as kissing, necking, petting, and sexual intercourse.

Attitudes of the patient toward heterosexual and homosexual fantasies and experiences are noted. The psychiatrist also records parental and sibling responses to the adolescent's activities.

The psychiatrist then explores adulthood attitudes and behaviors: the patient's choice of partner, how the couple met, their courting history, their engagement history, premarital sexual activities, their marriage, and (with traditional marriages) their honeymoon. Also recorded are the couple's expectations regarding children, as well as the couple's reactions to childbearing and child rearing and to different stages of development of their children. Marital crises and threats, or actual separations and/or divorces, are also subjects of inquiry. Similar inquiries are made for patients with nontraditional relationships.

Areas of sexual conflict or sexual dysfunctions are examined, such as loss of sexual desire, inability to perform, difficulties with erections and ejaculations, and problems of pain with intercourse or failure to achieve orgasm. The biological, psychological, and social factors influencing these dysfunctions are sought.

Patients will often be reluctant to discuss some, if not all, of these topics regarding sexuality because of accompanying shame, embarrassment, or discomfort. Psychiatrists learn to be nonjudgmental and supportive in exploring the sexual history of their patients.

Medical History

The psychiatrist reviews the patient's medical history, including common as well as chronic childhood illnesses, conditions leading to frequent medical consultation and treatment, and those requiring emergency department visits as well as those leading to hospitalizations. The psychiatrist also reviews the patient's surgical experiences, noting those requiring the administration of anesthesia. The history of accidents and orthopedic interventions is recorded. In addition to the nature and course of each illness, the psychiatrist reviews the impact of these illnesses on the child's growth and development. Inquiries are made about the patient's attitudes toward the professionals who cared for him or her as a child as well as family attitudes toward his or her medical problems.

The psychological meaning of illnesses and interventions is explored in terms of the patient's feelings about injury to body parts, effects on body image, and fears and concerns about invalidism and death. The psychiatrist reviews adult-onset illnesses, medical interventions, and surgical and obstetrical events. The effects of these on the patient's functioning at work and at play, on the families, and on interpersonal relationships are noted. The psychiatrist also assesses the patient's motivations for and capacities to assist in recovery, his or her levels of denial of the effect of serious illnesses on functioning and longevity, and the coping mechanisms that the patient employs. Inquiries are made about support systems that the patient has used to aid in the recovery from past illnesses, including the availability of these systems and the willingness of the patient to use them to help with the current situation.

Mental Status Examination

The mental status examination is a description of all the areas of mental functioning of the patient (Table 2–8). It serves the same function for psychiatrists as the physical examination does for the primary care physician. Psychiatrists follow a structured format in recording their findings. These descriptive data are then used to support the psychiatrists' diagnostic conclusions. An outline of the component parts of the mental status examination follows (Engel 1979; Keller and Manschreck 1981; Lewis 1943; Masserman and Schwab 1974; Menninger 1952; Reiser and Schroder 1980; Small 1981; Stevenson 1969; Tilley and Hoffman 1981; Trzepacz and Baker 1993; Weitzel et al. 1973).

General Description

Appearance

The psychiatrist records in detail the prominent physical features of an individual such that a portrait of the person could be painted that highlights his or her unique aspects. Included are facial features; hair color, texture, styling, and grooming; height; weight; body shape; cleanliness; neatness; posture; bearing; clothing; jewelry; skin texture, scar formation, and tattoos; level of eye contact; eye movements; facial expressions and mobility; tearfulness; degrees of friendliness; and an estimate of how old the patient looks compared with chronological age. In the report of these findings, poetic license can be used in painting a picture of the person.

TABLE 2–8. The mental status examination

1. General description
   a. Appearance
   b. Motor behavior
   c. Speech
   d. Attitudes
2. Emotions
   a. Mood
   b. Affective expression
   c. Appropriateness
3. Perceptual disturbances
   a. Hallucinations
   b. Illusions
   c. Depersonalization
   d. Derealization
4. Thought process
   a. Stream of thought
   b. Thought content
   c. Abstract thinking
   d. Education and intelligence
   e. Concentration
5. Orientation
6. Memory
   a. Remote memory
   b. Recent past memory
   c. Recent memory
7. Impulse control
8. Judgment
9. Insight

Motor Behavior

The psychiatrist describes the patient's gait and freedom of movement, noting the firmness and strength of handshake. The psychiatrist observes any involuntary or abnormal movements such as tremors, tics, mannerisms, lip smacking, akathisias, or repeated stereotyped movements. The pace of movements, whether accelerated or retarded, is also noted. The psychiatrist comments on the purposefulness of movements and takes note of degrees of agitation of the patient as reflected in pacing and hand wringing.

Speech

The psychiatrist listens for the patient's rate of speech, the spontaneity of verbal-izations, the range of voice intonation patterns, the volume in terms of loudness, defects with verbalizations such as stammering or stuttering, and any aphasias.

Attitudes

The psychiatrist routinely summarizes how the patient related to him or her in the course of the interview. The psychiatrist not only notes general impressions such as "friendly and cooperative" but focuses on any shifts or changes in attitude during particular points in the interview. An example would be the psychiatrist's noting that when inquiring about a patient's relations with authority figures, the patient related in a "belligerent, hostile, and threatening manner."

It is also helpful for the psychiatrist to keep track of his or her own attitudes toward the patient, whether they be "warm, caring, concerned, and empathic" or "frustrated and angry." Such a summary of the psychiatrist's attitudes can often help in diagnostic formulations as well as in planning treatment strategies.

Emotions

Mood

Mood is the sustained feeling tone that prevails over time for a patient. At times the patient will verbalize this mood. At other times, the psychiatrist will have to inquire about it and even infer the patient's mood from observations of the patient's nonverbal body language. When describing a mood, the psychiatrist records how deeply it is felt, the length of time that it prevails, and how much it fluctuates. Anxious, panicky, terrified, sad, depressed, angry, enraged, euphoric, and guilty are moods frequently described.

Affective Expression

The psychiatrist records his or her observations regarding the range of expression of feeling tones. The predominant expression is described. This may include flat affect, in which there is virtually no visible expression of feelings during the relating of emotionally charged material. This mode of expression has been classically associated with schizophrenia. The incongruity of the expressions with the verbalizations is most striking in schizophrenia and other psychotic disorders. Constricted affects are often seen with depression, lability of mood may be associated with cognitive disorders, and blunting of affect is often seen with dementia. The psychiatrist observes and records the patient's nonverbal behaviors, such as facial mobility, voice intonation patterns, and body movements, to assess affective expression.

Appropriateness

The psychiatrist judges whether the affective tone and expression are appropriate to the subject matter being discussed in the context of the patient's thinking. Disharmonies between affective expression and thought content are worthy of exploration with the patient.

Perceptual Disturbances

Hallucinations and Illusions

A *hallucination* is a perceptual distortion that a patient experiences for which there is no external stimulus. These hallucinations may be auditory (hearing noises or voices that nobody else hears), visual (seeing objects that are not present), tactile (feeling sensations when there is no stimulus for them), gustatory (tasting sensations when there is no stimulus for them), or olfactory (smelling odors that are not present). Hallucinations during the hypnagogic state (the drowsy state that precedes sleep) and the hypnopompic state (the semiconscious state that precedes awakening) are experiences associated with normal sleep and with narcolepsy.

An *illusion* is a false impression that results from a real stimulus. An example of an illusion is driving down a dry road and observing "water patches" several hundred feet ahead of you, then driving closer and having them disappear.

Depersonalization and Derealization

Depersonalization describes patients' feelings that they are not themselves, that they are strange, or that there is something different about themselves that they cannot account for. The symptom is associated with a variety of psychiatric disorders.

Derealization expresses patients' feelings that the environment is somehow different or strange but they cannot account for these changes. This perceptual distortion is frequently seen in schizophrenic patients.

Thought Process

The psychiatrist assesses how well a patient formulates, organizes, and expresses his or her thoughts. Coherent thought is clear, easy to follow, and logical. A formal thought disorder includes all disorders of thinking that affect language, communication of thought, or thought content. Such disorder is often ascribed to the disordered thinking of schizophrenic patients.

Stream of Thought

The psychiatrist records the quantity and rate of the patient's thoughts. The psychiatrist looks for the two extremes, whether a paucity or a flooding of thoughts. He or she also notes whether there is retardation or slowing or whether there is acceleration or racing. When thoughts are so sped up that the psychiatrist has difficulty keeping up with the patient, it is termed a *flight of ideas*.

The psychiatrist also examines the patient for the goal directedness and continuity of the patient's thoughts. Disturbances include circumstantiality, tangential thinking, blocking, loose associations, and perseveration.

Thought Content (Delusions, Obsessions, Compulsions, Preoccupations, Phobias)

Thought content refers to what the patient talks about. There are specific areas that the psychiatrist inquires about if they are not brought up by the patient. One important area is whether the patient has suicidal thoughts. This is particularly important in patients who signal feelings of helplessness, hopelessness, worthlessness, or giving up.

Delusions are false fixed beliefs that have no rational basis in reality and are deemed unacceptable by the patient's culture. Delusions that cannot be understood by other psychological processes are referred to as *primary delusions*. Examples include thought insertion, thought broadcasting, and beliefs about world destruction. *Secondary delusions* are based on other psychological experiences. These include delusions derived from hallucinations, other delusions, and morbid affective states.

Types of delusions include those of persecution, of jealousy, of guilt, of love, of poverty, and of nihilism.

In addition to the description of delusions, the psychiatrist assesses the degrees of organization of the delusion. The psychiatrist notes ideas of reference and ideas of influence.

The psychiatrist notes any *obsessions* the patient may have. These are marked by repetitive, unwelcome, irrational thoughts that impose themselves on the patient's consciousness and over which he or she has no apparent control. These thoughts are accompanied by feelings of anxious dread and are ego-alien, unacceptable, and undesirable. They are strongly resisted by the patient.

Compulsions, a closely parallel phenomenon, are repetitive, stereotyped behaviors that the patient feels impelled to perform ritualistically, even though he or she recognizes the irrationality and absurdity of the behaviors. Although no pleasure is derived from performing such an act, there is a temporary sense of relief of tension when it is completed.

In addition to describing obsessions and compulsions, the psychiatrist discusses the degree of interference with the patient's functioning. *Preoccupations* are also noted. These reflect the patient's absorption with his or her own thoughts to such a degree that the patient loses contact with external reality. The degree of preoccupation is also observed. Mild forms are reflected in absentmindedness; severe forms can involve suicidal or homicidal ideation and the autistic thinking of the schizophrenic patient.

Phobias are morbid fears that are reflected by morbid anxiety. They are often not spontaneously conveyed in the interview, and the psychiatrist should make specific inquiries about their presence (Campbell 1996; Stone 1988; Thompson 1979).

Abstract Thinking

Abstract, or categorical, thinking is formed late in the development of thought and reflects the capacity to formulate concepts and to generalize. Several methods are used to test this capacity. These include testing similarities, differences, and the meaning of proverbs. The inability to abstract is referred to as concreteness, which in turn reflects an earlier childhood development of thought. Concreteness of responses on formal testing reflects intellectual impoverishment, cultural deprivation, and cognitive disorders such as dementia. Bizarre and inappropriate responses to proverbs reflect schizophrenic thinking.

Education and Intelligence

Intelligence is best measured in the clinical interview by the patient's use of vocabulary. The expectations of levels of intelligence are influenced by the level of education of the patient.

Concentration

Concentration reflects the patient's ability to focus and to maintain his or her attention on a task. In the interview, troubles with concentration are reflected in the patient's inability to pay attention to the questions that he or she is being asked. He or she may be distracted by external or internal stimuli. When the patient's concentration is impaired, the psychiatrist often has to repeat the questions.

Orientation (Time, Place, Person, Situation)

Orientation reflects patients' capacities to know who they are, where they are, what date and time it is, and what their present circumstances are. Patients who have deficits in three spheres are commonly suffering from cognitive disorders.

Memory

Remote Memory

Remote memory is the recollection of events from earlier in life. The psychiatrist tests for this function by asking where the patient grew up, where he or she went to school, and what his or her first job was and inquires about significant people from the past (e.g., naming of presidents) and also significant events (e.g., World War II, the Korean War, the Vietnam War).

Recent Past Memory

Recent past memory refers to recalling verifiable events from the past few days. To test for this, the psychiatrist inquires about what the patient ate for breakfast or what he or she read in the newspaper or asks for details about what the patient watched on television the night before.

Recent Memory

Recent or short-term memory is gauged by the patient's capacity to recount what he or she was told 5 minutes after hearing it and being coached to remember it. The psychiatrist tests this capacity by asking the patient to repeat the names of three unrelated objects, then informing him or her that they will go on to discuss other subjects and that in 5 minutes the patient will be asked to name the three objects (Albert 1984; Folstein et al. 1975; Gurland et al. 1976; Taylor et al. 1980; Yudofsky and Hales 1997).

Impulse Control

Impulse control is "the ability to control the expression of aggressive, hostile, fearful, guilty, affectionate, or sexual impulses in situations where their expression should be maladaptive" (MacKinnon and Yudofsky 1986, p. 74). Manifestations of this phenomenon are verbal and/or behavioral. A loss of control can reflect a low frustration tolerance (MacKinnon and Yudofsky 1986; Yudofsky et al. 1986).

Judgment

Judgment refers to the patient's capacity to make appropriate decisions and appropriately act on them in social situations. An assessment of this function is best made in the course of obtaining patient's history. There is no necessary correlation between intelligence and judgment. Formal testing is rarely helpful. An example of testing would be to ask the patient, "What would you do if you saw a train approaching a broken track?"

Insight

The capacity of the patient to be aware and to understand that he or she has a problem or illness and to be able to review its probable causes and arrive at tenable solutions is referred to as insight. Emotional insight refers to the patient's awareness of his or her motivations, and, in turn, his or her feelings, so that the patient can change long-standing, ingrained patterns of behavior. Self-observation alone is insufficient for insight. Emotional insight must be applied for change to occur (Donnelly et al. 1970; Ross and Leichner 1984).

Reliability

On completion of an interview, the psychiatrist assesses the reliability of the information that has been obtained. Factors affecting reliability include the patient's intellectual endowment, his or her honesty and motivations, the presence of psychosis or organic defects, and the patient's tendency to magnify or understate his or her problems.

Psychodynamic Formulation

At the conclusion of the interview, history taking, and mental status examination, the psychiatrist documents a psychodynamic formulation of the patient. The psychiatrist describes the key elements of the patient's personality structures, principal psychological conflicts, and healthier, adaptive abilities.

The psychiatrist assesses the ego functions of the patient, including defense mechanisms used, regulation and control of drives, relationships to others, self-representation, stimulus regulation, adaptive relaxation, reality testing, and synthetic integration. By reviewing the patient's developmental history, the psychiatrist assesses the patient's typical drives, impulses, wishes, and anxieties at each stage of development. The psychiatrist can then establish the origins of each of the patient's conflicts and how they carry over to successive periods of development. The psychiatrist focuses on the major adaptive problems of the patient and on how earlier developmental deficits help explain the patient's current difficulties (Freud 1936/1946; Pruyser 1979; Wallerstein 1983; Yudofsky et al. 1986).

Psychiatrists thus trace from early development to the present patients' major conflicts, evolving symptoms, character traits, and defenses. They then organize these data in a psychodynamic formulation (MacKinnon and Yudofsky 1986).

Conclusions

The psychiatric interview is unique among medical interviews in its potential to go beyond mere formulation of symptoms and assignment of a diagnosis. When properly conducted, the interview allows for a thorough understanding of a patient and of how presenting problems relate to this particular individual. The interview represents an opportunity to gain an understanding of the patient in multiple dimensions—psychological, social, and biological. The psychiatric interview allows the psychiatrist to understand the patient and his or her illness.

References

Albert M: Assessment of cognitive function in the elderly. Psychosomatics 25:310–313, 316–317, 1984

American Psychiatric Association: Diagnostic and Statistical Manual of Mental Disorders, 4th Edition, Text Revision. Washington, DC, American Psychiatric Association, 2000

American Psychiatric Association: The Principles of Medical Ethics With Annotations Especially Applicable to Psychiatry, 2001 Edition. Washington, DC, American Psychiatric Association, 2001

Balint M: The Doctor, His Patient and the Illness, 2nd Edition. New York, International Universities Press, 1972

Campbell RJ: Psychiatric Dictionary, 7th Edition. New York, Oxford University Press, 1996

Donnelly J, Rosenberg M, Fleeson WP: The evolution of the mental status—past and future. Am J Psychiatry 126:997–1002, 1970

Engel IM: The mental status examination in psychiatry: origin, use and content. Journal of Psychiatric Education 3:99–108, 1979

Folstein MF, Folstein SW, McHugh PR: "Mini-Mental State": a practical method of grading the cognitive state of patients for the clinician. J Psychiatr Res 12:189–198, 1975

Freud A: The Ego and the Mechanisms of Defense (1936). New York, International Universities Press, 1946

Garrett A: Interviewing: Its Principles and Methods. New York, Family Service Association of America, 1942

Gill M, Newman R, Redich FC: The Initial Interview in Psychiatric Practice. New York, International Universities Press, 1954

Greenspan SI, Greenspan NT: The Clinical Interview of the Child, 2nd Edition. Washington, DC, American Psychiatric Press, 1991

Group for the Advancement of Psychiatry: Initial Interviews. New York, Group for the Advancement of Psychiatry, 1961

Gurland BJ, Copeland L, Sharpe J, et al: The Geriatric Mental Status Interview (GMS). Int J Aging Hum Dev 7:303–311, 1976

Halleck SL: Evaluation of the Psychiatric Patient: A Primer. New York, Plenum, 1991

Keller MB, Manschreck TC: The bedside mental status examination—reliability and validity. Compr Psychiatry 22:500–511, 1981

Kestenbaum CJ: The clinical interview of the child, in Textbook of Child and Adolescent Psychiatry, 2nd Edition. Edited by Wiener JM. Washington, DC, American Psychiatric Press, 1997, pp 79–88

Leon RL: Psychiatric Interviewing: A Primer. New York, Elsevier/North Holland, 1982

Lewis NDC: Outlines for Psychiatric Examinations, 3rd Edition. Albany, NY, New York State Department of Mental Hygiene, 1943

Luborsky L: Principles of Psychoanalytic Psychotherapy: A Manual for Supportive-Expressive Treatment. New York, Basic Books, 1984

MacKinnon RA, Michels R: The Psychiatric Interview in Clinical Practice. Philadelphia, PA, WB Saunders, 1971

MacKinnon RA, Yudofsky SC: The Psychiatric Evaluation in Clinical Practice. Philadelphia, PA, JB Lippincott, 1986

Masserman JH, Schwab JJ: The Psychiatric Examination. New York, Intercontinental Medical Books, 1974

Menninger KA: A Manual for Psychiatric Case Study. New York, Grune & Stratton, 1952

Morrison J: The First Interview: A Guide for Clinicians. New York, Guilford, 1993

Nurcombe B, Fitzhenry-Coor I: How do psychiatrists think? Clinical reasoning in the psychiatric interview: a research and education project. Aust N Z J Psychiatry 16:13–24, 1982

Othmer E, Othmer SC: The Clinical Interview Using DSM-IV, Vol 1: Fundamentals. Washington, DC, American Psychiatric Press, 1994

Platt FW, McMath JC: Clinical hypocompetence: the interview. Ann Intern Med 91:898–902, 1979

Pruyser PW: The Psychological Examination: A Guide for Clinicians. New York, International Universities Press, 1979

Reiser DE, Schroder AK: Patient Interviewing: The Human Dimension. Baltimore, MD, Williams & Wilkins, 1980

Robson KS (ed): Manual of Clinical Child Psychiatry. Washington, DC, American Psychiatric Press, 1986

Ross CA, Leichner P: Residents training in the mental status examination. Can J Psychiatry 29:315–318, 1984

Rutter M, Cox A: Psychiatric interviewing techniques, I: methods and measures. Br J Psychiatry 138:273–282, 1981

Rutter M, Tuma AH, Lann IS: Assessment and Diagnosis in Child Psychopathology. New York, Guilford, 1988

Slaby AE, Lieb J, Tancredi LR: Handbook of Psychiatric Emergencies: A Guide for Emergencies in Psychiatry, 2nd Edition. Garden City, NY, Medical Examination Publishing, 1981

Small SM: Outline for Psychiatric Examination. East Hanover, NJ, Sandoz Pharmaceuticals, 1981

Stevenson I: The Psychiatric Examination. Boston, MA, Little, Brown, 1969

Stone EM: American Psychiatric Glossary, 6th Edition. Washington, DC, American Psychiatric Press, 1988

Strayhorn JM Jr: Talking It Out: A Guide to Effective Communication and Problem Solving. Champaign, IL, Illinois Research Press, 1977

Strupp HH, Binder JL: Psychotherapy in a New Key: A Guide to Time-Limited Dynamic Psychotherapy. New York, Basic Books, 1984

Sullivan HS: The Psychiatric Interview. Edited by Perry HS, Gawel ML. New York, WW Norton, 1954

Taylor MA, Abrams R, Faber R, et al: Cognitive tasks in the mental status examination. J Nerv Ment Dis 168:167–170, 1980

Thompson MGG (ed): A Resident's Guide to Psychiatric Education. New York, Plenum, 1979

Tilley DH, Hoffman JA: Mental status examination: myth or method? Compr Psychiatry 22:562–564, 1981

Trzepacz PT, Baker RW: The Psychiatric Mental Status Examination. New York, Oxford University Press, 1993

Wallerstein RS: Defenses, defense mechanisms, and the structure of the mind. J Am Psychoanal Assoc 31 (suppl):207–225, 1983

Weitzel WD, Morgan DW, Guyden TE, et al: Toward a more efficient mental status examination. Arch Gen Psychiatry 28:215–218, 1973

Whitehorn JC: Guide to interviewing and clinical personality study. Archives of Neurology and Psychiatry 52:197–216, 1944

Yudofsky SC, Hales RE (eds): American Psychiatric Press Textbook of Neuropsychiatry, 3rd Edition. Washington, DC, American Psychiatric Press, 1997

Yudofsky SC, Silver JM, Jackson W, et al: The Overt Aggression Scale for the objective rating of verbal and physical aggression. Am J Psychiatry 143:35–39, 1986

Suggested Readings

Cameron N: Personality Development and Psychopathology: A Dynamic Approach. Boston, MA, Houghton-Mifflin, 1963

Endicott J, Spitzer RL: A diagnostic interview: the Schedule for Affective Disorders and Schizophrenia. Arch Gen Psychiatry 35:837–844, 1978

CHAPTER 3

Delirium, Dementia, and Amnestic Disorders

James A. Bourgeois, O.D., M.D.

Jeffrey S. Seaman, M.S., M.D.

Mark E. Servis, M.D.

D elirium, dementia, and amnestic disorders are classified with other disorders of memory and other cognitive functions in DSM-IV-TR (American Psychiatric Association 2000). As a group, they represent psychiatric disturbances formerly described as exclusively due to "organic" as opposed to "functional" etiological factors. In addition, psychological factors may be of great importance in the patient's experience of symptoms and his or her behavioral and emotional response to illness. Delirium, dementia, and the amnestic disorders make clear the need for psychiatric evaluation based on the biopsychosocial model of psychiatric illness.

In the management of cognitive disorders, there is a high likelihood of psychiatrist involvement with other specialty physicians in the often-complex medical and surgical presentations of these patients. Thorough evaluation of psychiatric, neurological, general medical/surgical,

and psychosocial variables is essential to render appropriate care. Although delirium, dementia, and amnestic disorders are discussed in this chapter as separate pathological entities, the alert physician must be mindful of the possible comorbidity of more than one cognitive disorder in a given patient.

Recent research and clinical developments have enabled advances in pathophysiology, prevention efforts, and treatments for delirium, dementia, and amnestic disorders. Skill in management of these disorders is expected of all psychiatrists and is the sine qua non of those practicing consultation-liaison psychiatry.

Delirium

Definition

Delirium is an acute, potentially reversible brain dysfunction manifested by a

The author of the "Dementia" portion of this chapter (J.A.B.) is grateful to Michael G. Wise, M.D., for his thoughtful review and editorial suggestions.

syndromal array of neuropsychiatric symptoms. Engel and Romano (1959) called delirium a "syndrome of cerebral insufficiency," analogous to cardiac or renal insufficiency. They essentially proposed that delirium is both a disease and a syndrome—a "new" conceptualization fundamental to a full understanding of delirium.

Clinical Features

DSM-IV-TR Diagnosis of Delirium

The DSM-IV-TR diagnostic criteria for delirium require a disturbance in *consciousness/attention* and a change in *cognition* that develop *acutely* and tend to *fluctuate* (Table 3–1). Lipowski (1983, 1987) characterized delirium as a disorder of attention, wakefulness, cognition, and motor behavior. The disruption of attention is often considered the core symptom. Patients struggle to sustain attentional focus, are easily distracted, and often vary in their level of alertness. Sleep and wake cycles are disrupted as well. The impairment in cognition can be across a wide spectrum—from subtle to overt and from focal to global. Deficits can occur in perception, memory, language, processing speed, and executive functioning.

Delirium Subtypes

Consistent with the ancient descriptions of phrenitis and lethargis, hyperactive and hypoactive subtypes have been reported. Liptzin and Levkoff (1992) characterized delirious patients with restlessness, hypervigilance, rapid speech, irritability, and combativeness as *hyperactive*, whereas those showing slowed speech and kinetics, apathy, and reduced alertness were designated *hypoactive*. Hypoactive patients tend to have more severe cognitive disturbances (Koponen et al. 1989c) and a poorer prognosis (Liptzin and Levkoff 1992; Reyes et al. 1981). Meagher and

TABLE 3–1. DSM-IV-TR diagnostic criteria for delirium due to...*[indicate the general medical condition]*

A. Disturbance of consciousness (i.e., reduced clarity of awareness of the environment) with reduced ability to focus, sustain, or shift attention.
B. A change in cognition (such as memory deficit, disorientation, language disturbance) or the development of a perceptual disturbance that is not better accounted for by a preexisting, established, or evolving dementia.
C. The disturbance develops over a short period of time (usually hours to days) and tends to fluctuate during the course of the day.
D. There is evidence from the history, physical examination, or laboratory findings that the disturbance is caused by the direct physiological consequences of a general medical condition.

Coding note: If delirium is superimposed on a preexisting vascular dementia, indicate the delirium by coding 290.41 vascular dementia, with delirium.

Coding note: Include the name of the general medical condition on Axis I, e.g., 293.0 delirium due to hepatic encephalopathy; also code the general medical condition on Axis III.

Trzepacz (1998) further hypothesized that specific delirium subtypes portend different precipitants and causes. Two examples are the hypoactive presentation in hepatic encephalopathy and the hyperactive or mixed forms in alcohol and sedative withdrawal.

Etiopathogenesis

Comorbid systemic diseases may precipitate, but do not cause, delirium. A campfire analogy may help to clarify this proposed model. The flammability of the wood is the baseline vulnerability, the matches are the precipitants, the fire is the etiopathogenic engine, and finally, the light and heat are the cognitive and be-havioral manifestations of delirium. In this section, the "fire" of the disease is explored.

Neuronal Integrity

Engel and Romano (1959) initiated the search to understand the basis of delirium. In their view, the functional integrity of the neuron was paramount; they even hy-pothesized that disturbances in oxygen and glutamate metabolism could be key. More recently, two clinician-scientists, Trzepacz (1994) and Brown (2000), have led the effort to extend Engel and Ro-mano's work (American Psychiatric Asso-ciation 1999).

The cornerstone of the Brown (2000) theory is the notion that it is the relation-ship between the limited energy reserves of the neuron and the varying resilience of different neuronal populations that underlies the behavioral and cognitive changes seen in delirium. In other words, Brown hypothesized, the development of delirium is initiated and then sustained through the selective and progressive dysfunction of specific neurotransmit-ters and neural circuits. Fundamentally, Brown (2000) noted that cerebral insuf-ficiency is intimately linked to relative deficits in oxygen (O_2) and energy me-tabolism.

Role of Oxygen

The clinical importance of oxygen in the pathogenesis of delirium was demon-strated in several studies. Aakerlund and Rosenberg (1994) reported that post-thoracotomy patients who developed de-lirium had lower postoperative O_2 satura-tions, and supplemental O_2 successfully treated these cases. Another study (Ro-senberg and Kehlet 1993) found a strong correlation between postoperative men-tal function and the O_2 saturations on the second postoperative night. The impor-tance of oxidative metabolism is also evi-dent in patients with sepsis. These pa-tients have lower hemoglobin, lower cerebral blood flow (CBF), lower meta-bolic rate for O_2, and lower cerebral O_2 delivery than control subjects (Maekawa et al. 1991). Even among healthy young adults, concentration and short-term learning is degraded when the partial pressure of oxygen (PaO_2) drops to 45–60 mm Hg, and frank delirium reliably occurs at a PaO_2 of 35–45 mm Hg (Gib-son et al. 1981). Delirium would likely have developed at a higher PaO_2 had this study been in a less robust population such as the elderly, who have less com-pensatory reserves.

Cardiovascular and Respiratory Reserves

A broad decline in cardiovascular and res-piratory reserves occurs with age. Oxygen delivery to the brain in times of increased metabolic stress can also be limited by the reduced capacity for compensatory changes in carotid and vertebral vessel dy-namics. Due to in part to these factors, the frail elderly patient can be viewed as being exquisitely vulnerable to sliding into "brain insufficiency" (Tune 1991)—much like patients with "brittle" congestive heart failure.

Oxygen Demand and Anemia

Brown (2000) noted that the hospitalized patient's homeostasis is additionally threatened by the increased O_2 demand from acute illness and fever (Fink 1997; Weissman et al. 1984). Anemia, which further limits O_2 delivery to the brain, is also commonly encountered among hospi-talized surgery patients and the chroni-cally ill. As will be shown, keeping the brain alive but not at an adequate func-tional level can have dire consequences.

Anoxia

In further exploring the role of oxidative metabolism in the development of delirium, Brown (2000) referred to research on anoxic encephalopathy. He reviewed the consequences of inadequate aerobic metabolism, including abnormal neurotransmitter synthesis, release, and metabolism (Gibson et al. 1981); anoxic depolarization with depressed neuronal function (Balestrino et al. 1989); and increased production and decreased disposal of neurotoxins (Globus et al. 1988a; Kirsch et al. 1989). Brown (2000) hypothesized that delirium might share these events, and thus, addressing these consequences of inadequate aerobic metabolism could provide more precise targets for physiological interventions.

Additional Selective Mechanisms

Further support for the role of selective vulnerability in delirium comes from animal models. In one hypoxic encephalopathy model, dopamine release was shown to increase 500-fold, whereas GABA release was increased only fivefold (Globus et al. 1988a). This massive increase in dopamine results from a breakdown in ATP-dependent transporters (decreased reuptake) during anoxic depolarization (Pulsinelli and Duffy 1983) as well as decreases in metabolism through the reduced activity of the O_2-dependent catechol-O-methyltransferase (Gibson et al. 1981). Another potential mechanism underlying the increase in dopamine is reduced activity of dopamine-β-hydroxylase. This enzyme is also O_2 dependent; thus, in hypoxic conditions, less dopamine is converted to norepinephrine (Gibson et al. 1981). Another animal model of encephalopathy (sepsis) also demonstrated these higher dopamine levels (Freund et al. 1986).

In hypoxic conditions, the metabolism of dopamine, but not of other catecholamines, shifts to more toxic oxidative pathways, generating cytotoxic quinones (Graham 1978). Interestingly, preexisting lesions of the substantia nigra have been found to protect projection areas during hypoxia (Globus et al. 1986). For these toxic agents to injure neurons, they first must overwhelm the cell's protective mechanisms—for example, superoxide dismutase, catalase, glutathione peroxidase, and reduced glutathione (Graham 1984). It would be of clinical interest to examine whether these protective systems are reduced in patients at high risk for delirium and, as Brown (2000) posited, whether these toxic metabolites are related to the permanent cognitive sequelae of delirium.

Research in hepatic encephalopathy may also offer insight into the etiopathogenesis of delirium. Specifically, ATP and phosphocreatine depletion occur in this disease (Bluml et al. 1998; Kosenko et al. 1994; Schenker et al. 1967). The neurotoxicity of ammonia is also mediated by N-methyl-D-aspartate (NMDA) receptor activation, which in turn further increases ATP consumption. Additionally, dopamine excess may be necessary for glutamate to exert its toxic effect (Globus et al. 1988b).

Neurotransmitter Roles

Regarding specific changes in neurotransmitters in delirium, the two most accepted are a reduction in ACh activity and an excess of dopamine activity (Trzepacz 2000). ACh has long been known to be decreased in delirium (Itil and Fink 1966) as well as in hypoxia (Gibson and Blass 1976). Attention, cognitive functioning, and memory are heavily dependent on ACh (Trzepacz 2000). Both human (Itil and Fink 1966) and animal (Trzepacz et al. 1992) models of delirium have utilized anticholinergic medications to induce delirium with the resultant hyperactivity, psychosis (humans), cognitive impairment, and electroencephalogram (EEG) slowing.

Dopamine is considered to have important roles in attention, mood, motor activity, perception (Trzepacz 2000), and executive functioning. Agonists of dopamine have also been shown to cause EEG slowing despite motoric hyperactivity (Ongini et al. 1985). Moreover, interplay between dopamine and ACh exists, as evidenced experimentally by the finding that D_2 antagonists enhance ACh release (Ikarashi et al. 1997) and clinically by the utility of antipsychotics in reversing anticholinergic-precipitated delirium (Itil and Fink 1966).

Neuroanatomic Loci

Although there is no single neuroanatomic locus for delirium, studies and case reports consistently identify prefrontal and right-sided brain dysfunction (Doyle and Warden 1996; Koponen et al. 1989b; Trzepacz 2000). Nonetheless, in a recent prospective study comparing stroke patients who became delirious with those who did not, there were no differences found between lesion location and delirium rates (Henon et al. 1999). Delirium has thus been associated with damage to specific brain regions (i.e., bifrontal and right prefrontal cortex, right anterior thalamus, right posterior parietal cortex, basal ganglia, and lingual gyrus), yet lesions anywhere can precipitate delirium (Trzepacz 2000).

Epidemiology

Inpatient Studies

Delirium is epidemic among hospitalized patients, especially in the elderly. Inouye (1998) estimated that delirium annually complicated the hospitalizations of 2.3 million elderly Americans, was present for about 17 million inpatient days, and cost Medicare alone 4 billion dollars, excluding the substantial postdischarge morbidity costs. Inpatient studies have reported a delirium prevalence of 12%–40% among geriatric patients (Francis and Kapoor 1992; Hodkinson 1973; Inouye and Charpentier 1996; Inouye et al. 1993, 1998; Johnson et al. 1990; O'Keeffe and Lavan 1997; Rockwood 1989; Schor et al. 1992; Thomas et al. 1988), 10%–15% across patients of all ages (Cameron et al. 1987; Erkinjuntii et al. 1986), and 37% among postoperative patients (Dyer et al. 1995). Delirium has been found to be even more common in elderly patients with hip fractures (41%, Marcantonio et al. 2000; 61%, Gustafson et al. 1988), hospitalized AIDS patients (57%, Fernandez et al. 1989), terminally ill cancer patients (46%, Gagnon et al. 2000; 85%, Massie et al. 1983), and patients undergoing stem-cell transplantation (73%, Fann et al. 2000).

Diagnostic and Liaison Challenges

As consultation psychiatrists can attest, most delirium cases either are never diagnosed (Cameron et al. 1987; Elie et al. 2000; Francis et al. 1990; Levin 1951; Rockwood et al. 1994) or are misdiagnosed (Armstrong et al. 1997; Golinger et al. 1987; Nicholas and Lindsey 1995). Diagnosis can also be difficult because some delirious patients remain "fluent" despite marked cognitive impairment (C.A. Ross et al. 1991). Delirium, of course, can also fluctuate. A patient may be in a "lucid interval" for the physician's visit and yet be frankly delirious at other times. Lastly, it is often only the troublesome behavioral cases that generate consultation requests or receive delirium-specific treatment (Engel and Romano 1959; Meagher et al. 1996). Opportunities clearly exist, then, for consultation-liaison psychiatrists to actively educate and assist in the management of delirium (Table 3–2).

TABLE 3–2. Evaluation of delirium

Standard
Complete history
Medication review
Neurological examination
Vital signs
Bedside testing: Mini-Mental State Examination, Trails B, Clock drawing, a test for vigilance, days of the week backward
As clinically warranted
Laboratory work: Complete blood count,
electrolytes, blood urea nitrogen, creatinine,
glucose, calcium, pulse oximetry or arterial
blood gas, urinalysis, drug screens, liver function tests with serum albumin, cultures,
cerebrospinal fluid examination
Tests: Chest X ray, electrocardiogram, brain
imaging, electroencephalogram

Clinical Evaluation

History

A thorough history is fundamental and
provides the majority of the diagnostic
information. The referral problem may be
characterized as psychosis, depression,
noncompliance, or unruly behavior. The
perspective of the consultation psychiatrist may facilitate clarification of the clinical question. Furthermore, the consultant
may be called later in the course of a delirium and thus must retrospectively
search for history and hospital course
data. A good starting point is to understand the patient's premorbid baseline is,
whether a recent change occurred, and
when. Not only is this information key in
distinguishing delirium from dementia, it
may also identify precipitants. Prime
sources of information are those who have
known the patient for some time, such as
family members and outpatient physicians.
Review of the patient's current medical or
surgical illness is also essential. Assessment
of the treatment environment with a focus
on variables that could affect sensory dep-

rivation or disorientation is helpful as well
(Francis and Kapoor 1990).

Medication Review

Every delirium evaluation warrants a medication review that includes current and
recently discontinued drugs, whether prescription, over-the-counter, herbal, or illicit. Medications with anticholinergic
properties should be discontinued or substituted as possible. The potential for
drug–drug interactions should be reviewed on an individual basis. Similarly,
consideration of the unique metabolism
or medication sensitivity in special populations—such as the young, the old, and
the malnourished (Dickson 1991), as well
as those with HIV or with renal or liver
compromise—is a necessity.

Interview and Observation

The interview itself should focus on establishing a global image of the patient's cognitive functioning. It is helpful to observe
for decreased attention capacity, psychosis, short-term memory deficits, disorientation, executive dysfunction, and changes
in mood or kinetics. Bedside exams (e.g.,
the A test for vigilance) and tests sensitive
for frontal lobe dysfunction (e.g., Trails B,
clock drawing) are quick and easy to administer. In regard to Folstein et al.'s
(1975) Mini-Mental State Examination
(MMSE), one study (C.A. Ross et al.
1991) reported the mean MMSE score to
be 14.3 for delirious patients, versus 29.6
for control subjects. The most sensitive
items were the serial 7s, orientation, and
recall memory. Unfortunately, the MMSE
is not particularly sensitive (33%) in identifying delirium (Trzepacz et al. 1986), although it can be valuable for following the
course of a delirium. Indeed, Tune and
Folstein (1986) reported serial improvement in MMSE scores with delirium resolution.

Rating Scales

The use of diagnostic and rating tools may also be warranted. These tools are invaluable for research and are useful for psychiatrists (Zou et al. 1998), other physicians, and "physician extenders" (e.g., physician's assistants, nurse practitioners) as well. Several of the commonly used and validated instruments are the DRS and the Delirium Rating Scale—Revised—98 (DRS-R-98; Trzepacz et al. 1988b, 2001), the Confusion Assessment Method (CAM; Inouye et al. 1990), and the Memorial Delirium Assessment Scale (Breitbart et al. 1997).

Neurological Examination

Unexplained or new focal neurological signs beyond cognitive disturbances are atypical in delirium and warrant discussion with a neurologist. Neuroimaging should be considered for patients with head injuries, focal findings, cancer, stroke risk, AIDS, and atypical presentations (e.g., young, healthy, lack of identifiable precipitants). Abnormalities on neuroimaging are common among delirious elderly patients (Koponen et al. 1987, 1989b), although they are often described as "chronic, age-related changes." Cortical atrophy could be considered a marker of reduced cerebral reserve. Indeed, the degree of generalized cortical atrophy has been more closely linked to delirium risk than focal cortical lesions alone (Tsai and Tsuang 1979).

Laboratory Tests

Tests are warranted on an individually tailored basis (Inouye 1998). Evaluations may include a complete blood count, electrolytes, blood urea nitrogen, creatinine, glucose, calcium, pulse oximetry or arterial blood gas, and urinalysis. Other tests commonly obtained are urine drug screens, liver function tests with serum albumin, cultures, chest X ray, and electrocardiogram (ECG). CSF examination should also be considered for cases in which meningitis or encephalitis is suspected as well as for atypical cases of delirium.

Electroencephalogram

Utilizing the EEG, Romano and Engel (1944) first demonstrated delirious patients had progressive disorganization of rhythms and generalized slowing. Specifically, delirious patients have slowing of the peak and average frequencies, in addition to increased theta and delta but decreased alpha rhythms (Koponen et al. 1989d). This same pattern of EEG slowing has been elicited in an animal model of delirium (Trzepacz et al. 1992) by decreasing ACh or increasing dopamine activity (Keane and Neal 1981). The pattern is also seen in humans with hypoxic encephalopathy (Bauer 1982). Interestingly, the EEG changes correlate with cognitive dysfunction and memory and attention deficits, but not with psychomotor subtype (Koponen et al. 1989d; Trzepacz 1994).

Patients with sedative-withdrawal delirium are known to have a different EEG pattern with low-voltage fast activity (Kennard et al. 1945). Other than for drug intoxication or drug-withdrawal delirium, however, there are only very rare reports of low-voltage fast activity in hyperactive delirium (Pro and Wells 1977).

In clinical practice, the EEG is only rarely used, as it is not necessary for the diagnosis of delirium and has limited specificity. EEG changes normalize before cognitive dysfunction clears (Trzepacz et al. 1992), whereas cognitive testing remains sensitive throughout the course of the delirium (Trzepacz et al. 1988a). Additionally, nondelirious elderly patients can exhibit EEG slowing, particularly if they have dementia (Obrist 1979).

Differential Diagnosis

Frequently, delirium needs to be distinguished from dementia. Dementia has an insidious rather than an acute onset, features chronic memory and executive disturbances, and—unless it is Lewy body dementia or there is a superimposed delirium—tends not to fluctuate. A nondelirious patient with dementia typically has intact attention and alertness; in addition, dementia is characterized by impoverished speech and thinking, as opposed to the confused or disorganized pattern seen in delirium. "Beclouded dementia" describes delirium that develops in a patient who already has dementia. Beclouded dementia should be approached like any other case of delirium (Trzepacz et al. 1998), albeit with the understanding that such patients are highly sensitive to precipitants and medications, in part because of a diminished cerebral reserve.

Other possibilities to consider in the differential diagnosis include drug intoxication, schizophrenia, and Bell's mania. A thorough history, physical examination, and toxicology screen should identify most intoxication cases. Stimulants, hallucinogens, and dissociative drugs are commonly abused agents capable of mimicking delirium. The first episode of a psychotic disorder can also be difficult to differentiate from delirium, particularly if the mental status change developed acutely without a prolonged prodrome. Attentional difficulties, disorganization, and diffuse cognitive dysfunction can occur in both illnesses. Another rare possibility to consider is brief psychotic disorder, a poorly understood condition that can be associated with various stressors (e.g., sleep deprivation). Finally, Bell's mania is a syndrome presenting as an extreme manic episode that also has the cognitive and attentional disturbances of delirium. History gathering is essential in diagnosing this illness, which is best treated with both antipsychotics and mood-stabilizing agents or electroconvulsive therapy (ECT) (Fink 1999).

Risk Factors: Precipitants and Baseline Vulnerability

A measure of confusion exists in the literature regarding what constitutes a cause versus a risk factor of delirium. It is recommended that *cause* be reserved for the underlying cerebral etiopathology of the disease of delirium, even though that etiopathology has not yet been fully elucidated. *Precipitant* should be used to subsume risk factors that are generally transient or acute (e.g., a medication effect, a urinary tract infection). Finally, *baseline vulnerability* is best suited to describe risk factors that by definition are more chronic and innate to the patient (e.g., age, dementia). Thus, it is proposed that numerous and widely varying precipitants can activate the disease of delirium in susceptible (high baseline vulnerability) patients (O'Keeffe 1999).

One of the most common precipitants of delirium is medication. Indeed, numerous medications across many classes have been noted to precipitate delirium (Brown and Stoudemire 1998). The anticholinergic activity of a medication has been shown to correlate with its propensity to cause delirium (Beresin 1988; Blazer et al. 1983; Golinger et al. 1987). A 1992 study (Tune et al.) in fact, found that 14 of the 25 drugs most commonly prescribed for elderly patients had detectable anticholinergic effects. Moreover, 10 of those drugs result in anticholinergic levels sufficient to create memory and attentional deficits in healthy elderly subjects (Miller et al. 1988). A recent report noted that a serum level of anticholinergic activity (SAA) above 20 pmol/mL atropine equivalents confers a risk for delirium (Mussi et al. 1999). Therefore, although a single medi-

TABLE 3–3.   Prospectively identified risk factors for delirium

Risk factor	Study*
Dementia/preexisting cognitive impairment	3, 4, 5, 6, 7, 8, 10, 12
Elderly age	1, 3, 5, 6, 9, 10, 12
Alcohol/sedative withdrawal	7, 6, 9
Illness severity	4, 8
Blood urea nitrogen/creatinine > 18	8, 4
Abnormal sodium, potassium, or blood glucose levels	4, 6
Anticholinergics	11
Vision or hearing impairment	8
Hypoxia	1
Windowless intensive care unit	2
Use of a bladder catheter	13
More than 3 new medications begun	13
Malnutrition	13
Psychoactive medications used	4
Thoracic or aortic aneurysm surgery	6
Preexisting cerebral atrophy	3
Fever	4
Fracture or infection	5

*1 = Foy et al. 1995; 2 = L.M. Wilson 1972; 3 = Henon et al. 1999; 4 = Francis et al. 1990; 5 = Schor et al. 1992; 6 = Marcantonio et al. 1994; 7 = Pompei et al. 1994; 8 = Inouye et al. 1993; 9 = Williams-Russo et al. 1992; 10 = Rockwood 1989; 11 = M.P. Rogers et al. 1989; 12 = Gustafson et al. 1988; 13 = Inouye and Charpentier 1996.

cation may have a low SAA, the combined effect of several such medications (Tune et al. 1992) may precipitate delirium in a susceptible individual.

Prospective studies have identified many other precipitants and baseline risks for delirium (Table 3–3). Two of the most frequently reported are preexisting cognitive decline and advanced age. Inouye and Charpentier (1996) separated out baseline risks present at admission (e.g., poor vision, preexisting cognitive impairment) from precipitants affecting patients after admission (e.g., new medications, new-onset respiratory insufficiency). Robust patients with less baseline vulnerability ("more cerebral reserve") were more resilient to new precipitants following admission. The reverse was true as well: the more baseline vulnerability a patient had, the higher the likelihood that he or she would develop delirium if the fragile homeostasis ("less cerebral reserve") was stressed with additional precipitants.

Prognosis

Mortality

Lipowski (1983) described delirium as a "grave prognostic sign." When the most robust studies were combined in a meta-analysis (Cole and Primeau 1993), patients with delirium were reported to have an average 1-month mortality of 14.2% (vs. 4.8% in control subjects) and a 6-month mortality of 22.2% (vs. 10.6% in control subjects). One study found the mortality risk to be higher, even after multivariate analysis, for patients whose delirium failed to improve and/or was rated as severe (Kelly et al. 2001). Delirium also independently predicted a shorter survival time in cancer patients receiving palliative care (Caraceni et al. 2000). In contrast, several other studies have not found delirium to independently affect mortality (Dolan et al. 2000; Francis and Kapoor 1992; Levkoff et al. 1992; O'Keeffe and Lavan 1997).

Morbidity

Delirium independently leads to poor clinical outcomes. The length of hospital stay (LOS) was found to be longer (Francis et al. 1990; Levkoff et al. 1992), and the loss of independent living more common (Francis and Kapoor 1992; Marcantonio et al. 2000; O'Keeffe and Lavan 1997), among patients who had been delirious. In contrast, one study (Inouye et al. 1998) found that delirium independently predicted increased nursing home placements and decreased ability to perform ADL (as also noted by O'Keeffe and Lavan 1997; Marcantonio et al. 2000) but not increased LOS alone. Overall, a meta-analysis (Cole and Primeau 1993) found that patients with delirium had a mean LOS of 20.7 days (vs. 8.9 days for control subjects) and a rate of independent living 6 months after admission of 56.8% (vs. 91.7% in control subjects).

Patients who experience delirium during hospitalization have less functional improvement 2 years after orthopedic surgery, experience a higher rate of major postoperative and hospital-acquired complications, and do less well in rehabilitation compared with patients without delirium (Dolan et al. 2000; Gustafson et al. 1988; Marcantonio et al. 1994, 2000; O'Keeffe and Lavan 1997; M.P. Rogers et al. 1989). Thus, delirium is not just a marker of poor prognosis but is actually a vital determinant of hospital outcomes (Inouye et al. 1998).

Duration

Average delirium episodes of 3–13 days have been reported, although 20 days was the mean in a sample of patients with "beclouded" dementia (Koponen et al. 1989c). Patients with hypoactive delirium have been shown to have longer episodes than those with the mixed or hyperactive subtypes (Kelly et al. 2001). Studies have also noted that some delirium symptoms persist at time of discharge in as many as 60%–96% of elderly patients who experienced delirium during their stay (Levkoff et al. 1992; Kelly et al. 2001; Rockwood 1993). Furthermore, in a recent study, stem cell transplant patients who had previously been delirious were later found to have more residual or new cognitive impairment well after the delirium had resolved (Fann et al. 2001). These findings suggest that delirium can resolve completely, resolve gradually, or transition to a more permanent cognitive disorder.

Persistent Cerebral Damage

Some investigators have suggested that the long-term morbidity and incomplete symptom resolution could be due to cerebral damage from the disease of delirium (Engel and Romano 1959; O'Keeffe 1999; O'Keeffe and Lavan 1997). Others have speculated that delirium may unmask a subtle, previously unidentified dementia that would account for most of the functional and progressive decline (Francis and Kapoor 1992; Koponen et al. 1989c). To examine this question, a recent prospective study followed elderly patients without preexisting diagnoses of dementia for 2 years after their initial episode of delirium (Rahkonen et al. 2000). Dementia was newly diagnosed in 27% after the resolution of their delirium, and by the 2-year point, a total of 57% of the patients had been diagnosed with dementia. Alternatively, Inouye et al. (1998) argued that the residual symptoms of delirium might themselves contribute to the observed morbidity (institutionalization, functional decline). All of these theories are potentially valid, and they may well function together to explain delirium's permanent sequelae.

Treatment and Prevention

Ideally, therapies can be matched more precisely to the neuropathology once the basis of delirium is better understood. Although new approaches can be proposed, traditional treatments remain the mainstay in the management of delirium.

Nonpharmacological Interventions

Among traditional treatments, nonpharmacological techniques clearly have a role in the management of delirium. Interventions have included reorientation, maintenance of circadian cycles, enhancement of communication, minimization of sensory deprivation and depersonalization, and reinforcement of cognitive functioning (American Psychiatric Association 1999; Inouye 1998; McCartney and Boland 1993). A recent effort, "The Elder Life Program," used nonpharmacological interventions targeted specifically toward delirium precipitants (Inouye et al. 1999). In this preventive model, delirium developed in 9.9% of the treatment group versus 15% of the usual-care control group.

Pharmacotherapy

Although environmental manipulations and supportive care are important, medications offer further advantages. First, interventions directed at delirium precipitants should be instituted (e.g., antibiotics for urinary tract infection). Unless the delirium clears very rapidly or is mild, the concurrent use of delirium-specific treatments is also recommended. Antipsy-

chotic medications are not just for behavioral management, as some have suggested, but rather are disease-specific treatments for delirium. Elevated dopamine levels are known to occur in delirium; thus, the use of dopamine-receptor antagonists is logical. Although further study is needed, patients with the nonagitated, hypoactive subtype of delirium may be among the most important to treat with delirium-specific medication (Platt et al. 1994), considering their poor prognosis (Liptzin and Levkoff 1992; Reyes et al. 1981).

Haloperidol is the most studied and most widely accepted treatment for delirium. The APA practice guideline (American Psychiatric Association 1999) supports haloperidol as a first-line agent for delirium because of its minimal anticholinergic effects, minimal sedation or orthostasis, low likelihood of extrapyramidal side effects (EPS) with intravenous use, and flexibility in dosing and administration with oral, intramuscular, and intravenous routes. Both oral and intravenous forms have been used for more than 40 years and have an extensive track record of safety and efficacy in even the most ill medical and surgical patients (Ayd 1978; Cassem and Sos 1978; Fernandez et al. 1989; Massie et al. 1983; Stiefel and Holland 1991). Haloperidol has also been proven clearly superior to benzodiazepines alone in delirium (Breitbart et al. 1996).

Oral haloperidol peaks in 4–6 hours, whereas intravenous doses offer onset of action within 5–20 minutes (Settle and Ayd 1983). The recommended dose (American Psychiatric Association 1999) is 1–2 mg every 2–4 hours as needed, with further titration until desired effects are seen. Once stabilized, patients are often transitioned to a twice-daily or a daily bedtime oral dose, which is then continued or slowly tapered until the delirium has resolved. AIDS patients are sensitive to developing EPS (Breitbart et al. 1988; Swenson et al. 1989); thus, low doses of haloperidol or atypical antipsychotics with lower EPS risk are recommended. Doses of 0.25–1 mg twice a day are recommended when haloperidol or risperidone are used in the elderly (Zayas and Grossberg 1998).

In severe delirium refractory to boluses, continuous haloperidol infusions of 3–25 mg/hour have been used safely (Fernandez et al. 1988; Riker et al. 1994), although the APA practice guideline suggested a ceiling of 5–10 mg/hour. ECG monitoring is recommended with continuous infusion because of concerns about torsades des pointes, although no specific dose threshold has been designated (American Psychiatric Association 1999; Hunt and Stern 1995; Sharma et al. 1998; Zee-Cheng et al. 1985). Awareness and management of risk factors for QTc (hypokalemia, hypomagnesemia, bradycardia, congenital long-QT syndrome, preexisting cardiac disease, and drug–drug interactions) is advised (Gury et al. 2000). Therefore, even though the association between haloperidol use and torsades des pointes is unclear (Trzepacz and Wise 1997), QTc intervals beyond 450 msec or 25% over baseline should prompt a cardiology consultation, a dosage reduction, or discontinuation of the antipsychotic agent (American Psychiatric Association 1999). Another agent that has been used for intractable hyperactive delirium is propofol. It decreases CBF and is associated with hypotension; its use requires intubation and artificial ventilation (Mirenda and Broyles 1995).

Of the atypical antipsychotics, risperidone (Sipahimalani and Masand 1997), quetiapine (Torres et al. 2001), and olanzapine (Passik and Cooper 1999; Sipahimalani and Masand 1998) have been reported to treat delirium successfully and safely in small case series.

Among other potential medications for delirium, droperidol has also been used (Frye et al. 1995). This faster-acting butyrophenone is more sedating, more hypotensive, and has more effect on QTc lengthening than does haloperidol (Gury et al. 2000). Most other antipsychotics (e.g., chlorpromazine, thioridazine) can be used to treat delirium; however, in general, these antipsychotics are not the best choices because of their associated anticholinergic, hypotensive, and excess sedation effects in addition to concerns about EPS and QTc lengthening.

Cholinergic agents would seem to be a logical treatment option as well, although little research has been done with them. Physostigmine has been successfully used to treat anticholinergic toxicity, including the associated delirium, although its side effects preclude routine use (American Psychiatric Association 1999). Among newer agents, rivastigmine was described as reversing a nonanticholinergic delirium in a single case report (Fischer 2001). On the other hand, tacrine toxicity was reported to precipitate delirium in a patient with Alzheimer's disease (AD; Trzepacz et al. 1996).

Prevention

An attractive intervention in the management of delirium is prevention (Inouye 1998; Lipowski 1983). Several studies have identified and tracked risk factors with which to develop predictive instruments, also called risk-stratification models (Eden et al. 1998; Francis et al. 1990; Inouye and Charpentier 1996; Inouye et al. 1993; Marcantonio et al. 1994). Four risk factors—vision impairment, severe illness, preexisting cognitive impairment, and dehydration—were used in one predictive model (Inouye et al. 1993). Nine percent of the low-risk patients (i.e., those with none of the four factors) later developed delirium, compared with 23%

of those with one or two factors and 83% of those with three or four factors.

Ideally, patients could be quickly screened for delirium in the emergency department (Monette et al. 2001) and also scored with a predictive model. Patients would be eligible for prophylactic interventions if judged to be at high risk for developing delirium. Such screening practices would be much like what is currently done to reduce the risks of other illnesses (e.g., subcutaneous heparin for pulmonary-embolus prophylaxis, benzodiazepines for alcohol-withdrawal prophylaxis). Candidates for preventive interventions would include low-dose antipsychotics, targeted protocols such as those employed in the Elder Life Program (Inouye et al. 1999), supplemental oxygen (Aakerlund and Rosenberg 1994), or close monitoring for and correction of hypoxemia, hypotension, electrolyte imbalance, and anemia (Marcantonio et al. 1994). Such preventive efforts could lessen the substantial morbidity and mortality associated with delirium and reduce associated costs as well.

Finally, as interventions for cerebral ischemia advance, it would seem reasonable to explore their use in delirium as well. Efforts to decrease brain metabolic requirements, as well as levels of glutamate inhibitors, NMDA receptor antagonists, calcium antagonists, and free-radical scavengers, have also been suggested (Kirsch et al. 1989; Kornhuber and Weller 1997).

Summary

Delirium is both a neuropsychiatric syndrome and a disease. Many different precipitants can trigger delirium in susceptible populations. New hypotheses suggest that specific, recurring pathological changes in neuronal metabolism occur in delirium. Clarifying the etiopathogenesis of delirium and then directly applying this knowledge with targeted interventions and preventive strategies are the next steps in improving the care of delirious patients.

Dementia

The dementias are a heterogeneous group of psychiatric disorders characterized by loss of previous levels of cognitive, executive, and memory (anterograde and/or retrograde) function in a state of full alertness. Dementia is most common in the elderly; with the increasing age of the population, the prevalence of dementia is expected to double by 2030 (Doraiswamy et al. 1998).

Dementia directly increases health care expenditures and complicates the management of comorbid medical conditions (Weiner et al. 1998). The average duration from diagnosis to death is 3–10 years (Doraiswamy et al. 1998).

Dementia uniquely challenges the psychiatrist's diagnostic, psychopharmacological, and psychotherapeutic skills. Because of the progressive nature of most dementias, the likelihood of physician involvement in medicolegal matters such as institutionalization and determination of decreased cognitive capacity for decision making is high. Contemporary advances in psychopharmacology have equipped the physician with a greater range of medications that can be used to maximize function, delay disease progression, and minimize disruption to patients and caregivers. Early identification of cases is now imperative, given that prompt evaluation and diagnosis facilitates early use of cognition-enhancing and neuroprotective therapies and supportive care to the patient and his or her family (Doraiswamy et al. 1998; Haley 1997).

TABLE 3–4.   Diagnostic features of the dementias

Features common to all dementias:
Multiple cognitive deficits that do not occur exclusively during the course of delirium, including
    memory impairment and aphasia, apraxia, agnosia, or disturbed executive functioning that
    represent a decline from previous level of functioning and impair role functioning
Dementia of the Alzheimer's type, additional features:
Gradual onset and continuing cognitive decline, deficits are not due to other central nervous
    system, systemic, or substance-induced conditions and not better attributed to another Axis I
    disorder
Vascular dementia, additional features:
Focal neurological signs and symptoms or laboratory/radiological evidence indicative of
    cerebrovascular disease etiologically related to deficits
Dementia due to other general medical conditions, additional features:
Clinical evidence that cognitive disturbance is direct physiological consequence of one of the
    following: HIV, head trauma, Parkinson's disease, Huntington's disease, Pick's disease, Creutz-
    feldt-Jakob disease, or another general medical condition (includes Lewy body dementia)
Substance-induced persisting dementia, additional features:
Deficits persist beyond usual duration of substance intoxication or withdrawal with clinical
    evidence that deficits are etiologically related to the persisting effects of substance use
Dementia due to multiple etiologies, additional feature:
Clinical evidence that the disturbance has more than one etiology
Dementia not otherwise specified, additional feature:
Dementia that does not meet criteria for one of the specified types above

Source.   Adapted with permission from American Psychiatric Association: *Diagnostic and Statistical Manual of Mental Disorders*, 4th Edition, Text Revision. Washington, DC, American Psychiatric Association, 2000. Copyright 2000, American Psychiatric Association.

Clinical Features of the Dementias

DSM-IV-TR Classification of Dementias

According to DSM-IV-TR, core features of the dementias include multiple cognitive deficits that cause impairment in role functioning and represent a significant decline (American Psychiatric Association 2000). Dementia subtypes specified in DSM-IV-TR are shown in Table 3–4.

Cortical and Subcortical Dementias

A distinction is made between dementias with primarily cortical and those with primarily subcortical pathology (Table 3–5). Whereas all dementias exhibit the same core clinical features, cortical and sub-

cortical dementias often differ in their specific clinical presentation. Cortical dementia is characterized by prominent memory impairment (recall and recognition), language deficits, apraxia, agnosia, and visuospatial deficits (Doody et al. 1998; Meyer et al. 1995; Paulsen et al. 1995b). Subcortical dementia features greater impairment in recall memory, decreased verbal fluency without anomia, bradyphrenia (slowed thinking), depressed mood, affective lability, apathy, and decreased attention/concentration (Doody et al. 1998; Paulsen et al. 1995a, 1995b). The cortical–subcortical dichotomy is not absolute, however, because aphasia, apraxia, and agnosia (in isolation) have a low sensitivity in distinguishing cortical from subcortical dementia, and several dementia types may express both cortical and sub-

TABLE 3–5.   Cortical and subcortical dementia types

Cortical dementias
    Dementia of the Alzheimer's type
    Frontotemporal dementia, including
       dementia due to Pick's disease
    Dementia due to Creutzfeldt–Jakob
       disease
Subcortical dementias
    Dementia due to HIV
    Dementia due to Parkinson's disease
    Dementia due to Huntington's disease
    Dementia due to multiple sclerosis
Dementias with cortical and subcortical
    features
    Vascular dementia (formerly multi-infarct
       dementia)[a]
    Vascular dementia (poststroke dementia)[a]
    Lewy body variant of Alzheimer's disease[a]
    Lewy body dementia[a]

[a]Relative amount of cortical and subcortical features is dependent on location of neuropathology.

cortical features at some point during the course of the illness (Kramer and Duffy 1996).

Cortical Dementias

Dementia of the Alzheimer's type (DAT), the most common dementia, is estimated to affect nearly 2 million white Americans (Hy and Keller 2000). There is an important conceptual and semantic distinction between the DSM-IV-TR diagnoses of DAT and AD (Rabins et al. 1997). DAT is a clinical diagnosis, based on the findings of insidious onset and gradual, steady progression of cognitive deficits. Because symptoms and signs consistent with DAT may be present with *other* types of neuropathology, a clinical diagnosis of AD should only be made after medical evaluation fails to reveal other causes for the dementia symptoms (Rabins et al. 1997). Even so, the clinical diagnosis of AD can only be *definitively* validated by microscopic examination of neural tissue, typi-

cally at autopsy, for characteristic AD neuropathology (Rabins et al. 1997). A *clinical* diagnosis of AD (after ruling out other dementia causes) is pathologically validated in 70%–90% of cases (Rabins et al. 1997). These distinctions should be kept in mind by the reader, because many literature references use the terms *Alzheimer's disease* or *Alzheimer's dementia* interchangeably and somewhat presumptively to describe cases that have not yet gone to autopsy. For simplicity, in this chapter the abbreviation DAT is used to refer to the clinical illness that is not yet validated by autopsy, and AD is used for literature addressing neuropathologically validated Alzheimer's disease. Established and proposed risk factors for DAT are shown in Table 3–6 (Evans et al. 2000; Guo et al. 2000; Hall et al. 2000; Helmer et al. 1999; Merchant et al. 1999; Moceri et al. 2000; Ott et al. 1999; Plassman et al. 2000; Whalley et al. 2000; Zubenko et al. 1996, 1999).

Amnesia and other cognitive symptoms may be present early in the disease, although poor insight regarding memory loss is common. The patient may become spatially disoriented and wander aimlessly. Apraxias for self-care behaviors may be evident. Deficits in memory, concentration, attention, and executive functions eventually render the patient unable to maintain employment or safely operate a motor vehicle.

Mood symptoms that occur before cognitive deficits may represent a prodromal state (Berger et al. 1999). Depressive disorders have been reported in up to 86% of patients with DAT, with a median estimate of 19% (Katz 1998). Depression is more common in mild DAT, whereas psychosis is more common in moderate to severe DAT (Mega et al. 1996; Rabins et al. 1997; Rao and Lyketsos 1998). Apathy, agitation, dysphoria, and aberrant motor behavior all increase

TABLE 3–6. Established and proposed risk factors for dementia of the Alzheimer's type

Increased age
Female gender
Head trauma
Small head size
Family history
Low childhood intelligence
Limited education
Childhood rural residence
Large sibships
Smoking
Never having married
Depression
Diabetes mellitus
Increased total cholesterol
Increased platelet membrane fluidity
Apolipoprotein E (APOE) ε4 allele on chromosome 19
Abnormalities on chromosomes 1, 6, 12, 14, and 21
Trisomy 21

with illness progression and increasing cognitive impairment (Kuzis et al. 1999; Mega et al. 1996). Disinhibited social and sexual behavior, assaultiveness, and inappropriate laughter or tearfulness are common. Evening agitation ("sundowning") may be a notably disruptive symptom. Other motor symptoms include motor slowing, EPS, gait disturbances, dysarthria, myoclonus, and seizures (Goldman et al. 1999; Rabins et al. 1997).

Psychosis is present in up to 40% of patients with DAT (Mega et al. 1996; Paulsen et al. 2000). The early appearance of psychosis or EPS correlates with more rapid cognitive decline (Levy et al. 1996; Paulsen et al. 2000). Visual hallucinations are the most common perceptual disturbance (Class et al. 1997). The prevalence of delusions in DAT is high as 73%; delusions of persecution, theft, reference, and jealousy are common (Rao and Lyketsos 1998).

The neuropathology of AD includes β-amyloid deposits, neuritic plaques, and neurofibrillary tangles (NFTs) (Felician and Sandson 1999; Jellinger 1996). Amyloid precursor protein (APP) is cleaved by proteases (β and γ secretases), producing insoluble β-amyloid (Felician and Sandson 1999; Haass and De Strooper 1999; Jellinger 1996). Inhibition of β and γ secretases and presenilin proteins 1 and 2 may decrease cleavage of APP, thereby decreasing production of insoluble β-amyloid (Haass and De Strooper 1999).

β-Amyloid activates macrophages and microglia, producing inflammation that accelerates neuronal damage (Breitner 1996; Smits et al. 2000). Oxidative stress appears to increase the rate of neuronal death; this process may be blocked by vitamin E (Felician and Sandson 1999). Increased CSF prostaglandin E2 (PGE2) has been found in AD, supporting the possibility that prostaglandin production may play a significant role in the pathogenesis of AD; this process might be blocked by the use of nonsteroidal anti-inflammatory drugs (NSAIDs) (Montine et al. 1999). Amyloid deposition in cerebral vessels is also seen (Cummings et al. 1998a).

Diffuse plaques are β-amyloid depositions without surrounding neuronal degeneration (Felician and Sandson 1999). Neuritic plaques (a core of β-amyloid encircled by dystrophic neurites) are surrounded by immune-activated microglia and reactive astrocytes (Felician and Sandson 1999; Smits et al. 2000). Neuritic plaque density is increased in several regions of the cortex, hippocampus, entorhinal cortex, amygdala, and cerebral vessels in AD (Felician and Sandson 1999; Haroutunian et al. 1998).

NFTs, intraneuronal bundles of phosphorylated tau proteins, are an early pathological change in the hippocampus, amygdala, and entorhinal cortex (Felician and Sandson 1999).

The apolipoprotein E (APOE) ε4 allele on chromosome 19 affects the rate of β-amyloid production and the clinical manifestations of AD in a dose-dependent fashion; homozygotes have a higher risk and faster rate of decline than heterozygotes and noncarriers (Caselli et al. 1999; Craft et al. 1998; Felician and Sandson 1999). The APOE ε2 allele may confer protection against AD, whereas the APOE ε3 allele appears to not affect AD risk (Rebeck and Hyman 1999).

The hippocampus is an early locus of pathology in AD. There is a correlation between hippocampal neuron and volume loss and an increase in hippocampal NFTs (Bobinski et al. 1996). Volumetric measurements of the hippocampus on magnetic resonance imaging (MRI) predict memory loss in both normal aging and AD (Jack et al. 2000; Petersen et al. 2000).

Central cholinergic hypofunction follows neuronal loss in the nucleus basalis of Meynert, medial septum, and diagonal band of Broca, clinically correlating with decreased attention and memory (Felician and Sandson 1999; Small 1998b; Whitehouse 1998). With progression of AD, a deficiency in central cholinergic function leads to a relative hyperdopaminergic condition correlating with the emergence of psychotic symptoms (Rao and Lyketsos 1998).

Other neurotransmitter systems affected in AD include serotonin (neuronal loss and NFTs in the dorsal raphe and central septal nucleus) and norepinephrine (similar changes in the locus coeruleus) (Felician and Sandson 1999). In one study, acute depletion of tryptophan led to an abrupt further decrease in cognitive function in AD, suggesting that cognitive deficits follow decreased cholinergic and serotonergic function (Porter et al. 2000). Depressed AD patients have a more dramatic loss of norepinephrine (Small 1998b).

Later stages of AD affect various areas of the cortex, forming the anatomic substrates for clinical deficits in construction, language, and problem solving (Paulsen et al. 1995b). Delacourte et al. (1999) demonstrated a temporal and spatial sequence of neurofibrillary degeneration in AD as follows: initial changes in the transentorhinal cortex; then the entorhinal cortex, hippocampus, anterior inferior and medium temporal cortex, polymodal association areas, unimodal areas, and primary motor or sensory areas; and, finally, all remaining neocortical areas.

In the parietal cortex, patients with AD were found to have decreased glucose metabolism both at rest and following stimulation, whereas the relatively more preserved areas of the visual and auditory cortex showed decreased glucose metabolism only under stimulation (Pietrini et al. 1999). Functional impairment of the parietal-occipital cortex has been demonstrated in a study examining visuospatial perception in AD (Tetewsky and Duffy 1999).

Higher educational attainment may lead to cognitive reserve that operates to forestall the clinical onset of memory decline in incipient AD (Stern et al. 1999). The "cognitive reserve" concept was also supported in a study using PET scanning (Alexander et al. 1997). Among patients with equal levels of dementia severity, those with higher levels of premorbid intellectual function showed greater decreases in cerebral metabolism in the prefrontal, premotor, and left superior parietal association areas.

Frontotemporal dementia (FTD), including dementia due to Pick's disease, features an earlier age at onset, executive dysfunction, attentional deficits, and personality changes with relatively spared memory and visuospatial functions (Duara et al. 1999; Perry and Hodges 2000). Consensus criteria for the diagnosis of

FTD have been developed that include the following core diagnostic features: insidious onset and gradual progression, early decline in social interpersonal conduct, early impairment in regulation of personal conduct, early emotional blunting, and early loss of insight (Neary et al. 1998). Neuropathological findings in FTD are restricted to the frontal and anterior temporal lobes (Jellinger 1996; H.R. Morris et al. 1999).

Dementia due to Creutzfeldt–Jakob disease (CJD), also called "spongiform encephalopathy," is a prion-mediated infection. It manifests as a rapidly progressive cortical dementia accompanied by myoclonus and may first appear with psychosis (Dunn et al. 1999; Zerr et al. 2000). In patients with CJD, the EEG shows a characteristic pattern of repetitive sharp waves or slow spikes followed by synchronous triphasic sharp waves (Dunn et al. 1999; Zerr et al. 2000).

Subcortical Dementias

Dementia due to HIV initially manifests as decreased psychomotor and information-processing speed, verbal memory, learning efficiency, and fine motor function with later cortical symptoms of decreased executive function, aphasia, apraxia, and agnosia (Maldonado et al. 2000). In advanced stages, ataxia, spasticity, increased muscle tone, and incontinence may develop (Maldonado et al. 2000). Dementia has been reported in up to 30% of HIV-positive patients, may present early in the course of illness, increases suicide risk, and may compromise compliance with antiviral regimens (Cohen and Jacobson 2000; Maldonado et al. 2000). Recent estimates of the incidence of dementia due to HIV are somewhat lower, possibly due to the neuroprotective effects of early, aggressive antiviral treatment (d'Arminio Monforte et al. 2000; Goodkin et al. 2001). Dementia due to HIV results from neurotoxicity mediated by HIV-infected macrophages (which serve as the site for viral replication) (McDaniel et al. 2000; Smits et al. 2000).

Dementia due to Parkinson's disease (PD) is seen in as many as 60% of patients with PD and features bradyphrenia, apathy, poor retrieval memory, decreased verbal fluency, and attention deficits (Levy and Cummings 2000; Marsh 2000). Cortical symptoms of executive dysfunction, visuospatial impairment, agnosia, anomia, aphasia, and apraxia may be seen in patients with PD dementia who develop cortical Lewy bodies (Hurtig et al. 2000; Levy and Cummings 2000; Marsh 2000). Increased age, greater severity of neurological symptoms, and the APOE ε2 allele have been associated with an increased risk of dementia in patients with PD (Harhangi et al. 2000; Hughes et al. 2000). Cognition may improve with treatment for the common comorbid mood disorders (Levy and Cummings 2000). Dementia due to PD features deposition of α-synuclein or tau protein in the substantia nigra and commonly involves Lewy bodies in the substantia nigra, cortex, and subcortex (Levy and Cummings 2000; Marsh 2000; H.R. Morris et al. 1999).

Dementia due to Huntington's disease (HD) features impairments in retrieval memory, cognitive speed, concentration, verbal learning, and cognitive flexibility (Ranen 2000). With progression, more global impairment in memory, visuospatial function, and executive function may follow (Ranen 2000). These patients have a high risk for personality change, irritability, aggressive behavior, and suicide (Ranen 2000; Rosenblatt and Leroi 2000). Dementia due to HD carries a high risk for comorbid depression (Rosenblatt and Leroi 2000). HD dementia results from cell loss in primary sensory and association areas, entorhinal cortex, caudate nucleus, and putamen (Jellinger 1996; Ranen 2000).

Dementia due to multiple sclerosis is seen in as many as 65% of multiple sclerosis patients (Schwid et al. 2000). Clinical features include deficits in memory, attention, information-processing speed, learning, and executive functions (Schwid et al. 2000). Cognitive impairment may present early in the course of multiple sclerosis, and progression is roughly proportional to the number of central nervous system (CNS) demyelinating lesions (Schwid et al. 2000).

Dementias With Cortical and Subcortical Features

Vascular dementia (VaD) broadly includes dementias resulting from vascular pathology that have as a final common pathway the loss of functional cortex. Because VaD exists on a continuum extending from the essentially subcortical pathology formerly described as "multi-infarct dementia" to the primarily cortical pathology in "poststroke dementia," it is problematic to attempt to fit all vascular dementias into the "cortical versus subcortical" dichotomy. This already problematic distinction between multi- and single-infarct dementias is further obscured by the inclusion of dementia following a single stroke within the classification of VaD in much clinical literature (Kaye 1998). In other literature, the term *vascular dementia* generally refers to dementia following multiple infarcts. A reasonable (albeit cumbersome) solution would be for clinicians to describe all dementias due to vascular pathology as "vascular dementia," with further specification as "multi-infarct" or "poststroke" as appropriate to the clinical situation.

Additionally, the boundary between AD and the broad category of VaD is itself quite permeable. Cerebral infarcts in established AD are associated with greater overall severity of dementia and poorer neuropsychological testing performance (Heyman et al. 1998).

Multi-infarct VaD is characterized by abrupt onset, decreased executive functioning, gait disturbance, affective lability, and parkinsonian symptoms (Choi et al. 2000; Patterson et al. 1999). Risk factors include increased age, hypertension, diabetes mellitus, atherosclerotic heart disease, hypertriglyceridemia, and hyperlipidemia (Curb et al. 1999; G.W. Ross et al. 1999). Because the cognitive deficits follow a series of discrete lesions, progression is "stepwise" with relative stability of cognitive status between vascular insults. The progression of multi-infarct VaD may be affected by risk factor modification and antiplatelet therapy (Rabins et al. 1997). Lesions are generally located in the subcortical nuclei, frontal lobe white matter, thalamus, and internal capsule and are associated with a characteristic appearance on MRI of periventricular hyperintensities on the T2 images (Choi et al. 2000; Doody et al. 1998). However, periventricular hyperintensities are also seen in normal aging and in other types of dementia and thus, in isolation, represent a nonspecific finding (Smith et al. 2000).

Poststroke VaD—dementia occurring as the acute or subacute consequence of a single stroke—may be difficult to clearly distinguish from multi-infarct VaD that follows a series of vascular events. Poststroke dementia is associated with apraxia, neglect, hemianopsia, facial paralysis, and extremity weakness (de Koning et al. 1998). Poststroke VaD was found to independently increase the risk of stroke recurrence (Moroney et al. 1997). Poststroke dementia was found in 24% of a series of 300 stroke patients (de Koning et al. 1998). Of the dementias seen in this study, 25% were AD plus VaD (inclusively defined) and the remaining 75% were probable VaD. Major depression is common with poststroke dementia, with anterior left-hemisphere stroke posing the highest risk (Robinson 1998).

Lewy body variant (LBV) of AD and Lewy body dementia (LBD) have a significant degree of overlap and may be difficult to differentiate clinically (Hansen et al. 1990). The more general term *dementia with Lewy bodies* is often used to denote the continuum of LBV, LBD, and dementia due to PD (Gomez-Isla et al. 1999; Jellinger 1996).

Clinically, LBV and LBD share the common features of fluctuation of mental status, visual hallucinations, delusions, depression, and EPS (Hansen et al. 1990; Heyman et al. 1999; Lopez et al. 2000a; Weiner et al. 1996). Visual hallucinations occur even with mild levels of cognitive impairment (Ballard et al. 2001). In comparison with AD, LBV exhibits greater deficits in attention, verbal fluency, and visuospatial functioning and increased parkinsonian symptoms (Hansen et al. 1990; Heyman et al. 1999; Lopez et al. 2000a; McKeith et al. 2000; Weiner et al. 1996). LBV has also been associated with more rapid cognitive decline, earlier institutionalization, and shorter survival time (Lopez et al. 2000a; Olichney et al. 1998). LBD also features impaired executive functioning, disinhibited social behavior, syncope, and increased sensitivity to antipsychotic agents (Litvan and McKee 1999; McKeith et al. 2000). Progression is usually more rapid in LBD than in AD, although psychotic symptoms in LBV and LBD may be improved by treatment with cholinesterase inhibitors (Ballard et al. 2001; Levy and Cummings 2000).

A similar degree of overlap is seen in the neuropathology of LBV and LBD. LBV is characterized by the presence of Lewy bodies (intraneuronal eosinophilic inclusion bodies) in subcortical and cortical structures in addition to AD neuropathology (Gomez-Isla et al. 1999; Hansen et al. 1990; Rabins et al. 1997). LBD also fea-

tures subcortical and cortical Lewy bodies, with a relative absence of NFTs and other AD neuropathology (Gomez-Tortosa et al. 1999; Litvan and McKee 1999). Occipital lobe metabolic rates in LBD have been found to be lower than those in AD, a finding that correlates with the prominence of visual hallucinations in LBD (Ishii et al. 1998). Both LBV and LBD are characterized by a marked loss of choline acetyltransferase (ChAT) activity and show more ChAT activity loss than does pure AD (Tiraboschi et al. 2000).

Epidemiology

Dementia Types

The risk of dementia increases exponentially with age, from 1% under age 65 years to 25%–50% over age 85 (Rabins et al. 1997; Jorm and Jolley 1998). The annual risk of dementia is 0.5% between ages 60 and 69 years, 1% between 70 and 74 years, 2% between 75 and 79 years, 3% between 80 and 84 years, and 8% thereafter (Rabins et al. 1997). Estimates of the relative frequency of the different dementia types in study populations of dementia patients include 50%–90% DAT, 8%–20% VaD, and 7%–26% LBD, with other subtypes less common (Lyketsos et al. 2000b; Parnetti 2000; Small 1998a). There is an estimated overlap of 20% between DAT and VaD, referred to as *mixed dementia* (Small 1998a). Reversible dementias are estimated to account for 1%–10% of dementias; examples of potentially reversible dementias are shown in Table 3–7 (Gliatto and Caroff 2001; Rabins et al. 1997; Small 1998a; Tager and Fallon 2001).

Comorbidity and Differential Diagnosis

The patient with cognitive impairment may have psychiatric illnesses other than or in addition to dementia. Clinical his-

TABLE 3–7. Potentially reversible etiologies of dementia

Structural central nervous system factors
   Vascular dementia
   Head trauma
   Subdural hematoma
   Normal-pressure hydrocephalus
   Multiple sclerosis
Psychiatric illness
   Major depression
   Substance dependence
Systemic/metabolic factors
   Hypothyroidism
   Hypercalcemia
   Hypoglycemia
   Thiamine, niacin, B_{12} deficiency
   Renal failure
   Hepatic failure
   Medications
Infectious diseases
   HIV
   Central nervous system infection

TABLE 3–8. Psychiatric differential diagnosis of dementia

Delirium
Mood disorders
Amnestic disorders
Substance use disorders
Psychotic disorders
Mental retardation

tory and examination need to be focused to consider these other diagnostic possibilities. The psychiatric differential diagnosis of dementia is shown in Table 3–8.

Delirium

Dementia increases the risk for delirium from numerous systemic conditions, both after surgery and as a side effect of medications (Rabins et al. 1997). Delirium in the elderly patient with dementia may present with decreased psychomotor activity (Daniel 2000). Given that aberrant

motor behaviors, such as repetitive pacing, are uncommon in early dementia, their presence in a patient with mild dementia is suggestive of a superimposed delirium (Mega et al. 1996). Hallucinations are more common in delirium than in dementia. EEG may be helpful in differentiating delirium from dementia, because an abnormal EEG is more suggestive of delirium.

Mood Disorders

Depressed patients may appear to have cognitive impairment, a phenomenon described as "pseudodementia." Such patients will often have a history of mood disorders (Raskind 1998). Depressed dementia patients may communicate their mood state indirectly, with agitation and insomnia, rather than through specific mood complaints (Small 1998a).

Amnestic Disorders

Amnestic disorders can be profoundly impairing, but the diagnosis of dementia requires impairment in other spheres of mental activity beyond loss of memory function. Conditions characterized by "pure" amnesia (e.g., carbon monoxide poisoning, Wernicke's encephalopathy, transient global amnesia) should be considered.

Substance Abuse/Dependence

Substance use disorders can lead to dementia, especially following a long history of alcohol dependence. Active management of substance abuse and dependence should be accomplished in the context of other psychiatric interventions for substance-dependent dementia patients.

Psychotic Disorders and Mental Retardation

Schizophrenia will very rarely be first diagnosed in an elderly patient and will feature prominent psychotic symptoms at the onset of illness. Mental retardation, while increasing the risk for dementia (e.g., trisomy 21), represents a stable state of decreased cognitive function.

Clinical Evaluation

History

A clinical history should first be obtained from the patient directly, initially without the presence of other family members (Doraiswamy et al. 1998). History taking should address recent cognitive function; examples include function at work, at home, while driving, and while performing other high-risk activities (Patterson et al. 1999). A personal and family history of psychiatric illness should be obtained, specifically to include dementia and neurological illness with high risk for dementia. Because the patient is most reliable in the early stages of illness, the physician should then separately interview family members and synthesize the separate histories obtained to derive the most balanced view of the patient's functioning (Cummings and Masterman 1998).

The medical history should address all chronic illnesses, with particular attention to systemic conditions that increase risk for DAT, VaD, and other dementia types. The medication history should address both psychotropic and nonpsychotropic medications taken before the onset of the cognitive and behavioral symptoms (Doraiswamy et al. 1998). The use of nonprescription medications (especially antihistamines and sedatives) and herbal preparations also needs to be explored.

The social history should address the patient's living circumstances, presence of supportive family members and/or of other significant persons living nearby, financial and insurance resources, participation in social activities, and personal relationships. Problematic symptoms such as

paranoia, agitation, physical violence, and inattentive and dangerous operation of dangerous machinery need to be addressed, as well as access to weapons and any threats made to self or others. Any complaint of neglect or abuse, or any physical examination findings suggestive of inappropriate care, should be reported promptly to the agency responsible for performing onsite evaluation of neglect or abuse of adults. Dementia patients are also at increased risk for syncope. Any report of falls in dementia patients requires a full evaluation for injuries.

Mental Status Examination

Formal assessment of cognitive function must be added to routine evaluation of mood and affect, level of consciousness, psychomotor activity, speech production, thought content, and thought processes. It is recommended that the clinician use a cognitive assessment instrument such as the MMSE. A score of 24 or less on the MMSE, when correlated with clinical findings, is highly suggestive of dementia, but education and other patient-specific variables must be taken into close account (Patterson et al. 1999). Serial administrations of the MMSE can quantify the progress or stability of dementia; a typical decline in MMSE scores in DAT is 2–4 points per year (Folstein et al. 1975; Rabins et al. 1997). An alternative dementia rating scale is the Alzheimer's Disease Assessment Scale (ADAS; Mohs and Cohen 1988; Rosen et al. 1984), a 21-item scale that scores both cognitive and noncognitive items to derive the degree of impairment. Depression rating scales (e.g., the Hamilton Rating Scale for Depression [Hamilton 1960]) are recommended to assist in distinguishing dementia from depression and in monitoring response to antidepressants (Katz 1998). Suicide risk increases in the elderly population, and clinical assessment of other suicide risk factors needs to be integrated into the physician's clinical examination.

Physical Examination

Relative sensory deprivation due to uncorrected vision and/or hearing deficits can cause spuriously poor performance on formal cognitive testing. Neurological examination should include assessment of gait, frontal lobe release signs, movement disorders, sensory function, and focal neurological deficits (Doraiswamy et al. 1998; Grossberg and Lake 1998). Physical examination should address signs of metabolic illnesses, marginal hygiene, poor nutritional status, weight loss, and dehydration.

Laboratory Tests

Laboratory tests may be modified on a case-by-case basis. Tests to consider are shown in Table 3–9 (Doraiswamy et al. 1998; Grossberg and Lake 1998; Patterson et al. 1999; Rabins et al. 1997). Serum drug levels of medications associated with altered mental status should be obtained if clinically indicated. A 12-lead ECG should be considered, especially if there is a history of cardiac and/or vascular disease.

When CJD is suspected, CSF samples should be obtained for testing for the neuronal proteins 14-3-3 and γ-enolase (Dunn et al. 1999; Zerr et al. 2000). CJD is characterized by a classic EEG appearance of repetitive sharp waves or slow spikes followed by synchronous triphasic sharp waves (Dunn et al. 1999; Zerr et al. 2000). Lumbar puncture should also be considered if there is a clinical suspicion of normal-pressure hydrocephalus, metastatic carcinoma, or unusually early onset and/or rapid progression of deficits (Small 1998a). Other laboratory tests to consider in specific cases include serum ammonia, heavy metals, and cortisol; carotid Doppler studies; chest X ray; and mammog-

TABLE 3–9. Laboratory tests for dementia workup

Electrolytes, blood urea nitrogen, creatinine, calcium
Liver-associated enzymes
Glucose
Complete blood count
Thyroid profile with thyroid-stimulating hormone assay
Erythrocyte sedimentation rate, antinuclear antibody panel
Prothrombin time/partial thromboblastin time
B_{12} and folate
Syphilis serology
Urinalysis and urine toxicology
Pulse oximetry
Medication levels (e.g., tricyclic antidepressants, anticonvulsants, digitalis, antiarrhythmics)

raphy (Patterson et al. 1999; Rabins et al. 1997).

Neuroimaging

It is recommended that computed tomography (CT) or MRI be considered to evaluate dementia (Doraiswamy et al. 1998; Small and Leiter 1998). One consensus panel recommends CT in the presence of age younger than 60 years, rapid cognitive decline, less than a 2-year duration of illness, head trauma and associated neurological symptoms, history of cancer, history of bleeding disorder and/or anticoagulant therapy, incontinence, gait disturbance, atypical cognitive symptoms, or localizing neurological signs (Patterson et al. 1999). In cases of suspected DAT, hippocampal atrophy may serve as a sensitive early marker for cognitive decline (Bottino and Almeida 1997; Jack et al. 2000; Petersen et al. 2000; Scheltens 1999).

Cortical atrophy and ventriculomegaly do not by themselves confirm dementia and, in isolation, are not specific findings (Doraiswamy et al. 1998; Small 1998a). If initial neuroimaging reveals hippocampal and/or cortical atrophy that correlates with the clinical presentation and gradual course of DAT, then serial neuroimaging to follow progress is not routinely necessary. Periventricular hyperintensities on MRI may be seen in DAT as well as in VaD; their significance in DAT is unclear, as they may not correlate independently with cognitive changes (Doody et al. 1998; Smith et al. 2000). If initial imaging shows white matter lesions typical of VaD that correlate with clinical findings, a follow-up CT or MRI could be considered if the patient later presents with an abrupt decrease in mental status suggestive of delirium and/or a new CVA. Functional neuroimaging (e.g., single photon emission computed tomography [SPECT], PET scanning), although not currently widely available, holds promise in the evaluation of the cortical pathology of dementia (Small 1998a).

Multidisciplinary Referrals

Neuropsychological consultation may be helpful in early dementia cases when cognitive deficits are subtle on clinical examination (Tschanz et al. 2000). Neuropsychological assessment may be especially useful in patients in whom the capacity for autonomy (e.g., driving, medical informed consent) appears equivocal on interview alone.

Social work intervention may be of substantial benefit. Family therapy can assist the patient and family to adjust to the reduced social expectations and impairments of the patient. Social workers may facilitate patient and family access to supportive social services to assist the patient in staying with his or her family, to secure institutional placement, and to explore funding sources for institutional care.

Psychiatric nurses may be invaluable in the area of home visitation and outreach.

A system of care in which the psychiatric nurse calls on the patient at home may be established for patients with dementia. The psychiatric nurse assesses mental status, helps with the management of psychotropic medications, and evaluates the residence for safe living circumstances.

Management

Clinical Management

Attention to comorbid systemic and neuropsychiatric illnesses is the first priority in clinical management of the dementia patient. Close collaboration with the patient's other physician(s) is essential for managing medical illnesses that increase the risk for cognitive deficits. Management of pain may decrease agitated behavior in patients with dementia (Geda and Rummans 1999). Psychopharmacological approaches to anxiety, psychotic, and mood disorders are discussed in detail below (see "Pharmacotherapy" later in this section). Substance abuse interventions consisting of medical detoxification, participation in Alcoholics Anonymous or other 12-Step recovery programs and close attention to comorbid substance-induced mood and anxiety disorders is necessary in the dementia patient with comorbid substance abuse or dependence.

Early, frank discussion of diagnosis, prognosis, and management, with clinical follow-ups scheduled at least every 3 months, are advised. Every visit should include an evaluation of whether the patient can still safely live at home. Admission to a psychiatry inpatient unit skilled in dealing with dementia patients may be needed for severely regressed, suicidal, violent, or psychotic patients (Rabins et al. 1997).

Psychoeducation can be very valuable, especially for family caregivers (Grossberg and Lake 1998). *The 36-Hour Day: A Family Guide to Caring for Persons With*

Alzheimer's Disease, Related Dementing Illnesses, and Memory Loss in Later Life (Mace and Rabins 1981) is often helpful to both patients and families. Support and advocacy groups are available through the Alzheimer's Association (1-800-621-0379; www.alz.org) (Rabins et al. 1997). The Alzheimer's Association can facilitate patient enrollment in the Safe Return Program, a nationwide program that assists in the identification and return of dementia patients who wander. The patient should always carry and/or wear identification (e.g., a MedicAlert bracelet) and can be registered with the local police department. Physicians should inform caregivers of the increased risk of depression in primary caregivers of dementia patients and facilitate respite opportunities for caregivers (Grossberg and Lake 1998; Haley 1997).

Environmental and behavioral management may include provision of adequate lighting, music, access to pets, and appropriate levels of psychological stimulation. The home should be organized to allow for simplicity of routines, with prominent display of calendars, schedules, and the photographs and names of people close to the patient. Events that trigger problematic behaviors should be identified and minimized (Parnetti 2000). For safety, childproofing devices may be considered. Vehicle keys, power tools, and sharp household objects should be secured. Weapons should be removed from the home or at least be secured in a locked cabinet.

Institutional placement is often a painful decision for the family, patient, and physician. To many patients, the loss of the home environment, even when clearly necessary to preserve safety, is a devastating experience that usually leads to further confusion, behavioral regression, and increased risk of depression. The physician should make every reasonable effort to maintain the patient in his or her home environment. An important intervention is respite care for caregivers. Various respite models to consider include in-home caregivers and adult day care centers/senior centers.

However, the patient may ultimately regress to a point at which life without 24-hour supervision is not safe. Specific examples of behaviors that cannot safely be managed at home include assaultive or threatening behavior, leaving dangerous appliances on inappropriately, continuing to drive despite prohibitions, and an inability to maintain feeding, drinking, dressing, and toileting functions. When placement is necessary, an institution that specializes in the care of dementia patients is advised. A secured unit may be required to prevent wandering.

Legal issues should be addressed early in the course of the illness, while the patient can still direct his or her wishes. These matters include the completion of medicolegal documents such as living wills, durable powers of attorney, and advance directives (Grossberg and Lake 1998). The patient's capacity for medical decision making needs to be considered as well. The physician is advised to thoroughly evaluate the patient's clinical status at the time a medical decision is needed to ensure that the patient understands the implications of his or her medical choices.

Driving and the operation of other dangerous machinery is often a point of great contention. Many patients will maintain the motor skills for driving despite showing substantial cognitive deficits (Rabins 1998). Even in mild dementia, the statistical risk of motor vehicle accidents is increased (Dubinsky et al. 2000). Physicians are advised to acquaint themselves with the disclosure laws regarding notification of dementia diagnoses to state motor vehicle departments

(Rabins 1998). A useful clinical guideline to consider is that driving is not advised whenever a dementia diagnosis leads the clinician to institute pharmacotherapy for dementia and/or when the MMSE score is less than 24. Other contraindications could be the presence of paranoia, agitation, or assaultive behavior.

Pharmacotherapy

Anticholinesterase agents act through inhibition of AChE, increasing the net amount of synaptic ACh available for neurotransmission (Table 3–10) (Taylor 1998). Anticholinesterase agents are advised early in the course of DAT and may reduce the rate of cognitive decline (Farlow 2000). Although their effects may be relatively modest, more often involving a slowing of decline than a reversal of cognitive losses, they represent a major breakthrough in psychopharmacology.

Anticholinesterase agents should also be considered (along with antipsychotics) in managing dementia-related psychotic symptoms (Rao and Lyketsos 1998). These agents can also be safely combined with antidepressants (Tune and Sunderland 1998). Cholinergic side effects seen with anticholinesterase agents include nausea, abdominal discomfort, vomiting, loose stools, muscle cramps, muscle weakness, increased sweating, and bradycardia (Ringman and Cummings 1999).

Anticholinesterase agents may also be used for other dementing illnesses (e.g., dementia due to PD, LBV, LBD, and CJD; mixed VaD and DAT); they may be particularly helpful with the psychotic symptoms of LBV and LBD (Cummings and Masterman 1998). Combination regimens consisting of an anticholinesterase agent and other agents more directly protective against neuronal degeneration (e.g., antioxidants, anti-inflammatory agents, hormones) with psychotropic medications are emerging as treatment for DAT (Cummings et al. 1998a; Farlow and Evans 1998). Tacrine, donepezil, rivastigmine, and galantamine are U.S. Food and Drug Administration (FDA)–approved for DAT.

Tacrine is taken four times daily, from an initial dose of 10 mg four times a day with dose increases every 6 weeks to a maximum of 160 mg/day (Felician and Sandson 1999). Dosages greater than 80 mg/day may delay nursing home placement (Knopman et al. 1996). About 50% of patients taking tacrine develop increases in liver-associated enzymes, usually within 12 weeks after starting treatment; 25% of patients have increases above three times the upper limit of the reference range (Soares and Gershon 1995). Weekly monitoring of liver-associated enzymes for the first 18 weeks of therapy and every 3 months thereafter is recommended (Class et al. 1997; Soares and Gershon 1995). Because of concerns about increased liver-associated enzymes, tacrine is now used infrequently.

Donepezil is started at 5 mg/day, which may be increased to 10 mg/day in 1–6 weeks. It has been shown to slow the rate of decline of or to improve cognitive performance in mild to moderate DAT (S.L. Rogers et al. 1998). Donepezil has been found to maintain improvements in cognition when continued for up to 98 weeks (S.L. Rogers and Friedhoff 1998). In addition, emotional and behavioral symptoms of dementia may improve (Weiner et al. 2000). Donepezil may help to delay higher-cost interventions associated with disease progression (Neumann et al. 1999).

Rivastigmine is a cholinesterase inhibitor with effects on both AChE and butyrylcholinesterase (BuChE) (Spencer and Noble 1998; Stahl 2000). Rivastigmine is highly selective for the hippocampus and cortex (Spencer and Noble 1998). Because it is not metabolized through the hepatic cytochrome P450 isoenzyme system, it has

TABLE 3–10. Dementia pharmacotherapy

Medication class	Target symptom(s)	Starting dose	Maximum dose
Cholinesterase inhibitors	Decreased cognition, delusions, hallucinations		
Tacrine		10 mg four times a day	40 mg four times a day
Donepezil		5 mg/day	10 mg/day
Rivastigmine		1.5 mg twice a day	6 mg twice a day
Galantamine		4 mg twice a day	12 mg twice a day
Antioxidants	Decreased cognition		
Alpha-tocopherol		1,000 IU twice a day	
Selegiline		5 mg/day	10 mg/day
Antidepressants	Depression, irritability, anxiety		
Fluoxetine		10 mg/day	40 mg/day
Paroxetine		10 mg/day	40 mg/day
Sertraline		25 mg/day	200 mg/day
Citalopram		10 mg/day	40 mg/day
Venlafaxine (extended release)		37.5 mg/day	350 mg/day
Nefazodone		50 mg/day	300 mg twice a day
Trazodone		25 mg/day at bedtime	400 mg/day at bedtime
Bupropion		37.5 mg twice a day	200 mg twice a day
Anxiolytic	Anxiety, irritability		
Buspirone		5 mg three times a day	20 mg three times a day
Anticonvulsants	Irritability, agitation		
Carbamazepine		100 mg/day	a
Valproate		125 mg/day	b
Antipsychotics	Delusions, hallucinations, disorganized thoughts, agitation		
Risperidone		0.25 mg/day at bedtime	3 mg/day at bedtime
Olanzapine		2.5 mg/day at bedtime	10 mg/day at bedtime
Quetiapine		25 mg/day at bedtime	100 mg twice a day

TABLE 3–10. Dementia pharmacotherapy (*continued*)

Medication class	Target symptom(s)	Starting dose	Maximum dose
Additional medications (consider as adjunctive therapy on case-by-case basis)			
Psychostimulants			
Nonsteroidal anti-inflammatory drugs			
Antiplatelet agents			
Hormones			
Highly active antiretroviral therapy (HAART)			

[a]Upper limit of dose to give serum drug level of 8–12 ng/mL; [b]Upper limit of dose to give serum drug level of 50–60 ng/mL.

little likelihood of problematic drug–drug interactions (Spencer and Noble 1998). Rivastigmine is started at 1.5 mg twice daily for 2 weeks; the dosage may be gradually raised every 2 weeks to a maximum recommended dose of 6 mg twice daily. Doses from 3 to 6 mg twice a day have a beneficial effect on cognitive and functional status (Spencer and Noble 1998).

Galantamine is a cholinesterase inhibitor that also allosterically modulates nicotine cholinergic receptors, theoretically further enhancing ACh release (Raskind et al. 2000; Stahl 2000). Galantamine is initially started at 4 mg twice a day, with dosage increases to 8 mg twice daily and 12 mg twice daily after 4-week intervals. A 6-month study of galantamine showed that a 24-mg daily dose was associated with improved cognitive and global function (Raskind et al. 2000).

The antioxidants selegiline and α-tocopherol (vitamin E) are used for their neuroprotective effects. Selegiline (a selective monoamine oxidase B [MAO-B] inhibitor) 5–10 mg/day is used in mild to moderate DAT (Sano et al. 1997; Tolbert and Fuller 1996). Selegiline may have a positive effect on both cognition and behavior (Lawlor et al. 1997; Tolbert and Fuller 1996). A tyramine-restricted diet is not required at doses up to 10 mg/day. Selegiline must be used cautiously because of its risk of drug–drug interactions and orthostatic hypotension (Sano et al. 1997). Its use is contraindicated with selective serotonin reuptake inhibitors (SSRIs), TCAs, and meperidine (Rabins et al. 1997).

α-Tocopherol 1,000 IU twice daily may slow the progression of moderate DAT, as its antioxidant properties may protect against neuronal damage caused by amyloid deposition (Felician and Sandson 1999). In addition, it has been associated with decreased coagulation function in patients with vitamin K deficiency (Rabins et al. 1997). Either selegiline or α-tocopherol may delay a poor outcome in dementia (Sano et al. 1997).

Antipsychotics are indicated for paranoid thinking, hallucinations, delirium, and agitation (Alexopoulos et al. 1998; Lanctot et al. 1998; Rabins 1998). Initial doses in elderly patients with dementia should be less than those used in younger patients because of the risks of sedation and further cognitive decline.

The atypical antipsychotic agents risperidone, olanzapine, and quetiapine are recommended in dementia with agitation and psychosis because of their greater tolerability and lower risk of EPS and neuroleptic malignant syndrome (Daniel 2000; De Deyn et al. 1999). Reduced starting and maximum dosages (e.g., risperidone dosage range of 0.25–3 mg/day at bedtime) are recommended to minimize side effects (Class et al. 1997; Daniel 2000). Risperidone dosages ranging from 0.75 to 1.75 mg/day were associated with only a 2.6% risk of tardive dyskinesia at 1-year follow-up (Jeste et al. 2000). In patients with feeding tubes or other limitations affecting their use of solid medications, risperidone elixir can be considered. Suggested dosages for olanzapine are 2.5–10.0 mg/day at bedtime; quetiapine dosages can range from 25 mg/day at bedtime to 100 mg twice daily (Daniel 2000).

Follow-up monitoring should include examination for medication-induced movement disorders with the Assessment of Involuntary Movements Scale. If problems with compliance lead the physician to consider depot antipsychotics, reduced doses (e.g., fluphenazine decanoate 1.25–3.75 mg im monthly) can be considered (Rabins et al. 1997). In the United States, the use of antipsychotic medication in nursing home patients with dementia is regulated by the Omnibus Budget Reconciliation Act of 1987, which requires clear documentation of clinical indications and consideration of alternative interventions (Rabins et al. 1997). Dosage decreases or trial discontinuations of antipsychotics should be considered as the illness progresses. Atypical antipsychotics may still be indicated even in severe dementia (Katz et al. 1999).

Antidepressants should be used for comorbid depressive disorders, depressive and anxiety symptoms that do not qualify for a full depressive or anxiety disorder diagnosis, sleep disturbances, and agitation (Borson and Raskind 1997; Raskind 1998). Because of their generally benign side-effect profile and their effectiveness, SSRIs are the preferred class of antidepressants in dementia patients and should be started at lower doses than in healthy adults (Alexopoulos et al. 1998; Katz 1998). Initial doses can be doubled after 2–4 weeks if necessary, and a trial should continue for at least 12 weeks once the usual adult dose has been reached (Class et al. 1997).

Other antidepressants to consider include bupropion, trazodone, and venlafaxine extended release (Alexopoulos et al. 1998; Class et al. 1997). Blood pressure must be monitored in patients using venlafaxine because of the risk of hypertension. TCAs should be used with caution in dementia because of the cognitive toxicity that may result from anticholinergic side effects (Katz 1998; Petracca et al. 1996).

Psychostimulants as adjunctive therapy with antidepressants may be considered for refractory mood symptoms and/ or apathy; methylphenidate 2.5–5 mg/day is a recommended starting dose (Rabins et al. 1997). ECT should be considered for cases of treatment-refractory depression; however, because of the risk for post-ECT delirium and amnesia, ECT treatments should be given no more frequently than twice per week with unilateral electrode placement (Rabins et al. 1997).

Anxiolytics may be used for anxiety or agitation. Because of the high risk of further memory impairment, sedation, and falls, physicians should avoid the use of benzodiazepines in dementia patients (Rabins et al. 1997). The clinician might consider buspirone 5 mg thrice daily and increase doses gradually to an upper limit of 20 mg three times a day (Alexopoulos et al. 1998; Class et al. 1997).

Anticonvulsants may be indicated for agitated and aggressive behavior or for emotional lability (Class et al. 1997). A recommended starting dose of carbamazepine for the elderly patient with dementia is 100 mg/day, which can be titrated to achieve a serum drug level of 8–12 ng/mL (Rabins et al. 1997).

Divalproex sodium can be started at 125 mg/day and titrated upward to yield a serum drug level of 50–60 ng/mL (Rabins et al. 1997). Monitoring of complete blood count and of liver-associated enzymes is recommended with the use of carbamazepine and valproate (Rabins et al. 1997).

NSAIDs (e.g., indomethacin 100–150 mg/day) may delay disease progression in dementia, based on the lower risk for DAT in patients with rheumatoid arthritis and/or chronic NSAID use (Anthony et al. 2000; Breitner 1996).

Antiplatelet therapy and/or ergot mesylates (e.g., hydergine 3 mg/day initially to a maximum of 9 mg/day) may be considered for cases of VaD and may stabilize or improve cognitive function (Meyer et al. 1995). Hydergine may be associated with nausea and other gastrointestinal symptoms; its use is contraindicated in patients with psychotic symptoms (Rabins et al. 1997).

Estrogen may improve blood flow in cerebral vessels and may also have more direct neuroprotective effects (Birge 1997). Female patients with DAT have been shown to have lower levels of endogenous estrogen (Manly et al. 2000). A large meta-analysis of the effects of post-menopausal hormone replacement on cognition concluded that hormone replacement therapy produced improvement in verbal memory, vigilance, reasoning, and motor speed in women with menopausal symptoms (LeBlanc et al. 2001).

Future exploration in pharmacotherapy will likely target DAT but would be expected to have applicability to other dementia types as well. Areas of active interest include neurotrophic factors (e.g., nerve growth factor), modification of amyloid metabolism (likely targeting the activities of APP), and reduction of oxidative stress and inflammation (Aisen and Davis 1997).

Highly active antiretroviral therapy (HAART) for the underlying HIV infection is an essential part of the management of HIV dementia and can reverse cognitive losses (Cohen and Jacobson 2000; Maldonado et al. 2000; McDaniel et al. 2000). Psychostimulants may be helpful in HIV-associated fatigue and decreased concentration and memory (Maldonado et al. 2000; McDaniel et al. 2000).

Summary

The dementias are a heterogeneous group of clinical syndromes, unified by their common findings of deterioration in cognitive and executive functions. Physicians need to be alert to the need for a thorough history, targeted evaluation, and psychopharmacological and psychosocial management in patients with these clinical syndromes. Modern clinical interventions, including anticholinesterase agents in conjunction with other psychopharmacological agents, should be aggressively used early in the disease process to maintain the patient's cognitive functional status. Advances in basic science research point

to possible new directions in the pathophysiology and psychopharmacological management of this major public health problem.

Amnestic Disorders

Amnestic disorders are characterized by a loss of memory due to the direct physiological effects of a general medical condition or due to the persisting effects of a substance. The amnestic disorders share a common symptom presentation of memory impairment but are differentiated by etiology. Amnestic disorders are secondary syndromes caused by systemic medical illness, primary cerebral disease or trauma, substance use disorders, or adverse medication effects. The impairment must be sufficient to compromise social and occupational functioning, and it should represent a significant decline from the previous level of functioning.

Epidemiology

Memory impairment due to head trauma is probably the most common etiology, with more than 500,000 patients hospitalized annually in the United States for head injury. Alcohol abuse and associated thiamine deficiency is a historically common etiology, but recent studies suggest that the incidence of alcohol-induced amnestic disorders is decreasing, whereas that of amnestic disorders due to head trauma is increasing (Kopelman 1995).

Etiology

The DSM-IV-TR diagnostic classification for amnestic disorders is based on etiology. Amnestic disorders can be diagnosed as resulting from a general medical condition (Table 3–11), as due to the effects of a substance (Table 3–12), or as "not otherwise specified." The most common etiol-

TABLE 3–11. DSM-IV-TR diagnostic criteria for amnestic disorder due to…*[indicate the general medical condition]*

A. The development of memory impairment as manifested by impairment in the ability to learn new information or the inability to recall previously learned information.
B. The memory disturbance causes significant impairment in social or occupational functioning and represents a significant decline from a previous level of functioning.
C. The memory disturbance does not occur exclusively during the course of a delirium or a dementia.
D. There is evidence from the history, physical examination, or laboratory findings that the disturbance is the direct physiological consequence of a general medical condition (including physical trauma).
   Specify if:
      Transient: if memory impairment lasts for 1 month or less
      Chronic: if memory impairment lasts for more than 1 month
Coding note: Include the name of the general medical condition on Axis I, e.g., amnestic disorder due to head trauma; also code the general medical condition on Axis III.

TABLE 3–12. DSM-IV-TR diagnostic criteria for substance-induced persisting amnestic disorder

A. The development of memory impairment as manifested by impairment in the ability to learn new information or the inability to recall previously learned information.
B. The memory disturbance causes significant impairment in social or occupational functioning and represents a significant decline from a previous level of functioning.
C. The memory disturbance does not occur exclusively during the course of a delirium or a dementia and persists beyond the usual duration of substance intoxication or withdrawal.
D. There is evidence from the history, physical examination, or laboratory findings that the memory disturbance is etiologically related to the persisting effects of substance use (e.g., a drug of abuse, a medication).
Code [Specific substance]–induced persisting amnestic disorder: (291.1 alcohol; 292.83 sedative, hypnotic, or anxiolytic; 292.83 other [or unknown] substance)

TABLE 3–13. Causes of amnestic disorders

Head trauma
Wernicke-Korsakoff syndrome
Alcohol-induced blackouts
Benzodiazepines
Barbiturates
Intrathecal methotrexate
Methylenedioxymethamphetamine
  (MDMA; "Ecstasy")
Seizures
Herpes simplex encephalopathy
Kluver-Bucy syndrome
Electroconvulsive therapy
Carbon monoxide poisoning
Heavy metal poisoning
Hypoxia
Hypoglycemia
Cerebrovascular disorders
Cerebral neoplasms

ogies are listed in Table 3–13 and usually involve bilateral damage to areas of the brain involved in memory. Unilateral damage may sometimes be sufficient to produce memory impairment, particularly in the case of left-sided temporal lobe and thalamic structures (Benson 1978).

Clinical Features

Patients with amnestic disorders either are impaired in their ability to learn and recall new information (anterograde amnesia) or are unable to recall previously learned material (retrograde amnesia). The deficits in short-term or recent memory seen in anterograde amnesia can be assessed by asking the patient to recall three objects after a 5-minute distraction. Whereas anterograde amnesia is nearly always present, retrograde amnesia is more variable and depends on the location and severity of brain damage. Both immediate recall (as tested by digit span) and remote memory for distant past events are usually preserved. Memory for the physical traumatic event that caused the deficit is often lost. Orientation may be impaired. The patient may therefore present as confused and disoriented, but without the fluctuation in level of consciousness associated with delirium. Orientation to self is nearly always preserved in amnestic disorders.

Most patients with amnestic disorders lack insight into their deficits and may vehemently deny the presence of memory impairment despite clear evidence to the contrary. More commonly, patients present with apathy, lack of initiative, and diminished affective expression suggestive of altered personality function.

Confabulation is often associated with amnestic disorders. Confabulation is characterized by responses to questions that not only are inaccurate but also are often so bizarre and unrealistic as to appear psychotic. Confabulation in amnestic disorders is usually seen during the early stages of the illness and tends to disappear over time.

Head trauma, vascular events, and specific neurotoxic exposures such as carbon monoxide poisoning are associated with acute mental status changes. Prolonged substance use, sustained nutritional deficiency, and chronic neurotoxic exposures may produce a more gradual and sustained decline in memory function.

Selected Amnestic Disorders
Head Injury

Severe neurological and psychiatric symptoms can result from head injury, even in the absence of radiological evidence of structural damage. Amnesia following head injury typically includes both anterograde (or ongoing) amnesia and retrograde amnesia for a period ranging from a few minutes to several years before the injury. As anterograde amnesia fades and the patient regains the ability to learn and recall new information, retrograde amnesia "shrinks," usually remaining only for the very short period (seconds to minutes) before the injury. A prolonged retrograde amnesia is an indication of ongoing anterograde amnesia, whereas a short period of retrograde amnesia is associated with recovery (Benson and McDaniel 1991).

Korsakoff's Syndrome

Korsakoff's syndrome is an amnestic disorder caused by thiamine deficiency, usually associated with excessive, prolonged ingestion of alcohol. It can also occur in other malnourished conditions (Kopelman 1995). Korsakoff's syndrome is associated with an acute phase of illness—known as Wernicke's encephalopathy—that presents with ophthalmoplegia, peripheral neuropathy, ataxia, nystagmus, and delirium. Although these acute neurological symptoms respond to aggressive thiamine repletion, a residual, persistent amnestic syndrome usually remains. Given the high prevalence of missed diagnoses of Wernicke-Korsakoff syndrome and the insidious, progressive course of the illness, in which each episode gives rise to cumulative damage, all alcohol-dependent patients should be treated with thiamine (Blansjaar and van Dijk 1992).

Transient Global Amnesia

Transient global amnesia is a form of amnestic disorder characterized by an abrupt episode of profound anterograde amnesia and a variable inability to recall events that occur during the episode. These episodes typically last for only a few minutes or hours, ending with a rapid, spontaneous restoration of intact cognitive function. Mean duration of the amnestic period is 4.2 hours; periods greater than 12 hours are exceptional. The patient's level of consciousness and orientation to self are unaffected during the episode (Fisher and Adams 1958; Shuping et al. 1980). Patients are often bewildered and confused during the episodes and may ask repeated questions about their circumstances. No data are available to suggest that transient global amnesia is associated with focal neurological features or with any comorbid psychiatric illness. Transient global amnesia is more common in men and usually occurs after age 50. The etiology is unclear, but most experts believe that it is associated with cerebrovascular disease and episodic vascular insufficiency of the mesial temporal lobe. The most common angiographic findings are in the vertebrobasilar system, specifically occlusion or stenosis of the posterior cerebral artery (Matthew and Meyer 1974). Transient global amnesia generally has a good prognosis, with only 8% of patients experiencing a second episode (Hodges and Warlow 1990b).

Benzodiazepine Persisting Amnestic Disorder

Benzodiazepines can cause anterograde amnesia and may interfere with memory consolidation and retrieval. Risk factors include high dose, intravenous administration, and use of high-potency, short-half-life agents such as triazolam (Scharf et al. 1987). These effects may be enhanced by the concurrent use of alcohol (Linnoila 1990; Roth et al. 1984).

Differential Diagnosis

Memory deficits seen in amnestic syndromes are frequently a feature of delirium and dementia. In delirium, the memory disturbance is accompanied by a disturbed level of consciousness and usually fluctuates with time. More pervasive signs of cerebral dysfunction, such as difficulty focusing or sustaining attention, are present. In dementia, memory impairment is accompanied by additional cognitive impairments.

In dissociative or psychogenic forms of amnesia, the memory loss usually does not involve deficits in learning and recalling new information. Patients typically present with a circumscribed inability to recall previously learned and personal information, often regarding the patient's own identity or a traumatic or stressful event. Patients with malingering or factitious disorders can present with amnestic symptoms that also fit the profile for dissociative amnesia. Systematic memory testing of these patients will often yield inconsistent results.

Treatment

As in delirium and dementia, the primary goal of treatment in amnestic disorders is to identify and treat the underlying cause or pathological process. There are no definitively effective treatments for amnestic disorder that are specifically aimed at reversing apparent memory deficits. Fortunately, these deficits are often temporary—as in transient amnestic syndromes—or are partially or completely reversible—as in head trauma, thiamine deficiency, or anoxia. Acute management should include continuous reorientation of the patient by means of verbal redirection, clocks, calendars, and familiar stimuli. Chronic reversible amnestic syndromes may be managed with cognitive rehabilitation and therapeutic milieus intended to promote recovery from brain injury (Kashima et al. 1999). More severe and permanent deficits may require supervised living environments to ensure appropriate care.

Conclusions

The cognitive disorders represent a heterogeneous group of clinical syndromes with the common denominator of disturbances in memory and other cognitive functions. Psychiatrists need to be mindful of the broad differential diagnosis of patients presenting with cognitive impairment. Thorough history taking; directed mental status testing; use of laboratory tests, EEG, and neuroimaging; and a willingness to creatively employ psychopharmacological and behavioral interventions based on an application of the biopsychosocial model are advised for the care of these patients. It is likely that future neuroscientific, pharmacological, and neuroimaging research will yield further options for diagnosis, treatment, and prevention of cognitive impairment.

References

Aakerlund LP, Rosenberg J: Postoperative delirium: treatment with supplemental oxygen. Br J Anaesth 72:286–290, 1994

Aisen PS, Davis KL: The search for disease-modifying treatment for Alzheimer's disease. Neurology 48 (suppl 6):S35–S41, 1997

Alexander GE, Furey ML, Grady CL, et al: Association of premorbid intellectual function with cerebral metabolism in Alzheimer's disease: implications for the cognitive reserve hypothesis. Am J Psychiatry 154:165–172, 1997

Alexopoulos GS, Silver JM, Kahn DA, et al: Treatment of agitation in older patients with dementia. A Postgraduate Medicine Special Report. Minneapolis, MN, McGraw-Hill, 1998, pp 1–88

American Psychiatric Association: Practice guideline for the treatment of patients with delirium. Am J Psychiatry 156 (suppl):1–20, 1999

American Psychiatric Association: Diagnostic and Statistical Manual of Mental Disorders, 4th Edition, Text Revision. Washington, DC, American Psychiatric Association, 2000

Anthony JC, Breitner JCS, Zandi PP, et al: Reduced prevalence of AD in users of NSAIDs and H2 receptor antagonists. Neurology 54:2066–2071, 2000

Armstrong SC, Cozza KL, Watanabe KS: The misdiagnosis of delirium. Psychosomatics 38:433–439, 1997

Ayd FJ: Intravenous haloperidol therapy. International Drug Therapy Newsletter 13:20–23, 1978

Balestrino M, Aitken PG, Somjen CG: Spreading depression-like hypoxic depolarization in CA1 and fascia dentata of hippocampal slices: relationship to selective vulnerability. Brain Res 497:102–107, 1989

Ballard CG, O'Brien JT, Swann AG, et al: The natural history of psychosis and depression in dementia with Lewy bodies and Alzheimer's disease: persistence and new cases over 1 year of follow-up. J Clin Psychiatry 62:46–49, 2001

Bauer G: Cerebral anoxia, in Electroencephalography: Basic Principles, Clinical Applications and Related Fields. Edited by Niedermayer E, Lopes da Silva F. Baltimore, MD, Urban & Schwarzenberg, 1982, pp 319–324

Benson DF: Amnesia. South Med J 71:1221–1228, 1978

Benson DF, McDaniel KD: Memory disorders, in Neurology in Clinical Practice, Vol 2. Edited by Bradley WG, Daroff RB, Fenichel GM, et al. Boston, MA, Butterworth-Heinemann, 1991, pp 1389–1406

Beresin E: Delirium in the elderly. J Geriatr Psychiatry Neurol 1:127–143, 1988

Berger A-K, Fratiglioni L, Frosell Y, et al: The occurrence of depressive symptoms in the preclinical phase of AD: a population-based study. Neurology 53:1998–2002, 1999

Birge SJ: The role of estrogen in the treatment of Alzheimer's disease. Neurology 48 (suppl 7): S36–S41, 1997

Blansjaar BA, Van Dijk JG: Korsakoff minus Wernicke syndrome. Alcohol Alcohol 27: 435–437, 1992

Blazer DG, Federspiel CF, Ray WA, et al: The risk of anticholinergic toxicity in the elderly: a study of prescribing practices in two populations. J Gerontol 38:31–35, 1983

Bluml S, Zuckerman E, Tan J, et al: Proton-decoupled 31P magnetic resonance spectroscopy reveals osmotic and metabolic disturbances in human hepatic encephalopathy. J Neurochem 71:1564–1576, 1998

Bobinski M, Wegel J, Wisniewski HM, et al: Neurofibrillary pathology-correlation with hippocampal formation atrophy in Alzheimer disease. Neurobiology of Aging 17:909–919, 1996

Borson S, Raskind MA: Clinical features and pharmacologic treatment of behavioral symptoms of Alzheimer's disease. Neurology 48 (suppl 6):S17–S24, 1997

Bottino CM, Almeida OP: Can neuroimaging techniques identify individuals at risk of developing Alzheimer's disease? Int Psychogeriatr 9:389–403, 1997

Breitbart W, Marotta R, Call P: AIDS and neuroleptic malignant syndrome. Lancet 2 (8626–8627):1488–1489, 1988

Breitbart W, Marotta R, Platt MM, et al: A double-blind trial of haloperidol, chlorpromazine, and lorazepam in the treatment of delirium in hospitalized AIDS patients. Am J Psychiatry 153:231–237, 1996

Breitbart W, Rosenfeld B, Roth A, et al: The memorial delirium assessment scale. J Pain Symptom Manage 13:128–137, 1997

Breitner JCS: The role of anti-inflammatory drugs in the prevention and treatment of Alzheimer's disease. Ann Rev Med 47: 401–411, 1996

Brown TM: Basic mechanisms in the pathogenesis of delirium, in The Psychiatric Care of the Medical Patient, 2nd Edition. Edited by Stoudemire A, Fogel BS, Greenberg DB. New York, Oxford University Press, 2000, pp 571–580

Brown TM, Stoudemire A: Psychiatric Side Effects of Prescription and Over-the-Counter Medications. Washington, DC, American Psychiatric Press, 1998

Cameron DJ, Thomas RI, Mulvihill M, et al: Delirium: a test of the Diagnostic and Statistical Manual III criteria on medical inpatients. J Am Geriatr Soc 35:1007–1010, 1987

Caraceni A, Nanni O, Maltoni M, et al: Impact of delirium on the short term prognosis of advanced cancer patients. Italian Multicenter Study Group on Palliative Care. Cancer 89:1145–1149, 2000

Caselli RJ, Graff-Radford NR, Reiman EM, et al: Preclinical memory decline in cognitively normal apolipoprotein E epsilon-4 homozygotes. Neurology 53:201–207, 1999

Cassem NH, Sos J: Intravenous use of haloperidol for acute delirium in intensive care settings. Paper presented at 131st Annual Meeting of the American Psychiatric Association, Washington, DC, May 1978

Choi SH, Na DL, Chung CS, et al: Diffusion-weighted MRI in vascular dementia. Neurology 54:83–89, 2000

Class CA, Schneider L, Farlow MR: Optimal management of behavioural disorders associated with dementia. Drugs Aging 10:95–106, 1997

Cohen MAA, Jacobson JM: Maximizing life's potential in AIDS: a psychopharmacologic update. Gen Hosp Psychiatry 22:375–388, 2000

Cole MG, Primeau FJ: Prognosis of delirium in elderly hospital patients. Can Med Assoc J 149:41–46, 1993

Craft S, Teri L, Edland SD, et al: Accelerated decline in apolipoprotein E-epsilon 4 homozygotes with Alzheimer's disease. Neurology 51:149–153, 1998

Cummings JL, Masterman DL: Assessment of treatment-associated changes in behavior and cholinergic therapy of neuropsychiatric symptoms in Alzheimer's disease. J Clin Psychiatry 59 (suppl 13):23–30, 1998

Cummings JL, Vinters HV, Cole GM, et al: Alzheimer's disease: etiologies, pathophysiology, cognitive reserve, and treatment opportunities. Neurology 51 (suppl 1):S2–S17, 1998a

Curb JD, Rodriguez BL, Abbott RD, et al: Longitudinal association of vascular and Alzheimer's dementia, diabetes, and glucose tolerance. Neurology 52:971–975, 1999

Daniel DG: Antipsychotic treatment of psychosis and agitation in the elderly. J Clin Psychiatry 61 (suppl 14):49–52, 2000

d'Arminio Monteforte A, Duca PG, Vago L, et al: Decreasing incidence of CNS AIDS-defining events associated with antiretroviral therapy. Neurology 54:1856–1859, 2000

De Deyn PP, Rabheru K, Rasmussen A, et al: A randomized trial of risperidone, placebo, and haloperidol for behavioral symptoms of dementia. Neurology 53:946–955, 1999

de Koning I, van Kooten F, Dippel DWJ, et al: The CAMCOG: a useful screening instrument for dementia in stroke patients. Stroke 29:2080–2086, 1998

Delacourte A, David JP, Sergeant N, et al: The biochemical pathway of neurofibrillary degeneration in aging and Alzheimer's disease. Neurology 52:1158–1165, 1999

Dickson LR: Hypoalbuminemia in delirium. Psychosomatics 32:317–323, 1991

Dolan MM, Hawkes WG, Zimmerman SI, et al: Delirium on hospital admission in aged hip fracture patients: prediction of mortality and 2-year functional outcomes. J Gerontol 55:M527–M534, 2000

Doody RS, Massman PJ, Mawad M, et al: Cognitive consequences of subcortical magnetic resonance imaging changes in Alzheimer's disease: comparison to small vessel ischemic vascular dementia. Neuropsychiatry Neuropsychol Behav Neurol 11: 191–199, 1998

Doraiswamy PM, Steffens DC, Pitchumoni S, et al: Early recognition of Alzheimer's disease: What is consensual? What is controversial? What is practical? J Clin Psychiatry 59 (suppl 13):6–18, 1998

Doyle M, Warden D: Use of SPECT to evaluate postcardiotomy delirium (letter). Am J Psychiatry 153:838–839, 1996

Duara R, Barker W, Luis CA: Frontotemporal dementia and Alzheimer's disease: differential diagnosis. Dement Geriatr Cogn Disord 10 (suppl 1):37–42, 1999

Dubinsky RM, Stein AC, Lyons K: Practice parameter: risk of driving and Alzheimer's disease (an evidence-based review). Neurology 54:2205–2211, 2000

Dunn NR, Alfonso CA, Young RA, et al: Creutzfeldt-Jakob disease appearing as paranoid psychosis. Am J Psychiatry 156: 2016–2017, 1999

Dyer CB, Ashton CM, Teasdale TA: Postoperative delirium: a review of 80 primary data-collection studies. Arch Intern Med 155:461–465, 1995

Eden BM, Foreman MD, Sisk R: Delirium: comparison of four predictive models in hospitalized critically ill elderly patients. Applied Nursing Research 11:27–35, 1998

Elie M, Rousseau F, Cole M, et al: Prevalence and detection of delirium in elderly emergency room department patients. Can Med Assoc J 163:977–981, 2000

Engel GL, Romano J: Delirium: a syndrome of cerebral insufficiency. J Chronic Dis 9: 260–277, 1959

Erkinjuntii T, Wikstrom J, Palo J, et al: Dementia among medical inpatients: evaluation of 2000 consecutive admissions. Arch Intern Med 146:1923–1926, 1986

Evans RM, Emsley CL, Gao S, et al: Serum cholesterol, APOE genotype, and the risk of Alzheimer's disease: a population-based study of African Americans. Neurology 54:240–242, 2000

Fann JR, Roth-Roemer S, Burington B, et al: Delirium in patients undergoing hematopoietic stem cell transplantation: epidemiology, risk factors, and outcomes. Symposium presented at the annual meeting of the Academy of Psychosomatic Medicine, Palm Springs, CA, November 2000

Fann JR, Burington B, Roth-Roemer S, et al: Delirium and affective and cognitive outcomes in patients undergoing stem cell transplantation. Ann Behav Med 23 (suppl): S064, 2001

Farlow M: New approaches in assessing delay of progression of Alzheimer's disease (pp 795–798), in Geula C, Farlow M, chairs: Alzheimer's disease: translating neurochemical insights into clinical benefits (Academic Highlights). J Clin Psychiatry 61:791–802, 2000

Farlow MR, Evans RM: Pharmacologic treatment of cognition in Alzheimer's dementia. Neurology 51 (suppl 1):S36–S44, 1998

Felician O, Sandson TA: The neurobiology and pharmacotherapy of Alzheimer's disease. J Neuropsychiatry Clin Neurosci 11:19–31, 1999

Fernandez F, Holmes VF, Adams F, et al: Treatment of severe, refractory agitation with a haloperidol drip. J Clin Psychiatry 49:239–241, 1988

Fernandez F, Levy JK, Mansell PW: Management of delirium in terminally ill AIDS patients. Int J Psychiatry Med 19:165–172, 1989

Fink M: Cytopathic hypoxia in sepsis. Acta Anaesthesiol Scand 110 (suppl):87–95, 1997

Fink M: Delirious mania. Bipolar Disord 1:54–60, 1999

Fischer P: Successful treatment of nonanticholinergic delirium with a cholinesterase inhibitor (letter). J Clin Psychopharmacol 21:118, 2001

Fisher CM, Adams RD: Transient global amnesia. Trans Am Neurol Assoc 83:143–146, 1958

Folstein MF, Folstein SE, McHugh PR: "Mini-Mental State": a practical method for grading the cognitive state of patients for the clinician. J Psychiatr Res 12:189–198, 1975

Foy A, O'Connell D, Henry D, et al: Benzodiazepine use as a cause of cognitive impairment in elderly hospital inpatients. J Gerontol 50A:M99–M106, 1995

Francis J, Kapoor WN: Delirium in hospitalized elderly. J Gen Intern Med 5:65–79, 1990

Francis J, Kapoor WN: Prognosis after hospital discharge of older medical patients with delirium. J Am Geriatr Soc 40:601–606, 1992

Francis J, Martin D, Kapoor WN: A prospective study of delirium in hospitalized elderly. JAMA 263:1097–1101, 1990

Freund HR, Muggia-Sullam M, LaFrance R, et al: Regional brain amino-acid and neurotransmitter derangements during abdominal sepsis and septic encephalopathy in the rat. Arch Surg 121:209–216, 1986

Frye MA, Coudreaut MF, Hakeman SM, et al: Continuous droperidol infusion for management of agitated delirium in an intensive care unit. Psychosomatics 36:301–305, 1995

Gagnon P, Allard P, Masse B, et al: Delirium in terminal cancer: a prospective study using daily screening, early diagnosis, and continuous monitoring. J Pain Symptom Manage 19:412–426, 2000

Geda YE, Rummans TA: Pain: cause of agitation in elderly individuals with dementia. Am J Psychiatry 156:1662–1663, 1999

Gibson GE, Blass JP: Impaired synthesis of acetylcholine in brain accompanying mild hypoxia and hypoglycemia. J Neurochem 27:37–42, 1976

Gibson GE, Pulsinelli W, Blass JP, et al: Brain dysfunction in mild to moderate hypoxia. Am J Med 70:1247–1254, 1981

Gliatto MF, Caroff SN: Neurosyphilis: a history and clinical review. Psychiatr Ann 31:153–161, 2001

Globus MY, Ginsberg M, Dietrich WD, et al: Substantia nigra lesion protects against ischemic damage in the striatum. Neurosci Lett 68:169–174, 1986

Globus MY, Busto R, Dietrich WD, et al: Effect of ischemia on the in vivo release of striatal dopamine, glutamate, and gamma-aminobutyric acid studied by intracerebral microdialysis. J Neurochem 51:1455–1464, 1988a

Globus MY, Busto R, Martinez E, et al: Intraischemic extracellular release of dopamine and glutamate is associated with striatal vulnerability to ischemia. Neurosci Lett 91:36–40, 1988b

Goldman WP, Baty JD, Buckles VD, et al: Motor dysfunction in mildly demented AD individuals without extrapyramidal signs. Neurology 53:956–962, 1999

Golinger R, Peet T, Tune L: Association of elevated plasma activity with delirium in surgical patients. Am J Psychiatry 144:1218–1220, 1987

Gomez-Isla T, Growdon WB, McNamara M, et al: Clinicopathologic correlates in temporal cortex in dementia with Lewy bodies. Neurology 53:2003–2009, 1999

Gomez-Tortosa E, Newell K, Irizarry MC, et al: Clinical and quantitative pathologic correlates of dementia with Lewy bodies. Neurology 53:1284–1291, 1999

Goodkin K, Baldewicz TT, Wilkie FL, et al: Cognitive-motor impairment and disorder in HIV-1 infection. Psychiatr Ann 31:37–44, 2001

Graham DG: Oxidative pathways for catecholamines in the genesis of neuromelanin and cytotoxic quinones. Molecular Pharmacology 14:633–643, 1978

Graham DG: Catecholamine toxicity: a proposal for the molecular pathogenesis of manganese neurotoxicity and Parkinson's disease. Neurotoxicology 5:83–96, 1984

Grossberg GT, Lake JT: The role of the psychiatrist in Alzheimer's disease. J Clin Psychiatry 59 (suppl 9):3–6, 1998

Guo Z, Cupples LA, Kurz A, et al: Head injury and the risk of AD in the MIRAGE study. Neurology 54:1316–1323, 2000

Gury C, Canceil O, Iaria P: Antipsychotic drugs and cardiovascular safety: current studies of prolonged QT interval and risk of ventricular arrhythmia (abstract). Encephale 26:62–72, 2000

Gustafson K, Berggren D, Brannstrom B, et al: Acute confusional states in elderly patients treated for femoral neck fractures. J Am Geriatr Soc 36:525–530, 1988

Haass C, De Strooper B: The presenilis in Alzheimer's disease: proteolysis holds the key. Science 286:916–919, 1999

Haley WE: The family caregiver's role in Alzheimer's disease. Neurology 48 (suppl 6): S25–S29, 1997

Hall KS, Gao S, Unverzagt FW, et al: Low education and childhood rural residence: risk for Alzheimer's disease in African Americans. Neurology 54:95–99, 2000

Hamilton M: A rating scale for depression. J Neurol Neurosurg Psychiatry 23:51–56, 1960

Hansen L, Salmon D, Galasko D, et al: The Lewy body variant of Alzheimer's disease: a clinical and pathologic entity. Neurology 40:1–8, 1990

Harhangi BS, de Rijk MC, van Duijn CM, et al: APOE and the risk of PD with or without dementia in a population-based study. Neurology 54:1272–1276, 2000

Haroutunian V, Perl DP, Dushyant DP, et al: Regional distribution of neuritic plaques in the nondemented elderly and subjects with very mild Alzheimer disease. Arch Neurol 55:1185–1191, 1998

Helmer C, Damon D, Letenneur L, et al: Marital status and risk of Alzheimer's disease: a French population-based study. Neurology 53:1953–1958, 1999

Henon H, Lebert F, Durieu I, et al: Confusional state in stroke: relation to preexisting dementia, patient characteristics, and outcome. Stroke 30:773–779, 1999

Heyman A, Fillenbaum GG, Welsh-Bohmer KA, et al: Cerebral infarcts in patients with autopsy proven Alzheimer's disease: CERAD, part XVIII. Neurology 51:159–162, 1998

Heyman A, Fillenbaum GG, Gearing M, et al: Comparison of Lewy body variant of Alzheimer's disease with pure Alzheimer's disease. Neurology 52:1839–1844, 1999

Hodges JR, Warlow CP: Syndromes of transient global amnesia: towards a classification. A study of 153 cases. J Neurol Neurosurg Psychiatry 53:834–843, 1990b

Hodkinson HM: Mental impairment in the elderly. J R Coll Physicians Lond 7:305–317, 1973

Hughes TA, Ross HF, Musa S, et al: A 10-year study of the incidence of and factors predicting dementia in Parkinson's disease. Neurology 54:1596–1602, 2000

Hunt N, Stern TA: The association between intravenous haloperidol and torsades de pointes. Psychosomatics 36:541–549, 1995

Hurtig HI, Trojanowski JQ, Galvin J, et al: Alpha-synuclein cortical Lewy bodies correlate with dementia in Parkinson's disease. Neurology 54:1916–1921, 2000

Hy LX, Keller DM: Prevalence of AD among whites: a summary by levels of severity. Neurology 55:198–204, 2000

Ikarashi Y, Takahashi A, Ishimaur H, et al: Regulation of dopamine D1 and D2 receptors on striatal acetylcholine release in rats. Brain Res Bull 43:107–115, 1997

Inouye SK: Delirium in hospitalized older patients. Acute Hospital Care 14:745–764, 1998

Inouye SK, Charpentier PA: Precipitating factors for delirium in hospitalized elderly persons: predictive model and interrelationship with baseline vulnerability. JAMA 275:852–857, 1996

Inouye SK, VanDyck CH, Alessi CA, et al: Clarifying confusion: the confusion assessment method: a new method for detection of delirium. Ann Intern Med 113:941–948, 1990

Inouye SK, Viscoli CM, Horwitz RI, et al: A predictive model for delirium in hospitalized elderly medical patients based on admission characteristics. Ann Intern Med 119:474–481, 1993

Inouye SK, Rushing JT, Foreman MD, et al: Does delirium contribute to poor hospital outcomes? A three-site epidemiologic study. J Gen Intern Med 13:234–242, 1998

Inouye SK, Bogardus ST, Charpentier PA, et al: A multicomponent intervention to prevent delirium in hospitalized older patients. N Engl J Med 340:669–676, 1999

Ishii K, Imamura T, Sasaki M, et al: Regional cerebral glucose metabolism in dementia with Lewy bodies and Alzheimer's disease. Neurology 51:125–130, 1998

Itil T, Fink M: Anticholinergic drug-induced delirium: experimental modification, quantitative EEG and behavioral correlations. J Nerv Ment Dis 6:492–507, 1966

Jack CR, Petersen RC, Xu YC, et al: Prediction of AD with MRI-based hippocampal volume in mild cognitive impairment. Neurology 54:1397–1403, 2000

Jellinger KA: Structural basis of dementia in neurodegenerative disorders. J Neural Transm 47 (suppl):1–29, 1996

Jeste DV, Okamoto A, Napolitano J, et al: Low incidence of persistent tardive dyskinesia in elderly patients with dementia treated with risperidone. Am J Psychiatry 157:1150–1155, 2000

Johnson JC, Gottlieb GL, Sullivan E, et al: Using DSM-III criteria to diagnose delirium in elderly general hospital medical patients. J Gerontol 45:113–116, 1990

Jorm AF, Jolley D: The incidence of dementia: a meta-analysis. Neurology 51:728–733, 1998

Kashima H, Kato M, Yoshimasu H, et al: Current trends in cognitive rehabilitation for memory disorders. Keio J Med 48:79–86, 1999

Katz IR: Diagnosis and treatment of depression in patients with Alzheimer's disease and other dementias. J Clin Psychiatry 59 (suppl 9):38–44, 1998

Katz IR, Jeste DV, Mintzer JE, et al: Comparison of risperidone and placebo for psychosis and behavioral disturbances associated with dementia: a randomized, double-blind trial. J Clin Psychiatry 60:107–115, 1999

Kaye JA: Diagnostic challenges in dementia. Neurology 51 (suppl 1):S45–S52, 1998

Keane PE, Neal H: The effect of injections of dopaminergic agonists into the caudate nucleus on the electrocorticogram of the rat. J Neurosci Res 6:237–241, 1981

Kelly KG, Zisselman M, Cutillo-Schmitter T, et al: Severity and course of delirium in medically hospitalized nursing facility residents. Am J Geriatr Psychiatry 9:72–77, 2001

Kennard MA, Bueding E, Wortis WB: Some biochemical and electroencephalographic changes in delirium tremens. Q J Stud Alcohol 6:4–14, 1945

Kirsch J, Diringer M, Borel C, et al: Brain resuscitation: medical management and innovations. Crit Care Nurs Clin North Am 1:143–154, 1989

Knopman D, Schneider L, Davis K, et al: Long-term tacrine (Cognex) treatment: effects on nursing home placement and mortality. Neurology 47:166–177, 1996

Kopelman MD: The Korsakoff syndrome. Br J Psychiatry 166:154–173, 1995

Koponen H, Hurri L, Stenback U, et al: Acute confusional states in the elderly: a radiological evaluation. Acta Psychiatr Scand 76:726–731, 1987

Koponen H, Hurri L, Stenback U, et al: Computed tomography findings in delirium. J Nerv Ment Dis 177:226–231, 1989b

Koponen H, Stenback U, Mattila E, et al: Delirium among elderly persons admitted to a psychiatric hospital: clinical course during the acute stage and one-year follow-up. Acta Psychiatr Scand 79:579–585, 1989c

Koponen H, Partanen J, Paakkonen A, et al: EEG spectral analysis in delirium. J Neurol Neurosurg Psychiatry 52:980–985, 1989d

Kornhuber J, Weller M: Psychogenicity and N-methyl-D-aspartate receptor antagonism: implications for neuroprotective pharmacology. Biol Psychiatry 41:135–144, 1997

Kosenko E, Kaminsky Y, Grau E, et al: Brain ATP depletion induced by acute ammonia intoxication in rats is mediated by activation of NMDA receptor and Na+, K+ AT-Pase. J Neurochem 63:2172–2178, 1994

Kramer JH, Duffy JM: Aphasia, apraxia, and agnosia in the diagnosis of dementia. Dementia 7:23–26, 1996

Kuzis G, Sabe L, Tiberti C, et al: Neuropsychological correlates of apathy and depression in patients with dementia. Neurology 52:1403–1407, 1999

Lanctot KL, Best TS, Mittman N, et al: Efficacy and safety of neuroleptics in behavioral disorders associated with dementia. J Clin Psychiatry 59:550–561, 1998

Lawlor BA, Aisen PS, Green C, et al: Selegiline in the treatment of behavioural disturbance in Alzheimer's disease. Int J Geriatr Psychiatry 12:319–322, 1997

LeBlanc ES, Janowsky J, Chan BKS, et al: Hormone replacement therapy and cognition: systematic review and meta-analysis. JAMA 285:1489–1499, 2001

Levin M: Delirium: a gap in psychiatric teaching. Am J Psychiatry 107:689–694, 1951

Levkoff SE, Evans DA, Liptzin B, et al: Delirium: the occurrence of and persistence of symptoms among elderly hospitalized patients. Arch Intern Med 152:334–340, 1992

Levy ML, Cummings JL: Parkinson's disease, in Psychiatric Management in Neurological Disease. Edited by Lauterbach EC. Washington, DC, American Psychiatric Press, 2000, pp 41–70

Levy ML, Cummings JL, Fairbanks LA, et al: Longitudinal assessment of symptoms of depression, agitation, and psychosis in 181 patients with Alzheimer's disease. Am J Psychiatry 153:1438–1443, 1996

Linnoila MI: Benzodiazepines and alcohol. J Psychiatr Res 24 (suppl 2):121–127, 1990

Lipowski ZJ: Transient cognitive disorders (delirium, acute confusional states) in the elderly. Am J Psychiatry 140:1426–1436, 1983

Lipowski ZJ: Delirium (acute confusional states). JAMA 258:1789–1792, 1987

Liptzin B, Levkoff SE: An empirical study of delirium subtypes. Br J Psychiatry 161:843–845, 1992

Litvan I, McKee A: Clinicopathologic case conference. J Neuropsychiatry Clin Neurosci 11:107–112, 1999

Lopez OL, Wisniewski S, Hamilton RL, et al: Predictors of progression in patients with AD and Lewy bodies. Neurology 54:1774–1779, 2000a

Lyketsos CG, Steinberg M, Schantz JT, et al: Mental and behavioral disturbances in dementia: findings from the Cache County Study on Memory in Aging. Am J Psychiatry 157:708–714, 2000b

Mace NL, Rabins PV: The 36-Hour Day: A Family Guide to Caring for Persons with Alzheimer's Disease, Related Dementing Illnesses, and Memory Loss in Later Life. Baltimore, MD, The Johns Hopkins University Press, 1981

Maekawa T, Fujii Y, Sadamitsu D, et al: Cerebral circulation and metabolism in patients with septic encephalopathy. Am J Emerg Med 9:139–143, 1991

Maldonado JL, Fernandez F, Levy JK: Acquired immunodeficiency syndrome, in Psychiatric Management in Neurological Disease. Edited by Lauterbach EC. Washington, DC, American Psychiatric Press, 2000, pp 271–295

Manly JJ, Merchant CA, Jacobs DM, et al: Endogenous estrogen levels and Alzheimer's disease among postmenopausal women. Neurology 54:833–837, 2000

Marcantonio ER, Goldman L, Mangione CM, et al: A clinical predictive rule for delirium after elective noncardiac surgery. JAMA 271:134–139, 1994

Marcantonio ER, Flacker JM, Michaels M, et al: Delirium is independently associated with poor functional recovery after hip fracture. J Am Geriatr Soc 48:618–624, 2000

Marsh L: Neuropsychiatric aspects of Parkinson's disease. Psychosomatics 41:15–23, 2000

Massie MJ, Holland J, Glass E: Delirium in terminally ill cancer patients. Am J Psychiatry 140:1048–1050, 1983

Matthew RJ, Meyer JS: Pathogenesis and natural history of transient global amnesia. Stroke 5:303–311, 1974

McCartney JR, Boland R: Understanding and managing behavioral disturbances in the ICU. J Crit Illn 8:87–97, 1993

McDaniel JS, Chung JY, Brown L, et al: Practice guideline for the treatment of patients with HIV/AIDS. Work Group on HIV/AIDS. American Psychiatric Association. Am J Psychiatry 157 (11 suppl):1–62, 2000

McKeith IG, Ballard CG, Perry RH, et al: Prospective validation on consensus criteria for the diagnosis of dementia with Lewy bodies. Neurology 54:1050–1058, 2000

Meagher DJ, Trzepacz PT: Delirium phenomenology illuminates pathophysiology, management, and course. J Geriatr Psychiatry Neurol 11:150–156, 1998

Meagher DJ, O'Hanlon D, O'Mahony E, et al: A study of environmental strategies in the study of delirium. Br J Psychiatry 168:512–515, 1996

Mega M, Cummings JL, Fiorello T, et al: The spectrum of behavioral changes in Alzheimer's disease. Neurology 46:130–135, 1996

Merchant C, Tang M-X, Albert S, et al: The influence of smoking on the risk of Alzheimer's disease. Neurology 52:1408–1412, 1999

Meyer JS, Muramatsu K, Mortel KF, et al: Prospective CT confirms differences between vascular and Alzheimer's dementia. Stroke 26:735–742, 1995

Miller PS, Richardson JS, Jyu CA, et al: Association of low serum anticholinergic levels and cognitive impairment in elderly presurgical patients. Am J Psychiatry 145:342–345, 1988

Mirenda J, Broyles G: Propofol as used for sedation in the ICU. Chest 108:539–548, 1995

Moceri VM, Kukull WA, Emanuel I, et al: Early life risk factors and the development of Alzheimer's disease. Neurology 54:415–420, 2000

Mohs RC, Cohen L: Alzheimer's Disease Assessment Scale (ADAS). Psychopharmacol Bull 24:627–628, 1988

Monette J, Galbaud du Fort G, Fung SH, et al: Evaluation of the Confusion Assessment Method (CAM) as a screening tool for delirium in the emergency room. Gen Hosp Psychiatry 23:20–25, 2001

Montine TJ, Sidell KR, Crews BC, et al: Elevated CSF prostaglandin E2 levels in patients with probable AD. Neurology 53:1495–1498, 1999

Moroney JT, Bagiella E, Tatemichi TK, et al: Dementia after stroke increases the risk of long term stroke recurrence. Neurology 48:1317–1325, 1997

Morris HR, Lees A, Wood NW: Neurofibrillary tangle parkinsonian disorders—tau pathology and tau genetics. Mov Disord 14:731–736, 1999

Mussi C, Ferrari R, Ascari S, et al: Importance of serum anticholinergic activity in the assessment of elderly patients with delirium. J Geriatr Psychiatry Neurol 12:82–86, 1999

Neary D, Snowden JS, Gustafson L, et al: Frontotemporal lobar degeneration: a consensus on clinical diagnostic criteria. Neurology 51:1546–1554, 1998

Neumann PJ, Hermann RC, Kuntz KM, et al: Cost-effectiveness of donepezil in the treatment of mild or moderate Alzheimer's disease. Neurology 52:1138–1145, 1999

Nicholas LM, Lindsey BA: Delirium presenting with symptoms of depression. Psychosomatics 36:471–479, 1995

Obrist WD: Electroencephalographic changes in normal aging and dementia, in Brain Function in Old Age. Edited by Hoffmeister F, Mhuller C. New York, Springer-Verlag, 1979, pp 102–111

O'Keeffe ST: Delirium in the elderly. Age Ageing 28:5–8, 1999

O'Keeffe ST, Lavan J: The prognostic significance of delirium in older hospital patients. J Am Geriatr Soc 45:174–178, 1997

Olichney JM, Galasko D, Salmon DO, et al: Cognitive decline is faster in Lewy body variant than in Alzheimer's disease. Neurology 51:351–357, 1998

Ongini E, Caporali MG, Massotti M: Stimulation of dopamine D1 receptors by SKF 38393 induces EEG desynchronization and behavioral arousal. Life Sci 37:2327–2333, 1985

Ott A, Stolk RP, van Harskamp F, et al: Diabetes mellitus and the risk of dementia: the Rotterdam study. Neurology 53:1937–1942, 1999

Parnetti L: Therapeutic options in dementia. J Neurol 247:163–168, 2000

Passik SD, Cooper M: Complicated delirium in a cancer patient successfully treated with olanzapine. J Pain Symptom Manage 17:219–223, 1999

Patterson CJS, Gauthier S, Bergman H, et al: The recognition, assessment, and management of dementing disorders: conclusions form the Canadian Consensus Conference on Dementia. Can Med Assoc J 160 (suppl):S1–S14, 1999

Paulsen JS, Salmon DP, Monsch AU, et al: Discrimination of cortical from subcortical dementias on the basis of memory and problem-solving tests. J Clin Psychol 51:48–58, 1995a

Paulsen JS, Butters N, Sadek JR, et al: Distinct cognitive profiles of cortical and subcortical dementia in advanced illness. Neurology 45:951–956, 1995b

Paulsen JS, Salmon DP, Thal LJ, et al: Incidence of and risk factors for hallucinations and delusions in patients with probable AD. Neurology 54:1965–1971, 2000

Perry RJ, Hodges JR: Differentiating frontal and temporal variant frontotemporal dementia from Alzheimer's disease. Neurology 54:2277–2284, 2000

Petersen RC, Jack CR, Xu Y-C, et al: Memory and MRI-based hippocampal volumes in aging and AD. Neurology 54:581–587, 2000

Petracca G, Teson A, Chemerinski E, et al: A double-blind placebo-controlled study of clomipramine in depressed patients with Alzheimer's disease. J Neuropsychiatry Clin Neurosci 8:270–275, 1996

Pietrini P, Furey ML, Alexander GE, et al: Association between brain functional failure and dementia severity in Alzheimer's disease: resting versus stimulation PET study. Am J Psychiatry 156:470–473, 1999

Plassman BL, Havlik RJ, Stefens DC, et al: Documented head injury in early adulthood and risk of Alzheimer's disease and other dementias. Neurology 55:2258–2266, 2000

Platt MM, Breitbart W, Smith M, et al: Efficacy of neuroleptics for hypoactive delirium. J Neuropsychiatry 6:66, 1994

Pompei P, Foreman M, Rudberg MA, et al: Delirium in hospitalized older persons: outcomes and predictors. J Am Geriatr Soc 42:809–815, 1994

Porter RJ, Lunn BS, Walker LLM, et al: Cognitive deficit induced by acute tryptophan depletion in patients with Alzheimer's disease. Am J Psychiatry 157:638–640, 2000

Pro JD, Wells CE: The use of the electroencephalogram in the diagnosis of delirium. Diseases of the Nervous System 38:804–808, 1977

Pulsinelli WA, Duffy TE: Regional energy balance in rat brain after transient forebrain ischemia. J Neurochem 40:1500–1503, 1983

Rabins PV: Alzheimer's disease management. J Clin Psychiatry 59 (suppl 13):36–38, 1998

Rabins PV, Blacker D, Bland A, et al: Practice guideline for the treatment of patients with Alzheimer's disease and other dementias of late life. American Psychiatric Association. Am J Psychiatry 154 (suppl): 1–39, 1997

Rahkonen T, Luukkainen-Markkula R, Paanila S, et al: Delirium episode as a sign of undetected dementia among community dwelling elderly subjects: a 2 year follow up study. J Neurol Neurosurg Psychiatry 69:519–521, 2000

Ranen NG: Huntington's disease, in Psychiatric Management in Neurological Disease. Edited by Lauterbach EC. Washington, DC, American Psychiatric Press, 2000, pp 71–92

Rao V, Lyketsos CG: Delusions in Alzheimer's disease: a review. J Neuropsychiatry Clin Neurosci 10:373–382, 1998

Raskind MA: The clinical interface of depression and dementia. J Clin Psychiatry 59 (suppl 10):9–12, 1998

Raskind MA, Peskind ER, Wessel T, et al: Galantamine in AD: a 6-month randomized, placebo controlled trial with a 6-month extension. The Galantamine USA-1 Study Group. Neurology 54:2261–2268, 2000

Rebeck GW, Hyman BT: Apolipoprotein E and Alzheimer disease, in Alzheimer Disease, 2nd Edition. Edited by Terry RD, Katzman R, Bick KL, et al. Philadelphia, PA, Lippincott Williams & Wilkins, 1999, pp 339–346

Reyes RL, Bhattacharyya AK, Heller D: Traumatic head injury: restlessness and agitation as prognosticators of physical and psychological improvement in patients. Arch Phys Med Rehabil 62:20–23, 1981

Riker RR, Fraser GL, Cox PM: Continuous infusion of haloperidol controls agitation in critically ill patients. Crit Care Med 22: 433–440, 1994

Ringman JM, Cummings JL: Metrifonate: update on a new antidementia agent. J Clin Psychiatry 60:776–782, 1999

Robinson RG: The Clinical Neuropsychiatry of Stroke: Cognitive, Behavioral, and Emotional Disorders Following Vascular Brain Injury. New York, Cambridge University Press, 1998

Rockwood K: Acute confusion in elderly medical patients. J Am Geriatr Soc 37:150–154, 1989

Rockwood K: The occurrence and duration of symptoms in elderly patients with delirium. J Gerontol 48:M162–M166, 1993

Rockwood K, Cosway S, Stolee P, et al: Increasing the recognition of delirium in elderly patients. J Am Geriatr Soc 42: 252–256, 1994

Rogers MP, Liang MH, Daltroy LH, et al: Delirium after elective orthopedic surgery: risk factors and natural history. Int J Psychiatry Med 19:109–121, 1989

Rogers SL, Friedhoff LT: Long-term efficacy and safety of donepezil in the treatment of Alzheimer's disease: an interim analysis of the results of a US multicentre open label extension study. Eur Neuropsychopharmacol 8:67–75, 1998

Rogers SL, Farlow MR, Doody RS, et al: A 24-week, double-blind, placebo-controlled trial of donepezil in patients with Alzheimer's disease. Neurology 50:136–145, 1998

Romano J, Engel GL: Delirium, part 1: electroencephalographic data. Archives of Neurology and Psychiatry 51:356–377, 1944

Rosen WG, Mohs RC, Davis KL: A new rating scale for Alzheimer's disease. Am J Psychiatry 141:1356–1364, 1984

Rosenberg J, Kehlet H: Postoperative mental confusion-association with postoperative hypoxemia. Surgery 114:76–81, 1993

Rosenblatt A, Leroi I: Neuropsychiatry of Huntington's disease and other basal ganglia disorders. Psychosomatics 41:24–30, 2000

Ross CA, Peyser CE, Shapiro I, et al: Delirium: phenomenologic and etiologic subtypes. Int Psychogeriatr 3:135–147, 1991

Ross GW, Petrovich H, White LR, et al: Characterization of risk factors for vascular dementia: the Honolulu-Asia Aging Study. Neurology 53:337–343, 1999

Roth T, Roehrs R, Wittig R, et al: Benzodiazepines and memory. Br J Clin Pharmacol 18:45–49, 1984

Sano M, Ernesto C, Thomas RG, et al: A controlled trial of selegiline, alpha-tocopherol, or both as treatment for Alzheimer's disease. The Alzheimer's Disease Cooperative Study. N Engl J Med 336: 1216–1222, 1997

Scharf MB, Saskin P, Fletcher K: Benzodiazepine-induced amnesia: clinical laboratory findings. J Clin Psychiatry Monogr 5:14–17, 1987

Scheltens P: Early diagnosis of dementia: neuroimaging. J Neurol 246:16–20, 1999

Schenker S, McCandless DW, Brophy E, et al: Studies on intracerebral toxicity of ammonia. J Clin Invest 46:838–848, 1967

Schor JD, Levkoff SE, Lipsitz LA, et al: Risk factors for delirium in hospitalized elderly. JAMA 267:827–831, 1992

Schwid SR, Weinstein A, Wishart HA, et al: Multiple sclerosis, in Psychiatric Management in Neurological Disease. Edited by Lauterbach EC. Washington, DC, American Psychiatric Press, 2000, pp 249–270

Settle EC, Ayd FJ: Haloperidol: a quarter century of experience. J Clin Psychiatry 44: 440–448, 1983

Sharma ND, Rosman HS, Padhi D, et al: Torsades de pointes associated with intravenous haloperidol in critically ill patients. Am J Cardiol 81:238–240, 1998

Shuping JR, Rollinson RD, Toole JF: Transient global amnesia. Ann Neurol 7:281–285, 1980

Sipahimalani A, Masand PS: Use of risperidone in delirium: case reports. Ann Clin Psychiatry 9:105–107, 1997

Sipahimalani A, Masand PS: Olanzapine in the treatment of delirium. Psychosomatics 39:422–430, 1998

Small GW: Differential diagnosis and early detection of dementia. Am J Geriatr Psychiatry 6:S26–S33, 1998a

Small GW: The pathogenesis of Alzheimer's disease. J Clin Psychiatry 95 (suppl 9):7–14, 1998b

Small GW, Leiter F: Neuroimaging for diagnosis of dementia. J Clin Psychiatry 59 (suppl 11):4–7, 1998

Smith CD, Snowdon DA, Wang H, et al: White matter volumes and periventricular white matter hyperintensities in aging and dementia. Neurology 54:838–842, 2000

Smits HA, Boven LA, Pereira CF, et al: Role of macrophage activation in the pathogenesis of Alzheimer's disease and human immunodeficiency virus type I–associated dementia. Eur J Clin Invest 30:526–535, 2000

Soares JC, Gershon S: THA: historical aspects, review of pharmacological properties and therapeutic effects. Dementia 6:225–234, 1995

Spencer CM, Noble S: Rivastigmine: a review of its use in Alzheimer's disease. Drugs Aging 13:391–411, 1998

Stahl SM: The new cholinesterase inhibitors for Alzheimer's disease, part I: their similarities are different. J Clin Psychiatry 61: 710–711, 2000

Stiefel F, Holland J: Delirium in cancer patients. Int Psychogeriatr 3:333–336, 1991

Stern Y, Albert S, Tang M-X, Tsai W-Y: Rate of memory decline in AD is related to education and occupation: cognitive reserve? Neurology 53:1942–1947, 1999

Swenson JR, Erman M, Labell J, et al: Extrapyramidal reactions: neuropsychiatric mimics in patients with AIDS. Gen Hosp Psychiatry 11:248–253, 1989

Tager FA, Fallon BA: Psychiatric and cognitive features of Lyme disease. Psychiatr Ann 31:173–181, 2001

Taylor P: Development of acetylcholinesterase inhibitors in the therapy of Alzheimer's disease. Neurology 51 (suppl 1):S30–S35, 1998

Tetewsky SJ, Duffy CJ: Visual loss and getting lost in Alzheimer's disease. Neurology 52:958–965, 1999

Thomas RI, Cameron DJ, Fahs MC: A prospective study of delirium and prolonged hospital stay. Arch Gen Psychiatry 45: 937–940, 1988

Tiraboschi P, Hansen LA, Alford M, et al: Cholinergic dysfunction in diseases with Lewy bodies. Neurology 54:407–411, 2000

Tolbert SR, Fuller MA: Selegiline in treatment of behavioral and cognitive symptoms of Alzheimer disease. Ann Pharmacother 30: 1122–1129, 1996

Torres R, Mittal D, Kennedy R: Use of quetiapine in delirium: case reports. Psychosomatics 42:347–349, 2001

Trzepacz PT: The neuropathogenesis of delirium: a need to focus our research. Psychosomatics 35:374–391, 1994

Trzepacz PT: Is there a final common neural pathway in delirium? Focus on acetylcholine and dopamine. Seminars in Clinical Neuropsychiatry 5:132–148, 2000

Trzepacz PT, Wise MG: Neuropsychiatric aspects of delirium, in The American Psychiatric Press Textbook of Neuropsychiatry, 3rd Edition. Edited by Yudofsky SC, Hales RE. Washington, DC, American Psychiatric Press, 1997, pp 447–470

Trzepacz PT, Maue FR, Coffman G, et al: Neuropsychiatric assessment of liver transplantation candidates: delirium and other psychiatric disorders. Int J Psychiatry Med 7:101–111, 1986

Trzepacz PT, Brenner RP, Coffman G, et al: Delirium in liver transplantation candidates: discriminant analysis of multiple test variables. Biol Psychiatry 24:3–14, 1988a

Trzepacz PT, Baker RW, Greenhouse J: A symptom rating scale for delirium. Psychiatry Res 23:89–97, 1988b

Trzepacz PT, Leavitt M, Congioli K: An animal model for delirium. Psychosomatics 33:404–414, 1992

Trzepacz PT, Ho V, Mallavarapu H: Cholinergic delirium and neurotoxicity associated with tacrine for Alzheimer's dementia. Psychosomatics 37:299–301, 1996

Trzepacz PT, Mulsant BH, Amanda Dew M, et al: Is delirium different when it occurs in dementia? A study using the delirium rating scale. J Neuropsychiatry Clin Neurosci 10:199–204, 1998

Trzepacz PT, Mittal D, Torres R, et al: Validation of the Delirium Rating Scale—Revised—98: comparison with the delirium rating scale and cognitive test for delirium. J Neuropsychiatry Clin Neurosci 13: 229–242, 2001

Tsai L, Tsuang MT: The Mini-Mental State Test and computerized tomography. Am J Psychiatry 136:436–439, 1979

Tschanz JT, Welsh-Bohmer KA, Skoog I, et al: Dementia diagnosis from clinical and neuropsychological data compared: the Cache County study. Neurology 54: 1290–1296, 2000

Tune LE: Postoperative delirium. Int Psychogeriatr 3:325–332, 1991

Tune LE, Folstein MF: Post-operative delirium. Adv Psychosom Med 15:51–68, 1986

Tune LE, Sunderland T: New cholinergic therapies: treatment tools for the psychiatrist. J Clin Psychiatry 59 (suppl 13):31–35, 1998

Tune LE, Carr S, Hoag E, et al: Anticholinergic effects of drugs commonly prescribed for the elderly: potential means for assessing risk of delirium. Am J Psychiatry 149: 1393–1394, 1992

Weiner MF, Risser RC, Cullum M, et al: Alzheimer's disease and its Lewy body variant: a clinical analysis of postmortem verified cases. Am J Psychiatry 153:1269–1273, 1996

Weiner M, Powe NR, Weller WE, et al: Alzheimer's disease under managed care: implications from Medicare utilization and expenditure patterns. J Am Geriatr Soc 46:762–770, 1998

Weiner MF, Martin-Cook K, Foster BM, et al: Effects of donepezil on emotional/behavioral symptoms in Alzheimer's disease patients. J Clin Psychiatry 61:487–492, 2000

Weissman C, Kemper M, Damask M, et al: Effect of routine intensive care interactions on metabolic rate. Chest 86:815–818, 1984

Whalley LJ, Starr JM, Athawes R, et al: Childhood mental ability and dementia. Neurology 55:1455–1459, 2000

Whitehouse PJ: The cholinergic deficit in Alzheimer's disease. J Clin Psychiatry 59 (suppl 13):19–22, 1998

Williams-Russo P, Urquhart BL, Sharrock NE, et al: Post-operative delirium: predictors and prognosis in elderly orthopedic patients. J Am Geriatr Soc 40:759–767, 1992

Wilson LM: Intensive care delirium: the effect of outside deprivation in a windowless unit. Arch Intern Med 130:225–226, 1972

Zayas EM, Grossberg GT: The treatment of psychosis in late life. J Clin Psychiatry 59 (suppl):5–10, 1998

Zee-Cheng CS, Mueller CE, Siefert CF, et al: Haloperidol and torsades de pointes (letter). Ann Intern Med 102:418, 1985

Zerr I, Schultz-Schaeffer WJ, Giese A, et al: Current clinical diagnosis in Creutzfeldt-Jakob disease: identification of uncommon variants. Ann Neurol 48:323–329, 2000

Zou Y, Cole MG, Primeau FJ, et al: Detection and diagnosis of delirium in the elderly: psychiatric diagnosis, confusion assessment method, or consensus diagnosis? Int Psychogeriatr 10:303–308, 1998

Zubenko GS, Tepley I, Winwood E, et al: Prospective study of increased platelet membrane fluidity as a risk factor for Alzheimer's disease: results at 5 years. Am J Psychiatry 153:420–423, 1996

Zubenko GS, Hughes HB, Stiffler JS: Neurobiological correlates of a putative risk allele for Alzheimer's disease on chromosome 12q. Neurology 52:725–732, 1999

Substance Use Disorders

Avram H. Mack, M.D.

John E. Franklin Jr., M.D., M.Sc.

Richard J. Frances, M.D.

In the United States, substance use disorders constitute a tremendous medical and social challenge: 13.8% of all Americans will have an alcohol-related substance use disorder in their lifetimes, an estimated 14.8 million Americans were current users of illicit drugs in 1999, and the monetary cost to the nation, including the related aspects of crime, absenteeism, and treatment, is estimated to be greater than $275 billion annually. Health care providers are constantly faced with treatment choices and options that are critical to the care of patients with substance use disorders. Substance use disorders are significant conditions that can be understood via the biopsychosocial model.

The Disease Model of Addiction

In current mainstream models, three (probably intertwined) aspects of the addictions are seen as central to their understanding as diseases: 1) addiction is the compulsion to use the substance, 2) addiction is a "brain disease," and 3) addiction is a chronic medical disorder.

That addiction is a "compulsion" means that the individual uses the substance at all costs, even in the face of severe negative consequences. The evidence that there is a biological component to addiction is growing. There is a basis for a genetic vulnerability to abuse of particular substances; there are biological markers in such vulnerable persons. Furthermore, research is focusing on the long-term changes in synaptic architecture and alterations in neurotransmitter physiology that may form the basis of the position that the brain of the addicted patient is different as a result of his or her excessive use—a difference that creates and maintains the compulsion to use (Leshner 1997).

Another development is the conceptualization of addiction as a chronic medical disease. Addictions have chronic courses comparable with other medical disorders such as diabetes mellitus, arthritis, and asthma—diseases that we can treat but perhaps never entirely cure, and in which relapses are to be expected, especially as they relate to choices patients make. For example, the former cocaine abuser who relapses after entering the environment in which he previously used the drug is analogous to the child with asthma who walks into a smoky room and develops an attack (O'Brien and McLellan 1996).

Neurobiology of the Addictions: Clinical Implications of Research Findings

Advances in cellular and molecular biology and in psychiatry and the addictions have produced increasing evidence that craving and addiction to virtually all substances of abuse are related to the dopaminergic systems in the brain—especially the mesolimbic reward system and the areas to which it projects: the limbic system and the orbitofrontal cortex (Leshner and Koob 1999). This even has been seen in the case of cannabinoids (Diana et al. 1998), and it may be the result not simply of homeostatic adaptations of neurons but even of neural plasticity and synaptic rearrangement that follow from activation of particular signal transduction pathways between stimulus and gene expression. Thus, addiction is not only a degenerative disease or a lesion but also a learned process in which long-term memory occurs (pathologically) at the molecular level (O'Brien and McLellan 1996). A full discussion of the burgeoning science of addiction is beyond the scope of this clinically oriented chapter; the reader is referred to more extensive manuscripts on this topic (Kreek 2000; Volkow and Fowler 2000; Volkow et al. 2001).

General Epidemiology of Substance-Related Use Disorders

Substance-related use disorders are likely the most prevalent of all types of medical and mental disorders, and they cost society greatly. There are a number of studies from which most of the data on substance use disorders have been gathered: the Drug Abuse Warning Network (DAWN; Office of Applied Studies 2000), which provides ongoing surveillance data; the Monitoring the Future study, an ongoing study of substance abuse among American high school and college students and young adults (Johnston et al. 2003); the National Household Survey (NHS; Office of Applied Studies 2002); the Epidemiologic Catchment Area study (ECA; Regier et al. 1990); and the National Comorbidity Survey (NCS; Kessler et al. 1997).

Medical and psychiatric problems associated with substance use disorders produce morbidity and mortality that hamper efforts to treat these disorders. Such problems include the effects of intoxication, overdose, and withdrawal and the consequences of chronic use: malnutrition, poor self-care, injection of unknown substances, cognitive disorder, endocarditis, and HIV among intravenous drug users.

In 2001, 15.9 million Americans were users of illicit drugs in the preceding 30 days, an increase from 14.8 million in 1999 (Office of Applied Studies 2002). An estimated 16.6 million Americans met diagnostic criteria for dependence on illicit drugs in 2001 (Office of Applied Studies 2002). Between 1997 and 1998, drug abuse deaths reported to DAWN increased from 9,565 to 10,091 (Office of Applied Studies 2000). Use varies by age to a great degree, and the rates of use are changing. Use among youths is discussed later in the section on treatment in children and adolescents.

Measures of the monetary cost of the addictions include per capita consumption, lifetime and point prevalence, morbidity and mortality, fetal effects of drugs, health care costs, and total cost of lost work time. The actual monetary cost to the United States is estimated to be greater than $275 billion annually, which includes the related aspects of crime, absenteeism, and treatment. Also, 30%–55% of the mentally ill have a substance use disorder, a circumstance that greatly multiplies the cost of treating primary mental illness.

Alcohol

At least 9 million Americans are alcohol dependent, and another 6 million abuse alcohol. The ECA study concluded that 13.8% of Americans will have an alcohol-related substance use disorder at some time in their lives. The current annual costs attributed to alcohol abuse are $166.5 billion, almost double the annual cost of the late 1980s (Harwood et al. 1998). The rate of frequent drinking among pregnant women, even when controlled for social characteristics, was approximately 4 times higher in 1995 than in 1991 (3.5% in 1995 and 0.8% in 1991) (Centers for Disease Control and Prevention 1997a). Although consumption of alcoholic beverages is illegal for those under 21 years of age, 10.1 million current drinkers were ages 12–20 years in 2001 (Office of Applied Studies 2002). Of this group, the majority engaged in binge drinking, including many who would also be classified as heavy drinkers.

Morbidity and mortality secondary to alcohol depend on the culture and nationality of the user. In America, the average person over age 14 years consumes 2.77 gallons of absolute alcohol annually, an amount less than in Russia, France, Scandinavia, and Ireland but more than in Islamic and Mediterranean cultures or in China. In the United States, approximately 10% of persons who drink consume half of all the alcohol sold. With suicide ranking as the eighth leading cause of death in 1998 and liver disease the

tenth (Murphy 2000), the estimate that 100,000 deaths per year are alcohol related is of importance. Alcoholism is the leading risk factor for cirrhosis. About 25% of general hospital admissions involve problems related to chronic alcohol use (e.g., cirrhosis, cardiomyopathy) or withdrawal (e.g., seizures, pneumonia, liver failure, subdural hematomas).

There is a high association between alcohol and violence. The suicide rate in persons with alcoholism is about 5%–6%. Nearly 50% of violent deaths in the United States are linked with alcohol (Institute of Medicine 1999), and in Eastern European nations alcohol is involved in 33% of all deaths in the 15- to 29-year age group (World Health Organization 2001). In the United States the proportion of traffic fatalities that were alcohol related was 38.5% in 1997 (Centers for Disease Control and Prevention 1999a).

Sedatives, Hypnotics, and Anxiolytics

Since 1976 there has been a decline in the abuse of benzodiazepines and other sedative-hypnotics. Abuse of the substances in this category is often iatrogenically induced. Barbiturate overdoses have decreased with the declining popularity of barbiturate prescription.

Opioids

An estimated 149,000 persons used heroin for the first time in 1999. Between 1994 and 1999, the rate of initiation for youths was at its highest level since the early 1970s (Office of Applied Studies 2002). The estimated number of current heroin users was 68,000 in 1993; 117,000 in 1994; 196,000 in 1995; 216,000 in 1996; 325,000 in 1997; 130,000 in 1998; 200,000 in 1999; 130,000 in 2000; and 123,000 in 2001 (Office of Applied Studies 2002). Lifetime heroin prevalence estimates have ranged from 2.3 million in 1979 to 1.7 million in 1992, 2 million in 1997, and 2.4 million in 1998 (Office of Applied Studies 2002). The ECA study showed that opioid use was greater in males, with a male:female ratio of between 3:1 and 4:1. Heroin abuse is usually a problem in urban males and in the 18- to 25-year-old group. A higher incidence of nonmedical use of opioids other than heroin (e.g., "painkillers") is found among whites (12% versus 7% for minorities). The rate of heroin abuse among minorities is twice as high as that in the general population—a figure that may be skewed because whites account for fewer admissions to public facilities and because there may be many white middle-class addicts who do not respond to surveys. Greater psychopathology is found in cultural groups in which heroin is less endemic.

Cocaine

Cocaine use reached a peak of 5.7 million persons (3.0% of the population) in 1985. In 2001 an estimated 1.7 million (0.7%) Americans ages 12 and older were current users of cocaine and 406,000 (0.2%) were current users of crack (Office of Applied Studies 2002). Cocaine use is inversely related to education, and it is highest among the unemployed. More men than women use cocaine.

Amphetamines

The estimated number of Americans who have tried methamphetamine is 4.7 million (Office of Applied Studies 2002). A substantial increase in use occurred in the 1990s, especially in California. Amphetamine-related admissions to publicly funded treatment programs tripled from 1992 to 1997 (Office of Applied Studies 2002). Methamphetamine-related emergency department episodes more than tri-

pled from 1991 to 1994 (Centers for Disease Control and Prevention 1995). From 1991 to 1994, the number of methamphetamine-related deaths nearly tripled, and most were in persons who were 26–44 years old (66%), male (80%), and white (80%). Nearly all deaths involved at least one other drug (Office of Applied Studies 2000).

Phencyclidine and Ketamine

PCP abuse is epidemic in certain areas of the United States and is often associated with violent and bizarre behavior. It reached a nadir in the 1980s but has become more popular again.

Ketamine has quickly become a major substance of abuse, especially among youth and young adults. It was first added to the Monitoring the Future survey in 2000, when the prevalence of ketamine abuse was 1.6%, 2.1%, and 2.5% in grades 8, 10, and 12, respectively (Johnston et al. 2003).

Hallucinogens

In 2001 there were an estimated 1.3 million current hallucinogen users (Office of Applied Studies 2002). Lysergic acid diethylamide (LSD) is once again becoming popular in some high school communities. A steady flow of new ("designer") phenylalkylamine derivatives has appeared, including the ring-substituted amphetamines such as MDA, MDMA (old and new "Ecstasy"), and MDEA.

MDMA is mainly used among youth and young adults. Between 1999 and 2000, the prevalence of MDMA use increased by 3.1%, 5.4%, and 8.2% among students in grades 8, 10, and 12, respectively. The perceived availability of MDMA has risen dramatically, whereas the perception of risk or disapproval has changed little (Johnston et al. 2003). Among adults in 2001, an estimated 8.1

million (3.6%) Americans ages 12 years or older had tried MDMA, an increase over the rate in 2000. The estimated number of current adult users was 786,000 (0.3%) (Office of Applied Studies 2002).

Cannabis

Worldwide, cannabis may be the most widely abused illicit substance of all; in the United States it is used by 76% of all illicit drug users. The number of individuals using marijuana for the first time in the United States was estimated at 2.3 million in 1999. Frequent users were estimated to number 6.8 million in 1998, significantly more than in 1995 (5.3 million) (Office of Applied Studies 2002). Among females, the age at first use is declining even as the prevalence of secondary problems is rising (Greenfield and O'Leary 1999). The prevalence of marijuana use in youth peaked in 1979 at 14.2%, declined to 3.4% in 1992, then climbed to 8.2% in 1995 and has fluctuated near that point since then (7.1 in 1996, 9.4% in 1997, and 8.3% in 1998) (Office of Applied Studies 2002).

Nicotine

Tobacco is the leading cause of preventable morbidity and mortality in the United States. Approximately 430,000 deaths annually (Centers for Disease Control and Prevention 1999b) are attributable to tobacco use. The prevalence of use is increasing: in 1999 an estimated 30.2% of Americans (66.8 million) used cigarettes, an increase from the number in 1998 (27.7%, 60 million).

Tobacco use is tied to race and ethnicity: prevalence of use in 1999 was significantly higher among American Indians/Alaska Natives (43.1%) than among most other groups, including non-Hispanic blacks (26.6%), non-Hispanic whites (31.9%), Hispanics (24.4%), and Asians/Pacific Islanders (18.6%). Use is higher among persons living below the poverty level (33.3%) than among those at or above that level (24.6%). Although cigarette use is decreasing in men, it has increased in women.

Of the 2.1 million Americans who began smoking cigarettes in 1997, more than 50% were younger than age 18 years (Office of Applied Studies 2002). In a 1999 Centers for Disease Control and Prevention survey, 70.4% of all students reported having smoked at least once in their life (Centers for Disease Control and Prevention 2000). In 1999 youths ages 12–17 who currently smoked cigarettes were 7.3 times more likely to use illicit drugs and 16 times more likely to drink heavily than were their nonsmoking peers.

Inhalants

Inhalant use stabilized in 1996 after increasing for 4 years, according to the National High School Senior and Young Adult Survey (Johnston et al. 1997). Fortunately, annual prevalence has declined in grades 8 through 12 as the view that these agents are dangerous has concurrently increased. Inhalants tend to be used by socioeconomically deprived males 13–15 years old and in certain subcultures (e.g., American and Mexican Indians). Inhalant intoxication has been linked with aggressive, disruptive, antisocial behavior as well as with poor performance in school, increased family disruption, and abuse of other drugs. Amyl nitrate abuse was popular in the 1970s in the homosexual population. Nitrous oxide abuse may be prevalent among certain health care workers.

Polysubstance Problems

Polysubstance abuse—with combined use of alcohol, heroin, cocaine, methadone, and/or tobacco—is on the rise. In the ECA study, 30% of alcoholic individuals also met criteria for another substance use disorder. The ECA study found that the most common comorbid psychiatric condition was another substance use disorder: nicotine dependence.

Use of combinations of substances has been especially noted in young and female patients. Teenagers tend to progress from alcohol and tobacco use to marijuana use and use of barbiturates, codeine, or other opioids before abusing heroin. Deaths related to overdose are more commonly associated with combinations of alcohol, depressants, and heroin than with cocaine, which has recently received greater public attention. Of note, treatment for one substance usually has the effect of lowering the use of others (e.g., a methadone maintenance program reduces comorbid cocaine abuse).

Substance-Related Disorders: DSM-IV-TR Definitions and Diagnostic Categories

In DSM-IV (American Psychiatric Association 1994) and DSM-IV-TR (American Psychiatric Association 2000), substance-related disorders are divided into two groups. The *substance use disorders* include substance dependence and substance abuse, and the *substance-induced disorders* include substance intoxication and substance withdrawal as well as other cognitive or psychiatric symptoms that are judged to be a direct physiological consequence of a substance.

DSM-IV-TR provides generic definitions of *dependence, abuse, intoxication,* and *withdrawal,* as well as various specific definitions for substance-induced syndromes. The reader is referred to DSM-

IV-TR for full and detailed definitions of each diagnostic category. This section discusses particular issues in the definition of the more complex conditions.

The following general points are important when considering a DSM-IV-TR substance-related disorder diagnosis:

1. In DSM-IV-TR, the term *substance* can refer to a drug of abuse, a medication, or a toxin, and it need not be limited to those that are "psychoactive."
2. "Organic" is a term absent from DSM-IV-TR. The conditions previously designated "substance-induced organic mental disorders" are now classified in the substance use disorders section. DSM-IV-TR does distinguish substance-induced *mental* disorders from substance-induced disorders that are due to a general medical condition and those that have no known etiology.
3. DSM-IV-TR diagnoses require the presence of "clinically significant distress and impairment in social, occupational, or other important areas of functioning."
4. DSM-IV-TR diagnoses require that the symptoms not be due to a general medical condition and not be better accounted for by another mental disorder.

Substance Use Disorders

Substance Dependence

Dependence is a state of cognitive, behavioral, and physiological features that, together, signify continued use despite significant substance-related problems. It is a pattern of repeated self-administration that can result in tolerance, withdrawal, and compulsive drug-taking behavior. In DSM-IV-TR a patient must exhibit at least 3 behaviors from a 7-item, polythetic criteria set over a 12-month period (Table 4–1). Although neither tolerance nor withdrawal is necessary or sufficient

---

TABLE 4–1. DSM-IV-TR diagnostic criteria for substance dependence

A maladaptive pattern of substance use, leading to clinically significant impairment or distress, as manifested by three (or more) of the following, occurring at any time in the same 12-month period:

(1) tolerance, as defined by either of the following:
    (a) a need for markedly increased amounts of the substance to achieve intoxication or desired effect
    (b) markedly diminished effect with continued use of the same amount of the substance
(2) withdrawal, as manifested by either of the following:
    (a) the characteristic withdrawal syndrome for the substance (refer to Criteria A and B of the criteria sets for withdrawal from the specific substances)
    (b) the same (or a closely related) substance is taken to relieve or avoid withdrawal symptoms
(3) the substance is often taken in larger amounts or over a longer period than was intended
(4) there is a persistent desire or unsuccessful efforts to cut down or control substance use
(5) a great deal of time is spent in activities necessary to obtain the substance (e.g., visiting multiple doctors or driving long distances), use the substance (e.g., chain-smoking), or recover from its effects
(6) important social, occupational, or recreational activities are given up or reduced because of substance use
(7) the substance use is continued despite knowledge of having a persistent or recurrent physical or psychological problem that is likely to have been caused or exacerbated by the substance (e.g., current cocaine use despite recognition of cocaine-induced depression, or continued drinking despite recognition that an ulcer was made worse by alcohol consumption)

Specify if:
    With Physiological Dependence: evidence of tolerance or withdrawal (i.e., either Item 1 or 2 is present)
    Without Physiological Dependence: no evidence of tolerance or withdrawal (i.e., neither Item 1 nor 2 is present)

Course specifiers:
    Early Full Remission
    Early Partial Remission
    Sustained Full Remission
    Sustained Partial Remission
    On Agonist Therapy
    In a Controlled Environment

---

for a diagnosis of substance dependence, a past history of tolerance or withdrawal is usually associated with a more severe clinical course. *Tolerance*—the need for greatly increased amounts of a substance to produce a desired effect or a greatly diminished effect with constant use of the same amount of the substance—may be difficult to discern by history when the substance used is of unknown purity. In such situations, quantitative laboratory tests may help. *Withdrawal* occurs when blood or tissue concentrations of a substance decline in an individual who had maintained prolonged heavy use of the substance. In this state, the person will likely take the substance to relieve or to avoid unpleasant withdrawal symptoms.

According to DSM-IV-TR, dependence can be further specified as mild, moderate, or severe, and remission may be noted to be early partial, early full, sustained full, or sustained partial. The presence or absence of tolerance or withdrawal, other signs of

TABLE 4–2.   DSM-IV-TR diagnostic
criteria for substance abuse

A. A maladaptive pattern of substance use
   leading to clinically significant impairment
   or distress, as manifested by one (or more)
   of the following, occurring within a
   12-month period:
   (1) recurrent substance use resulting in a
       failure to fulfill major role obligations
       at work, school, or home (e.g., repeated
       absences or poor work performance
       related to substance use; substance-
       related absences, suspensions, or
       expulsions from school; neglect of
       children or household)
   (2) recurrent substance use in situations
       in which it is physically hazardous
       (e.g., driving an automobile or operat-
       ing a machine when impaired by sub-
       stance use)
   (3) recurrent substance-related legal
       problems (e.g., arrests for substance-
       related disorderly conduct)
   (4) continued substance use despite hav-
       ing persistent or recurrent social or
       interpersonal problems caused or
       exacerbated by the effects of the sub-
       stance (e.g., arguments with spouse
       about consequences of intoxication,
       physical fights)
B. The symptoms have never met the criteria
   for substance dependence for this class of
   substance.

TABLE 4–3.   DSM-IV-TR diagnostic
criteria for substance intoxication

A. The development of a reversible substance-specific syndrome due to recent
   ingestion of (or exposure to) a substance.
   Note: Different substances may produce
   similar or identical syndromes.
B. Clinically significant maladaptive behavioral or psychological changes that are
   due to the effect of the substance on the
   central nervous system (e.g., belligerence,
   mood lability, cognitive impairment,
   impaired judgment, impaired social or
   occupational functioning) and develop
   during or shortly after use of the substance.
C. The symptoms are not due to a general
   medical condition and are not better
   accounted for by another mental disorder.

tently during the same 12 months. The
criteria for abuse do not include tolerance,
withdrawal, or compulsive use (Table 4–2).
Substance abuse can be applied to neither
caffeine nor nicotine. The term *abuse*
should not be used as a blanket term for
"use," "misuse," or "hazardous use."

Substance-Induced Disorders

Substance Intoxication

Substance *intoxication* (Table 4–3) is a reversible syndrome caused by recent exposure to a substance. It is often associated,
and may be concurrently diagnosed, with
substance abuse or dependence. The category does not apply to nicotine. Different
substances (sometimes even different
substance classes) may produce identical
symptoms during intoxication. DSM-IV-
TR allows specification of the presence of
"perceptual disturbances" in intoxication
by some substances.

Substance Withdrawal

Substance *withdrawal* (Table 4–4) is a behavioral, physiological, and cognitive state

"physiological dependence," current use of
agonist therapy, and placement in a controlled environment may also be specified.

Substance Abuse

In DSM-IV-TR, substance *abuse* includes
continued use despite significant problems caused by the use in those who do
not meet criteria for substance dependence. "Failure to fulfill major role obligations" is a criterion. To fulfill an abuse
criterion, the substance-related problem
must have occurred repeatedly or persis-

TABLE 4–4. DSM-IV-TR diagnostic criteria for substance withdrawal

A. The development of a substance-specific syndrome due to the cessation of (or reduction in) substance use that has been heavy and prolonged.
B. The substance-specific syndrome causes clinically significant distress or impairment in social, occupational, or other important areas of functioning.
C. The symptoms are not due to a general medical condition and are not better accounted for by another mental disorder.

---

caused by cessation of, or reduction in, heavy and prolonged substance use. Perhaps all withdrawing individuals crave the substance to reduce withdrawal symptoms. Signs and symptoms vary according to the substance used; most symptoms are the opposite of those observed in intoxication by the same substance. Withdrawal is usually associated with substance dependence. DSM-IV-TR allows for specification of "perceptual disturbances" in withdrawal from some substances.

Substance-Induced Mental Disorders

Diagnosis of a substance-induced mental disorder requires evidence of intoxication or withdrawal. Some disorders can persist after the substance has been eliminated from the body, but symptoms lasting more than 4 weeks after acute intoxication or withdrawal are considered manifestations either of a primary mental disorder or of a substance-induced persisting disorder. The differential diagnosis is complicated: withdrawal from some substances (e.g., sedatives) may partially mimic intoxication with others (e.g., amphetamines). That a syndrome (e.g., depression with suicidal ideation) is caused by a substance (e.g., cocaine)

in no way diminishes its clinical import. In most cases, intoxication and withdrawal are distinguished from substance-induced disorders of the same class because symptoms in the latter disorders are in excess of those usually associated with intoxication or withdrawal from the substance and are severe enough to warrant independent clinical attention.

Alcohol

Alcohol Use Disorders

It is important to distinguish alcohol abuse from dependence because the prognostic consequences of the two are different: the alcohol-abusing person has some chance of drinking in a controlled manner, the alcohol-dependent person *must* become abstinent. It is difficult to predict which abusers will go on to dependence. Abstinence is the safest course and prevents progression to dependence.

Alcohol Dependence

The DSM-IV-TR diagnostic criteria for alcohol dependence follow those for other substance disorders (Table 4–1). Specifying the presence of physiological dependence has prognostic value because it indicates a more severe clinical course (Schuckit et al. 1998), especially when withdrawal rather than tolerance is the basis on which physiological dependence is diagnosed.

Alcohol Abuse

Alcohol abuse requires fewer symptoms than does dependence and is diagnosed only if dependence has been ruled out. *Abuse* requires use that jeopardizes a person's ability to fulfill major role obligations. The development of medical and psychiatric complications related to alcohol use also helps in making the diagnosis.

TABLE 4–5. Blood alcohol level (BAL) and typical clinical presentation in the nontolerant, alcohol-intoxicated patient

BAL (mg/dL)	Clinical presentation
30	Attention difficulties (mild), euphoria
50	Coordination problems, driving is legally impaired
100	Ataxia, drunk driving
200	Confusion, decreased consciousness
>400	Anesthesia, ?coma, ?death

Alcohol-Induced Disorders

Alcohol Intoxication

Alcohol intoxication is time-limited and reversible, with onset depending on tolerance, amount ingested, and amount absorbed. It is affected by interactions with other substances, by medical status, and by individual variation. Table 4–5 lists blood alcohol levels and corresponding clinical features of a nonhabituated patient. Relative to degree of tolerance, increasing blood alcohol levels can lead to euphoria, mild coordination problems, ataxia, confusion, and decreased consciousness, and then to anesthesia, coma, and death. Alcohol intoxication may affect heart rate and electroencephalogram (EEG) readings and may cause nystagmus; slowed reaction times; and behavioral changes such as mood lability, impaired judgment, impaired social or occupational functioning, cognitive problems, and disinhibition of sexual or aggressive impulses. Alcohol intoxication closely resembles sedative, hypnotic, or anxiolytic intoxication. Individual and cultural variations of tolerance may influence symptom presentation. Other neurological conditions, such as cerebellar ataxia from multiple sclerosis, may mimic some of the physiological signs and symptoms of alcohol intoxication. "Alcohol idiosyncratic intoxication" is not present in DSM-IV-TR.

Alcohol Withdrawal

Any relative drop in an individual's blood alcohol level can precipitate withdrawal, even during continued alcohol consumption. Features of withdrawal include coarse tremor of hands, tongue, or eyelids; nausea or vomiting; malaise or weakness, autonomic hyperactivity; orthostatic hypotension; anxiety, depressed mood, or irritability; transient hallucinations (generally poorly formed) or illusions; headache; and insomnia. The generalized tremor, which is coarse and of intermediate frequency (5–7 Hz), can worsen with motor activity or emotional stress; it is most likely to be observed on extension of the hands or tongue. Often patients complain only of feeling shaky inside. Careful attention should be paid to vital signs in a suspected alcoholic individual. Symptoms peak 24–48 hours after the last drink and subside in 5–7 days even without treatment. Insomnia and irritability may last 10 days or longer. The withdrawal symptoms may precipitate a relapse.

Alcohol Intoxication Delirium or Withdrawal Delirium

Delirium tremens (DTs) can result from alcohol withdrawal or intoxication. It is a condition that differs from uncomplicated withdrawal in that it is a delirium that may include abnormal perceptions, agitation, terror, insomnia, mild fever, autonomic instability, or even simple peculiar behavior. Hallucinations may be auditory and of a persecutory nature, or they may be kinesthetic, such as tactile sensations of crawling insects. DTs can appear suddenly, but it usually occurs gradually 2–3 days after cessation of drinking, with peak intensity on day 4 or 5. It is usually benign and short-lived: the majority of cases subside after 3 days; subacute symptoms may last 4–5 weeks. The fatality rate may be less than 1%. DTs is associated with infections, subdural hematomas, trauma, liver disease, and metabolic disorders, and if death occurs amid DTs, the cause is usually infectious fat emboli or cardiac arrhythmias (usually associated with hyperkalemia, hyperpyrexia, and poor hydration).

Alcohol Withdrawal Seizures

Alcohol lowers the seizure threshold. Alcohol withdrawal seizures that are not a part of DTs generally occur between 7 and 38 hours after the last alcohol use in chronic drinkers; the average is about 24 hours after the last drink. Half of these seizures occur in bursts of two to six generalized grand mal seizures. A total of 10% of all chronic drinkers endure a grand mal seizure; of these, one-third go on to DTs and 2% go on to status epilepticus. Focal seizures suggest a prior focal lesion. Hypomagnesemia, respiratory alkalosis, hypoglycemia, and increased intracellular sodium have been associated with these seizures. These seizures predict a complicated withdrawal period.

Alcohol-Induced Persisting Dementia

Prolonged and heavy use of alcohol may be followed by dementia. Diagnosis is confirmed by its presence at least 3 weeks after ending alcohol intake. In this condition, unlike alcohol-induced persisting amnestic disorder, cognitive impairment affects more than memory function and no other cause is known.

Alcohol-Induced Persisting Amnestic Disorder (Korsakoff's Syndrome)

Thiamine (vitamin B_1) deficiency associated with prolonged heavy use of alcohol produces alcohol-induced persisting amnestic disorder (i.e., Korsakoff's syndrome) with its associated neurological deficits (peripheral neuropathy, cerebellar ataxia, and myopathy). Korsakoff's syndrome often follows acute Wernicke's encephalopathy (confusion, ataxia, nystagmus, ophthalmoplegia, and other neurological signs). Usually, as Wernicke's subsides, severe impairment of anterograde and retrograde memory persists; confabulation is common. Early treatment of Wernicke's encephalopathy with large doses of thiamine may prevent Korsakoff's syndrome. Unlike the case with other dementias, intellectual function is preserved in alcohol-induced persisting amnestic disorder.

Alcohol-Induced Psychotic Disorder With Delusions or Hallucinations

The hallucinatory form of alcohol-induced psychotic disorder is far more common than the delusional form. Hallucinosis presents with vivid and persistent hallucinations usually within 48 hours after reduction of alcohol in dependent patients. Auditory or visual hallucinations can occur. The disorder may last several weeks or months. Hallucinations may range from sounds (e.g., clicks, roaring, humming, ringing bells, chanting) to threatening or derogatory voices. Patients usually respond with fear, anxiety, and agitation. Diagnosis requires the absence of formal thought disorder. In the majority of cases, the symptoms recede in a few hours to days. Rarely, patients develop a quiet, chronic, paranoid delusional state indistinguishable from schizophrenia, from which remission would not be expected after 6 months. Differential diagnosis includes DTs, withdrawal syndrome, paranoid psychosis, and borderline transient psychotic episodes. In contrast to DTs, these hallucinations usually occur in a clear consciousness. Lack of autonomic symptoms differentiates the syndrome from withdrawal.

Alcohol-Induced Sexual Dysfunction

Alcohol broadly affects reproductive function, generally in proportion to the magnitude of use. Contrary to myth, both men and women have decreased sexual function when alcohol dependent.

Blackouts

Blackouts are periods of amnesia during periods of intoxication despite a state of consciousness that seems normal. They may occur in nonalcoholic persons during heavy drinking or at any time during alcohol dependence. Severity and duration of use correlate with blackout occurrence.

Sedatives, Hypnotics, and Anxiolytics

The sedative, hypnotic, and anxiolytic substances include the benzodiazepines, the carbamates, the barbiturates, and the barbiturate-like hypnotics. This class includes all prescription sleeping medications and almost all prescription anxiolytics. The nonbenzodiazepine anxiolytics are not included. Polysubstance abusers frequently self-medicate with sedatives to treat undesirable effects of cocaine or amphetamine. Definitions for this class of drugs follow the generic DSM-IV-TR definitions of abuse and dependence. This class of substances produces secondary clinical syndromes that generally parallel those secondary to alcohol, but their pharmacokinetics differ from alcohol in important ways.

Sedative, Hypnotic, or Anxiolytic Use Disorders

Sedative, Hypnotic, or Anxiolytic Dependence

A diagnosis of dependence should be considered only when, in addition to having physiological dependence, the individual using the substance shows evidence of a range of social or personal problems. In this substance class, degree of physical dependence is closely related to dosage and length of use. An individual who abruptly discontinues medically prescribed benzodiazepines at therapeutic doses may have evidence of tolerance and withdrawal in the absence of a diagnosis of substance dependence.

Sedative-, Hypnotic-, or Anxiolytic-Induced Disorders

Sedative, Hypnotic, or Anxiolytic Intoxication

Memory impairment is a prominent feature of sedative, hypnotic, or anxiolytic intoxication and is most often characterized by an anterograde amnesia. One (or more) of the following signs develop during, or shortly after, intoxicating sedative, hypnotic, or anxiolytic use: slurred speech, incoordination, unsteady gait, nystagmus, impairment in attention or memory, or stupor or coma.

Sedative, Hypnotic, or Anxiolytic Withdrawal

This characteristic syndrome develops in response to a relative decrease in intake after regular use. As with alcohol, withdrawal here includes two or more symptoms such as autonomic hyperactivity, tremor, insomnia, anxiety, nausea, vomiting, and psychomotor agitation. Relief on administration of any sedative–hypnotic agent supports a diagnosis of withdrawal. Grand mal seizures occur in 20%–30% of untreated withdrawing individuals. The withdrawal syndrome produced by substances in this class may present as a life-threatening delirium or with perceptual disturbances. The timing and severity of the syndrome depends on the substance and its pharmacokinetics and pharmacodynamics. Symptoms may develop more slowly for drugs with longer half-lives than for those with shorter half-lives. As with alcohol, lingering withdrawal symptoms (e.g., anxiety, moodiness, insomnia) can be mistaken for non–substance-induced anxiety or depressive disorders.

Sedative, hypnotic, or anxiolytic withdrawal delirium is characterized by disturbances in consciousness and cognition, with visual, tactile, or auditory hallucinations. When delirium is present, withdrawal delirium should be diagnosed instead of withdrawal.

Opioids

Opioid Use Disorders

Opioid Dependence

Most individuals with opioid dependence have significant tolerance. The diagnosis requires the presence of features that reflect either compulsive use without legitimate medical purpose or use of doses that are greatly in excess of those needed for pain relief.

Opioid Abuse

Dependence, rather than abuse, should be considered when problems related to opioid use are accompanied by evidence of tolerance, withdrawal, or compulsive behavior related to the use of opioids.

Opioid-Induced Disorders

Opioids are less likely than most other drugs of abuse to produce psychiatric symptoms and in fact may reduce such symptoms.

Opioid Intoxication

The magnitude of the behavioral and physiological changes that result from opioid use depends on the dose of the drug as well as the characteristics of the user.

Symptoms of intoxication usually last as long as the half-life of the drug. Intoxication is marked by miosis or, if severe, by mydriasis (due to anoxia). Drowsiness, slurred speech, and impairment in attention and memory are other signs. Aggression and violence are rarely seen. When hallucinations occur in the absence of intact reality testing, a diagnosis of opioid-induced psychotic disorder, with hallucinations, should be considered. Intoxication by alcohol, sedatives, hypnotics, or anxiolytics resembles opioid intoxication but produces neither miosis nor a response to a naloxone challenge.

Opioid overdose is an emergent situation that can be quickly diagnosed: It presents as coma, shock, and pinpoint pupils (dilation in severe cases) and depressed respiration that may lead to death. It rapidly responds to naloxone (Narcan), an opioid receptor antagonist; thus, a lack of response to naloxone undermines a presumed diagnosis of opioid overdose. However, if other classes of drugs are responsible for the altered mental state, naloxone will produce only partial improvement. Opioid intoxication is best distinguished from alcohol and sedative intoxication by the presence of pupillary constriction and laboratory studies.

Opioid Withdrawal

Opioid withdrawal is a syndrome that follows a relative reduction in heavy and prolonged use (see Table 4–6 for the DSM-IV-TR criteria set). The syndrome begins within 6–8 hours after the last dose and peaks at 48–72 hours; symptoms disappear in 7–10 days. It includes signs and symptoms that are opposite the acute agonist effects: lacrimation, rhinorrhea, pupillary dilation, piloerection, diaphoresis, diarrhea, yawning, mild hypertension, tachycardia, fever, and insomnia. A flulike syndrome subsequently develops, with complaints, demands, and drug seeking.

TABLE 4–6. DSM-IV-TR diagnostic
criteria for opioid withdrawal

A. Either of the following:
   (1) cessation of (or reduction in) opioid
       use that has been heavy and prolonged
       (several weeks or longer)
   (2) administration of an opioid antagonist
       after a period of opioid use
B. Three (or more) of the following, developing within minutes to several days after
   Criterion A:
   (1) dysphoric mood
   (2) nausea or vomiting
   (3) muscle aches
   (4) lacrimation or rhinorrhea
   (5) pupillary dilation, piloerection, or
       sweating
   (6) diarrhea
   (7) yawning
   (8) fever
   (9) insomnia
C. The symptoms in Criterion B cause clinically significant distress or impairment in
   social, occupational, or other important
   areas of functioning.
D. The symptoms are not due to a general
   medical condition and are not better
   accounted for by another mental disorder.

Although intense, uncomplicated withdrawal is usually not life-threatening unless a severe underlying disorder, such as
cardiac disease, is present. The anxiety
and restlessness associated with opioid
withdrawal resemble symptoms seen in
sedative, hypnotic, or anxiolytic withdrawal. However, opioid withdrawal is
also accompanied by rhinorrhea, lacrimation, and mydriasis, which are not seen in
sedative-type withdrawal.

Neonatal Opioid Withdrawal

Withdrawal occurs in 60%–94% of neonates of opioid-addicted mothers. The
baby may appear normal at birth, but signs
may appear 12–24 hours later and may
persist for months. The syndrome can include hyperactivity, tremors, seizures, hyperactive reflexes, gastrointestinal dysfunction, respiratory dysfunction, and
autonomic signs (yawning, sneezing,
sweating, nasal congestion, increased lacrimation, and fever). Over months, infants
may appear anxious, hard to please, hyperactive, and emotionally labile.

Cocaine

Cocaine can be administered in the form of
coca leaves (chewed); coca paste (smoked);
cocaine hydrochloride powder (inhaled
or injected); and cocaine alkaloid, "freebase," or "crack" (smoked). "Speedballing"—mixing cocaine and heroin—is particularly dangerous due to potentiation of
respiratory depressant effects. Cocaine-
induced states should be distinguished
from the symptoms of schizophrenia
(paranoid type), bipolar and other mood
disorders, generalized anxiety disorder,
and panic disorder.

Cocaine Use Disorders
Cocaine Dependence

Exposure to cocaine can quickly produce
dependence. An early sign is a growing difficulty resisting the drug. With cocaine's
short half-life, frequent use is needed to
keep "high." Complications of chronic use
are common and include paranoia, aggression, anxiety, depression, and weight loss.

Cocaine Abuse

The intensity and frequency of cocaine
use are less in abuse than in dependence.
Dependence, rather than abuse, should be
considered when use is accompanied by
tolerance, withdrawal, or compulsive behavior related to obtaining and using the
drug.

Cocaine-Induced Disorders
Cocaine Intoxication

Cocaine intoxication is a state that develops during or shortly after cocaine use.

After an initial "high," intoxication produces one or more of the following behavioral or psychological changes: euphoria with enhanced vigor, gregariousness, hyperactivity, restlessness, hypervigilance, interpersonal sensitivity, talkativeness, anxiety, tension, alertness, grandiosity, stereotyped or repetitive behavior, anger, and impaired judgment, and, in the case of chronic intoxication, affective blunting with fatigue or sadness and social withdrawal. These features occur with two or more of the following signs and symptoms: tachycardia or bradycardia; mydriasis; elevated or lowered blood pressure; perspiration or chills; nausea or vomiting; evidence of weight loss; psychomotor agitation or retardation; muscular weakness, respiratory depression, chest pain, or cardiac arrhythmias; and confusion, seizures, dyskinesias, dystonias, or coma. Cocaine's stimulant effects (e.g., euphoria, tachycardia, hypertension, psychomotor activity) are seen more commonly than its depressant effects (e.g., sadness, bradycardia, hypotension, psychomotor retardation), which emerge only with chronic high-dose use. In humans, binges are highly reinforcing and may lead to psychosis or death. Cocaine's effects on the noradrenergic system are significant and in the overdose setting are associated with muscular twitching, rhabdomyolysis, seizures, cerebrovascular accidents, myocardial infarctions, arrhythmias, and respiratory failure.

Intravenous or freebase use greatly intensifies cocaine's rush. Used intravenously, cocaine's half-life is less than 90 minutes, with euphoric effects lasting 15–20 minutes. Metabolism is slowed when cocaine is combined with alcohol, in which case there is a 18- to 25-fold greater chance of death than with cocaine alone.

Tolerance to cocaine's euphoric effects develops during a binge. With prolonged cocaine administration, a transient delusional psychosis simulating paranoid schizophrenia can be seen. Usually the symptoms remit, although heavy, prolonged use or predisposing psychopathology may lead to persisting psychosis. Often, amphetamine or phencyclidine intoxication can be distinguished from cocaine intoxication only through toxicological studies.

Cocaine Withdrawal

Cocaine withdrawal is accompanied by dysphoric mood (perhaps with suicidal ideation), irritability, anxiety, fatigue, insomnia or hyposomnia, vivid and unpleasant dreams, and psychomotor agitation. Anhedonia and drug craving may be present. Withdrawal occurs more than 24 hours after cessation of use and generally peaks in 2–4 days (although irritability and depression may continue for months). EEG abnormalities may be present.

Cocaine Intoxication Delirium

Cocaine intoxication delirium may occur within 24 hours of use. It may produce tactile or olfactory hallucinations; violent or aggressive behavior is frequent. It is self-limited and usually resolves after 6 hours.

Cocaine-Induced Psychotic Disorder, With Delusions

Cocaine-induced psychotic disorder with delusions is characterized by rapidly developing persecutory delusions that may be accompanied by body-image distortion, misperception of people's faces, formication, and aggression or violence.

Amphetamines

This drug class includes substances with a substituted-phenylethylamine structure (e.g., amphetamine, dextroamphetamine, methamphetamine ["speed"]) and those that have amphetamine-like action but are structurally different (e.g., methylphenidate and most appetite suppressants). Peripheral sympathomimetic effects may be quite potent.

Amphetamine Use Disorders

Patterns of use, abuse, and dependence on amphetamines parallel those of cocaine, although effects may last longer than in cocaine. Patterns of use involve oral administration (predominantly in pill form) and resemble those for cocaine, with binge episodes alternating with "crash" symptoms.

Amphetamine-Induced Disorders

Amphetamine Intoxication

Amphetamine intoxication follows use of amphetamine or a related substance. Behavioral and psychological changes are accompanied by at least two of the following: tachycardia or bradycardia, mydriasis, hyper- or hypotension, perspiration or chills, nausea or vomiting, weight loss, psychomotor agitation or retardation, muscular weakness, respiratory depression, and chest pain. Confusion, arrhythmias, seizures, dyskinesias, dystonias, or coma may follow. The state begins no more than 1 hour after use, depending on the drug and method of delivery. "Perceptual disturbances" should be specified when hallucinations or illusions occur without delirium and with intact reality testing. If hallucinations or illusions are accompanied by impaired reality testing, the diagnosis "amphetamine-induced psychotic disorder, with hallucinations" should be considered. Amphetamine psychosis can resemble acute paranoid schizophrenia, frequently with visual hallucinations.

Differential Diagnosis of Amphetamine-Induced Disorders

Amphetamine-induced disorders may resemble primary mental disorders. A very difficult differential diagnosis is that between amphetamine-induced psychosis and schizophrenia (Flaum and Shultz 1996). Intoxication with cocaine, hallucinogens, or phencyclidine may cause a similar picture and sometimes can only be distinguished from amphetamine intoxication by urine or serum toxicology, although mydriasis, history of recent drug use, and speed of onset are giveaways. Dependence or abuse involving amphetamines should be distinguished from dependence or abuse involving cocaine, phencyclidine, or hallucinogens.

Phencyclidine and Variants

Originally an anesthetic, phencyclidine (PCP; "angel dust," the "PeaCe" pill) has become a street drug with epidemic use in some urban areas. Variations include ketamine (Ketalar) and the thiophene analogue of PCP (TCP). These substances can be used orally or intravenously and can be smoked and inhaled. PCP is often mixed with other substances such as amphetamines, cannabis, cocaine, or hallucinogens.

Phencyclidine Use Disorders
Phencyclidine Dependence

PCP dependence may have a rapid onset, and its effects are generally unpredictable. Although the DSM-IV-TR diagnostic criteria for PCP dependence include the first 7 items of the generic definition of substance dependence, criteria 2a and 2b may not apply, given that a clear-cut withdrawal pattern is difficult to establish.

Phencyclidine Abuse

PCP abusers may fail to fulfill important role obligations because of intoxication. They may use the drug in situations where its use is physically hazardous. There may be recurrent social or interpersonal problems (due to intoxicated behavior or due to a chaotic lifestyle), legal problems, or arguments with significant others.

Phencyclidine-Induced Disorders

Phencyclidine Intoxication

PCP intoxication produces sympathetic and cholinergic effects. Intoxication begins by 5 minutes and peaks within 30 minutes. It produces affective instability, stereotypies, bizarre aggression, altered perception, disorganization, and confusion. Signs include hypertension, numbness, muscular rigidity, ataxia, and, at high dosages, hyperthermia and involuntary movements, followed by amnesia and coma, analgesia, seizures, and respiratory depression at the highest doses (i.e., >20 mg). Milder intoxication usually resolves after 8–20 hours; however, because of PCP's fat solubility, this state may persist for many days. Mydriasis and nystagmus (vertical more than horizontal) are characteristic of PCP use and help confirm the diagnosis. Perceptual disturbances should be specified if present. As with hallucinogens, adverse reactions to PCP may be more common among individuals with preexisting mental disorders.

Phencyclidine-Induced Psychotic Disorder

Psychosis, the most common PCP-induced disorder, may occur in predisposed individuals. It may be indistinguishable from a psychotic episode. Chronic psychosis may occur, along with long-term neuropsychological deficits.

Differential Diagnosis of Phencyclidine-Induced Disorders

PCP-induced disorders may resemble primary mental disorders. Recurring episodes of psychotic or mood symptoms due to PCP may mimic schizophrenia or mood disorders. The fact of PCP use establishes a role for the substance in producing the mentally disordered state but does not rule out the co-occurrence of other primary mental disorders (including conduct disorder or antisocial personality disorder). PCP users often use other drugs; thus, comorbid abuse or dependence on other substances must be considered.

Hallucinogens

This diverse group of substances includes indoleamine derivatives (LSD, morning glory seeds); phenylalkylamine derivatives (mescaline, "STP" [2,5-dimethoxy-4-methylamphetamine], and ring-substituted amphetamines—MDA [methylenedioxyamphetamine; old "ecstasy"], MDMA [methylenedioxymethamphetamine; new "Ecstasy"], MDEA [methylenedioxyethamphetamine]); indole alkaloids (psilocybin, DMT [dimethyltryptamine]); and miscellaneous other compounds. Excluded from this group are PCP and cannabis/delta-9-tetrahydrocannabinol (THC). Hallucinogens are usually taken orally, although dimethyltryptamine is smoked, and use by injection does occur.

Hallucinogen Use Disorders

Hallucinogen Dependence

No specific criteria exist for hallucinogen dependence; in addition, some of the generic DSM-IV-TR substance dependence criteria do not apply; others require qualification. Hallucinogen use is often limited to only a few times a week, even among individuals who meet the full criteria for hallucinogen dependence. Although tolerance to the euphoric and psychedelic effects of hallucinogens develops rapidly, tolerance to the autonomic effects (mydriasis, hyperreflexia, hypertension, increased body temperature, piloerection, and tachycardia) does not. Cross-tolerance exists between LSD and other hallucinogens (e.g., psilocybin, mescaline). Withdrawal has not been demonstrated, but clear reports of "craving" after stopping hallucinogens are known. Some MDMA users describe a "hangover" the day after use that includes insomnia, fatigue, drowsiness, sore jaw muscles from teeth clenching, loss of balance, and headaches.

Hallucinogen-Induced Disorders

Hallucinogen Intoxication

In hallucinogen intoxication, perceptual changes occur alongside full alertness during or shortly after hallucinogen use. Changes include subjective intensification of perceptions, depersonalization, derealization, illusions, hallucinations, and synesthesias. DSM-IV-TR criteria require the presence of at least two of the seven listed physiological signs. Synesthesias may occur. Hallucinations are usually visual, often involving geometric forms, sometimes involving persons and objects. Auditory or tactile hallucinations are rare. Reality testing is usually preserved. Hallucinogen intoxication should be differentiated from amphetamine or PCP intoxication. Intoxication with anticholinergics (e.g., trihexyphenidyl) can produce hallucinations, but such states are often associated with the usual anticholinergic effects.

Hallucinogen-Induced Psychotic Disorder

Hallucinogen-induced psychotic disorder may be brief or may lead into a long-lasting psychotic episode that is difficult to distinguish from schizophreniform disorder.

Hallucinogen Persisting Perception Disorder

Hallucinogen persisting perception disorder ("flashbacks") following cessation of hallucinogen use involves the reexperiencing of one or more of the same perceptual symptoms experienced while originally intoxicated. The disorder is usually fleeting, but in rare cases it may be more lasting and persistent. Symptoms may be triggered by stress, drug use (including that of other drugs such as cannabis), emergence into a dark environment, or even by intention. If the person's interpretation of the etiology of the state is delusional, the diagnosis is psychotic disorder NOS. In hallucinogen persisting perception disorder, the individual does not believe that the perception represents external reality, whereas a person with a psychotic disorder often believes that the perception is real.

Cannabis

The most commonly used substances in this class are marijuana, hashish, and purified THC. Although usually smoked, these substances may also be mixed with food and eaten.

Cannabis Use Disorders

Cannabis Dependence

Dependence is marked by daily, or almost daily, compulsive cannabis use. Tolerance to most of the effects of cannabis has been reported in chronic users, but these patients do not generally develop physiological dependence, and this is not a criterion for diagnosis in DSM-IV-TR. Withdrawal after heavy use is not clinically significant.

Cannabis Abuse

Abuse is characterized by episodic cannabis use with maladaptive behavior. When significant levels of tolerance are present or when psychological or physical problems are associated with cannabis in the context of compulsive use, dependence should be considered rather than abuse.

Cannabis-Induced Disorders

Cannabis Intoxication

Cannabis intoxication peaks 10–30 minutes after smoking cannabis and lasts about 3 hours; metabolites may have a half-life of approximately 50 hours. Because most cannabinoids are fat soluble, their effects may persist for 12–24 hours. Intoxication includes euphoria, anxiety, suspiciousness or paranoid ideation, sensation of slowed time, impaired judgment, and social withdrawal. Inappropriate laughter, panic attacks, and dysphoric affect may occur. Adverse reactions may be more common in those with psychiatric disorders or those frightened about the drug-taking situation. At least two of the following signs develop within 2 hours of use: 1) conjunctival infection, 2) increased appetite, 3) dry mouth, and 4) tachycardia. For differentiation, note that intoxication with alcohol or with a sedative, hypnotic, or anxiolytic substance usually decreases appetite, increases aggressive behavior, and produces nystagmus or ataxia. At low doses, hallucinogen intoxication may resemble cannabis intoxication. PCP intoxication is much more likely to cause ataxia and aggressive behavior. DSM-IV-TR provides a specifier for intoxication "with perceptual disturbances," although if hallucinations occur without intact reality testing, "substance-induced psychotic disorder, with hallucinations" should be diagnosed.

Cannabis-Induced Delusional Disorder

Cannabis-induced delusional disorder is a syndrome (usually with persecutory delusions) that develops shortly after cannabis use. It may be associated with marked anxiety, depersonalization, and emotional lability. Subsequent amnesia for the episode can occur.

Cannabis-Induced Mental Disorders

Cannabis-induced mental disorders are clinically diverse. Chronic cannabis use can cause a syndrome resembling dysthymic disorder. Acute adverse reactions to cannabis should be differentiated from panic, major depressive disorder, delusional disorder, bipolar disorder, or paranoid schizophrenia.

Nicotine

Nicotine has euphoric effects and reinforcement properties similar to those of cocaine and opioids. Its effects can follow use of all forms of tobacco, including prescription medications (nicotine gum and patch).

Nicotine Use Disorder

Nicotine Dependence

For nicotine, some of the generic DSM-IV-TR dependence criteria do not apply, and others need qualification. *Tolerance* can refer either to the absence of nausea, dizziness, and other characteristic symptoms despite the use of substantial amounts or to a diminished effect observed with continued use of the same amount of the substance. Spending a great deal of time attempting to procure nicotine is generally rare. An example of giving up important social, occupational, or recreational activities is the avoidance of an activity because it occurs in a smoking-restricted area.

Nicotine-Induced Disorders

Nicotine Withdrawal

Nicotine withdrawal develops after abrupt cessation of, or reduction in, nicotine use following a prolonged period of daily use. The withdrawal syndrome includes four or more of the following: dysphoric or depressed mood; insomnia; irritability, frustration, or anger; anxiety; difficulty concentrating; restlessness or impatience; decreased heart rate; and increased appetite or weight gain. Heart rate decreases by 5–12 beats per minute in the first few days after cessation, and weight increases an average of 2–3 kg in the year after cessation. Mild withdrawal may occur after switching to low-tar/low-nicotine cigarettes or after discontinuing the use of chewing tobacco, nicotine gum, or patches.

Differential Diagnosis of Nicotine-Induced Mental Disorders

The symptoms of nicotine withdrawal overlap with those of other withdrawal syndromes; caffeine intoxication; anxiety, mood, and sleep disorders; and medication-induced akathisia. Symptom reduction in response to replacement of nicotine confirms the diagnosis.

Inhalants

This class of inhaled substances includes the aliphatic and aromatic hydrocarbons found in substances such as gasoline, glue, paint thinners, and spray paints. Less commonly used are the halogenated hydrocarbons (in cleaners, correction fluid, spray-can propellants) and other volatile compounds containing esters, ketones, and glycols.

Inhalant Use Disorders

All of the substances in this class are capable of producing dependence, abuse, and intoxication. There are no specific criteria sets for dependence or abuse of inhalants, in part because of uncertainty in regard to the existence of tolerance or withdrawal syndromes. A possible withdrawal syndrome beginning 24–48 hours after cessation of use and lasting from 2 to 5 days has been described, with symptoms including sleep disturbances, tremor, irritability, diaphoresis, nausea, and fleeting illusions.

Inhalant-Induced Disorders

Inhalant Intoxication

Inhalant intoxication involves clinically significant maladaptive behavioral or psychological changes. These are accompanied by signs that include dizziness or visual disturbances (blurred vision or diplopia), nystagmus, incoordination, slurred speech, unsteady gait, tremor, or euphoria. Higher doses of inhalants may lead to the development of lethargy and psychomotor retardation, generalized muscle weakness, depressed reflexes, stupor, or coma.

Differential Diagnosis of Inhalant-Induced Disorders

Inhalant-induced disorders may be characterized by symptoms that resemble primary mental disorders. Mild to moderate intoxication from inhalants can be similar to intoxication caused by alcohol, sedatives, hypnotics, or anxiolytics. Chronic users are likely to use other substances frequently and heavily, further complicating the diagnosis. Rapid onset and resolution may also differentiate inhalant intoxication from other mental disorders and neurological conditions. Industrial workers may occasionally be accidentally exposed to volatile chemicals and suffer physiological intoxication, in which case the category "Other Substance-Related Disorders" should be used.

Caffeine

Caffeine is widely used in the form of coffee, tea, cola, chocolate, and cocoa and also through use of over-the-counter analgesics, cold preparations, and stimulants.

Caffeine Use Disorders

There is no DSM-IV-TR diagnosis for caffeine dependence or abuse. Although withdrawal headaches may occur, they are usually not severe enough to require treatment.

Caffeine-Induced Disorders

Caffeine Intoxication

Caffeine intoxication can lead to restlessness, nervousness, excitement, insomnia, flushing, diuresis, and gastrointestinal complaints. Doses leading to intoxication can vary. At high doses, there can be psychosis, arrhythmias, and psychomotor agitation. At massive doses, grand mal seizures and respiratory failure can result. In persons who have developed tolerance, intoxication may not occur.

DSM-IV-TR recognizes other caffeine-induced disorders such as anxiety disorder and sleep disorder, and there is a category for caffeine-related disorder NOS.

Differential Diagnosis of Caffeine-Induced Disorders

Caffeine-induced mental disorders must be differentiated from medical conditions. Manic episodes; panic disorder or generalized anxiety disorder; amphetamine intoxication; sedative, hypnotic, or anxiolytic withdrawal or nicotine withdrawal; sleep disorders; and medication-induced side effects (e.g., akathisia) can appear similar to caffeine intoxication.

Other (or Unknown) Substance-Related Disorders

The DSM-IV-TR category of other (or unknown) substance-related disorders encompasses symptoms of dependence, abuse, intoxication, withdrawal, delirium, psychosis with delusions, psychosis with hallucinations, persisting dementia or amnesia, mood disturbance, anxiety, sexual dysfunction, or disordered sleep that result either from use of a substance whose identity is unknown at the time of the patient's presentation or from use of a substance belonging to a group not large enough to warrant its own category. Examples of the latter include amyl nitrate, anticholinergics, γ-hydroxybutyrate (GHB), corticosteroids, anabolic steroids, antihistamines, antiparkinsonian agents, and others.

GHB, a schedule I substance, is structurally related to γ-aminobutyric acid (GABA). It is increasingly used worldwide as a recreational drug by party and nightclub attendees and bodybuilders and even as a "date rape" drug. GHB increases CNS dopamine levels and has effects in the endogenous opioid system. GHB toxicity includes coma, seizures, respiratory depression, vomiting, anesthesia, and amnesia (Centers for Disease Control and Prevention 1997b). The drug is missed by routine diagnostic urine screens. Although full recovery usually occurs, the toxic state is life-threatening and may be complicated by severe muscular pathology leading to rhabdomyolysis and myoglobinuria (Graeme 2000). An increasing number of reports have described clinically significant states of withdrawal from GHB (Craig et al. 2000).

Polysubstance Dependence

The DSM-IV-TR category of polysubstance dependence is used when, within the past year, the individual has repeatedly used at least three classes of substances (excepting nicotine and caffeine) without one predominating. Dependence is global and not for any one drug.

Often one drug is used to counterbalance the side effects or to potentiate the effects of another drug. "Speedballing"—the intravenous combination of heroin and cocaine—is known to mitigate cocaine dysphoria. Glutethimide (Doriden) and cocaine are often combined, potentiating respiratory depression. Pentazocine (Talwin) and diphenhydramine (Benadryl)—the "T's and Blues"—are prescription medications that produce intoxication when combined.

Clinical Diagnosis of Substance Use Disorder

Substance-abusing patients present with medical, neurological, and psychiatric disturbances that require careful, systematic assessment. The extreme complexity of differential diagnosis in this population should instill some degree of humility and conservatism. Cautious management with a careful review of the medical, psychiatric, and substance abuse histories; physical and mental status examinations; laboratory tests; and third-party information can clarify the diagnoses. In some cases, however, etiology can be elucidated only with time and observation.

Signs and Symptoms

Diagnosing and caring for substance-abusing patients requires attention to physical signs and symptoms, especially gait problems, nystagmus, tachycardia, bradycardia, mydriasis, miosis, or change in body temperature. At the outset it should be noted that when attempting to differentiate among overdose, withdrawal, chronic brain disease, and psychiatric diagnoses, one should rule out or treat life-threatening conditions first. Physical examination can detect fresh needle marks, recent alcohol intake, or nasal irritation from cocaine or inhalant abuse.

Countertransference and Diagnosis

Because of the strong countertransference reactions evoked by substance-abusing patients who use primitive defenses, inappropriate diagnostic and treatment decisions may ensue. Before making an unusual treatment decision or participating in uncharacteristic behavior with a patient, consultation with another expert may be useful, and sometimes a team approach is especially helpful. Frequently, obnoxious, uncooperative, or destructive behavior or apparent personality problems are time limited and related to the substance-induced state. Such behavior may reflect the patient's fear and low self-esteem or may quickly resolve on detoxification.

Psychiatric Comorbidity

Dual-diagnosis patients have a substance abuse disorder and another major psychiatric diagnosis. The causal connections between the two may be manifold (Vaillant 1993), and psychiatric disorders and substance abuse may present as independent conditions. Thus, it is difficult at any one time to differentiate symptoms of withdrawal, intoxication, and secondary psychopathology from underlying psychiatric disorders. Among the major psychopathologies, the reported odds ratios for comorbid substance use were 2 for major depressive disorder, 3 for panic disorder,

5 for schizophrenia, and 7 for bipolar illness (Regier et al. 1990).

Affective Disorders

Chronic major depression occurs late in the course of many addictions. This depression may be the result of altered neurochemistry, hormonal or metabolic changes, chronic demoralization, or grief from personal losses, or it may result from the stresses of the addictive lifestyle. Chronic heroin use often leads to lethargy and social withdrawal. Sustained alcohol use generally produces depression and anxiety, although brief periods of euphoria may still occur.

It is vitally important to differentiate alcohol-induced depressive disorder from primary depressive disorder (Schuckit et al. 1997). The presence of untreated major depression in a patient with primary alcoholism or of secondary alcoholism in a patient with primary depressive disorder worsens prognosis. Although most individuals with alcoholism will not have an independent diagnosis of major depressive disorder, other less severe depressive disorders may persist in a large proportion of alcoholic persons after cessation of drinking. In most cases, depressive symptomatology subsides after 3–4 weeks of abstinence and usually needs no pharmacological intervention. Use of antidepressants is indicated after a drug-free period.

The prevalence of major depression ranges from 17% to 30% in heroin-addicted persons and is considerably higher among methadone clients. Affective disorders have ranged as high as 60% among opioid abusers. Depressive episodes often are mild, may be related to treatment seeking, and frequently are stress related. Depression may be a poor prognostic sign in non-antisocial opioid-addicted patients (Brooner et al. 1997).

Affective disorders have been concurrently diagnosed in 30% of persons addicted to cocaine, with a significant proportion of these patients having bipolar or cyclothymic disorder. During manic episodes, patients may use cocaine to heighten feelings of grandiosity. The profound dysphoric mood related to cocaine binges will resolve in the majority of cocaine addicts. A minority of patients may have underlying unipolar or bipolar disorder, which needs to be treated separately. Some authors suggest that comorbid cocaine abuse constitutes a robust predictor of poor outcome among depressed alcoholic persons.

Psychosis

Psychotic symptomatology can result from the use of a wide range of psychoactive substances: alcohol, cocaine, PCP, hallucinogens, stimulants, and inhalants. Opioids have shown some antipsychotic properties.

The relationship between schizophrenia and substance abuse is complex. Various studies have shown that 50%–60% of schizophrenia patients and 60%–80% of bipolar patients abuse substances (Schneier and Siris 1987). The role of substance abuse in precipitating or altering the course of an underlying schizophrenic disorder is unclear. Substance abuse may trigger the reappearance of symptoms that were previously well controlled by medication. Alcohol, marijuana, hallucinogen, or cocaine abuse may produce psychotic symptoms that persist only in vulnerable individuals. It may be that schizophrenia patients seek out certain types of drugs for self-medication and for self-treatment of medication side effects. Persons with schizophrenia also use tobacco and caffeine more often than do control populations. Tobacco use has been associated with lowering of blood levels of neuroleptics and leads to a need for higher-than-average doses of neuroleptics for symptom control.

Anxiety Disorders

Generalized anxiety disorder, posttraumatic stress disorder, panic disorder, and phobic disorder are overrepresented in substance abuse patients, especially abusers of CNS depressants. One study of alcoholic patients reported general anxiety disorder in 9% and phobias in 3%, prevalences significantly higher than those in the general population (Ross et al. 1988). Panic disorder has been found in 5% of alcoholic inpatients (Kushner et al. 1990). Use of high doses of benzodiazepines (up to 1,000 or 1,500 mg diazepam equivalent) has been reported in patients with underlying anxiety disorders and very high tolerance to benzodiazepines. In the treatment of substance-addicted patients with anxiety disorders, benzodiazepines should be avoided if possible. Specific treatment of underlying anxiety disorders in abusers of CNS depressants may include typical and low-dose atypical antipsychotics, antidepressants, monoamine oxidase inhibitors (MAOIs), buspirone, gabapentin, or propranolol (see "Treatment of Substance Use Disorders").

Neuropsychiatric Impairment

Chronic abuse of alcohol, sedatives, or inhalants has been correlated with chronic brain damage and neuropsychological impairment. These impairments may be obvious (as in alcohol dementia or Korsakoff's syndrome) or relatively mild and detectable only by neuropsychological testing. Cognitive impairment may be short lived and recede after 3–4 weeks of abstinence, may improve gradually over several months or years of abstinence, or be permanent.

Natural Histories of Substance Abuse

Alcohol

The signs and symptoms of alcoholism can be strikingly consistent among individuals in the late stages of the disease, but there appear to be subtypes of alcoholics that may present with different ages at onset, underlying etiologies, degrees of hereditary influence, social and cultural backgrounds, and natural outcomes. Thus, it is important to understand alcoholism as a disease that assumes many different patterns and is characterized by relapses. Vaillant's (1996) longitudinal studies of alcoholic patients found that some drink until death, others stop drinking, and still others display a pattern of long abstinence followed by relapses. Large-scale outcome studies suggest that approximately 30% of alcoholic persons will at some point in the course of their illness achieve stable abstinence without any form of treatment (Armor et al. 1978). This percentage improves in some studies to approximately 70% with some form of treatment.

Types of Alcoholism

Cloninger et al. (1988) described two subtypes of alcoholism. In persons with type I alcoholism, heavy drinking generally starts after age 25 years and is reinforced by external circumstances. These individuals have greater ability to abstain for long periods of time and frequently feel loss of control, guilt, and fear about their alcohol dependency. In contrast, individuals with type II alcoholism generally have an early onset—before age 25 years—and show spontaneous alcohol-seeking behavior regardless of external circumstances. Fights and arrests are common with these individuals, and they rarely experience feelings of loss of control, guilt, or fear about their alcohol dependency.

Medical Complications

Gastrointestinal. Alcohol use can promote hepatic pathology. Fatty liver deposits occur in anyone with sufficient alcohol intake. Alcoholic hepatitis has a 5-year mortality rate of 50%. Cirrhosis occurs in only 10% of alcoholic persons. Of patients with chronic pancreatitis, 75% have an alcohol use disorder. Alcohol dissolves mucus and irritates the gastric lining, which contributes to bleeding. (Every alcoholism patient should have a stool guaiac as part of a complete physical examination [Lieber 1995]). In the acute, subacute, and chronic stages of alcohol use, hepatic dysregulation is present, albeit in differing patterns: in the acute (intoxicated) stage, there is inhibition of the metabolism of other molecules, such as medications (including substances of overdose); in the subacute phase, there is induction of liver cytochrome P450 (CYP) enzymes, increasing the metabolism of other molecules; and finally, in the cirrhotic state with portacaval shunting, there is again reduced metabolism of other systemic molecules (Weller and Preskorn 1984).

Hematological.   Alcoholism is part of the differential diagnosis for anemia, especially megaloblastic anemia. Alcohol impairs immune function and promotes oropharyngeal, esophageal, gastric, hepatic, and pancreatic cancer. Patients with oral cancer tend to delay seeking treatment longer than most other cancer patients. Early detection is particularly crucial in these diseases.

Endocrinological.   Sexual function is affected indirectly through alcohol's impact on the limbic system and the hypothalamic-pituitary-adrenal axis. Alcohol affects male sexual function and fertility both directly via effects on testosterone levels and indirectly through testicular atrophy. Relatively increased levels of estrogen lead to gynecomastia and body-hair loss in men. In women there may also be severe gonadal failure, affecting secondary sexual characteristics, reducing menstruation, and producing infertility.

Neurological.   Alcoholism increases blood pressure and is associated with increased risk of cerebrovascular accidents. Alcoholic cerebellar degeneration is a slowly evolving condition encountered in patients with a long-standing history of excessive use. Alcoholic peripheral neuropathy is characterized by a stocking-and-glove paresthesia with decreased reflexes and autonomic nerve dysfunction. Other long-term neurological effects of alcoholism include central pontine myelinolysis, Marchiafava-Bignami disease, and muscular pathology. Interestingly, some CT studies have shown that brain changes resulting from alcohol use may be reversible in as little as 3 weeks' time (Trabert et al. 1995).

Cardiovascular.   The relationship between alcohol and cardiovascular health and disease is complex. Alcoholic cardiomyopathy can develop after 10 or more years of drinking. For heavy drinkers, alcohol increases the risk of cardiomyopathy, heart failure, and poor postmyocardial infarction survival. Moderate (defined as 1–20 ounces per month) use of alcohol, on the other hand, may have beneficial effects on both the risk of heart failure in the elderly (Abramson et al. 2001) and postinfarction survival in the general population (Mukamal et al. 2001). However, these effects may be brittle (moderate, beneficial use might quickly become pathological), and no consensus recommendation yet exists for moderate use of alcohol.

Genetics: Familial Studies and High-Risk Populations

Alcoholism occurs in families, yet neither the mode of transmission nor the genotype or phenotype transmitted is known. Some studies have suggested that tolerance to alcohol is the transmitted trait. Others have proposed that what is trans-

TABLE 4–7. Possible markers of alcoholism in biological sons of alcoholics

Decreased subjective feelings of intoxication
Less impairment of motor performance
Less body sway
Less static ataxia
Less change in cortisol and prolactin findings
Low P3 amplitude (electroencephalogram)
Increased alpha-wave activity

mitted is a vulnerability to a particular substance (Schuckit et al. 1998).

Biological Markers

Biological markers are physiological findings associated with alcoholism that may help us to identify high-risk individuals before the onset of abuse, recognize dependence when it exists, and follow the course of the disease. Several promising markers have been found (Table 4–7). A finding among abstinent alcoholics and sons of alcoholics is an alteration of normal auditory brain-stem potentials. The p300 event-related potential (ERP) is of low amplitude in alcoholic persons and abstinent young sons of alcoholic men. Increased alpha-wave activity with alcohol exposure in alcoholic versus control subjects has also been reported. Controversy exists regarding whether alcoholic individuals have low platelet MAO-B activity (which may be even more apparent in type II alcoholism than in type I).

Finally, prospective longitudinal studies of sons of alcoholic parents have reported some evidence of poor neuropsychological performance in areas such as categorizing, organization, planning, abstracting, and problem-solving ability. Tarter and Edwards (1988) suggested that childhood ADHD or conduct disorder may predispose toward alcoholism and may be an expression of an underlying inherited temperament (although this has been disputed by epidemiological data [Biederman et al. 1997]). Risk taking, sensation-seeking individuals are thought to be at particularly high risk for alcoholism.

Sedatives, Hypnotics, and Anxiolytics

The course of CNS depressant abuse/dependence varies from long prodromal periods of use with benzodiazepines or hypnotics to more rapid onset of addiction with barbiturates to episodic abuse with other CNS depressants such as methaqualone (Quaalude) or ethchlorvynol (Placidyl). Combinations of CNS depressants with alcohol or opioids can potentiate the level of intoxication, leading to respiratory depression and mortality. Chronic sedative abuse can produce "blackouts" and neuropsychological damage similar to that experienced by alcoholic patients (Tonne et al. 1995). In patients originally using sedatives for anxiety, there will be an initial anxiety rebound on discontinuation that typically is similar to sedative withdrawal in terms of course and symptomatology.

Opioids

Psychosocial Features

Opioid abuse is often endemic to economically disadvantaged communities with high unemployment, low family stability, and increased tolerance of criminality. Alienation from social institutions such as school, increased social deviancy, and impulsivity are high-risk characteristics. The overwhelming majority of inner-city community members, however, are not opioid users.

Adverse Physical Effects

Impurities and contaminated needles may lead to endocarditis, septicemia, pulmonary emboli, pulmonary hypertension, skin infections, hepatitis B, and HIV. Death rates in young addicts are increased 20-fold by infection, homicide, suicide, overdose, and AIDS. Opioid overdose should be suspected in any undiagnosed coma patient.

Progression

The course of heroin addiction generally involves a 2- to 6-year interval between regular use of heroin and seeking of treatment. Early experimentation with opioids may not lead to addiction, but once addiction develops, a lifelong pattern of use and relapse frequently ensues. A preexisting personality disorder may be a factor in drug use progression. The need to secure the drug predisposes the addict to participate in crime.

The Self-Medication Hypothesis

The self-medication hypothesis suggests that the individual self-selects drugs on the basis of preexisting personality and ego impairments. Khantzian (1997) found a strong interaction between dominant dysphoric feelings and drug preference, and he emphasized an "antirage property to opioids" that provides a pharmacological solution or defense against overwhelming anger resulting from either deficient ego defenses or low frustration tolerance.

Cocaine

Natural Course

The time from first intranasal use to cocaine addiction is about 4 years in adults, but it may be only 1.5 years in adolescents. Both groups may progress faster with more potent cocaine derivatives (e.g., "crack"). Most addicts describe initial use as fun. At some point in the experience, however, it becomes joyless and compulsive. The activating properties of the drug become more prominent as the euphoria wanes. Consumption of cocaine may become an isolated, alienating experience, associated with considerable paranoia. Most casual cocaine users do not become dependent.

Cocaine is associated with violence. In 20% of suicides in New York City in the 1990s, it had been used immediately prior to death (Marzuk et al. 1992), and other studies have found cocaine in the urine of homicide victims, in those arrested for murder, and in overdose deaths. In cocaine-induced fatalities, the average blood concentration is 6.2 mg/L (Spiehler and Reed 1985).

Adverse Medical Effects

Chronic cocaine use depletes all neurotransmitters and leads to increased receptor sensitivity to dopamine and norepinephrine, which is associated with depression, fatigue, poor attention to self-care, poor self-esteem, poor libido, and mild parkinsonism. Tolerance to cocaine occurs. Psychosis, an attention-deficit syndrome, and/or stereotypies may result from continued use. There is evidence of cerebrovascular disease secondary to chronic use (Bartzokis et al. 1999).

Death may occur even in recreational, low-dose users. Other acute complications include agitation, diaphoresis, tachycardia, subarachnoid hemorrhage, metabolic and respiratory acidosis, arrhythmias, grand mal seizures, and respiratory arrest. Myocardial infarction is produced by coronary vasoconstriction with tachycardia. Malnutrition, severe weight loss, and dehydration often result from cocaine binges. Chronic complications of intranasal abuse include nasoseptal defects due to vasoconstriction, nasal stuffiness or "the runs" due to vasodilation, and dental neglect due to cocaine's anesthetic properties. Intravenous use may produce endocarditis, septicemia, HIV spread, local vasculitis, hepatitis B, emphysema, pulmonary emboli, and granulomas. Cocaine injection sites are characterized by prominent ecchymoses; opioid users more frequently show needle marks. Freebase cocaine has been associated with decreased pulmonary exchange and with persisting pulmonary dysfunction.

Pregnant women who use cocaine may have increased risks for abruptio placenta and neonatal tachycardia (Volpe 1992), and babies of cocaine-using mothers have been shown to have decreased interactive behavior on Brazelton scales. Further research is being conducted to study the teratogenicity of cocaine in infants. Fortunately, there have been few long-term developmental effects ascribed to cocaine itself (Frank et al. 2001).

Amphetamines

Amphetamine abuse may start as attempts at weight loss or energy enhancement. Amphetamine abuse by intravenous administration can present with the same medical complications seen with other drugs. Amphetamines are similar to cocaine in regard to signs, symptoms, and long-term sequelae.

Phencyclidine and Ketamine

Chronic psychotic episodes are reported following use of PCP. Use of PCP may lead to chronic neuropsychological deficits. PCP use may occur in conjunction with other substances, and its abuse may be associated with similar risk factors. Cases of "pure" PCP abuse have been reported in individuals with significant psychopathology; however, it is difficult to distinguish drug effects from premorbid personality.

Ketamine, originally used as an anesthetic, and its active metabolite norketamine act at many CNS receptor sites, including the NMDA receptor. The drug is taken intranasally or orally and has a fast

effect to get to "K land," as its dissociative effects are called. With the drug's elimination half-life of 2 hours, its effects last approximately 30 minutes. Ketamine has been known to produce psychosis in normal individuals (Krystal et al. 1994). The acute effects can be serious. Neurological toxicity includes nystagmus, mydriasis, agitation, delirium, hypertonus, rigidity, hallucinations, and seizures. Movement disturbances are common and include dystonia, ataxia, and bizarre posturing of limbs and facial expression. Rhabdomyolysis can ensue. Cardiovascular toxicity is consistent with sympathetic stimulation and includes tachycardia, palpitations, and hypertension. Respiratory arrest or apnea can occur, and there is a risk of aspiration. In cases of death from overdose, pulmonary edema has been noted.

Although long-term sequelae have not been well studied, flashbacks and cognitive disorder are known to occur in ketamine abuse (Jansen 1993).

Hallucinogens

Most hallucinogens can produce acute adverse effects. Hallucinogen use can also lead to chronic effects, including prolonged psychotic states that resemble psychosis or mania. However, syndromes that last longer than 4–6 weeks are generally thought to represent underlying primary psychiatric disease rather than conditions secondary to these substances. Flashbacks are another potential chronic sequelae of hallucinogens that occur in 15%–30% of chronic users. Prevalence of flashbacks increases with the number of times the individual seeks medical attention except during acute intoxication or disturbing flashbacks that may be precipitated by other substances such as marijuana. Most strikingly, some of the drugs in this class have produced permanent parkinsonism in users by selective destruction of the substantia nigra.

MDMA ("Ecstasy")

MDMA, a serotonin releaser and serotonin uptake inhibitor, is metabolized by CYP 2D6. MDMA can produce a state that resembles cocaine toxicity: fulminant hepatotoxicity, disseminated intravascular coagulation, cardiotoxicity, hyperthermia, rhabdomyolysis, and acute respiratory distress syndrome (Jonas and Graeme-Cook 2001). Over the long term, cognitive deficits do occur, especially in terms of memory (McCann et al. 1999).

Cannabis

Marijuana abuse tends to begin in adolescence. The use of alcohol, nicotine, or cocaine may be associated with marijuana abuse. Marijuana is described as a stepping stone to other illegal drugs. Although many people experiment with marijuana, actual abuse patterns tend to be associated with introduction to youth drug subcultures, low parental monitoring, parental substance abuse, and abuse of drugs by peers.

Chronic Psychological Effects

Generally, the adverse effects of marijuana are not treated in the medical setting. Mild anxiety, depression, and paranoia are frequent occurrences. Several neuropsychological changes and deficits have been identified with marijuana intoxication. Decreases in complex reaction-time tasks, digit-code memory tasks, fine-motor function, time estimation, the ability to track information over time, tactual form discrimination, and concept formation have been found. Undesirable physical effects include conjunctivitis, dry mouth, and lightheadedness. Emotional symptoms of anxiety, confusion, fear, and increased dependency can progress to panic or frank paranoid pathology. Marijuana can also exacerbate depression.

Chronic Physical Effects

There is increasing evidence that marijuana abuse creates at least some long-term adverse physical effects. Marijuana has been studied in relationship to human male and female fertility, cell metabolism and protein synthesis, normal cell division, and spermatogenesis. Cannabis smoke contains carcinogens similar to those in tobacco smoke, and chronic marijuana abuse may predispose the user to chronic obstructive lung disease and pulmonary neoplasm. Cannabis also increases heart rate and blood pressure, an effect that may be critical in patients with cardiovascular disease. Chronic marijuana abuse may lead to gynecomastia in men. There is some evidence of a marijuana withdrawal syndrome; however, this requires further investigation.

Nicotine

Course

Nicotine addiction frequently presents as a relapsing condition. Experimentation usually begins in adolescence. Environmental influences are important; peer tobacco use, parental tobacco use, and use of other substances are contributing factors. Relapse may be evident during periods of high stress, anxiety or maladjustment, poor social support, or low confidence. There is a strong association between alcohol and smoking. Often, alcoholic individuals can stop drinking but cannot stop smoking at the same time. Many substance treatment programs essentially ignore tobacco; however, it is a major health risk and should be addressed at some point. Factors associated with poor long-term outcomes include poor overall adjustment, low social support, environmental stress, exposure to people who continue to smoke, ignorance of the dangers of cigarette smoking, and higher use or tolerance.

Adverse Medical Sequelae

The associations between tobacco use and coronary vascular disease, chronic obstructive lung disease, lung cancer, oral cancers, and hypertension are well known. There is growing evidence of nicotine's dose-dependent link to cataracts in men. Nicotine tends to increase hepatic CYP450 drug metabolism and thus may lower the levels of medications, including neuroleptics and antidepressants, metabolized by the liver.

Inhalants

Course

Most inhalant users tend to cease their use after a relatively short period of time and may go on to abuse other psychoactive substances. There is a fairly strong association between aggressive, disruptive, and antisocial behavior and inhalant intoxication.

Adverse Medical Effects

Deaths have been reported from CNS respiratory depression, cardiac arrhythmia, and accidents. Long-term damage to bone marrow, kidneys, liver, neuromuscular tissue, and the brain have been reported. Evidence from CNS single photo emission computed tomography (SPECT) studies show the presence of abnormal perfusion in the brains of former users (Kucuk et al. 2000).

Laboratory Tests and Diagnostic Instruments

Laboratory Testing

There are many reasons to use laboratory studies in the treatment of substance use disorders, including the need to supplement an incomplete or missing drug history, to correlate clinical state with drug levels, to make a differential diagnosis, as part of follow-up or assessment, for forensic purposes, in athletic competition, to ensure public safety, for detection of relapse, and the fact that drug use declines when serious testing is in place.

Selection of Toxicological Tests and Pharmacokinetics

The choice of test requires consideration of what to sample, the half-life of the suspected substance, the significance of biotransformation of the suspected substance, and the test's sensitivity, specificity, and cost. Knowledge of the half-life of various drugs is helpful in interpreting results.

Urine Drug Screens

Urine drug screen results usually are reported as either positive or negative for any particular drug. Most routine urine screens cover the major drugs of abuse. Specificity and sensitivity are lower with thin-layer chromatography and immunoassay techniques. More sophisticated and sensitive quantitative testing with gas chromatography/mass spectrometry (GC/MS) can be done with certain drugs (e.g., marijuana) if urine from the original sample is positive. Urine drug screens generally are not useful in court because they do not answer the question of degree of intoxication. Urine drug screening should be routine in cases of coma of unknown cause, in atypical psychiatric presentations, with agitated and confused patients, in persons with known drug histories, or in those with physical evidence of substance abuse.

Blood Screening Tests

Suspicion of alcoholism or substance abuse may be heightened with corroborating laboratory evidence from blood studies (Table 4–8). Elevated serum gamma-

TABLE 4–8. Laboratory findings associated with alcohol abuse

Blood alcohol level
Positive breathalyzer
Elevated mean corpuscular volume
Elevated SGOT, SGPT, LDH
Elevated SGGT (particularly sensitive)
Elevated carbohydrate-deficient transferrin
Decreased albumin, B_{12}, folic acid (due to malnutrition)
Increased uric acid, elevated amylase, and evidence of bone marrow suppression

Note. LDH = lactate dehydrogenase; SGGT = serum gamma-glutamyl transpeptidase; SGOT = serum glutamic-oxaloacetic transaminase; SGPT = serum glutamic-pyruvic transaminase.

glutamyl transpeptidase (SGGT) is a particularly sensitive indicator of alcoholic liver disease. Alcoholic patients have a 4- to 10-times-higher rate of abnormal SGGT when they are actively drinking than when they are abstinent. As an indicator of heavy alcohol consumption, SGGT has a sensitivity of 70% and a specificity of 90%. Increased MCV is found in 45%–90% of alcoholics, whereas only 1%–5% of nonalcoholics demonstrate elevated MCVs (Holt et al. 1981) (and should be differentiated from B_{12} or folate deficiencies). Laboratory findings consistent with pancreatitis, hepatitis, bone marrow suppression, or certain types of infection may be clues to underlying alcoholism.

The detection of carbohydrate-deficient transferrin (CDT) will be increasingly important in detecting relapse as well as heavy alcohol use. The test is superior to SGGT in detecting relapse or recent heavy use (Schmidt et al. 1997). Since their pathogeneses differ, concurrent abnormal CDT and SGGT results are powerful indicators of alcohol abuse or dependence. Nonetheless, even that combination may be less sensitive than the CAGE alone when applied in the emergency department (Reynaud et al. 2001).

Other Studies

Although experience is accumulating with the use of sweat, hair, and saliva as laboratory specimens, their clinical reliability remains unknown. Breathalyzer tests are simple, do not require an invasive procedure, provide immediate results, and are widely used. Imaging studies of the liver, spleen, and brain and an EEG may be useful in the diagnosis of substance abuse as well.

Meaning of Test Results

Reaching the truth about a test result involves asking questions like the following:

- What test method was used?
- Did the assay analyze for the drug, its metabolite, or both?
- What is the cutoff threshold? (The laboratory should be called if this is unclear.)
- Was the time of sample collection close to the time of exposure?

False positives. A false positive is almost impossible when using thin-layer chromatography (TLC), because this technique has high specificity (although poor sensitivity) for both drugs and their metabolites, and because color dyes increase specificity. In radioimmunoassay (RIA) or enzyme multiplied immunoassay technique (EMIT), both sensitive tests, chemically similar compounds may cross-react, producing false positives. Immunoassays can be confirmed by chromatography, and vice versa. False-positives for cocaine can be produced by fluconazole and local anesthetics, for opioids by chlorpromazine, poppy seeds, dextromethorphan, ofloxacin, and rifampin, for cannabis by dronabinol and naproxen, and for benzodiazepines by oxaprozin (Ellenhorn 1997; Shearer et al. 1998).

False negatives. False negatives occur more easily than do false positives. Cutoffs may be too high for RIA or enzyme immunoassay (EIA). When the suspicion for substance use is strong, the clinician should repeat the test and should consult the laboratory regarding whether more sensitive drug-screening procedures, such as GC/MS, are available.

Diagnostic Instruments

No one personality causes any substance use disorder; thus, screening instruments are of high importance in identifying diagnoses.

Diagnostic Research Instruments

The need for better standardized diagnostic research instruments in psychiatry has produced structured interviews that have been helpful in identifying alcoholism in large epidemiological studies. Instruments proven to be fairly reliable in establishing DSM-IV and RDC substance abuse diagnoses include the Schedule for Affective Disorders and Schizophrenia (SADS; Endicott and Spitzer 1978), which is based on the Research Diagnostic Criteria (RDC; Feighner et al. 1972), and the Structured Clinical Interview for DSM-IV Axis II Personality Disorders (SCID-II; First et al. 1997). However, the anxiety, antisocial, and depression sections of these diagnostic instruments may be less useful in the substance-using population.

Instruments designed for research purposes sensitively measure attributes of alcohol abuse and include the Alcohol Use Inventory (AUI; Horn et al. 1986), a 17-item, self-administered questionnaire (Warburg and Horn 1985), and the Alcohol Dependence Scale (ADS; Skinner and Horn 1984), a brief 10-question instrument assessing physical dependence.

Dimensional Scales

Dimensional personality profile scales such as the Minnesota Multiphasic Personality Inventory (MMPI; Hathaway and McKinley 1967) and the Symptom Checklist–90 (SCL-90; Derogatis et al. 1973) have been useful in substance abuse populations. A markedly elevated schizophrenia scale score or evidence of male or female identity confusion may occasionally be expected. Although its usefulness is limited to augmentation of a good clinical diagnostic interview, the MMPI may be helpful in charting improvement over time. Personality subscales may improve as the acquired substance abuse–related personality attributes abate. Conversely, serious psychiatric problems may also be unmasked following drug removal. The MacAndrew Alcoholism Scale (MacAndrew 1965) is a subset scale of the MMPI that has been widely used in identifying alcoholism.

Diagnostic Screening Devices

Several instruments are available that are designed to measure various aspects of alcohol and other substance abuse. These have been found to be clinically useful in identifying psychoactive substance abuse. Two widely used alcoholism screening tests are the Michigan Alcoholism Screening Test (MAST) and the CAGE questionnaire. These tests have the advantage of being self-administered, brief screens that can point the way for further study. The MAST has a test–retest reliability in excess of .85. The sensitivities of the MAST and the SMAST are approximately .90 and .70, respectively.

Addiction Severity Index

The Addiction Severity Index (ASI, McLellan et al. 1981) has proven to be a useful instrument in the substance abuse population, particularly in treatment outcome research. The ASI establishes a dimensional scale and scoring system for the severity of need for treatment in seven major areas: 1) medical status, 2) employment–support status, 3) drug use, 4) alcohol use, 5) legal status, 6) family social relationships, and 7) psychiatric status. An ASI geared for teenagers is now available as well (Kaminer et al. 1991).

Treatment of Substance Use Disorders

Except for some overdose, intoxication, and withdrawal states that require very specific pharmacological and supportive measures, there is much overlap among the treatments for substance use disorders. Notwithstanding the standards contained in the American Psychiatric Association's "Practice Guideline for the Treatment of Patients With Substance Use Disorders" (American Psychiatric Association 1995), the American Society of Addiction Medicine's *Patient Placement Criteria for the Treatment of Substance-Related Disorders* (American Society of Addiction Medicine 1996), and the National Institute on Drug Abuse's "Principles of Drug Addiction Treatment" (National Institute on Drug Abuse 1999), facts about optimal treatment combinations await valid and well-constructed outcome research.

As in any part of the practice of medicine, the clinician's choices of treatment are enhanced by a careful history, by mental status and physical examinations, by diagnostic formulation, and by confirmatory evidence from laboratory tests and third-party sources.

Treatment of substance use disorders can be extremely difficult. Helping the patient to acknowledge that he or she has a problem and to accept help are the two most important steps in treatment. These steps are frequently difficult to take because of the nature of addictive disorders, which leads to denial, lying, and neuropathology. Most patients will wish to achieve controlled use and will have difficulty accepting abstinence as the goal for treatment. Patients frequently feel hopeless about ever achieving sustained abstinence and need to be encouraged that the goal is attainable. However, seeing others who are recovering and accumulating personal experience of increasing periods of abstinence can bring renewed hope. Harm-avoidance approaches such as needle exchange, relapse prevention, and continuance of pharmacological and psychotherapeutic modalities for patients with comorbidity can be combined with a long-range goal of abstinence.

General Principles

The following points are general principles to provide the basis for treatment of substance use disorders:

- *Case heterogeneity:* Patients are individuals and vary in terms of substance(s) used, pattern of use, clinical severity, functional impairment, secondary medical conditions, psychiatric comorbidity, strengths, vulnerabilities, and social and environmental context. Thus, no one treatment works for all individuals.
- *Phases of treatment:* Active treatment progresses; it does not all happen at once. Begin with comprehensive assessment and move to treatment of intoxication or withdrawal, development of treatment plan, and enactment of plan. The amount of time in treatment is a critical prognostic factor.
- *Comprehensive treatment:* Assessment and treatment must both take into account all aspects of the individual's life and illness. Collateral sources of information are extremely important in assessment. Coexisting psychiatric and medical conditions should be treated concurrently in an integrated manner.

Treatment programs should assess for HIV, hepatitis, tuberculosis, and other infectious diseases and should provide education to help patients to reduce their risk of contracting communicable diseases.

- *Treatment plans:* Goals should include the reduction of use, the achievement of abstinence, the reduction of relapse, and rehabilitation and recovery. Treatment status must be continually reviewed, reassessed, and updated.
- *Viewing relapse:* Relapses occur, and all treatment plans must assess for them. They do not always imply a treatment failure. Treatment must continue, but it must address the need for increased surveillance. Abstinence may sometimes seem an impossible goal (e.g., in the elderly), but reductions in morbidity and mortality follow any reduction in substance use, making the effort worthwhile (Marlatt and Gordon 1985).

Maintaining the Therapeutic Alliance

The therapeutic alliance may be one of the clinician's most important tools. Given that patients with substance problems often grew up in families with substance disorders, their propensity to have typical transference resistances to treatment and to evoke countertransference reactions in the therapist is not surprising. These countertransference reactions can either facilitate or negate treatment, depending on how they are handled (Group for the Advancement of Psychiatry 1998). Therapists who are well informed and well trained and who understand and are in touch with their own feelings are more helpful to patients and less likely to experience "burnout" (Frances and Alexopoulos 1982b). We can think of 10 attributes and attitudes that are helpful in maintain-

ing the therapeutic alliance with substance disorder patients (Table 4–9). (For further reading, see Frances et al. 2001 and Mack et al. 2001.)

TABLE 4–9. Attributes and attitudes helpful in working with patients with substance disorders

---

1. Respect for the provision of a caring and compassionate relationship
2. Informed optimism
3. The capacity to tolerate one's own anxiety, pain, frustration, and depression
4. Flexibility and open-mindedness
5. Good knowledge of general psychiatry; resourcefulness and creativity
6. Intellectual curiosity
7. Wisdom
8. Persistence and patience
9. The capacity to listen, to hear both what is and what is not said, and to act accordingly
10. Honesty and integrity (in the therapist and in the treatment team)

Potential Abuses in the Treatment of Substance Disorders

Table 4–10 presents examples of more or less subtle forms of corruption that individual therapists and treatment programs must attempt to avoid and to manage if they occur.

Abstinence

The importance of complete abstinence from all substances (except for maintenance replacement and substitution therapies) in the treatment of substance use disorders cannot be overestimated as a goal. Partial abstinence, although not ideal, does reduce morbidity and mortality and may be considered an improvement. Nevertheless, although many recovering patients want to continue using alcohol, it is impossible to identify those few for whom controlled drinking is safe. Total abstinence from all substances provides the best prognosis, and all treatment plans should include means of detecting relapse.

Recovery

The concept of abstinence is different from the concept of recovery or sobriety. Recovery implies a process in which the individual is not only abstaining from drug use but also developing a normal, balanced lifestyle, healthy self-esteem, healthy intimacy, and a sense of meaningful living. For addiction patients, recovery is a never-ending process; the term *cure* is avoided.

TABLE 4–10. Abuses in the treatment of substance use disorders

---

1. Preferential treatment influenced by VIP pressures, resulting in mistakes and splitting in the team
2. Distortions of diagnosis (e.g., underdiagnosis of alcoholism because of fears or pressure)
3. Premature discharge to save money
4. Ordering of excessive laboratory tests or diagnostic measures and overcharging for services
5. Excessively punitive or critical approaches, with constant threats of discharge for patients who are resistant to treatment
6. Breaches of confidentiality, leading to major problems in trust

---

Relapse

It is extremely important that those who have made commitments to recovery understand and anticipate relapse. Relapse is a process of attitudinal change that usually results in reuse of alcohol or drugs. In any one 12-month period after initiating abstinence, more than 90% of patients will likely use substances; of these, 45%–50%

will return to pretreatment levels of use (Armor et al. 1978). Patients need to develop coping strategies and contingency plans to thwart relapse, to minimize the extent of damage, and to quickly reestablish abstinence. The patient must understand his or her own unique set of high-risk relapse situations and avoid them or employ coping techniques so as to not relapse when offered substances. Marlatt and Gordon (1985) identified eight categories of high-risk drinking situations that could be applicable to other types of substance abuse: 1) unpleasant emotions, 2) physical discomfort, 3) pleasant emotions, 4) testing personal control, 5) urges and temptations, 6) conflict with others, 7) social pressure to drink, and 8) pleasant times with others. The degree to which a specific situation constitutes a high risk for relapse can vary among individuals or drug classes. For example, young, early abusers may be more susceptible to use when experiencing positive feelings. Older, more chronic users may relapse more often when experiencing depression or guilt. Abuse of opioids and cocaine may be more heavily tied to environmental cues than is abuse of other substances. Adolescents may be more susceptible to peer pressure compared with adults. The following are two important approaches to relapse prevention:

- *Reduction of guilt and shame:* Relapse is a fact of everyday life. Understanding this may prevent the patient's feeling that he or she has totally failed and that all is lost if a return to use occurs. Marlatt and Gordon (1985) coined the term *abstinence-violation effect* to describe the view that once use occurs, it must inevitably lead to pretreatment levels of use. Guilt, shame, a sense of lack of control, feelings of being trapped, and the absence of a contingency plan to minimize damage may escalate a return to drug use. The immediate benefits of drug use may overshadow the realization of the negative long-term consequences.

- *Practicing of social skills:* Identifying personal strengths, past coping behaviors, and environmental supports is important. Relapse prevention may require complete avoidance of high-risk situations and cues, especially in the early stages of recovery. Later on in the process, some avoidable high-risk situations can be mastered with alternative coping skills. In some situations, however, it may be advisable to avoid cues at all cost.

Predictors of Successful Treatment Outcome

Treatment outcome is better in those with high socioeconomic stability, antisocial personality, a lack of psychiatric and medical problems, and a negative family history for alcoholism. A history of Alcoholics Anonymous (AA) participation, a stable work and marriage history, and a lack of legal history are correlated with better outcome. Most studies of treatment settings have not differentiated outcome by treatment setting.

Differential Therapeutics

Choice of the most appropriate treatments for addicted patients is largely based on clinical considerations. The selection should fit the unique needs of the patient. Factors to be considered include medical and psychiatric illness, illness severity, individual patient characteristics, culture, availability of treatment resources, and awareness of the differential therapeutics of concomitant psychiatric disorders.

Matching Treatments to Patients

The finding that longer inpatient stays are more likely to lead to full or partial absti-

nence of alcohol follow-up and reduced relapse rates is untenable today. Specific efficacious treatments are needed for each patient. McLellan et al. (1997) found that matching problems to treatment services improved treatment effectiveness and led to good overall effectiveness for alcohol treatment. Patients with severe psychiatric problems did poorly regardless of modality or treatment setting. Patients with legal problems did poorly in inpatient programs. Patients with the least severe psychiatric problems did well in both inpatient and outpatient settings. Those patients with psychiatric problems in the middle range of severity usually also had employment or family problems, needed inpatient care, and improved when psychiatric services were also provided.

Treatment Settings

Inpatient Treatment

Inpatient treatment is indicated in the presence of major medical and psychiatric problems and their complications; severe withdrawal symptoms such as DTs or seizures; failure to benefit from trials of outpatient treatment; inability of family, friends, or AA members to provide an adequate social support network for abstinence; or polysubstance addiction requiring medical management. For most other patients, a trial of outpatient treatment is indicated before hospitalization unless complications are present. Most patients prefer outpatient treatment because it is less disruptive and more cost-effective than inpatient treatment. Inpatient detoxification is followed by outpatient treatment or by inpatient rehabilitation. Patients with the most severe psychiatric illness may need to be treated on a locked general hospital inpatient psychiatric unit.

Patients who complete day hospital substance abuse rehabilitation and then go on to participate in self-help groups are likely to have lower rates of alcohol and cocaine use during follow-up.

Outpatient Treatment

Outpatient treatment delivery ranges from the individual substance abuse therapist to a day or evening addiction treatment program to the primary care provider; all may utilize techniques employed in inpatient treatment programs. Indications for outpatient alcohol detoxification include high motivation and good social support, no previous history of DTs or seizures, brief or nonsevere recent binges, no severe medical or psychiatric problems or polyaddiction, and previous successful outpatient detoxifications.

Treatment of Clinical Situations

Overdose

Overdose is properly treated in the emergency department by a medical team. Table 4–11 outlines the major medical complications and treatment approaches to various drug overdoses (The Medical Letter 1996). The minimal time for observation of a suspected drug overdose should be 4 hours, because several drugs are slowly absorbed. Exact time of ingestion is often difficult to ascertain reliably. If there is good evidence that a specific drug was ingested, a call to the poison control center is suggested, and transfer to an emergency department is the next step. The first clinical task is to ensure the adequacy of airway patency, respiratory rate, blood pressure, and pulse. Outside of the hospital, cardiopulmonary resuscitation (CPR) may be lifesaving. In the medical setting, almost every overdose with loss of consciousness or any case of coma with unknown etiology should receive 50 mg

of dextrose 5% in water (D5W) and 0.4 mg of naloxone, which may need to be repeated. Prompt response provides evidence for hypoglycemia, opioid overdose, or alcohol overdose. D5W should not be given first in Wernicke's encephalopathy because glucose can further suppress thiamine stores. Other basic measures include diazepam treatment for status epilepticus and treatment of metabolic acidosis.

Elimination Methods

Our emphasis here is on general parameters (Table 4–12); the reader is referred elsewhere for technical information on elimination (Goldberg et al. 1986). Gastric emptying is appropriate only for orally ingested drugs. One absolute contraindication to gastric emptying is in cases of caustic ingestion. Dialysis is generally a heroic measure to save a life. It is more likely to be successful if the ingested drug is one that is in the plasma, minimally bound to tissue, or cleared poorly through the kidney. Dialysis has been especially valuable with alcohol, amphetamine, and aspirin overdose. Hypoperfusion is an extracorporeal blood-filtering technique similar to dialysis that uses a different type of membrane filtration. This technique has been especially useful in barbiturate overdose; it may, however, lead to thrombocytopenia.

Intoxication

Although most simple intoxication does not come to medical attention, those cases that do present to the emergency department should be screened carefully for medical problems such as subdural hematoma, meningitis, HIV, or endocarditis with embolization. Support measures include interrupting substance absorption, providing a safe environment, decreasing sensory stimulation, and allowing the safe passage of time. A calm, nonthreatening

TABLE 4–11. Management of overdose

Drug	Major complications[a]	Antidote or specific treatment	Potential lethal dose
Acetaminophen	Hepatotoxicity peaks at 72–96 hours. Complete recovery generally in 4 days, but injury worse for alcoholic patients. Mortality: 1%–2%	Acetylcysteine	140 mg/kg
Alcohol	Respiratory depression	None	350–700 mg (serum)
Amphetamines	Seizures	None; avoid neuroleptics	20–25 mg/kg
Short-acting barbiturates	Respiratory depression	None	>3 g
Long-acting barbiturates	Respiratory depression	None	>6 g
Benzodiazepine	Sedation, respiratory depression, hypotension, coma	Flumazenil reverses effects (but it may induce withdrawal in the dependent)	—
Carbon monoxide	Headaches, dizziness, weakness, nausea, vomiting, diminished visual acuity, tachycardia, tachypnea, ataxia, and seizures are all possible. Other manifestations include hemorrhages (cherry red spots on the skin), metabolic acidosis, coma, and death.	Hyperbaric oxygen	—
Cocaine	Peak toxicity 60–90 minutes after use leads to systemic sympathomimesis and seizures, acidosis. Followed by cardiopulmonary depression, perhaps pulmonary edema. Treatment of acidosis, seizures, and hypertension is imperative.	Naloxone (empirically)	—
Nonbenzodiazepine hypnotics	Delirium, extrapyramidal side effects	None	Varies with tolerance
Hydrocarbons	Gastrointestinal, respiratory, and central nervous system compromise	None	—

TABLE 4-11. Management of overdose *(continued)*

Drug	Major complications[a]	Antidote or specific treatment	Potential lethal dose
Opioids	Miosis, respiratory depression, obtundation, pulmonary edema, delirium, death	Naloxone Nalmefene helpful	Varies with tolerance
Phencyclidine/ ketamine	Hypertension, nystagmus, rhabdomyolysis	None; forced diuresis should not be attempted in cases of phencyclidine overdose with suspected rhabdomyolysis.	
Phenothiazines	Anticholinergic effects, extrapyramidal side effects, cardiac effects	Phenothiazine overdose should be monitored for 48 hours for cardiac arrhythmia. Lidocaine may be necessary for treatment of cardiac arrhythmia, norepinephrine for hypotension, sodium bicarbonate for metabolic acidosis, and phenytoin for seizures.	150 mg/kg
Salicylates	Central nervous system, acidosis	None	500 mg/kg
Tricyclic anti-depressants	Cardiac effects, hypotension, anticholinergism	None	35 mg/kg
Hallucinogens	Ring-substituted amphetamines, even lysergic acid diethylamide/mescaline, may lead to rhabdomyolysis, hyperthermia, hyponatremia	Temperature reduction, dantrolene	
Inhalants	Cardiotoxicity—arrhythmias	Cardiac monitoring	

[a]See "Overdose" for descriptions of overdose states.

TABLE 4–12. Overdose-elimination methods

Drug	Ipecac syrup	Forced diuresis	Gastric lavage	Activated charcoal	Hemodialysis	Hemoperfusion
Acetaminophen	Yes	Yes (alkaline)	Yes	No	No	No
Alcohol	No	No	Yes	Yes	Yes	No
Amphetamines	Yes	Yes (acid)	Yes	Yes	Yes	NA
Barbiturates	NA	Only for long-acting	NA	Yes	NA	Yes
Benzodiazepines	Yes	No	Yes	Repeated	NA	NA
Carbon monoxide	No	No	No	No	No	No
Cocaine	No	No	No	No	No	No
Nonbenzodiazepine hypnotics	Yes	No	Yes	Yes	NA	NA
Hydrocarbons	Yes	NA	Yes	NA	NA	NA
Opioids	NA	NA	Yes if orally ingested	NA	NA	NA
Phencyclidine/ ketamine	Only severe	Not in rhabdomyolysis (avoid in renal failure)	Only severe	Yes	NA	NA
Phenothiazines	Yes	NA	Yes	Yes	NA	NA
Salicylates	Yes	Yes (alkaline)	Yes	Yes	Yes	NA
Tricyclic antidepressants	NA	NA	NA	Repeated	No	No

Note. NA = not applicable.

manner should be employed, with clear communication and reality orientation. Attempts to reason with most intoxicated patients will not be fruitful except in cases of hallucinogen intoxication.

Alcohol

There is no proven amethystic (i.e., anti-drunkenness) agent that can hasten the cessation of alcohol intoxication. The safe passage of time is currently the only effective measure to reverse acute intoxication.

Opioids

No specific measures are generally needed to treat opioid intoxication. If a life-threatening overdose is suspected, prompt treatment with naloxone is necessary (see previous "Overdose" section and Table 4–11).

Cocaine and Amphetamines

For severe agitation, benzodiazepines such as diazepam or lorazepam may be helpful. If frank psychosis persists, low-dose haloperidol (2–5 mg) may be helpful, and the dose should be adjusted as necessary to control symptoms; however, haloperidol will also decrease the seizure threshold and should be used with caution. MAOIs should be avoided, as they inhibit the degradation of cocaine and can produce a hypertensive crisis.

Phencyclidine

The fundamental goal in treating the violence associated with PCP intoxication is to ensure the safety of all parties. When a patient becomes threatening, strong physical presence of at least five people is needed for physical containment. Benzodiazepines (e.g., diazepam) are superior to neuroleptics in the treatment of nonpsychotic agitation, but neuroleptics such as haloperidol are better for PCP toxic psychosis. Enhancement of excretion is help-ful with gastric lavage if the drug was taken orally, or by acidification of the urine if systemically administered. For lasting problems, ECT may be indicated.

Ketamine

As previously discussed, ketamine intoxication is a serious state and can include psychosis; delirium; dissociation; neuromuscular, peripheral, and CNS manifestations; respiratory dysfunction; cardiotoxicity; and movement abnormalities. In severe cases, intensive and supportive care is needed. For milder cases, monitoring for and treatment of rhabdomyolysis is necessary, and sedation with a short-acting benzodiazepine is helpful (Graeme 2000).

Cannabis

Cannabis intoxication generally needs no formal treatment. The occasional severe anxiety attacks or acute paranoid episodes can be handled with reality orientation. In rare cases, severe anxiety may warrant treatment with a benzodiazepine, and low-dose haloperidol or olanzapine may be helpful for cannabis-induced psychosis.

Hallucinogens

For most hallucinogens, patients can be "talked down" with reality orientation and reassurance. Benzodiazepines may help to provide sedation. This approach is adequate for mild cases of intoxication with MDMA; however, overdose, especially with MDMA, can lead to hyperpyrexia, dehydration, tachycardia, and even neuroleptic malignant syndrome, arrhythmias, seizures, cerebrovascular accidents, coma, disseminated intravascular coagulation, or death and should be treated in a medical setting.

The dangerous amphetamine-like state caused by ring-substituted amphetamine hallucinogens (MDMA, MDA) should be closely monitored. Supportive treatment should include hydration and monitoring for hyperpyrexia, and perhaps administration of dantrolene. The sympathomimetic state produced by LSD and mescaline calls for similar monitoring and support. Anxiety in patients experiencing these states requires reassurance and reorientation. Usually restraint can be avoided. To treat the psychological sequelae of hallucinogens, benzodiazepines are superior to typical neuroleptics.

Inhalants

Inhalant intoxication can vary in its presentation and need for active treatment. The main principle is protection of the individual from harm and from harming others; symptoms are usually time limited.

For inhalant-induced psychosis, carbamazepine has efficacy comparable to that of haloperidol but lacks haloperidol's risk of extrapyramidal side effects or lowering of seizure threshold (Hernandez-Avila et al. 1998).

Gamma-Hydroxybutyrate

GHB may be the cause of many unidentified emergency cases in which the presentation may include CNS depression, aggressive behavior, seizures, myoclonus, nystagmus, tunnel vision, incontinence, bradycardia followed by tachycardia, respiratory depression, apnea, nausea or vomiting, hypothermia, flushing, or diaphoresis. In most cases, all signs resolve in 2–7 hours and improve with supportive care (Graeme 2000).

Withdrawal

Alcohol Withdrawal/Detoxification

Setting: inpatient versus outpatient. For treatment of alcohol use disorders, patients with delirium, low IQ, Wernicke's encephalopathy, trauma history, neurolog-

ical symptoms, medical complications, psychopathology requiring medication, DTs, or alcoholic seizures or hallucinosis are probably best evaluated and treated in an inpatient setting. Polysubstance abuse, poor compliance, poor family support, inability to get from home to place of treatment, a chaotic or unstable home situation, and an environment in which the patient is continually exposed to others who abuse substances all predict a poor outcome for outpatient detoxification. Yet outpatient detoxification can be appropriate for the approximately 95% of patients with only mild-to-moderate withdrawal symptoms for whom supportive care with or without pharmacological intervention is adequate.

Treatment: pharmacological versus nonpharmacological. Pharmacological detoxification is warranted for those with significant signs of withdrawal, a clear history of severe daily dependence or high tolerance, codependence on other CNS depressants, or a past history of DTs or seizures. Medical complications (e.g., infections, trauma, metabolic or hepatic disorders) indicate pharmacological treatment. Pharmacological care enhances compliance and provides an alcohol-free interval that may help the patient commit to treatment. Nonpharmacological detoxification is for patients with mild symptoms or a withdrawal history and mild-to-moderate dependence. Close monitoring of patients for complications and adequate medical backup are needed for any detoxification.

For all patients withdrawing from alcohol, careful monitoring of vital signs, physical signs, and subjective symptoms must be done at least every 4 hours while the patient is awake (Table 4–13). Several objective rating scales and some subjective scales (e.g., Clinical Institute Withdrawal Assessment [CIWA; Sullivan et al. 1989]

TABLE 4–13. Medical workup for alcohol withdrawal

Routine lab tests	Complete blood count with differential, serum electrolytes, liver function tests including bilirubin, blood urea nitrogen, creatinine, fasting blood sugar, prothrombin time, cholesterol, triglycerides, calcium, magnesium, albumin, total protein, hepatitis B surface antigen, B_{12}, folate, stool guaiac, urinalysis, serum and urine toxic screens, chest X ray, electrocardiogram
Ancillary tests	Computed tomography, electroencephalogram, gastrointestinal series, HIV test, Venereal Disease Research Laboratory test

for those without general medical complications) are used to monitor the withdrawal state.

Pharmacological detoxification essentially involves substituting a drug that is cross-tolerant with alcohol and slowly withdrawing it from the body. For withdrawing patients with mental status alterations due to conditions other than alcohol (e.g., other substances, general medical or surgical conditions), detoxification remains a priority. Indeed, for those withdrawing from both opioids and alcohol, benzodiazepines might be given in preference to methadone in order to substitute for the alcohol while avoiding excessive sedation.

Benzodiazepine treatment. The benzodiazepines are the best medications for alcohol detoxification. With adequate benzodiazepine dosage, complications of alcohol withdrawal are extremely rare. At usual doses, benzodiazepines produce little respiratory depression and a have good margin of safety between effective dose and overdose. Long acting agents chlordiazepoxide (Librium) and diazepam (Valium) are the most commonly used benzodiazepines. Once a sufficient dose has been given, these drugs can be expected to "self-taper" without the need for further dosing. The intermediate-half-life benzodiazepines (e.g., lorazepam [Ativan], oxazepam [Serax]), which have a lesser risk of accumulation and overdose, are useful in patients with hepatic disease, delirium, dementia, or pulmonary disease or those who are older. Lorazepam also has the advantages of primarily renal clearance and reliable intramuscular absorption. Table 4–14 shows treatment protocols for benzodiazepine treatment of alcohol withdrawal. In all cases, thiamine 100 mg orally or intramuscularly, folic acid 1–3 mg, and multivitamins should also be added on a daily basis. When indicated, naltrexone or disulfiram can be added after medical workup is completed and after at least 72 hours since last ingestion of alcohol.

Outpatient detoxification for uncomplicated alcohol dependence can be accomplished with chlordiazepoxide 25 mg administered four times a day decreasing to zero within 4–5 days. Inpatient withdrawal from alcohol is accomplished with chlordiazepoxide (Librium) orally 25–100 mg four times daily, with 25–50 mg every 2 hours as needed for positive withdrawal signs. Doses can be held if the patient appears intoxicated. Both regimens should include thiamine 50–100 mg orally or intramuscularly, multivitamins, and folate 1–3 mg/day. Naltrexone is usually added 5 days after detoxification.

Adjuncts to benzodiazepines. The direct GABA agonism of benzodiazepines may be insufficient in the treatment of three important potential features of alcohol withdrawal:

TABLE 4–14. Benzodiazepine treatment for alcohol withdrawal

Outpatient	Chlordiazepoxide 25–50 mg po qid on first day, 20% decrease over 5 days, daily visits
Inpatient	1. Choose agent: diazepam or chlordiazepoxide—Give initial loading dose then monitor objectively every 2–4 hours using vital signs or Clinical Institute Withdrawal Assessment (CIWA) scale or both
	2. Give additional dose every 2–4 hours as needed: chlordiazepoxide 25–50 mg (maximum 400 mg/24 hours), diazepam 5–10 mg (maximum 100 mg/24 hours), oxazepam 15–30 mg, or lorazepam 1 mg
	3. Count total dose needed for stabilization of signs
	4. Total divided by 4 is amount to give four times a day
	5. Taper daily total about 25% over 3 days—continue no more than 10 days
	6. Use adjunctive treatments
	7. And: thiamine 100 mg 4 times a day, folate 1 mg 4 times a day, multivitamin each day, $MgSO_4$ 1 g IM every 6 hours for 2 days if seizures occur (or carbamazepine or valproate).

- *Protection from seizures:* Consideration of patients at imminent risk of withdrawal seizures or DTs should be a part of all detoxification strategies. Do not automatically provide patients with prophylactic doses of antiepileptics unless they have a history of a seizure disorder. Even those who have previously had seizures during withdrawal do not routinely receive preventive anticonvulsants. Gabapentin, which is renally excreted and which lacks significant drug–drug interactions, cognitive effects, and abuse potential, is an ideal medication for this indication. Phenytoin or magnesium sulfate (1 g four times a day for 2 days) were previously used for this purpose; valproate is the current first-line choice.

- *Alleviation of autonomic nervous system (ANS) signs:* Both β-blockers and α-blockers (e.g., clonidine) may alleviate ANS signs and symptoms that occur during withdrawal. The usual dose of propranolol is 10 mg every 6 hours as needed; that for clonidine is 0.5 mg two to three times a day as needed.

- *Treatment of psychotic features:* Neuroleptics are helpful for delirium, delu-

sions, and hallucinations. Haloperidol 0.5–2.0 mg can be administered intramuscularly every 2 hours.

Withdrawal From Other CNS Depressants

Withdrawal from benzodiazepines, barbiturates, and other depressants often requires pharmacological detoxification similar to that from alcohol. Conservative treatment requires slow withdrawal over many days or weeks. The effects of benzodiazepine withdrawal generally can be covered with chlordiazepoxide or diazepam. A standard benzodiazepine detoxification regimen is outlined in Table 4–15. If the abuse history is unreliable or difficult to ascertain, a pentobarbital tolerance test can be used to find a starting dose (Table 4–16). For most patients with benzodiazepine addictions, detoxification is best done on an inpatient unit. However, for those who have used low doses of benzodiazepines for long periods, detoxification can be accomplished on an outpatient basis with 6–12 weeks of gradual reduction, during which time added support and education are helpful. Offering the option of an as-needed dose to avoid feeling trapped is acceptable. The worst symptoms occur at the lowest doses and during the first week without any medication.

TABLE 4–15. Benzodiazepine detoxification

---

1. Establish usual maintenance dose from history or via pentobarbital tolerance test (Table 4–16).
2. Divide maintenance dose into equivalent as-needed doses of diazepam and administer first 2 days.
3. Decrease diazepam dose 10% each day thereafter.
4. Administer diazepam 5 mg every 6 hours as needed for signs of increased withdrawal.
5. When diazepam dose approaches 10% of original dose, reduce dose slowly over 3–4 days, then discontinue.

After detoxification, referral should be made to AA/NA and Al-Anon. For those who originally presented with anxiety, rebound can be expected. Nonbenzodiazepine alternatives for anxiety such as CBT, exercise, relaxation, or psychotherapy should be applied.

Some CNS depressants (e.g., glutethimide [Doriden]) are abused episodically and do not require formal detoxification. Detoxification is necessary for barbiturate or methaqualone abuse. Barbiturates can be detoxified with either a long-acting benzodiazepine or a long-acting barbiturate, such as phenobarbital.

In some cases there is a need to substitute one CNS depressant for another. Most such "cross-tapers" occur over 3 weeks and use clonazepam. In week 1, use clonazepam 0.5 mg at bedtime and the previously used drug on an as-needed basis. In week 2, discontinue the previously used drug. In week 3, reduce the clonazepam to zero. This regimen requires inpatient admission in the case of barbiturate use, polysubstance abusers, or outpatient failures. The pentobarbital tolerance test (see Table 4–16) should be used to set the initial dose when dosage of use is unknown.

Alprazolam (Xanax) is uniquely less amenable to drug substitution; breakthrough seizures have been reported despite adequate coverage with chlordiazepoxide. Alprazolam detoxification should include an estimation of daily use and a slow withdrawal over a several-week period. Clonazepam has also been successfully used in alprazolam detoxification.

Opioid Withdrawal/Detoxification

Opioid detoxification may be needed to interrupt an opioid use disorder. Patients with these disorders rarely bring themselves to treatment; rather, their presentation for treatment may coincide with a supply interruption, an overdose, or an attempt at self-detoxification. Methadone detoxification can be difficult due to its long half-life and chronic place in patients' lives.

The detoxification approach most commonly used for opioids involves the substitution and tapering of a long-acting opioid. An equivalent dose of methadone is substituted for the drug. For most heroin addicts, 20 mg of methadone is adequate as an initial dose, and the patient should be reevaluated every 2–4 hours for additional dosage. Ratios of pure drug to methadone are as follows: heroin:methadone, 2:1; morphine sulfate:methadone, 4:1; oxycodone:methadone, 12:1; meperidine:methadone, 20:1; and codeine:methadone, 50:1. Once a stable dose is achieved, methadone should be decreased over 4–14 days, usually by 5 mg/day.

Another approach is to slowly taper the abused drug over time. A low dose

TABLE 4–16.   Pentobarbital tolerance test (see clinical response 1 hour after 200-mg test dose of pentobarbital)

Patient condition after test dose	Degree of tolerance	Estimated 24-hour pentobarbital requirement (mg)
Asleep but arousable	None or minimal	None
Drowsy; slurred speech; ataxia; marked intoxication	Definite but mild	400–600
Comfortable; fine lateral nystagmus only	Marked	600–1,000
No signs of effect; abstinence signs persist	Extreme	1,000–1,200 or more: In this case, give 100 mg pentobarbital every 2 hours until mild intoxication is produced (to a maximum of 500 mg). Multiply the amount that produced mild intoxication by 4 to obtain the estimated 24-hour dose of pentobarbital, and convert this amount tophenobarbital equivalents (100 mg of pentobarbital is equivalent to 30 mg phenobarbital). Give that phenobarbital dose for 2 days, then taper by 30 mg per day or 10% per day, whichever is less.

Note.   Perform only in setting with available respiratory support. Patient should not be in an active withdrawal state, and no sedative agents should be already present in patient.

(25–50 mg) of thioridazine (Mellaril) concentrate can be added to reduce subjective discomfort.

Opioid detoxification can be accomplished with clonidine as the sole agent. Clonidine suppresses signs and symptoms of autonomic sympathetic activation during withdrawal (although it is less successful in decreasing the subjective discomfort of withdrawal). Clonidine detoxification is likely successful with mild dependence, higher motivation, and inpatient treatment. It is given orally on the first day at a dosage range of 0.1–0.3 mg three times a day (maximum 1.2 mg) and increased on the third day to 0.4–0.7 mg three times a day for a total detoxification period of 10–14 days. In appropriate patients, naltrexone can be started during the clonidine detoxification, as described in Table 4–17 (O'Connor et al. 1995). Outpatient detoxification with clonidine may be per-

formed with highly motivated patients (O'Connor et al. 1997).

Rapid and ultra rapid detoxification methods employ opioid antagonists as well as adjuncts such as clonidine, sedation, and even general anesthesia. Offered at few institutions, these approaches are used for patients in transition to antagonist therapy. Unfortunately, ultrarapid detoxification involves the increased risks of anesthesia, is performed without rehabilitation, and is expensive.

Opioid detoxification adjuncts.
Detoxification using clonidine as an adjunct should take 5–6 days; it is unlikely to help beyond 14 days. Clonidine can be administered transdermally via a patch. Use of clonidine at night should be avoided. Benzodiazepines are helpful for insomnia. At low doses (2–4 mg/day), buprenorphine is useful as a partial agonist because

TABLE 4–17. Ambulatory opioid detoxification medication protocols

9-Day clonidine detoxification ending with induction of naltrexone 50 mg/day

9-Day protocol	Day 1	Days 2, 3, and 4	Days 5, 6, and 7	Days 8 and 9
Clonidine	0.1–0.2 mg Maximum dose: 1 mg	0.1–0.2 mg po four times a day as needed Maximum dose: 1.4 mg	Taper to zero	Zero
Naltrexone				Day 8: 25 mg Day 9: 50 mg

5-Day clonidine detoxification ending with induction of naltrexone 50 mg/day

5-Day protocol	Days 1 and 2	Days 3, 4, and 5
Clonidine	Preload: 0.2–0.4 mg three times a day Maximum dose: 1.2 mg	Taper to zero
Oxazepam	Preload: 30–60 mg	Zero
Naltrexone	Day 1: 12.5 mg Day 2: 25 mg	50 mg po each day

it blocks withdrawal, but at larger doses it decreases respiratory drive. Other drugs helpful during withdrawal include dicyclomine (Bentyl) for gastrointestinal pain, nonsteroidal anti-inflammatory drugs for myalgias, and antiemetics.

Cocaine, Cannabis, Hallucinogen, and Inhalant Detoxification

There are no specific pharmacological detoxification strategies for these substances. General support measures are usually adequate (see "Intoxication" section). Benzodiazepines may help the cocaine-withdrawing patient but have the potential for abuse. Other medications that may help alleviate the symptoms of cocaine abstinence include desipramine, which is superior to lithium, carbamazepine, and other antidepressants; and perhaps buprenorphine, when opioids are part of the problem. Suicide precautions should be taken for patients who are depressed or psychotic.

Nicotine Withdrawal

A number of guidelines for smoking cessation have been produced (American Psychiatric Association 1996). Relapse, unfortunately, is the rule within 3 months. The primary care provider's assistance is essential. Compliance with the nicotine patch is greater than for nicotine chewing gum. Bupropion SR (Zyban) is helpful. Scheduled dosing may be better than as-needed dosing. A nasal spray is also available but is not first line. Neither fluoxetine nor clonidine is helpful.

Opioid Maintenance Treatment

Opioid agonist substitution is the key to maintenance treatment. Methadone is the standard, but new agents such as buprenorphine and levo-alpha acetyl methadol (LAAM) are effective as well. Given once daily, methadone provides a struc-ture for rehabilitation. Starting doses are usually 20–40 mg, depending on the degree of dependence, and may require an increase to 120 mg/day. Maintenance at doses of 70 mg and above leads to fewer relapses. NA-oriented rehabilitation approaches or therapeutic communities may exclude patients on methadone. Debate surrounds the substitution model, but the positive effects of methadone are vital to a subset of patients.

Methadone maintenance is primarily indicated for "hard-core addicts" and for patients who are HIV-positive, pregnant, or have a history of legal problems. Methadone maintenance is contraindicated for persons less than age 16 years, those scheduled to be jailed within 30–45 days, and those with a history of abusing the medicine. Methadone may be contraindicated with severe liver damage. When termination of methadone maintenance is indicated, it should be done slowly to minimize discomfort. Generally, the medication should not be decreased more than 10% per week. Below 10–20 mg of methadone, worsening subjective symptoms may necessitate a further decrease in the rate of withdrawal to 3% per week.

LAAM and buprenorphine are two agents that are used like methadone but that may be superior because they require less frequent dosing. One large study found that methadone, LAAM, and buprenorphine produced similar results in terms of both opioid and cocaine relapse prevention and patient ratings of severity of opioid craving, and also relapse on cocaine (R.E. Johnson et al. 2000). LAAM 60–100 mg three times weekly is equivalent to methadone 50–100 mg daily. LAAM may become rarely used in the coming years due to its adverse cardiovascular effects. Buprenorphine, a mixed agonist–antagonist that has lower addictive properties, fewer withdrawal symptoms, and lower overdose risk (because of its antagonist properties) relative to methadone, has proven efficacy in reducing illicit opioid use (Ling et al. 1998).

Antagonist Maintenance

As an opioid antagonist (see "Psychopharmacological Modalities"), naltrexone can lead to gradual extinction of drug-seeking behavior and to opioid relapse prevention. Naltrexone is usually given as a 25- to 50-mg/day dose over the initial 5–10 days, then gradually increased to 50–100 mg daily or thrice weekly. High rates of treatment refusal and treatment dropout limit its use to highly motivated individuals with a good prognosis who are likely to do well in a variety of treatment options and with whom there is a good treatment alliance. It is valuable in abstinence-oriented treatment.

Polysubstance Detoxification

In the case of concurrent withdrawal from CNS depressants and opioids, detoxification of the former is the priority because of the life-threatening nature of CNS-depressant withdrawal and the long duration of opioid detoxification. Also, combining benzodiazepines and methadone creates a risk for overdose and requires close patient monitoring and dose adjustments as needed. Simultaneous detoxification from different substance classes can greatly increase physical or psychological discomfort and lead to higher rates of elopement or relapse.

Treatment Modalities

The finding in other areas of psychiatry that combination psychotherapy and pharmacotherapy is more effective long term than either modality alone has been replicated in the field of substance abuse treatment, specifically with regard to the positive effects of naltrexone in the treatment of alcoholism (S.S. O'Malley et al. 1996) and the negative effects of discontinuing methadone maintenance in opioid addiction (Sees et al. 2000). Cognitive-behavioral therapy (CBT) is an effective treatment for depression in alcoholism (R.A. Brown et al. 1997).

Psychosocial Treatments

Addiction treatment is not simply "counseling." CBT, interpersonal therapy (IPT), dialectical behavior therapy (DBT), motivational interviewing, and psychodynamically oriented psychotherapy are specific modalities used for specific patients. There are data that show that psychotherapy combined with certain psychopharmacological treatments is more efficacious than either alone (Anton et al. 1999). There are some cases in which medication is essential.

Individual Therapy

Individual therapy can be conducted alone or with other modalities such as pharmacotherapy, 12-Step programs, and family and group treatments. Abstinence is an important measure of efficacy and should be considered a goal and a means to treatment success. Individual treatments are especially indicated when patients face bereavement, loss, or social disruption and have targeted problems (e.g., anxiety disorders, panic disorders).

At the outset, the therapist should concentrate on helping the patient accept that he or she has a problem and that treatment is needed to achieve and maintain sobriety. A contract with the patient should specify a clear goal of abstinence; specify treatment frequency and modality, including psychopharmacological treatment if indicated; set limits regarding the continuation of treatment despite continued substance use; and specify the participation of significant others in the patient's social network and arrangements regarding fees and time.

The Individual Psychotherapies

Psychodynamically oriented therapy. Psychodynamically-oriented individual treatment is for patients with problems relating to identity, separation and individuation, affect regulation, self-governance, and self-care. It requires psychological mindedness; a capacity for honesty, intimacy, and identification with the therapist; average to superior intelligence; economic stability; high motivation; and a willingness to discuss conflict. In such patients, expressive psychotherapy may lead to deepening of the capacity to tolerate depression and anxiety without substance use. When patients are not abstinent, however, exploratory treatment may do more harm than good, with reactivation of painful conflicts leading to further drinking and regression (Frances et al. 2001). Formal psychoanalysis is contraindicated in early phases of addictive treatment, especially in those who are actively drinking. With abstinence, however, some patients respond well to insight-oriented psychotherapy.

Cognitive-behavioral therapy. CBT has been modified for treatment of substance use disorders (Wright et al. 1993). The assumption is that abuse and dependence on substances is a learned and changeable behavior. It is a treatment in which the patient works to identify and modify maladaptive thought patterns resulting in feelings that lead to use. CBT is very helpful for relapse prevention (especially for cocaine), as well as for patients who are substance dependent or sociopathic or who suffer from primary psychiatric symptoms.

Dialectical behavior therapy. DBT is a comprehensive, behaviorally oriented treatment designed for highly dysfunctional patients who meet the criteria for borderline personality disorder. The basic challenge of the DBT therapist is in balancing validation and acceptance treatment strategies with problem-solving procedures, including contingency management, exposure-based techniques, cognitive modification, and skills training. DBT has been shown to be more effective than treatment-as-usual in treating drug abuse in women with borderline personality disorder (Linehan et al. 1999).

Motivational enhancement therapy. Motivational enhancement therapy is a directive, empathic, patient-centered counseling approach that addresses the patient's ambivalence and denial. Ideally, it will help motivate the patient and will make brief interventions more effective by taking the patient through stages of denial and cooperation. Implemented at the right stage, motivational interventions by primary care physicians can substantially contribute to recovery (Samet et al. 1996).

Group Therapy

Group therapy is frequently the principal treatment modality used for addictive disorders. Groups offer opportunities for resocialization, practicing of social skills and object relatedness, and impulse control; they foster an identity as a recovering person and facilitate acceptance of abstinence. They support self-esteem and reality testing. Groups for addicted patients have the advantage of providing a homogeneous issue—dealing with addictions—that can be used as a jumping-off point for discussing other problems that members may share.

Various group formats have been found useful in treatment of substance use disorders, including assertiveness training groups; couples groups; and groups for self-control, for ego strength, for self-concept, and for mood problems (e.g., anxiety, depression). Groups may be used to assist in problem solving, to focus on specific behavioral problems, and to help patients see that others have similar issues. They may be psychodynamically oriented, problem solving, or confrontational; they may offer couples therapy or occupational counseling. Although group modalities have primarily been used for alcohol problems, they may be especially effective for relapse prevention in cocaine dependence.

Network Therapy

Network therapy involves creation of a support group—consisting of family and friends who are not themselves addicted—that is tailored to the patient's needs. It uses a CBT approach regarding environmental triggers, makes use of community reinforcement, and emphasizes the support of the patient's social network as essential to recovery (Galanter et al. 1993). Network therapy can be a useful adjunct to individual therapy or AA.

Family Evaluation and Therapy

A family evaluation is warranted for all substance use disorder patients; information and aid from the family is crucial for both diagnosis and treatment. In many cases, it is confrontation by family members that brings the patient to treatment and helps the patient remain in treatment.

Family treatment is frequently indicated in substance abuse treatment, especially for families in which considerable support is available to the patient. Children of alcoholic parents may benefit from family evaluation and treatment. Family treatments based on the concept of "the alcoholic system" focus on the correction of dysfunctional patterns of interactional behavior within the family and

measure success not only by the achievement of abstinence but also by improvement in the family's level of functioning.

Self-Help

Every clinician needs to be thoroughly familiar with the work of the 12-Step self-help programs: AA, Al-Anon, NA, Cocaine Anonymous, Gamblers Anonymous, and Overeaters Anonymous (this includes having personally attended meetings of both AA and Al-Anon so as to be in touch with their patients' experiences). There is a small but growing body of evidence documenting the efficacy of AA. Self-help may also be very important for cocaine abuse and dependence. Peer-led groups have been helpful as well (Galanter 2000).

The major message of AA is that people with alcohol problems can help one another achieve sobriety through a spiritual program that includes recognition of alcoholism as an illness, acceptance of one's powerlessness over alcohol, and dependence on some source of change beyond the self. Al-Anon is a program parallel to AA that includes self-help for the family. Other family-oriented programs include Alateen, for teenage users and teenage children of alcoholics, and groups for adult children of alcoholics (see Mack et al. 2001).

How It Works

Although a 12-Step program is frequently recommended in conjunction with a variety of other treatment approaches, for many patients the program may suffice as the sole treatment for a substance use disorder. On average, members attend approximately 4 meetings per week, although in the early stages many attend daily meetings for 3 months. Patients with multiple addictions may attend several different 12-Step programs or groups.

A system of sponsorship of new members by veteran AA attendees and the creation of a support network of exchanged telephone numbers are important aspects of AA membership. AA provides an opportunity for people to experience relatedness, gain structure, test values, exercise judgment, practice honesty, find acceptance, and regain hope. Subgroups have developed for alcoholic persons who are gay or lesbian, physicians, adult children of alcoholics, atheists or agnostics, HIV-positive, or dually diagnosed. Meetings can be found in most major cities throughout the world and are essential for alcoholics who travel. Information about AA is easily obtainable from the Online Intergroup of Alcoholics Anonymous (http://www.aa-intergroup.org/) or the official AA web site (http://www.alcoholics-anonymous.org).

Referrals to 12-Step Programs

The therapist may take an active role in referring patients to 12-Step programs as well as in monitoring and interpreting resistances to regular attendance. The physician can have the patient call AA directly from his or her office or may make the call for the patient in order to select a meeting. Clinicians should address concerns or negative responses experienced by patients in their first AA meetings. Initially patients may be socially avoidant or may have difficulty understanding AA. Patients who react negatively to the spirituality elements of AA or who feel criticized or unaccepted in AA because of their use of psychiatric medications or their polysubstance abuse will need support. Patients should be encouraged to obtain an AA sponsor.

Counseling

Certified alcohol and drug addiction counselors have increasingly played prom-

inent roles in substance treatment programs. They are involved in every phase of treatment, including evaluation, psycho-education, individual and group counseling, and aftercare. For relapse prevention, counselors frequently provide support, advice, and valuable information regarding treatment and 12-Step programs.

Education

Most programs include education about the effects of alcohol and drugs on the abusing person and on the family, treatment alternatives, and relapse prevention. Education reduces fear, guilt, and shame; supports the medical model; and provides hope. Lectures, discussion groups, films, books, and homework assignments are an important part of the work of treatment and help keep patients productively engaged during treatment.

Psychopharmacological Modalities

In the treatment of substance use disorders, medications may be prescribed for detoxification, for treatment of comorbid psychiatric disorders or of complicating neuropsychological and medical disorders, for aversive treatment (e.g., disulfiram in alcoholic patients), for attenuation of craving or euphoria (e.g., naltrexone), or for psychological ego support. Generally, these medications are used as adjuncts to psychosocial treatment and education. Physicians should have a clear understanding of the differential diagnosis and natural history of substance abuse disorder and of the limitations of medication, as well as knowledge of drug–drug interactions and medication side effects.

Naltrexone

The superior efficacy of naltrexone (ReVia) for alcohol relapse prevention is well documented (Volpicelli et al. 1992). It is administered at 50 mg/day for 3 months. In fact, opioid μ-receptor antagonists reduce alcohol use in general. This is likely by blocking release of dopamine in the nucleus accumbens.

Naltrexone's primary indication is opioid relapse prevention, for which the usual dose is 50 mg/day. As an opioid-receptor antagonist, it causes withdrawal symptoms in persons with opioid intoxication. Because of these effects, many opioid detoxification protocols employ slow induction of naltrexone in conjunction with outpatient clonidine treatment (summarized in Table 4–17).

Methadone and Levo-Alpha Acetyl Methadol (LAAM)

Methadone has a dose-dependent effect on concurrent use of opioids and cocaine. High doses (65 mg/day) may be the most effective. A stable dose need not be altered except in the case of changes in pharmacokinetics. LAAM is a long-acting opioid agonist with used, like methadone, for maintenance. It has a longer half-life than methadone and thus may have the advantage of needing to be taken only 3 times a week. A warning about the arrhythmogenic properties of LAAM from the U.S. Food and Drug Administration has been followed by guidelines for cardiac monitoring of patients taking the drug.

Buprenorphine

Buprenorphine (Buprenex/Subutex) is a mixed opioid μ agonist–antagonist that has been demonstrated to be more effective than placebo in the treatment of opioid dependence (R.E. Johnson et al. 1995). Buprenorphine shows promise for both opioid detoxification and opioid maintenance. Suboxone is a buprenorphine–naloxone 4:1 combination sublingual tablet. The naloxone in Suboxone discourages illegal injection street use because it precipitates withdrawal. Buprenorphine's long duration of action means that it can be given three times a week instead of daily. A number of strategies for detoxification from buprenorphine have been established (Bickel et al. 1997).

Disulfiram

Disulfiram (Antabuse) is an aversive treatment used as a medication adjunct in the treatment of recovering alcoholic individuals. It enhances motivation for continued abstinence by making the "high" unavailable, thus discouraging impulsive alcohol use. Disulfiram is a potent reversible inhibitor of aldehyde dehydrogenase, an enzyme that metabolizes acetaldehyde, the first metabolite of alcohol. A buildup of acetaldehyde results in toxicity, which consists of nausea, vomiting, cramps, flushing, and vasomotor collapse. Disulfiram has relatively mild side effects, including sedation, halitosis, skin rash, and temporary impotence. More-serious side effects—such as peripheral neuropathy, seizures, optic neuritis, and psychosis—occur only rarely. Disulfiram appears to have a catecholamine effect, which may contribute to the alcohol reaction and make its use contraindicated with MAOI use. It also may inhibit the metabolism of other medications, including anticoagulants, phenytoin, and isoniazid, leading to higher-than-expected serum levels of these medications. In addition, disulfiram has adverse interactions with cough syrups. Its use should be avoided in patients with hepatic disease, peripheral neuropathy, renal failure, and cardiac disease, as well as in pregnancy. Other contraindications include medical conditions that would be greatly exacerbated by a disulfiram–alcohol reaction, such as liver disease, esophageal varices, heart disease, heart failure, emphysema, and peptic ulcer disease. Disulfiram should be avoided by anyone who is likely to become pregnant. Psychiatric contraindications include psychosis and severe depression. Disulfiram can exacerbate psychosis; depressed suicidal patients may deliberately precipitate a disulfiram reaction.

Initial doses of disulfiram are 250–500 mg/day. It can be administered in an oral suspension. Doses can be adjusted downward to 125 mg if sedation or other side effects are excessive or in those with relative contraindications. Patients should be informed about the rationale of disulfiram use, the disulfiram–alcohol reaction, and common side effects.

Although there has not been convincing evidence that disulfiram use affects long-term outcomes globally, disulfiram has been shown to be useful in certain subtypes of alcoholism, often when it can be administered by a patient's significant other. Socially stable alcoholic adults and affluent, married, less-sociopathic individuals with compulsive tendencies have the best results with disulfiram.

Lithium

Lithium is an integral component in the treatment of substance use disorders in the presence of an underlying comorbid primary bipolar or cyclothymic disorder. Its use may dampen or abort extreme mood swings or indirectly affect substance intake. Patients with lithium-responsive depression have a propensity to abuse alcohol or cocaine. Lithium has also been associated with decreased subjective experience of intoxication, exacerbation of deficits in cognitive and motor function during intoxication, and reduced alcohol consumption. Caution should be exercised when prescribing lithium to those who are actively abusing substances or who demonstrate poor compliance with treatment. Such patients need to be hospitalized to ensure abstinence and to manage titration of proper doses. Lithium has no documented usefulness in uncomplicated alcohol abuse or dependence. For

adolescents with bipolar disorder and secondary substance dependence, lithium is efficacious for both disorders (Geller et al. 1998).

Antidepressants

Antidepressants do not directly alter substance use disorders but are important adjuncts in the treatment of patients with primary mood disorders. Determination of which antidepressant to use follows consideration of the type of depression present and the side-effect profile of the medications, as well as recognition that judgment, impulse control, and cognition may be impaired in alcoholic patients in early recovery. Extreme caution should be used when prescribing MAOIs for depression in alcoholic patients, especially because wine contains tyramine. There is evidence that fluoxetine is not helpful for primary cocaine dependence. Venlafaxine, a broad-spectrum antidepressant, may be a safe, well-tolerated, rapidly acting, and effective treatment for patients with a dual diagnosis of depression and cocaine dependence.

Dopamimetics

Although few data support their effectiveness, dopamimetic agents are commonly used to treat cocaine dependence and withdrawal. It had previously been hypothesized that because cocaine's effects are dopamine-related, and because dopamine depletion is associated with cocaine craving, a dopamimetic substance such as bromocriptine might diminish cocaine craving. However, studies have failed to justify such application of bromocriptine, amantadine, or pergolide (a mixed D_1–D_2 agonist) (Malcolm et al. 2000).

Clonidine

Clonidine's use in opioid detoxification was discussed earlier (see "Opioid Withdrawal/Detoxification" subsection earlier in this chapter). Clonidine has also been reported to be helpful in alcohol withdrawal and in patients with hallucinogen persisting perception disorder (Lerner et al. 1998).

Valproate

Valproate is used in the treatment of bipolar disorder and in detoxification from alcohol. Moderate doses of valproate in alcoholic patients without significant hepatic disease do not cause significant adverse effects on white blood cell count, platelet count, or liver transaminase level (Sonne and Brady 1999). Liver function should be established prior to onset of therapy with this medicine.

Carbamazepine

Although previously felt to be helpful for symptoms of cocaine withdrawal, more recent studies have failed to find carbamazepine to be effective for this indication (Cornish et al. 1995). However, it may effectively treat ketamine intoxication.

Gabapentin

Gabapentin had been heralded as a major advance in alcohol relapse prevention, but this promise has not been realized in studies. It is efficacious as a mood stabilizer or an anticonvulsant and is useful in alcoholism because it is not hepatically metabolized, does not bind to plasma proteins, does not induce liver enzymes, and is renally eliminated without any metabolism.

Adrenergic Blockers

Using β-blockers to reduce β-adrenergic signs in alcohol withdrawal is controversial and not routinely advocated. β-Blockers are contraindicated in cocaine intoxication and withdrawal.

Neuroleptics

Neuroleptics have no place in the treatment of primary alcoholism or in alcohol detoxification. They lower the seizure threshold and carry the long-term risk of tardive dyskinesia. However, they can be very helpful in managing psychosis across a wide spectrum of toxic drug reactions. Neuroleptics can be used adjunctively with benzodiazepines in the treatment of delirium, including DTs. They are the primary treatment of choice in alcohol hallucinosis. Among the newer neuroleptics, olanzapine appears to be as effective as haloperidol in the treatment of cannabis-induced psychotic disorder and is associated with a lower rate of extrapyramidal side effects (Berk et al. 1999).

Benzodiazepines

Benzodiazepines are the treatment of choice for alcohol, barbiturate, or benzodiazepine detoxification. In fact, benzodiazepines are generally contraindicated in any substance use disorder except when used for detoxification, for manic patients acutely, or very selectively in compliant abstinent patients with anxiety disorders in whom other treatments have failed.

A common clinical dilemma involves the substance use disorder patient who has an underlying anxiety disorder, often in conjunction with high-dose benzodiazepine abuse. These patients may experience a relapse of their anxiety disorder symptoms following detoxification from CNS depressants. Such an anxiety disorder is often difficult to distinguish from other underlying disorders, anxiety symptoms associated with chronic subacute withdrawal, reactive fear, and anxiety about withdrawal. The impulse to relieve this suffering may lead clinicians to reinstate addictive substances, which can lead to a poor outcome. Effective use of other, perhaps more specific, treatment modalities, including selective serotonin reuptake inhibitors (SSRIs), desipramine, or MAOIs for panic and a neuroleptic for psychotic disorders or SSRIs, buspirone, gabapentin, or adrenergic blockers for generalized anxiety may be helpful.

Buspirone

Buspirone, an anxiolytic with no CNS depressant activity or abuse potential, is a useful adjunct in the treatment of generalized anxiety or transient anxiety in some substance abusers. However, it has the disadvantage of slow onset of efficacy (up to 3 weeks) and is thus of little use in transient anxiety disorders.

Acamprosate

Acamprosate is a new medication, not yet approved for use in the United States, that has great promise in alcohol relapse prevention (Kiefer et al. 2003). It crosses the blood–brain barrier, is chemically similar to amino-acid neurotransmitters, and acts at the NMDA receptor to reduce withdrawal's glutamatergic hyperactivity. It is dose dependent and has no abuse potential. Giving acamprosate to those dependent on alcohol will not lead to an acute withdrawal syndrome. Acamprosate is not metabolized but rather is renally excreted and should be given with caution to those with renal disease. A starting dose is 2–3 g/day in divided doses, and common side effects include diarrhea and headache.

Ondansetron

Ondansetron, a selective 5-HT$_3$ receptor antagonist, has shown promise in reducing overall alcohol intake, specifically among those with type I alcoholism (see Cloninger et al. 1988), and in diminishing the subjective positive effects of alcohol (B.A. Johnson et al. 2000). Its widespread use awaits further study.

Special Issues in Treatment

Rehabilitation

The rehabilitation model combines self-help, counseling, education, relapse prevention, group treatment, a warm and supportive environment, and emphasis on a medical model geared toward reducing stigma and blame. Most treatment units are highly structured, insist on an abstinence goal, and offer lectures, films, and discussion groups as part of a complete cognitive and educational program. Patients frequently become active 12-Step members and are encouraged to continue in aftercare.

Portions of these treatment components are often done in halfway houses in outpatient settings, and hospital stays of 3–12 days are common. Longer stays are indicated for adolescents and for patients with greater severity of illness, dual diagnoses, or severe medical problems.

The rehabilitation model emphasizes the provision of opportunities for patients to practice social skills and gain control over impulses, using the highly structured program as an auxiliary superego. Self-honesty and expression of feelings are encouraged. The program promotes the use of higher-level defenses (e.g., intellectualization) and actively confronts more primitive defenses (e.g., denial, splitting, projection), especially when these defenses are used in relation to the issue of abstinence (Frances and Alexopoulos 1982a).

Aftercare

On discharge from an inpatient or an organized outpatient program, aftercare must be part of the follow-up plan. Referral to a 12-Step program often complements other treatment, although self-help groups may suffice for some faithfully attending individuals. We recommend at least 2 years of follow-up care after the start of abstinence.

Treatment and Consultation in the Medical Setting

It has been estimated that 25%–50% of general hospital admissions are related to complications of substance use (Moore et al. 1989). A high index of suspicion may assist the health care provider in detecting hidden substance use disorders. There may be further advantages in confronting the addictive process during a medical crisis, when denial may be lessened or can be easily counteracted by irrefutable medical evidence. Alcoholism may be diagnosed on the basis of its associated medical problems, which include liver disease, pancreatitis, anemia, certain types of pneumonia, delirium, dementia, gastric ulcers, esophageal varices, tuberculosis, or symptoms mimicking psychiatric syndromes.

Admission Workup

Detailed alcohol and substance histories should be taken on admission from every patient in the general hospital setting. Information should be gathered in a straightforward manner in concert with the rest of the medical history. Health professionals should be knowledgeable regarding the components of a basic alcohol and substance history (Table 4–18). The history should include the type of liquor or the specific drug, the amount, the pattern or frequency of use, and time of last use; such historical information may be very important in distinguishing various organic mental states. The route of administration (oral, intravenous, or via pulmonary inhalation) may have important health consequences. Third-party sources

such as family or friends may be necessary to obtain crucial information. The psychoactive substance abuse history should involve a systematic review of all the major drug classes, including prescription medication. Often, patients will not consider a particular substance a "drug."

TABLE 4–18. Components of a basic alcohol and substance use history

Chief complaint

Current medical signs and symptoms

Substance abuse review of systems for all substances of abuse

Dates of first use, regular use, longest period of sobriety and overall life condition during sobriety, pattern, amount, frequency, time of last use, route of administration, circumstances of use, reactions to use

Medical history, medications, HIV and tuberculosis status

History of past substance abuse treatment, response to treatment, history of complications secondary to substances

Psychiatric history

Family history of psychiatric disease and substance use

Legal history

Object relations history

Personal and social history

Review of collected data (chart, family, primary care physician)

A history of early-morning tremors or shakes, a subjective need for a drink to calm the nerves, elevated pulse and blood pressure, or a known past history of alcohol-related seizures or DTs should signal the need for pharmacological detoxification. Polysubstance abuse may mask underlying physical dependence on one prominent psychoactive substance (e.g., opioids in "speedballing" or "hits," alcohol dependence secondary to cocaine addiction). Past history of hospitalization for motor vehicle accidents, accidental injuries, or substance-related violence should be sought in addition to any history of treatment for alcohol or other substance abuse problems.

Psychiatric Consultation in the General Hospital

Consultation requests from general hospital departments may involve straightforward requests for a substance abuse evaluation or more cryptic requests for evaluation of brain pathology, mood disorders, or acting-out behavior. Often, the patients for whom an evaluation is being requested are perceived as being manipulative, demanding, and unappreciative. In reality, they can indeed present as such. It is important not to disavow the staff's real feelings but rather to provide a framework for an understanding of the addictive process that can make those feelings meaningful and tolerable. In affective illnesses, the presence of overwhelming affects may focus attention away from a concomitant addictive process. In cases of organicity, important historical information may simply be forgotten. Table 4–19 offers general guidelines for approaching this patient population.

Each consultation request should be reviewed to clearly ascertain what is being requested. Frequently, such review requires a call to the referring physician. Reviewing the medical chart in detail is essential, not only to elicit important information about admitting signs and symptoms, third-party statements, and mental status, but also to piece together divergent clues of substance abuse in a fresh manner. Pertinent laboratory work, X rays, EEG, CT scans, and the like should be reviewed. Suggestions for additional laboratory work (e.g., magnesium levels in a patient with a history of DTs) should be made.

If the consultation request is for assessment of a substance abuse problem, that purpose should be clearly stated to

TABLE 4–19.   General considerations in approach to consultation

Have a high suspicion for drug abuse and obtain collected data

Obtain serum and urine toxicology screens as soon as possible to admission

Know general principles of detoxification and its differential therapeutics

Realize that detoxification often needs to be tailored to individual medical patients

Recall that when treating polysubstance dependence, sedative withdrawal occurs first

Use challenge tests or estimate conservatively when considering initial detoxification dose

Recognize drug–drug interactions and effects of medications on mental status examination

Always differentiate psychopathology, substance-induced disorders, and medical disorders

the patient early in the interview. The referring physician can be asked to join the interview if that seems appropriate. The consultant's impressions and recommendations should be prominent and the focus of the report. Often this message is the only one read.

Treatment Planning

Specific recommendations for treatment range from inpatient substance abuse or psychiatric treatment to outpatient substance abuse treatment to no further intervention. Often, active treatment must be postponed until the acute medical problems are stabilized. For patients exhibiting early abuse patterns, simple counseling, education, and appropriate reassurance may be all that is necessary. If a patient is motivated and has no marked medical or psychiatric complications, a less-serious abuse pattern, and little prior treatment exposure, outpatient referral is preferable. Inpatient psychiatric treatment may be indicated when major psychiatric illnesses (e.g., psychosis, major depression) require treatment or if suicidal or homicidal ideation is present. Transfer to an inpatient rehabilitation unit, when indicated, should be a direct transfer from the hospital to the treatment facility. All detoxification regimens should be clearly and explicitly spelled out.

Making the Referral

It is often best that the patient make the initial call to a rehabilitation or detoxification program. It is also important that all such calls be made while in the hospital setting and that appointments be scheduled before discharge. In cases in which substance abuse treatment facilities are connected with a general hospital, in-house contact is advised, as is attendance at in-house meetings, such as AA, when feasible.

Other Factors of Importance During Consultation

Drug Interactions

Special attention should be given to drug interactions in the general hospital setting because some psychoactive drugs adversely interact with prescribed medications. Alcohol interacts with other medi-

cations (Table 4–20). It has a bimodal effect on the CYP system. Initially, alcohol can inhibit the metabolism of other drugs, thus increasing serum levels of oral anticoagulants, diazepam, and phenytoin. After chronic use, however, alcohol can induce CYP enzymes, leading to decreased levels of these medications. Chlorpromazine, chloral hydrate, and cimetidine all inhibit alcohol dehydrogenase. Finally, alcohol increases the absorption of diazepam and increases the potency of all CNS depressants.

Management of Pain

A major concern of staff in treating substance abuse patients in the general hospital setting is iatrogenic contributions to addiction. This is most notable in intravenous drug users for whom pain medication is truly required. Many staff members are schooled to be very cautious and suspicious when prescribing pain medication for these patients, yet excessive caution can lead to undermedication. When offensive patients evoke too much rage and anger in treatment personnel, those staff members may be driven unconsciously to punish the patients by undermedicating them.

TABLE 4–20. Medication interactions with alcohol

Disulfiram	Flushing, diaphoresis, vomiting, confusion
Oral anticoagulants	Increased effect with acute intoxication, decreased effect after chronic use
Antimicrobials	Minor disulfiram reaction
Sedatives, hypnotics, narcotics, antihistamines	Increased central nervous system depression
Diazepam	Increased absorption
Phenytoin	Increased anticonvulsant effect with acute intoxication; alcohol intoxication or withdrawal may lower seizure threshold after chronic alcohol abuse
Salicylates	Gastrointestinal bleeding
Chlorpromazine	Increased levels of alcohol, lowered seizure threshold
Monoamine oxidase inhibitors	Adverse reactions to tyramine in some alcoholic beverages

In certain abusers, even larger-than-normal doses of pain medications are indicated because of tolerance. Each patient should be evaluated carefully, looking at past history, pattern of abuse, personality, and physical pathology. In some cases, the staff member should voluntarily remove him- or herself from the patient's care before a spiral develops that will lead to the abandonment of the patient.

Chronic pain patients do have a high risk for abusing drugs. Maintaining continuity of care and promoting realistic expectations are prominent treatment goals for such patients. It is necessary to avoid intramuscular medication and as-needed dosage scheduling and to ensure adequate coverage (i.e., selection of medications that have adequate half-lives for dosage scheduling, appropriate administration, and the right medication for type of pain) (Bouckoms and Hackett 1997).

Burn Patients

Alcohol and other substance use are risk factors for burns. In addition, preexisting substance use is associated with a worse prognosis for the burn patient. Alcohol is an independent predictor of death in such patients (McGill et al. 1995). This population requires important attention from both psychiatric and substance use standpoints in coping with present loss and in treatment planning for the future.

Organ Transplants

Mental health personnel are increasingly asked to assess patients' psychological readiness to receive organ transplants. Active alcoholism is considered a contraindication for liver transplantation, although controversy surrounds this issue. The evaluation of recovering alcoholics is a complicated issue. Care must be taken not to discriminate against a stable recovering individual who might well be a good candidate for transplant. Careful evaluation and application of certain criteria may diminish the risk of relapse. Such criteria include at least 6 months of sobriety from alcohol, no other active substance abuse, and good family support. Organ and patient survival among selected recovering alcoholic patients who receive transplants is as good as those for patients who receive a liver for non–alcohol-related diseases (Berlakovich et al. 1994). For patients on methadone maintenance in need of hepatic transplant, the state-of-the-art practice is to not discontinue the methadone (Koch and Banys 2001).

Prevention of Substance Use Disorders

Efforts at interdiction, education, and social planning in law enforcement have led to few changes in the magnitude of the problem of substance abuse. It is difficult to achieve changes in attitudes toward alcohol and drugs, and changes in drinking behavior have been modest or difficult to demonstrate. Advances in our understanding of addictions in terms of description, etiology, pathogenesis, course, and epidemiology provide hope that prevention strategies may be successful.

Along with interdiction, primary prevention efforts have focused on school- and work-based education programs and mass media campaigns. "Life skills" training is one model that focuses on value-clarification abilities, decision making, and drug refusal (Botvin et al. 1995). Other student-focused programs include education and groups (especially targeting children of alcoholics); treatment or referral for abusing students; early screening of students who evidence behavioral changes; and work with parents and community groups. Self-help groups such as AA, Al-Anon, Alateen, Adult Children of

Alcoholics, and Mothers Against Drunk Driving provide support and distribute educational materials.

Treatment Approaches to Specific Populations

Women

There are differences between sexes in the epidemiology, course, treatment, and stigma of substance use disorders. In the United States, the ratio of alcoholism in males compared with females is 3:1. This ratio is equal to that for most other substances, with the exception of prescription drugs, which women disproportionately abuse (Warner et al. 1995). Women suffer greater secondary medical morbidity from substance abuse than do men (Ashley et al. 1977). The dangers of fetal alcohol syndrome and HIV transmission add to the clinical significance of substance use disorders in women.

Women more frequently present with coexisting panic, anxiety, mood, and eating disorders than do men (Kessler et al. 1995). Female alcohol abusers also have a later onset of abuse, have a more rapid progression of abuse, abuse less total alcohol, and have higher rates of comorbid psychopathology; furthermore, in comparison with male alcohol abusers, they are more likely to have a "significant other" who is also a substance abuser. They also tend to have a history of sexual or physical abuse and to date the onset of their substance use disorder to a stressful event.

Women with alcohol use disorders are more likely to attempt and less likely to complete suicide than are men with these disorders. Among these women there is a higher mortality rate by all causes. For cocaine use disorders, the disease progresses more rapidly in women than in men, women's use is less than that of men,

women more often have a spouse who is also an abuser, and there is a greater likelihood of a suicide attempt.

Biological Effects

Compared with men, women have a higher blood alcohol level per pound of body weight per alcoholic drink; in addition, blood alcohol level effects in women fluctuate over the course of the menstrual cycle (the perimenstrual time is often marked by heavier consumption). In addition to having a lower tolerance for alcohol, women tend to have a more "telescoped" course of the chronic effects of excessive drinking, including cirrhosis of the liver, compared with men. These differences may be partially explained by the fact that men have greater amounts of alcohol dehydrogenase in the gastric mucosa. Thus, alcohol's neurotoxic effects may be greater in women than in men (Hommer et al. 2001).

Treatment Issues

Treatment for women must be tailored to address pathophysiological differences and to provide a perception of safety. Special programs and residences for women in rehabilitation programs are beneficial because women in traditional treatment programs may feel intimidated and outnumbered by men, especially when talking about sexual abuse and sexual issues. Special treatment considerations include watching especially closely for sedative–hypnotic dependence, anxiety disorders and depression, and hypersensitivity to stigma; helping women deal with abusive spouses; and instilling an awareness of fetal alcohol and drug effects. Having contact with recovered alcoholic women role models and working with female professionals may also facilitate improved self-esteem.

Inpatient treatment poses special problems for young mothers, and few programs exist in which women can have their children with them during hospitalization. There are also increased fears of loss of custody in alcoholic women and increased needs for child care services. Women frequently have economic problems that can make it more difficult for them to obtain good treatment, and women with alcoholism are often married to addicted men, who may not facilitate—or who may actively hinder—their efforts to achieve recovery. General guidelines for the care of addicted women are presented in Table 4–21 (Blume 1998).

Problems Secondary to Addiction in Women

General medical conditions.   Women who abuse substances are at risk of developing a number of specific general medical conditions, and, compared with men, when they develop such secondary conditions (e.g., alcoholic cardiomyopathy, cirrhosis) (Urbano-Marquez et al. 1995), the conditions progress more quickly and have higher morbidity, a phenomenon known as "telescoping." Women alcohol abusers are at greater risk than nonabusers of developing breast cancer (Singletary and Gapstur 2001). Thus, female substance use disorder patients need comprehensive primary care assessment (Table 4–21).

Sexual and reproductive function. Sexual function is affected by almost all drugs of abuse. Despite its reputation, alcohol is not an aphrodisiac; sexual function improves with sobriety (Gavaler et al. 1995). Heroin disrupts ovulation. The treatment of neonates for methadone withdrawal is a common procedure; thus, methadone use is not an absolute contraindication to pregnancy (H.L. Brown et al. 1998).

Fetal alcohol syndrome.   The incidence of fetal alcohol syndrome is approxi-

TABLE 4–21.   Special considerations in women's substance use treatment

Psychiatric assessment for comorbid disorders; date of onset for each (primary/secondary)
Attention to past history and present risk of physical and sexual assault
Assessment of prescription drug abuse/dependence
Comprehensive physical examination for physical complications and comorbid disorders
Need for access to health care (including obstetric care)
Psychoeducation to include information on substance use in pregnancy
Child-care services for women in treatment
Parenting education and assistance
Evaluation and treatment of significant others and children
Positive female role models (among treatment staff; friends, self-help)
Attention to guilt, shame, and self-esteem issues
Assessment and treatment of sexual dysfunction
Attention to the effects of sexism in the previous experience of the patient (e.g., underemployment, lack of opportunity, rigid sex roles)
Avoidance of iatrogenic drug dependence
Special attention to the needs of minority women, lesbian women, and those in the criminal justice system

mately 1–3 in 1,000 live births in the United States overall and as high as 1 in 100 births in some Eskimo villages (Institute of Medicine 1995). Typical signs of fetal alcohol syndrome include low birthweight, growth deficiency with delayed motor development, mental retardation and learning problems, and other, less severe fetal alcohol behavioral effects. No safe alcohol level during pregnancy has been established, and dangers are dose dependent.

Children and Adolescents

The prevalence of substance disorders is rising, the age at first use is dropping, and the morbidity and mortality of youth with substance use disorders is increasing. Substance abuse can interfere with natural growth and normal interaction and development, including relationships with peers, performance in school, and attitudes toward law and authority, and can have both acute and chronic systemic effects.

It is difficult to diagnose substance dependence in adolescents because of the reduced likelihood of observing signs and symptoms of withdrawal, which typically occur later in addiction. Compared with adult substance abusers, adolescents are less likely to report withdrawal symptoms, have shorter periods of addiction, and may recover more rapidly from withdrawal. Specific practice parameters have been developed for the treatment of substance use disorders in children and adolescents (Bukstein 1997).

Epidemiology

According to the latest figures from the Substance Abuse and Mental Health Services Administration (SAMHSA) National Household Survey, there was a slight decrease in drug abuse by adolescents (12–17 years old) during 1997, 1998, and 1999, from 11.4% to 9.9% to 9.0%, respectively. This trend reversed, going from 9.7% in 2000 to 10.8% in 2001 (Office of Applied Studies 2002). The trends may depend on the drug: Data from the 2002 Monitoring the Future study found statistically significant reductions in alcohol use among eighth, tenth, and twelfth graders (Johnston et al. 2003). Overall, this follows a stark increase in abuse that began in 1992, when the rate of past-month usage among youth ages 12–17 years reached a low of 5.3%

(from a high of 16.3% in 1979). Furthermore, the age at which drugs or alcohol is first used has dropped, such that as of 1994, more than 50% of students in grade 6 reported having tried alcohol or other illicit substances (P.M. O'Malley et al. 1995). Racial and ethnic differences are apparent among child and adolescent substance abusers: in one report, African American students had the lowest rates of illicit substance use in general, Hispanic students had the highest usage rates at grade 8, and white students had the highest at grade 12. However, Hispanic adolescents were found to use more cocaine, heroin, and steroids at grade 12 compared with the other groups (Bachman et al. 1991). Thus, the problem is wide, growing, and complex.

Early Detection in Adolescents

Signs of adolescent drug use include a drop in school performance, irritability, apathy, mood change (including depression), poor self-care, weight loss, oversensitivity to questions about drinking or drugs, and sudden changes in friends. Substance use screening in adolescents should include routine medical examinations before camp or in school. A younger age at onset of addiction is associated with a poorer outcome, including alcohol-related harm (physical damage, illness, or violence), and a greater potential for clinically significant use (DeWit et al. 2000).

Contributing Factors

Peer group, school environment, age, geography, race, values, family attitudes toward substance abuse, risk-seeking temperament, and biological predisposition are all contributing factors to adolescent substance abuse. Nonusing adolescents are more likely to describe close relationships with their parents than are users. They are more likely to be comfortably dependent on their parents and are closer to their families than are users, who report themselves as independent and distant. Users more frequently indicate that they do not want to be like their parents and do not feel they need their parents' approval; they may disavow a desire for affection from their parents. Frequently, adolescents with substance abuse problems have a positive family history for chemical dependence. Genetic studies indicate a strong hereditary predisposition to alcoholism. However, if offspring of alcoholic parents do not abuse substances by age 21, they are unlikely to do so after that point.

Families

Families play a more important role for adolescents than for adult substance abusers and are an important part of treatment. Parents and family members of adolescent abusers may be less resistant to being involved in treatment because the adolescent usually resides with them and the parents may feel responsible for their child's behavior. When parents themselves are actively addicted, the challenges of treatment are greater. Compared with adults, adolescents are less likely to enter treatment to avoid incarceration; rather, they are usually pushed into treatment by their families, by schools, and by pediatricians and family physicians. Children of divorced parents have a particularly high risk for substance abuse.

Mentally Ill Adolescents With Substance Abuse Disorders

To some extent, all childhood psychiatric disorders are associated with substance use disorders. Likewise, most adolescents in substance treatment programs have mental health problems, which can include conduct disorder, affective disorder, ADHD, anxiety disorders, eating disorders, and other Axis I conditions as well

as frequent Axis II diagnoses of passive-aggressive personality or borderline or narcissistic personality disorder. Of note, methylphenidate treatment of ADHD in adolescents significantly reduces the risk of developing substance abuse in later life (Biederman et al. 1997).

The risk of morbidity and mortality by various avenues must be assessed in this population. Careful history taking in regard to thoughts of and attempts at suicide as well as impulsive, thrill-seeking, or risk-taking behavior is crucial. In the presence of a family history of suicide or depression, psychosis, isolation from family and friends, previous suicide attempts, clear-cut plans of suicide, or a violent means of carrying out the plan, the risk of suicide is increased. Substance abuse in adolescents is frequently associated with risk-taking behavior linked to the spread of HIV infection. Substance use in adolescents may also directly and indirectly affect the immune system. Sexual abuse of children and adolescents is not uncommon in families with substance use disorders and may also increase the risk of HIV infection in families where an HIV-positive substance user is present.

Clinical Settings

Clinical management issues. The treatment of adolescents requires both structure and flexibility. Awareness of the possibility of contraband stashes and the necessity for intermittent urine screening are important in inpatient treatment programs to monitor compliance. Adolescent programs rely heavily on peer-support groups, family therapy, organized education, education on drug abuse, 12-Step programs such as AA and Alateen, vocational programs, patient–staff meetings, and activity therapy. Programs that do best with adolescents encourage openness and spontaneous expression of feelings, allow patients to engage in independent de-

cision making, have counselors help patients solve their real problems, use
cognitive and behavioral approaches and
relaxation techniques, have experienced
counselors and staff, and frequently employ the support of volunteers. Cognitive-
behavioral approaches have been modified
for adolescents, and treatment manuals
are available for guidance in the use of this
efficacious modality (Kaminer 1994).

**Substance intoxication or substance-
induced psychosis.** Intoxication with
drugs or alcohol in adolescents may lead
to disinhibition, violence, and medical
complications. One should generally avoid
the use of sedatives in adolescents, because benzodiazepines lead to greater disinhibition and increase the possibility of
violent acting out. Clinical support staff
may be needed to approach potentially
violent adolescents and to have an additional quieting effect. Emergency-room
checks for weapons are very important
with adolescents, and police should be
involved if the adolescent is carrying a
weapon.

Treatment settings. Inpatient or residential treatment is indicated for adolescents who have a drug problem that has
interfered with their ability to function in
school, work, and home environments and
who have been unable to maintain abstinence through outpatient treatment. Low
motivation for change, a disruptive home
life, frequent acting out, involvement
with the juvenile justice system, and additional psychiatric or medical problems all
may be reasons for inpatient treatment.
Depression, suicidality, hyperactivity,
chemical dependence, and overdoses of
drugs are additional indications. Adolescents frequently require longer hospital
stays than adults because of greater problems with creating dispositions, more resistance to treatment, greater difficulty of

controlling acting out in outpatient therapy, and greater severity of family problems.

Treatment outcome for adolescents is
worse than for adults. Predictors of treatment completion include greater severity
of alcohol abuse; worse abuse of drugs
other than alcohol, nicotine, or cannabis; a
higher degree of internalizing problems;
and lower self-esteem (Blood and Cornwall 1994).

Psychopharmacology

When considering pharmacological interventions in this population, great care and
attention are essential. Disulfiram is seldom used in adolescents. Although withdrawal from alcohol is rarely clinically significant in this population, it should be
monitored and treated as in adults. Methadone is generally avoided in adolescents
(Hopfer et al. 2001).

Relapses

Relapse prevention with adolescents is often more difficult than with adults, and
total abstinence is difficult to achieve.
Tough rules regarding relapse are less
likely to be effective in adolescent treatment services, where adolescents may
be looking for a means of escaping treatment. With adolescents, a slip needs to be
understood as a symptom of the problem;
the patient should not be rejected because
of a relapse. Relapses may lead to adjustment of treatment plans and may require
rehospitalization.

To prevent relapses, discharge planning must include outpatient treatment
for drug abuse and frequent attendance
at self-help support groups. Family or
group treatments may be added to individual treatment, depending on need.
Urine screens for drugs and alcohol are often part of a comprehensive outpatient
plan. Adolescents may also need halfway

houses, residential treatment centers, and, in some instances, long-term inpatient psychiatric care.

The Elderly

Substance abuse in the elderly may be the continuation of a lifelong pattern or a reaction to losses of ego or bodily integrity. The scope of substance use disorders in this population is poorly studied, and cultural factors likely create differences among groups. The incidence of alcoholism is lower (perhaps because persons with chronic alcoholism die prematurely), but the abuse of prescription drugs is common. Finally, age-related changes in the pharmacokinetics of prescribed medications compound the severe consequences of substance abuse in the elderly.

Special Problems in Detection

Diagnosis is difficult in the elderly for many reasons. Denial is common, and impairments in social and occupational functioning (including legal problems) may be hard to discern in retirees. It may be difficult to distinguish the consequences of substance use, such as cognitive impairments, from aging or from neurodegenerative disease. The adverse effects of heavy alcohol use on sleep, sexual functioning, and cognitive ability augment the changes that usually occur with aging or with the use of multiple medications. It is essential to keep in mind at all times that elderly alcoholics (especially males) are at a very high risk of suicide. Regular screening for alcohol-related disorders should be instituted. The MAST is a valid measure among elderly outpatients (Hirata et al. 2001).

Complications

The usual pharmacokinetic changes that accompany aging include a relatively in-

creased volume of distribution, greater CNS sensitivity to toxic substances, alterations in protein binding, and changes in hepatic and renal metabolism and excretion (Salzman 1998). Alcohol complicates these problems. Its hepatic effects may lead to either higher or lower bioavailability of medications. Alcohol's depressant effects may further contribute to major depression and cognitive impairment. For some elderly drinkers, there is a loss of tolerance, which leads to greater effects with smaller doses. Alcohol-induced persisting dementia is not reversible but does not progress further on cessation of drinking (Saunders et al. 1991). Thiamine deficiency is a common etiology of dementia in elderly alcoholic persons, and thiamine repletion should be instituted promptly to prevent Wernicke's encephalopathy.

Treatment Issues

Substance abuse treatment for the elderly requires greater creativity, flexibility, and sensitivity to the needs of this population. Geriatric patients may need to be protected from threatening and acting-out behaviors of younger patients. Older patients also require somewhat less confrontation and a higher degree of support, and more attention should be given to work with family members. The consequences of divorce are likely to also be greater in this group, and spouses are less likely to do well if left because of a drinking problem rather than for some other reason. Table 4–22 offers general guidelines for treatment of substance abuse in elderly persons.

Prescription Drug Abuse

Abuse of prescription drugs is common in the elderly (Abrams and Alexopoulos 1988). Abuse of benzodiazepines and of other hypnotics is common among women. Cognitive decline may lead to un-

TABLE 4–22. Guidelines for care of the elderly substance abuser

Avoid disulfiram
Use short-acting benzodiazepines
Remember that elderly patients are less likely to achieve full abstinence
Consider the patient's life experiences
Institute thiamine repletion

intentional misuse. Nursing home patients are sometimes overmedicated to reduce disruptiveness. Abusers of prescription medications may require hospitalization to discontinue use.

References

Abrams RC, Alexopoulos GS: Substance abuse in the elderly: over-the-counter and illegal drugs. Hosp Community Psychiatry 39: 822–823, 1988

Abramson JL, Williams SA, Krumholz HM, et al: Moderate alcohol consumption and risk of heart failure among older persons. JAMA 285:1971–1977, 2001

American Psychiatric Association: Diagnostic and Statistical Manual of Mental Disorders, 4th Edition. Washington, DC, American Psychiatric Association, 1994

American Psychiatric Association: Practice guideline for the treatment of patients with substance use disorders: alcohol, cocaine, opioids. Am J Psychiatry 152 (suppl):1–59, 1995

American Psychiatric Association: Practice guideline for the treatment of patients with nicotine dependence. Am J Psychiatry 153(suppl):1–31, 1996

American Psychiatric Association: Diagnostic and Statistical Manual of Mental Disorders, 4th Edition, Text Revision. Washington, DC, American Psychiatric Association, 2000

American Society of Addiction Medicine: Patient Placement Criteria for the Treatment of Substance-Related Disorders, 2nd Edition. Chevy Chase, MD, American Society of Addiction Medicine, 1996

Anton RF, Moak DH, Waid LR, et al: Naltrexone and cognitive behavioral therapy for the treatment of outpatient alcoholics: results of a placebo-controlled trial. Am J Psychiatry 156:1758–1764, 1999

Armor DJ, Polish SM, Stambul HB: Alcoholics and Treatment. New York, Wiley, 1978

Ashley MJ, Olin JS, LeRiche WH, et al: Morbidity in alcoholics: evidence for accelerated development of physical disease in women. Arch Intern Med 137:883–887, 1977

Bachman JG, Wallace JM Jr, O'Malley PM: Racial/ethnic differences in smoking, drinking, and illicit drug use among American high school seniors, 1976–89. Am J Public Health 81:372–377, 1991

Bartzokis G, Beckson M, Hance DB, et al: Magnetic resonance imaging evidence of "silent" cerebrovascular toxicity in cocaine dependence. Biol Psychiatry 45: 1203–1211, 1999

Berk M, Brook S, Trandafir AI: A comparison of olanzapine with haloperidol in cannabis-induced psychotic disorder: a double-blind randomized controlled trial. Int Clin Psychopharmacol 14:177–180, 1999

Berlakovich GA, Steininger R, Herbst F, et al: Efficacy of liver transplantation for alcoholic cirrhosis with respect to recidivism and compliance. Transplantation 58:560–565, 1994

Bickel WK, Amass L, Higgins ST, et al: Effects of adding behavioral treatment to opioid detoxification with buprenorphine. J Consult Clin Psychol 65:803–810, 1997

Biederman J, Wilens T, Mick E, et al: Is ADHD a risk factor for psychoactive substance use disorders? Findings from a four-year prospective follow-up study. J Am Acad Child Adolesc Psychiatry 36:21–29, 1997

Blood L, Cornwall A: Pretreatment variables that predict completion of an adolescent substance abuse treatment program. J Nerv Ment Dis 182:14–19, 1994

Blume S: Addictive disorders in women, in Clinical Textbook of Addictive Disorders, 2nd Edition. Edited by Frances RJ, Miller SI. New York, Guilford, 1998

Botvin GJ, Baker E, Dusenbury L, et al: Long-term follow-up results of a randomized drug abuse prevention trial in a white middle-class population. JAMA 273:1106–1112, 1995

Bouckoms A, Hackett TP: Pain patients, in MGH Handbook of General Hospital Psychiatry, 4th Edition. Edited by Cassem NH. St Louis, MO, Mosby-Year Book, 1997, pp 367–415

Brooner RK, King VL, Kidorf M, et al: Psychiatric and substance use comorbidity among treatment seeking opioid abusers. Arch Gen Psychiatry 54:71–80, 1997

Brown HL, Britton KA, Mahaffey D, et al: Methadone maintenance in pregnancy: a reappraisal. Am J Obstet Gynecol 179:459–463, 1998

Brown RA, Evans DM, Miller IW, et al: CBT for depression in alcoholism. J Consult Clin Psychol 65:715–726, 1997

Bukstein O: Practice parameters for the assessment and treatment of children and adolescents with substance use disorders. J Am Acad Child Adolesc Psychiatry 36:140S–156S, 1997

Centers for Disease Control and Prevention: Increasing morbidity and mortality associated with abuse of methamphetamine: United States, 1991–1994. MMWR Morb Mortal Wkly Rep 44:882–886, 1995

Centers for Disease Control and Prevention: Alcohol consumption among pregnant and childbearing-aged women: United States, 1991 and 1995. MMWR Morb Mortal Wkly Rep 46:346–350, 1997a

Centers for Disease Control and Prevention: Gamma hydroxybutyrate use: New York and Texas, 1995–1996. JAMA 277:1511, 1997b

Centers for Disease Control and Prevention: Alcohol involvement in fatal motor-vehicle crashes—United States, 1997–1998. MMWR Morb Mortal Wkly Rep 48: 1086–1087, 1999a

Centers for Disease Control and Prevention: Cigarette smoking among adults—United States, 1997. MMWR Morb Mortal Wkly Rep 48:993–996, 1999b

Centers for Disease Control and Prevention: Trends in cigarette smoking among high school students, United States, 1991–1999. MMWR Morb Mortal Wkly Rep 49:755–758, 2000

Cloninger CR, Sigvardsson S, Bohman M: Childhood personality predicts alcohol abuse in young adults. Alcoholism: Clinical and Experimental Research 12:494–505, 1988

Cornish JW, Maany I, Fudala PJ, et al: Carbamazepine treatment for cocaine dependence. Drug Alcohol Depend 38:221–227, 1995

Craig K, Gomez HF, McManus JL, et al: Severe gamma-hydroxybutyrate withdrawal: a case report and literature review. J Emerg Med 18:65–70, 2000

Derogatis LR, Lipman RS, Covi L: The SCL-90: an outpatient psychiatric rating scale. Psychopharmacol Bull 9:13–28, 1973

DeWit DJ, Adlaf EM, Offord DR, et al: Age at first alcohol use: a risk factor for the development of alcohol disorders. Am J Psychiatry 157:745–750, 2000

Diana M, Melis M, Muntoni AL, et al: Mesolimbic dopaminergic decline after cannabinoid withdrawal. Proc Natl Acad Sci U S A 95:10269–10273, 1998

Ellenhorn MJ: Ellenhorn's Medical Toxicology, Diagnosis, and Treatment of Human Poisoning, 2nd Edition. Baltimore, MD, Williams & Wilkins, 1997

Endicott J, Spitzer RL: A diagnostic interview: the Schedule for Affective Disorders and Schizophrenia. Arch Gen Psychiatry 35: 837–844, 1978

Feighner JP, Robins E, Guze SB, et al: Diagnostic criteria for use in psychiatric research. Arch Gen Psychiatry 26:57–63, 1972

First MB, Gibbon M, Spitzer RL, et al: User's Guide for the Structured Clinical Interview for DSM-IV Axis II Personality Disorders (SCID-II). Washington, DC, American Psychiatric Press, 1997

Flaum M, Schultz SK: When does amphetamine-induced psychosis become schizophrenia? Am J Psychiatry 153:812–815, 1996

Frances RJ, Alexopoulos GS: The inpatient treatment of the alcoholic patient. Psychiatr Ann 12:386–391, 1982a

Frances RJ, Alexopoulos GS: Patient management and education; getting the alcoholic into treatment. Physician and Patient 1:9–14, 1982b

Frances R, Borg L, Mack A, et al: Individual treatment: psychodynamics and the treatment of substance-related disorders, in Treatments of Psychiatric Disorders, 3rd Edition. Edited by Gabbard GO. Washington, DC, American Psychiatric Press, 2001, pp 827–838

Frank DA, Augustyn M, Knight WG, et al: Growth, development, and behavior in early childhood following prenatal cocaine exposure: a systematic review. JAMA 285:1613–1625, 2001

Galanter M: Self help treatment for combined addiction and mental illness. Hosp Community Psychiatry 51:877–879, 2000

Galanter M, Keller D, Dermatis H: Network therapy for addiction: assessment of the clinical outcome of training. Am J Psychiatry 150:28–36, 1993

Gavaler JS, Rizzo A, Rossaro L, et al: Sexuality of alcoholic women with menstrual cycle function: effects of duration of alcohol abstinence. Alcohol Clin Exp Res 17:778–781, 1995

Geller B, Cooper TB, Sun K, et al: Double-blind and placebo-controlled study of lithium for adolescent bipolar disorders with secondary substance dependency. J Am Acad Child Adolesc Psychiatry 37:171–178, 1998

Goldberg MJ, Spector R, Park GD, et al: An approach to the management of the poisoned patient. Arch Intern Med 146:1381–1385, 1986

Graeme KA: New drugs of abuse. Emerg Med Clin North Am 18:625–636, 2000

Greenfield SF, O'Leary G: Sex differences in marijuana use in the United States. Harv Rev Psychiatry 6:297–303, 1999

Group for the Advancement of Psychiatry: Addiction treatment; avoiding pitfalls: a case approach. GAP Report 142. Washington, DC, American Psychiatric Press, 1998

Harwood H, Fountain D, Livermore G, et al: The Economic Costs of Alcohol and Drug Abuse in the United States, 1992. Washington, DC, National Institute on Drug Abuse and National Institute on Alcohol Abuse and Alcoholism, 1998

Hathaway SR, McKinley JC: Minnesota Multiphasic Personality Inventory Manual, Revised Edition. New York, Psychological Corporation, 1967

Hernandez-Avila CA, Ortega-Soto HA, Jasso A, et al: Treatment of inhalant-induced psychotic disorder with carbamazepine versus haloperidol. Psychiatr Serv 49:812–815, 1998

Hirata ES, Almeida OP, Funari RR, et al: Validity of the Michigan Alcoholism Screening Test (MAST) for the detection of alcohol-related problems among male geriatric outpatients. Am J Geriatr Psychiatry 9:30–34, 2001

Holt S, Skinner M, Israel Y: Early identification of alcohol abuse, II: clinical and laboratory indicators. Can Med Assoc J 124:1279–1294, 1981

Hommer DW, Momenan R, Kaiser E, et al: Evidence for a gender-related effect of alcoholism on brain volumes. Am J Psychiatry 158:198–204, 2001

Hopfer CJ, Mikulich SK, Crowley TJ: Heroin use among adolescents in treatment for substance use disorders. J Am Acad Child Adolesc Psychiatry 39:1316–1323, 2001

Horn JL, Warburg KW, Foster FM: Alcohol Use Inventory. Minneapolis, MN, National Computer Systems, 1986

Institute of Medicine: Fetal alcohol syndrome: research base for diagnostic criteria, epidemiology, prevention, and treatment. Washington, DC, National Academy Press, 1995

Institute of Medicine: Workshop Summary. The Role of Co-Occurring Substance Abuse and Mental Illness in Violence: Division of Neuroscience and Behavioral Health, Institute of Medicine. Washington, DC, National Academy Press, 1999

Jansen KLR: Nonmedical use of ketamine. BMJ 306:601–602, 1993

Johnson BA, Roache JD, Javors MA, et al: Ondansetron for reduction of drinking among biologically predisposed alcoholic patients: a randomized controlled trial. JAMA 284:963–971, 2000

Johnson RE, Eissenberg T, Stitzer ML, et al: A placebo controlled clinical trial of buprenorphine as a treatment for opioid dependence. Drug Alcohol Depend 40:17–25, 1995

Johnson RE, Chutuape MA, Strain E, et al: A comparison of levomethadyl acetate, buprenorphine, and methadone for opioid dependence. N Engl J Med 343:1290–1297, 2000

Johnston LD, O'Malley PM, Bachman JG: National Annual High School Senior and Young Adult Survey. Washington, DC, U.S. Government Printing Office, 1997

Johnston LD, O'Malley PM, Bachman JG: Monitoring the Future National Survey Results on Adolescent Drug Use: Overview of Key Findings, 2002 (NIH Publ No 03-5374). Bethesda, MD, National Institute on Drug Abuse, 2003

Jonas MM, Graeme-Cook FM: A 17-year-old girl with marked jaundice and weight loss. N Engl J Med 344:591–599, 2001

Kaminer Y: Adolescent Substance Abuse: A Comprehensive Guide to Theory and Practice. New York, Plenum, 1994

Kaminer Y, Bukstein O, Tarter RE: The Teen-Addiction Severity Index: rationale and reliability. Int J Addict 26:219–226, 1991

Kessler RC, Sonnega A, Bromet E, et al: Posttraumatic stress disorder in the National Comorbidity Survey. Arch Gen Psychiatry 52:1048–1060, 1995

Kessler RC, Crum RM, Warner LA, et al: Lifetime co-occurrence of DSM-III-R alcohol abuse and dependence with other psychiatric disorders in the National Comorbidity Survey. Arch Gen Psychiatry 54:313–321, 1997

Khantzian EJ: The self-medication hypothesis of substance use disorders: a reconsideration and recent applications. Harv Rev Psychiatry 4:231–244, 1997

Kiefer F, Jahn H, Tarnaske T, et al: Comparing and combining naltrexone and acamprosate in relapse prevention of alcoholism: a double-blind, placebo-controlled study. Arch Gen Psychiatry 60:92–99, 2003

Koch M, Banys P: Liver transplantation and opioid dependence. JAMA 285:1056–1058, 2001

Kreek MJ: Methadone-related opioid agonist pharmacotherapy for heroin addiction. History, recent molecular and neurochemical research and future in mainstream medicine. Ann N Y Acad Sci 909:186–216; 2000

Krystal JH, Karper LP, Seibyl JP, et al: Subanesthetic effects of the noncompetitive NMDA antagonist, ketamine, in humans: psychotomimetic, perceptual, cognitive, and neuroendocrine responses. Arch Gen Psychiatry 51:199–214, 1994

Kucuk NO, Kilic EO, Ibis E, et al: Brain SPECT findings in long term inhalant abuse. Nucl Med Commun 21:769–773, 2000

Kushner MG, Sher KJ, Beitman BD: The relation between alcohol problems and the anxiety disorders. Am J Psychiatry 147:685–695, 1990

Lerner AG, Finkel B, Oyfee I, et al: Clonidine treatment for hallucinogen persisting perception disorder. Am J Psychiatry 155:1460, 1998

Leshner AI: Addiction is a brain disease and it matters. Science 278:45–47, 1997

Leshner AI, Koob GF: Drugs of abuse and the brain. Proc Assoc Am Physicians 111:99–108, 1999

Lieber CS: Medical disorders of alcoholism. N Engl J Med 333:1058–1065, 1995

Linehan MM, Schmidt H 3rd, Dimeff LA, et al: Dialectical behavior therapy for patients with borderline personality disorder and drug-dependence. Am J Addict 8:279–292, 1999

Ling W, Charuvastra C, Collins JF, et al: Buprenorphine maintenance treatment of opiate dependence: a multicenter, randomized clinical trial. Addiction 93:475–486, 1998

MacAndrew C: The differentiation of male alcohol outpatients from nonalcoholic psychiatric patients by means of the MMPI. Q J Stud Alcohol 26:238–246, 1965

Mack AH, Franklin JE Jr, Frances RJ: Concise Guide to Treatment of Alcoholism and Addictions, Second Edition. Washington, DC, American Psychiatric Publishing, 2001

Malcolm R, Kajdasz DK, Herron J, et al: A double-blind, placebo-controlled outpatient trial of pergolide for cocaine dependence. Drug Alcohol Depend 60:161–168, 2000

Marlatt GA, Gordon JR: Relapse Prevention: Maintenance Strategies in the Treatment of Addictive Behaviors. New York, Guilford, 1985

Marzuk PM, Tardiff KL, Leon AC, et al: Prevalence of cocaine use among residents of New York City who committed suicide during a one-year period. Am J Psychiatry 149:371–375, 1992

McCann UD, Mertl M, Eligulashvili V, et al: Cognitive performance in (+/–) 3,4-methylenedioxymethamphetamine (MDMA, "ecstasy") users: a controlled study. Psychopharmacology (Berl) 143:417–425, 1999

McGill V, Kowal-Vern A, Fisher SG: The impact of substance use on mortality and morbidity from thermal injury. J Trauma 38:931–934, 1995

McLellan AT, Luborsky L, Woody GE, et al: Are the "addiction-related" problems of substance abusers really related? J Nerv Ment Dis 169:232–239, 1981

McLellan AT, Grissom GR, Zanis D, et al: Problem-service matching in addiction treatment: a prospective study in 4 programs. Arch Gen Psychiatry 54:730–735, 1997

Moore RD, Bone LR, Geller G, et al: Prevalence, detection, and treatment of alcoholism in hospitalized patients. JAMA 261:403–407, 1989

Mukamal KJ, Maclure M, Muller JE, et al: Prior alcohol consumption and mortality following acute myocardial infarction. JAMA 285:1965–1970, 2001

Murphy SL: Deaths: Final Data for 1998: National Vital Statistics Reports, 48(11). Hyattsville, MD, National Center for Vital Statistics, 2000

National Institute on Drug Abuse: Principles of Drug Addiction Treatment: A Research-Based Guide (NIH Publication 00-4180). Rockville, MD, National Institute on Drug Abuse, 1999

O'Brien CP, McLellan AT: Myths about the treatment of addiction. Lancet 347:237–240, 1996

O'Connor PG, Waugh ME, Carrol KM, et al: Primary care-based ambulatory opioid detoxification: the results of a clinical trial. J Gen Intern Med 10:255–260, 1995

O'Connor PG, Carroll KM, Shi JM, et al: Three methods of opioid detoxification in a primary care setting. A randomized trial. Ann Intern Med 127:526–530, 1997

Office of Applied Studies: Drug Abuse Warning Network, Annual Medical Examiner Data, 1998. Rockville, MD, Substance Abuse and Mental Health Services Administration, 2000

Office of Applied Studies: National Household Survey on Drug Abuse, 2001. Rockville, MD, Substance Abuse and Mental Health Services Administration, 2002

O'Malley PM, Johnston LD, Bachman JG: Adolescent substance use. Epidemiology and implications for public policy. Pediatr Clin North Am 42:241–260, 1995

O'Malley SS, Jaffe AJ, Chang G, et al: Six-month follow-up of naltrexone and psychotherapy for alcohol dependence. Arch Gen Psychiatry 53:217–224, 1996

Regier DA, Farmer ME, Rae DS, et al: Comorbidity of mental disorders with alcohol and other drug abuse: results from the Epidemiologic Catchment Area study. JAMA 264:2511–2518, 1990

Reynaud M, Schwan R, Loiseaux-Meunier M-N, et al: Patients admitted to emergency services for drunkenness: moderate alcohol users or harmful drinkers? Am J Psychiatry 158:96–99, 2001

Ross HE, Glaser FB, Germanson T: The prevalence of psychiatric disorders in patients with alcohol and other drug problems. Arch Gen Psychiatry 45:1023–1031, 1988

Salzman C: Clinical Geriatric Psychopharmacology, 3rd Edition. Baltimore, MD, Williams & Wilkins, 1998

Samet JH, Rollnick S, Barnes H: Beyond CAGE: a brief clinical approach after detection of substance abuse. Arch Intern Med 156:2287–2293, 1996

Saunders PA, Copeland JRM, Dewey ME, et al: Heavy drinking as a risk factor for depression and dementia in elderly men. Br J Psychiatry 159:213–216, 1991

Schmidt LG, Schmidt K, Dufeu P, et al: Superiority of carbohydrate-deficient transferrin to gamma-glutamyltransferase in detecting relapse in alcoholism. Am J Psychiatry 154:75–80, 1997

Schneier FR, Siris SG: A review of psychoactive substance use and abuse in schizophrenia: patterns of drug choice. J Nerv Ment Dis 175:641–652, 1987

Schuckit MA, Tipp JE, Bergman M, et al: Comparison of induced and independent major depressive disorders in 2,945 alcoholics. Am J Psychiatry 154:948–957, 1997

Schuckit MA, Smith TL, Daeppen JB, et al: Clinical relevance of the distinction between alcohol dependence with and without a physiological component. Am J Psychiatry 155:733–740, 1998

Sees KL, Delucci KL, Masson C, et al: Methadone maintenance versus 180-day psychosocially enriched detoxification for treatment of opioid dependence. JAMA 283:1303–1310, 2000

Shearer DS, Baciewicz GJ, Kwong TC: Drugs of abuse testing in an outpatient psychiatry service. Clin Lab Med 18:713–725, 1998

Singletary KW, Gapstur SM: Alcohol and breast cancer: review of epidemiologic and experimental evidence and potential mechanisms. JAMA 286:2143–2151, 2001

Skinner HA, Horn JL: Alcohol Dependence Scale: Users Guide. Toronto, Ontario, Canada, Addiction Research Foundation, 1984

Sonne S, Brady KY: Valproate for alcoholics with bipolar disorder. Am J Psychiatry 156:1122, 1999

Spiehler VR, Reed D: Brain concentrations of cocaine and benzoylecgonine in fatal cases. J Forensic Sci 30:1003–1011, 1985

Sullivan JT, Sykora K, Schneiderman J, et al: Assessment of alcohol withdrawal: the revised clinical institute withdrawal assessment for alcohol scale (CIWA-Ar). Br J Addict 84:1353–1357, 1989

Tarter RE, Edwards K: Psychological factors associated with the risk for alcoholism. Alcohol Clin Exp Res 12:471–480, 1988

The Medical Letter: Acute reactions to drugs of abuse. Med Lett Drugs Ther 38:43–46, 1996

Tonne U, Hiltunen AJ, Vilkander B, et al: Neuropsychological changes during steady-state drug use, withdrawal and abstinence in primary benzodiazepine-dependent patients. Acta Psychiatr Scand 91:299–304, 1995

Trabert W, Betz T, Niewald M, et al: Significant reversibility of alcoholic brain shrinkage within 3 weeks of abstinence. Acta Psychiatr Scand 92:87–90, 1995

Urbano-Marquez A, Ramon E, Fernandez-Sola J, et al: The greater risk of alcoholic cardiomyopathy and myopathy in women compared with men. JAMA 274:149–154, 1995

Vaillant GE: Is alcoholism more often the cause or result of depression? Harv Rev Psychiatry 1:94–99, 1993

Vaillant GE: A long-term follow-up of male alcohol abuse. Arch Gen Psychiatry 53:243–249, 1996

Volkow ND, Fowler JS: Addiction, a disease of compulsion and drive: involvement of the orbitofrontal cortex. Cereb Cortex 10:318–325; 2000

Volkow ND, Chang L, Wang G-J, et al: Association of dopamine transporter reduction with psychomotor impairment in methamphetamine abusers. Am J Psychiatry 158:377–382, 2001

Volpe JJ: Effect of cocaine use on the fetus. N Engl J Med 327:399–407, 1992

Volpicelli JR, Alterman AI, Hayashida M, et al: Naltrexone in the treatment of alcohol dependence. Arch Gen Psychiatry 49:876–887, 1992

Warburg K, Horn J: The Alcohol Use Inventory. Port Logan, CO, Multivariate Measurement Consultants, 1985

Warner LA, Kessler RC, Hughes M, et al: Prevalence and correlates of drug use and dependence in the United States. Arch Gen Psychiatry 52:219–228, 1995

Weller R, Preskorn S: Psychotropic drugs and alcohol: pharmacokinetic and pharmacodynamic interactions. Psychosomatics 25:301–309, 1984

World Health Organization: Global Burden of Disease 2000. Cambridge, MA, Harvard University Press, 2001

Wright FD, Beck AT, Newman CF, et al: Cognitive therapy of substance abuse: theoretical rationale, in Behavioral Treatments for Drug Abuse and Dependence (NIDA Res Monogr 137). Edited by Onken LS, Blaine JD, Boren JJ. Rockville, MD, National Institute on Drug Abuse, 1993, pp 123–146

CHAPTER 5

Schizophrenia and Other Psychotic Disorders

Beng-Choon Ho, M.R.C.Psych.

Donald W. Black, M.D.

Nancy C. Andreasen, M.D., Ph.D.

Schizophrenia is perhaps the most enigmatic and tragic disease that psychiatrists treat, and perhaps also the most devastating. It is one of the leading causes of disability among young adults. Schizophrenia strikes at a young age so that, unlike patients with cancer or heart disease, patients with schizophrenia usually live many years after onset of the disease and continue to suffer its effects, which prevent them from leading fully normal lives—attending school, working, having a close network of friends, marrying, or having children. In a study commissioned by the World Health Organization and the World Bank, schizophrenia ranked as the ninth leading cause of disability in people ages 15–44 years worldwide, and fourth in developed countries (Murray and Lopez 1996).

Diagnosis

According to DSM-IV-TR, schizophrenia consists of the presence of characteristic positive or negative symptoms of at least 1 month in duration (unless successfully treated); deterioration in work, interpersonal relations, or self-care; continuous signs of the disturbance for at least 6 months; the ruling out of schizoaffective disorder and mood disorder with psychotic features; the determination that the disturbance is not due to a general medical condition or the direct physiological effects of a substance; and, finally, if autistic disorder or another pervasive developmental disorder is present, prominent hallucinations or delusions have also been present for at least 1 month. Schizophrenia is further classified according to course of illness, as shown in Table 5–1.

If an illness otherwise meets the criteria but has a duration of at least 1 month but less than 6 months, it is termed a *schizophreniform disorder*. If it has lasted less than 4 weeks, it may be classified as either a brief psychotic disorder or a psychotic disorder not otherwise specified, which is a residual category for psychotic disturbances that cannot be better classified.

TABLE 5–1. DSM-IV-TR diagnostic criteria for schizophrenia

A. *Characteristic symptoms:* Two (or more) of the following, each present for a significant portion of time during a 1-month period (or less if successfully treated):
   (1) delusions
   (2) hallucinations
   (3) disorganized speech (e.g., frequent derailment or incoherence)
   (4) grossly disorganized or catatonic behavior
   (5) negative symptoms, i.e., affective flattening, alogia, or avolition
   Note: Only one Criterion A symptom is required if delusions are bizarre or hallucinations consist of a voice keeping up a running commentary on the person's behavior or thoughts, or two or more voices conversing with each other.

B. *Social/occupational dysfunction:* For a significant portion of the time since the onset of the disturbance, one or more major areas of functioning such as work, interpersonal relations, or self-care are markedly below the level achieved prior to the onset (or when the onset is in childhood or adolescence, failure to achieve expected level of interpersonal, academic, or occupational achievement).

C. *Duration:* Continuous signs of the disturbance persist for at least 6 months. This 6-month period must include at least 1 month of symptoms (or less if successfully treated) that meet Criterion A (i.e., active-phase symptoms) and may include periods of prodromal or residual symptoms. During these prodromal or residual periods, the signs of the disturbance may be manifested by only negative symptoms or two or more symptoms listed in Criterion A present in an attenuated form (e.g., odd beliefs, unusual perceptual experiences).

D. *Schizoaffective and Mood Disorder exclusion:* Schizoaffective disorder and mood disorder with psychotic features have been ruled out because either (1) no major depressive, manic, or mixed episodes have occurred concurrently with the active-phase symptoms; or (2) if mood episodes have occurred during active-phase symptoms, their total duration has been brief relative to the duration of the active and residual periods.

E. *Substance/general medical condition exclusion:* The disturbance is not due to the direct physiological effects of a substance (e.g., a drug of abuse, a medication) or a general medical condition.

F. *Relationship to a Pervasive Developmental Disorder:* If there is a history of autistic disorder or another pervasive developmental disorder, the additional diagnosis of schizophrenia is made only if prominent delusions or hallucinations are also present for at least a month (or less if successfully treated).

Classification of longitudinal course (can be applied only after at least 1 year has elapsed since the initial onset of active-phase symptoms):
   Episodic With Interepisode Residual Symptoms (episodes are defined by the reemergence of prominent psychotic symptoms); *also specify if:*   **With Prominent Negative Symptoms**
   Episodic With No Interepisode Residual Symptoms
   Continuous (prominent psychotic symptoms are present throughout the period of observation); *also specify if:*   **With Prominent Negative Symptoms**
   Single Episode In Partial Remission; *also specify if:*   **With Prominent Negative Symptoms**
   Single Episode In Full Remission
   Other or Unspecified Pattern

Differential Diagnosis

Schizophrenia remains a clinical diagnosis that rests on historical information and a careful mental status examination, and there are no predictable laboratory abnormalities that are diagnostic of the disorder. The first step in diagnosis is to take a careful history and perform a physical examination to exclude psychoses with known medical causes. Psychotic symptoms have been found to result from substance abuse (e.g., hallucinogens, phencyclidine, amphetamines, cocaine, alcohol); intoxication due to commonly prescribed medications (e.g., corticosteroids, anticholinergics, levodopa); infectious, metabolic, and endocrine disorders; tumors and mass lesions; and temporal lobe epilepsy. Atypical presentations such as a relatively acute onset, clouding of the sensorium, or onset occurring after age 30 years demand careful investigation.

Routine laboratory tests may be helpful in ruling out potential medical causes. Common screening tests include a complete blood count (CBC), urinalysis, liver enzymes, serum creatinine, blood urea nitrogen (BUN), thyroid function tests, and serological tests for evidence of an infection with syphilis or HIV. Other tests will be indicated in selected patients, such as a serum ceruloplasmin to rule out Wilson's disease. Electroencephalography (EEG), computed tomography (CT), or magnetic resonance imaging (MRI) may be useful in selected cases to rule out alternate diagnoses, such as a tumor or mass lesion or epilepsy.

The major task in differential diagnosis involves separating schizophrenia from schizoaffective disorder, mood disorder with psychotic features, delusional disorder, or a personality disorder. To rule out schizoaffective disorder and psychotic mood disorders, major depressive or manic episodes should have been absent during the active phase, or the mood episode should have been brief relative to the total duration of the psychotic episode. Unlike delusional disorder, schizophrenia is characterized by bizarre delusions, and hallucinations are common. Patients with personality disorders, particularly those in the "eccentric" cluster (e.g., schizoid, schizotypal, and paranoid personality), may be indifferent to social relationships and display restricted affect, may have bizarre ideation and odd speech, or may be suspicious and hypervigilant, but they do not have delusions, hallucinations, or grossly disorganized behavior. Furthermore, patients with schizophrenia may develop other symptoms, such as a profound thought disorder, behavioral disturbances, and enduring personality deterioration. These symptoms are uncharacteristic of the mood disorders, delusional disorder, or the personality disorders.

Depersonalization disorder and sometimes panic disorder are accompanied by feelings of unreality, such as that one's mind and body are separate; however, insight is generally well preserved, and hallucinations and delusions are absent. The rituals occurring in a patient with obsessive-compulsive disorder may result in bizarre behavior, but they are performed to relieve anxiety, and not in response to delusional beliefs.

Other psychiatric disorders also must be ruled out, including schizophreniform disorder, brief psychotic disorder, factitious disorder with psychological symptoms, and malingering. If symptoms persist for more than 6 months, schizophreniform disorder can be ruled out. The history of how the illness presents will help to rule out brief psychotic disorder, since schizophrenia generally has an insidious onset and there are usually no precipitating stressors. Factitious disorder may be difficult to delineate from schizophre-

TABLE 5–2.   Differential diagnosis of schizophrenia

Psychiatric illness	General medical illness	Drugs of abuse
Psychotic mood disorders	Temporal lobe epilepsy	Stimulants (e.g., amphetamine, cocaine)
Schizoaffective disorder	Tumor, stroke, brain trauma	
Brief reactive psychosis	Endocrine/metabolic disorders (e.g., porphyria)	Hallucinogens (e.g., phencyclidine)
Schizophreniform disorder		
Delusional disorder	Vitamin deficiency (e.g., B_{12})	Anticholinergics (e.g., belladonna alkaloids)
Induced psychotic disorder	Infectious (e.g., neurosyphilis)	
Panic disorder	Autoimmune (e.g., systemic lupus erythematosus)	Alcohol withdrawal delirium
Depersonalization disorder		Barbiturate withdrawal delirium
Obsessive-compulsive disorder	Toxic (e.g., heavy metal poisoning)	
Personality disorders (e.g., "eccentric" cluster)		
Factitious disorder with psychological symptoms		
Malingering		

nia, especially when the patient is knowledgeable about mental illness or is medically trained, but careful observation should enable the clinician to make the distinction between real or feigned psychosis. Likewise, a malingerer could attempt to simulate schizophrenia, but careful observation will help to distinguish the disorders. With the malingerer, there will be evidence of obvious secondary gain, such as avoiding incarceration, and the history may suggest antisocial personality disorder. The differential diagnosis for schizophrenia is summarized in Table 5–2.

Clinical Findings

Clinical manifestations of schizophrenia and schizophreniform disorders are diverse and can change over time. Because of their variety, it has been said that to know schizophrenia is to know psychiatry.

Whereas many symptoms are obvious, such as hallucinations, others such as affective blunting or incongruity are relatively subtle and can be easily missed by a casual observer.

Various methods have been developed to describe and classify the multiplicity of symptoms in schizophrenia. Traditionally, schizophrenia is considered to be a type of "psychosis," yet the definition of psychosis has been elusive. Older definitions stressed the subjective and internal psychological experience and defined psychosis as an "impairment in reality testing." More recently, psychosis has been defined objectively and operationally as the occurrence of hallucinations and delusions. Because schizophrenia is characterized by so many different types of symptoms, clinicians and scientists have tried to simplify the description of the clinical presentation by dividing the symptoms into subgroups. The most widely used subdivision classifies the symptoms as positive and negative.

Positive and Negative Symptoms

The concept of positive and negative symptoms was originally formulated by the British neurologist John Hughlings-Jackson (1931). Jackson believed that positive symptoms reflected release phenomena occurring in more phylogenetically advanced brain regions, due to injury to the brain at a more primitive level. Negative symptoms, on the other hand, simply represented a "dissolution," or a loss of brain function. Current definitions of positive and negative symptoms are an amplification of these earlier ideas.

Positive symptoms, including hallucinations, delusions, marked positive formal thought disorder (manifested by marked incoherence, derailment, tangentiality, or illogicality), and bizarre or disorganized behavior reflect a distortion or exaggeration of functions that are normally present. For example, hallucinations are a distortion or exaggeration of the function of the perceptual systems of the brain: the person experiences a perception in the absence of an external stimulus.

Negative symptoms reflect a deficiency of a mental function that is normally present. For example, some patients display *alogia* (i.e., marked poverty of speech, or poverty of content of speech). Others show *affective flattening, anhedonia/asociality* (i.e., inability to experience pleasure, few social contacts), *avolition/apathy* (i.e., anergia, impersistence at work or school), and *attentional impairment*. These negative or deficit symptoms not only are difficult to treat and respond less well to neuroleptics than do positive symptoms, but they are also the most destructive because they render the patient inert and unmotivated. The schizophrenic patient with prominent negative symp-

toms may be able to raise his or her performance under supervision but cannot maintain it when supervision is withdrawn.

Crow (1980) proposed a method for classifying schizophrenic patients on the basis of the presence of positive or negative symptoms. He has designated schizophrenic patients with mostly positive symptoms as Type I and those with mostly negative symptoms as Type II. However, in practice patients generally display a mixture of both positive and negative symptoms (Andreasen et al. 1990b).

The Psychotic Dimension

This symptom dimension refers to two classic "psychotic" symptoms that reflect a patient's confusion about the loss of boundaries between himself or herself and the external world: hallucinations and delusions. Both symptoms reflect a "loss of ego boundaries": the patient is unable to distinguish between his or her own thoughts and perceptions and those that he or she obtains by observing the external world.

Hallucinations have sometimes been considered the hallmark of schizophrenia. Although hallucinations may occur in a variety of other disorders, including mood and organic disorders, they remain important symptoms of schizophrenia and schizophreniform disorders. *Hallucinations* are perceptions experienced without an external stimulus to the sense organs that have qualities similar to a true perception (e.g., intensity, location). They are usually experienced as originating in the outside world, or within one's own body, but not within the mind as through imagination. Hallucinations vary in complexity and in sensory modality. Schizophrenic patients commonly have auditory, visual, tactile, gustatory, or olfactory hallucinations, or a combination of several types.

Auditory hallucinations are the most frequent type observed in schizophrenia and may be experienced as noises, music, or more typically "voices." Voices may be mumbled or may sound clear and distinct, and words, phrases, or sentences may be heard. Hallucinations may be inferred when the patient appears to be talking in response to the voices and may whisper, mutter incomprehensibly, talk normally, or shout out loud. Visual hallucinations may be simple or complex and include flashes of light or the image of persons, animals, or objects; they may be smaller or larger than a true perception. They may be experienced as being located outside the field of vision such as being behind the head and are usually reported in normal color. Olfactory and gustatory hallucinations are often experienced together, leading to unpleasant tastes and odors. Tactile hallucinations (or *haptic* hallucinations) may be experienced as sensations of being touched or pricked, electrical sensa-

tions, or even a sensation of insects crawling under the skin, which is called *formication*. Tactile hallucinations may occur as feelings of body organs being pulled upon and distended, and sexual stimulation may be experienced. Schizophrenic patients in all cultures experience hallucinations, although they may differ in frequency and type, depending on the patient's experience and background (Ndetei and Vadher 1984).

Delusions involve a disturbance in inferential thinking rather than perception. Delusions are firmly held beliefs that are untrue; the judgment of "untrueness" must always be made within the context of the person's educational and cultural background. Delusions occurring in patients with schizophrenia may have somatic, grandiose, religious, nihilistic, or persecutory themes (Table 5–3). None is specific to schizophrenia, and like hallucinations, delusions tend to be culturally based.

TABLE 5–3. Varied content in delusions

Delusions	Foci of preoccupation
Grandiose	Possessing wealth or great beauty or having a special ability (e.g., extrasensory perception); having influential friends; being an important figure (e.g., Napoleon, Hitler)
Nihilistic	Belief that one is dead or dying; belief that one does not exist or that the world does not exist
Persecutory	Being persecuted by friends, neighbors, or spouses; being followed, monitored, or spied on by the government (e.g., the FBI, the CIA) or other important organizations (e.g., the Catholic Church)
Somatic	Belief that one's organs have stopped functioning (e.g., that the heart is no longer beating) or are rotting away; belief that the nose or other body part is terribly misshapen or disfigured
Sexual	Belief that one's sexual behavior is commonly known; that one is a prostitute, a pedophile, or a rapist; that masturbation has led to illness or insanity
Religious	Belief that one has sinned against God; that one has a special relationship to God or some other deity; that one has a special religious mission; that one is the Devil or is condemned to burn in Hell

The Disorganization Dimension

The disorganization dimension includes disorganized speech, disorganized or bizarre behavior, and incongruous affect.

Disorganized speech, or *thought disorder*, was regarded by Bleuler as the most important symptom of schizophrenia. Historically, types of thought disorder have included associative loosening, illogical thinking, overinclusive thinking, and loss of ability to engage in abstract thinking. A standard set of definitions for various types of thought disorder has been developed (Andreasen 1979) that stresses objective aspects of language and communication (which are empirical indicators of "thought"), such as derailment, poverty of speech, poverty of content of speech, or tangential replies. All have been found to occur frequently in both schizophrenia and mood disorders. Manic patients often have a thought disorder characterized by tangentiality, derailment (loose associations), and illogicality. Depressed patients manifest thought disorder less frequently than manic patients, but often display a poverty of speech, tangentiality, or circumstantiality. Other types of formal thought disorder include perseveration, distractibility, clanging, neologisms, echolalia, and blocking; with the possible exception of clanging in mania, none appears to be disorder specific. Because these various forms of thought disorder are inferred from listening to patients speak, the concept of disorganized speech has evolved and appears as such in the diagnostic criteria.

Disorganized or *catatonic motor behavior* is another aspect of this dimension. Many patients with schizophrenia display various motor disturbances and changes in social behavior. Abnormal motor behaviors range from catatonic stupor to excitement. In a catatonic stupor, the patient may be immobile, mute, and unresponsive, and yet remain fully conscious. A patient may exhibit uncontrolled and aimless motor activity while in a state of catatonic excitement. Some patients manifest *waxy flexibility* (flexibilitas cerea), in which they allow themselves to be placed in uncomfortable positions, which are maintained without apparent distress. Schizophrenic patients sometimes assume bizarre or awkward postures and maintain them for long periods, such as squatting for hours, which would cause obvious discomfort to most people.

Several disorders of movement that occur in schizophrenia need to be distinguished from drug-induced extrapyramidal side effects of antipsychotics and tardive dyskinesia (Manschreck et al. 1982). These include *stereotypies*, which are repeated movements that are not goal directed such as rocking; *mannerisms*, which are normal goal-directed activities that appear to have social significance but are either odd in appearance or out of context, such as grimacing or repeatedly running a hand through one's hair. *Mitgehen* is seen when the slightest pressure causes the patient's limbs to move in the direction of the push, despite being told to resist the pressure. Less common symptoms are *echopraxia*, which is imitating the movements and gestures of another person; *automatic obedience*, which is carrying out simple commands in a robotlike fashion; and *negativism*, which is refusing to cooperate with simple requests for no apparent reason. Many schizophrenic patients display ritualistic behaviors resembling those seen in obsessive-compulsive disorder, such as repetitive hand washing, checking, arranging, or counting (Fenton and McGlashan 1986). Some schizophrenic patients develop compulsive water drinking, which can lead to water intoxication necessitating careful attention to fluid and electrolyte balance (deLeon et al. 1994).

Antipsychotic medications are often associated with various extrapyramidal side effects (EPS) as well as tardive dyskinesia, all of which are discussed in Chapter 18. Many schizophrenic patients were reported to display EPS or spontaneous involuntary movements before antipsychotics became available (Chatterjee et al. 1995). The presence of spontaneous EPS has been linked to poorer treatment response and negative symptoms. When tardive dyskinesia is present, schizophrenic patients are often unaware of their involuntary movements. Even when the abnormal movements are pointed out, the patient may remain unconcerned (Caracci et al. 1990).

Deterioration of social behavior often develops along with social withdrawal. Patients may neglect themselves and become messy or unkempt; wear dirty, unmended, or inappropriate clothing; and ignore or neglect their cluttered, untidy surroundings. Patients may develop other odd behaviors, breaking social conventions by exhibiting crude table manners, foraging through garbage bins, or shouting obscenities. It has been estimated that between one-third and one-half of today's "homeless" persons have schizophrenia (Susser et al. 1989).

Incongruity of affect is the third component of the disorganization dimension. Patients may smile inappropriately when speaking of neutral or sad topics, or giggle for no apparent reason. This symptom should not be confused with the nervous smiling or giggling that sometimes occurs in anxious patients. Affective incongruity should only be considered a symptom of schizophrenia when it occurs in the context of other characteristic symptoms.

The Negative Dimension

DSM-IV-TR lists three negative symptoms as characteristic of schizophrenia: alogia, affective blunting, and avolition.

Other negative symptoms that are common in schizophrenia include anhedonia and attentional impairment (Andreasen 1982; Andreasen and Olson 1982).

Alogia is characterized by a diminution in the amount of spontaneous speech, a tendency to produce speech that is empty or impoverished in content when the amount is adequate. It is the external expression in language of the impoverishment of thought that occurs in many patients with schizophrenia. Patients may have great difficulty in producing fluent responses to questions. Instead, they tend to say little or reply concretely. For example, if asked, "What brought you to the hospital?" the patient may reply, "A car."

Affective flattening or blunting is a reduced intensity of emotional expression and response. It is manifested by unchanging facial expression, decreased spontaneous movements, poverty of expressive gestures, poor eye contact, lack of vocal inflections, and slowed speech.

Anhedonia, or the inability to experience pleasure, is also very common. Many patients describe themselves as feeling emotionally empty. They are no longer able to enjoy activities that previously gave them pleasure, such as playing sports or seeing family or friends. Their awareness that they have lost the capacity to enjoy themselves may be a source of great psychological pain.

Avolition is a loss of the ability to initiate goal-directed behavior and carry it through to completion. Patients seem to have lost their will or drive. They may initiate a project and then abandon it for no apparent reason. They may take a job, go to work for a few days or weeks, and then fail to appear or wander aimlessly away while at work. This symptom is sometimes interpreted as laziness, but in fact it represents the loss or diminution of basic drives and the capacity to formulate and pursue long-range plans.

Attentional impairment is reflected in the inability to concentrate or focus on a task or a question. Patients may complain of feeling bombarded by stimuli that they cannot process or filter; this in turn causes them to feel confused or to experience fragmented thoughts.

The negative symptoms of schizophrenia and the symptoms of depression are somewhat similar, making differential diagnosis of depression and schizophrenia difficult in some patients. Significant depressive symptoms occur in up to 60% of patients with schizophrenia (Guze et al. 1983), leading to substantial distress, prompting suicidal behavior in some patients, and compromising what little energy and motivation the patient has. Antipsychotic medication itself may induce what appears to be depression but is actually a drug-induced akinesia. This "depression" may go away when the dosage of antipsychotic is reduced or an anticholinergic medication is added (King et al. 1995). The International Classification of Diseases, Tenth Revision (ICD-10; World Health Organization 1992), recognizes a category called "post-psychotic depression," defined as a full-blown depression occurring after the acute-phase symptoms have fully resolved. In DSM-IV-TR, a postpsychotic depression, or a major depression occurring in a patient with well-established schizophrenia, is diagnosed as a depressive disorder not otherwise specified.

Cognitive Impairment as the Fundamental Deficit

Many thinkers, beginning with both Kraepelin and Bleuler, have considered schizophrenia to be a neurocognitive disorder, with the various signs and symptoms reflecting the downstream effects of a fundamental cognitive deficit. This fundamental cognitive deficit was highlighted in the original name *dementia praecox* and in the later name *schizophrenia* ("fragmented mind"). Schizophrenia poses special challenges to the development of cognitive models because of its breadth and diversity of symptoms. The symptoms include nearly all cognitive domains: perception (hallucinations), inferential thinking (delusions), fluency of thought and speech (alogia), clarity and organization of thought and speech ("formal thought disorder"), motor activity (catatonia), emotional expression (affective blunting), ability to initiate and complete goal-directed behavior (avolition), and ability to seek out and experience emotional gratification (anhedonia). Not all these symptoms are present in any given patient, however, and none is pathognomonic of the illness. An initial survey of the diversity of symptoms might suggest that multiple brain regions are involved, in a spotty pattern much as once occurred in neurosyphilis. In the absence of visible lesions and known pathogens, however, investigators have turned to the exploration of models that could explain the diversity of symptoms by a single cognitive mechanism. Several leading cognitive neuroscientists and psychiatrists have developed models that can explain the symptoms based on a fundamental cognitive deficit. The convergent conclusions of these different models are striking.

The common thread in these observations, gleaned from very different starting points, is that schizophrenia reflects a disruption in a fundamental cognitive process that affects a specific circuitry in the brain. Various research teams may use different terminology and somewhat different concepts—meta-representations, representationally guided behavior, information processing/attention, cognitive dysmetria—but they convey a common theme. The cognitive dysfunction in schizophrenia is an inefficient temporal and spatial referencing of information and experience as the individual attempts to determine boundaries between self and not-self and to formulate effective decisions or plans that will guide him or her through the small-scale (speaking a sentence) or large-scale (finding a job) maneuvers of daily living. This capacity is sometimes referred to as *consciousness*.

Clinical Validity of Cognitive Models

The clinical validity of these cognitive models of schizophrenia is supported by a variety of studies using neuropsychological testing. One crucial question addressed by these studies is whether patients with schizophrenia experience cognitive deterioration over time, as occurs in patients with Alzheimer's disease, or whether the cognitive impairment is stable. The bulk of the evidence supports the latter.

Neuropsychological impairment is not restricted to a small subset of patients; measurable impairment is present in 40%–60% of schizophrenic patients (Goldberg et al. 1988). Cognitive impairment tends to be generalized but is most pronounced for cognitive tasks involving attention, memory, and executive functions (Mohamed et al. 1999).

Other Symptoms

Lack of Insight

Lack of insight is common in schizophrenia. Patients often deny they are ill or abnormal, and insist their hallucinations and delusions are real. Poor insight is one of the most difficult symptoms to treat and often persists even when other symptoms (e.g., hallucinations) respond to medication. Orientation and memory are generally preserved, unless impaired by the patient's psychotic symptoms, inattention, or distractibility.

Soft Signs

Nonlocalizing *soft signs* occur in a substantial proportion of patients with schizophrenia and include abnormalities in stereognosis, graphesthesia, balance, and proprioception (Gupta et al. 1995a). Although the clinical significance of these signs is unclear, their presence may reflect dysfunction in areas of motor coordination, integrative sensory function, and ordering complex motor tasks. In one study (Krakowski et al. 1989), violent schizophrenic patients were more likely to exhibit neurological soft signs than were nonviolent patients.

Vegetative Functions

Some patients display disturbances of sleep, sexual interest, or other bodily functions. Various disrupted sleep measures have been reported in schizophrenia, but decreased delta sleep with diminished stage 4 is the most consistent finding (Neylan et al. 1992). Schizophrenic patients often have little interest in sexual activity and may derive little or no pleasure from sexual experiences (Lyketsos et al. 1983).

Immune System Function

Disturbed immune functioning has been reported in schizophrenia and includes abnormalities of circulating lymphocytes, peripheral and/or cerebrospinal fluid immunoglobulin and interferon levels, and the production of antibrain antibodies (Rothermundt et al. 2000).

Premorbid Personality

Several early writers including Kraepelin and Bleuler observed that patients with schizophrenia often had abnormal premorbid personalities. In a review of early studies of personality and schizophrenia, Cutting (1985) reported that premorbid schizoid traits were present in one-fourth of schizophrenic patients, but one-sixth had a range of other personality disturbances. Consistent with this review, a study of 52 chronic schizophrenic patients from the Iowa 500 sample (Pfohl and Winokur 1983) found 35% to meet criteria for a DSM-III personality disorder premorbidly; 44% of these personality disorders were schizoid, and the rest were a mixture of avoidant, paranoid, histrionic, compulsive, and other personality disorders.

Substance Abuse and Smoking

Comorbid alcohol and drug abuse is common in patients with schizophrenia and occurs at rates exceeding that found in the community (Dixon et al. 1991). Drug-taking schizophrenic patients tend to be younger and are more likely to be male than non–drug-taking schizophrenic patients. They also have poorer medication compliance, higher rates of rehospitalization, and poorer adjustment and treatment response than patients without such abuse or dependence (Drake et al. 1989). Some researchers believe that schizophrenic patients abuse drugs in an attempt to self-medicate, to treat their medication side effects (i.e., drug-induced akinesia), or to lessen their amotivation and avolition. Cigarette smoking is also very common, and in one study nearly three out of four schizophrenic patients smoke (Goff et al. 1992). Smoking increases neuroleptic metabolism and consequently may be associated with the need for higher neuroleptic dosages.

Subtypes of Schizophrenia

DSM-IV-TR recognizes five classic subtypes of schizophrenia: 1) paranoid, 2) disorganized, 3) catatonic, 4) undifferentiated, and 5) residual. The main purposes of subtyping are to improve predictive

validity, to help the clinician select treatments and predict outcome, and to help the researcher delineate homogeneous subtypes. However, these goals remain largely unfulfilled. The reliability and validity of the classic subtypes are poor. Data from the International Pilot Study of Schizophrenia also failed to substantiate their usefulness (Strauss and Carpenter 1981). Furthermore, many patients seem to fit several of these subtypes during the course of their illness.

Paranoid Schizophrenia

The paranoid subtype is characterized by a preoccupation with one or more delusions and/or frequent auditory hallucinations; disorganized speech/behavior, catatonic behavior, and flat or inappropriate affect are not prominent.

In contrast to other subtypes, patients with paranoid schizophrenia have an older age at onset, better premorbid functioning, and a better outcome. They are more likely to marry and have better occupational functioning than patients with other subtypes (Fenton and McGlashan 1991; Winokur et al. 1974).

Disorganized Schizophrenia

This subtype is characterized by disorganized speech and behavior and flat or inappropriate affect; it does not meet criteria for catatonic schizophrenia. Generally, delusions and hallucinations, if present, are fragmentary, unlike the well-systematized delusions of the paranoid schizophrenic. Hebephrenia typically has an early onset that begins with the insidious development of avolition, affective flattening, deterioration of habits, and cognitive impairment, as well as delusions and hallucinations (Winokur et al. 1974). Hebephrenic patients are also reported to have a greater family history of psychopathology, poorer premorbid functioning, and poorer long-term prognosis with continuous illness than patients with paranoid schizophrenia (Fenton and McGlashan 1991). Clinically, hebephrenic patients often seem silly and childlike. They sometimes grimace or giggle inappropriately or appear self-absorbed. Mirror gazing is commonly described in these patients.

Catatonic Schizophrenia

In DSM-IV-TR catatonic schizophrenia is defined as a type of schizophrenia dominated by at least two of the following: motoric immobility as evidenced by catalepsy or stupor, extreme agitation, extreme negativism or mutism, peculiarities of voluntary movement (e.g., stereotypies, mannerisms, grimacing), and echolalia or echopraxia. Compared with other subtypes, patients with catatonic schizophrenia tend to have the earliest age at onset, the most chronic course, and the poorest social and occupational functioning (Kendler et al. 1994b). This subtype of schizophrenia is reportedly less common than in the past, at least in developed countries (Sartorius et al. 1986).

Undifferentiated and Residual Subtypes

DSM-IV-TR also includes the undifferentiated subtype of schizophrenia, which is a residual category for patients meeting criteria for schizophrenia but not meeting criteria for the paranoid, disorganized, or catatonic subtypes. This subtype is the most widely diagnosed.

The residual subtype as described in DSM-IV-TR is applied to patients who no longer have prominent psychotic symptoms but who once met criteria for schizophrenia and have continuing evidence of illness. Ongoing illness may be indicated by the presence of negative symptoms or of two or more symptoms listed in criterion A for schizophrenia, present in an attenuated form (e.g., odd beliefs, unusual perceptual experiences).

Other Subtypes Not in DSM-IV-TR

Simple schizophrenia is characterized by the insidious development of odd behavior, inability to meet societal demands, and decline in performance, but the absence of true delusions or hallucinations. In a recent epidemiological study in Ireland, Kendler et al. (1994a) estimated the lifetime prevalence at 5.3 per 10,000. From a family perspective, the disorder appears related to typical schizophrenia.

A schizoaffective subtype was included in DSM-II. This diagnosis is used with individuals who have pronounced manic or depressive features commingled with schizophrenic symptoms. DSM-IV-TR recognizes schizoaffective disorder as a separate and distinct illness (see the "Schizoaffective Disorder" section later in this chapter).

Schizophreniform Disorder

The current DSM-IV-TR definition of schizophreniform disorder requires more than 1 month but less than 6 months of characteristic symptoms of schizophrenia (criterion A of schizophrenia) that are not due to schizoaffective disorder, mood disorders, direct physiological effects of drugs or medications, or a general medical condition (Table 5–4). Besides a shorter illness duration, schizophreniform disorder differs from schizophrenia in that it does not require impairment in social or occupational functioning, although such impairments may occur. The diagnosis changes to schizophrenia if symptoms extend past 6 months, even if the symptoms are residual. The disorder can be further subdivided into cases with and without good prognostic features (e.g., acute onset).

Most studies have not supported the validity of schizophreniform disorder as a distinct diagnosis. In a review, Strakowski (1994) reported that the diagnosis identifies a heterogeneous group of patients. Follow-up studies show that most patients with schizophreniform disorder eventually develop other psychiatric syndromes, including schizophrenia, mood disorders, or schizoaffective disorder. Results from family studies have been contradictory, some finding an increased rate of schizophrenia in relatives, others finding an increased rate of mood disorders. Neurobiological studies have generally failed to show any difference between patients with schizophreniform disorder and control subjects. In one intriguing study (DeLisi et al. 1992), ventriculomegaly occurring in patients with schizophreniform disorder was associated with poor outcome and progression to schizophrenia. Perhaps in a subset of these patients, enlarged ventricles may provide useful prognostic information.

Neuroendocrine challenge studies suggest that some patients with schizophreniform disorder exhibit abnormalities similar to those shown in patients with mood disorders. For example, Targum (1983) concluded that patients with schizophreniform disorder can be separated into those with atypical mood disorders and those with early schizophrenia by virtue of their neuroendocrine challenge test results including the dexamethasone suppression test. Outcome studies show that overall, patients with schizophreniform disorder have better outcomes than patients with schizophrenia (Coryell and Tsuang 1986), although outcome depends primarily on whether or not the patient subsequently developed schizophrenia or a mood disorder.

Clearly, the proper boundaries for schizophreniform disorder have not been established, so that the main use of the diagnosis is to guard against a premature

TABLE 5–4. DSM-IV-TR diagnostic criteria for schizophreniform disorder

A. Criteria A, D, and E of schizophrenia are met.
B. An episode of the disorder (including prodromal, active, and residual phases) lasts at least 1 month but less than 6 months. (When the diagnosis must be made without waiting for recovery, it should be qualified as "Provisional.")

Specify if:
   Without Good Prognostic Features
   With Good Prognostic Features: as evidenced by two (or more) of the following:
   (1) onset of prominent psychotic symptoms within 4 weeks of the first noticeable change in usual behavior or functioning
   (2) confusion or perplexity at the height of the psychotic episode
   (3) good premorbid social and occupational functioning
   (4) absence of blunted or flat affect

diagnosis of schizophrenia. Treatment of schizophreniform disorder is similar to that of an acute episode of schizophrenia, which is described later in this chapter.

Course and Outcome

The course of schizophrenia can follow various patterns, although schizophrenia is typically viewed as a chronic disorder that begins in late adolescence and has a poor long-term outcome. The overt manifestations of schizophrenia are often preceded by subtle, nonspecific behavioral and neuromotor cues that are observable as early as childhood (Bleuler 1950; Kraepelin 1919; Meares 1959; Walker and Lewine 1990; N.F. Watt 1978).

It has been estimated that these childhood behavioral and neuromotor antecedents are present in approximately one-third of schizophrenia patients. Onset of the schizophrenia syndrome itself may be insidious or abrupt, although schizophrenia generally begins with a *prodromal phase* characterized by social withdrawal and other subtle changes in behavior and emotional responsiveness. A patient may be seen as remote, aloof, emotionally detached, or even odd or eccentric. The onset of subtle thought disturbances and impaired attention may also occur at this stage. The prodrome varies in length, but typically lasts from months to years (Carpenter and Buchanan 1994).

The prodrome is followed by an *active phase* in which psychotic symptoms predominate. At this point, clinical disorder becomes evident, and a diagnosis of schizophrenia can usually be made. This phase is characterized by florid hallucinations and delusions, which alarm friends and family members and often lead to medical intervention. A *residual phase* follows the resolution of the active phase and is similar to the prodrome. Psychotic symptoms may persist during this phase, but at a lower level of intensity, and they may not be as troublesome to the patient. Active-phase symptoms may occur episodically ("acute exacerbations"), with variable levels of remission seen between episodes. The frequency and timing of these episodes is unpredictable, although stressful situations may precede these relapses, or in some instances, drug abuse (Linszen et al. 1994). Relapses are often preceded by changes in thought, feeling, or behavior noticed by the patient and family members. Symptoms preceding relapse include dysphoria, seclusiveness, sleep disturbance, anxiety, and ideas of reference (Herz 1985). Through this process, patients accrue increased levels of morbidity in the form of residual or persistent symptoms and decrements in function from their premorbid status. Relatively severe psychosis is continuous and unrelenting in some patients.

Outcome

The clinical course and outcome in schizophrenia has been studied and debated since Kraepelin first described dementia praecox as chronic and progressive, leading inevitably to severe impairment. Hegarty et al. (1994) summarized the outcome of 51,800 schizophrenic patients from 320 studies reported in the psychiatric literature between 1895 and 1992. Followed for an average of nearly 6 years, 40% of the patients were considered improved. Improvement was essentially defined as recovery, remission, or being well with minimal symptoms. They reported that outcome was much better when patients were diagnosed according to diagnostic symptoms with broad criteria (47% improved), rather than narrow criteria (27% improved). Further, the proportion of patients who improved was greater after the midcentury mark than before (49% versus 35%), perhaps reflecting a broadened concept of schizophrenia as well as improved treatment. Since 1975 the rate of favorable improvement has fallen to 36%, perhaps reflecting the impact of the reemergence of narrowed diagnostic criteria.

Several long-term follow-up studies have been published using contemporary American definitions of schizophrenia. The two best known are the Iowa 500, which used the St. Louis criteria, and the Chestnut Lodge study, which used the DSM-III criteria. The findings of these studies are remarkably similar (McGlashan 1984; Tsuang et al. 1979). In the Iowa 500 study, 186 schizophrenic patients admitted to the University of Iowa Psychiatric Hospital between 1934 and 1944 were followed up in the early 1970s. Twenty percent of patients with schizophrenia were reported to be psychiatrically well at follow-up, but 54% had incapacitating psychiatric symptoms; 21% were married or widowed, but 67% had never married; 34% lived in their own home or with a relative, but 18% were in mental institutions; 35% were economically productive, but 58% had never worked. The group experienced excess mortality from both natural and unnatural causes, and more than 10% committed suicide. In a recent reanalysis of this seminal study, Winokur and Tsuang (1996) reported that only two of the schizophrenic patients followed up were completely free of symptoms (i.e., had "zero symptoms"). They concluded that whereas a patient may be considered improved and is able to work and to live independently, he or she is unlikely to be free of all symptoms.

In the Chestnut Lodge study, 163 schizophrenic patients discharged from the private hospital between 1950 and 1975 were followed up in the early 1980s. Whereas 37% were living in a hospital or sheltered environment, only 28% were living independently; 26% had been employed 50% of the follow-up period or better; 41% were considered continuously incapacitated, and only 6% had recovered. McGlashan (1984) noted that roughly two-thirds of the schizophrenic patients were functioning marginally or worse at follow-up and that 7% had killed themselves during the interim.

However, Riecher-Rossler and Rossler (1998) contend that many of these outcome studies have major methodological problems, particularly with regard to sample selection biases that lead to underrepresentation of patients with both the best and the worst outcomes. Therefore, findings from such studies may not generalize to the real world. In their literature review, which focused on five prospective studies that used representative catchment-area-based first-admitted or first-contact samples, Riecher-Rossler and Rossler concluded that whereas the course of schizophrenia is far from uniform, many patients with schizophrenia have a relatively

good outcome and will avoid progressive deterioration. Significant improvement is possible, albeit years or decades after the first manifestations of psychosis. The illness process begins with nonspecific signs that occur long before first hospitalization and before the first occurrence of psychotic symptomatology.

Predicting Outcome

Although a variety of prognostic factors have been reported (Jonsson and Nyman 1984; McCabe et al. 1972; McGlashan 1986; Vaillant 1964), prediction of outcome remains a difficult task. Research has shown that definitions of schizophrenia that exclude patients with mood symptoms or those having a duration of illness under 6 months generally predict a poor prognosis. This is because these relatively restrictive definitions exclude patients with mood disorder, schizophreniform disorder, or schizoaffective disorders, who tend to have better outcomes. Perhaps the best study of outcome prediction was the International Pilot Study of Schizophrenia (World Health Organization 1975), in which psychiatrists in nine different countries participated. Regression analysis showed the five most powerful predictors of poor outcome to be social isolation, long duration of episode, history of past psychiatric treatment, being unmarried, and having a history of behavioral problems in childhood such as truancy and tantrums. The investigators also found that all 47 potential predictors accounted for only 38% of the variance. A summary of commonly reported prognostic factors is shown in Table 5–5.

Other Factors That Affect Outcome

Cultural Factors

Cross-cultural studies have shown that schizophrenic patients living in less developed countries tend to have better outcomes than those in more developed

TABLE 5–5.   Features associated with good and poor outcome in schizophrenia

Feature	Good outcome	Poor outcome
Age	Older	Younger
Gender	Female	Male
Social class	High	Low
Marital history	Married	Never married
Family history of schizophrenia	Negative	Positive
Perinatal complications	Absent	Present
Transcultural factors	Developing nations	Industrialized nations
Premorbid functioning	Good	Poor
Onset	Acute	Insidious
Duration	Short	Chronic
Sensorium	Clouded	Clear
Symptoms/subtypes	Paranoid subtype	Deficit syndrome
Affective symptoms	Present	Absent
Neurological functioning	Normal	Soft signs present
Neurocognition	Normal	Abnormal
Structural brain abnormalities	None	Present

countries. This unexpected finding was reported in the International Pilot Study of Schizophrenia (World Health Organization 1975), which demonstrated that the average outcome was considerably better in the developing countries (Colombia, India, and Nigeria) than in the industrialized countries (Czechoslovakia, Denmark, United Kingdom, United States, and the former Soviet Union). Despite extensive follow-up treatment available in industrialized countries, a high proportion of their patients had additional psychotic episodes not seen in the patients in developing countries. Although there were no important differences in the initial symptoms and other characteristics of the patients at the nine study sites, the possibility cannot be dismissed that these differences in outcome were due to unrecognized differences in the types of patients seeking treatment. One explanation is that the schizophrenic patient is better accepted in less developed countries, has fewer external demands, and is more likely to be taken care of by interested family members. The same finding emerged from a comparison of outcomes of schizophrenia in London and Mauritius (Murphy and Raman 1971).

Gender

Women with schizophrenia appear to have a more favorable outcome than men in treatment response, social functioning, and overall prognosis. A study of 121 schizophrenic patients in England (D.C. Watt et al. 1983) found that at a 5-year follow-up, 62% of women had a good outcome as compared with 35% of men. Women also had better housing, probably due to the fact that they were less likely than men to live alone or to be institutionalized. A similar study of 278 schizophrenic patients in Germany (Angermeyer et al. 1989) found women to have fewer rehospitalizations and shorter lengths of stay.

Epidemiology

Schizophrenia presents a challenge to the epidemiologist, due to disagreements about the definition of its core features and the breadth of its spectrum. The development of operational criteria, such as those in DSM-IV-TR, has provided greater specificity for the diagnosis of schizophrenia and has resulted in a more cautious use of the concept. This has led to a reassessment of earlier epidemiological studies that generated rates based on older conceptualizations of schizophrenia. Despite these advances, case identification remains an ongoing problem among epidemiologists. Efforts to standardize the diagnosis have met with some success, such as with the Present State Examination used in the International Pilot Study of Schizophrenia and the Composite Interview Diagnostic Instrument used in the National Comorbidity Study (Kessler et al. 1994).

Prevalence and Incidence

In a comprehensive review, Eaton et al. (1988) reported that the median point prevalence of schizophrenia was 3.2 per 1,000 (range 0.6–8.3). The median lifetime prevalence rate was 4.4 per 1,000 (range 1.7–7.0). *Point prevalence* includes all identified cases at a given point in time. *Lifetime prevalence*, or "disease expectancy," includes the proportion of persons studied who have ever experienced the disorder up to the time of assessment. The type of prevalence measure reported (i.e., point, lifetime) appears not to strongly influence the rate, presumably due to the chronic nature and low incidence of schizophrenia (Eaton 1985). In the National Comorbidity Study, in which lay-interviewed patients evidencing symptoms of psychosis were reinterviewed by a psychiatrist, the lifetime rate for schizophrenia was 0.14% (Bromet et al. 1995). This rate is much lower than the rate reported in the Epidemiologic Catchment Area study (1.3% lifetime; Robins et al. 1984). That finding

was based on results of the lay-administered Diagnostic Interview Schedule, an instrument with relatively poor reliability for the diagnosis of schizophrenia (Anthony et al. 1985).

A review of annual incidence rates of schizophrenia (Eaton et al. 1988) show a median rate of 0.20 per 1,000 (range 0.11–0.70). *Incidence* is the number of new cases that arise in a given time per unit of population. (A simple formula, prevalence = incidence × duration, shows the relationship between these two parameters.) Because incidence does not confound the rate of occurrence with duration, many investigators find it a more useful measure for etiological studies, although both measures are helpful for planning health services. A World Health Organization study (Jablensky et al. 1992) involving 10 research sites showed that incidence rates were remarkably similar across the various sites. A reported decline in the incidence rate of schizophrenia has been debated, as some researchers believe that new cases are less frequent than many decades ago (Eaton 1991). It is likely that any apparent rate decline is tied to changing diagnostic practices that favor more restrictive definitions such as that in DSM-IV-TR.

Age at Onset and Sex Ratio

Schizophrenia typically begins in early adulthood, but can develop at any age including early childhood (Beitchman 1985). Both Bleuler and Kraepelin reported an earlier onset for men than women, a finding confirmed by subsequent research. In one study (Loranger 1984), mean age at onset was 21.4 years for men and 26.8 years for women. Mean age at first treatment occurred 5 and 7 years later, respectively. A total of 9 of 10 males, but only 2 of 3 females, had developed schizophrenia by age 30. Onset after age 35 occurred in 17% of women, but in only 2% of men. The reason women develop schizophrenia later than men remains a mystery, but it is apparently not an artifact resulting from women having a more sheltered existence that conceals their illness. Kendler et al. (1996) concluded that environmental or developmental factors probably account for the variation seen in the age at onset in schizophrenia.

Early epidemiological studies showed approximately equal rates of schizophrenia for men and women, but the broad concept of schizophrenia used in the past may have led to the inclusion of a disproportionate number of women with mood disorders. Lewine et al. (1984) analyzed the effect of using six different diagnostic systems on the male-to-female ratio of schizophrenia among 387 inpatients. Diagnostic criteria that present a broad concept of schizophrenia, such as the New Haven schizophrenia index, yielded equal rates of schizophrenia among men and women. Diagnostic systems with more stringent criteria, such as the Research Diagnostic Criteria, yielded a greater male-to-female ratio.

Marital Status and Reproduction

Patients with schizophrenia are more likely to remain single than are patients in other diagnostic groups. This is particularly true in male patients (Eaton 1985), which can probably be explained by the fact that women tend to be younger than men when first married and are less likely to have experienced an initial psychotic episode. From a cultural perspective, women have traditionally been less active in initiating relationships, which may account for some of the difference.

Early researchers tended to find low rates of fertility and reproduction among patients with schizophrenia (Kallman

1938). This finding can probably be explained by several factors including lack of interest in social relations, general apathy, low sex drive, and lack of opportunity for a sexual relationship due to hospitalization or institutionalization. Rates of reproduction in patients with schizophrenia have probably increased since deinstitutionalization, although they remain lower than those found in the general population (Nimgaonkar 1998). Lower fecundity affects males more than females with schizophrenia.

Socioeconomic Status

Patients with schizophrenia generally have low social status. Eaton (1985) reviewed 17 studies of incidence of treated schizophrenia that included indicators of social class. The highest rate of schizophrenia was found in the lowest social class in 15 of the studies. Earlier studies suggested that the lower socioeconomic status seen in schizophrenic patients probably results from the "downward drift" in socioeconomic status they experience due to the debilitating effects of their symptoms, which impair social and occupational functioning.

Ethnicity and Race

Jablensky and Sartorius (1975) concluded from a literature review that except for a high rate found by Böök in north Sweden (10.8 per 1,000) and a low rate reported by Eaton and Weil for the Hutterite sect in the United States (1.1 per 1,000), prevalence rates for schizophrenia are relatively similar worldwide. Although early studies in the United States suggested a higher rate of schizophrenia in African Americans than in whites, this finding was probably due to a systematic bias to overdiagnose schizophrenia in blacks (Mukherjee et al. 1983).

Mortality and Morbidity

Research has long shown increased mortality in patients with schizophrenia (Simpson and Tsuang 1996). In the past, high death rates were attributed to both natural and unnatural causes. Before modern medical and psychiatric treatments were available, many patients suffered the ill effects of prolonged psychiatric symptoms leading to malnutrition or dehydration or were exposed to tuberculosis and other infectious diseases in large institutions. Because general medical and psychiatric care has improved, high death rates in patients with schizophrenia are now due primarily to suicide and accidents. In one study (Black and Fisher 1992), schizophrenic patients showed a near threefold increase over expected mortality. Those at risk for premature death were patients younger than 40 years and who were in their first few years of follow-up.

Based on early epidemiological studies, patients with schizophrenia were once thought to have some immunity from cancer. Recent research shows that although cancer death rates in general are not different than expected, there is evidence of lower risk for lung cancer despite high rates of smoking in those patients (Black and Winokur 1986; Gulbinat et al. 1992). There is evidence, too, that rheumatoid arthritis is less common in patients with schizophrenia (Eaton et al. 1992) than among persons in the general population, although the reason for this association is unknown.

Suicide and Suicidal Behavior

Patients with schizophrenia are at high risk for suicidal behavior. Nearly one-third will attempt suicide (Allebeck et al. 1987), and about 1 in 10 will complete suicide (Tsuang 1978). Between 2% and 3% of suicide completers have schizophrenia (Barraclough et al. 1974). Risk factors for suicide include male gender, age less than 30 years, living alone, unemployment, chronic relapsing course, prior depression, past treatment for depression, depression during the last episode of illness, history of substance abuse, and recent hospital discharge (Allebeck et al. 1987; A. Roy 1982). Schizophrenic patients with the paranoid subtype and those with a high level of education appear to be at greater risk for suicide (Fenton and McGlashan 1991), perhaps due to the patients' feelings of inadequacy and hopelessness, fear of disintegration, and a realization that desired expectations will never be met. Unlike other psychiatric patients who commit suicide, patients with schizophrenia may fail to communicate their suicidal intentions and may act impulsively, complicating any effort at intervention (Breier and Astrachan 1984).

Violence and Criminality

Until quite recently it was thought that mentally ill persons were not predisposed to violent behavior (Teplin 1985). In the Epidemiologic Catchment Area study (Swanson et al. 1990), however, patients with schizophrenia had rates of violent behavior five times higher than persons without mental illness, although the rate was about one-half that seen in individuals with alcohol abuse or dependence. Schizophrenic patients with coexisting alcoholism are even more likely to commit violent acts, including homicide, than patients not abusing substances (Modestin and Ammann 1996). The severely mentally ill have high rates of conviction for criminal offenses and incarceration, although many of the offenses have been called "survival crimes," such as shoplifting and petty thievery thought due to homelessness or deinstitutionalization (Csillag 1993). To some extent, violent behavior may be a function of the stage of a schizophrenic patient's illness (e.g., in response to persecutory delusions) and remains one of the primary reasons for hospitalization.

Treatment Delays and Utilization of Health Services

Studies of first-episode psychosis from around the world have consistently shown that there is a time lag averaging 1–2 years between the onset of psychotic symptoms and initiation of treatment (McGlashan 1999). Although the reasons for the treatment delay remain unclear (Ho and Andreasen 2001), its implications for service delivery and outcome are increasingly being recognized (Lieberman and Fenton 2000). Based on the pioneering work of Falloon (1992) and McGorry et al. (1996), programs dedicated to detecting patients at the prodrome stage of the disorder and reducing treatment delays have shown much promise. However, currently available methods of screening for schizophrenia still have moderately high false-positive rates. Furthermore, whether earlier treatment leads to better outcome has yet to be established (Ho and Andreasen 2001). More research is still needed before the potential of secondary prevention can be realized.

National Institute of Mental Health data show schizophrenia to be the first or second most frequent diagnosis for admissions to various types of psychiatric inpatient services, ranging from 21% for private hospitals to 38% for state and county hospitals, with a length of stay averaging 18–42 days, respectively. There were over 1.6 million admissions of schizophrenic patients to inpatient facilities in 1980 (Taube and Barrett 1985). Results from the Epidemiologic Catchment Area study (Shapiro et al. 1984) showed that nearly 78% of schizophrenic patients surveyed

had health care visits during the previous 6 months; 45% of visits were for mental health care. Patients with schizophrenia tended to obtain mental health care from specialists rather than from general medical providers, which indicates the severity of the illness, since the opposite was true for most nonpsychotic disorders.

Pathophysiology and Etiology

Consensus now exists among many investigators that schizophrenia is best conceptualized as a "multiple-hit" illness similar to cancer. Individuals may carry a genetic predisposition, but this vulnerabilty is not "released" unless other factors also intervene. Although most of these factors are considered environmental, in the sense that they are not encoded in DNA and could potentially produce mutations or influence gene expression, most are also biological rather than psychological and include factors such as birth injuries or nutrition. Current studies of the neurobiology of schizophrenia examine a multiplicity of factors, including genetics, anatomy (primarily through structural neuroimaging), functional circuitry (through functional neuroimaging), neuropatholgy, electrophysiology, neurochemistry and neuropharmacology, and neurodevelopment.

Genetics

Evidence for a hereditary contribution to schizophrenia is based on family studies, twin studies, and studies of adoptees. As early as 1916, Rudin reported an increased prevalence of dementia praecox among the siblings of affected probands. Subsequent family studies have confirmed an increased prevalence of schizophrenia and related disorders in family members, with risk related to the number of shared genes of family members with the schizophrenic proband. Summaries of individual family studies have shown siblings of schizophrenic patients to have a near 10% lifetime risk of developing schizophrenia, while children who have one parent with schizophrenia have a 5%–6% lifetime risk (Gottesman and Shields 1982). The risk of a family member developing schizophrenia markedly increases when two or more family members have the illness, with a lifetime expectancy of schizophrenia of 17% for those with one sibling and one parent with schizophrenia and up to 46% in children of two parents with schizophrenia. Although these findings strongly support the familial nature of schizophrenia, they do not confirm a genetic over a familial environmental cause.

Twin studies and adoption studies allow a natural experimental paradigm to separate the genetic and environmental effects of familial associations. Despite varying methods, twin studies have been remarkably consistent in demonstrating high concordance rates for monozygotic twins (Farmer et al. 1987; Gottesman and Shields 1982). Rates have averaged 46% as compared with 14% in dizygotic twins across multiple studies, with only one negative twin study (Tienari 1963). However, the failure of monozygotic twins to be 100% concordant suggests that a hereditary component may be necessary but is insufficient to cause schizophrenia and that environmental factors are also important.

Adoption studies present another paradigm for evaluating genetic influences in familial illness. Heston (1966) examined grown children of mothers with schizophrenia who had been adopted and compared them with control adoptees whose mothers had no psychiatric disorder. He found a nearly 17% age-corrected morbid-

ity risk of schizophrenia in the adoptees of schizophrenic mothers, a figure similar to those reported family studies of children of mothers with schizophrenia not given up for adoption; no control adoptees had schizophrenia. The best-known adoption study was conducted in Denmark using a national psychiatric case register and a register of adoptions. Kety et al. (1975) reported that schizophrenia and *schizophrenia spectrum disorders* were more common in the biological relatives of index adoptees who had schizophrenia than in the biological relatives of mentally healthy control adoptees. Schizophrenia spectrum disorders include personality disorders that share certain characteristics with schizophrenia, such as paranoid ideas or eccentric behavior, without meeting full syndromal criteria.

Mode of inheritance of schizophrenia has also been studied, mainly by using mathematical modeling of pedigrees and twin and adoption study data. Proposed modes of inheritance include a single-gene model and a polygenic model. However, polygenic models of inheritance are consistent with published family and twin data (Gottesman and Shields 1982); they are also consistent with genetic studies finding increased risk in families with more than one schizophrenic member and increased risk in first-degree relatives of more severely ill probands compared with less severely ill probands (Rice and McGuffin 1985).

Some evidence also suggests that schizophrenia may show the phenomenon of *anticipation:* increasingly severe onset at earlier ages within multigeneration affected families (Gorwood et al. 1996). Anticipation has been observed in other neuropsychiatric disorders, including Huntington's disease, fragile X syndrome, and myotonic dystrophy. In these disorders, increasing proliferation of trinucleotide repeats at the disease locus in successive generations correlated with anticipation. Although there is no evidence of large trinucleotide repeats in schizophrenia (Petronis et al. 1996), the occurrence of anticipation in schizophrenia may provide some clues as to its specific genetic loci and mechanisms (Petronis and Kennedy 1995).

Neuroanatomy and Structural Neuroimaging

The finding of ventricular enlargement in schizophrenia has now been confirmed by numerous CT studies and is perhaps the best-replicated finding in psychiatry (Andreasen et al. 1982, 1990c; Weinberger et al. 1979, 1980). This early work with CT, conducted during the 1980s, firmly established that schizophrenia is a brain disorder with a measurable structural component that can be observed at the gross anatomic level when groups of patients are pooled together, averaged, and compared with healthy volunteer control subjects.

Cerebral ventricular enlargement is the most consistently replicated finding, but sulcal enlargement or abnormalities in cortical or subcortical subregions are also reported. Although these findings cannot be explained on the basis of such factors as treatment with medications, they may be explained in part by gender, because it may be predominantly a male effect (Flaum et al. 1990). Examination of ventricular size in patients with schizophrenia and healthy subjects over a broad age range suggest that enlargement does not progress over time at a greater rate in schizophrenic patients than normally and that structural brain abnormalities are present from the outset (Andreasen et al. 1990a; Nopoulos et al. 1995a). Although not all studies show exactly the same correlates, there is substantial evidence to suggest that ventricular enlargement is

associated with poor premorbid functioning, negative symptoms, poor response to treatment, and cognitive impairment. CT scan abnormalities may have some clinical significance, but they are not diagnostically specific; similar abnormalities are seen in other disorders such as Alzheimer's disease or alcoholism.

MRI has now largely supplanted CT as a clinical and research tool. Its particular advantage lies in its ability to distinguish gray and white matter, allowing the size of particular brain regions and structures to be measured. MRI has permitted investigators to move from asking, "Is there a grossly measurable brain abnormality in schizophrenia?" to asking, "Is a specific region or group of regions affected?" Many candidate regions have been explored, but none has been conclusively confirmed. The conflicting reports appear to largely reflect the growing maturity of this method of study. Early reports used relatively primitive techniques such as area measurements on single slices and manual tracing. More recent studies apply automated volumetric measures that have greater power and sophistication.

The earliest MRI study reported a selective decrease in the frontal cortex, in addition to smaller cerebral and intracranial size, and it suggested that this combination of findings was consistent with a neurodevelopmental process in which the brain failed to grow normally, rather than with a neurodegenerative process (Andreasen et al. 1986). Many subsequent studies examined the issue of brain size; a recent meta-analysis examining all available studies of intracranial size ($N = 18$) and brain volume ($N = 27$) has confirmed a small but highly statistically significant difference between patients and control subjects in both brain and intracranial volume (Ward et al. 1996).

A decrease in frontal lobe size has been less consistently replicated, although hypotheses about a dysfunction of the frontal cortex continue to be widely discussed, particularly in functional imaging studies (see "Functional Circuitry and Functional Neuroimaging"). The prefrontal cortex performs a large array of higher cortical functions that are disrupted in schizophrenia (e.g., "executive functions," abstract thinking, working memory), making it an attractive candidate for study. Yet it is also a large and functionally diverse brain region that was difficult to measure accurately prior to the recent development of three-dimensional acquisition procedures with MRI and volume-rendering techniques that permit visualization of cortical surface anatomy and parcellation of the frontal lobe into functionally distinct areas (Crespo-Facorro et al. 1999a). Studies that used relatively sophisticated measurement techniques have shown decreased frontal size in both chronic and first-episode patients (Andreasen et al. 1994a; Breier et al. 1992; Nopoulos et al. 1995a). If all studies are pooled, however, negative studies are as frequent as positive ones (for a review, see Shenton et al. 1997). More recent studies have examined specific subregions within the frontal cortex, and both volumetric and morphological differences between schizophrenia patients and healthy control subjects have been reported (Crespo-Facorro et al. 2000; Szeszko et al. 1999).

MRI has also been used to explore possible abnormalities in other specific brain subregions, such as the thalamus, amygdala/hippocampus, temporal lobes, or basal ganglia. Several studies have indicated that the size of temporal regions is decreased in schizophrenia and that there may even be a relatively specific abnormality in the superior temporal gyrus or planum temporale that is correlated with the presence of hallucinations or formal thought disorder (Barta et al. 1990; Shenton et al. 1992).

Finally, longitudinal MRI assessment studies of brain morphology in first-episode schizophrenia patients have revealed that structural abnormalities are present by the time that patients present for treatment. The literature on progressive volumetric brain changes during the longitudinal course of schizophrenia is conflicting (Weinberger and McClure 2002). However, findings from recent longitudinal MRI studies provide increasingly convergent evidence that there may be ongoing structural brain changes after the diagnosis of schizophrenia (DeLisi et al. 1997; Gur et al. 1998; Ho et al., in press; Lieberman et al. 2001; Rapoport et al. 1997). These progressive changes seem most evident in the frontal lobes and are correlated with poor outcome (K.L. Davis et al. 1998; Ho et al., in press; Lieberman et al. 2001).

Functional Circuitry and Functional Neuroimaging

Beginning with the work of Ingvar and Franzen (1974), studies of regional cerebral blood flow (rCBF) have been used to explore the possibility of functional or metabolic abnormalities in schizophrenia (Andreasen et al. 1992). Data from these studies suggested that patients with schizophrenia had a relative "hypofrontality," which was associated with prominent negative symptoms. Since that early work, functional imaging studies have become more sophisticated, and it is now clear that PET can be used to explore the functional circuitry used by healthy individuals while they perform a variety of mental tasks and to identify circuits that are dysfunctional in schizophrenia. Much of this research has been facilitated by the maturation of the ^{15}O H_2O technique with PET. ^{15}O H_2O is a tracer with a very short half-life (around 2 minutes), which permits investigators to perform multiple repeated scans (usually 6–12) with differing cognitive tasks during a short time period (around 2 hours). This permits the dissection of the components of cognitive activities (e.g., memory encoding versus retrieval) and visualization of their associated circuitry.

Current thinking about the mechanisms of schizophrenia, based on functional imaging, postulates a disruption in distributed functional circuits rather than a single abnormality in a single brain region such as the prefrontal cortex or one of its specific subregions such as the dorsolateral prefrontal cortex. Although no single group of regions has definitively emerged as the "schizophrenia circuit," a consensus is developing concerning some of the nodes that may be involved. They include various subregions within the frontal cortex (orbital, dorsolateral, medial), the anterior cingulate gyrus, the thalamus, several temporal lobe subregions, and the cerebellum.

Neuropathology

Schizophrenia, once called the "graveyard of neuropathologists," continues to vex researchers in their efforts to establish its characteristic pathological changes. Although many of the neuropathological findings in schizophrenia remain controversial, histological abnormalities with the strongest evidence include smaller cortical and hippocampal neurons, fewer neurons in the dorsal thalamus, reduced synaptic and dendritic markers in the hippocampus, and an absence of gliosis (Harrison 1999).

Neurophysiology

Schizophrenia patients frequently display abnormal smooth-pursuit eye movements (SPEM). This is a disorder of the visual tracking of smoothly moving targets and has been consistently observed in schizo-

phrenic patients for nearly 90 years. Some experts believe that abnormal SPEM may represent a biological marker for schizophrenia, because it has been observed in patients with remitted schizophrenia and schizotypal personality disorder and is more frequently found in relatives of schizophrenic patients than in the general population (Holzman et al. 1984; Thacker et al. 1996).

Neurodevelopment

Several lines of evidence support the thesis that schizophrenia is a neurodevelopmental disorder resulting from neuronal injury occurring early in life that interferes with normal brain maturation (Andreasen et al. 1986; Feinberg 1982; Weinberger 1987). As described earlier, MRI studies have shown an increased rate of neurodevelopmental brain anomalies in this illness. The observation that perinatal complications often precede the development of severe neurological and psychological disorders, such as cerebral palsy and mental retardation, have led investigators to explore the role of perinatal and obstetrical complications in the etiology of schizophrenia. Patients with schizophrenia are more likely to have a history of obstetrical complications than are patients with other psychiatric disorders or healthy control subjects (Geddes and Lawrie 1995). Prematurity, oxygen deprivation, and long labor are especially common complications. Minor physical anomalies (slight anatomic defects of the head, hands, feet, and face) are relatively common in schizophrenia patients and are themselves believed to reflect abnormal neurodevelopment (Green et al. 1994).

Throughout the temperate northern latitudes, the birth dates of patients with schizophrenia tend to cluster in the winter months (Hare et al. 1973; Mortensen et al. 1999). This finding suggests that a seasonally varying influence (a viral infection, for example) is acting in utero or in early life to cause neurological injury. Thus, children born during the winter months would be more vulnerable to brain injury due to the increased frequency of viral infections.

Neurochemistry and Neuropharmacology

For many years, the most widely accepted explanation for the biochemical pathophysiology of schizophrenia was the *dopamine hypothesis*, which suggests that the disorder is primarily caused by a functional hyperactivity in the dopamine system (Carlsson 1988; K.L. Davis et al. 1991). Much of the support for the dopamine hypothesis arose from the observation that the efficacy of many of the neuroleptic drugs used to treat schizophrenia was highly correlated with their ability to block dopamine D_2 receptors (Creese et al. 1976; Seeman et al. 1976). Conversely, drugs that enhance dopamine transmission, such as the amphetamines, tend to worsen the symptoms of schizophrenia (Snyder 1972). Therefore, the dopamine hypothesis also suggested that the abnormality in this illness might specifically lie in the D_2 receptors. For many years, the "ideal drug" was thought to be a highly specific D_2 blocker.

Recent work in neuropharmacology and chemical anatomy has demonstrated that there are five types of dopamine receptors, which differ in their cerebral distribution. The D_1 receptor is linked to adenylate cyclase and is located in the cortex and basal ganglia. The D_2 receptor is not linked to adenylate cyclase and is prominent in the striatum. The D_3 and D_4 receptors have a higher distribution in limbic regions. This distribution raises questions about the classic dopamine hypothesis, because limbic regions (or, alternately, frontal or temporal regions)

have been the presumed target for neuroleptic drug action, yet D_2 receptors are not densely concentrated in these target regions.

Postmortem brain research has documented an increase in D_2 receptors in the caudate and nucleus accumbens in postmortem brains (Clardy et al. 1993). Other postmortem studies have documented increased dopamine or homovanillic acid in these regions as well as the left amygdala in schizophrenic patients (K.L. Davis et al. 1991). There is a concern, however, that these findings may be an artifact of treatment with antipsychotics. Animal work has shown that antipsychotics produce receptor supersensitivity in response to receptor blockade by increasing the number of D_2 receptors available. Consequently, an increase in D_2 receptors in postmortem brains could be a direct consequence of neuroleptic treatment itself.

Alternative biochemical hypotheses have been advanced, in part because of the difficulty in confirming the dopamine hypothesis and in the realization that antidopaminergic agents are not always effective. More recent hypotheses also include the role of other neurotransmitter systems (e.g., norepinephrine, serotonin, glutamate, γ-aminobutyric acid [GABA]), neuropeptides, and neuromodulatory substances in the pathophysiology of schizophrenia (Meltzer 1987; VanKammen et al. 1990). The development of the new atypical neuroleptics, which have potent effects on serotonin, provides partial confirmation of the importance of additional neurotransmitter systems in schizophrenia, because they not only cause fewer extrapyramidal side effects than do conventional antipsychotics but are more effective as well. The observation that phencyclidine intoxication leads to schizophrenia-like manifestations has also stimulated interest in the NMDA receptor

complex and the possible role of glutamate in the pathophysiology of schizophrenia (Javitt and Zukin 1991; Olney
and Farber 1995).

Social and Family Factors

Theories about the role of society, urban-
ization, and stress on the development of
mental illness, including schizophrenia,
were popular during the 1930s and 1940s.
In an early study, Faris and Durham (1939)
found higher rates for mental hospital admissions, including admissions for schizophrenia, in central slums than in the sub-
urbs. This finding was replicated in other
cities in both the United States and Europe. The conclusion was drawn that
schizophrenia was caused by the ill effects
of a slum environment, where people
were faced with enormous stress from
social disorganization, poverty, and the
general adversity imposed by poor living
conditions. These conditions were believed to produce or "breed" schizophrenia (Hare 1956).

Another explanation soon developed
to explain the finding of geographic isolation of the severely mentally ill. The drift
hypothesis stated that living in poor areas
resulted from schizophrenia and was not
causal (Wender et al. 1973). Rather,
because schizophrenia leads to amotivation, cognitive impairment, poor hygiene,
and other symptoms that make it impossible for the person with schizophrenia to
maintain employment and survive in middle and upper class structures, persons
with schizophrenia drift down in social
class as their illness progresses. Subsequent research has supported this view.

Clinical Management

Antipsychotic Medication

Antipsychotic medication has been the
mainstay of treatment for schizophrenia

since chlorpromazine was introduced in
1952. In fact, these agents are probably
responsible in large measure for the deinstitutionalization that occurred in the
1950s and 1960s. Because these medications were so effective, large numbers of
patients were able to leave psychiatric
hospitals. In 1955, for instance, over one-
half million hospital beds were filled by
the chronic mentally ill, mainly schizophrenic patients; by the early 1990s the
number of beds had been reduced to
103,000 (Lamb 1993).

All antipsychotics are superior to placebo in the treatment of schizophrenia.
Controlled studies have not supported use
of a specific agent for a specific subtype of
schizophrenia, nor is there any benefit
from prescribing more than a single antipsychotic at a time. Although these drugs
are effective in controlling acute psychosis
and provide long-term relapse prevention,
they are not curative. The putative mechanism of action of antipsychotic drugs is
their ability to block postsynaptic dopamine D_2 receptors in the limbic forebrain.
This blockade is thought to initiate a series of events responsible for both acute
and chronic therapeutic actions. Whereas
these drugs block dopamine D_2 receptors
almost immediately, onset of antipsychotic action takes weeks to develop. Recent research findings suggest that clinical
response corresponds with the degree of
D_2 receptor occupancy (Farde et al.
1992), with increased likelihood of symptomatic improvement when D_2 occupancy exceeds 65% (Kapur et al. 2000).
Besides being dopamine-receptor antagonists, these drugs also block noradrenergic,
cholinergic, histaminic, and serotonergic
receptors to differing degrees, accounting
for the unique side-effect profile of each
agent.

During the 1990s, several second-
generation or "atypical" antipsychotics
have been introduced that represent the

most important advance in the treatment of schizophrenia since the introduction of chlorpromazine. Clozapine, risperidone, olanzapine, quetiapine, ziprasidone, and aripiprazole are now available for clinical use in the United States, and some (except clozapine) have become first-line therapy for schizophrenia. Not only do these second-generation antipsychotics appear to be more effective than first-generation antipsychotics in reducing positive and negative symptoms, but they may also be superior in improving depression (Tollefson et al. 1998) and decreasing cognitive dysfunction in schizophrenia (Keefe et al. 1999). However, two recent meta-analyses have raised questions about the superior efficacy of these newer antipsychotics. Although Leucht et al. (1999) found that olanzapine- and risperidone-treated patients showed greater overall improvement than patients who received conventional antipsychotics, the authors questioned the clinical relevance of the improvement because the effect sizes were modest. Geddes et al. (2000) reported that the advantage for atypical antipsychotics was observed only when the doses of comparative conventional antipsychotics (haloperidol or chlorpromazine) were relatively high. When the authors analyzed studies in which the mean doses of haloperidol were less than 12 mg/day, the efficacy and dropout rates of the newer atypical antipsychotics were no better than those of lower doses of haloperidol.

Nevertheless, these second-generation antipsychotics still represent a major advance in the treatment of schizophrenia. They are clearly more tolerable than conventional antipsychotics, especially because of their lower propensity to induce extrapyramidal side effects and possibly tardive dyskinesia. Extrapyramidal side effects result from blockade of the nigrostriatal D_2 receptors, and the likelihood of extrapyramidal side effects increases when receptor occupancy exceeds 78% (Kapur et al. 2000). The atypical antipsychotics also block serotonin 5-HT$_{2A}$ receptors in the frontal cortex and striatal system, which may help protect against the development of extrapyramidal side effects as well (Meltzer et al. 1989). However, more recent data from neuroimaging and animal studies suggest that the lower propensity to cause extrapyramidal side effects in this group of antipsychotics may be related to their fast dissociation from D_2 receptors (Kapur and Seeman 2001). Although the atypical antipsychotics are associated with fewer extrapyramidal side effects, other side effects, including weight gain (Allison et al. 1999), impaired glucose tolerance, and dyslipidemia (Goldstein et al. 1999; Henderson et al. 2000), have come to attention. This information poses new challenges for the pharmacotherapy of schizophrenia. The type and severity of these side effects vary among the various second-generation medications.

Another challenge in the treatment of schizophrenia is that approximately 10%–20% of patients respond poorly to antipsychotic drugs, with the quality of response varying from patient to patient (Carpenter and Buchanan 1994). Clozapine remains the "gold standard" in treatment-refractory patients (Chakos et al. 2001). Clozapine was first used in the mid-1970s, but early reports of agranulocytosis in 1%–2% of patients delayed its introduction in the United States. A multicenter clinical trial (Kane et al. 1988) found that about 30% of inpatients with schizophrenia who had failed to respond to traditional antipsychotics responded to clozapine within 4–6 weeks; up to 60% may respond within 4–6 months (Schooler et al. 1995). There is preliminary evidence to suggest that risperidone and olanzapine may also be more effective than conventional antipsychotics in treatment-refractory patients (Conley et al. 1998; Wirshing et al. 1999).

Treatment of Acute Psychosis

Most acutely psychotic schizophrenic patients will respond to a daily dose between 10 and 15 mg of haloperidol (or its equivalent) within several days or weeks (Kane and Marder 1993). Higher dosages of conventional antipsychotics may be needed in some patients, but controlled studies have not shown an advantage to either rapid loading or sustained high dosages. Furthermore, higher dosages will increase the likelihood of adverse side effects. For example, in one study (McEvoy et al. 1991), acutely psychotic schizophrenic patients were given relatively low doses (generally from 2 to 6 mg) of haloperidol for 2 weeks, then randomly assigned to a dosage 2–10 times higher or to the same dosage for another 2 weeks. Higher dosages caused significantly more extrapyramidal side effects, but not greater improvement in measures of psychosis. In another study, Rifkin et al. (1991) found no difference in the response of newly admitted schizophrenic patients given 10 mg, 30 mg, or 80 mg of oral haloperidol for 6 weeks. High dosages of atypical antipsychotics also appear unnecessary. In a fixed-dose trial of risperidone (Marder and Meibach 1994), doses of 2 mg, 6 mg, 10 mg, and 16 mg were compared with doses of 20 mg of haloperidol and placebo. All doses of risperidone were effective in relieving the symptoms of schizophrenia, but the 6-mg dose was the most effective and also proved superior to haloperidol.

Measuring plasma levels of antipsychotic drugs can be helpful in selected cases, but there is little to be gained from routine monitoring. Plasma levels are most useful 1) in patients who have failed to respond to conventional doses, 2) when antipsychotic medications are combined with other drugs that can affect their pharmacokinetics (e.g., carbamazepine), and 3) to assess compliance. The very young, the elderly, or the medically compromised patient with schizophrenia may also benefit from plasma level monitoring. Because of the difficulties involved in correlating plasma levels and response, research results are not entirely consistent. Nonetheless, levels of haloperidol between 5 and 18 ng/mL (P.J. Perry and Smith 1993), levels of fluphenazine between 0.6 and 1.5 ng/mL (Levinson et al. 1995), and levels of clozapine approaching 350 ng/mL (VanderZwaag et al. 1996) appear effective for most patients. Plasma levels of many other antipsychotic drugs can be reliably measured, but attempts to correlate responses with levels have not been successful.

A high-potency conventional antipsychotic (e.g., haloperidol), risperidone (i.e., 4–6 mg daily), or olanzapine (10–20 mg daily) has been recommended as the initial choice for treatment of acute psychosis (American Psychiatric Association 1997). Recent controlled trials have indicated that lower doses of risperidone (2–4 mg daily) are efficacious and are associated with reduced rates of extrapyramidal side effects. The initial starting dose for ziprasidone is 20 mg twice daily with adjustment up to 80–160 mg daily, depending on individual clinical status. The dose–efficacy relationship for quetiapine has been less clear, although 400–600 mg daily is recommended as the therapeutic dose for most patients. The recommended therapeutic dose for aripiprazole is 15–30 mg/day. If no response is observed after 3–8 weeks, one of the other drugs should be tried. If a patient shows a partial response to the initial antipsychotic at 3 weeks, the trial should be extended another 2–9 weeks (Expert Consensus Guideline Series Steering

Committee 1996). In this algorithm, clozapine is a second-line choice because of its expense and propensity to cause agranulocytosis.

Highly agitated patients require rapid control of their symptoms and should be given frequent, equally spaced doses of an antipsychotic drug. High-potency antipsychotic medications (e.g., haloperidol) may be given every 30–120 minutes orally or intramuscularly until the agitation is under control (Dubin et al. 1985). Rarely is more than 20–30 mg of haloperidol required in a 24-hour period, and lower doses are optimal. It is likely that haloperidol's effectiveness in subduing patients results from sedation rather than from any specific antipsychotic effect. Because sedation is desired, a combination of antipsychotic medication and a benzodiazepine may work even better for the rapid control of agitated psychotic patients. In one study (Garza-Trevino et al. 1989), doses of haloperidol (5 mg) and lorazepam (4 mg) were administered and repeated every 30 minutes. Most patients achieved tranquilization after the initial dose. The average time required to achieve a satisfactory response was 60 minutes. Once the patient has calmed down, the benzodiazepine can be gradually withdrawn. Although rapid sedation may also be achieved with administration of droperidol (5–10 mg im) (Slaby and Moreines 1990), the potential side effects of severe hypotension and QT prolongation necessitate caution when using this agent.

Maintenance Therapy

Patients benefiting from short-term treatment with antipsychotic medications are candidates for long-term prophylactic treatment, which has as its goal the sustained control of psychotic symptoms. To minimize the risk of side effects, particularly tardive dyskinesia, an often irreversible movement disorder, the lowest effective antipsychotic dose should be used. In a review of 35 well-designed studies of relapse rates, J.M. Davis et al. (1993) concluded that patients receiving placebo relapsed at a rate of 55%, whereas only 21% of patients with schizophrenia relapsed when maintained on antipsychotic drugs. Furthermore, they concluded that all patients not receiving antipsychotic medication will relapse within about 3 years, essentially guaranteeing multiple relapses and disrupted lives. Patients who experience a temporary worsening of psychotic symptoms in response to methylphenidate administration and those with tardive dyskinesia may be more likely to relapse when off medication (Lieberman et al. 1987).

Although duration of treatment for relapse prevention has not been established, the following guidelines were developed at an international consensus conference (Kissling 1991):

1. Prevention of relapse is more important than risk of side effects, since most side effects are reversible and the consequences of relapse may be irreversible.
2. At least 1–2 years of treatment are recommended after the initial episode due to the high risk of relapse and the possibility of social deterioration from further relapses.
3. At least 5 years of treatment is recommended for multiepisode patients, given that high risk of relapse remains. Beyond this, data are incomplete, but indefinite, perhaps lifelong, treatment is recommended for those patients who pose a danger to themselves or to others.

Clinicians should periodically reassess whether the patient requires continued maintenance treatment. When it is time to reassess the need for medication, an attempt should be made to withdraw the drug slowly over weeks or months. Should symptoms reoccur, the drug should be immediately reinstituted and the dosage increased. Because many patients develop increased negative symptoms and decreased positive symptoms over time, they may have less need for antipsychotic medication (Carpenter 1996). Some research suggests that the risk of relapse remains greater on oral than on intramuscular antipsychotics, probably because of patient noncompliance (J.M. Davis et al. 1993). Although drug holidays have been recommended by some investigators as a means of lowering the risk of tardive dyskinesia, we cannot endorse this recommendation; targeted medication leads to more decompensation and rehospitalization than does continuous medication, without lowering risk for tardive dyskinesia (Carpenter et al. 1990). For patients who are unable to take oral medication on a regular basis or are noncompliant, long-acting preparations are available, such as fluphenazine decanoate or haloperidol decanoate. There is no universally accepted method for converting a patient from oral to long-acting forms, and dosing with sustained-released preparations must be individualized. Further information about antipsychotic drugs and their rational use is found in Chapter 18.

Adjunctive Pharmacological Treatments

Medications other than antipsychotics are occasionally useful in patients with schizophrenia, but their role has not been clearly defined. Conventional agents primarily used for the treatment of other psychiatric disorders such as benzodiazepines, propranolol, lithium carbonate, carbamazepine, sodium valproate, and antidepressants have been used with varying degrees of success.

Benzodiazepines have been used alone and in combination with antipsychotic medications (Christison et al. 1991). High doses have been used with the intent of relieving agitation, thought disorder, delusions, and hallucinations. The theoretical justification supporting the use of benzodiazepines is that they facilitate GABA neurotransmission, which may inhibit dopamine neurotransmission. Individual response to these agents is highly variable, and the greatest use for benzodiazepines may be as an adjunct to antipsychotic medications in the acute management of psychotic agitation (Wolkowitz and Pickar 1991). Benzodiazepines have also been used to relieve the akathisia associated with antipsychotic medications. In a double-blind, randomized clinical trial, Carpenter et al. (1999b) found that diazepam was equivalent to fluphenazine but superior to placebo in treating the early warning signs of symptom exacerbation. Diazepam treatment may therefore be helpful in preventing symptom progression in patients who refuse antipsychotic treatment.

Propranolol and other β-blockers have been used to treat schizophrenia, alone and in conjunction with antipsychotic drugs (Christison et al. 1991). One of propranolol's actions may be to raise plasma antipsychotic levels, but it has been reported to reduce aggressive behaviors and temper outbursts (Peet et al. 1981). It has also been used to relieve neuroleptic-induced akathisia (Lipinsky et al. 1984). However, a recent review of randomized placebo-controlled trials did not find evidence to support the use of β-blockers as an adjunct to antipsychotic medications in the treatment of schizophrenia (Wahlbeck et al. 2000).

Lithium carbonate, which has a clear role in bipolar affective disorder, has been used mainly in an attempt to reduce impulsive and aggressive behaviors, hyperactivity, or excitation, as well as to stabilize mood (Delva and Letemendia 1982). Carbamazepine and sodium valproate have also been used in patients with schizophrenia. Their main benefit, too, has probably been to reduce aggressive behavior and to modulate mood (Johns and Thompson 1995). Nonetheless, the effectiveness of the mood stabilizers in schizophrenia has not been adequately determined and requires further study.

Antidepressants have also been used in the treatment of patients with schizophrenia, primarily in those who have developed a serious depression. Although early research suggested that antidepressants could cause worsening of a thought disorder, more recent work suggests that they have a legitimate role in treating the depressed patient with schizophrenia (Levinson et al. 1999). When used, antidepressants should be prescribed with an antipsychotic to prevent worsening of psychosis and should not be routinely used in floridly psychotic patients. Continuation treatment appears to be safe and effective in patients who respond to adjunctive antidepressants (Siris et al. 1987, 1994).

Other Treatments

Although electroconvulsive therapy (ECT) has been found primarily to benefit those with mood disorders, it is still widely used in the treatment of schizophrenia. Early uncontrolled studies were generally enthusiastic, but later studies failed to show a strong therapeutic effect of ECT in schizophrenia. It is now generally acknowledged that ECT is effective in acute and subacute forms of schizophrenia, but is rarely helpful in chronic cases (Johns and Thompson 1995). Its primary usefulness is in the treatment of a few specific syndromes and in patients not responding to antipsychotic medication.

Catatonia and depression secondary to schizophrenia have both been recognized as indications for ECT. In these situations, ECT appears to be rapidly effective based on clinical reports, although neither its use in catatonia nor its use in depression secondary to schizophrenia has been carefully studied.

Psychosocial and Programmatic Intervention

Psychosocial interventions play an important role in the management of schizophrenic patients and should be integrated with pharmacotherapy. Like antipsychotic medication, psychosocial treatments should be tailored to fit the schizophrenic patient's needs. The fit will depend on the individual, the phase of illness, and the living situation. For example, patients living with their families might benefit from family therapy, whereas patients living alone might benefit from the social stimulation provided in a day hospital program or contact with a visiting home nurse. Some patients may be self-sufficient and employed, whereas others may require around-the-clock care for extended periods in the hospital. Furthermore, patients may require one type of intervention early in the course of illness and different interventions in later stages, when clinical symptoms have changed. Clinicians must work actively to ensure that patients with schizophrenia receive adequate mental health care and community benefits and are encouraged to develop a close working relationship with their local social service agencies. Although optimal care necessitates the availability of a range of services to fit the needs of the patient, including social, vocational, and housing needs, these services are inadequate in many communities (Lamb 1986).

Newer psychosocial treatment models have been developed that emphasize the practical resolution of common social and psychological difficulties seen in schizophrenic patients. Meanwhile, older models involving family therapy have received greater prominence. Family interventions are especially important because they have a direct impact on relapse rates. It is now clear that combining pharmacological treatment with psychosocial interventions offers advantages beyond the power of any single approach. Most clinicians understand the importance of integrated treatment approaches. For example, common sense tells us that although medication will not teach patients social skills, or to budget and shop for themselves, it may facilitate learning by diminishing psychotic symptoms.

Locus of Care

Patients with schizophrenia are rarely placed in long-term custodial institutions today, because the locus of care has shifted to outpatient clinics and the community. Patients, their families, and society at large have benefited from this shift, as greater emphasis has been placed on outpatient management and brief hospital stays. Patients are able to achieve greater degrees of independence and have more opportunities to participate in community life. But many communities have been unable to provide the kind of integrated and coordinated system of care that patients need to reduce risk of relapse and enhance functioning.

Hospitalization

Hospitalization is reserved for patients with schizophrenia who pose a danger to themselves or others; patients who refuse to properly care for themselves (e.g., refuse food or fluids); and patients requiring special medical observation, tests, or treatments. When a patient is a danger to himself or others and refuses to enter the

hospital, it is usually necessary to obtain a court order for hospitalization. When hospitalized, schizophrenic patients stay briefly in special psychiatric hospitals or in psychiatric units found in general hospitals. Stays are short (e.g., days to weeks), and the patient is generally returned to the community.

An active ward milieu is superior to a custodial one in the hospital, especially if well structured and not overly stimulating (Maxmen 1984). The following characteristics have been found optimal: small units, short stays, high staff-to-patient ratio, low staff turnover, low percentage of psychotic patients, broad delegation of responsibility with clear lines of authority, low perceived levels of anger and aggression, high levels of support, and a practical problem-solving approach (Ellsworth 1983).

Partial Hospitalization/ Day Treatment

Partial hospitalization programs may provide an alternative to inpatient treatment for acutely psychotic patients or allow for further stabilization following inpatient care. Day treatment programs, on the other hand, provide more continuous structure and support for the more severely impaired patients and assist such patients in maintaining stability within the community and in relapse prevention. Both types of programs generally operate on weekdays, with patients returning home on evenings and weekends. Psychopharmacological management is provided along with psychosocial rehabilitation. With most programs, the services provided and frequency of attendance will be individualized to fit the needs of the patient (Gudeman et al. 1983).

Outpatient Care

The outpatient clinic will be the locus of treatment for most schizophrenic patients and is the most appropriate setting in which to coordinate care. A well-equipped clinic should be able to provide close monitoring of patients for relapse detection and prevention through careful medication management, to provide both individual or group counseling and psychoeducation, to arrange family interventions, and to arrange special programmatic interventions such as social skills training or cognitive rehabilitation. Case managers should be available to help coordinate the patients' care and to help them access governmental programs to which they may be entitled.

Assertive Community Treatment

A treatment modality available in some areas is assertive community treatment (ACT; Stein 1993), which consists of careful monitoring of patients, the availability of mobile mental health teams, and aggressive programming individually tailored to each patient. ACT programs operate 24 hours a day and have been shown to reduce hospital admission rates and to improve quality of life for many patients with schizophrenia (i.e., patients report greater satisfaction and are more likely to be employed and living independently). ACT involves teaching patients basic living skills, helping patients to work with community agencies, and assisting patients in developing a social support network. Voluntary job placement and supported work settings (i.e., sheltered workshops) are an important part of the program.

Supportive Housing

Appropriate and affordable housing is a major concern for many patients, and depending on the community, options may range from supervised shelters and group homes ("halfway houses") to boarding homes to supervised apartment living. Group homes provide peer support and companionship, along with on-site staff supervision. Supervised apartments offer greater independence with the availability and support of trained staff. Clearly, not all patients with schizophrenia will be able to take advantage of sheltered care residences. Persons with greater levels of impairment may need round-the-clock supervision in a nursing home (Lamberti and Tariot 1995).

Self-Help Organizations

In addition to more formal family interventions, self-help organizations for family members can be enormously beneficial. They provide a forum for family members to obtain information about schizophrenia, to gain encouragement from others, and to learn how to cope with its manifestations. The best-known group in the United States is the Alliance for the Mentally Ill (AMI), and local chapters can be found in many communities. Many other countries have similar national organizations (e.g., the Schizophrenia Fellowship of Canada or Great Britain) that emphasize education, advocacy, mutual support, and self-help.

Specific Psychosocial Interventions

Individual Psychotherapy

The treatment most commonly received by patients with schizophrenia may be the combination of antipsychotic medication with some form of "individual psychotherapy" (Dixon et al. 1999; Fenton 2000). Although intensive psychodynamic- and insight-oriented psychotherapy is generally not recommended, the form of individual psychotherapy that psychiatrists employ when providing pharmacological treatment typically involves a synthesis of various psychotherapeutic strategies and interventions. These include problem solving, reality testing, psychoeducation, and supportive and cognitive-behavioral techniques anchored on an empathetic therapeutic alliance with the patient. The specific approach or combination of approaches used often depends on the patient's clinical condition. The goals of such individual psychotherapy are to improve medication compliance, enhance social and occupational functioning, and prevent relapse. Although combining some form of individual psychotherapy with pharmacological management may seem clinically prudent, there is little to no evidential basis regarding its efficacy.

In contrast, there is a growing body of evidence of the efficacy of cognitive-behavioral therapy (CBT) in schizophrenia, particularly for ameliorating residual psychotic symptoms (Sensky et al. 2000; Tarrier et al. 1993). Initial CBT studies focused on changing the schizophrenic patient's abnormal thoughts (e.g., delusions) or his or her responses to them. Through structured and systematic reality testing, CBT allows patients to collaboratively test alternative explanations to their delusional beliefs and to work toward belief modification. Patients also learn various behavioral coping strategies, such as listening to music to mask auditory hallucinations. Recent randomized controlled trials have extended to testing other CBT techniques, including the use of paced activity scheduling and diary recording of mastery and pleasure to target negative symptoms.

Family Interventions

When combined with antipsychotic medication, family therapy has been demonstrated to reduce relapse rates in schizophrenia. Carpenter (1996) reviewed 14 controlled trials and reported that relapse rates ranged from 40% to 53% in the control condition, compared with 6%–23% in the experimental condition (i.e., family

therapy). Although family therapy may gain some of its impact through enhanced medication compliance, it may also help to protect the schizophrenic patient from the demands of the "real world" by providing improved social support, structure, and guidance.

Although the exact mechanism of improvement in family therapy is unknown, and no specific approach is better than another (Penn and Mueser 1996), several recommendations can be made. First, families can benefit from education about schizophrenia itself. This should include information about the chronic nature of the disorder and the need for long-term care based on realistic expectations. Education will improve cooperation and compliance of both patient and family. However, education needs to be combined with other family interventions aimed at improving communication and learning to minimize criticism and emotional over-involvement—interventions that will help to decrease the schizophrenic patient's level of stress. Gaining a more realistic appraisal of the patient's illness and future expectations will reduce expressed emotion, which, as discussed earlier in the chapter, has been shown to lead to schizophrenic relapse. Family therapy also benefits family members and can help to reduce their feelings of anger, frustration, and helplessness. In addition to education and family support, the Schizophrenia Patient Outcomes Research Team further recommends that family psychosocial interventions provide crisis intervention and training in problem-solving skills (Lehman et al. 1998b). Research shows that multiple-family groups may work even better than single-family interventions (McFarlane et al. 1995).

Group Therapy

Group therapy is frequently used with schizophrenic patients to provide emotional support in a setting where a patient can learn social skills and develop friendships. Groups that are most successful are highly structured and set limited goals (Yalom 1983). Traditional group-therapy approaches that encourage self-exploration and the seeking of insight are generally countertherapeutic (Kanas 1985). This is particularly true with psychotic or highly paranoid individuals, who might misinterpret situations that arise in group therapy.

Psychosocial Rehabilitation

Psychosocial rehabilitation is a term used to describe services that aim to restore the patient's ability to function in the community. It may include the medical and psychosocial treatments described above, but it may also involve ways to foster social interaction, to promote independent living, and to encourage vocational performance (Cook et al. 1996). Patients are encouraged to become involved in developing and implementing their rehabilitation plan, which has as its focus enhancing the patient's talents and skills. The goal of psychosocial rehabilitation is to integrate patients back into the community rather than segregating them in separate facilities, as has occurred in the past. In many locations, patient clubhouses are available to promote psychosocial rehabilitation, such as Fountain House, a program in New York City that patients help to run. The organization serves various functions, including providing job training, social and leisure-time activities, residential assistance, and skills training (Beard et al. 1982).

Social Skills Training

Because social and interpersonal skills are generally deficient in patients with schizophrenia, social skills training aims to help the patient develop more appropriate behaviors. This is accomplished by using modeling and social reinforcement and by providing opportunities, both individual and group, to practice the new behaviors. This could be as simple as helping the patient learn to maintain eye contact or as complicated as helping him learn conversational skills. Research has shown that social skills training can significantly enhance social functioning, but probably has little effect on risk of relapse (Marder et al. 1996). The best results appear to occur in patients with early-onset schizophrenia whose social development would have been disrupted by the emergence of illness and in persons who persist in a training program for more than 1 year (Penn and Mueser 1996). However, the generalizability of social skills training remains uncertain, because there has been limited evidence that patients are able to apply their acquired social skills in real-life situations (Heinssen et al. 2000).

Vocational Rehabilitation

Vocational training and support can also be of enormous benefit to patients with schizophrenia in helping to "mainstream" them back into the community. Research shows that vocational interventions can be effective in helping patients find and maintain paid jobs (Lehman 1995). Vocational rehabilitation may involve supported employment, competitive work in integrated settings, and more formal job training programs. The best initial setting may be a simple, repetitive job environment offering both interpersonal distance and on-site supervision, such as that found in a "sheltered workshop." Although some patients will not be employable in any setting because of apathy, amotivation, or chronic psychosis, employment should be encouraged in able patients. A job will serve to improve self-esteem, bring in additional income, and provide a social outlet for the patient (Mackota and Lamb

1989). Gradually, a patient may move toward a more demanding work setting, although the clinician should help the patient develop appropriate goals. Failure will only diminish a patient's already shaky self-esteem and reinforce the "sick" role. Assessment by a vocational guidance counselor will be helpful in matching patients with appropriate jobs by gaining a better understanding of the patient's abilities, aptitudes, and interests.

Cognitive Rehabilitation

Cognitive rehabilitation has as its goal the remediation of abnormal thought processes known to occur in schizophrenia (Penn and Mueser 1996) and uses techniques pioneered in the treatment of brain-injured individuals. Work with schizophrenic patients is focused on improving information-processing skills such as attention, memory, vigilance, and conceptual abilities. Early studies with cognitive rehabilitation have yielded mixed results but suggest that performance on specific tasks (e.g., Wisconsin Card Sorting Test) can be improved. Whether improvement on specific tasks can generalize to other situations and which cognitive deficits are most appropriate targets for rehabilitation still need further study (Bellack et al. 1999).

Alcohol/Drug Abuse Treatment

Alcohol and other drug abuse is a significant problem for many patients with schizophrenia and needs to be a focus of concern. Substance abuse or dependence aggravates the symptoms of schizophrenia, leads to medication noncompliance, and undermines other treatment interventions. Abstinence should be encouraged in all patients, and some will need referral for drug detoxification and rehabilitation (Ziedonis and Fisher 1994). Although these services may not be helpful in acutely psychotic or agitated patients,

they may be enormously beneficial once the patient has improved and the schizophrenic illness has stabilized. Disulfiram should be used with caution because it inhibits dopamine-β-hydroxylase, increasing the dopamine available to the central nervous system, and may exacerbate psychotic symptoms (Kingsbury and Salzman 1990).

Schizoaffective Disorder

Conceptual Issues

The concept of schizoaffective disorder attempts to define individuals who have features of both schizophrenia and affective disorders. Kasanin (1933) coined the term *acute schizoaffective psychosis* to describe patients with acute onset of "emotional turmoil" and distorted perceptions, usually precipitated by a "difficult environmental situation." Although Kasanin believed schizoaffective psychosis to be a subtype of dementia praecox, these patients were different in that they were well adjusted premorbidly, recovered following weeks or months of psychosis, and were able to attain good social and occupational functioning subsequently.

Schizoaffective disorder is an inherently difficult construct because it is an intermediate category that straddles the boundaries of schizophrenia and mood disorder. Confusion surrounding the term has persisted despite operationalized diagnostic criteria. In fact, profound shifts in its definition over the years (i.e., from the Research Diagnostic Criteria [Spitzer et al. 1978] to DSM-III [American Psychiatric Association 1980], DSM-III-R [American Psychiatric Association 1987], DSM-IV [American Psychiatric Association 1994], and ICD-10 [World Health Organization 1992]) may have added to the confusion. Within the current nomenclature, ICD-10 conceptualizes schizoaffective disorder as *episodic*, whereas DSM-IV-TR describes an *uninterrupted* illness in which the characteristic symptoms of schizophrenia are present concurrently with a depressive syndrome, a manic syndrome, or a mixed episode (Table 5–6). During the illness, more than 2 weeks of delusions or hallucinations in the absence of prominent affective symptoms are required, helping to set schizoaffective disorder apart from psychotic depression or mania. In addition, affective symptoms need to be present for a substantial portion of the total duration of the illness so as to differentiate it from schizophrenia, in which mood symptoms are generally present for brief periods. Investigators have found the interrater reliability of the DSM-IV schizoaffective disorder diagnostic category to be low (Maj et al. 2000). The validity of the schizoaffective disorder construct, as well as its division into depressive and bipolar subtypes, has also been questioned (Kendler et al. 1995; Maj et al. 2000).

At least five conceptual models have been proposed to explain the coexistence of schizophrenic and affective symptoms in the same person: 1) all schizoaffective patients have "true" schizophrenia with incidental affective symptoms; 2) all schizoaffective patients have "true" affective disorder with incidental schizophrenia symptoms; 3) schizoaffective disorder patients are a heterogeneous group consisting of "true" schizophrenia and "true" mood disorder patients; 4) all schizoaffective patients have both schizophrenia and affective disorder; and 5) schizoaffective disorder represents a distinct third psychotic illness (Brockington and Meltzer 1983). In all likelihood, schizoaffective disorder probably constitutes a heterogeneous group within which some patients have schizophrenia and others have mood disorders.

TABLE 5–6. DSM-IV-TR diagnostic criteria for schizoaffective disorder

A. An uninterrupted period of illness during which, at some time, there is either a major depressive episode, a manic episode, or a mixed episode concurrent with symptoms that meet Criterion A for schizophrenia. **Note:** The major depressive episode must include Criterion A1: depressed mood.

B. During the same period of illness, there have been delusions or hallucinations for at least 2 weeks in the absence of prominent mood symptoms.

C. Symptoms that meet criteria for a mood episode are present for a substantial portion of the total duration of the active and residual periods of the illness.

D. The disturbance is not due to the direct physiological effects of a substance (e.g., a drug of abuse, a medication) or a general medical condition.

Specify type:

Bipolar Type: if the disturbance includes a manic or a mixed episode (or a manic or a mixed episode and major depressive episodes)

Depressive Type: if the disturbance only includes major depressive episodes

Epidemiology

Relatively little is known about the incidence, prevalence, demographic factors, or risk factors associated with schizoaffective disorder. This is in part related to differing definitions of schizoaffective disorder used in various studies. The prevalence of schizoaffective disorder has been estimated to be less than 1% in the general population, but the prevalence in patient populations is often much higher. It appears to occur more often in women than in men. Family studies have shown an increased risk for both schizophrenia and mood disorders among the relatives of schizoaffective patients.

Course and Prognosis

The course of schizaffective disorder is variable, with recovery rates that range widely (between 29% and 83%). Approximately 20%–30% of patients show a deteriorating course with persistent psychotic symptoms, whereas in another 10% of patients the relative prominence of affective and schizophrenic symptoms may shift over time. Psychotic and affective symptoms can be present concurrently or in an alternating fashion. Psychosis can be either mood congruent or mood incongruent. In general, the prognosis of patients with schizoaffective disorder is intermediate between that of schizophrenia and that of affective disorder patients. Some studies have indicated that outcomes in patients with the bipolar subtype of schizoaffective disorder may be more similar to outcomes in those with bipolar affective disorder, whereas outcomes in the depressive subtype are more akin to those in schizophrenia. Predictors of poor outcome in schizoaffective disorder include poor premorbid functioning, insidious onset, absence of a precipitating factor, predominance of psychotic symptoms, early age at onset, poor interepisode recovery, and a family history of schizophrenia.

Pharmacological Management

Systematic pharmacological treatment studies of patients with schizoaffective disorder represent a relatively neglected area of research. Patients with schizoaffective disorder often end up with complex pharmacological regimens as clinicians attempt to target both psychotic and affective symptoms. There is no clear evidence that any one pharmacological strategy is superior to the others, whether during acute or maintenance treatment: antipsychotic monotherapy, mood-stabilizer monotherapy (lithium, carbamazepine, sodium valproate), antidepressant monotherapy, or combinations (antipsychotic with a mood stabilizer, antipsychotic with an antidepressant). Acute treatment usually requires antipsychotics, because most acutely ill patients have prominent psychotic symptoms. With little evidence from controlled studies, the choice of maintenance strategy is often guided by the subtype of schizoaffective disorder; for example, mood stabilizers may be used in patients with the bipolar subtype, antidepressants in those with the depressive subtype, and antipsychotics in patients with persistent psychosis. There is preliminary evidence that atypical antipsychotics may have mood-stabilizing properties, which suggests that this class may provide the ideal monotherapy for patients with schizoaffective disorder (Keck et al. 1999). In patients with treatment-refractory illness, a trial of clozapine should be considered.

Delusional Disorder

Delusional disorder is characterized by the presence of systematized, nonbizarre delusions accompanied by affect appropriate to the delusion. Personality is generally spared, but the delusion may preoccupy and dominate the patient's life.

Diagnosis

According to DSM-IV-TR (Table 5–7), delusional disorders are characterized by nonbizarre delusions lasting at least 1 month, behavior that is not obviously odd or bizarre apart from the delusion or its ramifications, absence of active phase symptoms that may occur in schizophrenia (e.g., hallucinations, disorganized speech, negative symptoms), and the determination that the disorder is not due to a mood disorder with psychotic features, is not substance induced, and is not

---

TABLE 5–7. DSM-IV-TR diagnostic criteria for delusional disorder

---

A. Nonbizarre delusions (i.e., involving situations that occur in real life, such as being followed, poisoned, infected, loved at a distance, or deceived by spouse or lover, or having a disease) of at least 1 month's duration.

B. Criterion A for schizophrenia has never been met. **Note:** Tactile and olfactory hallucinations may be present in delusional disorder if they are related to the delusional theme.

C. Apart from the impact of the delusion(s) or its ramifications, functioning is not markedly impaired and behavior is not obviously odd or bizarre.

D. If mood episodes have occurred concurrently with delusions, their total duration has been brief relative to the duration of the delusional periods.

E. The disturbance is not due to the direct physiological effects of a substance (e.g., a drug of abuse, a medication) or a general medical condition.

Specify type (the following types are assigned based on the predominant delusional theme):

Erotomanic Type: delusions that another person, usually of higher status, is in love with the individual

Grandiose Type: delusions of inflated worth, power, knowledge, identity, or special relationship to a deity or famous person

Jealous Type: delusions that the individual's sexual partner is unfaithful

Persecutory Type: delusions that the person (or someone to whom the person is close) is being malevolently treated in some way

Somatic Type: delusions that the person has some physical defect or general medical condition

Mixed Type: delusions characteristic of more than one of the above types but no one theme predominates

Unspecified Type

---

due to a medical condition. The core feature, however, is the presence of a well-systematized, often logical, nonbizarre delusion. The term *systematized* indicates that the delusion and its ramifications fit into an all-encompassing, complex scheme that makes sense to the patient. The term *nonbizarre* implies that the delusion involves situations that can occur in real life, such as being followed, and not implausible or impossible situations, such as having all of one's internal organs replaced by those of bug-eyed Martians. Auditory or visual hallucinations, if present, are not prominent. However, olfactory or tactile hallucinations may be present and prominent.

The diagnostic validity of delusional disorder still remains uncertain (Kendler 1980). It may not be a distinct disease entity that is separate from paranoid schizophrenia or from affective disorders. The symptoms of delusional disorder appear to separate into four independent factors: delusions, hallucinations, depressive symptoms, and irritability (Serretti et al. 1999). Although generally less impaired than patients with schizophrenia, patients with delusional disorder did not differ significantly in terms of clinical, demographic, or neuropsychological measures (Evans et al. 1996). Another study found that the diagnosis of delusional disorder was temporally consistent in only about 50% of the patients (Fennig et al. 1996). This suggests that an initial diagnosis of delusional disorder should be considered as provisional, and that patients need to be reassessed longitudinally.

Differential Diagnosis

A careful assessment is necessary in order to rule out other functional or medical causes for the delusions. This workup should include a physical examination to rule out alcohol-, amphetamine-, cocaine-, and other drug-induced conditions; dementia; and infectious, metabolic, and endocrine disorders (Manschreck 1996). Routine lab tests may be indicated depending on the results of the history and physical examination. CT or MRI may be helpful in selected cases, especially when mass lesions are suspected. Symptom onset, course, and associated features are also relevant. Abrupt changes in mood, mental state, or personality strongly suggest a medical origin. Disturbed consciousness, perceptual disturbances, or physical signs (e.g., fever) may point to specific causes. Isolated paranoid symptoms are often an early sign of medical illness and are especially common among elderly inpatients.

The major diagnostic task remains in separating delusional disorder from mood disorders, schizophrenia, and paranoid personality. The chief distinction is that in delusional disorder a full depressive or manic syndrome is absent, developed after the psychotic symptoms, or was brief in duration relative to the duration of the psychotic symptoms. Unlike schizophrenia, delusional disorder is characterized by nonbizarre delusions and generally either no hallucinations or hallucinations that are not prominent. Furthermore, patients with delusional disorder do not typically develop other schizophrenic symptoms such as incoherence or grossly disorganized behavior, and personality is generally preserved. Persons with paranoid personality are suspicious and hypervigilant, but are not delusional.

Associated features of delusional disorder include anger, social isolation and seclusiveness, eccentric behavior, suspiciousness, hostility, and sometimes violence prompted by the delusion (Kennedy et al. 1992). Winokur (1977) reported that patients with delusional disorders frequently develop sexual problems and depression, and described many as over-

talkative and circumstantial. Clinical wisdom suggests that many patients become litigious and end up as lawyers' clients rather than as psychiatrists' patients.

Delusional disorder includes the following DSM-IV-TR subtypes:

1. *Erotomanic type* (de Clerambault's syndrome), in which there is a belief that a person, usually of higher status, is in love with the patient
2. *Grandiose type*, in which there is a belief that one is of inflated worth, power, knowledge, or identity or has a special relation to a deity or famous person
3. *Jealous type*, in which the delusion is that one's sexual partner is unfaithful
4. *Persecutory type*, in which there is a belief that one is being malevolently treated in some way
5. *Somatic type*, in which the delusion is that a person has some physical defect, disorder, or disease, such as AIDS
6. *Mixed type*, in which there is more than one characteristic theme and no one theme predominates
7. *Unspecified type*, in which the patient does not fit any of the previous categories or the dominant delusional belief cannot be clearly determined

The DSM-IV-TR diagnosis of shared psychotic disorder is made when two or more persons share a delusion (*folie à deux*).

Epidemiology

Delusional disorder constitutes from 1% to 4% of psychiatric admissions and from 2% to 7% of admissions for functional psychosis (Kendler 1982). The incidence of first admissions for paranoia was estimated to fall between 1 and 3 per 100,000 per year and the prevalence to fall between 24 and 30 per 100,000 population. Delusional disorder occurs primarily in middle to late adult life, with a peak frequency of first admissions between 35 and 55 years of age. More women than men develop the disorder, and whereas 60%–75% of patients are married, up to one-third are widowed, divorced, or separated. Individuals with delusional disorder are economically and educationally disadvantaged, and immigrants seem especially prone to develop the disorder. Patients with delusional disorder are also more extroverted, dominant, and hypersensitive premorbidly than are schizophrenic patients, who, as discussed earlier in the chapter, are likely to be introverted and schizoid premorbidly. Once established, delusional disorder is generally chronic and lifelong. However, it appears to have a better long-term prognosis than schizophrenia (Opjordsmoen 1989; Winokur 1977). Remission is reported in one-third to one-half of cases (Jorgensen 1994).

Etiology

The cause of delusional disorder is unknown, although it is unlikely that delusional disorders are related to schizophrenia or the mood disorders. The relatives of probands with delusional disorder show increased rates of jealously, suspiciousness, paranoid personality, and delusional disorder over control relatives, but the families have no increase in schizophrenia or mood disorders (Kendler et al. 1982, 1985a; J.A.G. Watt 1985; Winokur 1985).

Other potentially relevant risk factors for delusional disorder include social isolation and immigration. *Prison psychosis* has been described in which persons placed in solitary confinement have developed a paranoid psychosis. *Migration psychoses*, which are often persecutory, have been described in persons migrating from one country to another (although it is reasonable to assume that persons in whom paranoia is prone to develop may be more likely to emigrate than others). *Querulent paranoia*, a special form of paranoia characterized by litigiousness, is believed by Scandinavian investigators to be a psychogenic disorder in which unlucky personal experiences precipitate paranoia in persons with deviant personalities (Astrup 1984).

Clinical Management

Clinical management of the patient with delusional disorder involves establishing the diagnosis, instituting appropriate interventions, and providing follow-up care. Because there are no systematic data comparing treatments in delusional disorder (Munro and Mok 1995), recommendations are based on clinical observation, not empirical evidence. Treatment will most often include both psychotherapy and medication.

Most patients have little insight about their illness and refuse to acknowledge a problem, so an initial obstacle is getting the patient to the physician. This fact might account for the low percentage of cases reported by physicians. Most patients can be treated as outpatients, but hospitalization is necessary if threats of self-harm or harm to others are present. Suicide is uncommon but may occur when the patient becomes depressed and despondent. The potential for violence may exist because some patients will act on their delusions, particularly jealous or erotomanic men. In these cases the target is not random, but specific to the delusional concern. Thus, a clinician caring for a patient with delusional disorder must carefully assess potential for harm to self or others.

Tact and skill are necessary to help persuade a delusional disorder patient to accept treatment. It may help to first convince the patient to receive treatment for depressive or anxiety symptoms and not the delusions. Once a therapeutic relationship is established, a clinician can begin to gently challenge the delusional beliefs by showing how they interfere with the patient's life, but must neither condemn nor collude in the beliefs. The patient should be assured of privacy, and the physician should take care not to discuss confidential matters with the patient's family without the patient's consent. Group therapy is usually not recommended; the patient's chronic suspiciousness and hypersensitivity may lead him or her to misinterpret situations that may arise in the context of group therapy.

Because delusional disorder is relatively uncommon, its treatment with antipsychotic medication has never been properly evaluated; anecdotal evidence suggests that response is poor (Winokur 1977). Antipsychotics may reduce the agitation, apprehension, and anxiety that accompany delusions, but leave the core delusion untouched. Any of the standard antipsychotics can be used, although there is some suggestion that pimozide may produce better results (Munro and Mok 1995). The selection of medication and dosage will depend on the patient's age and the drug's potential side effects. If the patient is helped by the antipsychotic, depot forms of several are available to ensure compliance (e.g., haloperidol decanoate, fluphenazine decanoate). Neuroleptics have been reported to specifically reduce the intensity of the delusions in erotomania and the associated ideas of reference (Segal 1989).

Conclusions

Tremendous progress has been made during the past two decades to better our understanding of schizophrenia, schizophreniform disorder, and delusional disorder. While the introduction of DSM-III criteria in 1980 narrowed the definition for schizophrenia and created a more homogeneous group of subjects for research, some experts believed the narrowing went too far. A reemphasis on negative symptoms of schizophrenia (Bleuler's "fundamental" symptoms) in DSM-IV-TR has added balance to the perhaps too-rigid emphasis on Schneiderian symptoms in the 1970s. Advances in classification and epidemiology have allowed us to reevaluate the distribution of schizophrenia and its risk factors.

During the 1990s, the "Decade of the Brain," the drive in psychiatry was to develop a comprehensive understanding of brain function at levels that range from mind to molecule and to determine how aberrations in these normal functions lead to the development of symptoms of mental illness. Progress in the coming decade will be to build on the foundation of current research and enhance our understanding of the pathophysiology and etiology of schizophrenia. Our ultimate goal is to give physicians more powerful tools to treat those who suffer from schizophrenia and, if possible, prevent its development.

References

Allebeck P, Varla A, Kristjansson E, et al: Risk factors for suicide among patients with schizophrenia. Acta Psychiatr Scand 76:414–419, 1987

Allison DB, Mentore JL, Heo M, et al: Antipsychotic-induced weight gain: a comprehensive research synthesis. Am J Psychiatry 156:1686–1696, 1999

American Psychiatric Association: Diagnostic and Statistical Manual of Mental Disorders, 3rd Edition. Washington, DC, American Psychiatric Press, 1980

American Psychiatric Association: Diagnostic and Statistical Manual of Mental Disorders, 3rd Edition, Revised. Washington, DC, American Psychiatric Press, 1987

American Psychiatric Association: Diagnostic and Statistical Manual of Mental Disorders, 4th Edition. Washington, DC, American Psychiatric Press, 1994

American Psychiatric Association: Practice guideline for the treatment of patients with schizophrenia. Am J Psychiatry 154 (suppl):1–63, 1997

Andreasen NC: Thought, language, and communication disorders, I: clinical assessment, definition of terms, and evaluation of their reliability. Arch Gen Psychiatry 36:1315–1321, 1979

Andreasen NC: Negative symptoms in schizophrenia: definition and reliability. Arch Gen Psychiatry 39:784–788, 1982

Andreasen NC, Olson S: Negative versus positive schizophrenia: definition and validation. Arch Gen Psychiatry 39:789–794, 1982

Andreasen NC, Smith MR, Jacoby CG, et al: Ventricular enlargement in schizophrenia: definition and prevalence. Am J Psychiatry 139:292–296, 1982

Andreasen NC, Nasrallah HA, Dunn V, et al: Structural abnormalities in the frontal system in schizophrenia: a magnetic resonance imaging study. Arch Gen Psychiatry 43:136–144, 1986

Andreasen NC, Ehrhardt JC, Swayze VW, et al: Magnetic resonance imaging of the brain in schizophrenia: the pathophysiologic significance of structural abnormalities. Arch Gen Psychiatry 47:35–44, 1990a

Andreasen NC, Flaum M, Swayze VW, et al: Positive and negative symptoms in schizophrenia: a critical reappraisal. Arch Gen Psychiatry 47:615–621, 1990b

Andreasen NC, Swayze VW, Flaum M, et al: Ventricular enlargement in schizophrenia: evaluation with computed tomographic scanning. Arch Gen Psychiatry 47:1008–1015, 1990c

Andreasen NC, Rezai K, Alliger R, et al: Hypofrontality in neuroleptic-naive patients and in patients with chronic schizophrenia: assessment with xenon 133 single-photon emission computed tomography and the Tower of London. Arch Gen Psychiatry 49:943–958, 1992

Andreasen NC, Flashman L, Flaum M, et al: Regional brain abnormalities in schizophrenia measured with magnetic resonance imaging. JAMA 272:1763–1769, 1994a

Angermeyer ML, Goldstein JM, Kuehn L: Gender differences in schizophrenia: rehospitalization and community survival. Psychol Med 19:365–382, 1989

Anthony JC, Folstein M, Romanoski AJ, et al: Comparison of the lay Diagnostic Interview Schedule and a standardized psychiatric diagnosis. Arch Gen Psychiatry 42: 667–675, 1985

Astrup C: Querulent paranoia: a follow-up. Neuropsychobiology 11:149–154, 1984

Barraclough B, Bunch J, Nelson B, et al: A hundred cases of suicide: clinical aspects. Br J Psychiatry 125:355–373, 1974

Barta PE, Pearlson GD, Powers RE, et al: Auditory hallucinations and smaller superior temporal gyral volume in schizophrenia. Am J Psychiatry 147:1457–1462, 1990

Beard JH, Propst RN, Malamud TJ: The Fountain House model of psychiatric rehabilitation. Psychosocial Rehabilitation Journal 5:47–54, 1982

Beitchman JH: Childhood schizophrenia: a review and comparison with adult onset schizophrenia. Pediatr Clin North Am 8: 793–814, 1985

Bellack AS, Gold JM, Buchanan RW: Cognitive rehabilitation for schizophrenia: problems, prospects, and strategies. Schizophr Bull 25:257–274, 1999

Black DW, Fisher R: Mortality in DSM-III-R schizophrenia. Schizophr Res 7:109–116, 1992

Black DW, Winokur G: Cancer mortality in psychiatric patients: the Iowa Record-Linkage Study. Int J Psychiatry Med 16: 189–198, 1986

Bleuler E: Dementia Praecox, or the Group of Schizophrenias (1911). Translated by Zinken J. New York, International Universities Press, 1950

Breier A, Astrachan BM: Characterization of schizophrenic patients who commit suicide. Am J Psychiatry 141:206–209, 1984

Breier A, Buchanan RW, Elkashef A, et al: Brain morphology and schizophrenia: a magnetic resonance imaging study of limbic, prefrontal cortex, and caudate structures. Arch Gen Psychiatry 49:921–926, 1992

Brockington IF, Meltzer HY: The nosology of schizoaffective psychosis. Psychiatr Dev 1:317–338, 1983

Bromet EJ, Dew MA, Eaton W: Epidemiology of psychosis with special reference to schizophrenia, in Textbook of Psychiatric Epidemiology. Edited by Tsuang MT, Tohen M, Zahner GEP. New York, Wiley-Liss, 1995, pp 283–300

Caracci G, Mukherjee S, Roth SD, et al: Subjective awareness of abnormal involuntary movements in chronic schizophrenic patients. Am J Psychiatry 147:295–298, 1990

Carlsson A: The current status of the dopamine hypothesis of schizophrenia. Neuropsychopharmacology 1:179–186, 1988

Carpenter WT Jr: Maintenance therapy of persons with schizophrenia. J Clin Psychiatry 57 (suppl 19):10–18, 1996

Carpenter WT Jr, Buchanan RW: Schizophrenia. N Engl J Med 330:681–690, 1994

Carpenter WT Jr, Hanlon TL, Heinrichs DW, et al: Continuous versus targeted medication in schizophrenic outpatients: outcome results. Am J Psychiatry 147:1138–1148, 1990

Carpenter WT Jr, Buchanan RW, Kirkpatrick B, et al: Diazepam treatment of early signs of exacerbation in schizophrenia. Am J Psychiatry 156:299–303, 1999b

Chakos M, Lieberman J, Hoffman E, et al: Effectiveness of second-generation antipsychotics in patients with treatment-resistant schizophrenia: a review and meta-analysis of randomized trials. Am J Psychiatry 158:518–526, 2001

Chatterjee A, Chako SM, Koreen A, et al: Prevalence and clinical correlates of extrapyramidal signs and spontaneous dyskinesia in never-medication schizophrenic patients. Am J Psychiatry 152:1724–1729, 1995

Christison GW, Kirch DG, Wyatt RJ: When symptoms persist: choosing among alternative somatic treatments for schizophrenia. Schizophr Bull 17:217–245, 1991

Clardy JA, Hyde TM, Kleinman JE: Postmortem neurochemical and neuropathological studies in schizophrenia, in Schizophrenia: From Mind to Molecule. Edited by Andreasen NC. Washington, DC, American Psychiatric Press, 1993, pp 123–146

Conley RR, Tamminga CA, Bartko JJ, et al: Olanzapine compared with chlorpromazine in treatment-resistant schizophrenia. Am J Psychiatry 155:914–920, 1998

Cook JA, Pickett SA, Razzano L, et al: Rehabilitation services for persons with schizophrenia. Psychiatr Ann 26:97–104, 1996

Coryell W, Tsuang MT: Outcome after 40 years in DSM-III schizophreniform disorder. Arch Gen Psychiatry 43:324–328, 1986

Creese R, Burt BR, Snyder SH: Dopamine receptor binding predicts clinical and pharmacologic potencies of antipsychotic drugs. Science 192:81–84, 1976

Crespo-Facorro B, Kim JJ, Andreasen NC, et al: Human frontal cortex: an MRI-based parcellation method. Neuroimage 10:500–519, 1999a

Crespo-Facorro B, Kim J, Andreasen NC, et al: Regional frontal abnormalities in schizophrenia: a quantitative gray matter volume and cortical surface size study. Biol Psychiatry 48:110–119, 2000

Crow TJ: Positive and negative schizophrenic symptoms and the role of dopamine. Br J Psychiatry 137:383–386, 1980

Csillag C: Denmark: psychiatric offenders. Lancet 341:683–684, 1993

Cutting J: The Psychology of Schizophrenia. London, England, Churchill Livingstone, 1985

Davis JM, Kane JM, Marder SR, et al: Dose response of prophylactic antipsychotics. J Clin Psychiatry 54(suppl 3):24–30, 1993

Davis KL, Kahn RS, Ko G, et al: Dopamine in schizophrenia: a review and reconceptualization. Am J Psychiatry 148:1474–1486, 1991

Davis KL, Buchsbaum MS, Shihabuddin L, et al: Ventricular enlargement in poor-outcome schizophrenia. Biol Psychiatry 43:783–793, 1998

deLeon J, Verghese C, Tracy JI, et al: Polydipsia and water intoxication in psychiatric patients: a review of the epidemiologic literature. Biol Psychiatry 35:519–530, 1994

DeLisi LE, Hoff Al, Kushner M, et al: Left ventricular enlargement associated with diagnostic outcome of schizophreniform disorder. Biol Psychiatry 32:199–201, 1992

DeLisi LE, Sakuma M, Tew W, et al: Schizophrenia as a chronic active brain process: a study of progressive brain structural change subsequent to the onset of schizophrenia. Psychiatry Res 74:129–140, 1997

Delva NJ, Letemendia FJJ: Lithium treatment in schizophrenia and schizoaffective disorders. Br J Psychiatry 141:387–400, 1982

Dixon L, Haas G, Weiden PJ, et al: Drug abuse in schizophrenic patients: clinical correlates and reasons for use. Am J Psychiatry 148:224–230, 1991

Dixon L, Lyles A, Scott J, et al: Services to families of adults with schizophrenia: from treatment recommendations to dissemination. Psychiatr Serv 50:233–238, 1999

Drake RE, Osher FC, Wallach MA: Alcohol use and abuse in schizophrenia: a prospective community study. J Nerv Ment Dis 177:408–414, 1989

Dubin WR, Waxman HM, Weiss KJ, et al: Rapid tranquilization: the efficacy of oral concentrate. J Clin Psychiatry 46:475–478, 1985

Eaton WW: Epidemiology of schizophrenia. Epidemiol Rev 7:105–126, 1985

Eaton WW: Update on epidemiology of schizophrenia. Epidemiol Rev 13:320–328, 1991

Eaton WW, Day R, Kramer M: The use of epidemiology for risk factor research in schizophrenia: an overview and methodologic critique, in Handbook of Schizophrenia, Vol 3: Nosology, Epidemiology, and Genetics. Edited by Tsuang MT, Simpson JC. Amsterdam, Elsevier Science, 1988, pp 169–204

Eaton WW, Hayward C, Ram R: Schizophrenia and rheumatoid arthritis: a review. Schizophr Res 6:181–192, 1992

Ellsworth RB: Characteristics of effective treatment milieu, in Principles and Practice of Milieu Therapy. Edited by Gunderson JG, Will OA, Mosher LF. New York, Jason Aronson, 1983, pp 87–123

Evans JD, Paulsen JS, Harris MJ, et al: A clinical and neuropsychological comparison of delusional disorder and schizophrenia. J Neuropsychiatry Clin Neurosci 8:281–286, 1996

Expert Consensus Guideline Series Steering Committee: Treatment of schizophrenia. J Clin Psychiatry 57 (suppl 12B):1–58, 1996

Falloon IR: Early intervention for first episodes of schizophrenia: a preliminary exploration. Psychiatry 55:4–15, 1992

Farde L, Nordstrom AL, Wiesel FA, et al: Positron emission tomographic analysis of central D1 and D2 dopamine receptor occupancy in patients treated with classical neuroleptics and clozapine: relation to extrapyramidal side effects. Arch Gen Psychiatry 49:538–544, 1992

Faris REL, Durham HL: Mental Disorder in Urban Areas. Chicago, IL, University of Chicago Press, 1939

Farmer AE, McGuffin P, Gottesman II: Twin concordance for DSM-III schizophrenia: scrutinizing the validity of the definition. Arch Gen Psychiatry 44:634–641, 1987

Feinberg I: Schizophrenia and late maturational brain changes in man. Psychopharmacol Bull 18:29–31, 1982

Fennig S, Craig TJ, Bromet EJ: The consistency of DSM-III-R delusional disorder in a first-admission sample. Psychopathology 29:315–324, 1996

Fenton WS: Evolving perspectives on individual psychotherapy for schizophrenia. Schizophr Bull 26:47–72, 2000

Fenton WS, McGlashan TH: The prognostic significance of obsessive-compulsive symptoms in schizophrenia. Am J Psychiatry 143:437–441, 1986

Fenton WS, McGlashan TH: Natural history of schizophrenia subtypes, I: longitudinal study of paranoid, hebephrenic, and undifferentiated schizophrenia. Arch Gen Psychiatry 48:969–977, 1991

Flaum M, Arndt S, Andreasen NC: The role of gender in studies of ventrical enlargement in schizophrenia: a predominantly male effect. Am J Psychiatry 147:1327–1332, 1990

Garza-Trevino ES, Hollister LE, Overall JE, et al: Efficacy of combinations of intramuscular antipsychotics and sedative-hypnotics for control of psychotic agitation. Am J Psychiatry 146:1598–1601, 1989

Geddes JR, Lawrie SM: Obstetrical complications and schizophrenia: a meta-analysis. Br J Psychiatry 167:786–793, 1995

Geddes J, Freemantle N, Harrison P, et al: Atypical antipsychotics in the treatment of schizophrenia: systematic overview and meta-regression analysis. BMJ 321:1371–1376, 2000

Goff DC, Henderson DC, Amico E: Cigarette smoking and schizophrenia: relationship to psychopathology and medication side effects. Am J Psychiatry 149:1189–1194, 1992

Goldberg TE, Kelsoe JR, Weinberger DR, et al: Performance of schizophrenic patients on putative neuropsychological tests of frontal lobe function. Int J Neurosci 42:51–58, 1988

Goldstein LE, Sporn J, Brown S, et al: New-onset diabetes mellitus and diabetic ketoacidosis associated with olanzapine treatment. Psychosomatics 40:438–443, 1999

Gorwood P, Leboyer M, Falissard B, et al: Anticipation in schizophrenia: new light on a controversial problem. Am J Psychiatry 153:1173–1177, 1996

Gottesman II, Shields J: Schizophrenia: The Epigenetic Puzzle. Cambridge, England, Cambridge University Press, 1982

Green MF, Satz P, Christensen C: Minor physical remedies in schizophrenia patients, bipolar patients, and their siblings. Schizophr Bull 20:433–440, 1994

Gudeman JE, Shore MF, Dickey B: Day hospitalization and an inn instead of inpatient care for psychiatric patients. N Engl J Med 308:749–753, 1983

Gulbinat W, Dupont A, Jablensky A, et al: Cancer incidence in schizophrenic patients: results of record linkage studies in three countries. Br J Psychiatry Suppl 18:75–83, 1992

Gupta S, Andreasen NC, Arndt S, et al: Neurological soft signs in neuroleptic-naïve and neuroleptic treated schizophrenic patients and in normal comparison subjects. Am J Psychiatry 152:191–196, 1995a

Gur RE, Cowell P, Turetsky BI, et al: A follow-up magnetic resonance imaging study of schizophrenia: relationship of neuroanatomical changes to clinical and neurobehavioral measures. Arch Gen Psychiatry 55:145–152, 1998

Guze SB, Cloninger CR, Martin RL, et al: A follow-up and family study of schizophrenia. Arch Gen Psychiatry 40:1273–1276, 1983

Hare EH: Mental illness and social conditions in Bristol. J Ment Sci 102:349–357, 1956

Hare EH, Price JS, Slater E: Mental disorder and season of birth. Nature 241:480, 1973

Harrison PJ: The neuropathology of schizophrenia. A critical review of the data and their interpretation. Brain 122:593–624, 1999

Hegarty JD, Baldessarini RJ, Tohen M, et al: One hundred years of schizophrenia: a meta-analysis of the outcome literature. Am J Psychiatry 151:1409–1415, 1994

Heinssen RK, Liberman RP, Kopelowicz A: Psychosocial skills training for schizophrenia: lessons from the laboratory. Schizophr Bull 26:21–46, 2000

Henderson DC, Cagliero E, Gray C, et al: Clozapine, diabetes mellitus, weight gain, and lipid abnormalities: a five-year naturalistic study. Am J Psychiatry 157:975–981, 2000

Herz M: Prodromal symptoms and prevention of relapse in schizophrenia. J Clin Psychiatry 46:22–25, 1985

Heston LL: Psychiatric disorders in foster home reared children of schizophrenic mothers. Br J Psychiatry 112:819–825, 1966

Ho BC, Andreasen NC: Long delays in seeking treatment for schizophrenia. Lancet 357: 898–900, 2001

Ho BC, Andreasen NC, Nopoulos P, et al: Progressive structural brain abnormalities and their significance to clinical outcome: a longitudinal magnetic resonance imaging study early in schizophrenia. Arch Gen Psychiatry, in press

Holzman PS, Soloman CM, Levin S, et al: Pursuit eye movement dysfunctions in schizophrenia: family evidence for specificity. Arch Gen Psychiatry 41:136–139, 1984

Hughlings-Jackson J: Selected Writings. London, England, Hodder & Stoughton, 1931

Ingvar DH, Franzen G: Abnormalities of cerebral blood flow distribution in patients with chronic schizophrenia. Acta Psychiatr Scand 50:425–462, 1974

Jablensky A, Sartorius N: Culture and schizophrenia. Psychol Med 5:113–124, 1975

Jablensky A, Sartorius N, Ernberg G, et al: Schizophrenia: manifestation, incidence, and course, in Different Cultures: A World Health Organization Ten-Country Study—Psychological Medicine Monograph Supplement 20. Cambridge, England, Cambridge University Press, 1992

Javitt DC, Zukin SR: Recent advances in the phencyclidine model of schizophrenia. Am J Psychiatry 148:1301–1308, 1991

Johns CA, Thompson JW: Adjunctive treatments in schizophrenia: pharmacotherapies and electroconvulsive therapy. Schizophr Bull 21:607–619, 1995

Jonsson H, Nyman AK: Prediction of outcome in schizophrenia. Acta Psychiatr Scand 69: 274–291, 1984

Jorgensen P: Course and outcome in dimensional disorders. Psychopathology 27:79–88, 1994

Kallman FJ: The Genetics of Schizophrenia. New York, Augustin, 1938

Kanas N: Inpatient and outpatient group therapy for schizophrenic patients. Am J Psychother 39:431–439, 1985

Kane JM, Marder SR: Psychopharmacologic treatment of schizophrenia. Schizophr Bull 19:287–302, 1993

Kane JM, Honigfeld G, Singer J, et al: Clozapine for the treatment-resistant schizophrenic: a double-blind comparison with chlorpromazine. Arch Gen Psychiatry 45:789–796, 1988

Kapur S, Seeman P: Does fast dissociation from the dopamine D2 receptor explain the action of atypical antipsychotics? A new hypothesis. Am J Psychiatry 158: 360–369, 2001

Kapur S, Zipursky R, Jones C, et al: Relationship between dopamine D2 occupancy, clinical response, and side effects: a double-blind PET study of first-episode schizophrenia. Am J Psychiatry 157:514–520, 2000

Kasanin J: The acute schizoaffective psychoses. Am J Psychiatry 13:97–126, 1933

Keck PE, McElroy SL, Strakowski SM: Schizoaffective disorder: role of atypical antipsychotics. Schizophr Res 35:S5–S12, 1999

Keefe RSE, Silva SG, Perkins DO, et al: The effects of atypical antipsychotic drugs on neurocognitive impairment in schizophrenia: a review and meta-analysis. Schizophr Bull 25:201–222, 1999

Kendler KS: The nosological validity of paranoia (simple delusional disorder): a review. Arch Gen Psychiatry 37:699–706, 1980

Kendler KS: Demography of paranoid psychosis (delusional disorder): a review and comparison with schizophrenia and affective illness. Arch Gen Psychiatry 39:890–902, 1982

Kendler KS, Gruenberg AM, Strauss JS: An independent analysis of the Copenhagen sample of the Danish Adoption Study of Schizophrenia, III: the relationship between paranoid psychosis (delusional disorder) and the schizophrenia spectrum disorders. Arch Gen Psychiatry 38:985–987, 1982

Kendler KS, Masterson CC, Davis KL: Psychiatric illness in first-degree relatives of patients with paranoid psychosis, schizophrenia, and medical illness. Br J Psychiatry 147:524–531, 1985a

Kendler KS, McGuire M, Gruenberg AM, et al: An epidemiologic, clinical, and family study of simple schizophrenia in County Roscommon, Ireland. Am J Psychiatry 151:27–34, 1994a

Kendler KS, McGuire M, Gruenberg AM, et al: Outcome and family study of the subtypes of schizophrenia in the west of Ireland. Am J Psychiatry 151:849–856, 1994b

Kendler KS, McGuire M, Gruenberg AM, et al: Examining the validity of DSM-III-R schizoaffective disorder and its putative subtypes in the Roscommon Family Study. Am J Psychiatry 152:755–764, 1995

Kendler KS, Karkowski-Shuman L, Walsh D: Age at onset in schizophrenia and risk of illness in relatives: results from the Roscommon Family Study. Br J Psychiatry 169:213–218, 1996

Kennedy HG, Kemp LI, Dyer DE: Fear and anger in delusional (paranoid) disorder: the association with violence. Br J Psychiatry 160:488–492, 1992

Kessler R, McGonagle K, Zhao S, et al: Lifetime and 12-month prevalence of DSM-III-R psychiatric disorders in the United States: results from the National Comorbidity Study. Arch Gen Psychiatry 51:8–19, 1994

Kety SS, Rosenthal D, Wender PH, et al: Mental illness in the biologic and adoptive families of adopted individuals who have become schizophrenic: a preliminary report based on psychiatric interviews, in Genetic Research in Psychiatry. Edited by Fieve R, Rosenthal D, Brill H. Baltimore, MD, Johns Hopkins University Press, 1975, pp 147–165

King DJ, Burke M, Lucas RA: Antipsychotic drug-induced dysphoria. Br J Psychiatry 167:480–482, 1995

Kingsbury SJ, Salzman C: Disulfiram in the treatment of alcoholic patients with schizophrenia. Hosp Community Psychiatry 41:133–134, 1990

Kissling W (ed): Guidelines for Neuroleptic Relapse Prevention in Schizophrenia. Berlin, Germany, Springer-Verlag, 1991

Kraepelin E: Dementia Praecox and Paraphrenia. Translated by Barkley RM. Edinburgh, Scotland, E & S Livingstone, 1919

Krakowski MI, Convit A, Jaeger J, et al: Neurologic impairment in violent schizophrenic inpatients. Am J Psychiatry 146: 849–853, 1989

Lamb HR: Some reflections on treating schizophrenics. Arch Gen Psychiatry 43:1007–1011, 1986

Lamb HR: Lessons learned from deinstitutionalization in the United States. Br J Psychiatry 162:587–592, 1993

Lamberti JS, Tariot PN: Schizophrenia in nursing home patients. Psychiatr Ann 25:441–448, 1995

Lehman AF: Vocational rehabilitation in schizophrenia. Schizophr Bull 21:645–656, 1995

Lehman AF, Steinwachs DM, and PORT coinvestigators: Translating research into practice: the Schizophrenia Patient Outcomes Research Team (PORT) treatment recommendations. Schizophr Bull 24:1–10, 1998

Leucht S, Pitschel-Walz G, Abraham D, et al: Efficacy and extrapyramidal side-effects of the new antipsychotics olanzapine, quetiapine, risperidone and sertindole compared to conventional antipsychotics and placebo: a meta-analysis of randomized controlled trials. Schizophr Bull 35:51–68, 1999

Levinson DF, Simpson GM, Lo ES, et al: Fluphenazine plasma levels, dosage, efficacy, and side effects. Am J Psychiatry 152:765–771, 1995

Levinson DF, Umapathy C, Musthaq M: Treatment of schizoaffective disorder and schizophrenia with mood symptoms. Am J Psychiatry 156:1138–1148, 1999

Lewine R, Burbach D, Melzer HY: Effect of diagnostic criteria on the ratio of male to female schizophrenic patients. Am J Psychiatry 141:84–87, 1984

Lieberman JA, Fenton WS: Delayed detection of psychosis: causes, consequences, and effect on public health. Am J Psychiatry 157:1727–1730, 2000

Lieberman JA, Kane JM, Sarantakos S, et al: Prediction of relapse in schizophrenia. Arch Gen Psychiatry 44:592–603, 1987

Lieberman JA, Chakos M, Wu H, et al: Longitudinal study of brain morphology in first episode schizophrenia. Biol Psychiatry 49:487–499, 2001

Linszen DH, Dingemans PM, Lenior ME: Cannabis abuse and the course of recent-onset schizophrenic disorders. Arch Gen Psychiatry 51:273–279, 1994

Lipinsky JF, Zubenko G, Cohen BM, et al: Propranolol in the treatment of neuroleptic-induced akathisia. Am J Psychiatry 141:412–415, 1984

Loranger AW: Sex difference in age at onset of schizophrenia. Arch Gen Psychiatry 41:157–161, 1984

Lyketsos GC, Sakka P, Mailis A: The sexual adjustment of chronic schizophrenics: a preliminary study. Br J Psychiatry 143:376–382, 1983

Mackota G, Lamb HR: Vocational rehabilitation. Psychiatr Ann 19:548–552, 1989

Maj M, Pirozzi R, Formicola AM, et al: Reliability and validity of the DSM-IV diagnostic category of schizoaffective disorder: preliminary data. J Affect Disord 57:95–98, 2000

Manschreck TC: Delusional disorder: the recognition and management of paranoia. J Clin Psychiatry 57(suppl 3):32–38, 1996

Manschreck TC, Maher BA, Rucklos ME, et al: Disturbed voluntary motor activity in schizophrenic disorder. Psychol Med 12:73–84, 1982

Marder SR, Meibach RC: Risperidone in the treatment of schizophrenia. Am J Psychiatry 151:825–835, 1994

Marder SR, Wirshing WC, Mintz J, et al: Two-year outcome of social skills training and group psychotherapy for outpatients with schizophrenia. Am J Psychiatry 153:1585–1592, 1996

Maxmen JS: Delivery of after care services, in Management of Chronic Schizophrenia. Edited by Caton CLM. New York, Oxford University Press, 1984

McCabe MS, Fowler RC, Cadoret RJ, et al: Symptom differences in schizophrenics with good and poor prognosis. Am J Psychiatry 128:1239–1243, 1972

McEvoy JP, Hogarty GE, Steingard S: Optimal dose of neuroleptic in acute schizophrenia. Arch Gen Psychiatry 48:734–745, 1991

McFarlane WR, Lukens E, Link B, et al: Multiple family groups and psychoeducation in the treatment of schizophrenia. Arch Gen Psychiatry 52:679–687, 1995

McGlashan TH: The Chestnut Lodge Follow-Up Study, II: long-term outcome of schizophrenia and the affective disorders. Arch Gen Psychiatry 41:586–601, 1984

McGlashan TH: The prediction of outcome in chronic schizophrenia, IV: the Chestnut Lodge Follow-Up Study. Arch Gen Psychiatry 43:167–176, 1986

McGlashan TH: Duration of untreated psychosis in first-episode schizophrenia: marker or determinant of course? Biol Psychiatry 46:899–907, 1999

McGorry PD, Edwards J, Mihalopoulos C, et al: EPPIC: an evolving system of early detection and optimal management. Schizophr Bull 22:305–326, 1996

Meares A: The diagnosis of prepsychotic schizophrenia. Lancet 1:55–58, 1959

Meltzer HY: Biological studies in schizophrenia. Schizophr Bull 13:77–100, 1987

Meltzer HY, Matsubara S, Lee JC: Classification of typical and atypical antipsychotic drugs on the basis of dopamine D1, D2 and serontonin2 pKi values. J Pharmacol Exp Ther 251:238–246, 1989

Modestin T, Ammann R: Mental disorders and criminality: male schizophrenia. Schizophr Bull 22:69–82, 1996

Mohamed S, Paulsen JS, O'Leary D, et al: Generalized cognitive deficits in schizophrenia. Arch Gen Psychiatry 56:749–754, 1999

Mortensen PB, Pedersen CB, Westergaard T, et al: Effects of family history and place and season of birth on the risk of schizophrenia. N Engl J Med 340:603–608, 1999

Mukherjee S, Shukla S, Woodle J, et al: Misdiagnosis of schizophrenia in bipolar patients: a multiethnic comparison. Am J Psychiatry 140:1571–1574, 1983

Munro A, Mok H: An overview of treatment in paranoia/delusional disorder. Can J Psychiatry 40:616–622, 1995

Murphy HBM, Raman AC: The chronicity of schizophrenia in indigenous tropical people: results of a twelve-year follow-up survey in Mauritius. Br J Psychiatry 118:489–497, 1971

Murray CJL, Lopez AD: The Global Burden of Disease: A Comprehensive Assessment of Mortality and Disability From Diseases, Injuries, and Risk Factors in 1990 and Projected to 2020. Cambridge, MA, Harvard University Press, 1996

Ndetei DM, Vadher A: A comparative cross-cultural study of the frequencies of hallucinations in schizophrenia. Acta Psychiatr Scand 70:545–549, 1984

Neylan TC, van Kammen DP, Kelley ME, et al: Sleep in schizophrenic patients on and off haloperidol therapy: clinically stable versus relapsed patients. Arch Gen Psychiatry 49:643–649, 1992

Nimgaonkar VL: Reduced fertility in schizophrenia: here to stay? Acta Psychiatr Scand 98:348–353, 1998

Nopoulos P, Torres I, Flaum M, et al: Brain morphology in first-episode schizophrenia. Am J Psychiatry 152:1721–1723, 1995a

Olney JW, Farber NB: Glutamate receptor dysfunction and schizophrenia. Arch Gen Psychiatry 52:998–1007, 1995

Opjordsmoen S: Delusional disorders, I: comparative long-term outcome. Acta Psychiatr Scand 80:603–612, 1989

Peet M, Middlemiss DN, Yates RA: Propranolol in schizophrenia, II: clinical and biochemical aspects of combining propranolol with chlorpromazine. Br J Psychiatry 139:112–117, 1981

Penn DL, Mueser KT: Research update on the psychosocial treatment of schizophrenia. Am J Psychiatry 153:607–617, 1996

Perry PJ, Smith DA: Neuroleptic plasma concentrations: an estimate of their sensitivity and specificity as predictors of response, in Clinical Use of Neuroleptic Plasma Levels. Edited by Marder SR, Davis JM, Janicak PG. Washington, DC, American Psychiatric Press, 1993, pp 113–135

Petronis A, Kennedy JL: Unstable genes—unstable mind? Am J Psychiatry 152:164–172, 1995

Petronis A, Bassett AS, Honer WG, et al: Search for unstable DNA in schizophrenia families with evidence for genetic anticipation. Am J Hum Genet 59:905–911, 1996

Pfohl B, Winokur G: The micropsychopathology of hebephrenic/catatonic schizophrenia. J Nerv Ment Dis 171:296–300, 1983

Rapoport JL, Giedd J, Kumra S, et al: Childhood-onset schizophrenia: progressive ventricular change during adolescence. Arch Gen Psychiatry 54:897–903, 1997

Rice JP, McGuffin P: Genetic Etiology of Schizophrenia and Affective Disorders in Psychiatry, Vol 1. Edited by Michels R, Cavenar JO. Philadelphia, PA, JB Lippincott, 1985

Riecher-Rossler A, Rossler W: The course of schizophrenic psychoses: what do we really know? A selective review from an epidemiological perspective. Eur Arch Psychiatry Clin Neurosci 248:189–202, 1998

Rifkin A, Doddi S, Karajgi B, et al: Dosage of haloperidol for schizophrenia. Arch Gen Psychiatry 48:166–170, 1991

Robins LN, Helzer JE, Weissman MM, et al: Lifetime prevalence of specific psychiatric disorders in three sites. Arch Gen Psychiatry 41:949–958, 1984

Rothermundt M, Arolt V, Leadbeater J, et al: Cytokine production in unmedicated and treated schizophrenic patients. Neuroreport 11:3385–3388, 2000

Roy A: Suicide in chronic schizophrenia. Br J Psychiatry 141:171–177, 1982

Rudin E: Studien uber Vererbung und Entstehung geistiger storungen I: Zur vererbung und Neuenstehung der Dementia Praecox. Berlin, Germany, Springer-Verlag, 1916

Sartorius N, Jablensky A, Korten A: Early manifestations and first contact incidence of schizophrenia in different cultures: a preliminary report on the evaluation of the WHO Collaborative Study in Determinants of Outcome of Severe Mental Disorders. Psychol Med 16:909–928, 1986

Schooler NR, Kane JM, Marder SR, et al: Efficacy of clozapine vs. haloperidol in a long-term clinical trial: preliminary findings (abstract). Schizophr Bull 15:165, 1995

Seeman P, Lee T, Chau-Wong M, et al: Antipsychotic drug doses and neuroleptic-dopamine receptors. Nature 261:717–719, 1976

Segal JH: Erotomania revisited: from Kraepelin to DSM-III-R. Am J Psychiatry 146:1261–1266, 1989

Sensky T, Turkington D, Kingdon D, et al: A randomized controlled trial of cognitive-behavioral therapy for persistent symptoms in schizophrenia resistant to medication. Arch Gen Psychiatry 57:165–172, 2000

Serretti A, Lattuada E, Cusin C, et al: Factor analysis of delusional disorder symptomatology. Compr Psychiatry 40:143–147, 1999

Shapiro S, Skinner EA, Kessler LG, et al: Utilization of health and mental health services: three Epidemiologic Catchment Area sites. Arch Gen Psychiatry 41:971–978, 1984

Shenton ME, Kikinis R, Jolesz FA, et al: Abnormalities of the left temporal lobe and thought disorder in schizophrenia: a quantitative magnetic resonance imaging study. N Engl J Med 327:604–612, 1992

Shenton ME, Wible CG, McCarley RW: A review of magnetic resonance imaging studies of brain anomalies in schizophrenia, in Brain Imaging in Clinical Psychiatry. Edited by Krishnan KRR, Doraiswamy PM. New York, Marcel Dekker, 1997, pp 297–380

Simpson JC, Tsuang MT: Mortality among patients with schizophrenia. Schizophr Bull 22:485–499, 1996

Siris SG, Morgan V, Fagerstrom R, et al: Adjunctive imipramine in the treatment of postpsychotic depression: a controlled trial. Arch Gen Psychiatry 44:533–539, 1987

Siris SG, Bermanzohn PC, Mason SE, et al: Maintenance imipramine therapy for secondary depression in schizophrenia: a controlled trial. Arch Gen Psychiatry 51:109–115, 1994

Slaby AE, Moreines R: Emergency room evaluation and management of schizophrenia, in Handbook of Schizophrenia, Vol 4: Psychosocial Treatment of Schizophrenia. Edited by Herz MI, Keith SJ, Docherty JP. New York, Elsevier, 1990, pp 247–268

Snyder SH: Catecholamines in the brain as mediators of amphetamine psychosis. Arch Gen Psychiatry 27:169–179, 1972

Spitzer RL, Endicott J, Robins E: Research diagnostic criteria: rationale and reliability. Arch Gen Psychiatry 35:773–782, 1978

Stein L: A system approach to reducing relapse in schizophrenia. J Clin Psychiatry 54 (suppl 3):7–12, 1993

Strakowski SM: Diagnostic validity of schizophreniform disorder. Am J Psychiatry 151:815–824, 1994

Strauss JS, Carpenter WJ: Schizophrenia. New York, Plenum, 1981

Susser E, Struening EL, Conover S: Psychiatric problems in homeless men: lifetime psychosis, substance use, and current disorders in new arrivals at New York City shelters. Arch Gen Psychiatry 46:845–850, 1989

Swanson JW, Holtzer CE, Ganju VK, et al: Violence and psychiatric disorder in the community: evidence from the Epidemiologic Catchment Area Surveys. Hosp Community Psychiatry 41:761–770, 1990

Szeszko PR, Bilder RM, Lencz T, et al: Investigation of frontal lobe subregions in first-episode schizophrenia. Psychiatry Res 90:1–15, 1999

Targum SD: Neuroendocrine dysfunction in schizophreniform disorder: correlation with 6-month clinical outcome. Am J Psychiatry 140:309–313, 1983

Tarrier N, Beckett R, Harwood S, et al: A trial of two cognitive-behavioral methods of treating drug-resistant residual psychotic symptoms in schizophrenic patients, I: outcome. Br J Psychiatry 162:524–532, 1993

Taube CA, Barrett SA (eds): Mental Health United States 1985 (DHHS Publ No ADM 85–1378). Rockville, MD, National Institute of Mental Health, 1985

Teplin LA: The criminality of the mentally ill: a dangerous misconception. Am J Psychiatry 142:593–599, 1985

Thacker GK, Cassady S, Adami H, et al: Eye movements in spectrum personality disorders: comparison of community subjects and relatives of schizophrenic patients. Am J Psychiatry 153:362–368, 1996

Tienari P: Psychiatric illness in identical twins. Acta Psychiatr Scand Suppl, No 171, 1963

Tollefson GD, Sanger TM, Lu Y, et al: Depressive signs and symptoms in schizophrenia: a prospective blinded trial of olanzapine and haloperidol. Arch Gen Psychiatry 55:250–258, 1998

Tsuang MT: Suicide in schizophrenics, manics, depressives, and surgical controls: a comparison with general population suicide mortality. Arch Gen Psychiatry 35:153–155, 1978

Tsuang MT, Woolson RF, Fleming JA: Long-term outcome of major psychoses, I: schizophrenia and affective disorders compared with psychiatrically symptom-free surgical conditions. Arch Gen Psychiatry 36:1295–1304, 1979

Vaillant GE: Prospective prediction of schizophrenic remission. Arch Gen Psychiatry 11:509–518, 1964

VanderZwaag C, McGee M, McEvoy JP, et al: Response of patients with treatment-refractory schizophrenia to clozapine with three serum level ranges. Am J Psychiatry 153:1579–1584, 1996

VanKammen DP, Peters J, Yao J, et al: Norepinephrine in acute exacerbations of chronic schizophrenia: negative symptoms revisited. Arch Gen Psychiatry 47:161–168, 1990

Wahlbeck K, Cheine MV, Gilbody S, et al: Efficacy of beta-blocker supplementation for schizophrenia: a systematic review of randomized trials. Schizophr Res 41:341–347, 2000

Walker E, Lewine RJ: Prediction of adult-onset schizophrenia from childhood home movies of the patients. Am J Psychiatry 147:1052–1056, 1990

Ward KE, Friedman L, Wise A, et al: Meta-analysis of brain and cranial size in schizophrenia. Schizophr Res 22:197–123, 1996

Watt DC, Katz K, Shepard M: The natural history of schizophrenia: a five-year prospective follow-up of a representative sample of schizophrenics by means of a standardized clinical and social assessment. Psychol Med 13:663–670, 1983

Watt JAG: The relationship of paranoid states to schizophrenia. Am J Psychiatry 142:1456–1458, 1985

Watt NF: Patterns of childhood social development in adult schizophrenics. Arch Gen Psychiatry 35:160–165, 1978

Weinberger DR: Implications of normal brain development for the pathogenesis of schizophrenia. Arch Gen Psychiatry 44:660–669, 1987

Weinberger DR, McClure RK: Neurotoxicity, neuroplasticity, and magnetic resonance imaging morphometry: what is happening in the schizophrenic brain? Arch Gen Psychiatry 59:553–558, 2002

Weinberger DR, Torrey EF, Neophytides AN, et al: Lateral cerebral ventricle enlargement in chronic schizophrenia. Arch Gen Psychiatry 36:735–755, 1979

Weinberger DR, Bigelow LB, Kleinman JE, et al: Cerebral ventricular enlargement in chronic schizophrenia: an association with poor response to treatment. Arch Gen Psychiatry 37:11–13, 1980

Wender PH, Rosenthal D, Kety SS, et al: Social class and psychopathology in adoptees: a natural experimental method for separating the roles of genetic and experimental factors. Arch Gen Psychiatry 28:318–325, 1973

Winokur G: Delusional disorder (paranoia). Compr Psychiatry 18:511–521, 1977

Winokur G: Familial psychopathology in delusional disorder. Compr Psychiatry 26:241–248, 1985

Winokur G, Tsuang MT: The Natural History of Mania, Depression, and Schizophrenia. Washington, DC, American Psychiatric Press, 1996

Winokur G, Morrison J, Clancy J, et al: Iowa 500: the clinical and genetic distinction of hebephrenic and paranoid schizophrenia. J Nerv Ment Dis 159:12–19, 1974

Wirshing DA, Marshall BD Jr, Green MF, et al: Risperidone in treatment-refractory schizophrenia. Am J Psychiatry 156:1374–1379, 1999

Wolkowitz OM, Pickar D: Benzodiazepines in the treatment of schizophrenia: a review and reappraisal. Am J Psychiatry 148:714–726, 1991

World Health Organization: Schizophrenia: The International Pilot Study of Schizophrenia, Vol 1. Geneva, Switzerland, World Health Organization, 1975

World Health Organization: International Statistical Classification of Diseases and Related Health Problems, Tenth Revision (ICD-10). Geneva, Switzerland, World Health Organization, 1992

Yalom ID: Inpatient Group Psychotherapy. New York, Basic Books, 1983

Ziedonis DM, Fisher W: Assessment and treatment of comorbid substance abuse in individuals with schizophrenia. Psychiatr Ann 24:477–483, 1994

Mood Disorders

Steven L. Dubovsky, M.D.

Robert Davies, M.D.

Amelia N. Dubovsky, B.A.

Mood disorders can be relatively straightforward or they can assume complex forms that are difficult to treat. In this chapter, we review the epidemiology, diagnosis, comorbidity, biological and psychological concomitants, etiology, and treatment of the wide variety of affective syndromes that are encountered in psychiatric practice.

Epidemiology

Estimates of the incidence and prevalence of mood disorders vary. In the United States, the lifetime risk of a major depressive episode is said to be around 6%, and the lifetime risk of any mood disorder is said to be around 8% (Cassem 1995). The prevalence of major depression ranges from 2.6% to 5.5% in men and from 6.0% to 11.8% in women. The prevalence of dysthymia is 3%–4%. Some reports suggest that as much as 48% of the United States population has had one or more lifetime mood episodes (Cassem 1995). Most studies have found unipolar depression in general to be twice as common in women as in men (Reynolds et al. 1990).

The meaning of the sex difference remains to be clarified. Gender does not appear to affect the prevalence of bipolar disorder (Reynolds et al. 1990). The incidence of major depression is higher in separated or divorced people than in married individuals, especially men, and in medically ill patients (Lehtinen and Joukamaa 1994; Reiger et al. 1988), and depression is associated with greater use of general health services (Weissman et al. 1988b). The prevalence of major depression in primary care practice is 4.8%–9.2%, and the prevalence of all depressive disorders is 9%–20%, which makes mood disorders the most common psychiatric problems in primary care (McDaniel et al. 1995).

The effects of culture and stress on the prevalence of depression were illustrated by the Cross-National Collaborative Group study of 10 countries, which used the Diagnostic Interview Schedule to make DSM-III (American Psychiatric Association 1980) diagnoses (Weissman et al. 1996). In this study, the lifetime rate for major depression varied from a low of 1.5 cases per 100 adults in Taiwan to as many as 19.0 per 100 in Beirut, and the annual rate of depression was as low as 0.8 cases per 100 in Taiwan and as high as 5.8 per 100 in New Zealand.

The prevalence of bipolar disorder generally is reported as being between 1% and 2.5% (Akiskal 1995; Angst 1995); however, some studies suggested rates for bipolar disorders of 3%–6.5% (Akiskal 1995; Angst 1995). The frequency with which bipolar disorder is diagnosed probably depends on how it is defined; broader definitions produce significantly higher rates (Akiskal 1995; Angst 1995). Most prevalence studies require the presence of mania for a bipolar diagnosis to be recorded, but the bipolar II variant, which is characterized by episodes of hypomania but not mania, is more common than the bipolar I variant (Cassano et al. 1989; Simpson et al. 1993). If bipolar spectrum disorders, or subsyndromal and complex forms of bipolar disorder (see "Masked and Subsyndromal Bipolar Disorder"), are also considered (Akiskal 1995), the incidence of bipolar mood disorder is substantially higher. About 10%–15% of patients with a diagnosis of unipolar depression will eventually receive a revised diagnosis of bipolar disorder (Olie et al. 1992).

When conservative criteria are used, between 5% and 15% of cases of adult depression are found to be bipolar (Geller et al. 1996). However, Akiskal's group (Cassano et al. 1989) found that one-third of patients with primary depression met their criteria for bipolar spectrum disorders. The risk of bipolarity is higher in juvenile major depression—at least 20% in depressed adolescents and 32% in depressed children younger than 11 years (Geller et al. 1996). The lifetime rate of classically defined bipolar I disorder is relatively consistent across cultures, ranging from 0.3 per 100 in Taiwan to 1.5 per 100 in New Zealand (Weissman et al. 1996).

In all industrialized countries in the world, the incidence of depression, mania, suicide, and psychotic mood disorders has been increasing with every generation born

after 1910 (Cross-National Collaborative Group 1992; Klerman 1988; Klerman et al. 1985). The risk of severe and moder depression increased 10-fold from 19 1957 to 1957–1972 (Khodorov et al. 19 For unknown reasons, there was an ab jump in the rate of increase for people born after 1940—a true increase in the incidence of mood disorders in subsequent generations (cohort effect) and not a function of better recognition or more help-seeking (Cross-National Collaborative Group 1992; Doris et al. 1999; Klerman 1988; Klerman et al. 1985). Mood disorders not only are becoming more common but also are appearing at an earlier age (especially bipolar mood disorders) (Lasch and Weissman 1990).

In worldwide surveys, depression is the fourth most important cause of disability (Figiel et al. 1998) and the fourth most costly medical illness. Depressed patients spend more time in bed than do patients with diabetes, hypertension, arthritis, or chronic lung disease (Martin et al. 1992) and have as much functional disability as do patients with heart disease (Martin et al. 1992). Primary care physicians spend more time treating depression than hypertension, arteriosclerotic heart disease, and diabetes mellitus.

Suicide is an obvious public health problem that complicates mood disorders more frequently than other conditions. The lifetime risk of suicide in mood disorders is 10%–15% (Barklage 1991; Guze and Robbins 1970), and the risk of attempted suicide was increased 41-fold in depressed patients compared with those with other diagnoses in the Epidemiologic Catchment Area (ECA) survey (Petronis et al. 1990). It is well known that women attempt suicide more frequently than men do, but men are more likely to succeed. In one study, the excess risk of completed suicide in men was entirely accounted for by a higher prevalence of substance abuse in men and a greater likelihood that women have primary responsibility for children younger than 18 (Young et al. 1994).

The risk of suicide is high in mania as well as in depression. Patients with mixed bipolar states characterized by a combination of depression, rage, and grandiosity may be more likely to involve others in a suicide attempt—for example, through gunfights with the police. As much as 4% of people who commit suicide murder someone else first. High levels of distress and hopelessness increase the risk of suicide attempts in adolescents (Fritsch et al. 2000). Neuropsychological deficits are more common in depressed patients who have made high-lethality suicide attempts than in those who have made low-lethality attempts and nonpatients, suggesting that impaired executive function may exist in people at risk for severe suicide attempts (Keilp et al. 2001).

Despite the demonstrated inability of mental health professionals to predict (or prevent) suicide in any systematic manner (H.L. Miller et al. 1984), patients, families, and courts expect them to be able to do so. In an evaluation of immediate suicide risk, factors summarized in Table 6–1 can be considered (Pokorny 1993; Young et al. 1994). However, these factors at best suggest increased immediate risk. In addition, the short-term risk tends to fluctuate, and it is not known whether one risk factor is more important than another or how risk factors may interact with one another. Given the current state of knowledge, it is probably impossible for anyone to predict with any certainty the long-term risk of completed suicide, although there is at least a consensus on immediate risk factors.

Mood Disorders in Special Populations

Postpartum depression occurs in about 10% of mothers; risk factors include a

TABLE 6–1. Factors suggesting an increased risk of suicide

Demographic factors
  Male sex
  Recent loss
  Never married
  Older age
Symptoms
  Severe depression
  Anxiety
  Hopelessness
  Psychosis, especially with command
    hallucinations
History
  History of suicide attempts, especially
    if multiple or severe attempts
  Family history of suicide
  Active substance abuse
Suicidal thinking
  Presence of a specific plan
  Means available to carry out the plan
  Absence of factors that would keep the
    patient from completing the plan
  Rehearsal of the plan

history of a mood disorder, unwanted pregnancy, unemployment of the mother, lack of breast-feeding, a past history of depression, and the mother as head of the household (J. Hopkins et al. 1984; Warner et al. 1996). Postpartum depression increases the chance of alcohol and illicit drug use in teenaged mothers (Barnet et al. 1995). Some evidence indicates that depression in a mother adversely affects temperament (C.T. Beck 1996) and cognitive development (Hay and Kumar 1995) in the infant. Depressed mothers of preschoolers have more negative perceptions of and interactions with their children (Lang et al. 1996). Depression that begins for the first time in the postpartum period is more likely to have a bipolar outcome; postpartum psychosis very frequently is a manifestation of bipolar disorder. In women, depression associated with one reproductive event (e.g., menarche) tends to recur with other reproductive events (e.g., pregnancy, menopause).

Estimates of the prevalence of major depression in elderly people range from 2%–4% in community samples to 12% of medically hospitalized older patients to 16% of geriatric patients in long-term care (Blazer and Koenig 1996). Late-onset depression is associated with an increased likelihood of cerebrovascular disease and enlarged ventricles and may be more likely than depression in younger patients to be accompanied by prominent cognitive complaints.

Major depressive disorder (MDD) is said to occur in as many as 18% of preadolescents, with no gender differences in prevalence. However, mood disorders are often underdiagnosed in this population because many clinicians still do not believe that depression occurs in children and because depression may be more difficult to recognize in children than in older patients. Among adolescents, the prevalence of MDD has been reported to be 4.7% in 14- to 16-year-olds. By this age, depression is more common in girls than in boys. In nonclinical samples, up to one-third of the adolescents reported some depressive symptoms. Major depression in adolescents is associated with substance abuse and antisocial behavior, both of which sometimes obscure the affective diagnosis. The lifetime prevalence of bipolar disorder was 0.6% in 150 adolescents who were not psychiatrically referred. As discussed later in this chapter (see section titled "Mood Disorders in Children and Adolescents"), many cases of bipolar disorder in younger patients may be overlooked because mania has not yet appeared or because, when mania is present, it is manifested by anxiety, irritability, and attentional and behavioral syndromes that mask the mood disorder.

Diagnosis

DSM-IV-TR

DSM-IV (and its recent update DSM-IV-TR [American Psychiatric Association 2000]) distinguishes between mood episodes and mood disorders. An episode is a period lasting at least 2 weeks during which there are enough symptoms for full criteria to be met for the disorder. The criteria for a major depressive episode are summarized in Table 6–2. Patients with or without a history of mania may have a major depressive episode if they fulfill these criteria, but MDD refers to one or more episodes of major depression in the absence of mania or hypomania (i.e., unipolar depression). A major depressive episode may be modified by additional specifiers for psychotic, melancholic (Table 6–3), and atypical features (Table 6–4).

The interpretation of studies of mood disorders is facilitated by familiarity with several common terms. In most treatment studies, *response* is defined as at least 50% improvement, whereas *partial response* is 25%–50% improvement, and *nonresponse* is less than 25% improvement. According to this terminology, patients who are still half as symptomatic as at the beginning of treatment will be considered responders at the end of a treatment study. This is not a trivial point, given that most studies consider improvement rather than remission as the end point. *Remission* is defined as the state of having few or no symptoms of a mood disorder for at least 8 weeks. *Recovery*, the period after remission, is present if no symptoms have been present for more than 8 weeks, and the term implies that the disorder is quiescent. A *relapse* is a return of symptoms during the period of remission, implying continuation of the original episode, whereas *recurrence* is a later return of symptoms (during recovery), suggesting that a new

---

TABLE 6–2. DSM-IV-TR diagnostic criteria for major depressive episode

---

A. Five (or more) of the following symptoms have been present during the same 2-week period and represent a change from previous functioning; at least one of the symptoms is either (1) depressed mood or (2) loss of interest or pleasure.

   Note: Do not include symptoms that are clearly due to a general medical condition, or mood-incongruent delusions or hallucinations.

   (1) depressed mood most of the day, nearly every day, as indicated by either subjective report (e.g., feels sad or empty) or observation made by others (e.g., appears tearful).
      Note: In children and adolescents, can be irritable mood.

   (2) markedly diminished interest or pleasure in all, or almost all, activities most of the day, nearly every day (as indicated by either subjective account or observation made by others)

   (3) significant weight loss when not dieting or weight gain (e.g., a change of more than 5% of body weight in a month), or decrease or increase in appetite nearly every day.
      Note: In children, consider failure to make expected weight gains.

   (4) insomnia or hypersomnia nearly every day

   (5) psychomotor agitation or retardation nearly every day (observable by others, not merely subjective feelings of restlessness or being slowed down)

   (6) fatigue or loss of energy nearly every day

   (7) feelings of worthlessness or excessive or inappropriate guilt (which may be delusional) nearly every day (not merely self-reproach or guilt about being sick)

   (8) diminished ability to think or concentrate, or indecisiveness, nearly every day (either by subjective account or as observed by others)

   (9) recurrent thoughts of death (not just fear of dying), recurrent suicidal ideation without a specific plan, or a suicide attempt or a specific plan for committing suicide

B. The symptoms do not meet criteria for a mixed episode.

C. The symptoms cause clinically significant distress or impairment in social, occupational, or other important areas of functioning.

D. The symptoms are not due to the direct physiological effects of a substance (e.g., a drug of abuse, a medication) or a general medical condition (e.g., hypothyroidism).

E. The symptoms are not better accounted for by bereavement, i.e., after the loss of a loved one, the symptoms persist for longer than 2 months or are characterized by marked functional impairment, morbid preoccupation with worthlessness, suicidal ideation, psychotic symptoms, or psychomotor retardation.

---

episode has developed. These distinctions can be difficult to make in clinical practice. For example, mild residual symptoms of an initial episode or persistent psychosocial dysfunction may be overlooked or may be attributed to character pathology after improvement of the more dramatic manifestations of an episode, leading to the mistaken conclusion that a return of more severe symptoms represents a new episode rather than an exacerbation of the original episode.

Unipolar and Bipolar Mood Disorders

One of the most important distinctions between mood disorders is the distinction between unipolar and bipolar categories (Leonhard 1987a, 1987b). Unipolar mood disorders are characterized by depressive symptoms in the absence of a history of pathologically elevated mood. In bipolar mood disorders, depression alternates or is mixed with mania or hypomania. Patients who have only had recur-

TABLE 6–3.   DSM-IV-TR diagnostic criteria for melancholic features specifier

Specify if:

With Melancholic Features (can be applied to the current or most recent major depressive episode in major depressive disorder and to a major depressive episode in bipolar I or bipolar II disorder only if it is the most recent type of mood episode)

A. Either of the following, occurring during the most severe period of the current episode:
  (1) loss of pleasure in all, or almost all, activities
  (2) lack of reactivity to usually pleasurable stimuli (does not feel much better, even temporarily, when something good happens)
B. Three (or more) of the following:
  (1) distinct quality of depressed mood (i.e., the depressed mood is experienced as distinctly different from the kind of feeling experienced after the death of a loved one)
  (2) depression regularly worse in the morning
  (3) early morning awakening (at least 2 hours before usual time of awakening)
  (4) marked psychomotor retardation or agitation
  (5) significant anorexia or weight loss
  (6) excessive or inappropriate guilt

TABLE 6–4.   DSM-IV-TR diagnostic criteria for atypical features specifier

Specify if:

With Atypical Features (can be applied when these features predominate during the most recent 2 weeks of a current major depressive episode in major depressive disorder or in bipolar I or bipolar II disorder when a current major depressive episode is the most recent type of mood episode, or when these features predominate during the most recent 2 years of dysthymic disorder; if the major depressive episode is not current, it applies if the feature predominates during any 2-week period)

A. Mood reactivity (i.e., mood brightens in response to actual or potential positive events)
B. Two (or more) of the following features:
  (1) significant weight gain or increase in appetite
  (2) hypersomnia
  (3) leaden paralysis (i.e., heavy, leaden feelings in arms or legs)
  (4) long-standing pattern of interpersonal rejection sensitivity (not limited to episodes of mood disturbance) that results in significant social or occupational impairment
C. Criteria are not met for with melancholic features or with catatonic features during the same episode.

rent mania ("unipolar mania") are given the diagnosis of bipolar mood disorder on the assumption that they will eventually develop an episode of depression. DSM-IV-TR criteria for a manic episode are summarized in Table 6–5. Hypomania, a milder form of pathologically elevated mood that can be present for a shorter period before it is diagnosed, is described in Table 6–6. Although most people think of *elation* as a defining characteristic of mania and hypomania, many patients experience only irritability, anxiety, or a dysphoric sense of increased energy, as if they were "crawling out of their skins." This kind of presentation may occur most frequently in women and younger patients with bipolar disorder and in antidepressant-induced hypomania. In DSM-IV-TR, it is noted that mania is a state of increased goal-directed behavior that is pleasurable and has obvious potential for

TABLE 6–5. DSM-IV-TR diagnostic criteria for manic episode

A. A distinct period of abnormally and persistently elevated, expansive, or irritable mood, lasting at least 1 week (or any duration if hospitalization is necessary).

B. During the period of mood disturbance, three (or more) of the following symptoms have persisted (four if the mood is only irritable) and have been present to a significant degree:
  (1) inflated self-esteem or grandiosity
  (2) decreased need for sleep (e.g., feels rested after only 3 hours of sleep)
  (3) more talkative than usual or pressure to keep talking
  (4) flight of ideas or subjective experience that thoughts are racing
  (5) distractibility (i.e., attention too easily drawn to unimportant or irrelevant external stimuli)
  (6) increase in goal-directed activity (either socially, at work or school, or sexually) or psychomotor agitation
  (7) excessive involvement in pleasurable activities that have a high potential for painful consequences (e.g., engaging in unrestrained buying sprees, sexual indiscretions, or foolish business investments)

C. The symptoms do not meet criteria for a mixed episode.

D. The mood disturbance is sufficiently severe to cause marked impairment in occupational functioning or in usual social activities or relationships with others, or to necessitate hospitalization to prevent harm to self or others, or there are psychotic features.

E. The symptoms are not due to the direct physiological effects of a substance (e.g., a drug of abuse, a medication, or other treatment) or a general medical condition (e.g., hyperthyroidism).
  Note: Manic-like episodes that are clearly caused by somatic antidepressant treatment (e.g., medication, electroconvulsive therapy, light therapy) should not count toward a diagnosis of bipolar I disorder.

harm; however, behavior in mania is often excessive, disorganized, and dysphoric but not clearly harmful or dangerous (American Psychiatric Association 2000). The physical hyperactivity of chronic hypomania may be characterized primarily by random increases in activity that shifts its focus from moment to moment, and some patients experience more mental than physical overstimulation.

Most authorities agree that the bipolar–unipolar distinction is dichotomous: a patient either is or is not manic. In addition, the course of bipolar disorders differs from that of unipolar disorders (Dubovsky et al. 1989, 1991a; Faedda et al. 1995; Leibenluft et al. 1995; Weissman et al. 1996; Winokur 1995); some of the differences are summarized in Table 6–7. On closer scrutiny, these distinctions may not be as obvious as they might seem at first. For example, unipolar depression can be psychotic with severe depressive symptoms, and unipolar depressive episodes may be highly recurrent without ever being associated with mania. Lithium can increase the effectiveness of antidepressants in unipolar depression, and electroconvulsive therapy (ECT) is effective in treating both mania and depression. Patients with unipolar depression may have symptoms generally associated with bipolar disorder such as agitation, racing thoughts, and overspending. Unipolar and bipolar disorders can aggregate in the same families, and some studies suggest that there are no significant differences between unipolar and bipolar disorder with regard to familial rates of bipolar illness (E.S. Gershon et al. 1982; Weissman et al. 1984; Winokur 1995). Unipolar and bipolar disorders may not be totally distinct because they coaggregate in families.

Given that mania and depression are opposites of each other, one would think that only one of the two disorders could

TABLE 6–6.   DSM-IV-TR diagnostic criteria for hypomanic episode

A. A distinct period of persistently elevated, expansive, or irritable mood, lasting throughout at least 4 days, that is clearly different from the usual nondepressed mood.
B. During the period of mood disturbance, three (or more) of the following symptoms have persisted (four if the mood is only irritable) and have been present to a significant degree:
  (1) inflated self-esteem or grandiosity
  (2) decreased need for sleep (e.g., feels rested after only 3 hours of sleep)
  (3) more talkative than usual or pressure to keep talking
  (4) flight of ideas or subjective experience that thoughts are racing
  (5) distractibility (i.e., attention too easily drawn to unimportant or irrelevant external stimuli)
  (6) increase in goal-directed activity (either socially, at work or school, or sexually) or psychomotor agitation
  (7) excessive involvement in pleasurable activities that have a high potential for painful consequences (e.g., the person engages in unrestrained buying sprees, sexual indiscretions, or foolish business investments)
C. The episode is associated with an unequivocal change in functioning that is uncharacteristic of the person when not symptomatic.
D. The disturbance in mood and the change in functioning are observable by others.
E. The episode is not severe enough to cause marked impairment in social or occupational functioning, or to necessitate hospitalization, and there are no psychotic features.
F. The symptoms are not due to the direct physiological effects of a substance (e.g., a drug of abuse, a medication, or other treatment) or a general medical condition (e.g., hyperthyroidism).
  Note: Hypomanic-like episodes that are clearly caused by somatic antidepressant treatment (e.g., medication, electroconvulsive therapy, light therapy) should not count toward a diagnosis of bipolar II disorder.

TABLE 6–7.   Differences between unipolar and bipolar depression

Unipolar	Bipolar
Later onset	Earlier onset
Fewer episodes	More episodes
More gradual onset	Acute onset
Female > male	Female = male
More psychomotor agitation	More psychomotor retardation and lethargy
Typical symptoms	Atypical symptoms
Insomnia	Hypersomnia
Lower risk of suicide	Greater risk of suicide
Less frequently accompanied by psychotic symptoms in younger patients	Greater likelihood of psychotic symptoms in younger patients
Antidepressants more effective	Antidepressants less effective
Lithium less effective	Lithium more effective
Family history of depression	Family history of mania and depression
Normal $[Ca^{2+}]_i$	Increased $[Ca^{2+}]_i$

Note. $[Ca^{2+}]_i$ = free intracellular concentration of calcium ions.

be present at a time. However, between 30% and 50% of manic episodes are accompanied by depressive symptoms (Bowden et al. 1995; McElroy et al. 1992). According to DSM-IV-TR, a mixed episode (dysphoric mania) should be diagnosed if the full criteria (with the exception of duration) are met for both mania and major depression. However, many more patients with one pole of the disorder have some symptoms of the other, as exemplified by exhibitionistic depression with outbursts of rage and a decreased need for sleep or by hypomania with suicide attempts and fatigue (McElroy et al. 1992). Dysphoric mania is more common in females and is associated with a greater risk of suicide and a poorer response to lithium (McElroy et al. 1992). There also may be an association between mixed states and very rapid mood swings (ultradian cycling).

Specific Mood Disorders

The identification of an episode of mania and/or depression is the first step in making a comprehensive diagnosis. The next steps are to decide which modifiers in addition to melancholia and atypical features apply to the episode and then to consider specific subtypes of mood disorders. Some of these subtypes meet criteria for DSM-IV-TR mood disorders with or without symptomatic or course specifiers, and some are commonly recognized syndromes that may not meet formal diagnostic criteria but are nonetheless clinically important.

Major Depressive Disorder

MDD is characterized by one or more major depressive episodes in the absence of mania or hypomania. Depressive syndromes caused by medical illnesses (mood disorder due to a general medical condition) and by medications or psychoactive substances (substance-induced mood disorder) are not considered to be primary mood disorders and do not qualify for a diagnosis of MDD. In DSM-IV-TR, several course specifiers can be applied to the current or most recent depressive episode.

Although MDD can consist of a single episode, recurrence is the rule rather than the exception. After a single major depressive episode, the risk of a second episode is about 50%; after a third episode, the risk of a fourth is about 90% (Thase 1990). Each new episode tends to occur sooner and to begin more abruptly, and new episodes often include the same symptoms that previous episodes included, along with new and more severe symptoms.

DSM-IV-TR specifiers are used to indicate whether a major depressive episode has remitted fully (i.e., no symptoms have been present for at least 2 months), partially (i.e., not enough ongoing depressive symptoms to qualify for a diagnosis of a major depressive episode or no symptoms for less than 2 months), or not at all (i.e., a chronic major depressive episode). Longitudinal course specifiers for MDD indicate whether recurrent major depressive episodes remit completely or partially in between episodes and whether major depressive episodes are superimposed on dysthymia. If one counts only the defining symptoms listed in Table 6–2, these kinds of distinctions may seem relatively uncomplicated. However, recall of depressive symptoms may be greater when a patient feels more depressed than when depression is less severe (i.e., recall is state dependent). Because the severity of depression tends to fluctuate in all but the most profoundly depressed patients, a history obtained when a patient feels worse may suggest a more chronic illness than may a history obtained when the same patient feels better.

TABLE 6–8. DSM-IV-TR diagnostic criteria for dysthymic disorder

A. Depressed mood for most of the day, for more days than not, as indicated either by subjective account or observation by others, for at least 2 years. **Note:** In children and adolescents, mood can be irritable and duration must be at least 1 year.
B. Presence, while depressed, of two (or more) of the following:
   (1) poor appetite or overeating
   (2) insomnia or hypersomnia
   (3) low energy or fatigue
   (4) low self-esteem
   (5) poor concentration or difficulty making decisions
   (6) feelings of hopelessness
C. During the 2-year period (1 year for children or adolescents) of the disturbance, the person has never been without the symptoms in Criteria A and B for more than 2 months at a time.
D. No major depressive episode has been present during the first 2 years of the disturbance (1 year for children and adolescents); i.e., the disturbance is not better accounted for by chronic major depressive disorder, or major depressive disorder, in partial remission.
   Note: There may have been a previous major depressive episode provided there was a full remission (no significant signs or symptoms for 2 months) before development of the dysthymic disorder. In addition, after the initial 2 years (1 year in children or adolescents) of dysthymic disorder, there may be superimposed episodes of major depressive disorder, in which case both diagnoses may be given when the criteria are met for a major depressive episode.
E. There has never been a manic episode, a mixed episode, or a hypomanic episode, and criteria have never been met for cyclothymic disorder.
F. The disturbance does not occur exclusively during the course of a chronic psychotic disorder, such as schizophrenia or delusional disorder.
G. The symptoms are not due to the direct physiological effects of a substance (e.g., a drug of abuse, a medication) or a general medical condition (e.g., hypothyroidism).
H. The symptoms cause clinically significant distress or impairment in social, occupational, or other important areas of functioning.
Specify if:
   Early Onset: if onset is before age 21 years
   Late Onset: if onset is age 21 years or older
Specify (for most recent 2 years of dysthymic disorder):
   With Atypical Features

Dysthymic Disorder

Dysthymic disorder (*dysthymia* means "ill-tempered") was introduced in DSM-III to indicate a nonepisodic chronic depression that was thought to be less severe than major depression. The cardinal feature of dysthymic disorder is a chronically depressed mood that is present most of the day, for more days than not, for at least 2 years.

In an attempt to distinguish between chronic MDD and dysthymic disorder, DSM-IV-TR (Table 6–8) stipulates that chronic depressive symptoms lasting less than 2 years after a major depressive episode and otherwise meeting criteria for dysthymic disorder be diagnosed as major depressive episode, in partial remission; if a full remission from a major depressive episode lasts at least 6 months and is then followed by dysthymia, a diagnosis of dysthymic disorder is justified.

What is the real difference between MDD and dysthymic disorder? Dysthymia begins insidiously and to be diagnosed must be present for at least 2 years, during which time criteria for a major depressive episode must not be met. However, retrospective accounts of the onset of a mood disorder years in the past are likely to be colored by patients' moods at the time of recall, making anything but prospective evaluation of patients who are at risk for depression unreliable in distinguishing between dysthymic disorder and chronic MDD. Another defining difference is that more depressive symptoms are required to diagnose MDD than dysthymic disorder (American Psychiatric Association 1994a). However, as Table 6–9 shows, if a dysthymic patient reports only two more symptoms, the diagnosis is changed to MDD (Kocsis and Frances 1987). This commonly occurs because most patients who meet criteria for dysthymic disorder exceed the minimum number of symptoms required for the diagnosis, regardless of the diagnostic method used (e.g., DSM-III, DSM-III-R, DSM-IV, DSM-IV alternative criteria). Indeed, 80% of patients with dysthymia also have a lifetime diagnosis of major depression, and most patients with dysthymic disorder seek treatment for superimposed major depression. If a patient with depression meeting criteria for MDD has barely the requisite number of symptoms, do the inevitable fluctuations in symptoms signify that a different disorder has developed? Does the advent of one particular additional symptom in a dysthymic patient have more significance than another for a new diagnosis of MDD? Is there any difference between severe dysthymia and mild major depression?

Dysthymic disorder produces as much impairment as MDD in work, leisure activities, relationships, general health, and ability to perform social roles (Frances 1993). Even minor depression (a Research Diagnostic Criteria [RDC] condition in which the number of depressive symp-

TABLE 6–9. Dysthymic disorder versus major depressive disorder

Dysthymic disorder	Major depressive disorder
2 years' duration	2 weeks' duration
Depressed mood plus two additional symptoms	Depressed mood plus four additional symptoms
More cognitive symptoms	More vegetative symptoms
Mild onset may be followed after 2 years by major depression	Onset may begin with more severe symptoms

toms is insufficient to meet criteria for dysthymic disorder or MDD) is associated with almost as much impairment as are dysthymic disorder and MDD (Broadhead et al. 1990). Comorbidity with other Axis I disorders and with personality disorders is about equally frequent in the two conditions. Despite dysthymic disorder's being defined as a less severe condition, the prognosis of dysthymic disorder is not substantially different from that of MDD (Wells et al. 1992). Both disorders respond to the same antidepressant and psychotherapeutic regimens (Frances 1993; Kocsis et al. 1989; J. Scott 1992).

Double Depression

Although it is not a separate DSM-IV-TR diagnosis, double depression, or dysthymic disorder with a superimposed major depressive episode, has been extensively discussed in the literature, and clinicians use the term frequently. The major depressive episode must appear 2 years or more (1 year in children and adolescents) after the onset of dysthymia for double depression to be diagnosed. Double depression is far from uncommon in dysthymic patients. Between 68% and 90% of dysthymic patients experience at least one major depressive episode (Thase 1992), and 25%–50% of patients with MDD have coexisting dysthymic disorder (Hirschfeld 1994; Levitt et al. 1991). It has been estimated that 22%–66% of all patients with unipolar depression have experienced a combination of dysthymia and major depression (Hirschfeld 1994). A 9-year prospective study found dysthymic disorder with superimposed MDD or recurrent brief depression in 3% of the general population (Hirschfeld 1994).

Compared with major depressive episodes alternating with euthymia (episodic MDD), MDD superimposed on dysthymia has an earlier onset of major depression (Levitt et al. 1991), more severe depressive symptoms (Belsher and Costello 1988; Wells et al. 1992), more psychosocial impairment (Belsher and Costello 1988), a greater risk of suicide, more treatment resistance (Barrett 1984), and more comorbidity (Klein et al. 1988), especially with avoidant and dependent personality disorders (Sanderson et al. 1992). The major depressive episode in double depression is less likely to remit (I.W. Miller et al. 1986; Wells et al. 1992) than that in episodic MDD (i.e., recurrent major depression not superimposed on dysthymia) and is more likely to recur (Levitt et al. 1991). In one report (Belsher and Costello 1988), the relapse rate of major depression after 8 weeks of recovery was 30% for double depression and 4% for episodic MDD. In this study, major depression recurred in 50% of the patients with double depression and 35% of the patients with episodic MDD after 1 year and in 65% and 37%, respectively, after 2 years. The risk of a bipolar outcome also appears greater in double depression: 29% of the patients with double depression in the National Institute of Mental Health Collaborative Study of the Psychobiology of Depression (NIMH-CS) developed hypomania, compared with 9% of the patients with episodic MDD.

Subsyndromal Depression

Subsyndromal disorders are conditions that partially meet diagnostic criteria for a particular disorder. Akiskal (1991, 1994) divided syndromes marked by depressive traits into *subaffective dysthymia*, in which depressive personality traits are caused by chronic subclinical depression, and *character spectrum disorder*, which he considered to be a type of personality disorder in which depressed mood is just one feature of a chronically unhappy and unfulfilled orientation of the personality. As a result of deliberations by the DSM-IV Personality Disorders Work Group, a version of character spectrum disorder is included in the Appendix to DSM-IV as *depressive personality disorder*. The DSM-IV field trials suggested that this condition "requiring further research" (Table 6–10) was associated with a passive, unassertive style, in the absence of current diagnosable dysthymia, in almost 50% of cases. Patients thought to have depressive personality disorder were noted to have a tendency to develop dysthymic disorder or MDD after the diagnosis of depressive personality disorder was made, which suggests that the apparent personality disorder might be an early-onset traitlike variant of other depressive disorders. This hypothesis is supported by the existence of a familial association between depressive personality disorder and other depressive disorders (American Psychiatric Association 1994a) and by earlier onset and more depressive episodes in patients with MDD and a premorbid depressive personality than in patients with major depression but without this premorbid temperament.

From a clinical standpoint, defining a personality disorder that overlaps with but is distinct from primary mood disorders has the theoretical benefit of identifying a group of patients who would be expected to have a poor response to typi-

TABLE 6–10. DSM-IV-TR research criteria for depressive personality disorder

A. A pervasive pattern of depressive cognitions and behaviors beginning by early adulthood and present in a variety of contexts, as indicated by five (or more) of the following:
 (1) usual mood is dominated by dejection, gloominess, cheerlessness, joylessness, unhappiness
 (2) self-concept centers around beliefs of inadequacy, worthlessness, and low self-esteem
 (3) is critical, blaming, and derogatory toward self
 (4) is brooding and given to worry
 (5) is negativistic, critical, and judgmental toward others
 (6) is pessimistic
 (7) is prone to feeling guilty or remorseful
B. Does not occur exclusively during major depressive episodes and is not better accounted for by dysthymic disorder.

cal treatments for depression and a better response to specialized psychotherapeutic approaches. However, the overlap between abnormal mood and stable personality traits is often so extensive that the two can be indistinguishable. Obviously, many people with diagnoses of MDD and dysthymia meet DSM-IV-TR symptomatic criteria for depressive personality disorder. In one study, 41% of the patients with a major depressive episode were found to meet all criteria for depressive personality disorder, including persistence of symptoms when the full mood disorder was not obviously present.

Psychotic Depression

The term *psychotic depression* (or *delusional depression*) refers to a major depressive episode accompanied by psychotic features (i.e., delusions and/or hallucinations). Most studies continue to report that 16%–54% of depressed pa-

tients have psychotic symptoms. Delusions occur without hallucinations in one-half to two-thirds of the adults with psychotic depression, whereas hallucinations are unaccompanied by delusions in 3%–25% of patients. Half of all psychotically depressed patients experience more than one kind of delusion. Hallucinations occur more frequently than delusions in younger depressed patients and in patients with bipolar psychotic depression (Chambers et al. 1982; Goodwin and Jamison 1991).

The classification of psychotic symptoms as mood congruent (i.e., consistent with a depressed or an elated mood) or mood incongruent is complex. Prominent mood-incongruent psychotic symptoms in depressed patients such as delusions of control, along with poor adolescent adjustment, may be associated with a somewhat worse prognosis of psychotic depression (K.S. Kendler 1991; Tsuang and Coryell 1993). The RDC, which were used in many earlier studies of psychotic depression, specify a diagnosis of schizoaffective disorder for depressed patients who have concurrent mood-incongruent psychotic features. However, bipolar psychotic depression is frequently associated with mood-incongruent psychotic symptoms, some of which may be bizarre and may be easily mistaken for typical "schizophrenic" symptoms (Akiskal et al. 1983, 1985; McGlashan 1988); a formal thought disorder is present in at least 20% of psychotically depressed patients (Goodwin and Jamison 1991). Because bipolar illness is overrepresented in psychotic depression (Coryell 1996; Weissman et al. 1988a), it may be bipolar illness rather than mood incongruence that contributes to a poorer treatment response in mood-incongruent psychotic depression. In recognition of the uncertain contribution of mood incongruence to the prognosis, DSM-IV-TR requires the existence of psychotic symptoms for 2 or more weeks in the absence of prominent mood symptoms for a diagnosis of schizoaffective disorder, a specifier that seems more consistently associated with a somewhat poorer prognosis of mixed affective and psychotic syndromes than the RDC (Coryell 1996).

Psychotic features tend to develop after several episodes of nonpsychotic depression. Once psychotic symptoms occur, they reappear with each subsequent episode, even if depression in later episodes is not as severe. With each recurrence, psychotic symptoms take the same form that they did in previous episodes (e.g., patients with hallucinations have them in the same modality and with the same content from episode to episode). Relatives of psychotically depressed patients have an increased risk for psychotic depression themselves; and when psychotic depression is present, the content of the psychosis tends to be similar to that of the proband. The families of psychotically depressed patients also have an elevated risk of schizophrenia.

Whereas treatment with both an antipsychotic drug and an antidepressant is usually necessary for a remission of psychotic depression, *antipsychotic* drugs may improve the *depression* and the *antidepressant* may improve *psychosis*. Furthermore, coaggregation of severe mood disorders and schizophrenia exists in families of patients with psychotic depression. These two observations suggest that psychotic depression is not a simple combination of psychosis and depression but rather a complex interaction between the capacity to become psychotic and the capacity to become severely depressed. Depression may have to reach a certain level of severity in order for psychosis to be expressed; but once psychosis develops, a unique disorder has evolved. Some features in addition to the unique treatment response that distinguish psychotic from

nonpsychotic depression include a greater rate of recurrence; a higher suicide risk; more nonsuppression on the dexamethasone suppression test (DST), with higher postdexamethasone cortisol levels; more prominent sleep abnormalities; a level of neuropsychological impairment similar to schizophrenia, and higher ventricular-to-brain ratios (Albus et al. 1996; Coryell 1996). The extent to which the symptoms, course, and treatment response of psychotic depression are a function of psychosis itself or the overrepresentation of bipolar disorder in psychotically depressed patients (Weissman et al. 1988a) has not been studied.

Recurrent Brief Depression

Both RDC and DSM-IV-TR criteria require 2 weeks of continuous symptoms for a diagnosis of a major depressive episode to be made. Researcher Jules Angst and colleagues (1990) described a depressive disorder called *recurrent brief depression*, in which depressive episodes meet DSM-IV-TR symptomatic but not duration criteria for major depression. Depressive episodes in recurrent brief depression have the same number and severity of symptoms as DSM-IV-TR major depressive episodes but last 1 day to 1 week. Depressive episodes must recur at least once per month over at least 12 months (not in association with the menstrual cycle) for recurrent brief depression to be diagnosed (Angst and Hochstrasser 1994). Although each acute depressive episode is short-lived, recurrent brief depression carries a high risk of suicide (Lepine et al. 1995), perhaps because of the inevitable return of depression and the repeated drastic contrast between the depressed and well states.

The appendix to DSM-IV listed recurrent brief depressive disorder defined by Angst's criteria as a condition requiring further study because it was thought that not enough data had accumulated to warrant its inclusion as an established diagnosis (American Psychiatric Association 1994a). In the DSM-IV mood disorders field trial, 1.5% of 524 subjects had a lifetime history of recurrent brief depression, and the 1-year prevalence of recurrent brief depressive disorder was 7% (American Psychiatric Association 1994a). Recurrent brief depression has been found to have rates of comorbidity with panic disorder, generalized anxiety disorder, and substance use disorders that are similar to comorbidity rates with MDD (Lepine et al. 1995). Recurrent brief depression also has been found often to have a seasonal pattern, with more recurrences in the winter (American Psychiatric Association 1994a).

Bipolar Subtypes

Bipolar disorder is a mood disorder that is accompanied by episodes of mania and/or hypomania (DSM-IV-TR criteria for manic, hypomanic, and mixed episodes are summarized in Tables 6–5 and 6–6). DSM-IV-TR includes two primary subtypes of bipolar disorder. Bipolar I disorder is characterized by manic episodes that occur with or without episodes of hypomania. In bipolar II disorder, one or more hypomanic episodes occur, but the patient never experiences mania; also, the hypomanic episodes may be milder than the depressive episodes (Akiskal 1995). Evidence that bipolar II disorder is distinct from bipolar I disorder comes from several sources (Bowden 1993; Bowden et al. 1995; Leibenluft 1996; Solomon et al. 1995). Patients with bipolar II disorder never become manic, despite experiencing multiple hypomanic episodes. In addition, the bipolar II diagnosis seems to "breed true" in that patients with this diagnosis have close relatives with hypomania but not mania, whereas patients with bipolar I disorder have some relatives who

have had mania and some who have had only hypomania.

Although bipolar III disorder is not a DSM-IV-TR diagnosis, the term has been used to describe patients with a history of depression who have at least one blood relative with a history of mania, on the grounds that such patients may have a bipolar diathesis that has not yet been expressed. In some circles, *bipolar III* refers to patients with antidepressant-induced mania, and *bipolar IV* is used to describe depressed patients with a family history of mania. In DSM-IV-TR, mania or hypomania that appears in response to treatment with an antidepressant is not counted toward a diagnosis of a bipolar mood disorder, but many clinicians consider antidepressant-induced mania to be an indication of the capacity to develop mania or hypomania spontaneously and therefore a sign of a type of bipolar mood disorder (this seems most likely to be true of children and adolescents [Strober and Carlson 1982]).

Brief hypomania. Angst (1995) defined a subtype of hypomania called *brief hypomania*. Although brief hypomania consists of the same symptoms as hypomania, the duration of symptoms is 1–3 days rather than the 4 days or more required by DSM-IV-TR for a diagnosis of hypomania. Angst found that despite the short duration of any episode, brief hypomania has a very high rate of recurrence and produces marked impairment. The prevalence of brief hypomania was 2.28% among patients with bipolar mood disorders in one study (Angst 1995), but further data are needed before diagnostic precision can be achieved for brief manic or hypomanic symptoms.

Bipolar depression. Depression in patients with bipolar mood disorders may alternate or be mixed with mania. Classical bipolar depression is characterized by "atypical" symptoms such as hypersomnia, anergia, carbohydrate craving, and psychomotor slowing (Goodwin and Jamison 1991). However, in contrast to atypical unipolar depression, mood in bipolar depression that is not mixed with hypomania usually is not reactive (Mitchell et al. 2001). Especially in younger patients, bipolar depression is more frequently associated with psychotic symptoms (Mitchell et al. 2001).

Cyclothymic Disorder

Cyclothymic disorder (cyclothymia) was originally classified as a personality disorder with mood swings that were not clearly manic or depressed. Although most investigators now consider cyclothymic disorder to be a mood disorder, it is still called *cyclothymic personality* in the RDC. As Table 6–11 indicates, DSM-IV-TR cyclothymia can be diagnosed in patients with recurrent hypomanic and depressive symptoms that may not permit a diagnosis of major depression or hypomania. In the RDC, cyclothymia is characterized by recurrent depressed mood lasting several days, alternating with elevated mood with at least two hypomanic symptoms. In both diagnostic schemes, the patient rarely experiences a normal mood.

Patients with cyclothymia typically experience mood states that alternate between depression, irritability, cheerfulness, and relative normality that last days, weeks, or months (Jamison 1993). Many complain of unpredictable changes in energy, vague physical symptoms, and a seasonal pattern of mood swings (e.g., depression in the winter). In some studies, 44% of the cyclothymic patients developed hypomania while taking antidepressants, and about one-third developed full-blown hypomanic, manic, or depressive episodes during drug-free follow-up. In addition, at least one-third of the time the onset of clear bipolar I or bipolar II mood disorder is preceded by cyclothymia, which usually begins in adolescence or early adulthood.

TABLE 6–11.   DSM-IV-TR diagnostic criteria for cyclothymic disorder

A. For at least 2 years, the presence of numerous periods with hypomanic symptoms and numerous periods with depressive symptoms that do not meet criteria for a major depressive episode.   **Note:** In children and adolescents, the duration must be at least 1 year.

B. During the above 2-year period (1 year in children and adolescents), the person has not been without the symptoms in Criterion A for more than 2 months at a time.

C. No major depressive episode, manic episode, or mixed episode has been present during the first 2 years of the disturbance.
    Note: After the initial 2 years (1 year in children and adolescents) of cyclothymic disorder, there may be superimposed manic or mixed episodes (in which case both bipolar I disorder and cyclothymic disorder may be diagnosed) or major depressive episodes (in which case both bipolar II disorder and cyclothymic disorder may be diagnosed).

D. The symptoms in Criterion A are not better accounted for by schizoaffective disorder and are not superimposed on schizophrenia, schizophreniform disorder, delusional disorder, or psychotic disorder not otherwise specified.

E. The symptoms are not due to the direct physiological effects of a substance (e.g., a drug of abuse, a medication) or a general medical condition (e.g., hyperthyroidism).

F. The symptoms cause clinically significant distress or impairment in social, occupational, or other important areas of functioning.

Rapid Cycling

In DSM-IV-TR, *rapid cycling* is a specifier that refers to a bipolar I or bipolar II mood disorder in which four or more episodes of depression and/or mania or hypomania occur per year, with either 2 weeks of normal mood between episodes or a shift directly from one pole to the other (e.g., from mania to depression) with no intervening period of normal mood (American Psychiatric Association 2000). Rapid-cycling bipolar disorder is probably not a separate illness but a phase in the evolution of bipolar disorder that may last years but may not be permanent (Tomitaka and Sakamoto 1994). Rapid cycling may have a lower response to lithium (Kilzieh and Akiskal 2000; Roy-Byrne et al. 1984). Rapid cycling is more common in women and in patients with bipolar II disorder (Leibenluft 1996; Lish et al. 1993) and is more likely to occur after an episode of mania or hypomania than after depression (Altschuler et al. 1995). Additional risk factors for the development of rapid cycling include hypothyroidism, right cerebral hemisphere disease, mental retardation, and use of alcohol and stimulants (Ananth et al. 1993; Leibenluft 1996; Sachs 1996). As many as 60%–90% of patients with rapid cycling have been found to have hypothyroidism, which often is too mild to produce medical morbidity even though it can contribute to mood instability (Bauer et al. 1990). Lithium itself may cause rapid cycling by inducing hypothyroidism (Terao 1993).

A causal role of antidepressants in mania and rapid cycling has been widely debated. A review of records of 535 patients admitted to a general psychiatric inpatient service found that 8.1% required hospitalization because of psychosis or mania that occurred within 16 weeks of starting an antidepressant and remitted rapidly with antidepressant withdrawal (Preda et al. 2001). Antidepressants may contribute to rapid cycling by inducing mania or by speeding up the inherent cyclicity of bipolar mood disorders (Altschuler et al. 1995; Goodwin et al. 1982; Kilzieh and Akiskal 2000; Post 1994; Sachs 1996; Wehr 1993). Although most patients with rapid-cycling bipolar disorder are taking antidepressants, it is difficult to prove that antidepressants are the cause of rapid cycling (Altschuler et al. 1995). Alternative explanations would be that antidepressants are administered more frequently to patients with rapid-cycling and other forms of deteriorating bipolar disorder because depression is prominent or because nothing else is helping or that rapid cycling would have developed with or without an antidepressant. The only way to prove a causal relation would be to follow prospectively matched patients with bipolar mood disorder who were randomly assigned to take antidepressants or placebos, an experiment that is too difficult technically and ethically to be performed. If assessment of the association between starting antidepressants and developing rapid cycling is retrospective, the results are subject to being skewed by state-dependent recall and difficulty remembering the exact onset of complex mood swings. Even in a prospective study, it is difficult to be certain whether rapid cycling that develops after prolonged treatment with an antidepressant was caused by the medication or simply reflected the natural history of the condition.

These issues were addressed to some extent by Altschuler et al. (1995), who defined antidepressant-induced mania and rapid cycling as a change in order of episodes or a first episode of severe mania or cycling appearing within 8 weeks of starting antidepressants. In a literature review, Altschuler et al. (1995) identified 158 patients with bipolar depression in 15 placebo-controlled antidepressant trials in patients with mostly unipolar depression. Within this subgroup, 35% had likely antidepressant-induced mania by the stringent criteria used, the risk being more than 2.5 times as great (72% vs. 28%) for patients who were not also taking lithium. Among the limitations of the literature review were the relatively small number of patients with bipolar mood disorders in each study reviewed, the lack of reliable data from trials of other antidepressants, and the lack of inclusion of hypomania as an antidepressant-induced event. In addition, patients in these studies were not identified as having bipolar mood disorders in the first place and might have had a different response to antidepressants than patients with more obvious bipolar disorder.

Altschuler and her colleagues (1995) then used a life-chart method to characterize affective episodes carefully in 51 patients with lithium-refractory bipolar mood disorders, 55% of whom had rapid cycling. Although 82% of the sample developed mania while taking an antidepressant, the investigators concluded that only one-third met their criteria for definite antidepressant-induced mania. One reason for this low rate may have been that their patients had such a high rate of spontaneous affective episodes and so many had taken antidepressants at some point, that it was not possible to detect increases attributable to an antidepressant. The authors found that antidepressant-induced mania increased the risk of rapid cycling 4.6-fold; 50% of the increase was directly attributable to the use of antidepressants and 50% was assumed to reflect the natural history of bipolar disorder. On the basis of their study and literature review, the authors suggested that continuing antidepressants aggravated rapid cycling, but withdrawing the antidepressant did not necessarily stop cycling. Most omi-

nously, antimanic drugs did not predictably prevent or treat rapid cycling. In a review of patients with refractory bipolar disorder that used a similar methodology, mania was thought to be attributable to antidepressant therapy in 35% of the patients and to rapid cycling in 26% (Roy-Byrne et al. 1985).

These results must be considered conservative for several reasons. First, hypomania and more subtle forms of pathologically elevated mood were not considered. Second, only classically defined rapid cycling was considered; other forms of mood cycling (described in the next subsection) may be even more common. Because there is no reason to think that antidepressants must take 8 weeks or less to induce hypomania or mood swings, use of this arbitrary cutoff value may result in overlooking many patients for whom months or even years of antidepressant therapy may be necessary to destabilize mood but who would not develop rapid cycling without antidepressants.

Ultradian Cycling

In a malignant form of rapid cycling called *ultradian cycling* (or *ultrarapid cycling*) (Roy-Byrne et al. 1984), patients appear chronically depressed. On close inspection, however, they are found to experience multiple recurrences of dysphoric hypomania and depression over the course of hours to days. For example, a patient may wake up feeling emotionally paralyzed and unable to get out of bed. A few hours later, the patient feels so energized that it is impossible to sit still and to refrain from acting impulsively; shortly thereafter, the patient sinks abruptly into suicidal despair. The patient briefly feels relatively well but then flies into a rage when criticized and experiences command hallucinations. Racing thoughts keep the patient from falling asleep; however, once the patient does fall asleep,

sleep lasts 14 hours, and the patient is exhausted the next day. Rather than having nonspecific "mood swings," the patient is experiencing distinct but very brief recurrences of bipolar depression, dysphoric hypomania, a mixture of depressive and hypomanic symptoms, and a psychotic energized state, with fleeting euthymia between episodes or an abrupt switch from one pole to the other.

It is not clear whether ultradian cycling represents a deteriorated form of rapid cycling or a different condition. However, no evidence exists to indicate that ultradian cycling is a separate bipolar subtype (Kilzieh and Akiskal 2000). The research that has been performed with patients with ultradian cycling suggests that it is even more refractory to treatment than traditionally diagnosed rapid cycling. Ultradian cycling, like rapid cycling, may be preceded by one or more hypomanic episodes (Post 1990b, 1994). Experience does suggest that the depression of ultradian cycling is aggravated rather than ameliorated by antidepressants (Akiskal 1991; J. Scott 1988).

Mixed Bipolar States

Almost half of bipolar patients experience depressive and manic symptoms at the same time (M.P. Freeman and McElroy 1999). Manic symptoms in mixed states usually are dysphoric, with irritability, anxiety, or unpleasant activation rather than elation. Such states can be difficult to distinguish from ultradian cycling, in which moods change so rapidly that they seem to blend into each other, and mixed states and ultrarapid cycling often accompany each other. Both conditions probably represent deterioration of a more organized mood disorder associated at least in some cases with chronic use of antidepressants, and both have similar treatments.

Seasonal Affective Disorder

Many people living in climates in which there are marked seasonal differences in the length of the day experience seasonal changes in mood, sleep, and energy (Kasper et al. 1989). Also, seasonal variations occur in most mood disorders. For example, unipolar depression is more likely to recur in the spring, whereas bipolar depression is more likely to recur in the fall, and mania is more likely to recur during the summer (Barbini et al. 1995). Contrary to popular wisdom, the time of greatest risk of suicide is not during the Christmas holidays but during the months of May and June. The time of the seasonal peak in the incidence of suicide is independent of latitude, but the amplitude of the peak is greatest where the seasonal variation in light is the greatest. Hospital admissions for unipolar depression peak in the spring, whereas admissions for mania peak in the summer. The observations that seasonal variations in mood disorders in the Southern Hemisphere are the reverse of those in the Northern Hemisphere (e.g., more admissions for mania during the winter) and that the pattern of seasonal affective disorder (SAD) is the reverse in the Northern and Southern Hemispheres support the hypothesis that these changes are dependent on variations in available daylight.

SAD has been defined as a condition that meets criteria for an RDC major affective disorder in which major depression occurs during the fall or winter for at least 2 consecutive years, with remission in the spring or summer. In SAD, depressive episodes cannot be associated with seasonal stressors, and no other Axis I diagnoses can be present. DSM-IV-TR criteria (Table 6–12), which are derived from the criteria of Rosenthal and colleagues (Rosenthal and Blehar 1989), include additional provisos that hypomania as well as

TABLE 6–12.   DSM-IV-TR diagnostic criteria for seasonal pattern specifier

Specify if:

With Seasonal Pattern (can be applied to the pattern of major depressive episodes in bipolar I disorder, bipolar II disorder, or major depressive disorder, recurrent)

A. There has been a regular temporal relationship between the onset of major depressive episodes in bipolar I or bipolar II disorder or major depressive disorder, recurrent, and a particular time of the year (e.g., regular appearance of the major depressive episode in the fall or winter).
    Note: Do not include cases in which there is an obvious effect of seasonal-related psycho-social stressors (e.g., regularly being unemployed every winter).

B. Full remissions (or a change from depression to mania or hypomania) also occur at a characteristic time of the year (e.g., depression disappears in the spring).

C. In the last 2 years, two major depressive episodes have occurred that demonstrate the temporal seasonal relationships defined in Criteria A and B, and no nonseasonal major depressive episodes have occurred during that same period.

D. Seasonal major depressive episodes (as described above) substantially outnumber the nonseasonal major depressive episodes that may have occurred over the individual's lifetime.

remission of depression may occur during the summer and that seasonal depressive episodes should substantially outnumber nonseasonal episodes (American Psychiatric Association 2000). In DSM-IV-TR, a seasonal pattern is considered to be not a separate diagnosis but an additional specifier of MDD with recurrent depression, bipolar I disorder, or bipolar II disorder.

In some samples, most patients with SAD have summer hypomania and therefore meet criteria for a diagnosis of bipolar II disorder; in other samples, the incidence of hypomania is low. Some of the discrepancy may be a function of the frequency with which increased energy, decreased sleep, and related experiences during the summer are viewed as hypomania or simply relief of depression. More data are needed to determine how frequently SAD is bipolar and how frequently it is unipolar. There is greater agreement about the presence of atypical depressive symptoms in the winter depressions of SAD, features that occur more frequently in bipolar depression.

Secondary Mood Disorders

In some circles, the term *secondary mood disorder* is used to indicate a mood disor-der having another cause—for example, a medical illness or substance. To other experts, a secondary mood disorder is a mood disorder that occurs in the context of another disorder, such as schizophrenia or an anxiety disorder, with etiology not necessarily being implied (Knesper 1995). DSM-IV-TR implies causality of secondary mood disorders with the phrases *mood disorder due to a general medical disorder* (mood disorder caused by a medical or surgical illness; see Table 6–13) and *substance-induced mood disorder* (mood disorder caused by a medication or a psychoactive substance).

The different connotations of secondary mood disorder have been addressed in two ways in DSM-IV-TR. Although it is permissible to make a diagnosis of a mood disorder in a patient with another Axis I disorder such as schizophrenia, chronic affective symptoms that occur exclusively during the course of a psychotic disorder such as schizophrenia and do not meet criteria for an independent mood disorder are not given a separate diagnosis of a depressive disorder. The purpose of this approach is to avoid implying meaningless comorbidity. It is also important to distinguish between symptoms that are a com-

TABLE 6–13. Some medical conditions that can cause manic or depressive syndromes

Neurological disease	Parkinson's disease, Huntington's disease, traumatic brain injury, stroke, dementias, multiple sclerosis
Metabolic disease	Electrolyte disturbances, renal failure, vitamin deficiencies or excess, acute intermittent porphyria, Wilson's disease, environmental toxins, heavy metals
Gastrointestinal disease	Irritable bowel syndrome, chronic pancreatitis, Crohn's disease, cirrhosis, hepatic encephalopathy
Endocrine disorders	Hypo- and hyperthyroidism, Cushing's disease, Addison's disease, diabetes mellitus, parathyroid dysfunction
Cardiovascular disease	Myocardial infarction, angina, coronary artery bypass surgery, cardiomyopathies
Pulmonary disease	Chronic obstructive pulmonary disease, sleep apnea, reactive airway disease
Malignancies and hematological disease	Pancreatic carcinoma, brain tumors, paraneoplastic effects of lung cancers, anemias
Autoimmune disease	Systemic lupus erythematosus, fibromyalgia, rheumatoid arthritis

ponent of another disorder and mood disorders that are truly secondary to another condition, which have a poorer treatment response than primary mood disorders (Knesper 1995).

Mood Disorders in Children and Adolescents

It is now known that depression can be diagnosed in children as young as 3 years old. Consequently, DSM-III-R criteria for juvenile mood disorders were similar to the criteria for adult mood disorders, except that irritability could substitute for depressed mood, failure to maintain expected weight gain could substitute for weight loss, decreased school performance could substitute for decreased occupational function, and loss of interest in friends and play could substitute for loss of interest or pleasure. Symptom duration for a diagnosis of dysthymia in children and adolescents was established as 1 year as opposed to the required duration of 2 years in adults. These criteria have not been changed substantially in DSM-IV-TR.

Because of continued disagreement about the nature of juvenile mood disorders, estimates of prevalence and incidence vary. When the Schedule for Affective Disorders and Schizophrenia for School-Aged Children (K-SADS) was administered to 1,710 adolescents age 14–18 years, almost 30% had at least one current depressive symptom, the most common symptoms being depressed mood, disturbed sleep, problems thinking, and anhedonia (Roberts et al. 1995). However, only 2.6% of the sample met full criteria for a current diagnosis of a mood disorder. Other reports suggested that childhood mood disorders have more familial loading than adult mood disorders and that when children from depressed families become depressed, the depression occurs earlier than does depression in children of families that are not depressed (ages 12–13 years vs. 16–17 years) (Geller et al. 1996). These kinds of findings suggest that inherited factors may be more important in juvenile mood disorders. The cumulative prevalence of suicide attempts in adolescents is as high as 3%.

One area of ongoing investigation is the presentation of bipolar disorder in children and adolescents. Compared with adult bipolar disorder, juvenile bipolar

disorder is characterized by more irritability, dysphoria, psychosis, schizophreniform symptoms, hyperactivity, mixed mania, rapid cycling, chronicity, and familial
loading (Ballenger et al. 1982; Faedda et
al. 1995; Geller et al. 1995). An important question is whether a first episode of
major depression in a younger patient is
more likely than a first episode in an adult
to be the initial presentation of a bipolar
mood disorder. Features that juvenile major depressive episodes share with bipolar
disorder include an early age at onset,
equal numbers of males and females affected, mood lability, a high rate of recurrence, prominent irritability and explosive
anger suggestive of mixed bipolar episodes, and a relatively poor response to
antidepressant medications.

Features of major depressive episodes
in younger patients listed in Table 6–14
have been found to increase the likelihood of the eventual occurrence of mania (Akiskal 1995; Strober and Carlson
1982). Although no predictive studies exist regarding the prognostic validity of
these features, their regular occurrence in
younger patients with bipolar disorder is
reason for caution in treating juvenile
major depression. One of these factors in
particular warrants additional discussion.
As we noted earlier, hypomania that occurs only when antidepressants are being
taken is excluded in DSM-IV-TR as a diagnostic criterion for bipolar disorder in
adults because not all patients with this
experience will become manic spontaneously. However, several small studies of
depressed adolescents and children indicate a very high rate of spontaneous mania
or hypomania following antidepressant-
induced hypomania (Akiskal 1995).

A controversial area of diagnostic confusion concerns attention-deficit/hyper-
activity disorder (ADHD). Some reports
suggest a familial link between juvenile bipolar disorder and ADHD, and these con-

TABLE 6–14. Features associated with a
bipolar outcome in juvenile major
depression

Early onset
Acute onset
Psychotic symptoms, especially hallucinations
Significant psychomotor slowing
Family history of bipolar disorder
Any mood disorder in three consecutive
   generations
Antidepressant-induced hypomania

ditions are frequently diagnosed together
(Biederman 1995). For example, in a
study in which 28% of 270 psychiatric inpatients age 5–18 years who were given
the K-SADS met criteria for ADHD, 36%
of the patients with ADHD met criteria
for nonpsychotic depression, 8% met criteria for an affective psychosis, and 22%
met criteria for bipolar disorder (Butler et
al. 1995); there was no follow-up to determine how many of the depressed patients developed mania.

Clinical experience also suggests that
ADHD and bipolar disorder are often
diagnosed in the same patient, but it is
not clear whether this means that the two
disorders are frequently comorbid or that
the symptoms of the two disorders overlap, so that patients who meet criteria for
one condition will regularly also meet criteria for the other (Butler et al. 1995).
The latter point is illustrated in Table 6–
15 (American Psychiatric Association
1994a).

Most patients with bipolar disorder
meet virtually all criteria for ADHD, but
patients with ADHD do not meet most
criteria for bipolar disorder (Geller et al.
1998). For example, elation, depression,
decreased need for sleep, hypersomnia,
grandiosity, psychosis, and rapid, pressured speech are not characteristic of
ADHD (Biederman 1995) except as manifestations of stimulant toxicity. Racing

TABLE 6–15. Common features of juvenile bipolar disorder and attention-deficit/ hyperactivity disorder

Attention-deficit/hyperactivity disorder	Bipolar disorder[a]
Mood lability, temper outbursts	Mood lability, temper outbursts
Fails to give close attention to detail	(Racing thoughts, impulsivity)
Difficulty sustaining attention	Racing thoughts
Does not listen when spoken to directly	Self-involvement
Does not follow through	(Impulsivity, distractibility, tangential thinking, changeable direction of effort driven by mood swings)
Difficulty organizing tasks and activities	(Disorganization, changeable focus of attention, impulsivity)
Loses things necessary for tasks	(Distractibility, impulsivity)
Easily distracted	Distractibility
Forgetful in daily activities	(Fluctuating interest and motivation)
Fidgets or squirms	(Increased levels of activity)
Leaves seat when remaining seated is expected	Increased energy
Runs about or climbs excessively	Increased activity
Difficulty playing quietly	Increased energy and activity
Often on the go or as if driven by a motor	Increased energy and activity
Talks excessively	Pressure of speech
Blurts out answers before questions have been completed	Racing thoughts
Difficulty awaiting turn	(Impulsivity, increased energy)
Interrupts or intrudes on others	(Impulsivity, grandiose self-centeredness)

[a]DSM-IV-TR symptoms of bipolar disorder; features of bipolar disorder not formally listed as diagnostic criteria for bipolar disorder are noted in parentheses.

and tangential thinking may be difficult to differentiate from the kind of talkativeness that is encountered in patients with ADHD, but an increased content of thought, especially with multiple coexisting complex ideas and plans, is more suggestive of bipolar disorder than of ADHD. Irritability, fighting, and thrill seeking can be encountered in both disorders, but attacks of rage that provoke prolonged organized attacks on others in response to threats to self-esteem and attempts to control the patient are more common in bipolar disorder, as is the kind of grandiosity that leads to fighting multiple opponents, fearlessness in the face of overwhelming odds, and jumping from extreme heights with the belief that one cannot be hurt and a response of hilarity to being injured. Patients with ADHD may become hyperfocused on television or on video games, but bipolar patients are more likely to become intensely preoccupied with projects, books, ideas, or other people. Historical elements listed in Table 6–14 are more common in bipolar disorder, although, as we noted earlier, bipolar disorder and ADHD may aggregate in the same families. Finally, bipolar disorder may be more common in tertiary care centers, given that uncomplicated ADHD is usually treated successfully in the offices of pediatricians, family physicians, and psychiatrists who consult to schools.

A study of 140 boys age 6–17 years with diagnoses of ADHD attempted to address the question of symptomatic overlap by rediagnosing patients after specific symptoms of ADHD listed in Table 6–15 had been subtracted (Milberger et al. 1995). Seventy-nine percent of the patients still met criteria for MDD, 56% met criteria for bipolar disorder, and 75% met criteria for generalized anxiety disorder. One interpretation of these findings is that other disorders may have a sufficient number of characteristics similar to those of ADHD (and each other) to result in diagnostic confusion between these conditions. A positive response to stimulants is often interpreted as evidence in favor of a diagnosis of ADHD, but the effect of stimulants in enhancing attention is not specific to ADHD. In addition, depressed patients with slowed thinking may show improvement of attention with stimulants, and some manic patients have been noted to experience calming and behavioral slowing in response to stimulants (Max et al. 1995). Although no controlled studies have addressed this issue, adolescent and young adult patients are encountered in practice who were apparently treated successfully with stimulants or antidepressants for ADHD, only to develop dysphoric manic symptoms such as increasing irritability, anxiety, impulsivity, thrill seeking, grandiose defiance, mood swings, and psychosis with continued treatment. It is impossible to know whether long-term treatment with stimulants eventually destabilized mood in patients with bipolar disorders misdiagnosed as ADHD or whether the adverse outcome represented the natural progression of bipolar disorder.

Comorbidity

Mood disorders are frequently comorbid with other psychiatric and medical conditions (Weissman et al. 1996), especially anxiety, substance-related, eating, soma-toform, and personality disorders and chronic medical illnesses. In one study of this issue, 11,701 medically ill patients were compared with 9,039 psychiatric patients in the Department of Veterans Affairs database (Moos and Mertens 1996). As many as 60% of the patients with mood disorders treated in mental health settings had a comorbid psychiatric diagnosis, as did 30% of the mood disorder patients treated in medical settings. Eighty percent of the psychiatric patients had comorbid medical conditions.

Medical Illness

The prevalence of major depressive episodes in patients with malignancies has been reported to be around 50% in those with pancreatic cancer, 22%–40% in those with cancer of the oropharynx, 10%–32% in patients with breast cancer, 13%–25% in those with colon cancer, and 23%, 17%, and 11%, respectively, in patients with gynecological cancer, lymphoma, and gastric carcinoma (McDaniel et al. 1995). Depression was found in 16% of bone marrow transplantation patients (Fann and Tucker 1995). Major depression occurs at increased rates in patients with myocardial infarction, ventricular arrhythmias, and congestive heart failure (Franco-Bronson 1996). Major depression has been found to increase the risk of developing coronary heart disease and to increase mortality after myocardial infarction (Barefoot and Schroll 1996). Hypothyroidism is very common in patients with depression, especially among those with treatment-refractory mood disorders and rapid-cycling bipolar disorder (Franco-Bronson 1996). Much of the hypothyroidism that occurs in depressed patients is caused by thyroiditis, which suggests a link between susceptibility loci for major depression and thyroiditis. In a subgroup analysis of the Baltimore ECA study, the lifetime risk of self-reported migraine headaches was elevated 3.14 times in persons with current major depression (Swartz et al. 2000). Additional medical conditions frequently associated with depression include irritable bowel syndrome, fibromyalgia, chronic fatigue syndrome, acquired immunodeficiency syndrome, renal failure, and autoimmune disease (Franco-Bronson 1996; Gruber et al. 1996).

Several neurological illnesses are also associated with an increased risk of mood disorders (Fann and Tucker 1995). Between 8% and 75% of patients with cerebrovascular accidents develop major depression; in one study, depressed stroke patients had an eightfold risk of mortality compared with matched nondepressed stroke patients (P.L.P. Morris et al. 1993). Anatomic location of the stroke appears to have a marked effect on the prevalence of associated depression: left prefrontal and basal ganglia lesions more frequently result in depressive disorders than do right hemisphere lesions (P.L.P. Morris et al. 1993). Conversely, right hemisphere lesions are often associated with development of secondary mania (Berthier et al. 1996). Cerebrovascular and degenerative disease on the left side of the brain is a common cause of late-onset depression, and disease on the right side of the brain is often associated with late-onset mania (Shulman and Hermann 1999; Simpson et al. 1999). Depression is the most frequent psychiatric complication of Parkinson's disease, possibly because of the participation of the basal ganglia in mood regulation (Klassen et al. 1995).

About 50% of patients with Alzheimer's disease meet criteria for major depression or dysthymia (Petracca et al. 1996). Approximately 2%–3.8% of Alzheimer's disease patients develop mania (Fann and Tucker 1995). Despite the fact that the pattern of dementia is cortical in Alzheimer's disease and subcortical in the dementia syndrome of depression, it can be impossible to distinguish one from the other clinically, and depression can aggravate the dementia of Alzheimer's disease. The incidence of depression is also increased in temporal lobe epilepsy, AIDS, Huntington's disease, traumatic brain injury, spinal cord injury, and multiple sclerosis, and AIDS and traumatic brain injury also can present as mania (Blumer et al. 1995; Fann and Tucker 1995; Kishi and Robinson 1996; T.F. Scott et al. 1996).

Anxiety Disorders

Anxiety is a prominent symptom in as many as 70% of depressed outpatients (Rosenbaum et al. 1995). In addition, comorbidity of specific mood and anxiety disorders has been found consistently in large studies (Weissman et al. 1996). The NIMH-CS, a community survey, found that 32% of depressed patients had phobias, 31% had panic attacks, and 11% had obsessions or compulsions (Glass et al. 1989). Conversely, major depressive episodes have been reported in 8%–39% of patients with generalized anxiety disorder, 50%–90% of patients with panic disorder, 35%–70% of patients with social phobia, and 33% of patients with obsessive-compulsive disorder (OCD) (Brawman-Mintzer and Lydiard 1996; Gorman and Coplan 1996). Social phobia has been reported in more than 40% of patients with MDD (Bruder et al. 1997). Bipolar illness is also more common in patients with panic disorder and OCD (Strakowski et al. 1994). Manic overstimulation may be expressed as panic attacks, which can be distinguished from panic disorder by the presence of racing thoughts and a sense of having too much energy. Conversely, comorbid anxiety disorders are associated with a worse prognosis of bipolar disorder.

Anxiety in depressed patients increases severity, chronicity, and impairment associated with depression and makes depression more refractory to treatment; anxiety also increases the risk of suicide in depressed patients, perhaps because it is a marker of higher levels of arousal (Keck et al. 1994; Rudd et al. 1993). Depressed people who are anxious have more anxious people in their families, and they also have more familial loading for depression (Breier et al. 1985; Clayton et al. 1991). In these families, anxiety may be a marker of a risk factor for more severe, treatment-resistant, and/or familial form of depression.

Substance Use Disorders

Major mood disorders have high rates of comorbidity with use of many substances, especially alcohol (Maier et al. 1995b; Weissman et al. 1996). Alcohol abuse or dependence occurs in 50% of patients with unipolar depression, 60% of patients with bipolar I disorder, and 50% of patients with bipolar II disorder (Feinman and Dunner 1996). The ECA study reported that about one-third of the individuals with mood disorders had a comorbid substance use disorder (McDowell and Clodfelter 2001). Comorbid alcoholism worsens the course of both unipolar depression (Hasin et al. 1996) and bipolar disorder (Feinman and Dunner 1996). Conversely, abstinence improves the response of the mood disorder to treatment (Hasin et al. 1996).

The prevalence of depression in individuals with substance dependence is higher in active drinkers, consistent with findings discussed earlier that certain substances can induce depression. In one study (Davidson 1995), prevalence rates for depression in alcohol-dependent patients decreased from 67% when they were actively drinking to 13% after detoxification. Such findings, as well as studies showing reduced response rates to antidepressants during active alcohol use, have led to the clinical practice of deferring treatment for depression until substance use has been curtailed. However, recent work with substance-dependent adolescents suggested that the presence of depression interferes with the patients' ability to engage in treatment for the substance use disorder (Rao et al. 2000; Riggs et al. 1997) and that antidepressant therapy improves depressive symptoms and may even reduce alcohol consumption in nonabstinent depressed alcoholic patients (McGrath et al. 1996). These observations may support an approach to some patients in which depression and substance use are treated concurrently or depression is treated before patients become fully abstinent.

Schizophrenia

Major depressive episodes occur in 25%–50% of cases of schizophrenia (American Psychiatric Association 1993). The traditional belief that most of these episodes are "postpsychotic" and involve reactions to awareness of having a severe illness is contradicted by the finding that half of the depressive episodes occurring during the course of schizophrenia develop in the midst of an acute psychotic episode, and the affective component may become apparent only after the psychosis resolves. Fears that administration of antidepressants may aggravate schizophrenia have been contradicted by observations that in all but the most acute psychotic exacerbations, treatment of depression improves the prognosis of comorbid schizophrenia.

Personality Disorders

Between 30% and 70% of depressed patients receive a concurrent diagnosis of a personality disorder (Thase 1996), usually in Cluster B (i.e., borderline, histrionic, and antisocial personality disorder)

(Corruble et al. 1996). Similar diagnoses, along with narcissistic personality disorder, are often made in patients with bipolar mood disorders. Thase's group (Thase 1996) found that when they reinterviewed depressed patients after successful treatment, the rate of personality disorder was half the rate before treatment.

Studies of Inherited Factors

When interpreting studies of etiological factors in mood disorders, it is important to be aware that it is not likely that there is a single cause of even the most rigidly defined mood disorder. There is no reason to think that any inborn factor causes mood disorders; such factors interact with experiential and other environmental influences to lead to illness. Etiologies considered in a single dimension are no less complex. One abnormal gene may produce an abnormal protein that contributes to a positive symptom, whereas another gene may fail to make a protein that regulates the emergence of the same symptom. A neurotransmitter may set in motion a chain of events that overlaps a second cascade initiated by another neurotransmitter, so that dysfunction of either transmitter can have the same end result. In the same manner, any one of a number of symptoms may be a cue for the entire symptom complex that is clinically called an *affective syndrome*. Bearing these limitations in mind, we consider several areas of research and then attempt to integrate the current state of knowledge about the causes of mood disorders.

Family Studies

Relatives of people with mood disorders are consistently two to three times as likely to have mood disorders as are relatives of control subjects (E.S. Gershon 1990). If one parent has a bipolar mood disorder, the risk that a child will have a unipolar or bipolar mood disorder is around 28%; if both parents have mood disorders, the risk is two to three times as great. Patients with mood disorders also have an elevated familial incidence of substance abuse (Geller et al. 1996), and patients who are depressed and anxious have more relatives who are depressed, anxious, or both (Breier et al. 1985; Gorman and Coplan 1996).

Wealth and political affiliation also run in families, but they are not genetic. One way to begin to determine a genetic contribution is to compare the concordance of mood disorders in first- and second-degree relatives of probands with mood disorders. Because first-degree relatives (parents, children, and siblings) share 50% of their genomes, whereas only 25% of the genes are identical in second-degree relatives (grandparents, uncles, aunts, nephews, and nieces), a greater rate of a mood disorder in first-degree relatives of individuals with the same disorder than in second-degree relatives of these individuals suggests a genetic influence. The expectation of a greater likelihood of mood disorders in first-degree relatives of patients with mood disorders than in second-degree relatives or control populations usually has been confirmed.

Most studies suggest a more prominent familial transmission of bipolar than of unipolar mood disorders, often with affected relatives in consecutive generations. In addition, the age at symptom onset is earlier in bipolar individuals with strongly positive family histories (Johnson et al. 2000). Family members of patients with bipolar disorder are more likely to have bipolar as well as unipolar mood disorders themselves than are family members of patients with unipolar disorder. However, the rate of bipolar disorder in the families of the patients with unipolar depression is as much as three to four times the rate in control subjects (E.S. Gershon et al. 1982; Weissman et al. 1984). According to published family studies (E.S. Gershon et al. 1982; Weissman et al. 1984), first-degree relatives of patients with unipolar depression have a risk of unipolar depression of 5.5%–28.4% and a risk of bipolar disorder of 0.7%–8.1%; and first-degree relatives of probands with bipolar disorder have a 4.1%–14.6% likelihood of having a bipolar disorder themselves and a 5.4%–14% likelihood of having unipolar depression.

Twin Studies

Another approach to investigating genetic contributions to mood disorders is to study differences in concordance between monozygotic (identical) and dizygotic (fraternal) twins. Monozygotic twins come from the same egg and have the same genes, whereas dizygotic twins come from different eggs and share 50% of their genes, like any other siblings. A greater concordance rate for a disorder in monozygotic twins than in dizygotic twins suggests a genetic influence because the role of intrauterine and postnatal environments is presumably similar for both kinds of twins. Concordance studies reliably confirm that the overall risk of mood disorders is three times as great in monozygotic as in dizygotic twins of probands with mood disorders. For bipolar disorder, concordance rates average 0.67–1.00 for monozygotic and 0.20 for dizygotic twins. Concordance rates for unipolar depression are generally 0.50 in monozygotic twins and 0.20 in dizygotic twins. The greater difference in concordance rates between monozygotic and dizygotic twins in bipolar disorder may reflect a greater genetic influence in bipolar disorder.

Because concordance rates for mood disorders in twin studies are less than 100%, any genetic factors that are present

must interact with environmental influences to create the risk for development of the actual disorder. Reviews of twin studies suggest that 21%–45% of the variance in the risk of depressive disorders can be attributed to genetic factors, and 55%–75% of the variance can be attributed to environmental factors (K.K. Kendler et al. 1992). Of stressful life events, losses seem to be most influential.

Adoption Studies

The influence of the environment on the development of mood disorders also can be assessed by examining rates of mood disorders in adoptive and biological families of the people who were adopted in infancy. Most of these studies report that adoptees with mood disorders are more likely to have biological than adoptive relatives with mood disorders. Because rates of bipolar disorder in adoptive families of probands with bipolar disorder are no greater than in the general population, whereas rates of bipolar disorder in the biological families of these adoptees are the same as those in bipolar individuals raised with bipolar family members, adoptive factors have little or no role in bipolar mood disorders. Adoptive studies suggest that genetic factors are also important in determining transmission of unipolar depression, but adoptive (i.e., environmental) mechanisms play an important role; similar findings have emerged for transmission of suicide risk.

Imaging Findings

A variety of findings have emerged from structural and brain imaging studies of depressed patients. One of the most consistent abnormalities in structural imaging studies of unipolar depression has been enlarged lateral ventricles, which are reported most frequently in late-onset

MDD. Subcortical white matter and periventricular hyperintensities have been found on magnetic resonance imaging (MRI) in older but not younger unipolar depressed patients. Regional abnormalities most consistently reported in unipolar depression have included decreased size of the caudate, putamen, and possibly the cerebellum. The basal ganglia receive input from medial temporal structures that regulate emotion, such as the amygdala and hippocampus, but there has not been any reliable evidence of abnormalities in the amygdala and hippocampus in mood disorders. Reduced frontal lobe volume has been variably reported. Loss of hippocampal volume is reversible after early, but not later, episodes of unipolar or bipolar mood disorders.

Imaging studies in patients with bipolar mood disorders (Geller et al. 1996; Woods et al. 1995) have noted enlarged third ventricles at all ages in adults (and in a small sample of children), as well as the same kinds of subcortical white matter and periventricular hyperintensities that are seen in older patients with unipolar depression. White matter hyperintensities on MRI increase with age in patients with bipolar mood disorders but not in control subjects, suggesting an interaction between age and diagnosis (Woods et al. 1995). Bipolar disorder is associated with more subcortical hyperintensities on MRI than is unipolar depression or no mood disorder (Dupont et al. 1995). Because the presence of psychotic symptoms may be correlated with enlarged lateral ventricles in depressed patients and because psychotic features are more frequent in bipolar depression than in unipolar depression, ventricular enlargement in bipolar patients at any age may be linked more closely to psychosis than to bipolarity. However, although enlarged lateral ventricles are more common in major depression with psychotic features, white matter

hyperintensities are not. In contrast to unipolar depression, no consistent MRI changes in the frontal lobes have been reported in bipolar mood disorders.

Cerebral Blood Flow Findings

Functional brain imaging with positron emission tomography (PET) and single photon emission computed tomography (SPECT) measures regional cerebral blood flow, which is closely related to regional brain metabolism (Gyulai et al. 1997). PET has shown reduced metabolic activity in the frontal lobes (i.e., hypofrontality) in unipolar (Buchsbaum et al. 1997) and bipolar (Gyulai et al. 1997) depression. Antidepressants were found to normalize frontal metabolic activity (Buchsbaum et al. 1997). Asymmetries in cerebral blood flow also have been found in depression, but such findings have been variable.

Electroencephalographic Findings

The same direction of cerebral asymmetry has been found in electroencephalographic studies of major depression, with less left frontal activation and greater right frontal activation (as measured by alpha suppression) in major depression. Bruder et al. (1997) found less left than right anterior cortical activation in depressed patients with comorbid anxiety disorders but not in depressed patients without anxiety disorders. In contrast, nonanxious depressed patients had less activation at right posterior sites than at left posterior sites. These patterns could reflect differences in mobilization of the stress response in anxious arousal compared with that in depression without anxiety. As is true of genetic studies, such findings illustrate the possibility that abnormalities are linked to specific dimensions of the mood disorder rather than to global diagnosis.

Biological Markers

Clear associations have been established between mood disorders and alterations in biological functioning measurable in the laboratory. Most biological markers are reported more frequently in severe, psychotic, and bipolar mood disorders and in inpatients, who are of course more severely ill. However, few markers have consistently distinguished between bipolar and unipolar mood disorders. Although there has been extensive theorizing on the issue, it is not certain whether well-replicated biological markers reflect a process that is the cause or a result of mood disorders.

Dexamethasone Suppression Test

In the DST, 1 mg of dexamethasone (a synthetic adrenal steroid) is given in the afternoon to provide feedback inhibition of cortisol production by the adrenal cortex, and serum cortisol levels are measured one or more times the following day. Because the assay for cortisol does not read dexamethasone, the level of cortisol the day after dexamethasone administration is a measure of how readily the pituitary-adrenal-cortical axis can be suppressed. Normally, cortisol levels decrease to 5 μg/dL or less with dexamethasone suppression. Hyperactivity at any point between the hypothalamus and the adrenal cortex can be associated with failure of dexamethasone suppression, indicated by higher postdexamethasone cortisol levels (i.e., nonsuppression).

Melancholic major depression is associated with a 40%–50% rate of dexamethasone nonsuppression. The frequency of nonsuppression is higher (80%–90%) in severe and psychotic unipolar depression, in major depression associated with more severe suicide attempts, in inpatients, and in those with a family history of affective disorder. Bipolar depression and mania have the same frequency of dexamethasone nonsuppression as melancholic unipolar depression. The DST has been found to be a state variable; DST results convert to normal 1–3 weeks before clinical remission and revert to nonsuppression within 1–3 weeks of clinical relapse.

The proximate cause of dexamethasone nonsuppression associated with mood disorders may be hypersecretion of corticotropin-releasing factor (CRF) (Gold et al. 1995), the hypothalamic hormone that stimulates the pituitary to release corticotropin, which in turn stimulates the adrenal cortex to release cortisol. Serotonergic input stimulates secretion of both CRF and corticotropin and participates in inhibition by corticosteroids of CRF and corticotropin. Noradrenergic influences inhibit CRF production but can stimulate release of corticotropin. An entirely different mechanism is suggested by findings of considerable variability in dexamethasone serum levels between patients taking the same dose of the steroid (Devanand et al. 1991b). This observation raises the possibility that in some patients, apparent dexamethasone nonsuppression may actually reflect faster metabolism of dexamethasone, with insufficient levels to provide feedback inhibition of CRF and cortisol production.

Although it may create a window into the physiology of arousal in mood disorders, the DST has not proved useful as a diagnostic tool (Carroll 1986; Pitts 1984). Dexamethasone nonsuppression can be a response to hospitalization, acute illness, dementia, and recent weight loss. Smoking, alcohol use, and medications that accelerate dexamethasone metabolism can make it more difficult to achieve levels of dexamethasone necessary to suppress cortisol and can therefore increase the number of false-positive results in actual clinical practice. Because the 50%–60% of endogenously depressed patients with normal DST results still have a depressive illness, without a clinical evaluation it is not possible to differentiate true-positive from false-positive results. On the other hand, persistent dexamethasone nonsuppression in a patient with remitted major depression may be a marker of increased risk of relapse if treatment is stopped, and very high postdexamethasone cortisol levels (>10 μg/dL) may be a marker of psychosis in depressed patients. The DST has a specificity of 87% and a sensitivity of 48% for distinguishing between melancholic and nonmelancholic depression, but this is not of great practical importance, given that a positive DST result does not inform treatment of depression.

Thyrotropin-Releasing Hormone Stimulation Test

The TRH stimulation test, an assay of the activity of the hypothalamic-pituitary-thyroid axis, involves measuring the increase in thyrotropin several times after the intravenous infusion of a standard dose (usually 500 IU) of protirelin. If thyrotropin increases by less than 5 IU/mL after TRH infusion, the TRH stimulation test result is said to be blunted, in which case feedback inhibition of the pituitary by a hyperactive thyroid gland is excessive or primary pituitary failure has occurred.

About one-third of otherwise euthyroid melancholic depressed patients have been found to have a blunted TRH stimulation test result. In some studies, this finding has been a state variable, reverting to normal with remission of depression, whereas in other studies, it has been a trait variable, remaining abnormal after mood normalizes. In most studies, there is at

most a modest likelihood that depressed patients with a nonsuppressed DST result will also have a blunted TRH stimulation test result.

A blunted TRH stimulation test in melancholic depression is not associated with changes in circulating levels of thyroid hormones, and therefore it is unlikely that the test is a marker of true hyperthyroidism. However, delivery of thyroid hormone to feedback systems in the pituitary and hypothalamus may be excessive. It is also possible that TRH receptors in the pituitary are hypoactive. Chronic overstimulation of these receptors by endogenous TRH might lead to their downregulation but also would result in elevated thyroid hormone levels, so a primary defect in cellular signaling seems more likely. The input of serotonergic and noradrenergic tracts to the pituitary could permit a functional deficiency of norepinephrine activity, or an excess of serotonin transmission could contribute to a blunted TRH stimulation test result.

Abnormal Sleep

Abnormal sleep is one of the most common symptoms of depression, and the most frequent cause of sleep disorders in patients evaluated at sleep centers is depression (Buysse et al. 1994). Well-replicated changes in sleep architecture in MDD include decreased sleep continuity, more awakenings, decreased rapid eye movement (REM) latency (i.e., decreased length of time between the onset of sleep to the first REM cycle), increased REM density (increased number of REMs per unit of time during REM sleep), increased length of time in REM sleep, and difficulty entering and remaining in slow-wave sleep (McDermott et al. 1997). Some of the decreased REM latency observed in melancholic depression is primary, and some is secondary to reduced slow-wave sleep, which allows REM sleep to shift to the earlier part of the night (Kupfer 1995). Deficiencies in sleep efficiency and slow-wave sleep may explain why depressed patients sometimes feel tired even if they appear to sleep excessively.

Abnormalities of sleep architecture have been most notable in melancholic depression and in bipolar and psychotic depression, the latter being accompanied by sleep-onset REM or a REM latency of less than 20 minutes. However, reduced REM latency has not been found in SAD. Some findings—such as decreased slow-wave sleep—are trait variables, whereas others—such as decreased sleep continuity, decreased REM latency, and increased phasic REM activity—are state variables.

Any single abnormality of sleep architecture is not strongly associated with major depression. However, the triad of reduced REM latency, increased REM density, and decreased sleep efficiency reliably discriminated between patients with MDD and control subjects in a carefully controlled study. Even in this study, however, 55% of the depressed outpatients had no abnormalities on any of the three measures, which makes the sleep electroencephalogram a poor diagnostic test.

Hypotheses regarding mechanisms of the complex changes in sleep architecture in major depression are incomplete. In cases of early-morning awakening and decreased REM latency, there appears to be a phase advance of the sleep–wake cycle, which is driven by the "weak oscillator" that also drives activity–rest cycles, and of the REM sleep cycle, which is dependent on the "strong oscillator" that also controls body temperature. Because muscarinic cholinergic systems increase REM sleep (Poland et al. 1997), cholinergic excess could be one cause of increased REM density and increased time in REM sleep. However, decreased REM latency also could be a function of noradrenergic

deficiency (Poland et al. 1997). Changes in REM sleep may be secondary to a disturbance of non-REM sleep, which is regulated by corticothalamic circuits.

Clinical Uses of Biological Tests

Laboratory tests are useful for examining the pathophysiology of mood disorders, but the large numbers of false-positive and false-negative results make them relatively ineffective for diagnosing mood disorders. In addition, no laboratory test can outperform the gold-standard clinical interview to which it is referenced (Somoza and Mossman 1990), and no studies exist in which diagnosis was prospectively predicted by laboratory test alone. A single laboratory test such as the DST can occasionally be used to predict the risk of a relapse if an antidepressant is withdrawn or to increase the index of suspicion of psychosis in refractory depression. However, studies of correlations between multiple tests may create a better window into the complex phenomenology of mood disorders.

Ultimately, biological tests may prove most useful in identifying specific dimensions of mood disorders that may indicate specific treatments or combinations of them. For example, inhibitors of the hypothalamic-pituitary-adrenal axis might be useful for patients with refractory depression and excessive release of CRF, whereas manipulations of the sleep–wake cycle might be effective for patients with prominent disruptions of the relation between slow-wave and REM sleep.

Etiology: Biological Factors and Theories

Biological Rhythms

Depressed mood often has a diurnal variation, and episodes may follow a monthly or seasonal pattern of recurrence. Some mood disorders, such as SAD and rapid-cycling bipolar disorder, are defined by their periodicity. Phase advances (i.e., peaking earlier in the day) have been noted in sleep onset, REM sleep, temperature, and hormonal and neurotransmitter rhythms, including those of concentrations of cortisol, serotonin, dopamine, and norepinephrine.

This kind of cyclicity has led to hypotheses of chronobiological causes of mood disorders (Goodwin et al. 1982; Teicher et al. 1997). One such hypothesis is that abnormalities of mood in MDD are related to a phase advance or at least desynchronization of the strong oscillator (which controls rhythms of body temperature, REM sleep, plasma cortisol, and melatonin) with respect to the weak oscillator (which controls the sleep–wake and activity–rest cycles). Loss of predictability of circadian rhythms—with reduced amplitude of rhythms of body temperature, norepinephrine, cortisol, and melatonin—could suggest impaired entrainment of these rhythms. Antidepressants restore normal organization of circadian rhythms and resynchronize the two oscillators, but it is not clear whether this is a therapeutic mechanism or one of a number of markers of overall improvement of psychobiology.

Neuroanatomical Factors

It is possible that subtle alterations in the structure or function of brain areas that participate in mood regulation could contribute to primary mood disorders. Relevant areas of the brain for this kind of formulation include the prefrontal cortex; subcortical structures such as the basal ganglia, thalamus, and hypothalamus; the brain stem; and the white matter pathways connecting these structures to one another and the cerebral cortex (e.g., the

limbic-thalamic-cortical circuit and the limbic-striatal-pallidal-thalamic-cortical circuit), and possibly the cerebellum. Abnormalities in these areas that could contribute to affective symptoms might be caused by abnormal brain development, vascular injury, aging, or degenerative disease.

Biogenic Amines

Biologically active (biogenic) amines such as norepinephrine, serotonin, dopamine, and acetylcholine (ACh) are neurotransmitters in brain systems that originate in the brain stem. These systems modulate background activity of multiple neuronal circuits, and abnormal function of biogenic amines has been proposed in mood disorders. The monoamine hypothesis, which was first proposed in 1965, holds that monoamines such as norepinephrine and serotonin are deficient in depression and that the therapeutic action of antidepressants depends on increasing synaptic availability of these monoamines (Schildkraut 1965).

Additional experience has not confirmed the monoamine depletion hypothesis. Monoamine precursors such as tyrosine or tryptophan by themselves do not improve mood. Depletion of serotonin can aggravate depression that has been in remission, but it does not predictably cause depression, and when it does cause depression, the depression is not sustained. Some substances that are monoamine reuptake inhibitors, such as amphetamines and cocaine, do not have reliable antidepressant properties, and antidepressant medications exist (e.g., iprindole, mianserin, mirtazapine, ketanserin) that have no effect on monoamine reuptake. In the case of monoamine reuptake inhibitors that are antidepressants, reuptake inhibition is immediate, whereas the onset of antidepressant effect is delayed a month or more.

Norepinephrine

Both relative deficiencies and excesses of
central noradrenergic activity have been
postulated to exist in depression. An early
hypothesis was that decreased activity
and motivation in depression was related
to reduced noradrenergic tone and that
hyperactivity in mania was related to noradrenergic excess (Schildkraut 1965).
However, reports of increased norepinephrine activity in depression have been
more frequent than reports of reduced
activity. This is consistent with evidence
of high levels of arousal such as the nonsuppressed DST or phase advance of circadian rhythms, which are present even in
behaviorally slowed depressed patients.

Drawing on studies of responsiveness
of noradrenergic measures such as plasma
MHPG, a norepinephrine metabolite, to
mild stresses, Siever and Davis (1985)
suggested that depression is associated not
with consistently elevated or reduced norepinephrine activity but with uneven
responsiveness to stresses that activate
noradrenergic stress response systems.
Like the heat produced by a furnace that
is controlled by a poorly regulated ther-
mostat, baseline noradrenergic activity is
excessive, but acute stresses that call for
mobilization of the stress response result
in inadequate mobilization of additional
noradrenergic transmission. The behavioral and affective correlates of this situation would be high levels of baseline
anxiety with a sense of "spinning one's
wheels" with inability to mount an organized response to important challenges.

Serotonin

Neurons using serotonin, which is phylogenetically the oldest neurotransmitter,
originate in raphe (midline) nuclei in the
brain stem and project throughout the
brain. These connections and interactions
make it possible for serotonin to interact

with other biogenic amines and to contribute to the regulation of many core psychobiological functions that are disrupted in
mood disorders, including mood, anxiety,
arousal, vigilance, irritability, thinking,
cognition, appetites, aggression, circadian
and seasonal rhythms, nociception, and
neuroendocrine functions (Coccaro 1989;
Grahame-Smith 1992; Leonard 1992;
Montgomery and Fineberg 1989; Murphy
et al. 1989). Serotonin may serve as a
"neurochemical brake" on certain innate
behaviors that are normally suppressed,
such as aggression, including aggression
turned against the self (Benkelfat 1993).
Therefore, it is not surprising that serotonergic dysfunction has been implicated in
mood disorders and that medications that
act on serotonin are useful in the treatment of mood disorders.

Serotonin mediates its diverse actions
through multiple receptors with different
second messenger signaling mechanisms.
At least 15 distinct serotonin receptor
subtypes have been identified, many with
further functional subtypes (e.g., 5-HT_{1A},
5-HT_{1D}) (Dubovsky and Thomas 1995;
Kroeze and Roth 1998). More is known
about some of these receptors than others
(Charney et al. 1990; Dubovsky 1994a;
Dubovsky and Thomas 1995).

Several studies have found lower concentrations of 5-hydroxyindoleacetic acid
(5-HIAA, the major serotonin metabolite) in the CSF of depressed patients
than in the CSF of control subjects. The
finding of reduced platelet serotonin uptake in unmedicated major depression
could represent hypofunction of a cellular
serotonin transporter. If a similar malfunction existed in the brain, it could
result in reduced serotonin stores, or reduction of serotonin uptake could be a
means of compensating for increased
serotonin availability. Decreased binding
of [³H]-imipramine, a marker of the serotonin uptake site, has been inconsistently

found in platelets of unmedicated depressed patients. Additionally, no change in platelet binding of [^{3}H]-paroxetine, which may be a better marker of the serotonin uptake site, has been found in major depression.

Reduction of central serotonin and its metabolites may not be a marker of depression so much as features that commonly accompany depression. Of seven studies, five reported modestly reduced brain-stem serotonin and 5-HIAA in persons who committed suicide, regardless of diagnosis (Mann et al. 1989). In 10 of 15 studies of CSF 5-HIAA, levels were lower in depressed patients who made a suicide attempt than in those who did not attempt suicide (Mann et al. 1989). Increased binding of labeled markers to 5-HT$_2$ and 5-HT$_{1A}$ receptors in the frontal cortex of individuals who committed suicide suggests that these receptors were upregulated to compensate for decreased synaptic availability of serotonin in suicide (Buchsbaum et al. 1997). A study of 22 drug-free depressed inpatients with a history of a suicide attempt found that current depressive episodes in patients whose past attempts caused more medical damage and were better planned were associated with lower CSF 5-HIAA (but no changes in other neurotransmitter metabolites) than were depressive episodes in patients who had made less lethal and less well planned suicide attempts, which suggests that reduced 5-HIAA may be a marker of seriousness of suicidal ideation (Mann and Malone 1997). In a study of 237 patients with mood disorders and 187 control subjects, a variant of the serotonin transporter gene was associated with violent but not other kinds of suicide attempts (Bellivier et al. 2000).

Considered together, studies of serotonin in major depression suggest both hypofunction and hyperfunction. Findings such as decreased serotonin and 5-HIAA levels in postmortem brain and CSF studies, brief relapse of depression with diets that deplete serotonin precursors, decreased postsynaptic serotonin receptor sensitivity in depression, and the existence of antidepressant properties of some medications that enhance serotonergic transmission suggest underactivity of serotonin systems. Conversely, decreased platelet serotonin uptake in depression, increased 5-HT$_2$ receptor binding in the frontal cortex of individuals who committed suicide, and reduction of postsynaptic 5-HT$_2$ binding and CSF 5-HIAA by chronic antidepressant treatment suggest increased serotonergic transmission in major depression.

One reason for this uncertainty is that neurobiological and pharmacological studies generally emphasize isolated aspects of serotonin function, although in the intact organism, the activity of this neurotransmitter cannot be separated from the action of other transmitters. For example, serotonin is a cotransmitter with γ-aminobutyric acid (GABA) (Kahn et al. 1990) and norepinephrine (Jaim-Etcheverry and Zieher 1982). Serotonergic and noradrenergic neurons can take up each other's transmitter, altering the functioning of the parent neuron (Jaim-Etcheverry and Zieher 1982). Serotonergic raphe neurons inhibit noradrenergic neurons in the locus coeruleus (Kahn et al. 1990) and regulate β-adrenergic receptor number and function (Charney et al. 1990). Conversely, agonists of α- and β-adrenergic receptors and GABA$_B$ receptors alter the function of several serotonin receptors (Grahame-Smith 1992).

Many other serotonin interactions have been identified. Raphe serotonergic neurons synapse with nigrostriatal and mesolimbic dopaminergic neurons (Bleich et al. 1990), and dopaminergic neurons have serotonin receptors that permit tonic control of dopamine release in the midbrain, striatum, and nucleus accumbens (Meltzer 1992). Depending on the circumstances, serotonin may facilitate dopamine release in the nucleus accumbens and inhibit dopaminergic activity in the striatum (Meltzer 1992). Serotonergic neurons have glucocorticoid receptors that alter gene transcription, perhaps providing a feedback loop between the stress response and resetting of serotonin function.

Dopamine

Some investigations have found that CSF concentrations of the dopamine metabolite homovanillic acid (HVA) are lower in patients with major depression than in control subjects and that lower CSF HVA levels are found in more severely depressed patients, but results have not been consistent. The dopamine reuptake inhibitors nomifensine (no longer available), amineptine (available in Europe), and bupropion are antidepressants. Dopaminergic agonists such as bromocriptine, pramipexole, and piribedil and the dopamine-releasing stimulants methylphenidate and dextroamphetamine have antidepressant properties that make them useful adjuncts in the treatment of depression.

As is true of serotonin, any apparent dopaminergic hypofunction may have a greater effect on dimensions of mood disorders than on specific diagnoses. Because mobilization of goal-directed behavior is mediated by dopamine, underactivity of dopaminergic systems may be related to decreased drive and motivation in depression. Unresponsive dopaminergic systems could be one reason that experience is unrewarding to depressed patients. Hyperactivity of dopaminergic motivational and action systems could be related to manic or psychotic symptoms in mood disorders.

GABA

GABA is the major inhibitory neurotransmitter in the central nervous system. Inadequate GABAergic input to noradrenergic arousal systems could lead to the kind of unrestrained arousal that characterizes mood disorders. Decreased CSF GABA levels have been reported in major depression, and some antidepressants increase the number of GABA$_B$ receptor sites in rat brain. Because GABA$_B$ receptors may act as heteroreceptors on serotonergic terminals in limbic regions, in addition to moderating noradrenergic output, any pathophysiological contribution of GABA and any therapeutic effect of GABAergic medications in mood disorders may ultimately be mediated by other neurotransmitter systems.

Acetylcholine

It has been hypothesized that cholinergic transmission, relative to noradrenergic transmission, is excessive in depression and inadequate in mania. Because ACh is a neurotransmitter in structures that mediate withdrawal and punishment such as the periventricular system, cholinergic hyperactivity could increase withdrawal behavior and contribute to depression (Poland et al. 1997). In support of this hypothesis are the findings that cholinergic input reduces REM latency (i.e., decreased REM latency is seen in depression); some antidepressants have anticholinergic properties; lecithin, an ACh precursor, and cholinesterase inhibitors such as physostigmine and donepezil, reduce mania in some patients and sometimes replace mania with depression; and cholinergic rebound following abrupt withdrawal of anticholinergic medications can cause a relapse of depression (Dilsaver and Coffman 1989; Janowsky and Risch 1984; Keshavan 1985). Objections raised against the cholinergic hypothesis include observations that not all anticholinergic medications are antidepressants; that none of the newer antidepressants is anticholinergic; and that muscarinic receptors were initially considered in testing the hypothesis, although most agents used to test the hypothesis act on nicotinic receptors (Dilsaver and Coffman 1989).

Substance P

Speculations have arisen that substance P could mediate the psychological pain of depression as well as physical pain, and increased circulating levels of substance P were recently reported in major depression. Some trials of antagonists of substance P receptors have suggested an antidepressant action, but this finding has not been confirmed, and additional studies are now under way.

Interactions of Neurotransmitter Systems

Early attempts to understand the role of neurotransmitters and their receptors involved the hypothesis that some depressions were characterized by functional norepinephrine deficiency, whereas others were associated with serotonin hypofunction. According to this hypothesis, low norepinephrine depression would respond preferentially to noradrenergic antidepressants, and low serotonin depressions would respond better to treatments that enhance serotonin availability. This prediction was never confirmed, and no evidence of differing "serotonergic" and "noradrenergic" depressive subtypes has emerged. The hypothesis was then revised (termed the *permissive amine hypothesis*) to include the concept that serotonergic deficiency contributed to most cases of depression, some of which had additional noradrenergic dysfunction and others of which did not. This hypothesis would predict that treatments that enhance seroto-

nergic transmission are antidepressants. However, tianeptine—an effective TCA available in France—enhances serotonin reuptake, reducing available synaptic serotonin.

These kinds of observations underscore the overlap of dimensional features of depression driven by dysfunction of one or more serotonin systems in interaction with other neurotransmitter systems (Lopez-Ibor 1988; O'Keane et al. 1992). When arousal associated with noradrenergic excess is sufficient to overwhelm regulation of aggression and impulsivity that has been impaired by suboptimally active serotonin systems, suicide, various forms of outwardly directed aggression, or generalized impulsivity may be the predominant problem, whether the primary diagnosis is a mood disorder, an anxiety disorder, schizophrenia, or a personality disorder. Inadequate function of serotonergic systems that regulate intrusive thought may interact with disturbances of mood to produce ruminative depressive states or racing thoughts that remain stuck on a particular idea. If the interaction is with the consequences of traumatic experiences, the intrusive recall of posttraumatic stress disorder may develop if serotonergic systems that regulate recurrent thoughts and arousal do not function normally. Dysregulation of thought processes is a feature of schizophrenia, and when this interacts with the psychobiology of mood, the same malfunction may figure in psychotic depression, bipolar illness, and schizoaffective disorder.

Traditional single neurotransmitter hypotheses ignore evidence of dysfunction of other neurotransmitters in mood disorders. In addition, none of these hypotheses is readily applicable to bipolar mood disorders. If mania is associated primarily with neurotransmitter changes (e.g., increased norepinephrine and dopaminergic activity) that are the opposites of changes in depression, for example, why are almost 50% of manic patients depressed at the same time they are manic (i.e., mixed mania)? And how could the direction of neurotransmitter activity change so abruptly and rapidly if such activity were driving ultradian cycling?

It is impossible to understand reported neurotransmitter changes in mood disorders without appreciating that all neurotransmitters and receptors that have been studied interact with and influence one another. Cotransmission using more than one neurotransmitter in the same neuron is the rule (Jaim-Etcheverry and Zieher 1982; McCormick and Williamson 1989). Most cerebral functions are the result of the converging action of many different neurotransmitters. For example, excitability in the human cortex is regulated by ACh, GABA, norepinephrine, histamine, and purines, in addition to serotonin (McCormick and Williamson 1989). Each of these transmitters may produce more than one postsynaptic signal in the same neuron by activating interacting receptors, and more than one transmitter may induce the same change in postsynaptic neurons. This kind of overlap provides a mechanism for fine-tuning of complex adaptations to multiple kinds of input (McCormick and Williamson 1989).

Such interactions make it unlikely that the pathophysiology of mood disorders can be linked to any single neurotransmitter. Instead, different aspects of the psychobiological malfunctions in mood disorders may be related to different kinds of neurotransmitter dysfunctions.

Etiology: Psychological Factors and Theories

As with biological data, there is less disagreement about whether specific psychological dimensions of mood disorders exist than about whether they are etiological. And as is true of biological factors, proving that a particular psychological factor is causal would require prospectively following up people at risk for depression to determine whether those with the factor are more likely to develop a mood disorder. A finding that patients who already have had an affective episode and who have the factor in question are more likely to have a recurrence could simply imply that the factor is a residual symptom of the index episode and not an independent risk factor. Even if expensive and difficult prospective studies of psychological risk factors were conducted, a positive finding would not guarantee that any factors identified were not markers of an underlying biological factor.

Because none of the psychological theories of mania (e.g., that it is a defense against depression) has ever been tested empirically, we focus on psychological hypotheses of depression.

Abnormal Reactions to Loss

Loss is the life event that has been most reliably linked to depression. In most studies comparing depressed patients with nondepressed control subjects, childhood loss—especially loss of a parent—has had a positive association with adult depression, which has been temporally associated with a recent loss, separation, or disappointment (Bemporad 1988; Paykel 1982). In primate studies, separation from a mother or from a peer in animals raised with peers reliably results in behavioral depression and in the physiology of human depression; separation depression can be prevented or reversed by use of antidepressants (Kaufman and Rosenblum 1967; Suomi et al. 1978). Separation during infancy from the mother or, in the case of animals raised with peers, from the peer group also notably increases the risk of adult separation depression (Kaufman and Rosenblum 1967; McKinney 1988). Similarly, experience with human infants has shown that early separation can produce a depressive syndrome that predisposes to later depression (Bowlby 1980). Early separations may sensitize arousal and withdrawal systems to react excessively to subsequent losses, whether real or symbolic.

Although the association between depression and loss seems reliable, it is not as strong as was originally thought. Not only does loss account for only a relatively small portion of the variance in the risk of depression (Paykel 1982), but losses of one kind or another precede many other medical and psychiatric illnesses (MagPhil and Thomas 1981). Loss, an event that is stressful in itself and that removes an important external source of regulation of disrupted psychology and physiology, may be a more severe instance of a range of stresses that predispose to mood disorders.

Other Psychodynamic Theories

Psychoanalyst Karl Abraham postulated that depression is a manifestation of aggression turned against the self in a patient who is unable to express anger against loved ones. Attacks on the introjected other, who psychologically has become a part of the self, undermine adaptive capacities and produce negative affect. In support of this hypothesis is the fact that many depressed patients have difficulty expressing anger openly, either because they lack self-confidence or because they are afraid of being abandoned by a loved one on whom they are excessively dependent. However, it seems unlikely that anger is converted directly into depression in such individuals because many depressed patients are openly irritable. A more likely explanation is that dependency, sensitivity to loss, and lack of assertiveness lead de-

pressed people to conceal anger, or even differences of opinion with others, until it becomes overwhelming, at which point it intrudes into everyday interactions. This problem may be compounded by intensification of all emotional experience in depression.

A hypothesis first clearly articulated by Edward Bibring is that the central psychological fault in depression is loss of self-esteem. According to this hypothesis, the depression-prone person is an over-ambitious, conventional individual with unrealistically high ego ideals. Depression represents deflation of self-confidence and vitality within the self that results from failing to live up to internalized standards that are essential to the patient's self-concept.

Interpersonal Theory

Interpersonal theory emphasizes four basic interpersonal issues: unresolved grief, disputes between partners and family members about roles and responsibilities in the relationship, transitions to new roles such as parent and retired person, and deficits in the social skills that are necessary to sustain a relationship (Klerman et al. 1984). As in other psychodynamic theories, depressed mood and altered biology are hypothesized to be responses to loss or the threat of loss. A psychotherapy derived from interpersonal theory (i.e., IPT), which is described later in this chapter (see subsection "Interpersonal Therapy"), has been found to be effective as a primary treatment for depression and an adjunct in the treatment of bipolar disorder, although this does not prove that the etiological concept behind the psychotherapy is accurate.

Cognitive Theory

Cognitive theory holds that negative thinking is a cause rather than a result of depression (A.T. Beck et al. 1985; Thase 1996). According to the cognitive model, early experience leads to the development of global negative assumptions called *schemata*. Depressive schemata involve all-or-nothing assumptions such as

- If I'm not completely happy, I'll be totally miserable.
- If something isn't done exactly right, it's worthless.
- If I'm not perfect, I'm a failure.
- If everyone doesn't love me unconditionally, then no one loves me at all.
- If I'm not in complete control, I'm helpless.
- If I depend on anyone for anything, I'm totally needy.

As long as experience seems to support a schema—for example, if everything a person does seems to work out or if a person never leans on anyone else—mood remains unambivalently positive. However, if something happens to contradict an all-or-nothing assumption, the negative side of the patient's thinking predominates. Failure in one endeavor makes the patient feel like a complete failure, or becoming ill or otherwise requiring assistance results in the patient's thinking, "I'm totally needy" or "I can't do anything for myself." These negative beliefs, or negative cognitions, are supported by self-fulfilling prophecies that reinforce negative thinking. For instance, the patient who feels helpless as a result of not having been able to influence the outcome of a complex and difficult situation stops trying to do anything to deal with later, simpler stresses. When this lack of effort results in subsequent failures, the patient's belief that nothing can be done to influence the environment seems to have been proven. Systematic errors in thinking lead to catastrophic thinking and generalization of single negative events to global

negative expectations of the self, the environment, and the future (the "cognitive triad").

Much of the evidence in favor of the cognitive theory of depression comes from demonstrations that psychotherapy based on the theory (i.e., cognitive therapy, discussed in the "Cognitive Therapy" section later in this chapter) is an effective treatment for major depression. However, cognitive therapy is effective even when patients do not express negative cognitions, and all-or-nothing thinking is characteristic of several conditions (e.g., personality disorders) in addition to depression.

Learned Helplessness

A concept related to cognitive theory is *learned helplessness*, which was first clearly shown experimentally by psychologist Martin Seligman (Abramson et al. 1978; Seligman 1975). The classic learned helplessness paradigm involves exposing an animal to an inescapable noxious but harmless stimulus such as a mild electrical shock. At first, the animal attempts to flee from the shock, but when escape is prevented, it lies down and accepts the shock passively. If the situation is changed so that the animal can escape the stimulus (e.g., if the investigator removes a barrier that was preventing the animal from leaving the portion of the cage where the shock is applied), the animal continues to act as though it cannot get away. The animal cannot be coaxed away from the shock; only forcibly dragging the animal to safety reverses the learned helpless behavior. A second instance of learned helplessness develops more readily than a first episode. Learned helplessness that develops in one situation may generalize to other situations.

Learned helplessness resembles the passive, withdrawn behavior of depression, and resistance to reversing a negative experience is reminiscent of the self-fulfilling negative expectations of depression. Learned helplessness can be demonstrated in humans—for example, by exposing normal subjects to an inescapable noxious sound—and subjects who score higher on depression rating scales develop learned helplessness more readily than do those without depressive symptoms (Abramson et al. 1978).

Experimental evidence in favor of the learned helplessness theory of depression may not be as strong as it might seem. It is not clear that learned helplessness in animals is equivalent to human depression. Human subjects with elevated depression scores have not had actual depressive disorders and have not sought treatment for any reason. In addition, depression involves symptoms beyond those of learned helplessness.

Behavioral Theories

Behavioral theories of depression, which are related to learned helplessness, hold that depression is caused by loss of reinforcement for nondepressive behaviors, resulting in deficits in adaptive social behaviors such as being assertive, responding positively to challenge, and otherwise seeking important reinforcers such as affection, caretaking, and attention. At the same time that environmental rewards are no longer forthcoming with positive behavior (this is known as *noncontingent reinforcement*), helplessness, expressions of distress, physical complaints, and other depressive behaviors may be rewarded, especially if significant others pay more attention to disability than to competence. Loss, in addition to rupturing an important attachment bond, removes a major social reinforcer and results in depressive behaviors if the patient has not developed an adequate repertoire of adaptive behaviors and does not have other sources of reinforcement. Like negative cognitions, depressive behaviors would be expected to drive a depressed mood.

There is little question that interpersonal rewards influence behavior. If important people pay more attention to expressions of helplessness and inadequacy than to expressions of competence, it may be more rewarding to be depressed than to be healthy. However, it remains to be proven that behavioral factors by themselves can induce depression or that treatment of clinically important depression by behavioral techniques alone is effective.

Course of Mood Disorders

The mean age at onset of unipolar depression is 24.8–34.8 years (Weissman et al. 1996). About 25% of patients have low-grade chronic or intermittent depression before developing a major depressive episode. There is a 50% chance of remission of depression that has been present for 3–6 months, but there is only a 5% likelihood of remission within the next 6 months of a major depressive episode that has been present for 2 years. Rates of partial remission in studies of antidepressants, psychotherapy, and/or behavior therapy have ranged from 5% to 42% (Fochtmann 1994).

Prospective follow-up studies lasting 2–20 years after an index major depressive episode suggest that 5%–27% (mean = 17%) of patients with MDD remain chronically ill (Keller et al. 1984; Piccinelli and Wilkinson 1994; Winokur and Morrison 1973). Coryell et al. (1994) found that patients who did not recover from an episode within 2 months had a one-in-three chance of recovery over the next 2 months. The odds of recovery in any 2 of the next 8 months declined to one in five to six. In the second year of depression, the likelihood of recovery in any 2-month period decreased to a little more than 7%. Such results confirm data indicating that the longer major depression has been present, the more likely it is to persist (Piccinelli and Wilkinson 1994). On the other hand, even patients who have been depressed for many years may eventually recover. Predictors of a chronic course that have emerged in these studies include a family history of mood disorder or psychosis; multiple losses; comorbid medical illness; substance dependence; a disabled spouse; agitation; anxiety; delusions; passive, dependent, or avoidant personality style; work impairment; and double depression (Fochtmann 1994).

Unipolar major depressive episodes have a tendency to recur, even with treatment (Thase 1992). The rates of recurrence after recovery from an episode of major depression have been found to range from 50% within 2 years to 90% in 6 years (Coryell et al. 1994). After having been depressed once, the average person has at least a 50% chance of becoming depressed again, but after two episodes, the risk of a third episode is 70%. After the third episode, the risk of a fourth is 80%, and after three episodes, the risk of another one is 90%. Overall, between 75% and 95% of patients with a major depressive episode will have at least one more episode over the course of their lives. On average, major depressive episodes recur every 5 years, the latency between episodes shortening from an average of 6 years after two episodes to just 2 years after three episodes. About 15% of unipolar patients have only one episode of major depression, whereas 13%–54% (mean = 27%) have three or more episodes. The average lifetime number of episodes of unipolar depression is four. The recurrence rates of both major depression and dysthymia are higher in

double depression than in episodic MDD or dysthymic disorder without MDD (J. Scott 1988).

Various factors have been found to increase the risk of relapse and recurrence of unipolar depression (Belsher and Costello 1988; Boyce et al. 1991; Coryell et al. 1991; Keitner and Miller 1990; Keitner et al. 1991; J. Scott 1988; Thase 1992). One of the most important of these is inadequate treatment. Because residual depressive symptoms increase the risk of a relapse fourfold, any depressive episode should be treated as completely as possible. Discontinuation of effective treatment often leads to relapse, especially if medications are withdrawn rapidly. The greater the number of previous recurrences, the higher the risk of future recurrences. High expressed emotion in the family, marital problems, and psychosis also increase the risk of a relapse of unipolar depression. Secondary depression, whether associated with medical or nonaffective psychiatric illness, increases the risk of relapse by 60% and reduces the length of time to relapse. Severity of a depressive episode does not affect the risk of relapse.

In the NIMH Treatment of Depression Collaborative Research Program, rates of recovery from a recurrence were similar to rates of recovery after an index episode. In this particular investigation, each time a patient had another episode, the chance of not recovering from that episode was 8% after 5 years. Preventing recurrence therefore is an important step toward reducing the accumulating risk of chronicity.

The average age at first onset of bipolar disorder is 6 years younger than that for unipolar depression (Weissman et al. 1996), usually by the second or third decade of life. However, first episodes of mania have been reported after age 50 years (Sachs 1996). The median duration of a manic episode is 5–10 weeks, and that of a bipolar depressive episode is 19 weeks. Mixed bipolar episodes have a median duration of 36 weeks. Fewer than one-third of patients with acute bipolar affective episodes remain euthymic for a year, and 20% of acute affective episodes in bipolar disorder become chronic, with the highest rate of chronicity occurring in mixed bipolar episodes (Sachs 1996).

In patients who experience discrete recurrences of bipolar affective episodes, cycle length shortens during the first three to six episodes and then stabilizes at one to two episodes per year, the frequency of depressive and manic recurrences being about the same (Sachs 1996). The average patient with a bipolar mood disorder has an onset of symptoms in adolescence and has had 10 or more acute affective episodes before age 35 (Sachs 1996). Residual hypomanic symptoms increase the risk of depressive recurrences in bipolar mood disorder even more than do residual depressive symptoms (Thase 1992). As with unipolar depression, the risk of bipolar relapse or recurrence decreases the longer a patient remains completely well (Coryell et al. 1994). By the same token, starting mood-stabilizing medications such as lithium earlier in the course of illness is associated with better prophylaxis of recurrences than if medications are started later in the course of illness (Franchini et al. 1999).

Functional Outcome

Functional outcome in depression is as poor as it is in chronic medical disorders such as diabetes mellitus and cardiovascular disease. In the prospective study of the Iowa 500, 17% of the depressed patients were unable to work because of depression, and 22% had incapacitating symptoms. The medical outcomes study of 22,462 outpatients in a health maintenance organization found that those with depressive disorders functioned more poorly in almost all areas measured than did patients with diabetes, cardiovascular disease, arthritis, or pulmonary disease. Similarly, in the NIMH-CS study, depressed patients were less likely to be employed, earned less money, were more likely never to have been married, had poorer spousal relationships when they were married, and were less satisfied with sexual activity compared with control subjects, even when the patients were not clinically ill.

Somatic Treatments

Antidepressant Medications

Antidepressants are traditionally classified according to their structure (e.g., tricyclic, tetracyclic) or their effect on neurotransmitter dynamics (e.g., norepinephrine reuptake inhibitors, serotonin reuptake inhibitors, MAOIs) or receptors (e.g., 5-HT$_2$ antagonists). As we mentioned earlier, it seems unlikely that any particular neurotransmitter action can account for the therapeutic effect of the antidepressants. However, neurotransmitter actions do predict side effects. For example, noradrenergic antidepressants can produce jitteriness, tremor, sweating, and insomnia; serotonergic antidepressants cause nausea, headaches, and sexual dysfunction; and dopaminergic antidepressants are activating.

All antidepressants produce about a 60% response rate in unipolar nonpsychotic depression, which is significantly higher than the 20%–40% rate of placebo response. Although antidepressants have been found to be effective for milder depression, the difference between active antidepressant and placebo diminishes in the case of less severe depression. The high placebo response rate in less severe forms of depression results in an overall effect size of only 0.5 in nonbipolar, nonpsychotic depression of mild to moderate severity (Doris et al. 1999). In severe and psychotic depression, placebo response rates approach zero and antidepressants are substantially superior.

Tricyclic and tetracyclic antidepressants (Table 6–16) have a three- or four-carbon ring structure (Bech 1993; Kasper et al. 1992; Osser 1993). All of these medications have similar properties. In most cases, either the parent drugs (e.g., desipramine) or their metabolites (e.g., desmethylclomipramine) block norepinephrine reuptake, and some parent drugs (e.g., chlorimipramine, imipramine) block serotonin reuptake. As was mentioned earlier, neurotransmitter reuptake inhibition mainly predicts adverse effects. For example, noradrenergic antidepressants are more likely to cause arousal, diaphoresis, tremor, and insomnia, and serotonergic antidepressants are more likely to produce headaches, gastrointestinal side effects, and sexual dysfunction. However, potent serotonin reuptake inhibition of clomipramine (chlorimipramine) makes it the only TCA that is effective in the treatment of OCD.

All TCAs have similar side-effect profiles. A quinidine-like effect makes the TCAs as effective as the type IA antiarrhythmics in the treatment of ventricular tachyarrhythmias; however, these medications can aggravate heart block and have a negative inotropic effect. Tertiary amine TCAs such as imipramine and amitriptyline have more anticholinergic and sedative side effects. The tertiary amines also produce more α_1-adrenergic blockade, resulting in postural hypotension, and more histamine H_1 antagonism, which contributes to sedation and weight gain. These kinds of adverse effects, along with the potential negative effect on memory

of anticholinergic side effects, make the tertiary amine TCAs poor choices for older patients and patients with dementia. Nortriptyline definitely has a therapeutic window, and desipramine probably has a therapeutic window. Aside from a sinusoidal correlation between serum level and clinical response for imipramine and possibly amitriptyline, no other correlations between antidepressant serum level and clinical response have been demonstrated (Perry et al. 1994).

Second-generation antidepressants (Table 6–17) are heterogeneous with respect to their structures and actions (Bech 1993; Kasper et al. 1992; Montgomery 1995). Trazodone is primarily a 5-HT_2 receptor antagonist with prominent sedative properties. It is frequently used as a hypnotic because its short elimination half-life results in less daytime impairment than that caused by some traditional hypnotics. The same feature means that multiple doses of trazodone are necessary to achieve steady-state concentrations. However, daytime sedation may limit this schedule. In 1 in 6,000 patients taking trazodone, α_1-adrenergic blockade causes priapism. Bupropion is not sedating and does not have anticholinergic or cardiotoxic effects. Unlike the serotonin reuptake inhibitors, bupropion does not have sexual side effects. However, divided doses are necessary, even with the sustained-release form, and doses greater than 450 mg/day are associated with a 5% incidence of seizures, which is a greater problem in bulimic patients.

Six serotonin reuptake inhibitors are available in the United States. Although these medications are called SSRIs, none is truly selective clinically or pharmacologically (Benkelfat 1993; Dubovsky 1994a; Grahame-Smith 1992; Jaim-Etcheverry and Zieher 1982; Lopez-Ibor 1988; McCormick and Williamson 1989; Meltzer 1989, 1992; van Praag et al.

TABLE 6–16. Tricyclic and tetracyclic antidepressants

Generic name	Trade name	Usual daily dose (mg)	Comments
Amitriptyline	Elavil	150–300	Sedating, anticholinergic; metabolized to nortriptyline
Nortriptyline	Pamelor, Aventyl	75–150	Therapeutic window 50–150 ng/mL
Protriptyline	Vivactil	15–60	Used for sleep apnea
Trimipramine	Surmontil	150–300	As potent as cimetidine as histamine H_2 antagonist
Imipramine	Tofranil	150–300	Reference antidepressant; metabolized to desipramine
Desipramine	Norpramin, Pertofrane	150–300	Therapeutic window in some studies 125–200 ng/mL
Doxepin	Sinequan, Triadapin	100–300	Like trimipramine; useful for treating allergies, esophagitis, peptic ulcer
Amoxapine	Asendin	150–600	A metabolite of loxapine, a neuroleptic; 7-OH metabolite of amoxapine has neuroleptic properties
Maprotiline	Ludiomil	150–225	A tetracyclic antidepressant between imipramine and desipramine in side-effect profile; doses above 225 mg/day associated with increased risk of seizures
Clomipramine	Anafranil	150–250	Only tricyclic effective for obsessive-compulsive disorder; doses above 250 mg/day can cause seizures

TABLE 6–17. Second- and third-generation antidepressants

Generic name	Trade name	Usual daily dose (mg)	Comments
Trazodone	Desyrel	200–600	Divided dose necessary for antidepressant effect
Bupropion	Wellbutrin	200–450	Sustained-release preparation still requires twice-daily dosing; drug can be used to treat SSRI-induced sexual dysfunction
Fluoxetine	Prozac	10–60	Therapeutic window may develop over time, requiring reduction in dose; parent drug has half-life of 3 days; biologically active metabolite has half-life of 6–9 days; drug can be more activating than other SSRIs
Sertraline	Zoloft	50–200	One metabolite with minimal activity
Paroxetine	Paxil	10–40	Anticholinergic properties equivalent to those of nortriptyline; may cause weight gain and withdrawal
Fluvoxamine	Luvox	100–300	Shorter half-life may necessitate twice-daily dosing for some patients
Citalopram	Celexa	10–40	Fewer pharmacokinetic interactions but similar side effects compared with other SSRIs
Escitalopram	Lexapro	10–40	The S-enantiomer of citalopram, this has greater affinity than citalopram for 5-hydroxytryptamine reuptake pump but does not have greater clinical efficacy
Venlafaxine	Effexor	75–375	Effective for refractory depression
Nefazodone	Serzone	200–600	Useful for sleep disorders
Mirtazapine	Remeron	15–45	Could have antiemetic properties; oversedation and weight gain are common

Note. SSRI = selective serotonin reuptake inhibitor.

1987). In addition to being equally effective treatments for major depression, the SSRIs have applications in anxiety disorders, OCD, posttraumatic stress disorder, eating disorders, and any condition associated with dysregulation of functions that are moderated by serotonergic systems, such as unpredictable, unprovoked aggression; recurrent, intrusive thinking; and excessive sexual or appetitive behavior. SSRIs all have similar side effects, including nausea, diarrhea, headache, activation, sedation, and sexual dysfunction. An action on 5-HT$_2$ heteroreceptors located on dopaminergic neurons in the basal ganglia can result in reduced dopaminergic transmission, which is sometimes manifested as emotional blunting and extrapyramidal side effects (Dubovsky and Thomas 1996). Fluoxetine and paroxetine inhibit the cytochrome P450 2D6 isoenzyme, whereas fluvoxamine inhibits the 3A4 isoenzyme. Some interactions that result are elevations of serum levels and elimination half-lives of TCAs, phenothiazines, warfarin, and many other medications by fluoxetine and paroxetine and of triazolobenzodiazepines, haloperidol, and astemizole by fluvoxamine. Additional P450 enzyme inhibitions occur with many of the SSRIs. Citalopram and escitalopram do not have significant effects on the cytochrome P450 system, and the effect of sertraline on this system usually is not clinically important.

Several third-generation antidepressants act on various neurotransmitters and receptors, with or without serotonin reuptake inhibition (Dubovsky 1994a; Montgomery and Fineberg 1989; G. Parker and Blennerhassert 1998; Poirier and Boyer 1999). Treatment with venlafaxine—which inhibits reuptake of serotonin, norepinephrine, and, to a lesser extent, dopamine—has been found to be efficacious in refractory depression, perhaps with a higher rate of remission than

the SSRIs. Norepinephrine reuptake inhibition is apparent only at higher doses (i.e., >75–150 mg) of this medication. The immediate-release form of venlafaxine requires divided dosing, which is also necessary with higher doses of the sustained-release (XR) form. Venlafaxine can have adverse effects related to all three neurotransmitters affected (e.g., headaches, jitteriness, activation). Mild elevation of diastolic blood pressure can occur; more severe hypertension develops rarely. Rapid discontinuation of venlafaxine has been associated with withdrawal symptoms, including headache, nausea, fatigue, dizziness, dysphoria, rebound depression, and occasionally hallucinations. Nefazodone has serotonin reuptake inhibition and 5-HT$_2$ antagonist properties. Unlike most antidepressants, nefazodone does not suppress REM sleep, and therefore the drug is associated with a lower incidence of disturbing dreams caused by REM rebound. The sedative properties of nefazodone and possibly its effect on slow-wave sleep make nefazodone a useful drug for treating patients with insomnia and fibromyalgia, but because of its short half-life, divided dosing is required, which can be difficult when patients experience daytime sedation or dizziness. Severe hepatotoxicity has been reported in 18 patients. Mirtazapine, which is related to the antidepressant mianserin, is an antagonist of 5-HT$_2$ and 5-HT$_3$ receptors and norepinephrine presynaptic α$_2$-adrenergic receptors. Antagonism of 5-HT$_2$ receptors could prove useful for treating psychotic depression (as could also be true of nefazodone), whereas 5-HT$_3$ receptor blockade could have an antiemetic effect. Sedation and weight gain are common adverse effects of mirtazapine.

The MAOIs (Priest et al. 1995) may be more frequently effective than TCAs for major depression with atypical features (SSRIs also appear to be more effective than the TCAs for atypical depression, although possibly less effective than the MAOIs). Four MAOIs are currently available in the United States. Phenelzine has more sedative and anticholinergic properties than do the other MAOIs but has probably been most widely used. Reports of the use of tranylcypromine, a more activating MAOI, in bipolar depression have been more consistently positive than those of the use of other antidepressants. L-Deprenyl (selegiline), which is used to treat Parkinson's disease in doses of 10 mg/day and may inhibit the progression of neurological damage as a result of an antioxidant effect, has antidepressant properties at doses of 30–50 mg/day. Isocarboxazid, which was recently re-released, is less activating than other MAOIs.

The most important limitations to the use of MAOIs have been hypertensive reactions when foods high in content of the pressor monoamine tyramine or sympathomimetic medications are ingested and serotonin syndrome when serotonergic substances such as SSRIs or dextromethorphan are used concurrently. These problems arise because inhibition of the A form of monoamine oxidase (MAO-A) in the small intestine leads to absorption of excessive amounts of tyramine, a pressor amine found in many foods. Systemic inhibition of MAO leads to accumulation of toxic levels of serotonin, another monoamine, when MAOIs are combined with serotonergic substances. Two approaches to minimizing this problem have emerged. The first involves developing medications that are selective for the B form of monoamine oxidase (MAO-B), which is present in high concentrations in the brain but not the gastrointestinal tract. Selegiline is an example of a selective MAOI, but at antidepressant doses, it loses its selectivity,

and dietary restrictions must be followed. Moclobemide is a reversible inhibitor of MAO-A that is displaced from the enzyme by tyramine, allowing the tyramine to be metabolized normally. Moclobemide is available in several countries but not in the United States because the manufacturer determined that the patent would expire before the cost of gaining Food and Drug Administration approval could be recovered.

Antipsychotic Medications

As we noted earlier, the response rate of psychotic depression to a combination of an antipsychotic drug and an antidepressant is significantly greater than the response to either one alone. Although most research into the use of antipsychotic medications in psychotic depression has involved the neuroleptics, especially perphenazine, the atypical antipsychotics are often medications of first choice because they are better tolerated and because they have antidepressant as well as antipsychotic properties.

Some patients with severe nonpsychotic depression respond to antidepressants as poorly as do patients with psychotic depression. In an 8-week double-blind, random-assignment trial in 28 patients with recurrent, nonbipolar, nonpsychotic depression that had been resistant to antidepressants, olanzapine or fluoxetine alone produced significantly less improvement than the combination of the two medications (Shelton et al. 2001b).

Novel Medications

In eight randomized controlled trials, St. John's wort (*Hypericum*) was more effective than placebo but less effective than TCAs in treating major depression of mild to moderate severity (Gaster and Holroyd 2000). A 6-week British study published after these studies randomly assigned

324 outpatients with mild major depression to 150 mg/day of imipramine or 500 mg/day of a standardized preparation of *Hypericum* extract (Remotiv/Imipramine Study Group 2000). Mean HRSD scores decreased by about 50% in both groups, but St. John's wort was better tolerated and more effective in reducing anxiety. The absence of a placebo group, the lack of a complete response in either group, and the relatively mild nature of the depression limited the interpretation of the data. One of these deficiencies was corrected in a more recent 8-week American multicenter study in outpatients with major depression and slightly higher baseline severity of depression who were randomly assigned to placebo or 1,200 mg/day of standardized *Hypericum* extract (Shelton et al. 2001a). Reductions in rating scale scores for depression and anxiety did not differ between the groups. Although St. John's wort usually is well tolerated, it may interact with highly serotonergic antidepressants and MAOIs, and occasional cases of apparent serotonin syndrome have been reported (V. Parker et al. 2001).

Observations of elevated activity of the hypothalamic-pituitary-adrenal axis in major depression noted earlier suggest that medications that inhibit cortisol production or action may be useful. In 28 reports of antiglucocorticoid treatment of Cushing's syndrome, depression improved in as many as 70% of the patients (Wolkowitz and Reus 1999). A few small open trials of CRF inhibitors in refractory and psychotic depression at least support the possibility that such approaches may reduce some depressive symptoms (Wolkowitz and Reus 1999), although this kind of treatment obviously is not without substantial risks. RU 486, which is a cortisol receptor antagonist at high doses, was a useful adjunct in several 1-week trials in psychotic depression.

S-Adenosylmethionine is a product of methionine metabolism that participates in transmethylation, transsulfuration, and transaminopropylation. Reports of reduced CSF levels of S-adenosylmethionine in depressed patients (Bottiglieri et al. 1990) led to a series of clinical trials of supplemental S-adenosylmethionine for depression. Double-blind comparisons of parenteral S-adenosylmethionine with placebo and several TCAs suggested efficacy in major depression (Janicak et al. 1988a). Comparisons of high doses of oral S-adenosylmethionine with imipramine and desipramine (Bell et al. 1994) in depressed inpatients found similar degrees of improvement in all groups, but in the absence of a placebo group, it is difficult to know whether this might have occurred with any substance.

Electroconvulsive Therapy

Unipolar Depression

ECT is the oldest and most reliable of the modern somatic therapies for mood disorders (Abrams 1988). ECT is most clearly useful in the case of acute major depressive episodes, especially when they are characterized by rapid onset, brief duration, severity, psychosis, motor retardation, catatonia, severe pseudodementia, lack of insight, and inability to tolerate antidepressants. ECT is also highly effective in mania and catatonia (Small et al. 1996).

Evidence has emerged of a relation between the dose of the electrical stimulus and response to unilateral ECT; stimulus intensities one to three times the seizure threshold appear to be more reliably effective in major depression (Devanand et al. 1991a; Lamy et al. 1994). In routine use, right (nondominant) unilateral ECT usually is used first in the treatment of a major depressive episode because it is associated with a lower risk of cognitive impairment. Bilateral ECT is used in cases of nonresponse to unilateral ECT and as an initial approach in severe depression, psychotic depression, catatonic stupor, Parkinson's disease, and depression in which a smaller number of ECT treatments is desirable (e.g., in cases of high anesthetic risk). Although 6–12 ECT treatments usually are sufficient for major depression, standard practice is to continue treatment until the patient responds; further treatment after this point is unnecessary and may produce intolerable cognitive impairment. An early practice of estimating the "dose" in ECT by the number of seizure seconds was not supported by later research.

ECT usually is recommended for depressed patients who are refractory to antidepressants because the expectation is that it will be effective when medications were not. Comparisons of patients who received adequate doses of antidepressants (or antidepressant-neuroleptic combinations for psychotic depression) with those who received inadequate medication doses found that about 90% of the latter responded to ECT, whereas the response rate was only about 50% for patients who received adequate antidepressant doses (Devanand et al. 1991a; Piper 1993; Sackeim 1994). The assumption that patients who were unresponsive to a particular antidepressant before ECT respond to that medication after ECT also was contradicted by the same research, which showed that antidepressants are no more effective after ECT than they were before it. However, a patient's ability to tolerate an antidepressant may be enhanced by ECT. Some form of maintenance therapy involving either adequate doses of antidepressants that have not been ineffective previously or continued periodic ECT treatments is necessary to prevent relapse and recurrence of depression (Sackeim 1994; Schwarz et al. 1995).

Maintenance ECT is safe and effective in preventing relapse and recurrence and is especially useful in the elderly, who tolerate maintenance pharmacotherapy poorly (Rabheru and Persad 1998).

The most common side effects of ECT are confusion and memory loss, and these effects are more pronounced after bilateral ECT (Aperia 1985; Calev et al. 1989, 1995; Krueger et al. 1992; Pettinati and Rosenberg 1984). Anterograde amnesia is most obvious within 45 minutes of a treatment, but loss of memory of events occurring from a few days to as long as 2 years before ECT (i.e., retrograde amnesia) also occurs. In some cases, personally significant memories from the recent or distant past (i.e., autobiographical memory) may be lost permanently. Most of the time, however, cognitive functioning after recovery from the acute effects of ECT is better than it was before the treatment, probably because of recovery from the cognitive impairment of depression (Calev et al. 1995; Krueger et al. 1992; Prudic et al. 2000; Sackeim et al. 1992). A small group of patients complain of severe cognitive disruption that cannot be demonstrated on objective testing (Prudic et al. 2000). Because these patients also have not had remission of depression, cognitive symptoms may represent residual depressive symptoms or perhaps awareness of subtle deficits that nondepressed individuals would ignore. No evidence from studies of cerebral structure or function shows that ECT as it is currently administered causes brain damage (Coffey et al. 1991; Weiner 1984).

Bipolar Disorder

ECT appears to be the most rapidly effective treatment for mania (H.S. Hopkins and Gelenberg 1994; Small et al. 1996) and the most effective treatment for bipolar depression (Bergsholm et al. 1992; H.S. Hopkins and Gelenberg 1994). In a review of the published literature on the efficacy of ECT for acute mania, Mukherjee et al. (1994) found that the overall rate of "remission or marked clinical improvement" was 80% (470 of 589 patients). Interpretation of these composite figures is limited by differences in methodology and outcome measures in the studies reviewed and by the secondhand assessment of data with a nonstandard method. Although some studies found that unilateral ECT was as effective as bilateral ECT (Black et al. 1987), others found bilateral ECT to be more frequently and more rapidly effective (Milstein et al. 1987; Small et al. 1985, 1996), possibly because of shunting of current through the scalp with the Lancaster right (nondominant) unilateral electrode placement, which was used in one study showing superiority of bilateral ECT (Mukherjee et al. 1994).

Repetitive Transcranial Magnetic Stimulation

Unipolar Depression

The hypothesis that the pathophysiology of depression involves in part hypoactivity of the left prefrontal cortex (Triggs et al. 1999) led to the application of a potent local magnetic field over the left prefrontal cortex (George et al. 1997; Mosimann et al. 2000), which induces a localized electrical current perpendicular to the magnetic field. Preliminary studies of motor evoked potential threshold suggested that changes in brain activity may occur at sites remote from the stimulus without a generalized electrical seizure in the brain (Triggs et al. 1999). High-frequency (10–20 Hz) repetitive transcranial magnetic stimulation (rTMS), which increases brain glucose metabolism and regional blood flow, has been found to be more effective in the treatment of major depression than low-frequency (1 Hz) rTMS and sham rTMS (Post et al. 1999).

Open studies have found that rTMS produces significant improvement in depressive symptoms in patients with refractory depression (Triggs et al. 1999) but has no effect on mood in nondepressed subjects (Mosimann et al. 2000). A random-assignment crossover comparison of active and sham high-frequency rTMS found that the active treatment reduced HRSD scores by 5 points, whereas HRSD scores increased by 3 points during sham treatment (George et al. 1997). ECT and rTMS were equivalently effective in a random-assignment trial in psychotic depression; this trial lacked a control group. On the other hand, a 2-week double-blind comparison of "real" and sham rTMS followed by 4 weeks of real rTMS failed to find a difference between the groups because of a high rate of spontaneous improvement in all subjects (C. Loo et al. 1999). Although rTMS is theoretically appealing because it does not have cognitive side effects (Kirkcaldie et al. 1997; Little et al. 2000), the only important adverse effects being headache and rare seizures, most studies are of very short duration and involve small numbers of subjects, limiting interpretation of the data. However, one study noted persistence of improvement 6 months after rTMS with maintenance antidepressant treatment.

Bipolar Disorder

Data on the potential efficacy of rTMS in bipolar disorder are very sparse, although it shows some promise (Post 1999). A comparison of fast left and right prefrontal rTMS in 16 manic patients found significantly more improvement with right than with left placement, which is the opposite of what has been found in unipolar depression (Grisaru et al. 1998).

Antimanic Drug Therapy

Medications that are used to treat mania (i.e., antimanic drugs) also are used to prevent or reduce the frequency of affective recurrences in bipolar disorder, in which case they are called *mood stabilizers*. A consensus panel involving 58 national experts produced strong agreement that antimanic drugs should be used in all phases of the treatment of bipolar disorder, including depression (Sachs et al. 2000).

Lithium

Lithium, the best studied of the antimanic drugs, has established efficacy as an antimanic and is prophylactic against recurrences of mania and depression in bipolar disorder (Schou 1997). Lithium may reduce depressive recurrences in highly recurrent unipolar depression (Schou 1995, 1997), and it reduces the risk of suicide in patients with mood disorders. Lithium appears to be most effective in patients with pure (i.e., not mixed) mania, complete remissions between episodes, the absence of rapid cycling, and no requirement for neuroleptics (Bowden 1995; Gelenberg and Hopkins 1993; H.S. Hopkins and Gelenberg 1994; Schou 1997). However, more than 50% of lithium-treated patients have another affective episode within 2 years (Goldberg et al. 1995), and the prophylactic effect of the drug is attenuated over time in 20%–40% of patients (Goldberg et al. 1995, 1996; Harrow et al. 1990; Post 1990b). Discontinuation of long-term use of lithium (and probably other mood stabilizers), especially if it is rapid, can result in rebound (i.e., worsening) of the mood disorder as well as refractoriness to the therapeutic effect of the medication when it is restarted in some (H.S. Hopkins and Gelenberg 1994; Post 1990a, 1990b) but not all (Berghofer and Miller-Oerlinghausen 2000) patients.

Lithium doses are adjusted by serum level. Although some studies suggest that trough levels greater than 0.8 mEq/L (0.8 mM) are associated with greater efficacy if more side effects, other research suggests that levels greater than 0.8 mM may not be more effective than levels of 0.5–0.8 mM, possibly because of greater dropout rates at the higher level (Vestergaard et al. 1998). Common adverse effects of lithium at therapeutic levels include polydipsia, polyuria, hypothyroidism, hyperparathyroidism, tremor, impaired cognitive function, nausea, and weight gain. The last-named side effect, along with interference with signaling of insulin receptors, makes lithium therapy problematic for diabetic patients.

On the other hand, lithium reduces excitotoxicity through an action on NO and increases expression of genes for neuroprotective proteins such as brain-derived neurotrophic factor. Lithium toxicity, which becomes more likely as serum levels exceed 1.5 mM, causes a coarse tremor, ataxia, vertigo, dysarthria, vomiting, delirium, muscle fasciculations, cardiotoxicity, and death. Debate continues about whether chronic lithium therapy causes nephrotoxicity (Schou 1997), but permanent neurotoxicity after lithium intoxication has been reported (Saxena and Maltikarjuna 1988). The 24-hour elimination half-life of chronically administered lithium permits once-daily dosing, which may reduce the frequency of adverse effects.

Anticonvulsants

The anticonvulsants carbamazepine and valproate (divalproex) also have been widely studied as antimanic drugs and mood stabilizers (Bowden 1995; Bowden et al. 1994; Chou 1991; Keck et al. 1992, 1993; McElroy et al. 1996b; Okuma et al. 1990; Post et al. 1993; Simhandl et al. 1993). Alone or in combination with each other or with lithium, the anticonvulsants may be more frequently effective than lithium in mixed mania, rapid-cycling bipolar disorder, and refractory bipolar disorder.

One study suggested that the therapeutic level of valproate in the treatment of acute mania may be around 100 μg/mL, which is achieved with daily doses of 750–5,000 mg (Bowden et al. 1994). Therapeutic levels can be achieved quickly through rapid oral loading (Keck et al. 1993). The dosage of carbamazepine (usually 400–1,200 mg/day) is frequently adjusted on the basis of serum level, but no scientific evidence indicates a specific therapeutic level for carbamazepine in epilepsy, let alone mood disorders (Chen 1931; Froscher 1992; Schoenenberger et al. 1995). On the other hand, higher serum levels are associated with more psychomotor impairment from the anticonvulsant (Thompson and Trimble 1983). The practice of obtaining periodic complete blood counts and of withdrawing carbamazepine if the white blood cell count drops below 3,000 will not prevent agranulocytosis because this extremely rare (2 cases in 525,000 patients) event occurs abruptly and is not correlated with the benign gradual decrease in white blood cell count that takes place during the first few months of carbamazepine treatment and then remits in one-third of patients. Use of anticonvulsants during pregnancy may be associated with fetal neural tube defects and cognitive deficits (Lindhout and Omtzigt 1992).

Two newer anticonvulsants, lamotrigine and gabapentin, which have been approved in the United States as adjuncts in the treatment of refractory epilepsy (Mattson 1995; M.J. McLean 1995), have been used in clinical settings to treat bipolar illness (Walden and Hesslinger 1995). A few case reports and open series have been published in which gabapentin was associated with improvement of mood in bipolar disorder (Cabras et al. 1999; Letterman and Markowitz 1999). However,

controlled studies have not confirmed this impression (Ghaemi and Gaughan 2000).

Lamotrigine was found in controlled trials to be useful in bipolar depression (Ghaemi and Gaughan 2000), and a small controlled study suggested efficacy in mania. In a 48-week open trial of lamotrigine as adjunctive treatment ($n = 60$) or monotherapy ($n = 15$) in patients with bipolar I and bipolar II disorder (Calabrese et al. 1999b), depressed patients had a mean reduction in depression scores of 42%, and patients with hypomania, mania, or a mixed state had on average a 74% reduction in mania rating scores. A group treated with a comparison medication and a placebo group would be necessary to be confident of the long-term efficacy of lamotrigine. In an open study of lamotrigine as an adjunctive (in 60 patients) or primary (in 15 patients) medication, patients with rapid cycling entering the study while depressed had a better response than did patients with predominantly manic symptoms (Bowden et al. 1999). A double-blind study by the same group found that 200 mg/day of lamotrigine monotherapy had a significant antidepressant effect in patients with bipolar depression compared with placebo (Calabrese et al. 1999a). A comparison of lamotrigine and lithium found the former to be better at lengthening the time to depressive recurrences and found lithium to be more effective at increasing the latency to manic recurrences.

The most frequent adverse effects of lamotrigine and gabapentin have been dizziness, headache, diplopia, ataxia, nausea, amblyopia, somnolence, fatigue, ataxia, rash, weight gain, and vomiting (Beydoun et al. 1995; Matsuo et al. 1996; M.J. McLean 1995; G.L. Morris 1995). The manufacturer raised concerns about dangerous allergic rashes with use of lamotrigine, but the risk is lower than originally reported. Gabapentin has been reported to induce mania (Hauck and Bhaumik 1995; Lweeke et al. 1999) and was associated with aggressive behavior, hyperactivity, and tantrums in some children, most of whom had ADHD (Lee et al. 1996; Tallian et al. 1996).

Calcium Channel Blockers

Increasing experience with refractory bipolar syndromes has created pressure for the development of alternative treatments for patients who do not tolerate or respond to lithium and the anticonvulsants. Of the various innovative therapies that have been proposed, the best studied are the calcium channel blockers. Double-blind trials of verapamil in manic or hypomanic individuals (Dose et al. 1986; Dubovsky et al. 1986; Garza-Trevino et al. 1992; Giannini et al. 1984, 1985, 1987; Hoschl and Kozemy 1989) and a blinded trial of nimodipine in 11 rapidly cycling patients (Post et al. 1993) have been reported. In two 4- to 5-week double-blind trials (Garza-Trevino et al. 1992; Hoschl and Kozemy 1989), equivalent antimanic efficacy of verapamil and lithium was found. Verapamil and nimodipine have been noted to have mood-stabilizing properties in some manic and rapidly cycling patients (Barton and Gitlin 1987; Giannini et al. 1987; Manna 1991; Wehr et al. 1988). One trial has been reported in which verapamil appeared to be less effective than lithium in the treatment of acute mania (Walton et al. 1996), but the results were limited by small absolute numerical differences between groups in rating scale scores, P values that usually would not be considered significant with the statistical measures used in the study, and the absence of any differences between mania rating scale scores in the lithium and verapamil groups.

The dosage of verapamil that has most frequently been found to be effective in bipolar mood disorders is 360–480 mg/day. A short elimination half-life requires dosing four times daily; the sustained-release formulation of verapamil is not predictably effective for mood disorders. The most common side effects are related to vasodilation and include dizziness, skin flushing, tachycardia, and nausea (Bigger and Hoffman 1991; Gerber and Nies 1991; Murad 1991). In randomized trials of calcium channel blockers for maternal hypertension, premature labor, and fetal arrhythmias during pregnancy, no evidence of teratogenicity was found, nor were there significant effects on uterine or placental blood flow (Byerly et al. 1991; Carbonne et al. 1993; Ulmsten et al. 1980; Wide-Swensson et al. 1996). In two published reports of the use of verapamil in pregnant patients, good control of mania and uneventful delivery of normal infants occurred (Goodnick 1993).

Antipsychotic Drugs

Case reports, studies, and reviews have suggested that chlorpromazine, haloperidol, pimozide, thiothixene, and thioridazine have applications alone or as adjuncts to lithium in maintenance as well as acute treatment of bipolar disorder (Ahlfors et al. 1981; Bigelow et al. 1981; Chou 1991; Esparon et al. 1986; Littlejohn et al. 1994; Lowe 1985; McCabe and Norris 1977; McElroy et al. 1996a; Prien et al. 1972; Rifkin et al. 1994). A critical review concluded that randomized controlled trials show that all neuroleptics have antimanic properties, especially as adjuncts; however, their efficacy as maintenance treatments is not well demonstrated.

Common problems that occur when bipolar disorder is treated with neuroleptics include increased risks of tardive dyskinesia and neuroleptic malignant syndrome (Bowden et al. 1994; Mukherjee et al. 1986) and neurotoxic interactions with lithium (Small et al. 1996). In addition, continuing neuroleptics for too long could make manic patients prone to more severe and prolonged depressive episodes and rapid cycling (Kukopulos et al. 1980; McElroy et al. 1996a). Naturalistic follow-up studies found that 34%–95% of patients continue to take neuroleptics alone or in combination with lithium 6–12 months after an index manic episode (Harrow et al. 1990). In some of these cases, continued neuroleptic therapy may be necessary for prevention of affective recurrence even if psychosis has remitted (Aronson et al. 1988). Such a possibility is supported by a finding that lithium alone ameliorated bipolar psychotic depression in 10 patients, but 8 patients required the addition of a neuroleptic to prevent relapses (Aronson et al. 1988).

Published reports suggest that clozapine, an atypical antipsychotic drug with complex actions, may have an antimanic effect in nonpsychotic as well as psychotic patients with bipolar and schizoaffective disorders (Banov et al. 1994; Calabrese et al. 1991; Frye et al. 1996; Klapheke 1991; McElroy et al. 1991; Privitera et al. 1993; Small et al. 1996; Suppes et al. 1992, 1994). Clozapine has been found useful for treating nonrapid- and rapid-cycling bipolar disorder (Calabrese et al. 1991, 1996) and refractory bipolar disorder (Green et al. 2000). Experience is insufficient to ascertain whether observations of better prophylaxis against recurrent mania than depression (Banov et al. 1994) are reliable, but this observation has been made about most effective mood-stabilizing treatments. In contrast, clozapine has not been reported to induce mania or rapid cycling.

Adverse effects of clozapine and the need for frequent laboratory monitoring, as well as potential enhancement of a crowded market for antipsychotic drugs, have stimulated interest in the newer atypical antipsychotic agents as possible adjunctive mood stabilizers. Impressions of a positive effect of risperidone in bipolar mood disorders (Madhusoodanan et al. 1995; Singh and Catalan 1994; Tohen et al. 1996a, 1996b) have involved low doses and trials that were probably too brief for any antidepressant properties of risperidone to predominate over the sedating and antipsychotic effects. The manufacturer sponsored two double-blind comparisons of placebo and olanzapine in an average dose of about 20 mg/day in manic inpatients. In the first trial, which lasted 3 weeks, 49% of the olanzapine-treated patients responded (50% reduction in Young Mania Rating Scale scores), compared with only 25% of the placebo patients (Tohen et al. 1999). In the second 4-week trial, olanzapine-treated patients had a mean 15-point reduction in Young Mania Rating Scale scores compared with an 8-point reduction with placebo (Tohen et al. 2000). However, at the end of both studies, patients who were improved (or defined arbitrarily as euthymic) in the second study were still symptomatic. In addition, reduction of Young Mania Rating Scale scores on items such as racing thoughts and decreased sleep that would be expected to be ameliorated by nonspecific sedative effects of the active medication was not held constant in the data analysis. Olanzapine was as effective as divalproex in a random-assignment trial in mania, but neither drug improved depressive symptoms.

Because other antipsychotic medications (e.g., haloperidol), benzodiazepines, and clonidine all have been found to be effective for acute mania, it remains to be shown that a putative antimanic action of atypical antipsychotics is specific to these medications. One issue that requires further study is the possibility that even if sedative and antipsychotic properties may be helpful for mania, antidepressant properties identified in multicenter schizophrenia trials (Anonymous 1998) could eventually overcome any potential anti-manic effect and lead to mood destabilization. This concern is supported to some extent by several reports of mania apparently induced by medications in this class (Benazzi 1999a; Borysewicz and Borysewicz 2000; Simon et al. 1999; Solhkhah et al. 2000). There have been a number of reports of increased manic symptoms specifically associated with treatment with risperidone (Dwight et al. 1994; Koek and Kessler 1996; Sajatovic 1996; Sajatovic et al. 1996; Schaffer and Schaffer 1996) and olanzapine (Benazzi 1999b; Fitz-Gerald et al. 1999; John et al. 1998; Lindenmayer and Klebanov 1998; London 1998; Pozo and Aleantara 1998; Reeves et al. 1998; Simon et al. 1999). An analysis of acute-mania olanzapine trials described earlier that found no increase in manic symptoms did not exclude the risk of a more gradual onset of an antidepressant effect.

Benzodiazepines

In the treatment of acute mania, addition to antipsychotic drugs of benzodiazepines, especially lorazepam and clonazepam, appears to provide more rapid control of agitation than do neuroleptics alone (Chouinard et al. 1983; Garza-Trevino et al. 1989; Salzman et al. 1986)—as well as a reduction in neuroleptic requirement—but not necessarily with fewer extrapyramidal side effects (Busch et al. 1989). Benzodiazepines have not been shown to have benefits other than improving sleep, agitation, or anxiety in patients with bipolar mood disorder. Benzodiazepines can have neurotoxic interactions with lithium (Aronson et al. 1989; Colwell and Lopez 1987; Freinhar and Alvarez 1985; Santos and Morton 1987). Tolerance may develop to the psychotropic (Post 1990b) and antiepileptic (Colwell and Lopez 1987) effects of clonazepam.

Omega-3 Fatty Acids

Because omega-3 fatty acids, like mood-stabilizing medications such as lithium, reduce hyperactive turnover of membrane phospholipids (Kinsella 1990), a possible advantage of these substances in bipolar disorder has been investigated. In the only published double-blind study (Stoll et al. 1999), patients who received slightly less than 10 g/day of omega-3 fatty acids in addition to their standard treatment had significantly longer periods of remission than did control subjects who received placebo (Severus and Ahrens 2000). Until more data are accumulated, the use of omega-3 fatty acids as adjunctive mood stabilizers must be considered experimental.

Thyroid Hormone

In patients treated openly, L-thyroxine in doses of 0.025–0.5 mg/day added to lithium or taken alone appeared to reduce or totally eliminate rapid affective recurrences in patients with bipolar mood disorders (Stancer and Persad 1982). Most of these patients had laboratory evidence of hypothyroidism (usually in the form of an elevated thyrotropin level), whereas in some cases, results of thyroid testing, including a TRH stimulation test, were normal. Bauer et al. (1990) prospectively studied 11 patients with rapid-cycling bipolar I or bipolar II illness who were taking lithium (6 patients); lithium and carbamazepine (2 patients); antidepressants alone (2 patients); a benzodiazepine alone (1 patient); neuroleptics as needed combined with other medications (4 patients); or thyroxine with other medications (3 patients). At the beginning of the study, only 3 patients had normal thyroid function, as indicated in part by normal results of a TRH stimulation test. In all patients, open addition of 0.15–0.4 mg/day of thyroxine (or increase of the existing thyroxine dose for patients already taking thyroxine) resulted in increases in serum thyroxine and decreases in thyrotropin concentrations into the hyperthyroid range. Of the 11 patients, 10 had significant decreases in depression and mania ratings and increases in ratings of quality of life for 78–370 days of follow-up. Of the 4 patients in whom a placebo was then substituted for thyroxine in a single-blind protocol, 3 experienced a return of cycling. Although these findings are provocative, the study was complicated by the open method in most patients, a single-blind discontinuation protocol in only 4 patients, a diverse group of patients likely to have had highly variable courses, and different lengths of thyroxine trials in different patients. To the extent that these high doses of thyroxine did in fact enhance the therapeutic effect of the thymoleptics, it is not clear whether this involved a primary action of the hormone or correction of central hypothyroidism in patients with poor delivery of thyroid hormone to the brain. There is no reason to think that thyroxine by itself has antimanic or mood-stabilizing properties in euthyroid patients. Risks of excessive thyroid replacement include anxiety, atrial fibrillation, and osteoporosis in menopausal women.

Psychotherapy for Mood Disorders

Certain psychotherapies have been found to be as effective as antidepressants, especially in less severe cases of unipolar depression (Sotsky et al. 1991). Two psychotherapies designed specifically for major depression—cognitive therapy (and a variant, CBT) and IPT—have been subjected to controlled research and have been compared with reference antidepressants. However, most studies have involved mildly to moderately depressed nonpsy-

chotic, nonbipolar patients. In addition, comparisons of psychotherapy with medication use imipramine, the standard reference antidepressant, in a fixed-dose protocol. The dropout rate in such protocols is undoubtedly greater than it is for patients taking antidepressants in clinical practice because newer, better-tolerated antidepressants are used and because a component of pharmacotherapy includes increasing the dose in the case of nonresponse, treating side effects, and encouraging compliance. In addition, antidepressant medications and psychotherapies may not be directly comparable because they act on different symptoms, psychotherapy working faster to improve social function and suicidal thinking and medications resulting in a faster onset of improvement of disturbed mood, sleep, and appetite.

In the NIMH Collaborative Research Program, unipolar, nonpsychotically depressed patients received a 16-week course of placebo plus "clinical management" (i.e., nonspecific supportive psychotherapy), imipramine plus clinical management, IPT, or CBT. For mildly depressed patients, no active treatment was any more effective than placebo plus clinical management, probably reflecting a high rate of spontaneous improvement or at least fluctuation of symptoms in this population. As depression became more severe, imipramine plus clinical management was found to be consistently superior on the broadest range of outcome measures. IPT was better than a placebo but not as effective as imipramine. CBT was only slightly less effective than IPT, but it was not significantly better than a placebo (Hollon et al. 1992). The results suggested that support and no medication might be effective for mild acute depression, whereas more severely depressed patients appear to require antidepressants.

Cognitive Therapy

Cognitive therapy is based on the premise that the negative emotions of depression are reactions to negative thinking derived from dysfunctional global negative attitudes. The patient and therapist work together to identify automatic negative thoughts, correct the pervasive beliefs that generate these thoughts, and develop more realistic basic assumptions (A.T. Beck et al. 1985). Treatment involves systematically monitoring negative cognitions whenever the patient feels depressed; recognizing the association between cognition, affect, and behavior; generating data that support or refute the negative cognition; generating alternative hypotheses to explain the event that precipitated the negative cognition; and identifying the negative schemata predisposing to the emergence of global negative thinking when one side of an all-or-nothing assumption is disappointed. In the course of examining dysfunctional attitudes, the patient learns to label and counteract information-processing errors such as overgeneralization, excessive personalization, all-or-nothing thinking, and generalization from single negative events.

The best studied of the psychotherapies for major depression, cognitive therapy has been compared with nonpharmacological-control conditions for the acute-phase treatment of depression in at least 21 randomized controlled clinical trials (Shea et al. 1988). In a meta-analysis of 12 suitable studies, cognitive therapy had an overall efficacy rate of 46.6% and was 30.1% more effective than no therapy in waiting-list control subjects (two studies) but was only 9.4% more effective than placebo plus clinical management in the collaborative study mentioned earlier. Although early studies reported superiority of cognitive therapy over pharmacotherapy provided by a primary care physi-

cian, comparisons with more rigorous pharmacological treatment provided by psychiatrists suggest equivalence of the two treatments for depression of moderate severity (Hollon et al. 1992).

Although some studies suggest that starting treatment with an antidepressant and then adding cognitive therapy (sequential combined therapy) may improve efficacy more than adding antidepressants to cognitive therapy (Bowers 1990; Hollon et al. 1992), in clinical practice, patients who have a poor response to cognitive therapy (or any psychotherapy) alone often respond to addition of antidepressants. Rates of response to individual cognitive therapy exceed those to group cognitive therapy (50.1% vs. 39.2%).

Monthly cognitive therapy achieved the same level of prophylaxis as continuation pharmacotherapy in one study (Blackburn et al. 1986). In a naturalistic follow-up study of cognitive therapy responders compared with antidepressant responders who had been withdrawn from medication and antidepressant responders treated with continuation pharmacotherapy, cognitive therapy–treated patients relapsed significantly less often than did patients treated initially with antidepressants who were withdrawn from antidepressant monotherapy (21% vs. 50% at 2 years) and at a rate comparable to that for antidepressant-treated patients who continued to take medication (15%).

After recovering from at least a third episode of major depression with TCAs or SSRIs administered according to a standardized protocol similar to that in the Frank et al. (1990) study discussed in the next section, 40 patients continued for 3–5 months with full doses of antidepressants, after which they were randomly assigned to pharmacotherapy plus CBT or pharmacotherapy plus "clinical management." Antidepressants were then withdrawn from both groups at a rate of 25 mg of amitriptyline equivalent every other week. CBT included treatment of residual negative cognitions, exposure to reduce anxiety, lifestyle modification, and well-being therapy (a two- to three-session approach to changing attitudes that interfere with positive self-regard, relationships with others, environmental mastery, and personal growth).

In this study, CBT but not clinical management resulted in significant improvement of residual symptoms. After 4 years (total follow-up = 6 years after completion of CBT), 50% of the CBT patients and 73% of the clinical management patients had at least one relapse, a nonsignificant difference; however, CBT patients had significantly fewer total episodes (i.e., fewer multiple recurrences) than the clinical management group (mean 0.8 ± 0.95 episodes in CBT vs. 1.7 ± 1.3 for clinical management) (Beauchamp et al. 1993). Of course, the question of whether simply continuing the antidepressant would have had a similar prophylactic effect was not addressed. The authors speculated that the short course of CBT (10 vs. the usual 16–20 sessions) was effective because CBT was added after medications had established a remission, at which point CBT was only needed for residual symptoms that might otherwise progress to relapse (Akiyoshi et al. 1996).

Interpersonal Therapy

IPT is designed to improve depression by enhancing the quality of the patient's interpersonal world (Klerman et al. 1984). The treatment begins with an explanation of the diagnosis and treatment options, legitimizing depression as a medical illness. The acute course of treatment is conducted according to a manualized protocol over 12–16 weeks. A protocol for maintenance IPT also has been developed. Through structured assignments, IPT helps the patient to work toward explicit goals related to whichever of the four basic interpersonal problems (unresolved grief, role disputes, transitions to new roles, and social skills deficits) is believed to be important. Role-playing is used to help the patient acquire new interpersonal skills, and structured conjoint meetings are used to help partners to clarify their expectations of each other.

In initial randomized clinical trials involving outpatients with nonpsychotic major depression, IPT was superior to amitriptyline in producing improvement in mood, suicidal ideation, and interest, whereas the antidepressant was more effective for appetite and sleep disturbances (DiMascio et al. 1979; Weissman et al. 1979). In the collaborative study mentioned earlier comparing IPT, cognitive therapy, imipramine plus clinical management, and placebo plus clinical management, IPT was found to be equivalent to imipramine and cognitive therapy by the end of 16 weeks, but imipramine was more rapidly effective.

Efficacy as a maintenance treatment as well as acute therapy has been shown for IPT. In a prospective study of 128 patients, each of whom had had at least two previous episodes of recurrent unipolar depression, patients were randomized after remission with treatment with imipramine to one of five treatment conditions: 1) continued monthly IPT with imipramine, 2) monthly IPT with placebo, 3) monthly IPT without medication, 4) imipramine with supportive management, and 5) placebo with supportive management. Both active-medication conditions were associated with about 80% relapse-free rates at 3-year follow-up. In addition, IPT with or without a placebo more than doubled relapse-free survival rates compared with placebo and supportive management at 3 years (30%–40% vs. 10%). Blind independent ratings of the quality of IPT indicated that patients treated with higher-quality IPT had 2-year relapse-free survival rates comparable with rates among patients treated with imipramine, and 3-year survival rates for patients in the former group were about 40%. Patients receiving IPT of below-average quality had survival rates that were no better than rates for patients receiving a placebo (Frank et al. 1991).

A form of IPT called interpersonal and social rhythm therapy (IPSRT) is under study as an adjunct to thymoleptic medication therapy in the maintenance treatment of bipolar mood disorders (Frank et al. 1994). In addition to interpersonal techniques such as encouraging the expression of grief for the loss of the person the patient was before the illness began and resolving interpersonal conflicts, IPSRT includes a structured approach to normalizing circadian rhythms. The patient first keeps a log that records the timing of 17 *zeitgebers* (e.g., getting out of bed, eating meals, first interaction with another person, exercising, going to bed). Average times for each of these cues to circadian rhythms are computed, and the patient is helped to keep a regular schedule for each of them.

After 1 year of prospective comparison of IPSRT with supportive psychotherapy, using an education and medication compliance module (each psychotherapy added to standard pharmacotherapy protocols), in patients who had achieved a remission of mania or bipolar depression for at least 4 months, patients treated with IPSRT were significantly more likely to have normalized their schedules of the 17 circadian cues (i.e., their schedules were identical to those of control populations studied with the same instrument). No significant clinical differences were found between the IPSRT and the sup-

portive psychotherapy groups after half of this planned 2-year study of a relatively small population had been completed. However, another study found that social rhythm therapy plus psychoeducation reduced recurrences in bipolar patients taking mood stabilizers.

Family Therapy

Involvement of the family is a defining characteristic of IPT. Family-focused treatment is a manualized psychoeducational treatment for bipolar disorder, the goal of which is to alter family interactions that interfere with medication adherence and promote affective recurrences. Patients and their relatives are exposed to a series of modules that focus on education about bipolar illness in general and their own symptoms in particular, developing a relapse prevention plan, enhancing communication between patients and their relatives, and solving family problems (Craighead and Miklowitz 2000). A recent study of this adjunctive treatment showed that it was associated with fewer relapses and longer delays before relapses when added to open treatment with mood-stabilizing medications.

Behavior Therapy

Therapies for depression derived from principles of classic and operant conditioning, social learning theory, and learned helplessness include social learning approaches (Lewinsohn et al. 1984; P.D. McLean 1982), self-control therapy (Rehm 1977), social skills training, and structured problem-solving therapy. Behavior therapies use education, guided practice, homework assignments, and social reinforcement of successive approximations in a time-limited format, typically over 8–16 weeks. Depressive behaviors such as self-blame, passivity, and negativism are ignored, whereas behaviors that are inconsistent with depression, such as activity, experiencing pleasure, and solving problems, are rewarded. Rewards can include anything that the patient seems to seek out—from attention, to praise, to being permitted to withdraw or complain, to money. Learned helplessness is combated by the therapist's giving patients small, discrete tasks that very gradually become more demanding. Social skills training teaches self-reinforcement, assertive behavior, and the use of social reinforcers such as eye contact and compliments.

In a meta-analysis of 10 suitable studies by the Agency for Health Care Policy and Services Research (1993), behavior therapy had an overall intention-to-treat efficacy rate of 55.3% and appeared to have a small advantage in relation to comparison psychotherapies in six studies and to pharmacotherapy in two studies. However, the adequacy of the treatments to which behavior therapy was compared has been questioned (Crits-Christoph 1992; Meterissian and Bradwejn 1989). Behavior therapy has appeared to be as effective in depression as it is in other psychiatric disorders (Budman et al. 1988). Group and individual behavior therapies appear to have similar efficacy rates. Support for the efficacy of maintenance behavior therapy in preventing depressive recurrence is not as well developed as is support for its efficacy as an acute treatment.

Psychodynamic Psychotherapy

No controlled studies of prolonged psychodynamic psychotherapy or psychoanalysis in mood disorders have been done. Brief dynamic psychotherapies have been applied to depressive disorders (Davanloo 1982; Luborsky 1984; J. Mann 1973; Strupp and Binder 1984), but they have not been studied as rigorously as

TABLE 6–18. Characteristics of an effective psychotherapy for depression

Time limited
Explicit rationale for treatment shared by patient and therapist
Active and directive therapist
Focus on current problems
Emphasis on changing current behavior
Self-monitoring of progress
Involvement of significant others
Expression of cautious optimism
Problems divided into manageable units with short-term goals
Homework assignments

have cognitive therapy and IPT (American Psychiatric Association 1993).

Characteristics of an Effective Psychotherapy for Depression

Even though data from controlled studies of psychotherapy for depression are limited, the characteristics listed in Table 6–18 have repeatedly emerged as distinguishing effective treatments, regardless of the technical details of the therapy (Thase 1996). Extended, unstructured psychotherapies may be useful for treating associated problems such as personality disorders, but given the lack of data supporting the use of these therapies as primary treatments for depression, more focused, time-limited therapies seem appropriate, at least as initial approaches.

Combining Medications and Psychotherapy

Until more informative data become available about mild to moderate unipolar nonpsychotic depression, the recommendation that such depressive episodes be treated initially either with antidepressants or with one of the focused psychotherapies for depression (Klerman et al. 1974) seems reasonable. Some experts suggest that more severe major depressive episodes be treated first with antidepressants alone, so that time is not lost and the expense of psychotherapy is avoided for those patients who respond to a single treatment. These experts recommend combining medication and psychotherapy for patients with an inadequate response to either modality, with multiple symptom clusters that might respond differentially to psychotherapy and medication, or with a previously chronic course. More severe cases of depression may be more likely to have a better response to combined pharmacotherapy and psychotherapy than either treatment alone (Doris et al. 1999).

Because addition of IPT to antidepressants reduced the attrition rate from 21% to 8% in the continuation therapy study of patients with recurrent unipolar depression, psychotherapy should be included in the maintenance treatment of recurrent unipolar depression, even if the index episode was not severe. However, as mentioned earlier, adding psychotherapy to antidepressants may be more efficient than starting both treatments at the same time unless barriers to compliance with medications are identified at the start of treatment or the mood disorder is more severe or complex. Combining thymoleptic (mood-stabilizing) medications with IPSRT and behavioral techniques that reduce expressed emotion in the family shows promise of improving both medication compliance (Cochran 1984) and overall treatment response in bipolar mood disorders (Goodwin and Jamison 1991; Miklowitz 1992).

Integrated Treatment of Mood Disorders

Although psychotherapy and antidepressants are equally effective for mild depression (Martin et al. 1992), controlled outpatient studies of nonbipolar depression showed that combined pharmacotherapy and psychotherapy was significantly more effective than psychotherapy alone for severe depression (Martin et al. 1992). A "mega-analysis" involved a meta-analysis of original data of 595 patients with nonbipolar, nonpsychotic MDD enrolled in six standardized treatment protocols in which they received treatment for 16 weeks with either CBT or IPT alone ($n = 243$) or IPT plus an antidepressant ($n = 352$). In mild depression, combined therapy was not significantly more effective than psychotherapy alone. However, in more severe recurrent major depression, combined treatment was significantly more effective. In a comparison of monotherapy with nefazodone, a form of CBT alone, or the combination of the two, the combination was statistically and clinically significantly superior to either treatment alone in producing initial improvement and preventing relapse in patients with chronic depression (Keller et al. 2000).

The American Psychiatric Association (1993) "Practice Guideline for Major Depressive Disorder in Adults" states that successful treatment of mood disorders begins with a careful diagnostic, psychosocial, and medical evaluation and consideration of the patient's treatment preferences. The initial assessment of the patient with a mood disorder (and all subsequent treatment) occurs in the context of a relationship between doctor and patient. This interaction is crucial to the development of a therapeutic alliance (Sexton et al. 1996) in which the patient is engaged in a collaborative enterprise. In the NIMH Collaborative Study, the therapeutic alliance significantly affected outcomes of IPT, CBT, active pharmacotherapy, and placebo (Blatt et al. 1996; Krupnick et al. 1996). Treatment dropout rates are less than 10% when a collaborative alliance has been fostered.

Evaluation of risk factors for suicide is essential in all patients with mood disorders (Buzan and Weissberg 1992). Because suicidal patients, especially those with psychotic mood disorders, bipolar illness, or both, may kill someone else before they kill themselves, homicide risk also should be evaluated. Dangerousness is not a static issue but one that evolves with the mood disorder. It is therefore necessary to reevaluate dangerousness to self and others repeatedly throughout the treatment of a mood disorder.

Review of the patient's use of substances that can cause or aggravate depression and mania is another essential component of the evaluation of the patient with a mood disorder. Ongoing debate about the possibility of starting an antidepressant before abstinence has been achieved notwithstanding, it is much more difficult to treat a mood disorder in a patient who is actively using alcohol or illicit drugs.

The next important step is to decide whether the mood disorder is unipolar or bipolar. Such a distinction is crucial given the different treatment approaches to the two disorders. When a patient has a clear-cut history of mania, the diagnosis is straightforward; bipolar disorder may be more difficult to identify when a patient has had one or a few depressive episodes without obvious manic or hypomanic symptoms. Clues to bipolarity in a depressed patient are summarized in Table 6–19, although like all other aspects of mood disorders, the bipolar-unipolar distinction is one that may be clarified only with continued observation.

Unipolar Major Depressive Disorder

A mildly to moderately severe single major depressive episode without psy-

TABLE 6–19. Clues to bipolarity in depressed patients

Highly recurrent depression
Intense anger
Racing thoughts
Mood-incongruent psychotic symptoms
Hallucinations
Thrill seeking
Increased libido with severe depression
Family history of bipolar disorder
Three consecutive generations with mood disorders

chotic features can be treated with antidepressants or psychotherapy. However, the longer the duration of the episode or the greater its severity, the more likely an antidepressant is to be needed. Even if formal psychotherapy is not provided, antidepressant prescriptions should at least be accompanied by informed psychological management (Merriam and Karasu 1996). Because the presence of a comorbid personality disorder or perfectionism predicts a poorer response to antidepressants (Blatt 1995), as well as to briefer psychotherapies (Thase 1996), more intensive forms of psychodynamic psychotherapy may be appropriately added to antidepressants when these factors are present (Conte et al. 1986; I.W. Miller and Keitner 1996), although empirical support for this approach has not yet emerged.

As was mentioned earlier, all of the currently available antidepressants are equally effective (Bech 1993; Kasper et al. 1992). This is not to say that all antidepressants are equally effective for all patients; many patients who do not respond to one agent will respond to another (Rush and Kupfer 1995). The initial choice of an antidepressant generally depends on history and current symptoms. For example, patients who have had a good response to a particular antidepressant may respond to the same medication again, although an antidepressant that was effective at one point may not be as effective on a second trial. Insomnia associated with depression often improves with remission of depression, but more sedating antidepressants such as doxepin, imipramine, trazodone, mirtazapine, and nefazodone can produce more rapid relief of insomnia, whereas more activating antidepressants such as fluoxetine, bupropion, and tranylcypromine can aggravate insomnia (Neylan 1995).

Once recovery with antidepressant therapy begins, its time course is the same as spontaneous remission, suggesting that antidepressants may speed recovery but not change its natural course. One implication of this finding is that antidepressants should be continued acutely at least for at least as long as the depressive episode would be expected to last if it had remained untreated. It may take longer than anticipated in the acute treatment of major depression to produce a complete remission. For example, in a Dutch cohort of 56 patients with MDD treated with pharmacotherapy and psychotherapy (Van Londen et al. 1998), 49% of the patients had a full remission and 45% had a partial remission after 9 months. Over the next 3–5 years, 82% had full remission; 16% of the patients required 2 years to reach a full remission. Over the same period, 41% of the sample had recurrences.

Another investigation randomized patients with chronic major or double depression who were partial responders after 3 months of treatment with either imipramine or sertraline to continuation treatment with the same antidepressant. During the next 4 months, 50% of the sample had remissions, 30% remained partial responders, and 20% underwent a change from partial to no response. This result suggests that partial responders to treatment of chronic depression may

respond to an additional 4 months of treatment. After satisfactory responses for 7 months, the responders were randomized to maintenance with sertraline or placebo. Sertraline was clinically and statistically superior to placebo in preventing relapse.

Antidepressant overdose is the most common method of suicide in the United States (Buzan and Weissberg 1992). A large body of clinical experience contradicts a report of a small number of cases in which suicidal ideation was thought to be increased by SSRIs (Teicher et al. 1993) and indicates that the risk of suicide is reduced by all antidepressants, especially SSRIs, which decrease inwardly as well as outwardly directed impulsive aggression (Isacsson et al. 1996; Letizia et al. 1996; Warshaw and Keller 1996). Because the newer antidepressants are safer in overdose than TCAs, SSRIs, venlafaxine, mirtazapine, and nefazodone may be the best initial choices for suicidal patients (Montgomery 1995). If the risk of suicide is so great that the physician cannot trust the patient with an antidepressant, the patient should be hospitalized.

ECT is a particularly appropriate option for patients who are too severely depressed or suicidal to wait for an antidepressant to take effect, patients who cannot tolerate an antidepressant, and patients with associated illnesses that might benefit from ECT, such as delirium or Parkinson's disease (Devanand et al. 1991a).

A substantial amount of information has accumulated about the treatment of major depression with psychotic features. Psychotic depression has a very low rate of spontaneous recovery (Kettering et al. 1987) and virtually no response to placebo (Spiker and Kupfer 1988) or psychotherapy alone. Only 0%–46% (average, about 25%–35%) of patients with psychotic depression respond to TCAs (Avery and

Lubano 1979; W.H. Nelson et al. 1984), even in high doses (Avery and Lubano 1979; W.H. Nelson et al. 1984; Spiker et al. 1986b); MAOIs do not produce better results (Janicak et al. 1988b). Whereas 19%–48% of psychotically depressed patients recover with antipsychotic medications alone (Spiker et al. 1986a, 1986b), the combination of a neuroleptic and an antidepressant leads to improvement in an average of 70%–80% of patients (Anton and Burch 1986; Aronson et al. 1988; Spiker et al. 1986b). Higher neuroleptic doses than those used for schizophrenia may be needed for psychotic depression (Aronson et al. 1987; J.C. Nelson et al. 1986; Spiker et al. 1985, 1986b). Amoxapine, an antidepressant that is a metabolite of the neuroleptic loxatine and has neuroleptic properties of its own, is almost as effective as traditional neuroleptic–antidepressant combinations in psychotic depression (Anton and Burch 1986). Preliminary experience suggests that atypical antipsychotic drugs also may be effective as monotherapy (McElroy et al. 1991). The response rate of psychotic depression is greatest with ECT (Solan et al. 1988).

The antidepressant properties of atypical antipsychotic agents, and their lower risk of neurological side effects, make these medications appealing choices for treating psychotic depression. A review of records of 15 hospitalized patients with discharge diagnoses of unipolar or bipolar depression with psychotic features who were given olanzapine compared with matched patients who took neuroleptics (most in each group also taking antidepressants) found a higher rate of improvement in the patients who received olanzapine (Rothschild et al. 1999). Obviously, controlled prospective trials would be necessary to determine whether atypical antipsychotic drugs may be effective alone or in combination with antidepressants.

Following initial improvement, response to an antidepressant sometimes fades. A review of published double-blind, placebo-controlled trials with at least 20 patients reporting loss of antidepressant efficacy during maintenance treatment found this problem to be reported in 9%–33% of patients. Relapse during the first 12 weeks was thought to reflect loss of an initial placebo response, especially when features of a placebo response such as abrupt, fluctuating improvement were present initially. The authors found 75 reported cases that were thought to reflect tolerance to antidepressants following full remission rather than loss of a placebo effect. Tolerance to antidepressants has been reported with serotonin reuptake inhibitors, heterocyclic antidepressants, and MAOIs.

Certain varieties of treatment-emergent loss of antidepressant benefit require a more global reconsideration of the pharmacological strategy. The most important of these is bipolar depression masquerading as recurrent or fluctuating unipolar depression. The antidepressant is effective initially, but as it accelerates the tendency of bipolar depression to recur as well as its tendency to remit, another episode appears that is mistaken for loss of antidepressant efficacy. A change in the antidepressant produces another remission, but this is inevitably followed by another recurrence, often mixed with dysphoric hypomanic symptoms such as anxiety, intense irritability, racing thoughts, inability to shut one's mind off and get to sleep, overstimulation, or subtle psychotic symptoms. Whereas continuing to change the dose or preparation of the antidepressant produces more recurrences and sometimes more persistent depression, adding a mood-stabilizing medication and gradually withdrawing the antidepressant often eliminates depressive recurrences.

Dysthymic Disorder and Chronic Major Depression

Placebo-controlled trials show that dysthymia responds as well as major depression does to TCAs, SSRIs, MAOIs, and atypical antidepressants such as tianeptine, although rates of noncompliance related to demoralization and intolerance of adverse effects are high (Harrison and Stewart 1993; Kocsis et al. 1988, 1989). In a comparison of the effect of ECT in 25 patients with double depression and 75 patients with MDD only, Prudic et al. (1993) found that both groups had the same level of improvement in depression rating scale scores. However, patients with double depression had more residual symptoms and were more likely to relapse in the year following ECT, which suggests that the underlying dysthymia had been incompletely treated.

Psychotherapies that have been found useful for treating chronic depressive disorders, albeit creating a less robust response than in acute depression (Thase et al. 1994), include cognitive therapy, IPT, behavior therapy, CBT, supportive therapy, psychoeducation, and family and marital therapy (Akiskal 1994; Keitner and Miller 1990). Combining specific psychotherapies with antidepressants produces better results than medication therapy alone in dysthymic patients (J. Scott 1988). Maintenance pharmacotherapy and psychotherapy are particularly important in reducing the risk of recurrence of dysthymia, as well as that of chronic major depression and double depression.

Recurrent Brief Depression

Only a few studies of the treatment of recurrent brief depression have been done. The data that have emerged suggest that antidepressants are not particularly effective in preventing acute depressive recurrences (Angst et al. 1990). Lithium may reduce recurrences, even though no evidence has emerged of a bipolar outcome in recurrent brief depression (Angst and Hochstrasser 1994). It is not known whether other mood-stabilizing medications might reduce the rate of recurrence of this form of depression, but insofar as all of these medications have antirecurrence as well as antimanic properties, it seems reasonable to consider using them.

Seasonal Affective Disorder

Artificial bright light is an effective treatment for SAD in which rates of remission in published studies range from 36% to 75%. The minimal intensity of light that appears necessary for an antidepressant effect is 2,500 lux (1 lux = 10 foot candles) placed about 1 m from the patient. At greater intensities of light, a shorter duration of exposure to the light appears necessary. For example, remission rates with a 10,000-lux light unit for 30 minutes are similar to those with 2,500 lux for 2 hours. To be effective, light must enter the patient's eyes.

Although some patients respond exclusively to morning light and some respond equally well to light administered at any time of the day, few patients respond preferentially to evening light. Some authorities recommend that the patient start the treatment at whatever time of day is most convenient, so that compliance is increased, whereas others think that morning light should be tried first, especially in patients who tend to sleep late. Exposure to light too late in the day may make it difficult to fall asleep. There do not appear to be clinically significant differences in the effectiveness of any particular wavelength of light or of full-spectrum light versus cool-white fluorescent light.

Many patients respond to bright light within 3–5 days and relapse if they discontinue the light treatment for 3 days in a row during the winter. However, some patients who do not respond after 1 week of treatment will respond during the second week (Labbate et al. 1995). Patients with bipolar SAD may have a better response to artificial bright light than do patients with unipolar SAD (Deltito et al. 1991).

Several medications, including fluoxetine, moclobemide, tranylcypromine, bupropion, and alprazolam, appear to be at least as effective as bright light for treating SAD. Whereas some patients prefer bright light because it is not a medication and has no real interactions, others find antidepressants more convenient, especially if they travel frequently. In patients with yearly recurrences of seasonal depression, prophylactic bright light therapy usually is begun in the early fall and continued through the spring to prevent depressive recurrences. It is not known whether seasonal administration of antidepressants is as effective in preventing winter recurrences of depression or whether chronic antidepressants would be more appropriate. Patients with bipolar SAD can be treated with seasonal use of bright light with or without a thymoleptic, depending on the response to the light and whether thymoleptics alone prevent seasonal recurrences.

Unipolar Depression: Maintenance Treatment

It is commonly recommended that antidepressants be continued for 6–9 months after a single episode of unipolar major depression (Consensus Development Panel 1985). However, this recommendation is based on only observational data and a small number of discontinuation studies (Abernathy and Schwartz 2000) and does not take into account the capacity of antidepressants to prevent recurrence, which occurs within 2 years of remission of a first episode in 50% of the

patients not taking maintenance antidepressants (Consensus Development Panel 1985). The decision to withdraw an antidepressant after the first major depressive episode therefore is more complex than it might appear at first glance.

If the episode was relatively mild and easy to treat, the risk of discontinuing antidepressants is relatively low. Conversely, if the episode was severe or had major consequences such as a serious suicide attempt, inability to work, or disruption of the family, the risk of another episode may be substantially greater than the inconvenience of continuing antidepressant treatment. If depression responded only after multiple antidepressant trials, the benefit of continuing antidepressants may outweigh the risk of another long and difficult course of treatment. After improvement of depression with psychotherapy or pharmacotherapy, relapse and recurrence are up to five times more likely to occur after treatment withdrawal if residual symptoms are present (Blackburn et al. 1986; Thase et al. 1992). Slower antidepressant withdrawal may be less likely to be followed by relapse than rapid drug discontinuation.

After three or more episodes, withdrawal of the antidepressant within 5 years of remission has been found to be associated with an increased risk of recurrence. In view of reliable data indicating that relapse and recurrence of unipolar depression are reduced by continuation of the antidepressant (Devanand et al. 1991a; Fava and Kaji 1994; Frank et al. 1993), patients with recurrent unipolar depression should continue to take an effective antidepressant indefinitely. Of 23 prospective, double-blind, randomized studies of continuation and maintenance pharmacotherapy for depression, 22 found more recurrences in the placebo group, and the only study that detected no difference involved too small a sample to be reliable (Solomon and Bauer 1993). The same dose that produced a remission appears necessary to prevent recurrence (Blackburn 1994; Devanand et al. 1991a; Frank et al. 1993).

There have been at least 25 reports on the use of continuation/maintenance ECT since 1987 that suggest that such therapy can decrease rehospitalization rates by two-thirds or more (Petrides et al. 1994; Schwarz et al. 1995; Vanelle et al. 1994; Weiner 1995). Continuation/maintenance ECT is frequently administered on an outpatient basis, which increases patient acceptance (Association for Convulsive Therapy 1996). The frequency of maintenance treatments is based on symptom emergence as the time between ECT treatments is gradually increased.

Because cognitive therapy (Belsher and Costello 1988; Fava and Kaji 1994), CBT (J. Scott 1992), and IPT (Frank et al. 1991) have an additive effect with antidepressants in reducing the risk of recurrence of unipolar depression, there is good reason to assume that continuation, possibly at a reduced frequency, of one of these psychotherapies—or any other psychotherapeutic approach that has proven useful in acute depression—along with the antidepressant will reduce the risk of relapse or recurrence of major depression or dysthymia. A random assignment trial of 10 sessions of continuation cognitive therapy for 8 months after remission of an acute episode of unipolar depression with a standard course of 20 sessions of cognitive therapy found that 16 months after conclusion of the continuation phase, the risk of relapse and recurrence was significantly reduced in the group that received continuation cognitive therapy (Jarrett et al. 2001). This finding may suggest that the benefit of maintenance psychotherapy persists longer after the treatment is discontinued than is the case for maintenance pharmacotherapy, or the relatively

prolonged benefit of a continuation phase of psychotherapy may have been a function of patients in this trial being less severely ill than the patients in studies of maintenance pharmacotherapy.

One problem that might be particularly responsive to maintenance psychotherapy is nonadherence with continuation of antidepressants. Between 33% and 68% of depressed patients have been found to be noncompliant with antidepressants (Burrows 1992; Jacob et al. 1984; Overall et al. 1987). Compliance with psychotherapy usually is better than with pharmacotherapy (Basco and Rush 1995), probably because psychotherapy has fewer adverse effects and because there is more focus on the clinician–patient alliance.

Residual dysfunction commonly persists after remission of specific depressive symptoms. In addition to attenuated depressive symptoms, residual symptoms may include personality problems, social maladjustment, interpersonal friction, inhibited communication, poor work or school performance, and dysfunctional attitudes. Patients often overlook subsyndromal residual symptoms (Figiel et al. 1990), whereas physicians may mistake them for indications of a comorbid personality disorder.

It is not uncommon for patients and their physicians to discontinue treatment at this point, with important consequences. Over time, patients experience deterioration of self-esteem, an increase in dysfunctional attitudes, greater functional and role impairment, more utilization of medical services, a higher suicide risk, and an increased risk of recurrence and relapse. Like patients with residual depressive symptoms, patients with residual social dysfunction have a high risk of relapse and recurrence (Martin et al. 1992). Conversely, patients who are completely asymptomatic are less likely to have recurrences than are those with residual symptoms.

Preventing the negative effect of residual symptoms on current functioning and later liability to recurrence involves several principles. The finding that as many as 46% of patients with partial remissions ultimately had a full remission with continuation of aggressive treatment is an indication for continuing acute treatment for a longer time in chronically depressed patients if improvement has not reached a distinct plateau at a level lower than remission. However, it is important to use the most aggressive treatment possible to produce a remission rather than just a response.

Use of Antidepressants in Children and Adolescents

Experience with antidepressants has not been as positive in younger patients as it has been in adults. In placebo-controlled trials, the efficacy of TCAs has consistently been found to be equivalent to that of placebo in children with major depression and less than that of placebo in adolescents with this disorder (Ambrosini et al. 1993).

One of two controlled studies of fluoxetine in children and adolescents showed superiority of fluoxetine to placebo, and one study showed no difference between placebo and active drug. A controlled study of venlafaxine in 33 patients age 8–17 years showed no differences between active drug and placebo, but dosages were very low and patients given placebo as well as those given venlafaxine received psychotherapy in addition to medication. Phase IV studies found superiority to placebo of sertraline, paroxetine, and fluvoxamine in younger depressed patients. ECT is about as effective and safe in juvenile patients as it is in adults (Bertagnolli and Borchardt 1990; Fink

1993; Schneekloth et al. 1993; Walter and Rey 1997).

Given the current state of knowledge, children and adolescents with depression should first receive individual and/or family psychotherapy (Emslie et al. 1995); more intensive psychotherapies may be more likely to achieve full recovery. Nonresponders to psychotherapy might receive an SSRI before any other class of antidepressant. The high rate of bipolar outcome and the lack of any prospective studies of antidepressant maintenance therapy warrant discontinuation of antidepressants at some point after remission, but the timing of this intervention remains to be studied.

Mania

An expert consensus panel that compiled opinions of 58 national experts agreed that mood-stabilizing medications should be used in all phases of treatment of bipolar disorder (Sachs et al. 2000). The consensus panel suggested lithium or divalproex as initial treatments, with carbamazepine as the next choice. Antipsychotic medications were recommended for psychotic bipolar disorder and as adjuncts for severe nonpsychotic mania and mixed states. Anticonvulsants were preferred over lithium for mixed and rapid-cycling states.

Lithium, carbamazepine, valproate (divalproex), and verapamil appear to be equally effective in the treatment of acute mania; response rates range from 60% to 78% (Bowden 1995; Bowden et al. 1994; Delgado and Gelenberg 1995; Dubovsky 1994b, 1995). Lithium is the best studied and most clearly established of these agents, whereas verapamil has not been subjected to multicenter studies. Treatment with lithium may be less effective than treatment with the anticonvulsants in mixed (dysphoric) mania and rapid cycling (McElroy et al. 1992); however, a direct comparison of carbamazepine and lithium in rapid-cycling bipolar disorder found both drugs to be equally effective (Okuma et al. 1990). Treatment with combinations of antimanic drugs may be more effective than that with a single medication (Keck et al. 1992).

Until recently, neuroleptics, particularly haloperidol, were used routinely to control agitation until the antimanic drug took effect. However, not all manic patients are psychotic, and psychosis accompanying mania may remit with adequate treatment of the mania (Cohen and Lipinski 1986; Fennig et al. 1995; Goodwin and Jamison 1991; Prien et al. 1972). Supplementation of neuroleptics with the benzodiazepines lorazepam or clonazepam was introduced as a means of minimizing neuroleptic exposure with its attendant risks of side effects and adverse interactions with antimanic drugs (Sachs 1990; Salzman et al. 1986). The atypical antipsychotic drugs can be used with or without benzodiazepines as treatments of acute mania, but given the current state of knowledge, they should be considered supplements for established antimanic drugs because their mood-stabilizing properties (i.e., their capacity to reduce affective recurrences) have not been established. Benzodiazepines have been used without antipsychotic drugs in the initial treatment of mania (Bradwejn et al. 1990; Colwell and Lopez 1987; Lenox et al. 1986; Modell et al. 1985; Santos and Morton 1987). The benzodiazepine, with or without an antipsychotic drug, can be administered first to improve agitation and sleep. Once the patient's behavior is under better control, any antipsychotic medications that have been prescribed should be slowly withdrawn as an antimanic drug is gradually introduced. Although some patients, especially those with persistent severe depression, may

benefit from continuation of an atypical antipsychotic medication, the possibility that antidepressant actions of these medicines may eventually predominate should be kept in mind.

Bipolar Depression

Fewer controlled studies of the treatment of bipolar depression than of other forms of depression have been done (Brady et al. 1995; Post et al. 1997; Sachs et al. 2000). However, in view of the risk of antidepressant-induced mania and rapid cycling noted earlier, the American Psychiatric Association (1994b) "Practice Guideline for the Treatment of Patients With Bipolar Disorder," the Expert Consensus Guidelines (Sachs et al. 2000), and other expert opinions (Compton and Nemeroff 2000; Nolen and Bloenkolk 2000) recommend that treatment of bipolar depression begin with an antimanic drug. Lithium has been noted to be an effective antidepressant in 30%–79% of bipolar depressed patients (Sachs et al. 1994b). Valproate and carbamazepine have not been as well studied for treatment of bipolar depression, but experience suggests that they usually are not effective antidepressants as monotherapies (American Psychiatric Association 1994b). Lamotrigine has more obvious antidepressant properties (Sachs et al. 2000); however, because its capacity to stabilize mood at the same time remains to be clearly established, it is probably safer to combine it with a well-established antimanic drug.

When bipolar depression does not remit with treatment with an antimanic drug, the clinician must decide whether to add a second antimanic drug or an antidepressant. Antimanic drugs are not as effective as antidepressants for treating depression and have more adverse effects, but all antidepressants carry the risk of inducing mania and rapid cycling (Akiskal 1994; Peet and Peters 1995; Srisurapanont et al. 1995). In the absence of controlled data, only clinical experience and expert opinion are available to guide the choice between these two courses. Our experience has been that antidepressants do not produce a predictably positive response in bipolar depression with prominent mixed hypomanic symptoms such as profound irritability, decreased sleep without feeling tired during the day, racing thoughts, extreme interpersonal sensitivity, hallucinations, or increased libido. Instead, the antidepressant either provokes more dysphoric hypomania or produces initial improvement followed by more recurrences of mixed bipolar depression. Treatment with a combination of antimanic drugs may produce a remission, or it may at least convert a refractory mixed state to a more uncomplicated bipolar depression with hypersomnia, lethargy, slowed thinking, and lack of interpersonal sensitivity that may respond more predictably to addition of an antidepressant.

It seems clear that antidepressants normally should not be administered to patients with bipolar depression unless an antimanic drug is coadministered (Nolen and Bloenkolk 2000; Sachs et al. 2000). However, the choice of a specific antidepressant in treating bipolar depression is limited by lack of replicated data. The TCAs seem more likely to induce mania and rapid cycling than bupropion, the MAOIs, and the SSRIs (Akiskal 1994; Rosenbaum et al. 1995; Sachs et al. 1994a; Stoll et al. 1994). Stimulants generally are not used as primary antidepressants in unipolar depression because tolerance to their antidepressant action develops, but the rapid onset and short duration of antidepressant effect of stimulants can be useful for treating bipolar depression. Artificial bright light can be a rapidly effective and safe antidepressant for bipolar depression with a seasonal component or with lethargy and oversleeping (Papatheodorou and Kutcher 1995); as is true of stimulants, the short duration of action may make adverse effects on mood wear off more rapidly. The atypical antipsychotic drugs other than clozapine can be useful antidepressants, as can lamotrigine and gabapentin. The most reliable class of antidepressant medication for bipolar depression is probably the MAOIs, particularly tranylcypromine (Nolen and Bloenkolk 2000). ECT is the most effective treatment for bipolar depression, which is unlike other antidepressant therapies in that it rarely induces mania, and when it does, further ECT usually normalizes mood.

In contrast to unipolar depression, no evidence indicates that continuation of antidepressants after remission of bipolar depression prevents further depressive recurrences (H. Loo and Brochier 1995). In view of the risks of long-term antidepressant therapy, it seems prudent to attempt to withdraw the antidepressant once mood normalizes, while continuing the mood-stabilizing regimen (Sharma et al. 1997). Gradual discontinuation of antidepressants may reduce the risk of rebound of depression. If it becomes necessary to continue treatment with the antidepressant, lower doses may be less likely to destabilize mood. As described later in this chapter (see section titled "Bipolar Disorder: Maintenance Treatment"), maintenance ECT can prevent recurrences of bipolar depression as well as mania.

Mixed and Rapid-Cycling Bipolar Disorder

Although the response rate of uncomplicated mania to lithium in three recent trials ranged from 59% to 91%, response rates in patients with mixed states were only 29%–43% (S. Gershon and Soares 1997); similar results have been obtained in patients with rapid cycling. Patients with either form of complex mood disorder may have a better response to valproate or carbamazepine (T.W. Freeman et al. 1992; Post 1992). Valproate appears to be equally effective in rapid- and non-rapid-cycling bipolar disorder (Bowden et al. 1994). A consensus panel recommended valproate as the first choice for treating rapid cycling, followed by carbamazepine and then lithium (Expert Consensus Panel 1996). Additional treatments that have been reported to be useful for some patients with rapid-cycling bipolar disorder include ECT, antimanic combinations, nimodipine, clozapine, and supplementation with suprametabolic doses of thyroxine (Baumgartner et al. 1994; Calabrese et al. 1991, 1996; Expert Consensus Panel 1996; Frye et al. 1996; Stancer and Persad 1982; Suppes et al. 1994; Swann 1995; Terao 1993; Wehr et al. 1988). As we mentioned in the previous section, it may be necessary first to use a combination of mood-stabilizing medications, possibly with supplementation with an antipsychotic medication (clozapine can be useful in refractory cases) to eliminate cycling and mixed hypomanic symptoms, even if this produces stable bipolar depression without any mixed symptoms of activation. The next phase of treatment would involve introduction of an antidepressant, with an attempt to very slowly withdraw the antidepressant when the depression remits and an effort to slowly withdraw the antipsychotic medication, continuing the combination of mood-stabilizing medications.

Bipolar Disorder: Maintenance Treatment

The high rates of affective recurrence and the increasing severity and complexity and more rapid onset of each recurrence (Keller et al. 1993) are reasons to continue a mood-stabilizing regimen after remission of any acute episode of mania or bipolar depression. Treatment response can be assessed over time with the help of a structured mood chart. Post (1992; Post et al. 1988) and others (Altschuler et al. 1995; Roy-Byrne et al. 1984) developed a "life-charting" method that quantifies symptoms and important life events. However, life charting is time-consuming and relies on observations by nursing staff. In everyday outpatient practice, it may be equally helpful to construct with the patient a graph on which specific symptoms are rated one or more times per day on whatever scale makes the most sense (e.g., mood can be rated from −5 for very depressed to +5 for manic, with 0 signifying euthymia). Different symptoms can be indicated by different line colors or styles, and changes in treatment and important events can be noted on the same graph. However it is accomplished, some form of prospective mood charting can be essential in tracking mixtures of depressive, hypomanic, and psychotic symptoms to determine whether to add more mood-stabilizing medications, an antipsychotic drug, or an antidepressant or whether a particular treatment should be withdrawn.

At least 10 double-blind, placebo-controlled studies containing more than 200 patients each reported that lithium substantially reduces the number of manic and depressive recurrences (0%–44% of patients taking lithium had recurrences, compared with 38%–93% of patients taking placebo) (Goodwin and Jamison 1991; Solomon and Bauer 1993). More than 50% of patients experience an affective episode within 6 months of discontinuing lithium therapy, but the risk of recurrence is almost five times as great (median time in remission = 4 months) in patients who discontinue lithium therapy rapidly than in those who taper the drug over several months (median time in remission = 20 months) (Baldessarini et al. 1996). There is no reason to expect different results with discontinuation of other thymoleptics. The prophylactic effect of lithium results in a substantial decrease in suicide rates, which adds 7 years to life expectancy (National Institute of Mental Health 1995).

Carbamazepine was effective as a maintenance treatment in bipolar illness in four published trials; however, lack of a placebo control in three of these trials and only a trend toward superiority of carbamazepine in the only placebo-controlled trial limit the strength of this conclusion (Solomon et al. 1995). Retrospective studies suggest that valproate prevents affective recurrences in bipolar disorder, but only one prospective placebo-controlled study of maintenance with valproate—in which patients were randomized to lithium monotherapy, divalproex monotherapy, or placebo—has been conducted (Solomon et al. 1995). Verapamil and nimodipine have had mood-stabilizing effects in small numbers of cases of bipolar mood disorder with varying degrees of placebo control (Dubovsky 1995). We reviewed earlier data indicating that mood-stabilizing properties of lamotrigine and the atypical antipsychotic medications have not yet been confirmed.

Case series suggest that combinations of two or three mood stabilizers may provide better affective prophylaxis than can be achieved with monotherapy (Bowden 1996; Expert Consensus Panel 1996). ECT is a highly effective maintenance therapy (Karliner and Wehrheim 1965; Vanelle et al. 1994). Neuroleptics may be necessary adjuncts in the maintenance therapy of psychotic bipolar disorder, although as noted earlier, these medications are thought to increase depressive recurrences in some cases. Clozapine seems more consistently effective as a mood stabilizer (Calabrese et al. 1991; Puri et al. 1995; Zarate et al. 1995).

The efficacy of antimanic drugs in preventing recurrences (i.e., as mood stabilizers) has been noted to decline significantly from the first year to the fifth year of treatment (Peselow et al. 1994). Although the evolving physiology of bipolar disorder is probably one important factor in the increasing rate of recurrence with time, the fact that only one-third of outpatients are estimated to remain compliant is at least as important an issue (S. Gershon and Soares 1997). Noncompliance with mood stabilizers occurred in 64% of the patients in the month preceding hospitalization for acute mania in one study. On follow-up of 140 patients recently hospitalized for bipolar disorder, 51% were partially or totally noncompliant with medications (Keck et al. 1997).

Use of Antimanic Drugs in Children and Adolescents

Lithium has not consistently been found to be effective in mania or bipolar depression in younger patients (Kafantaris 1995). As is true of unipolar depression, higher rates of spontaneous improvement and a high placebo response rate may contribute to the apparent reduced rate of responsiveness to lithium in juvenile bipolar mood disorder. It is also possible that this population requires more frequent dosing or higher serum levels than are required for a thymoleptic response in adults. CSF levels of lithium with a given serum level are lower in children than in adults. Anticonvulsants have been the subject of open trials in childhood and adolescent bipolar disorder but not of placebo-controlled studies (Kafantaris 1995; Papatheodorou et al. 1995; Porter 1987). The results of these trials show that valproate and carbamazepine are well tolerated and possibly effective. Verapamil, which is used to treat childhood and adolescent cardiovascular disease, has been used successfully in a few cases of adolescent mania (Kastner and Friedman 1992). Case series and clinical experience indicate that ECT is as effective for treating mania in juvenile patients as it is in adults (Bertagnolli and Borchardt 1990; Carr et al. 1983; Kutcher and Robertson 1995). The course of juvenile bipolar disorder is more chronic than is that of adult bipolar disorder (Lewinsohn et al. 1995), but until empirical data are accumulated, decisions about the balance between potential positive and negative effects of maintenance medications on affective recurrence and intellectual and personality development are matters of opinion and personal experience.

Conclusions

Mood disorders are not unitary illnesses but complex syndromes with distinct etiologies, courses, and treatment responses that ultimately may be better understood through the addition of a more thorough dimensional analysis (e.g., early vs. late onset, comorbidity, disordered thinking, degree of intrusion into the personality) to existing categorical diagnoses and the DSM multiaxial approach. Even the most complete description of an affective episode at one point in time does not fully capture the picture of a mood disorder as it evolves over time. Mood disorders are not static but are dynamic conditions in which each new episode is a function of previous episodes with an evolving course and treatment response.

One important implication of the accumulating data about the course of mood disorders is that it is easier to treat early than later episodes of any mood disorder. Complete treatment of early episodes and continuation of effective therapy reduce the risk of later, more refractory episodes. Unfortunately, denial, reluctance to ac-

knowledge needing help because being helped feels like a sign of weakness, pressure from family members who themselves may have mood disorders, and acceptance of a good but incomplete remission make it difficult for people in the early stages of a mood disorder to recognize the seriousness of the illness, let alone treat it. Public education has reduced the stigma of seeking treatment for depression to some extent, but efforts to educate primary care physicians, who are more likely than mental health professionals to encounter patients with mood disorders for the first time, have not been successful in increasing rates of effective recognition, treatment, and, when necessary, referral of these patients for specialty care. Research into strategies for approaching mood disorders in primary care practice is therefore as important as research into new treatment technologies.

References

Abernathy DR, Schwartz JB: Calcium-antagonist drugs. N Engl J Med 341:1447–1457, 2000

Abrams RC: Electroconvulsive Therapy. New York, Oxford University Press, 1988

Abramson LY, Seligman MEP, Teasdale JD: Learned helplessness in humans: critique and reformulation. J Abnorm Psychol 87:49–74, 1978

Agency for Health Care Policy and Services Research: Clinical Practice Guideline: Depression in Primary Care, Vol 2: Treatment of Major Depression. Rockville, MD, U.S. Department of Health and Human Services, 1993

Ahlfors UG, Baastrup PC, Dencker SJ: Flupenthixol decanoate in recurrent manic-depressive illness: a comparison with lithium. Acta Psychiatr Scand 64:226–237, 1981

Akiskal HS: Chronic depression. Bull Menninger Clin 240:349–354, 1991

Akiskal HS: Dysthymic and cyclothymic depressions: therapeutic considerations. Compr Psychiatry 55 (suppl 4):46–52, 1994

Akiskal HS: Le spectre bipolaire: acquisitions et perspectives cliniques. Encephale 21 (Spec No 6):3–11, 1995

Akiskal HS, Walker P, Puzantian VR, et al: Bipolar outcome in the course of depressive illness. J Affect Disord 5:115–128, 1983

Akiskal HS, Downs J, Jordan P, et al: Affective disorders in referred children and younger siblings of manic-depressives. Arch Gen Psychiatry 42:996–1003, 1985

Akiyoshi J, Isogawa K, Yamada K, et al: Effects of antidepressants on intracellular Ca2+ mobilization in CHO cells transfected with the human 5-HT2C receptors. Biol Psychiatry 39:1000–1008, 1996

Albus M, Hubmann W, Wahlheim C, et al: Contrasts in neuropsychological test profile between patients with first-episode schizophrenia and first-episode affective disorders. Acta Psychiatr Scand 94:87–93, 1996

Altschuler LL, Post RM, Leverich GS: Antidepressant-induced mania and cycle acceleration: a controversy revisited. Am J Psychiatry 152:1130–1138, 1995

Ambrosini PJ, Bianchi MD, Rabinovich H, et al: Antidepressant treatments in children and adolescents, I: affective disorders. J Am Acad Child Adolesc Psychiatry 32:1–5, 1993

American Psychiatric Association: Diagnostic and Statistical Manual of Mental Disorders, 3rd Edition. Washington, DC, American Psychiatric Association, 1980

American Psychiatric Association: Practice guideline for major depressive disorder in adults. Am J Psychiatry 150 (suppl 4):1–26, 1993

American Psychiatric Association: Diagnostic and Statistical Manual of Mental Disorders, 4th Edition. Washington, DC, American Psychiatric Association, 1994a

American Psychiatric Association: Practice guideline for the treatment of patients with bipolar disorder. Am J Psychiatry 151 (suppl 12):1–36, 1994b

American Psychiatric Association: Diagnostic and Statistical Manual of Mental Disorders, 4th Edition, Text Revision. Washington, DC, American Psychiatric Association, 2000

Ananth J, Wohl M, Ranganath V: Rapid cycling patients: conceptual and etiological factors. Neuropsychobiology 27:193–198, 1993

Angst J: Epidémiologie du spectre bipolaire. Encephale 21(Spec No 6):37–42, 1995

Angst J, Hochstrasser B: Recurrent brief depression: the Zurich Study. Compr Psychiatry 55(suppl 4):3–9, 1994

Angst J, Merikangas K, Scheidegger P, et al: Recurrent brief depression: a new subtype of affective disorder. J Affect Disord 19:87–98, 1990

Anonymous: Atypical antipsychotics for treatment of depression in schizophrenia and affective disorders. Collaborative Working Group on Clinical Trial Evaluations. J Clin Psychiatry 59(suppl 12):41–45, 1998

Anton RF, Burch EA: Amoxapine versus amitriptyline combined with perphenazine in the treatment of psychotic depression. Am J Psychiatry 147:1203–1208, 1986

Aperia B: Effects of electroconvulsive therapy on neuropsychological function and circulating levels of ACTH, cortisol, prolactin, and TSH in patients with major depressive illness. Acta Psychiatr Scand 72:536–541, 1985

Aronson TA, Shukla S, Hoff A: Continuation therapy after ECT for delusional depression: a naturalistic study of prophylactic treatments and relapse. Convuls Ther 3:251–259, 1987

Aronson TA, Shukla S, Hoff A, et al: Proposed delusional depression subtypes: preliminary evidence from a retrospective study of phenomenology and treatment course. J Affect Disord 14:69–74, 1988

Aronson TA, Shukla S, Hirschowitz J: Clonazepam treatment of five lithium-refractory patients with bipolar disorder. Am J Psychiatry 146:77–80, 1989

Association for Convulsive Therapy: Ambulatory electroconvulsive therapy: report of a task force of the Association for Convulsive Therapy. Convuls Ther 12:42–55, 1996

Avery D, Lubano A: Depression treated with imipramine and ECT: the DeCarolis study reconsidered. Am J Psychiatry 136:559–562, 1979

Baldessarini RJ, Tondo L, Faedda GL, et al: Effects of the rate of discontinuing lithium maintenance treatment in bipolar disorders. Compr Psychiatry 57:441–448, 1996

Ballenger JC, Reus VI, Post RM: The "atypical" clinical picture of adolescent mania. Am J Psychiatry 139:602–606, 1982

Banov MD, Zarate CA, Tohen M, et al: Clozapine therapy in refractory affective disorders: polarity predicts response in long-term follow-up. Compr Psychiatry 55:295–300, 1994

Barbini B, Di Molfetta D, Gasperini M, et al: Seasonal concordance of recurrence in mood disorder patients. European Psychiatry 10:171–174, 1995

Barefoot JC, Schroll M: Symptoms of depression, acute myocardial infarction, and total mortality in a community sample. Circulation 93:1976–1980, 1996

Barklage NE: Evaluation and management of the suicidal patient. Emergency Care Quarterly 7:9–17, 1991

Barnet B, Duggan AK, Wilson MD, et al: Association between postpartum substance use and depressive symptoms, stress, and social support in adolescent mothers. Pediatrics 96:659–666, 1995

Barrett JE: Naturalistic change after 2 years in neurotic depressive disorders (RDC categories). Compr Psychiatry 25:404–418, 1984

Barton BM, Gitlin MJ: Verapamil in treatment-resistant mania: an open trial. J Clin Psychopharmacol 7:101–103, 1987

Basco MR, Rush AJ: Compliance with pharmacotherapy in mood disorders. Psychiatr Ann 25:269–279, 1995

Bauer MS, Whybrow PC: The effect of changing thyroid function on cyclic affective illness in a human subject. Am J Psychiatry 143:633–636, 1986

Bauer MS, Whybrow PC: Rapid cycling bipolar affective disorder. Arch Gen Psychiatry 47:435–440, 1990

Bauer MS, Whybrow PC, Winokur A: Rapid cycling bipolar affective disorder, I: association with grade I hypothyroidism. Arch Gen Psychiatry 47:427–432, 1990

Baumgartner A, Bauer M, Hellweg R: Treatment of intractable non-rapid cycling bipolar affective disorder with high-dose thyroxine: an open clinical trial. Neuropsychopharmacology 10:183–189, 1994

Beauchamp G, Lavoie P, Elie R: Effect of some stereoisomeric tricyclic antidepressants on 45Ca uptake in synaptosomes from rat hippocampus. Psychopharmacology 110:133–139, 1993

Bech P: Acute therapy of depression. Compr Psychiatry 54 (suppl 8):18–27, 1993

Beck AT, Jallon SD, Young JE: Treatment of depression with cognitive therapy and amitriptyline. Arch Gen Psychiatry 42:142–148, 1985

Beck CT: A meta-analysis of the relationship between postpartum depression and infant temperament. Nurs Res 45:225–230, 1996

Bell KM, Potkin SG, Carreon D, et al: S-Adenosylmethionine blood levels in major depression: changes with drug treatment. Acta Neurol Scand Suppl 154:15–18, 1994

Bellivier F, Szoke A, Henry C, et al: Possible association between serotonin transporter gene polymorphism and violent suicidal behavior in mood disorders. Biol Psychiatry 48:319–322, 2000

Belsher G, Costello CG: Relapse after recovery from unipolar depression: a critical review. Psychol Bull 104:84–96, 1988

Bemporad JR: Psychodynamic models of depression and mania, in Depression and Mania. Edited by Georgotas A, Cancro R. New York, Elsevier, 1988, pp 167–180

Benazzi F: Olanzapine-induced psychotic mania in bipolar schizo-affective disorder (letter). European Psychiatry 14:410–411, 1999a

Benazzi F: Olanzapine-induced psychotic mania in bipolar schizoaffective disorder. Can J Psychiatry 44:667–668, 1999b

Benkelfat C: Serotonergic mechanisms in psychiatric disorder: new research tools, new ideas. Int Clin Psychopharmacol 8 (suppl 2):53–56, 1993

Berghofer A, Miller-Oerlinghausen B: Is there a loss of efficacy of lithium in patients treated for over 20 years? Neuropsychobiology 42 (suppl 1):46–49, 2000

Bergsholm P, Martinsen EW, Svoen N, et al: Affective disorders: drug treatment and electroconvulsive therapy. Tidsskr Nor Laegeforen 112:2651–2656, 1992

Bertagnolli MW, Borchardt CM: A review of ECT for children and adolescents. J Am Acad Child Adolesc Psychiatry 29:302–307, 1990

Berthier ML, Kulisevsky J, Gironell A: Poststroke bipolar affective disorder: clinical subtypes, concurrent movement disorders, and anatomical correlates. J Neuropsychiatry Clin Neurosci 8:160–167, 1996

Beydoun A, Uthman BM, Sackellares JC. Gabapentin: pharmacokinetics, efficacy, and safety. Clin Neuropharmacol 18:469–481, 1995

Biederman J: Developmental subtypes of juvenile bipolar disorder. Sexual and Marital Therapy 3:227–230, 1995

Bigelow LB, Weinberger DR, Wyatt RJ: Synergism of combined lithium-neuroleptic therapy: a double-blind, placebo-controlled case study. Am J Psychiatry 138: 81–83, 1981

Bigger JT, Hoffman BF: Antiarrhythmic drugs, in Goodman and Gilman's The Pharmacological Basis of Therapeutics, 8th Edition. Edited by Gilman AG, Rall TW, Nies AS, et al. New York, Pergamon, 1991, pp 840–873

Black DW, Winokur G, Nasrallah A: Treatment of mania: a naturalistic study of electroconvulsive therapy versus lithium in 438 patients. Compr Psychiatry 48:132–139, 1987

Blackburn I-M: Psychology and psychotherapy of depression. Current Opinion in Psychiatry 7:30–33, 1994

Blackburn I-M, Eunson KM, Bishop S: A two-year naturalistic follow-up of depressed patients treated with cognitive therapy, pharmacotherapy, and a combination of both. J Affect Disord 10:67–75, 1986

Blatt SJ: The destructiveness of perfectionism: implications for the treatment of depression. Am Psychol 50:1003–1020, 1995

Blatt SJ, Sanislow CA, Zuroff DC, et al: Characteristics of effective therapists: further analyses of data from the National Institute of Mental Health Treatment of Depression Collaborative Research Program. J Consult Clin Psychol 64:1276–1284, 1996

Blazer DG, Koenig HG: Mood disorders, in Textbook of Geriatric Psychiatry. Edited by Busse EW, Blazer DG. Washington, DC, American Psychiatric Press, 1996, pp 235–264

Bleich A, Brown S-L, van Praag HM: A serotonergic theory of schizophrenia, in The Role of Serotonin in Psychiatric Disorders. Edited by Brown S-L, van Praag HM. New York, Brunner/Mazel, 1990, pp 183–214

Blumer D, Montouris G, Hermann B: Psychiatric morbidity in seizure patients on a neurodiagnostic monitoring unit. J Neuropsychiatry Clin Neurosci 7:445–456, 1995

Borysewicz K, Borysewicz W: A case of mania following olanzapine administration. Psychiatr Pol 34:299–306, 2000

Bottiglieri T, Godfrey P, Flynn T, et al: Cerebrospinal fluid S-adenosylmethionine in depression and dementia: effects of treatment with parenteral and oral S-adenosylmethionine. J Neurol Neurosurg Psychiatry 53:1096–1098, 1990

Bowden CL: The clinical approach to the differential diagnosis of bipolar disorder. Psychiatr Ann 23:57–63, 1993

Bowden CL: Predictors of response to divalproex and lithium (review). Compr Psychiatry 56(suppl 3):25–30, 1995

Bowden CL: Dosing strategies and time course of response to antimanic agents. Compr Psychiatry 57(suppl 13):4–9, 1996

Bowden CL, Brugger AM, Swann AC: Efficacy of divalproex vs lithium in the treatment of mania. JAMA 271:918–924, 1994

Bowden CL, Calabrese JR, Wallin BA, et al: Illness characteristics of patients in clinical drug studies of mania. Psychopharmacol Bull 31:103–109, 1995

Bowden CL, Calabrese JR, McElroy SL, et al: The efficacy of lamotrigine in rapid cycling and non-rapid cycling patients with bipolar disorder. Biol Psychiatry 45:953–958, 1999

Bowers WA: Treatment of depressed inpatients: cognitive therapy plus medication, relaxation plus medication, and medication alone. Br J Psychiatry 156:73–78, 1990

Bowlby J: Loss: Sadness and Depression. New York, Basic Books, 1980

Boyce P, Parker G, Barnett B, et al: Personality as a vulnerability factor to depression. Br J Psychiatry 159:106–114, 1991

Bradwejn J, Shriqui C, Kosczycki D, et al: Double-blind comparison of the effects of clonazepam and lorazepam in acute mania. J Clin Psychopharmacol 10:403–408, 1990

Brady KT, Sonne SC, Anton R, et al: Valproate in the treatment of acute bipolar affective episodes complicated by substance abuse: a pilot study. Compr Psychiatry 56:118–121, 1995

Brawman-Mintzer O, Lydiard RB: Generalized anxiety disorder: issues in epidemiology. Compr Psychiatry 57(suppl 7):3–8, 1996

Breier A, Charney DS, Heniger GR: The diagnostic validity of anxiety disorders and their relationship to depressive illness. Am J Psychiatry 142:787–797, 1985

Broadhead WE, Blazer DG, George LK, et al: Depression, disability days, and days lost from work in a prospective epidemiologic survey. JAMA 264:2524–2528, 1990

Bruder GE, Fong R, Tenke CE, et al: Regional brain asymmetries in major depression with or without an anxiety disorder: a quantitative electroencephalographic study. Biol Psychiatry 41:939–948, 1997

Buchsbaum MS, Wu J, Siegel BV, et al: Effect of sertraline on regional metabolic rate in patients with affective disorder. Biol Psychiatry 41:15–22, 1997

Budman SH, Demby A, Redondo JP, et al: Comparative outcome in time-limited individual and group psychotherapy. Int J Group Psychother 38:63–86, 1988

Burrows GD: Long-term clinical management of depressive disorders. Compr Psychiatry 53(suppl 3):32–35, 1992

Busch FN, Miller FT, Weiden PJ: A comparison of two adjunctive treatment strategies in acute mania. Compr Psychiatry 50:453–455, 1989

Butler SF, Arredondo DE, McCloskey V: Affective comorbidity in children and adolescents with attention deficit hyperactivity disorder. Ann Clin Psychiatry 7:51–55, 1995

Buysse DJ, Reynolds CF, Kupfer DJ, et al: Clinical diagnoses in 216 insomnia patients using the International Classification of Sleep Disorders (ICSD), DSM-IV and ICD-10 categories: a report from the APA/NIMH DSM-IV field trial. Sleep 17:630–637, 1994

Buzan RD, Weissberg M: Suicide: risk factors and prevention in medical practice. Annu Rev Med 43:37–46, 1992

Byerly WG, Hartmann A, Foster DE, et al: Verapamil in the treatment of maternal paroxysmal supraventricular tachycardia. Ann Emerg Med 20:552–554, 1991

Cabras PL, Hardoy MJ, Hardoy MC, et al: Clinical experience with gabapentin in patients with bipolar or schizoaffective disorder: results of an open-label study. J Clin Psychiatry 60:245–248, 1999

Calabrese JR, Meltzer HY, Markovitz PJ: Clozapine prophylaxis in rapid cycling bipolar disorder. J Clin Psychopharmacol 11:396–397, 1991

Calabrese JR, Kimmel SE, Woyshville MJ, et al: Clozapine for treatment-refractory mania. Am J Psychiatry 153:759–764, 1996

Calabrese JR, Bowden CL, Sachs GS, et al: A double-blind placebo-controlled study of lamotrigine monotherapy in outpatients with bipolar I depression. Lamictal 602 Study Group. J Clin Psychiatry 60:79–88, 1999a

Calabrese JR, Bowden CL, McElroy SL, et al: Spectrum of activity of lamotrigine in treatment-refractory bipolar disorder. Am J Psychiatry 156:1019–1023, 1999b

Calev A, Ben-Tzvi E, Shapira B, et al: Distinct memory impairments following electroconvulsive therapy and imipramine. Psychol Med 19:111–119, 1989

Calev A, Gaudino EA, Squires NK, et al: ECT and non-memory cognition: a review. Br J Clin Psychol 34:505–515, 1995

Carbonne B, Jannet D, Touboul C, et al: Nicardipine treatment of hypertension during pregnancy. Obstet Gynecol 81:908–914, 1993

Carr V, Dorrington C, Schrader G, et al: The use of ECT for mania in childhood bipolar disorder. Br J Psychiatry 143:411–415, 1983

Carroll BJ: Informed use of the dexamethasone suppression test. Compr Psychiatry 47 (suppl):10–12, 1986

Cassano GB, Akiskal HS, Musetti L, et al: Psychopathology, temperament, and past course in primary major depressions, 2: toward a redefinition of bipolarity with a new semistructured interview for depression. Psychopathology 22:278–288, 1989

Cassem EH: Depressive disorders in the medically ill: an overview. Psychosomatics 36: S2–S10, 1995

Chambers WJ, Puig-Antich J, Tabrizi MA, et al: Psychotic symptoms in prepubertal major depressive disorder. Arch Gen Psychiatry 39:921–927, 1982

Charney DS, Delgado PL, Price LH, et al: The receptor sensitivity hypothesis of antidepressant action: a review of antidepressant effects on serotonin function, in The Role of Serotonin in Psychiatric Disorders. Edited by Brown S-L, van Praag HM. New York, Brunner/Mazel, 1990, pp 27–56

Chen PJ: The efficacy and blood concentration monitoring of carbamazepine on mania [in Chinese]. Chung Hua Shen Ching Ching Shen Ko Tsa Chih 23:261–265, 1931

Chou JCY: Recent advances in treatment of acute mania. J Clin Psychopharmacol 11:3–21, 1991

Chouinard G, Young SN, Annable L: Antimanic effect of clonazepam. Biol Psychiatry 18:451–466, 1983

Clayton PJ, Grove WM, Coryell W, et al: Follow-up and family study of anxious depression. Am J Psychiatry 148:1512–1517, 1991

Coccaro EF: Central serotonin and impulsive aggression. Br J Psychiatry 155 (suppl 8):52–62, 1989

Cochran SD: Preventing medical noncompliance in the outpatient treatment of bipolar affective disorder. J Consult Clin Psychol 52:873–878, 1984

Coffey CE, Weiner RD, Djang WT, et al: Brain anatomic effects of electroconvulsive therapy: a prospective magnetic resonance imaging study. Arch Gen Psychiatry 48: 1013–1017, 1991

Cohen BM, Lipinski JF: Treatment of acute psychosis with non-neuroleptic agents. Psychosomatics 26 (suppl):7–16, 1986

Colwell BL, Lopez JR: Clonazepam in mania. Drug Intelligence and Clinical Pharmacy 21:794–795, 1987

Compton MT, Nemeroff CB: The treatment of bipolar depression. Compr Psychiatry 61(suppl 9):1–57, 2000

Consensus Development Panel: NIMH/NIH Consensus Development Conference statement: mood disorders—pharmacologic prevention of recurrences. Am J Psychiatry 142:469–476, 1985

Conte HR, Plutchik R, Wild K, et al: Combined psychotherapy and pharmacotherapy for depression. Arch Gen Psychiatry 43:471–479, 1986

Corruble E, Ginestet D, Guelfi JD: Comorbidity of personality disorders and unipolar major depression: a review. J Affect Disord 37:157–170, 1996

Coryell W: Psychotic depression. Compr Psychiatry 57(suppl 3):27–31, 1996

Coryell W, Endicott J, Keller MB: Predictors of relapse into major depressive disorder in a nonclinical population. Am J Psychiatry 148:1353–1358, 1991

Coryell W, Akiskal HS, Leon AC, et al: The time course of nonchronic major depressive disorder. Arch Gen Psychiatry 51:405–410, 1994

Craighead WE, Miklowitz DJ: Psychosocial Interventions for bipolar disorder. J Clin Psychiatry 61 (suppl 13):58–64, 2000

Crits-Christoph P: The efficacy of brief dynamic psychotherapy: a meta-analysis. Am J Psychiatry 149:151–158, 1992

Cross-National Collaborative Group: The changing rate of major depression: cross-national comparisons. JAMA 268:3098–3105, 1992

Davanloo H: Short-Term Dynamic Psychotherapy. New York, Jason Aronson, 1982

Davidson KM: Diagnosis of depression in alcohol dependence: changes in prevalence with drinking status. Br J Psychiatry 166:199–204, 1995

Delgado PL, Gelenberg AJ: Antidepressant and antimanic medications, in Treatment of Psychiatric Disorders. Edited by Gabbard GO. Washington, DC, American Psychiatric Press, 1995, pp 1131–1168

Deltito JA, Moline M, Pollak C, et al: Effects of phototherapy on non-seasonal unipolar and bipolar depressive spectrum disorders. J Affect Disord 23:231–237, 1991

Devanand DP, Sackeim HA, Prudic J: Electroconvulsive therapy in the treatment-resistant patient. Psychiatr Clin North Am 14:905–923, 1991a

Devanand DP, Sackeim HA, Lo E-S, et al: Serial dexamethasone suppression tests and plasma dexamethasone levels. Arch Gen Psychiatry 48:525–533, 1991b

Dilsaver SC, Coffman JA: Cholinergic hypothesis of depression: a reappraisal. J Clin Psychopharmacol 9:173–179, 1989

DiMascio A, Weissman MM, Prusoff BA: Differential symptom reduction by drugs and psychotherapy in acute depression. Arch Gen Psychiatry 36:1450–1456, 1979

Doris A, Ebmeier KP, Shajahan P: Depressive illness. Lancet 354:1369–1375, 1999

Dose M, Emrich HM, Cording-Tommel C: Use of calcium antagonists in mania. Psychoneuroendocrinology 11:241–243, 1986

Dubovsky SL: Beyond the serotonin reuptake inhibitors: rationales for the development of new serotonergic agents. Compr Psychiatry 55(suppl 2):34–44, 1994a

Dubovsky SL: Why don't we hear more about the calcium antagonists? An industry-academia interaction. Biol Psychiatry 35:149–150, 1994b

Dubovsky SL: Calcium channel antagonists as novel agents for manic-depressive disorder, in The American Psychiatric Press Textbook of Psychopharmacology. Edited by Schatzberg AF, Nemeroff CB. Washington, DC, American Psychiatric Press, 1995, pp 377–388

Dubovsky SL, Thomas M: Beyond specificity: effects of serotonin and serotonergic treatments on psychobiological dysfunction. J Psychosom Res 39:429–444, 1995

Dubovsky SL, Thomas M: Tardive dyskinesia associated with fluoxetine. Psychiatr Serv 47:991–993, 1996

Dubovsky SL, Franks RD, Allen S, et al: Calcium antagonists in mania: a double-blind study of verapamil. Psychiatry Res 18:309–320, 1986

Dubovsky SL, Christiano J, Daniell LC: Increased platelet intracellular calcium concentration in patients with bipolar affective disorders. Arch Gen Psychiatry 46:632–638, 1989

Dubovsky SL, Lee C, Christiano J: Elevated intracellular calcium ion concentration in bipolar depression. Biol Psychiatry 29:441–450, 1991a

Dupont RM, Jernigan TL, Heindel W, et al: Magnetic resonance imaging and mood disorders: localization of white matter and other subcortical abnormalities. Arch Gen Psychiatry 52:747–755, 1995

Dwight MM, Keck PE, Stanton SP, et al: Antidepressant activity and mania associated with risperidone treatment of schizoaffective disorder. Lancet 344:554–555, 1994

Emslie GJ, Kennard BD, Kowatch RA: Affective disorders in children: diagnosis and management. J Child Neurol 10 (suppl 1):S42–S49, 1995

Esparon J, Kolloori J, Naylor GJ: Comparison of the prophylactic action of flupenthixol with placebo in lithium treated manic-depressive patients. Br J Psychiatry 148: 723–725, 1986

Expert Consensus Panel: Treatment of bipolar disorder. Compr Psychiatry 57 (suppl 12A):1–88, 1996

Faedda GL, Baldessarini RJ, Suppes T, et al: Pediatric-onset bipolar disorder: a neglected clinical and public health problem. Sexual and Marital Therapy 3:171–195, 1995

Fann JR, Tucker GJ: Mood disorders with general medical condition. Curr Opin Psychiatry 8:13–18, 1995

Fava M, Davidson KG: Definition and epidemiology of treatment-resistant depression. Psychiatr Clin North Am 19:179–195, 1996

Fava M, Kaji J: Continuation and maintenance treatments of major depressive disorders. Psychiatr Ann 24:281–290, 1994

Feinman JA, Dunner DL: The effect of alcohol and substance abuse on the course of bipolar affective disorder. J Affect Disord 37:43–49, 1996

Fennig S, Craig TJ, Tanenberg-Karant M, et al: Medication treatment in first-admission patients with psychotic affective disorders: preliminary findings on research-facility diagnostic agreement and rehospitalization. Ann Clin Psychiatry 7:87–90, 1995

Figiel GS, Krishnan KRR, Doraiswamy PM: Subcortical structural changes in ECT-induced delirium. J Geriatr Psychiatry Neurol 3:172–176, 1990

Figiel GS, Epstein C, McDonald WM, et al: The use of rapid-rate transcranial magnetic stimulation (rTMS) in refractory depressed patients. J Neuropsychiatry Clin Neurosci 10:20–25, 1998

Fink M: Electroconvulsive therapy in children and adolescents. Convuls Ther 9:155–157, 1993

Fitz-Gerald MJ, Pinkofsky HB, Brannon G, et al: Olanzapine-induced mania (letter). Am J Psychiatry 156:1114, 1999

Fochtmann LJ: Animal studies of electroconvulsive therapy: foundations for future research. Psychopharmacol Bull 30:321–344, 1994

Franchini J, Zanardi R, Smeraldi E, et al: Early onset of lithium prophylaxis as a predictor of good long-term outcome. Eur Arch Psychiatry Clin Neurosci 249:227–230, 1999

Franco-Bronson K: The management of treatment-resistant depression in the medically ill. Psychiatr Clin North Am 19:329–350, 1996

Frank E, Kupfer DJ, Perel JM, et al: Three-year outcomes for maintenance therapies in recurrent depression. Arch Gen Psychiatry 47:1093–1099, 1990

Frank E, Kupfer DJ, Wagner EF, et al: Efficacy of interpersonal psychotherapy as a maintenance treatment of recurrent depression: contributing factors. Arch Gen Psychiatry 48:1053–1059, 1991

Frank E, Kupfer DJ, Perel JM, et al: Comparison of full-dose versus half-dose pharmacotherapy in the maintenance treatment of recurrent depression. J Affect Disord 27:139–145, 1993

Frank E, Kupfer DJ, Ehlers CL, et al: Interpersonal and social rhythm therapy for bipolar disorder: integrating interpersonal and behavioral approaches. Behav Ther 17:143–149, 1994

Freeman MP, McElroy SL: Clinical picture and etiologic models of mixed states. Psychiatr Clin North Am 22:535–546, 1999

Freeman TW, Clothier JL, Pazzaglia P, et al: A double-blind comparison of valproate and lithium in the treatment of acute mania. Am J Psychiatry 149:108–111, 1992

Freinhar JP, Alvarez WH: Use of clonazepam in two cases of acute mania. Compr Psychiatry 46:29–30, 1985

Fritsch S, Donaldson D, Spirito A, et al: Personality characteristics of adolescent suicide attempters. Child Psychiatry Hum Dev 30:219–235, 2000

Froscher W: Clinical relevance of the determination of antiepileptic drugs in serum. Wien Klin Wochenschr Suppl 191:15–18, 1992

Frye M, Altschuler LL, Bitran JE: Clozapine in rapid cycling bipolar disorder (letter). J Clin Psychopharmacol 16:87–90, 1996

Garza-Trevino ES, Hollister LE, Overall JE, et al: Efficacy of combinations of intramuscular antipsychotics and sedative-hypnotics for control of psychotic agitation. Am J Psychiatry 146:1598–1601, 1989

Garza-Trevino ES, Overall JE, Hollister LE: Verapamil versus lithium in acute mania. Am J Psychiatry 149:121–122, 1992

Gaster B, Holroyd J: St John's wort for depression: a systematic review. Arch Intern Med 24:152–156, 2000

Gelenberg AJ, Hopkins HS: Report on efficacy of treatments for bipolar disorder. Psychopharmacol Bull 29:447–456, 1993

Geller B, Sun K, Zimerman B, et al: Complex and rapid-cycling in bipolar children and adolescents: a preliminary study. J Affect Disord 34:259–268, 1995

Geller B, Williams M, Zimerman B, et al: Prepubertal and early adolescent bipolarity differentiate from ADHD by manic symptoms, grandiose delusions, ultrarapid or ultradian cycling. J Affect Disord 51:81–91, 1998

George MS, Wassermann EM, Kimbrell TA, et al: Mood improvement following daily left prefrontal repetitive transcranial magnetic stimulation in patients with depression: a placebo-controlled crossover trial. Am J Psychiatry 154:1752–1756, 1997

Gerber JS, Nies AS: Antihypertensive agents and the drug therapy of hypertension, in Goodman and Gilman's The Pharmacological Basis of Therapeutics, 8th Edition. Edited by Gilman AG, Rall TW, Nies AS, et al. New York, Pergamon, 1991, pp 784–813

Gershon ES: Genetics, in Manic-Depressive Illness. Edited by Goodwin FK, Jamison KR. New York, Oxford University Press, 1990, pp 373–401

Gershon ES, Hamovit J, Guroff I, et al: A family study of schizoaffective, bipolar I, bipolar II, unipolar and normal control probands. Arch Gen Psychiatry 39:1157–1167, 1982

Gershon S, Soares JC: Current therapeutic profile of lithium. Arch Gen Psychiatry 54:16–18, 1997

Ghaemi SN, Gaughan S: Novel anticonvulsants: a new generation of mood stabilizers? Harv Rev Psychiatry 8:1–7, 2000

Giannini AJ, Houser WL, Loiselle RH: Antimanic effects of verapamil. Am J Psychiatry 141:1602–1603, 1984

Giannini AJ, Loiselle RH, Price WA: Comparison of antimanic efficacy of clonidine and verapamil. J Clin Pharmacol 25:307–308, 1985

Giannini AJ, Taraszewski R, Loiselle RH: Verapamil and lithium as maintenance therapy of manic patients. J Clin Pharmacol 27:980–982, 1987

Glass DR, Pilkonis PA, Leber WR, et al: National Institute of Mental Health Treatment of Depression Collaborative Research Program. Arch Gen Psychiatry 46:971–982, 1989

Gold PW, Licinio J, Wong ML, et al: Corticotropin releasing hormone in the pathophysiology of melancholic and atypical depression and the mechanisms of action of antidepressant drugs. Ann N Y Acad Sci 77:716–729, 1995

Goldberg JF, Harrow M, Grossman LS: Course and outcome in bipolar affective disorder: a longitudinal follow-up study. Am J Psychiatry 152:379–384, 1995

Goldberg JF, Harrow M, Leon AC: Lithium treatment of bipolar affective disorders under naturalistic followup conditions. Psychopharmacol Bull 32:47–54, 1996

Goodnick PJ: Verapamil prophylaxis in pregnant women with bipolar disorder (letter). Am J Psychiatry 150:1560, 1993

Goodwin FK, Jamison KR: Manic Depressive Illness. New York, Oxford University Press, 1991

Goodwin FK, Wirz-Justice A, Wehr TA: Evidence that the pathophysiology of depression and the mechanism of antidepressant drugs both involve alterations in circadian rhythms. Adv Biochem Psychopharmacol 32:1–11, 1982

Gorman JM, Coplan JD: Comorbidity of depression and panic disorder. Compr Psychiatry 57(suppl 10):34–41, 1996

Grahame-Smith DG: Serotonin in affective disorders. Int Clin Psychopharmacol 6 (suppl 4):5–13, 1992

Green AI, Tohen M, Patel JK, et al: Clozapine in the treatment of refractory psychotic mania. Am J Psychiatry 157:982–986, 2000

Grisaru N, Chudakov B, Yaroslavosky Y, et al: Transcranial magnetic stimulation in mania: a controlled study. Am J Psychiatry 155:1608–1610, 1998

Gruber AJ, Hudson JI, Pope HG: The management of treatment-resistant depression in disorders on the interface of psychiatry and medicine. Psychiatr Clin North Am 19:351–369, 1996

Guze SB, Robbins E: Suicide and primary affective disorders. Br J Psychiatry 117:437–438, 1970

Gyulai L, Alavi A, Broich K, et al: I-123 iofetamine single-photon computed emission tomography in rapid cycling bipolar disorder: a clinical study. Biol Psychiatry 41:152–161, 1997

Harrison WM, Stewart JW: Pharmacotherapy of dysthymia. Psychiatr Ann 23:638–648, 1993

Harrow M, Goldberg JF, Grossman LS, et al: Outcome in manic disorders: a naturalistic follow-up study. Arch Gen Psychiatry 47:665–671, 1990

Hasin DS, Tsai W-Y, Endicott J, et al: Five-year course of major depression: effects of comorbid alcoholism: the effect of alcohol and substance abuse on the course of bipolar affective disorder. J Affect Disord 37:43–49, 1996

Hauck A, Bhaumik S: Hypomania induced by gabapentin (letter). Br J Psychiatry 167:549, 1995

Hay DF, Kumar R: Interpreting the effects of mothers' postnatal depression on children's intelligence: a critique and re-analysis. Child Psychiatry Hum Dev 25:165–181, 1995

Hirschfeld RMA: Guidelines for the long-term treatment of depression. Compr Psychiatry 55(suppl 12):61–69, 1994

Hollon SD, DeRubeis RJ, Evans MD, et al: Cognitive therapy and pharmacotherapy for depression: singly and in combination. Arch Gen Psychiatry 49:774–781, 1992

Hopkins HS, Gelenberg AJ: Treatment of bipolar disorder: how far have we come? Psychopharmacol Bull 30:27–38, 1994

Hopkins J, Marcus M, Campbell SB: Postpartum depression: a critical review. Psychol Bull 95:498–515, 1984

Hoschl C, Kozemy J: Verapamil in affective disorders: a controlled, double-blind study. Biol Psychiatry 25:128–140, 1989

Isacsson G, Bergman U, Rich CL: Epidemiological data suggest antidepressants reduce suicide risk among depressives. J Affect Disord 41:1–8, 1996

Jacob M, Turner L, Kupfer DJ, et al: Attrition in maintenance therapy for recurrent depression. J Affect Disord 6:181–189, 1984

Jaim-Etcheverry G, Zieher LM: Coexistence of monoamines in peripheral adrenergic neurones, in Co-Transmission. Edited by Cuello AC. London, England, Macmillan, 1982, pp 189–207

Jamison KR: Touched With Fire: Manic-Depressive Illness and the Artistic Temperament. New York, Free Press, 1993

Janicak PG, Lipinski JF, Davis JM, et al: S-Adenosylmethionine in depression: a literature review and preliminary report. Alabama Journal of Medical Science 25:306–313, 1988a

Janicak PG, Pandey GN, Davis JM, et al: Response of psychotic and nonpsychotic depression to phenelzine. Am J Psychiatry 145:93–95, 1988b

Janowsky DS, Risch SC: Adrenergic-cholinergic balance and affective disorders: a review of clinical evidence and therapeutic implications. Psychiatric Hospital 15:163–171, 1984

Jarrett RB, Kraft D, Doyle J, et al: Preventing recurrent depression using cognitive therapy with and without a continuation phase: a randomized clinical trial. Arch Gen Psychiatry 58:381–388, 2001

John V, Rapp M, Pies R: Aggression, agitation, and mania with olanzapine (letter). Can J Psychiatry 43:1054, 1998

Johnson L, Andersson-Lundman G, Aberg-Wistedt A, et al: Age of onset in affective disorder: its correlation with hereditary and psychosocial factors. J Affect Disord 59:139–148, 2000

Kafantaris V: Treatment of bipolar disorder in children and adolescents. J Am Acad Child Adolesc Psychiatry 34:732–741, 1995

Kahn RS, Kalus O, Wetzler S, et al: The role of serotonin in the regulation of anxiety, in The Role of Serotonin in Psychiatric Disorders. Edited by Brown S-L, van Praag HM. New York, Brunner/Mazel, 1990, pp 129–160

Karliner W, Wehrheim HK: Maintenance convulsive treatments. Am J Psychiatry 121: 1113–1115, 1965

Kasper S, Wehr TA, Bartko JJ, et al: Epidemiological findings of seasonal changes in mood and behavior. Arch Gen Psychiatry 46:823–833, 1989

Kasper S, Fuger J, Moller H-J: Comparative efficacy of antidepressants. Drugs 43(suppl 2):11–23, 1992

Kastner T, Friedman DL: Verapamil and valproic acid treatment of prolonged mania. J Am Acad Child Adolesc Psychiatry 31: 271–275, 1992

Kaufman IC, Rosenblum LA: The reaction to separation in infant monkeys: anaclitic depression and conservation-withdrawal. Psychosom Med 29:648–675, 1967

Keck PE, McElroy SL, Vuckovic A, et al: Combined valproate and carbamazepine treatment of bipolar disorder. J Neuropsychiatry Clin Neurosci 4:319–322, 1992

Keck PE, McElroy SL, Tugrul KC, et al: Valproate oral loading in the treatment of acute mania. J Clin Psychiatry 54:305–308, 1993

Keck PE, Merikangas KR, McElroy SL, et al: Diagnostic and treatment implications of psychiatric comorbidity with migraine. Ann Clin Psychiatry 6:165–171, 1994

Keck PE, McElroy SL, Strakowski SM, et al: Compliance with maintenance treatment in bipolar disorder. Psychopharmacol Bull 33:87–91, 1997

Keilp JG, Sackeim HA, Brodsky BS, et al: Neuropsychological dysfunction in depressed suicide attempters. Am J Psychiatry 158:735–741, 2001

Keitner GI, Miller IW: Family functioning and major depression: an overview. Am J Psychiatry 147:1128–1137, 1990

Keitner GI, Ryan CE, Miller IW, et al: 12-Month outcome of patients with major depression and comorbid psychiatric or medical illness (compound depression). Am J Psychiatry 148:345–350, 1991

Keller MB, Klerman G, Lavori PW: Long-term outcome of episodes of major depression. JAMA 252:788–792, 1984

Keller MB, Lavori PW, Coryell W, et al: Bipolar I: a five-year prospective follow-up. J Nerv Ment Dis 181:238–245, 1993

Keller MB, McCullough JP, Klein DN, et al: A comparison of nefazodone, the cognitive behavioral-analysis system of psychotherapy, and their combination for the treatment of chronic depression. N Engl J Med 342:1462–1470, 2000

Kendler KK, Neale MC, Kessler CC, et al: A population-based twin study of major depression in women: the impact of varying definitions of illness. Arch Gen Psychiatry 49:257–266, 1992

Kendler KS: Mood-incongruent psychotic affective illness. Arch Gen Psychiatry 48: 362–369, 1991

Keshavan MS: Benzhexol withdrawal and cholinergic mechanisms in depression. Br J Psychiatry 147:560–564, 1985

Kettering RL, Harrow M, Grossman L, et al: The prognostic relevance of delusions in depression: a follow-up study. Am J Psychiatry 144:1154–1160, 1987

Khodorov B, Pinelis V, Vinskaya N, et al: Li+ protects nerve cells against destabilization of Ca2+ homeostasis and delayed death caused by removal of external Na+. FEBS Lett 448:173–176, 1999

Kinsella JE: Lipids, membrane receptors, and enzymes: effects of dietary fatty acids. JPEN J Parenter Enteral Nutr 14:200S–217S, 1990

Kirkcaldie M, Pridmore S, Reid P: Bridging the skull: electroconvulsive therapy (ECT) and repetitive transcranial magnetic stimulation (rTMS) in psychiatry. Convuls Ther 13:83–91, 1997

Kishi Y, Robinson RG: Suicidal plans following spinal cord injury: a six-month study. J Neuropsychiatry Clin Neurosci 8:442–445, 1996

Klapheke MM: Clozapine, ECT, and schizoaffective disorder, bipolar type. Convuls Ther 7:36–39, 1991

Klassen T, Verhey FRJ, Rozendaal N: Treatment of depression in Parkinson's disease: a meta-analysis. J Neuropsychiatry Clin Neurosci 7:281–286, 1995

Klein DN, Taylor EB, Harding K, et al: Double depression and episodic major depression: demographic, clinical, family, personality, and socioenvironmental characteristics and short-term outcome. Am J Psychiatry 145:1225–1231, 1988

Klerman GL: The current age of youthful melancholia: evidence for increase in depression among adolescents and young adults. Br J Psychiatry 152:4–14, 1988

Klerman GL, DiMascio A, Weissman MM, et al: Treatment of depression by drugs and psychotherapy. Am J Psychiatry 131:186–191, 1974

Klerman GL, Weissman MM, Rounsaville BJ, et al: Interpersonal Psychotherapy of Depression. New York, Basic Books, 1984

Klerman GL, Lavori PW, Rice J, et al: Birth-cohort trends in rates of major depressive disorder among relatives of patients with affective disorder. Arch Gen Psychiatry 42:689–693, 1985

Knesper DJ: The depressions of Alzheimer's disease: sorting, pharmacotherapy, and clinical advice. J Geriatr Psychiatry Neurol 8 (suppl 1):S40–S51, 1995

Kocsis JH, Frances AJ: A critical discussion of DSM-III dysthymic disorder. Am J Psychiatry 144:1534–1542, 1987

Kocsis JH, Frances AJ, Voss C, et al: Imipramine treatment for chronic depression. Arch Gen Psychiatry 45:253–257, 1988

Kocsis JH, Mason BJ, Frances AJ, et al: Prediction of response of chronic depression to imipramine. J Affect Disord 17:255–260, 1989

Koek RJ, Kessler CC: Possible induction of mania by risperidone (letter). Compr Psychiatry 57:174, 1996

Kroeze WK, Roth BI: The molecular biology of serotonin receptors: therapeutic implications for the interface of mood and psychosis. Biol Psychiatry 44:1128–1142, 1998

Krueger RB, Sackeim HA, Gamzu ER: Pharmacological treatment of the cognitive side effects of ECT: a review. Psychopharmacol Bull 28:409–424, 1992

Krupnick JL, Sotsky SM, Simmens S, et al: The role of the therapeutic alliance in psychotherapy and pharmacotherapy outcome: findings in the National Institute of Mental Health Treatment of Depression Collaborative Research Program. J Consult Clin Psychol 64:532–539, 1996

Kukopulos A, Reginaldi D, Laddomada P: Course of the manic-depressive cycle and changes caused by treatment. Pharmakopsychiatry Neuropsychopharmakoly 13:156–167, 1980

Kupfer DJ: Sleep research in depressive illness: clinical implications—a tasting menu. Biol Psychiatry 36:391–403, 1995

Kutcher S, Robertson HA: Electroconvulsive therapy in treatment-resistant bipolar youth. J Child Adolesc Psychopharmacol 5:167–175, 1995

Labbate LA, Lafer B, Thibault A, et al: Influence of phototherapy treatment duration for seasonal affective disorder: outcome at one vs. two weeks. Biol Psychiatry 38:747–750, 1995

Lamy S, Bergsholm P, d'Elia G: The antidepressant efficacy of high-dose nondominant long-distance parietotemporal and bitemporal electroconvulsive therapy. Convuls Ther 10:43–52, 1994

Lang C, Field T, Pickens J, et al: Preschoolers of dysphoric mothers. J Child Psychol Psychiatry 37:221–224, 1996

Lasch K, Weissman MM: Birth cohort changes in the rate of mania. Psychiatry Res 33:31–37, 1990

Lee DO, Steingard RJ, Cesena M, et al: Behavioral side effects of gabapentin in children. Epilepsia 37:87–90, 1996

Lehtinen V, Joukamaa M: Epidemiology of depression: prevalence, risk factors and treatment situation. Acta Psychiatr Scand 89 (suppl):7–10, 1994

Leibenluft E: Women with bipolar illness: clinical and research issues. Am J Psychiatry 153:163–173, 1996

Leibenluft E, Clark CH, Myers FS: The reproducibility of depressive and hypomanic symptoms across repeated episodes in patients with rapid-cycling bipolar disorder. J Affect Disord 33:83–88, 1995

Lenox RH, Modell JG, Weiner S: Acute treatment of manic agitation with lorazepam. Psychosomatics 27 (suppl):28–31, 1986

Leonard BE: Sub-types of serotonin receptors: biochemical changes and pharmacological consequences. Int Clin Psychopharmacol 7:13–21, 1992

Leonhard K: Differential diagnosis and different aetiology of monopolar and bipolar depressions. Psicopatologia 7:277–285, 1987a

Leonhard K: Differential diagnosis and different etiology of monopolar and bipolar phasic psychoses [in German]. Psychiatrie, Neurologie und Medizinische Psychologie 39:524–533, 1987b

Lepine J, Pelissolo A, Weiller E, et al: Recurrent brief depression: clinical and epidemiological issues. Psychopathology 28 (suppl 1):86–94, 1995

Letizia C, Kapik B, Flanders WD: Suicidal risk during controlled clinical investigations of fluvoxamine. Compr Psychiatry 57:415–421, 1996

Letterman L, Markowitz JS: Gabapentin: a review of published experience in the treatment of bipolar disorder and other psychiatric conditions. Pharmacotherapy 19:565–572, 1999

Levitt AJ, Joffe RT, MacDonald C: Life course of depressive illness and characteristics of current episode in patients with double depression. J Nerv Ment Dis 179:678–682, 1991

Lewinsohn PM, Antonuccio DA, Steinmetz J, et al: The Coping With Depression Course: A Psychoeducational Intervention for Unipolar Depression. Eugene, OR, Castalia Press, 1984

Lewinsohn PM, Klein DN, Seeley JR: Bipolar disorders in a community sample of older adolescents: prevalence, phenomenology, comorbidity, and course. J Am Acad Child Adolesc Psychiatry 34:454–463, 1995

Lindenmayer JP, Klebanov R: Olanzapine-induced manic-like syndrome (letter). J Clin Psychiatry 59:318–319, 1998

Lindhout D, Omtzigt JG: Pregnancy and the risk of teratogenicity. Epilepsia 33(suppl 4):S41–S48, 1992

Lish JD, Gyulai L, Resnick SM, et al: A family history study of rapid-cycling bipolar disorder. Psychiatry Res 48:37–46, 1993

Little JT, Kimbrell TA, Wassermann EM, et al: Cognitive effects of 1- and 20-hertz repetitive transcranial magnetic stimulation in depression: preliminary report. Neuropsychiatry Neuropsychol Behav Neurol 13:119–124, 2000

Littlejohn R, Leslie F, Cookson J: Depot antipsychotics in the prophylaxis of bipolar affective disorder. Br J Psychiatry 165:827–829, 1994

London JA: Mania associated with olanzapine (letter). J Am Acad Child Adolesc Psychiatry 37:135–136, 1998

Loo C, Mitchell P, Sachdev P, et al: Double-blind controlled investigation of transcranial magnetic stimulation for the treatment of resistant major depression. Am J Psychiatry 156:946–948, 1999

Loo H, Brochier T: Long-term treatment with antidepressive drugs [in French]. Ann Med Psychol (Paris) 153:190–196, 1995

Lopez-Ibor JL: The involvement of serotonin in psychiatric disorders and behaviour. Br J Psychiatry 153(suppl 3):26–39, 1988

Lowe MR: Treatment of rapid cycling affective illness (letter). Br J Psychiatry 146:558, 1985

Luborsky L: Principles of Psychoanalytic Psychotherapy: A Manual for Supportive-Expressive Treatment. New York, Basic Books, 1984

Lweeke FM, Bauer J, Elger CE: Manic episode due to gabapentin treatment (letter). Br J Psychiatry 175:291, 1999

Madhusoodanan S, Brenner R, Araujo L, et al: Efficacy of risperidone treatment for psychoses associated with schizophrenia, schizoaffective disorder, bipolar disorder, or senile dementia in 11 geriatric patients: a case series. Compr Psychiatry 56:514–518, 1995

MagPhil PLG, Thomas CB: Themes of interaction in medical students' Rorschach responses as predictors of midlife health or disease. Psychosom Med 43:215–225, 1981

Maier W, Lichtermann D, Minges J, et al: The relationship between bipolar disorder and alcoholism: a controlled family study. Psychol Med 25:787–796, 1995b

Mann J: Time-Limited Psychotherapy. Cambridge, MA, Harvard University Press, 1973

Mann JJ, Malone KM: Cerebrospinal fluid amines and higher-lethality suicide attempts in depressed inpatients. Biol Psychiatry 41:162–171, 1997

Mann JJ, Arango V, Marzuk PM: Evidence for the 5-HT hypothesis of suicide: a review of post-mortem studies. Br J Psychiatry 155 (suppl 8):7–14, 1989

Manna V: Disturbi affettivi bipolari e ruolo del calcio intraneuronale: effetti terapeutici del trattamento con cali di litio e/o calcio antagonista in pazienti con rapida inversione di polarita. Minerva Med 82:757–763, 1991

Martin M, Figiel GS, Mattingly G, et al: ECT-induced interictal delirium in patients with a history of a CVA. J Geriatr Psychiatry Neurol 5:149–155, 1992

Matsuo F, Madsen J, Tolman KG, et al: Lamotrigine high-dose tolerability and safety in patients with epilepsy: a double-blind, placebo-controlled, eleven-week study. Epilepsia 37:857–862, 1996

Mattson RH: Efficacy and adverse effects of established and new antiepileptic drugs. Epilepsia 36(suppl 2):S13–S26, 1995

Max JE, Richards L, Hamdan-Allen G: Case study: antimanic effectiveness of dextroamphetamine in a brain-injured adolescent. J Am Acad Child Adolesc Psychiatry 34:472–476, 1995

McCabe MS, Norris B: ECT versus chlorpromazine in mania. Biol Psychiatry 12:245–254, 1977

McCormick DA, Williamson A: Convergence and divergence of neurotransmitter action in human cerebral cortex. Proc Natl Acad Sci U S A 86:8098–8102, 1989

McDaniel JS, Musselman DL, Proter MR: Depression in patients with cancer. Arch Gen Psychiatry 52:89–99, 1995

McDermott OD, Prigerson HG, Reynolds CF III, et al: Sleep in the wake of complicated grief symptoms: an exploratory study. Biol Psychiatry 41:710–716, 1997

McDowell DM, Clodfelter RC: Depression and substance abuse: considerations of etiology, comorbidity, evaluation, and treatment. Psychiatr Ann 31:244–251, 2001

McElroy SL, Dessain EC, Pope HG, et al: Clozapine in the treatment of psychotic mood disorders, schizoaffective disorder, and schizophrenia. Compr Psychiatry 52:411–414, 1991

McElroy SL, Keck PE, Pope HG, et al: Clinical and research implications of the diagnosis of dysphoric or mixed mania or hypomania. Am J Psychiatry 149:1633–1644, 1992

McElroy SL, Keck PE, Strakowski SM: Mania, psychosis, and antipsychotics. Compr Psychiatry 57 (suppl 3):14–26, 1996a

McElroy SL, Keck PE, Stanton SP, et al: A randomized comparison of divalproex oral loading versus haloperidol in the initial treatment of acute psychotic mania. Compr Psychiatry 57:142–146, 1996b

McGlashan TH: Adolescent versus adult onset of mania. Am J Psychiatry 145:221–223, 1988

McGrath PJ, Nunes EV, Stewart JW, et al: Imipramine treatment of alcoholics with primary depression: a placebo controlled clinical trial. Arch Gen Psychiatry 53:232–240, 1996

McKinney WT: Animal models for depression and mania, in Depression and Mania. Edited by Georgotas A, Cancro R. New York, Elsevier, 1988, pp 181–196

McLean MJ: Gabapentin. Epilepsia 36 (suppl 2):S73–S86, 1995

McLean PD: Behavior therapy: theory and research, in Short-Term Psychotherapies for Depression. Edited by Rush AJ. New York, Guilford, 1982, pp 19–49

Meltzer HY: Serotonergic dysfunction in depression. Br J Psychiatry 155 (suppl 8): 25–31, 1989

Meltzer HY: The importance of serotonin-dopamine interactions in the action of clozapine. Br J Psychiatry 160 (suppl 17): 22–29, 1992

Merriam AE, Karasu TB: The role of psychotherapy in the treatment of depression. Arch Gen Psychiatry 53:301–302, 1996

Meterissian GB, Bradwejn J: Comparative studies on the efficacy of psychotherapy, pharmacotherapy, and their combination in depression: was adequate pharmacotherapy provided? J Clin Psychopharmacol 9:334–339, 1989

Miklowitz DJ: Longitudinal outcome and medication noncompliance among manic patients with and without mood-incongruent psychotic features. J Nerv Ment Dis 180:703–711, 1992

Milberger S, Biederman J, Faraone SV, et al: Attention deficit hyperactivity disorder and comorbid disorder: issues of overlapping symptoms. Am J Psychiatry 152: 1793–1799, 1995

Miller HL, Coombs DW, Leeper JD, et al: An analysis of the effect of suicide prevention facilities on suicide rates in the United States. Am J Public Health 74:340–343, 1984

Miller IW, Keitner GI: Combined medication and psychotherapy in the treatment of chronic mood disorders. Psychiatr Clin North Am 19:151–171, 1996

Miller IW, Norman WH, Dow MG: Psychosocial characteristics of "double depression." Am J Psychiatry 153:1042–1044, 1986

Milstein V, Small JG, Klapper MH: Uni- versus bilateral ECT in the treatment of mania. Convuls Ther 3:1–9, 1987

Mitchell PB, Wilhelm K, Parker G, et al: The clinical features of bipolar depression: a comparison with matched major depressive disorder patients. J Clin Psychiatry 62:212–216, 2001

Modell JG, Lenox RH, Weiner S: Inpatient clinical trial of lorazepam for the management of manic agitation. J Clin Psychopharmacol 5:109–113, 1985

Montgomery SA: Selective serotonin reuptake inhibitors in the acute treatment of depression, in Psychopharmacology, The Fourth Generation of Progress. Edited by Bloom FE, Kupfer DJ. New York, Raven, 1995, pp 1043–1051

Montgomery SA, Fineberg N: Is there a relationship between serotonin receptor subtypes and selectivity of response in specific psychiatric illnesses? Br J Psychiatry 155 (suppl 8):63–70, 1989

Moos RH, Mertens JR: Patterns of diagnoses, comorbidities, and treatment in late-middle-aged and older affective disorder patients: comparison of mental health and medical sectors. J Am Geriatr Soc 44: 682–688, 1996

Morris GL: Efficacy and tolerability of gabapentin in clinical practice. Clin Ther 17: 891–900, 1995

Morris PLP, Robinson RG, Samuels J: Depression, introversion and mortality following stroke. Aust N Z J Psychiatry 27:443–449, 1993

Mosimann UP, Rihs TA, Engeler J, et al: Mood effects of repetitive transcranial magnetic stimulation of left prefrontal cortex in healthy volunteers. Psychiatry Res 94: 252–256, 2000

Mukherjee S, Rosen AM, Caracci G, et al: Persistent tardive dyskinesia in bipolar patients. Arch Gen Psychiatry 43:342–346, 1986

Mukherjee S, Sackeim HA, Schnur DB: Electroconvulsive therapy of acute manic episodes: a review of 50 years' experience. Am J Psychiatry 151:169–176, 1994

Murad F: Drugs used for the treatment of angina: organic nitrates, calcium-channel blockers, and β-adrenergic agents, in Goodman and Gilman's The Pharmacological Basis of Therapeutics, 8th Edition. Edited by Gilman AG, Rall TW, Nies AS, et al. New York, Pergamon, 1991, pp 764–783

Murphy DL, Zohar J, Benkelfat C: Obsessive-compulsive disorder as a 5-HT subsystem-related behavioural disorder. Br J Psychiatry 155(suppl 8):15–24, 1989

National Institute of Mental Health: Affective Disorders (Mood Disorders): Budget Estimate. Bethesda, MD, National Institute of Mental Health, 1995

Nelson JC, Price LH, Jatlow PI: Neuroleptic dose and desipramine concentrations during combined treatment of unipolar delusional depression. Am J Psychiatry 143:1151–1154, 1986

Nelson WH, Khan A, Orr WW: Delusional depression: phenomenology, neuroendocrine function and tricyclic antidepressant response. J Affect Disord 6:297–306, 1984

Neylan TC: Treatment of sleep disturbances in depressed patients. Compr Psychiatry 56 (suppl 2):56–61, 1995

Nolen WA, Bloenkolk D: Treatment of bipolar depression: a review of the literature and a suggestion for an algorithm. Neuropsychobiology 42(suppl 1):11–17, 2000

O'Keane V, Moloney E, O'Neill H, et al: Blunted prolactin responses to d-fenfluramine in sociopathy: evidence for subsensitivity of central serotonergic function. Br J Psychiatry 160:643–646, 1992

Okuma T, Yamashita I, Takahashi R, et al: Comparison of the antimanic efficacy of carbamazepine and lithium carbonate by double-blind controlled study. Pharmacopsychiatry 23:143–150, 1990

Olie JP, Brochier T, Bouvet O, et al: La conception actuelle des troubles de l'humeur: incidence sur la prise en charge thérapeutique. Encephale 18 (Spec No 1):55–63, 1992

Osser DN: A systematic approach to the classification and pharmacotherapy of nonpsychotic major depression and dysthymia. J Clin Psychopharmacol 13:133–144, 1993

Overall JE, Donachie ND, Faillace LA: Implications of restrictive diagnosis for compliance to antidepressant drug therapy: alprazolam versus imipramine. Compr Psychiatry 48:51–54, 1987

Papatheodorou G, Kutcher S: The effect of adjunctive light therapy on ameliorating breakthrough depressive symptoms in adolescent-onset bipolar disorder. J Psychiatry Neurosci 20:226–232, 1995

Papatheodorou G, Kutcher SP, Katic M, et al: The efficacy and safety of divalproex sodium in the treatment of acute mania in adolescents and young adults: an open clinical trial. J Clin Psychopharmacol 15:110–116, 1995

Parker G, Blennerhassett J: Withdrawal reactions associated with venlafaxine. Aust N Z J Psychiatry 32:291–294, 1998

Parker V, Wong AH, Boon HS, et al: Adverse reactions to St. John's wort. Can J Psychiatry 46:77–79, 2001

Paykel ES: Handbook of Affective Disorders. New York, Guilford, 1982, pp xii, 699

Peet M, Peters S: Drug-induced mania. Drug Saf 12:146–153, 1995

Perry PJ, Zeilmann C, Arndt S: Tricyclic antidepressant concentrations in plasma: an estimate of their sensitivity and specificity as a predictor of response. J Clin Psychopharmacol 14:230–235, 1994

Peselow ED, Fieve RR, Difiglia C, et al: Lithium prophylaxis of bipolar illness. Br J Psychiatry 164:208–214, 1994

Petracca G, Teson A, Chemerinski E: A double-blind placebo-controlled study of clomipramine in depressed patients with Alzheimer's disease. J Neuropsychiatry Clin Neurosci 8:270–275, 1996

Petrides G, Dhossche D, Fink M, et al: Continuation ECT: relapse prevention in affective disorders. Convuls Ther 10:189–194, 1994

Petronis KR, Samuels JF, Moscicki EK, et al: An epidemiologic investigation of potential risk factors for suicide attempts. Soc Psychiatry Psychiatr Epidemiol 25:193–199, 1990

Pettinati HM, Rosenberg J: Memory self-ratings before and after electroconvulsive therapy: depression versus ECT induced. Biol Psychiatry 19:539–548, 1984

Piccinelli M, Wilkinson G: Outcome of depression in psychiatric settings. Br J Psychiatry 164:297–304, 1994

Piper AJ: Tricyclic antidepressants versus electroconvulsive therapy: a review of the evidence for efficacy in depression. Ann Clin Psychiatry 5:13–23, 1993

Pitts FN: Recent research on the DST. Compr Psychiatry 45:380–381, 1984

Poirier MF, Boyer P: Venlafaxine and paroxetine in treatment-resistant depression: double-blind, randomised comparison. Br J Psychiatry 175:12–16, 1999

Pokorny AD: Suicide prevention revisited. Suicide Life Threat Behav 23:1–10, 1993

Poland RE, McCracken JT, Lutchmansingh P, et al: Differential response of rapid eye movement sleep to cholinergic blockade by scopolamine in currently depressed, remitted, and normal control subjects. Biol Psychiatry 41:929–938, 1997

Porter RJ: How to initiate and maintain carbamazepine therapy in children and adults. Epilepsia 28 (suppl 3):S59–S63, 1987

Post RM: Non-lithium treatment for bipolar disorder. Compr Psychiatry 51 (suppl 8): 9–16, 1990a

Post RM: Prophylaxis of bipolar affective disorders. International Review of Psychiatry 2:277–320, 1990b

Post RM: Anticonvulsants and novel drugs, in Handbook of Affective Disorders. Edited by Paykel ES. Edinburgh, Scotland, Churchill Livingstone, 1992, pp 387–417

Post RM: Mechanisms underlying the evolution of affective disorders: implications for long-term treatment. Washington, DC, American Psychiatric Press, 1994, pp 23–65

Post RM: Comparative pharmacology of bipolar disorder and schizophrenia. Schizophr Res 39:153–158, 1999

Post RM, Roy-Byrne PP, Uhde TW: Graphic representation of the life course of illness in patients with affective disorder. Am J Psychiatry 145:844–848, 1988

Post RM, Ketter TA, Pazzaglia PJ, et al: New developments in the use of anticonvulsants as mood stabilizers. Neuropsychobiology 27:132–137, 1993

Post RM, Leverich GS, Denicoff KD, et al: Alternative approaches to refractory depression in bipolar illness. Depress Anxiety 5:175–189, 1997

Post RM, Kimbrell TA, McCann UD, et al: Repetitive transcranial magnetic stimulation as a neuropsychiatric tool: present status and future potential. J ECT 15:39–59, 1999

Pozo P, Aleantara AG: Mania-like syndrome in a patient with chronic schizophrenia during olanzapine treatment (letter). J Psychiatry Neurosci 23:309–310, 1998

Preda A, MacLean RW, Mazure CM, et al: Antidepressant-associated mania and psychosis resulting in psychiatric admissions. Compr Psychiatry 62:30–33, 2001

Prien RF, Caffey EM, Klett CJ: Comparison of lithium carbonate and chlorpromazine in the treatment of mania. Arch Gen Psychiatry 26:146–153, 1972

Priest RG, Gimbrett R, Roberts M, et al: Reversible and selective inhibitors of monoamine oxidase A in mental and other disorders. Acta Psychiatr Scand Suppl 386:40–43, 1995

Privitera MR, Lamberti JS, Maharaj K: Clozapine in a bipolar depressed patient (letter). Am J Psychiatry 150:986, 1993

Prudic J, Sackeim HA, Devanand DP, et al: The efficacy of ECT in double depression. Depression 1:38–44, 1993

Prudic J, Peyser S, Sackeim HA: Subjective memory complaints: a review of patient self-assessment of memory after electroconvulsive therapy. J ECT 16:121–132, 2000

Puri BK, Taylor DG, Alcock ME: Low-dose maintenance clozapine treatment in the prophylaxis of bipolar affective disorder. Br J Clin Pract 49:333–334, 1995

Rabheru K, Persad E: A review of continuation and maintenance electroconvulsive therapy. Can J Psychiatry 42:476–484, 1998

Rao U, Daley SE, Hammen C: Relationship between depression and substance use disorders in adolescent women during the transition to adulthood. J Am Acad Child Adolesc Psychiatry 39:315–322, 2000

Reeves RR, McBride WA, Brannon GE: Olanzapine-induced mania (letter). J Am Osteopath Assoc 98:550, 1998

Rehm LP: A self-control model of depression. Behav Ther 8:787–804, 1977

Reiger DA, Boyd JH, Burke JD: One-month prevalence of mental disorders in the United States. Arch Gen Psychiatry 45:977–986, 1988

Remotiv/Imipramine Study Group: Comparison of St John's wort and imipramine for treating depression: randomised controlled trial. BMJ 321:536–539, 2000

Reynolds CF III, Kupfer DJ, Thase ME, et al: Sleep, gender and depression: an analysis of gender effects on the electroencephalographic sleep of 302 depressed outpatients. Biol Psychiatry 28:673–684, 1990

Rifkin A, Doddi S, Karajgi B, et al: Dosage of haloperidol for mania. Br J Psychiatry 165:113–116, 1994

Riggs PD, Mikulich S, Coffman L, et al: Fluoxetine in drug-dependent delinquents with major depression: an open trial. J Child Adolesc Psychopharmacol 7:87–95, 1997

Roberts RE, Lewinsohn PM, Seeley JR: Symptoms of DSM-III-R major depression in adolescence: evidence from an epidemiological survey. J Am Acad Child Adolesc Psychiatry 34:1608–1617, 1995

Rosenbaum JF, Fava M, Nierenberg AA, et al: Treatment-resistant mood disorders, in Treatment of Psychiatric Disorders. Edited by Gabbard GO. Washington, DC, American Psychiatric Press, 1995, pp 1275–1328

Rosenthal NE, Blehar MC (eds): Seasonal Affective Disorders and Phototherapy. New York, Guilford, 1989

Rothschild AJ, Bates KS, Boehringer KL, et al: Olanzapine response in psychotic depression. J Clin Psychiatry 60:116–118, 1999

Roy-Byrne PP, Joffe RT, Uhde TW, et al: Approaches to the evaluation and treatment of rapid-cycling affective illness. Br J Psychiatry 145:543–550, 1984

Roy-Byrne PP, Post RM, Uhde TW, et al: The longitudinal course of recurrent affective illness: life chart data from research patients at the NIMH. Acta Psychiatr Scand Suppl 317:1–34, 1985

Rudd MD, Dahm PF, Rajab MH: Diagnostic comorbidity in persons with suicidal ideation and behavior. Am J Psychiatry 150:928–934, 1993

Rush AJ, Kupfer DJ: Strategies and tactics in the treatment of depression, in Treatment of Psychiatric Disorders. Edited by Gabbard GO. Washington, DC, American Psychiatric Press, 1995, pp 1349–1368

Sachs GS: Use of clonazepam for bipolar disorder. Compr Psychiatry 51(suppl 5):31–34, 1990

Sachs GS: Treatment-resistant bipolar depression. Psychiatr Clin North Am 19:215–235, 1996

Sachs GS, Lafer B, Stoll AL, et al: A double-blind trial of bupropion versus desipramine for bipolar depression. Compr Psychiatry 55:391–393, 1994a

Sachs GS, Lafer B, Truman CJ, et al: Lithium monotherapy: miracle, myth and misunderstanding. Psychiatr Ann 24:299–306, 1994b

Sachs G, Printz DJ, Kahn DA, et al: The Expert Consensus Guideline Series: Medication Treatment of Bipolar Disorder 2000. Postgrad Med 108(Spec No):1–104, 2000

Sackeim HA: Continuation therapy following ECT: directions for future research. Psychopharmacol Bull 30:501–521, 1994

Sackeim HA, Freeman J, McElhiney M, et al: Effects of major depression on estimates of intelligence. J Clin Exp Neuropsychol 14:268–288, 1992

Sajatovic M: A pilot study evaluating the efficacy of risperidone in treatment-refractory, acute bipolar, and schizoaffective mania (abstract). Psychopharmacol Bull 31: 613, 1996

Sajatovic M, DiGiovanni SK, Bastani B, et al: Risperidone therapy in treatment refractory acute bipolar and schizoaffective mania. Psychopharmacol Bull 32:55–61, 1996

Salzman C, Green AI, Rodriguez-Villa F, et al: Benzodiazepines combined with neuroleptics for management of severe disruptive behavior. Psychosomatics 27 (suppl): 17–21, 1986

Sanderson WC, Wetzler S, Beck AT, et al: Prevalence of personality disorders in patients with major depression and dysthymia. Psychiatry Res 42:93–99, 1992

Santos AB, Morton WA: More on clonazepam in manic agitation. J Clin Psychopharmacol 7:439–440, 1987

Saxena S, Maltikarjuna P: Severe memory impairment with acute overdose lithium toxicity. Br J Psychiatry 152:853–854, 1988

Schaffer CB, Schaffer LC: The use of risperidone in the treatment of bipolar disorder (letter). Compr Psychiatry 57:136, 1996

Schildkraut JJ: The catecholamine hypothesis of affective disorders: a review of supporting evidence. Am J Psychiatry 122:509–514, 1965

Schneekloth TB, Rummans TA, Logan KM: Electroconvulsive therapy in adolescents. Convuls Ther 9:158–166, 1993

Schoenenberger RA, Tanasijevic MJ, Jha A, et al: Appropriateness of antiepileptic drug level monitoring. JAMA 274:1622–1626, 1995

Schou M: Prophylactic lithium treatment of unipolar and bipolar manic-depressive illness. Psychopathology 28(suppl 1):81–85, 1995

Schou M: Forty years of lithium treatment. Arch Gen Psychiatry 54:9–13, 1997

Schwarz T, Loewenstein J, Isenberg KE: Maintenance ECT: indications and outcome. Convuls Ther 11:14–23, 1995

Scott J: Chronic depression. Br J Psychiatry 153:287–297, 1988

Scott J: Chronic depression: can cognitive therapy succeed when other treatments fail? Behavioral Psychotherapy 20:25–36, 1992

Scott TF, Allen D, Price TRP: Characterization of major depression symptoms in multiple sclerosis patients. J Neuropsychiatry Clin Neurosci 8:318–323, 1996

Seligman MEP: Helplessness: On Depression, Development and Death. San Francisco, CA, WH Freeman, 1975

Severus WE, Ahrens B: Omega-3 fatty acids in psychiatry. Nervenarzt 71:58–62, 2000

Sexton HC, Hembre K, Kvarme G: The interaction of the alliance and therapy microprocess: a sequential analysis. J Consult Clin Psychol 64:471–480, 1996

Sharma V, Yatham LN, Haslam DR, et al: Continuation and prophylactic treatment of bipolar disorder. Can J Psychiatry 42 (suppl 2):92S–100S, 1997

Shea MT, Elkin I, Hirschfeld RMA, et al: Psychotherapeutic treatment of depression, in American Psychiatric Press Review of Psychiatry. Edited by Frances AJ, Hales RE. Washington, DC, American Psychiatric Press, 1988, pp 235–255

Shelton RC, Keller MB, Gelenberg AJ, et al: Effectiveness of St. John's wort in major depression: a randomized controlled trial. JAMA 285:1978–1986, 2001a

Shelton RC, Tollefson GD, Tohen M, et al: A novel augmentation strategy for treating resistant major depression. Am J Psychiatry 158:131–134, 2001b

Shulman KI, Hermann N: Bipolar disorder in old age. Can Fam Physician 45:1229–1237, 1999

Siever LJ, Davis KL: Overview: toward a dysregulation hypothesis of depression. Am J Psychiatry 142:1017–1025, 1985

Simhandl CA, Denk E, Thau K: The comparative efficacy of carbamazepine low and high serum level and lithium carbonate in the prophylaxis of affective disorders. J Affect Disord 28:221–231, 1993

Simon AE, Aubry JM, Malky L, et al: Hypomania-like syndrome induced by olanzapine. Int Clin Psychopharmacol 14:377–378, 1999

Simpson SG, Folstein SE, Meyers DA, et al: Bipolar II: the most common bipolar phenotype? Am J Psychiatry 150:901–903, 1993

Simpson S, Baldwin RC, Jackson A, et al: The differentiation of DSM-III-R psychotic depression in later life from nonpsychotic depression: comparisons of brain changes measured by multispectral analysis of magnetic resonance brain images, neuropsychological findings, and clinical features. Biol Psychiatry 45:193–204, 1999

Singh AN, Catalan J: Risperidone in HIV related manic psychosis. Lancet 344:1029–1030, 1994

Small JG, Small IF, Milstein V: Manic symptoms: an indication for bilateral ECT. Biol Psychiatry 20:125–134, 1985

Small JG, Klapper MH, Milstein V, et al: Comparison of therapeutic modalities for mania. Psychopharmacol Bull 32:623–627, 1996

Solan WJ, Khan A, Avery DH, et al: Psychotic and nonpsychotic depression: comparison of response to ECT. Compr Psychiatry 49: 97–99, 1988

Solhkhah R, Finkel J, Hird S: Possible risperidone-induced visual hallucinations (letter). J Am Acad Child Adolesc Psychiatry 39:1074–1075, 2000

Solomon DA, Bauer MS: Continuation and maintenance pharmacotherapy for unipolar and bipolar mood disorders. Psychiatr Clin North Am 16:515–540, 1993

Solomon DA, Keitner GI, Miller IW, et al: Course of illness and maintenance treatments for patients with bipolar disorder. Compr Psychiatry 56:5–13, 1995

Somoza E, Mossman D: Optimizing REM latency as a diagnostic test for depression using receiver operating characteristic analysis and information theory. Biol Psychiatry 27:990–1006, 1990

Sotsky SM, Glass DR, Shea MT, et al: Patient predictors of response to psychotherapy and pharmacotherapy: findings in the NIMH Treatment of Depression Collaborative Research Program. Am J Psychiatry 148:997–1008, 1991

Spiker DG, Kupfer DJ: Placebo response rates in psychotic and nonpsychotic depression. J Affect Disord 14:21–23, 1988

Spiker DG, Weiss JC, Dealy RS, et al: The pharmacological treatment of delusional depression. Am J Psychiatry 142:430–436, 1985

Spiker DG, Perel JM, Hanin I, et al: The pharmacological treatment of delusional depression: part II. J Clin Psychopharmacol 6:339–342, 1986a

Spiker DG, Dealy RS, Hanin I, et al: Treating delusional depressives with amitriptyline. Compr Psychiatry 47:243–246, 1986b

Srisurapanont M, Yatham LN, Zis AP: Treatment of acute bipolar depression: a review of the literature. Can J Psychiatry 40: 533–544, 1995

Stancer HC, Persad E: Treatment of intractable rapid-cycling manic-depressive disorder with levothyroxine: clinical observations. Arch Gen Psychiatry 39:311–312, 1982

Stoll AL, Mayer PV, Kolbrener M, et al: Antidepressant-associated mania: a controlled comparison with spontaneous mania. Am J Psychiatry 151:1642–1645, 1994

Stoll AL, Severus WE, Freeman MP, et al: Omega3 fatty acids in bipolar disorder: a preliminary double-blind, placebo-controlled trial. Arch Gen Psychiatry 56:407–412, 1999

Strakowski S, McElroy SL, Keck PW Jr: The co-occurrence of mania with medical and other psychiatric disorders. Int J Psychiatry Med 24:305–328, 1994

Strober M, Carlson G: Bipolar illness in adolescents with major depression. Arch Gen Psychiatry 39:549–555, 1982

Strupp HH, Binder JL: Psychotherapy in a New Key: A Guide to Time-Limited Dynamic Psychotherapy. New York, Basic Books, 1984

Suomi SJ, Seaman SF, Lewis JK: Effects of imipramine treatment of separation-induced social disorders in rhesus monkeys. Arch Gen Psychiatry 35:321–325, 1978

Suppes T, McElroy SL, Gilbert J, et al: Clozapine in the treatment of dysphoric mania. Biol Psychiatry 32:270–280, 1992

Suppes T, Phillips KA, Judd CR: Clozapine treatment of nonpsychotic rapid cycling bipolar disorder: a report of three cases. Biol Psychiatry 36:338–340, 1994

Swann AC: Mixed or dysphoric manic states: psychopathology and treatment. Compr Psychiatry 56 (suppl 3):6–10, 1995

Swartz KL, Pratt LA, Armenenian HK, et al: Mental disorders and the incidence of migraine headaches in a community sample: results from the Baltimore Epidemiologic Catchment Area Follow-up Study. Arch Gen Psychiatry 57:945–950, 2000

Tallian KB, Nahata MC, Lo W, et al: Gabapentin associated with aggressive behavior in pediatric patients with seizures. Epilepsia 37:501–502, 1996

Teicher MH, Glod CA, Cole JO: Antidepressant drugs and the emergence of suicidal tendencies. Drug Saf 8:186–212, 1993

Teicher MH, Glod CA, Magnus E, et al: Circadian rest-activity disturbances in seasonal affective disorder. Arch Gen Psychiatry 54:124–130, 1997

Terao T: Subclinical hypothyroidism in recurrent mania. Biol Psychiatry 33:853–854, 1993

Thase ME: Relapse and recurrence in unipolar major depression: short-term and long-term approaches. Compr Psychiatry 51 (suppl 26):51–57, 1990

Thase ME: Long-term treatments of recurrent depressive disorders. Compr Psychiatry 53 (suppl 9):32–44, 1992

Thase ME, Kupfer DJ: Recent developments in the pharmacotherapy of mood disorders. J Consult Clin Psychol 64:646–659, 1996

Thase ME, Simons AD, McGeary J, et al: Relapse after cognitive behavior therapy of depression: potential implications for longer courses of treatment. Am J Psychiatry 149:1046–1052, 1992

Thase ME, Reynolds CF, Frank E, et al: Response to cognitive-behavioral therapy in chronic depression. J Psychother Pract Res 3:204–214, 1994

Thompson PJ, Trimble MR: Anticonvulsant serum levels: relationship to impairments of cognitive functioning. J Neurol Neurosurg Psychiatry 46:227–233, 1983

Tohen M, Zarate CA, Centorrino F, et al: Risperidone in the treatment of mania. Compr Psychiatry 57:249–253, 1996a

Tohen M, Zarate CA, Centorrino F, et al: Risperidone in the treatment of mania (abstract). Psychopharmacol Bull 31:626, 1996b

Tohen M, Sanger TM, McElroy SL, et al: Olanzapine versus placebo in the treatment of acute mania. Am J Psychiatry 156:702–709, 1999

Tohen M, Jacobs TG, Grundy SL, et al: Efficacy of olanzapine in acute bipolar mania: a double-blind, placebo-controlled study. The Olanzapine HGGW Study Group. Arch Gen Psychiatry 57:841–849, 2000

Tomitaka S, Sakamoto K: Definition and prognosis of rapid cycling affective disorder (letter). Am J Psychiatry 151:1524, 1994

Triggs WJ, McCoy KJ, Greer R, et al: Effects of left frontal transcranial magnetic stimulation on depressed mood, cognition, and corticomotor threshold. Biol Psychiatry 48:1440–1446, 1999

Tsuang D, Coryell W: An 8-year follow-up of patients with DSM-III-R psychotic depression, schizoaffective disorder and schizophrenia. Am J Psychiatry 150:1182–1188, 1993

Ulmsten U, Anderson KE, Wingerup I: Treatment of premature labor with the calcium antagonist nifedipine. Arch Gynecol 229:1–5, 1980

Vanelle J-M, Loo H, Galinowski MD, et al: Maintenance ECT in intractable manic-depressive disorders. Convuls Ther 10:195–205, 1994

Van Londen L, Molenaar RPG, Goerkoop JG, et al: Three- to 5-year prospective follow-up of outcome in major depression. Psychol Med 28:731–735, 1998

van Praag HM, Kahn RS, Asnis GM: Denosologization of biological psychiatry or the specificity of 5-HT disturbances in psychiatric disorders. J Affect Disord 13:1–8, 1987

Vestergaard P, Licht RW, Brodersen A, et al: Outcome of lithium prophylaxis: a prospective follow-up of affective disorder patients assigned to high and low serum lithium levels. Acta Psychiatr Scand 98:310–315, 1998

Walden J, Hesslinger B: Value of old and new anticonvulsants in treatment of psychiatric diseases. Fortschr Neurol Psychiatr 63: 320–335, 1995

Walter G, Rey J: An epidemiological study of the use of ECT in adolescents. J Am Acad Child Adolesc Psychiatry 36:809–815, 1997

Walton SA, Berk M, Brook S: Superiority of lithium over verapamil in mania: a randomized, controlled, single-blind trial. Compr Psychiatry 57:543–546, 1996

Warner R, Appleby L, Whitton A, et al: Demographic and obstetric risk factors for postnatal psychiatric morbidity. Br J Psychiatry 168:607–611, 1996

Warshaw MG, Keller MB: The relationship between fluoxetine use and suicidal behavior in 654 subjects with anxiety disorders. Compr Psychiatry 57:158–166, 1996

Wehr TA: Can antidepressants induce rapid cycling? Arch Gen Psychiatry 50:495–496, 1993

Wehr TA, Sack DA, Rosenthal NE, et al: Rapid cycling affective disorder: contributing factors and treatment responses in 51 patients. Am J Psychiatry 145:179–184, 1988

Weiner RD: Does electroconvulsive therapy cause brain damage? Behav Brain Sci 7:1–13, 1984

Weiner RD: Electroconvulsive therapy, in Treatment of Psychiatric Disorders. Edited by Gabbard GO. Washington, DC, American Psychiatric Press, 1995, pp 1237–1273

Weissman MM, Prusoff BA, DiMascio A, et al: Efficacy of drugs and psychotherapy in the treatment of acute depressive episodes. Am J Psychiatry 136:555–558, 1979

Weissman MM, Prusoff BA, Gammon GD, et al: Psychopathology in the children (ages 6–18) of depressed and normal parents. J Am Acad Child Adolesc Psychiatry 23: 78–84, 1984

Weissman MM, Warner V, John K, et al: Delusional depression and bipolar spectrum: evidence for a possible association from a family study of children. Neuropsychopharmacology 1:257–264, 1988a

Weissman MM, Leaf PJ, Bruce ML: The epidemiology of dysthymia in five communities: rates, risks, comorbidity, and treatment. Am J Psychiatry 145:815–819, 1988b

Weissman MM, Bland RC, Canino GJ, et al: Cross-national epidemiology of major depression and bipolar disorder. JAMA 276: 293–299, 1996

Wells KB, Burnnam A, Rogers WH, et al: The course of depression in adult outpatients: results from the medical outcomes study. Arch Gen Psychiatry 49:788–794, 1992

Wide-Swensson DG, Ingemarsson I, Lunell N, et al: Calcium channel blockade (isradipine) in treatment of hypertension in pregnancy: a randomized placebo-controlled study. Am J Obstet Gynecol 173: 872–878, 1996

Winokur G: Manic-depressive disease (bipolar): is it autonomous? Psychopathology 28 (suppl 1):51–58, 1995

Winokur G, Morrison J: The Iowa 500: follow-up of 225 depressives. Br J Psychiatry 123:543–548, 1973

Wolkowitz OD, Reus VI: Treatment of depression with antiglucocorticoid drugs. Psychosom Med 61:698–711, 1999

Woods BT, Yurgelun-Todd D, Mikulis D, et al: Age-related MRI abnormalities in bipolar illness: a clinical study. Biol Psychiatry 38:846–847, 1995

Young MA, Fogg LF, Schefner WA, et al: Interaction of risk factors in predicting suicide. Am J Psychiatry 151:434–435, 1994

Zarate CA Jr, Tohen M, Banov MD, et al: Is clozapine a mood stabilizer? Compr Psychiatry 56:108–112, 1995

CHAPTER 7

Anxiety Disorders

Eric Hollander, M.D.

Daphne Simeon, M.D.

Anxiety disorders are the most common of all psychiatric illnesses and result in considerable functional impairment and distress. Recent research developments have had a broad impact on our understanding of the underlying mechanisms of illness and treatment response. Working with patients who have an anxiety disorder can be highly gratifying for the informed psychiatrist, because these patients, who are in considerable distress, often respond to proper treatment and return to a high level of functioning. The major anxiety disorders presented in this chapter are panic disorder, generalized anxiety disorder (GAD), social phobia, specific phobias, obsessive-compulsive disorder (OCD), and posttraumatic stress disorder (PTSD).

If pathological anxiety is induced either by psychoactive substance use or by an Axis III physical illness, it is classified in DSM-IV (American Psychiatric Association 1994) under the anxiety disorders (substance-induced anxiety disorder or anxiety disorder due to a general medical condition, respectively). DSM-IV also allowed specification of the subtype as generalized anxiety, panic attacks, or obsessive-compulsive symptoms.

Panic Disorder

The DSM-IV-TR (American Psychiatric Association 2000) definition of a panic attack is presented in Table 7–1. Panic disorder is subdivided into panic disorder with and panic disorder without agoraphobia, as in DSM-III-R, depending on whether any secondary phobic avoidance is present (Tables 7–2 and 7–3).

Clinical Description

Onset

In the typical onset of a case of panic disorder, a person is engaged in some ordinary aspect of life when suddenly his heart begins to pound and he cannot catch his breath. The person feels dizzy, lightheaded, and faint and is convinced he is about to die. Patients with panic disorder are usually young adults, most likely in the third decade; however, onset may be as late as the sixth decade.

Although the first attack generally strikes during some routine activity, several events are often associated with the early presentation of panic disorder. It is not uncommon for the initial panic attack

TABLE 7–1. DSM-IV-TR definition of panic attack

A discrete period of intense fear or discomfort in which four (or more) of the following symptoms developed abruptly and reached a peak within 10 minutes:

(1) Palpitations, pounding heart, or accelerated heart rate
(2) Sweating
(3) Trembling or shaking
(4) Sensations of shortness of breath or smothering
(5) Feeling of choking
(6) Chest pain or discomfort
(7) Nausea or abdominal distress
(8) Feeling dizzy, unsteady, lightheaded, or faint
(9) Derealization (feelings of unreality) or depersonalization (being detached from oneself)
(10) Fear of losing control or "going crazy"
(11) Fear of dying
(12) Paresthesias (numbness or tingling sensation)
(13) Chills or hot flushes

TABLE 7–2. DSM-IV-TR diagnostic criteria for panic disorder with agoraphobia

A. Both (1) and (2):
  (1) recurrent unexpected panic attacks
  (2) at least one of the attacks has been followed by 1 month (or more) of one (or more) of the following:
    (a) persistent concern about having additional attacks
    (b) worry about the implications of the attack or its consequences (e.g., losing control, having a heart attack, "going crazy")
    (c) a significant change in behavior related to the attacks
B. The presence of agoraphobia.
C. The panic attacks are not due to the direct physiological effects of a substance (e.g., a drug of abuse, a medication) or a general medical condition (e.g., hyperthyroidism).
D. The panic attacks are not better accounted for by another mental disorder, such as social phobia (e.g., occurring on exposure to feared social situations), specific phobia (e.g., on exposure to a specific phobic situation), obsessive-compulsive disorder (e.g., on exposure to dirt in someone with an obsession about contamination), posttraumatic stress disorder (e.g., in response to stimuli associated with a severe stressor), or separation anxiety disorder (e.g., in response to being away from home or close relatives).

to occur in the context of a life-threatening illness or accident, the loss of a close interpersonal relationship, or a separation from family (e.g., after starting college or accepting a job out of town). Patients developing either hypothyroidism or hyperthyroidism may experience the first flurry of attacks at this time. Attacks also begin during the immediate postpartum period. Finally, many patients have reported experiencing their first panic attacks while taking drugs of abuse, especially marijuana, lysergic acid diethylamide (LSD), sedatives, cocaine, and amphetamines. However, even when these concomitant conditions are resolved, the attacks often continue unabated. This situation gives the impression that some stressors may act as triggers to provoke the beginning of panic attacks in patients who are already predisposed.

Patients experiencing their first panic

attack generally fear that they are having a heart attack or losing their mind. Such patients often rush to the nearest emergency department, where routine laboratory tests, electrocardiography, and physical examination are performed. All that is found is an occasional case of sinus tachycardia, and the patients are reassured and sent home. These patients may indeed feel reassured, and at this point the diagnosis of panic disorder would be premature. However, perhaps a few days or even weeks later they will again have the sud-

TABLE 7–3. DSM-IV-TR diagnostic criteria for panic disorder without agoraphobia

A. Both (1) and (2):
  (1) recurrent unexpected panic attacks
  (2) at least one of the attacks has been followed by 1 month (or more) of one (or more) of the following:
    (a) persistent concern about having additional attacks
    (b) worry about the implications of the attack or its consequences (e.g., losing control, having a heart attack, "going crazy")
    (c) a significant change in behavior related to the attacks
B. Absence of agoraphobia.
C. The panic attacks are not due to the direct physiological effects of a substance (e.g., a drug of abuse, a medication) or a general medical condition (e.g., hyperthyroidism).
D. The panic attacks are not better accounted for by another mental disorder, such as social phobia (e.g., occurring on exposure to feared social situations), specific phobia (e.g., on exposure to a specific phobic situation), obsessive-compulsive disorder (e.g., on exposure to dirt in someone with an obsession about contamination), posttraumatic stress disorder (e.g., in response to stimuli associated with a severe stressor), or separation anxiety disorder (e.g., in response to being away from home or close relatives).

den onset of severe anxiety with all of the associated physical symptoms. Again, they seek emergency medical treatment. At this point, they may be told the problem is psychological, be given a prescription for a benzodiazepine tranquilizer, or be referred for extensive medical workup.

Symptoms

Typically, during a panic attack, a patient will be engaged in a routine activity—perhaps reading a book, eating in a restaurant, driving a car, or attending a concert—when he or she will experience the sudden onset of overwhelming fear, terror, apprehension, and a sense of impending doom. Several of a group of associated symptoms, mostly physical, are also experienced: dyspnea, palpitations, chest pain or discomfort, choking or smothering sensations, dizziness or unsteadiness, feelings of unreality (derealization and/or depersonalization), paresthesias, hot and cold flashes, sweating, faintness, trembling and shaking, and a fear of dying, going crazy, or losing control of oneself. It is clear that most of the physical sensations of a panic attack represent massive overstimulation of the autonomic nervous system.

Attacks usually last from 5 to 20 minutes and rarely as long as an hour. Patients who claim they have attacks that last a whole day may fall into one of four categories. 1) Some patients continue to feel agitated and fatigued for several hours after the main portion of the attack has subsided. 2) At times, attacks occur, subside, and occur again in a wavelike manner. 3) Alternatively, the patient with so-called long panic attacks often has some other form of pathological anxiety, such as severe generalized anxiety, agitated depression, or obsessional tension states. 4) Finally, in some cases, such severe anticipatory anxiety may develop with time in expectation of future panic attacks so that the two may blend together in the patient's description and be difficult to distinguish.

Although many people experience an occasional unexpected attack of panic, the diagnosis of panic disorder is only made when the attacks occur with some regularity and frequency. However, patients with occasional unexpected panic attacks may be genetically similar to patients with panic disorder. A twin study found the best results for genetic linkage when patients with regular panic attacks were included together with patients who had only occasional attacks (Torgersen 1983).

Some patients do not progress in their illness beyond the point of continuing to have unexpected panic attacks. Most patients develop some degree of anticipatory anxiety consequent to the experience of repetitive panic attacks. The patient comes to dread experiencing an attack and starts worrying about doing so in the intervals between attacks. This can progress until the level of fearfulness and autonomic hyperactivity in the interval between panic attacks almost approximates the level during the actual attack itself. Such patients may be mistaken for GAD patients.

Agoraphobia

Agoraphobia frequently develops in response to panic attacks, leading to the DSM-IV diagnosis of panic disorder with agoraphobia. The clinical picture in agoraphobia consists of multiple and varied fears and avoidance behaviors that center around three main themes: 1) fear of leaving home, 2) fear of being alone, and 3) fear of being away from home in situations in which one can feel trapped, embarrassed, or helpless. According to DSM-IV, the fear is one of developing distressing symptoms in situations in which escape is difficult or help is unavailable. Typical agoraphobic fears are of using public transportation (buses, trains, subways, planes); being in crowds, theaters, elevators, restaurants, supermarkets, or department stores; waiting in line; and of traveling a distance from home. In severe cases, patients may be completely housebound, fearful of leaving home without a companion or even of staying home alone.

Character Traits

It has not been clearly established whether particular character types are correlated with panic disorder, and studies are fur-

ther confounded because the presence of panic disorder may have secondary effects on personality. Noyes et al. (1991) conducted personality follow-up of patients with panic disorder who were treated for panic over 3 years and found that the initial avoidant and dependent traits were to a large extent state related, waning with the treatment of panic. On the other hand, experience leads many clinicians to feel that patients with agoraphobia and panic are more likely to have histories of dependent character traits that predate the onset of panic.

Epidemiology

The National Institute of Mental Health (NIMH) Epidemiologic Catchment Area (ECA) study examined the population prevalence of DSM-III–diagnosed panic disorder using the Diagnostic Interview Schedule (DIS; Regier et al. 1988). The 1-month, 6-month, and lifetime prevalence rates for panic disorder at all five study sites combined were 0.5%, 0.8%, and 1.6%, respectively. Women had a 1-month prevalence rate of 0.7%, which was significantly higher than the 0.3% rate found among men; women also tended to have a greater rise in panic disorder in the age range of 25–44 years, and their attacks tended to continue longer into older age (Regier et al. 1988). The epidemiology of panic disorder appears to be similar in whites and blacks (Horwath et al. 1993).

The relationship between panic disorder and major depression has been questioned in numerous studies because it is well known that the two commonly co-occur. A recent family study found that panic disorder and major depression are clearly distinct disorders, despite their substantial co-occurrence, and panic comorbid with major depression does not segregate in families as a distinct disorder (Weissman et al. 1993).

Etiology

Biological Theories

Several biological theories of panic disorder are prominent in the psychiatric literature. Here we summarize the evidence for or against some of the most promising of these. Certain agents have a powerful and specific capacity to induce panic, in contrast with other agents that produce prominent physiological changes but fail to induce panic. These findings argue strongly against the notion that panic is a reaction to nonspecific distressing stimuli and suggest more specific biological bases, even if these involve multiple neurochemicals and circuits. The various theories discussed in this subsection need not be viewed as mutually exclusive, but rather as potentially interlocking pieces of a larger puzzle. Neurochemical, imaging, and genetic research findings are described as well.

The sympathetic system. Some investigators have found anxiety reactions associated with increases in levels of urinary catecholamines, especially epinephrine. Studies of healthy individuals exposed to novel stress also demonstrate elevations in plasma catecholamine levels (Dimsdale and Moss 1980). Elevated plasma levels of epinephrine are not, however, a regular accompaniment of panic attacks induced in the laboratory (Liebowitz et al. 1985a).

Examination of various autonomic parameters seems to dispel the notion of simple autonomic dysregulation in panic (M.B. Stein and Asmundson 1994). Indeed, global sympathetic activation is not observed in panic disorder patients at rest, nor even during panic attacks in some patients (Wilkinson et al. 1998).

The locus coeruleus has been implicated in the pathogenesis of panic attacks. This nucleus is located in the pons and contains more than 50% of all noradrener-gic neurons in the entire central nervous system. It sends afferent projections to a wide area of the brain, including the hippocampus, amygdala, limbic lobe, and cerebral cortex. Electrical stimulation of the animal locus coeruleus produces a marked fear and anxiety response, whereas ablation of the animal locus coeruleus renders an animal less susceptible to fear response in the face of threatening stimuli. In humans, drugs known to be capable of increasing locus coeruleus discharge in animals are anxiogenic, whereas many drugs that curtail locus coeruleus firing and decrease central noradrenergic turnover are antianxiety agents.

Yohimbine challenge was reported to induce greater anxiety and a greater increase in plasma 3-methoxy-4-hydroxyphenyl-glycol (MHPG), a major noradrenergic metabolite, in patients with frequent panic attacks, compared with patients who have panic attacks less frequently or with healthy control subjects. Such a finding is suggestive of heightened central noradrenergic activity in panic (Charney and Heninger 1986). The results from challenge tests with the α_2-adrenergic agonist clonidine, although difficult to interpret, have suggested noradrenergic dysregulation in panic, with hypersensitivity of some and subsensitivity of other brain α_2-adrenoreceptors. Compared with control subjects, panic disorder patients had heightened cardiovascular responses (Charney et al. 1984; Nutt 1989) but blunted growth hormone (GH) responses (Nutt 1989; Tancer et al. 1993) to clonidine. Dysregulated noradrenergic function, in the form of markedly elevated MHPG volatility in response to clonidine challenge, has been described in patients with panic disorder; it normalizes after treatment with selective serotonin reuptake inhibitors (SSRIs) (Coplan et al. 1997).

The panicogen sodium lactate. Lactate-provoked panic is specific to patients with prior spontaneous attacks, closely resembles such attacks, and can be blocked by the same drugs that block natural attacks. Pitts and McClure (1967) first administered intravenous infusions of sodium lactate to patients with "anxiety" disorder; they found that most of the patients experienced an anxiety attack during the infusion. The subjects all believed that these attacks were quite typical of their naturally occurring attacks. Healthy control subjects did not experience panic attacks during the infusion.

Having been replicated on numerous occasions under proper experimental conditions, the finding that 10 mL/kg of 0.5 molar sodium lactate infused over 20 minutes will provoke a panic attack in most patients with panic disorder but not in healthy control subjects is now a well-accepted fact. The mechanism, however, that may account for the observed biochemical and physiological changes (Liebowitz et al. 1985a) has been the focus of much uncertainty and controversy. Theories have included nonspecific arousal that cognitively triggers panic; induction of metabolic alkalosis; hypocalcemia; alteration of the NAD:NADH ratio; and transient intracerebral hypercapnia. Of these, transient intracerebral hypercapnia has received considerable interest and validation in recent studies and is discussed later (see "Carbon dioxide hypersensitivity theory" subsection).

GABA–benzodiazepine system. Benzodiazepines have long been known to be a highly efficacious treatment for panic. The possibility is then raised that either aberrant production of an endogenous ligand or altered receptor sensitivity may occur in patients with panic, interfering with proper benzodiazepine receptor function and causing their symptoms.

There is support for such a theory, although findings in the literature to date

have been somewhat contradictory. One study found that patients with panic disorder, compared with healthy control subjects, demonstrated less reduced saccadic eye movement velocity in response to diazepam, suggesting hyposensitivity of the benzodiazepine receptor in panic (Roy-Byrne et al. 1990). The benzodiazepine antagonist flumazenil was found to be panicogenic in panic patients but not in normal control subjects, suggesting a deficiency in an endogenous anxiolytic ligand or altered benzodiazepine receptor sensitivity in panic (Nutt et al. 1990). However, results from another study of flumazenil responses in panic were negative (Strohle et al. 1999).

More recently, imaging studies have consistently revealed alterations in the GABA–benzodiazepine system. Decreased benzodiazepine receptor binding observed on single photon emission computed tomography (SPECT) scanning was found in the hippocampus of patients with panic disorder, and prefrontal cortex binding was also decreased in those subjects who experienced a panic attack during the scanning (Bremner et al. 2000). These findings could tie in neatly with the current "neurocircuitry of fear" model of panic (described later), in which the amygdala, hippocampus, and prefrontal cortex play a central role in modulating conditioned fear responses. Similarly, a global decrease in benzodiazepine receptor binding, most prominently in the prefrontal cortex and the insula (Malizia et al. 1998), has been observed on positron emission tomography (PET) scans. Finally, a 22% reduction in total occipital GABA levels was recently found in subjects with panic compared with control subjects (Goddard et al. 2001).

The serotonergic system. Although the serotonergic system has not been as extensively investigated in panic in comparison with other neurochemical systems, it is generally thought to be one of the systems that at least indirectly modulate dysregulated responses in panic disorder. Indirect evidence for this is provided by the high efficacy of serotonin reuptake inhibitors in treating panic. It has recently been proposed that serotonergic medications may act by desensitizing the brain's fear network via projections from the raphe nuclei to the locus coeruleus, inhibiting noradrenergic activation; to the periaqueductal gray region, inhibiting freeze/flight responses; to the hypothalamus, inhibiting corticotropin-releasing factor (CRF) release; and possibly directly at the level of the amygdala, inhibiting excitatory pathways from the cortex and the thalamus (Gorman et al. 2000). A recent study of tryptophan, a serotonin (5-hydroxytryptamine [5-HT]) precursor, found that its depletion resulted in increased anxiety and carbon dioxide (CO_2)–induced panic attacks in panic patients but not in comparison subjects (Miller et al. 2000).

Hypothalamic-pituitary-adrenal axis.
The hypothalamic-pituitary-adrenal (HPA) system, which is central to an organism's response to stress, would clearly be of interest in panic disorder, in which increased early-life stressful events such as separations, losses, and abuse have been described (Horesh et al. 1997; M.B. Stein et al. 1996; Tweed et al. 1989). However, HPA findings have been inconsistent. Cortisol responses in lactate-induced panic have suggested HPA axis involvement in anticipatory anxiety, as is known to occur in other anxiety and stress states, but not in the actual panic attacks (Hollander et al. 1989). There is some evidence for uncoupling of noradrenergic and HPA axis activity in patients with panic disorder (Coplan et al. 1995). In a recent study, adrenocorticotropic hormone (ACTH)

and cortisol responses to CRF challenge were not clearly altered in panic disorder patients compared with healthy subjects (Curtis et al. 1997).

Carbon dioxide hypersensitivity theory. Controlled hyperventilation and respiratory alkalosis do not routinely provoke panic attacks in most patients with panic disorder. Surprisingly, however, giving these patients a mixture of 5% CO_2 in room air to breathe causes panic almost as often as does a sodium lactate infusion (Gorman et al. 1984). This finding has been rather consistently replicated. Similarly, sodium bicarbonate infusion provokes panic attacks in patients with panic disorder at a rate comparable to that induced by CO_2 inhalation (Gorman et al. 1989a).

By what mechanism, then, does 5% CO_2 induce panic? Such a phenomenon may be partially explained by the findings of Svensson and colleagues, who showed that CO_2, when added to inspired air, causes a reliable dose-dependent increase in rat locus coeruleus firing (Elam et al. 1981). Alternatively, patients with panic disorder may have hypersensitive brainstem CO_2 chemoreceptors in the medulla.

Such a model is of interest because it could account for the generally well-established finding that hyperventilation does not cause panic, whereas CO_2, lactate, and bicarbonate do. Infused lactate is metabolized to bicarbonate, which is then converted in the periphery to CO_2. In other words, CO_2 constitutes the common metabolic product of both lactate and bicarbonate. This CO_2 selectively crosses the blood–brain barrier and produces transient cerebral hypercapnia. The hypercapnia then sets off the brain-stem CO_2 chemoreceptors, leading to hyperventilation and panic. Thus, a "false suffocation alarm" theory of panic has been formulated that proposes that patients with panic are hypersensitive to CO_2 because they have an overly sensitive brain-stem suffocation alarm system.

On the other hand, Gorman et al. (2000) argued, based on several lines of evidence, that brain-stem respiratory centers constitute a secondary mechanism by which panic attack symptoms relating to respiration become manifest, as one of several pathways that are activated by central excitation of the amygdala.

Neurocircuitry of fear. The most recently proposed model of panic attempts to integrate neurochemical, imaging, and treatment findings in the disorder, coupled with mostly preclinical work in the neurobiology of conditioned fear responses (Coplan and Lydiard 1998; Gorman et al. 2000). The model postulates that panic attacks are to a degree analogous to animal fear and avoidance responses and may be manifestations of dysregulation in the brain circuits underlying conditioned fear responses. Panic is speculated to originate in an abnormally sensitive fear network, centered in the amygdala. Input to the amygdala is modulated by both thalamic input and prefrontal cortical projections, and amygdalar projections extend to several areas involved in various aspects of the fear response, such as the locus coeruleus (involved in arousal), the brain stem (respiratory activation), the hypothalamus (activation of the HPA stress axis), and the cortex (cognitive interpretations). This model is thought to explain why a variety of biologically diverse agents have panicogenic properties (by acting at different pathways or neurochemical systems of this network); it is proposed that the respiratory brain-stem nucleus could not be directly triggered by such a variety of agents (Gorman et al. 2000). Thus, dysregulated "cross-talk" between the various neurotransmitter systems previ-

ously described, such as serotonergic, noradrenergic, GABAergic, CRF, and others, may underlie the pathogenesis of panic (Coplan and Lydiard 1998). This is a very comprehensive and theoretically exciting biological model of panic—which, however, is still in great need of empirical validation.

Genetics. Several family and twin studies of panic disorder have consistently supported the presence of a moderate genetic influence in the expression of panic disorder. Crowe et al. (1983) found a morbidity risk for panic disorder of 24.7% among relatives of patients with panic disorder, compared with a risk of only 2.3% among healthy control subjects. In a study of 32 monozygotic and 53 dizygotic twins, Torgersen (1983) found panic attacks to be five times more frequent in the former than in the latter group. However, the absolute concordance rate in monozygotic twins was 31%, which suggests that nongenetic factors play an important role in the development of the illness. Moderate heritability was also found in a female twin study (Kendler et al. 1993). Individuals with an early onset of the disorder appear to have a much higher familial aggregation of the disorder, possibly suggesting a stronger genetic component in a familial subtype of the disorder, which might better lend itself to molecular genetic studies (Goldstein et al. 1997).

Molecular genetic research on panic disorder has been quite active in recent years and holds promise for the future. However, a whole-genome scan in 23 panic pedigrees did not yield any evidence of linkage (Knowles et al. 1998). Also, there have been several negative studies of putative genetic markers and candidate genes for panic in the last decade, such as a linkage study of eight $GABA_A$ receptor genes (Crowe et al. 1997) and two studies of the serotonin transporter gene (Deckert et al. 1997; Ishiguro et al. 1997). Some studies have yielded positive results for a variety of candidate genes, including the X-linked monoamine oxidase A gene in females (Deckert et al. 1999), the cholecystokinin gene (Wang et al. 1998), the cholecystokinin receptor gene (Kennedy et al. 1999), and the adenosine A2a receptor gene (Deckert et al. 1998). These isolated genetic polymorphisms are best viewed as individual risk factors that possibly increase susceptibility to the disorder but that are not, in and of themselves, necessary or sufficient for phenotypic expression.

Psychodynamic Theories

In this subsection we present the major landmarks in the evolution of psychodynamic theories of anxiety and panic and their relationship to recent biological advances. More lengthy expositions and critiques of the psychoanalytic theories can be referred to by interested readers (A.M. Cooper 1985; Michels et al. 1985; Nemiah 1988).

Freud's first theory of anxiety neurosis (id or impulse anxiety). In his earliest concept of anxiety formation, Freud (1895 [1894]/1962b) postulated that anxiety stems from the direct physiological transformation of libidinal energy into the somatic symptoms of anxiety, without the mediation of psychic mechanisms. Freud termed such anxiety an "actual neurosis" as opposed to a psychoneurosis, because of the postulated absence of psychic processes. Such anxiety, originating from overwhelming instinctual urges, would today be referred to as id or impulse anxiety.

Structural theory and intrapsychic conflict. By 1926, with the advent of the structural theory of the mind, Freud's theory of anxiety had undergone a major transformation (Freud 1926/1959). According to Freud, anxiety is an affect belonging to the ego and acts as a signal alerting the ego to internal danger. The danger stems from intrapsychic conflict between instinctual drives from the id, superego prohibitions, and external reality demands. Anxiety acts as a signal to the ego for the mobilization of repression and other defenses to counteract the threat to intrapsychic equilibrium. Inhibitions and neurotic symptoms develop as measures designed to avoid the dangerous situation and to allow only partial gratification of instinctual wishes, thus warding off signal anxiety. In the revised theory then, anxiety leads to repression, instead of the reverse.

The intrapsychic conflict model of anxiety continues to constitute a major tenet of contemporary psychoanalytic theory. Psychoanalytic theorists after Freud, such as Melanie Klein (1948) and Joachim Flescher (1955), also made significant contributions to the understanding of the psychodynamic origins of anxiety. Whereas Freud concentrated on the role of sexual impulses and the oedipal conflict in the genesis of anxiety, these theorists drew attention to the role that aggressive impulses and preoedipal dynamics can also play in generating anxiety. Since Freud, the psychodynamic literature has to a degree shifted away from formulations that primarily emphasize libidinal wishes and castration fears in understanding phobias such as agoraphobia (Michels et al. 1985). For example, the significance of a trustworthy and safe companion in individuals with agoraphobia could be understood as a simultaneous expression of aggressive impulses toward the companion and a magical wish to protect the companion from such impulses by always being together. Alternatively, excessive fear of object loss and its concomitant separation anxiety could explain both the fear of being away from home alone and the alleviation of this fear when a companion is present.

It has been postulated that patients with unconscious conflict and a neural predisposition to panic may manifest their anxiety in the form of panic attacks, whereas individuals without this neural predisposition may manifest milder forms of signal anxiety (Nemiah 1981). Along these more contemporary lines of thinking, a recent psychodynamic study of patients with panic disorder proposed that in patients who are neurophysiologically predisposed to early fearfulness, exposure to parental behaviors that augment this fearfulness may result in disturbances of object relations and persistence of conflicts surrounding dependence and catastrophic fears of helplessness that can be addressed in psychodynamic treatment (Shear et al. 1993).

Research in infant and child development has brought to the forefront attachment theories and the importance of attachment disturbances in the genesis of psychopathology. Based on Bowlby's (1973) work on attachment and separation, D.F. Klein (1981) advanced the notion that the attachment of an infant animal or human to its mother is not simply a learned response but rather is genetically programmed and biologically determined. Indeed, 20%–50% of adults with panic disorder and agoraphobia recall manifesting symptoms of pathological separation anxiety, often taking the form of school phobia, when they were children. Furthermore, the initial panic attack in the history of a patient who goes on to develop panic disorder is sometimes preceded by the real or threatened loss of a significant relationship. One systematic study showed the number and severity of recent life events—especially events related to loss—were greater in patients

with new-onset panic than in control subjects (Faravelli and Pallanti 1989). A blinded psychodynamic study showed separation anxiety to be a significantly more prevalent theme in the dreams and screen memories of patients with panic disorder than in those of healthy control subjects. In a related finding, Weissman et al. (1984) found a threefold increase in risk for separation anxiety in children of parents with panic disorder.

Contemporary psychoanalysts, in response, have claimed that this neurophysiological and ethological model of a disrupted separation mechanism and panic may be unnecessarily reductionistic (Michels et al. 1985). They point out an inconsistency between the conceptualization of panic attacks as spontaneous and the frequently reported histories of childhood separation anxiety in patients with panic attacks and state that psychological difficulties with separation can also play a role in subsequent vulnerability to panic. On the other hand, contemporary psychoanalysts have also given more credence to the role of biological substrates in the genesis of anxiety symptoms in at least some patients who have developed their anxious personality structure secondary to a largely contentless biological dysregulation, so that although psychological triggers for anxiety may still be found, the anxiety threshold is so low in these patients that it is no longer useful to view the psychological event as etiologically significant (A.M. Cooper 1985).

Learning Theories

Anxiety attacks can be conceptualized as conditioned responses to fearful situations. For example, an infant learns that if his mother is not present (i.e., the conditioned stimulus), he will experience hunger (i.e., the unconditioned stimulus); thus, he learns to become anxious automatically whenever the mother is absent (i.e., the conditioned response). The anxiety may persist even after the child is old enough to feed himself. Or, to provide another example, a life-threatening situation in someone's life (e.g., skidding in a car during a snowstorm) is paired with the experience of rapid heartbeat (i.e., the conditioned stimulus) and tremendous anxiety. Long after the accident, a rapid heartbeat alone, whether during vigorous exercise or minor emotional upset, becomes capable by itself of provoking the conditioned response of an anxiety attack.

Several problems are posed by such a theory. First, no triggering traumatic event can be located. Second, given that clinical experience does not support the notion that anxiety disorder patients undergo repeated traumatic events, these patients should be able to extinguish their anxiety. Thus, despite their powerful basis in experimental animal research, learning theories do not seem to explain adequately, in and of themselves, the pathogenesis of human anxiety disorders. However, coupled with a dysregulated biological mechanism or vulnerability that may be linked to the process of fear conditioning in panic, such as altered functioning of the amygdala and related fear circuits (see "Biological Theories" section earlier in this chapter), heightened anxiety responses could conceivably persist over time.

It appears that particular types of information-processing biases contribute to the maintenance of panic, if not its genesis. Compared with control subjects, patients with panic disorder demonstrate an attentional bias toward threatening (versus positive) words (McNally et al. 1997). In addition, a bias in explicit but not implicit memory processes for words denoting physical threat has been demonstrated in patients with panic disorder

relative to healthy comparison subjects (Lundh et al. 1997).

Course and Prognosis

The course of illness without treatment is highly variable. At present, there is no reliable way to know which patients will develop, for example, agoraphobia. The illness seems to have a waxing and waning course in which spontaneous recovery occurs, only to be followed months to years later by a new outburst. At the extreme, some patients become completely housebound for decades.

A 7-year follow-up study examined prognostic factors in naturalistically treated patients with panic disorder. Although patients had generally good outcomes, there were several predictors of poorer outcome, including greater severity of panic attacks and agoraphobia, longer duration of illness, comorbid major depression, separation from a parent by death or divorce, high interpersonal sensitivity, low social class, and single marital status (Noyes et al. 1993). Another long-term outcome study, conducted over a 5-year period, had fairly optimistic findings: at follow-up, 34% of patients were recovered, 46% were minimally impaired, and only 20% remained moderately to severely impaired. The most significant predictor of poor outcome was an anxious–fearful personality type, followed by poor response to initial treatment (O'Rourke et al. 1996). Finally, another large outcome study showed that fewer than 20% of panic disorder patients remained seriously agoraphobic or disabled. Panic attack frequency at baseline, initial medication used, and continuous use of medication (versus intermittent use) were not related to outcome, whereas longer duration of illness and more severe initial avoidance were unfavorable predictors (Katschnig et al. 1995).

Diagnosis

Physical Signs and Behavior

The diagnosis of panic disorder is made when a patient experiences recurrent panic attacks that are discrete and unexpected and are followed by a month of persistent anticipatory anxiety or behavioral change. These panic attacks are characterized by a sudden crescendo of anxiety and fearfulness, in addition to the presence of at least four physical symptoms. Finally, the attacks cannot be secondary to a known organic factor or due to another mental disorder. However, these diagnoses are not always obvious, and a number of other psychiatric and medical disorders may mimic these conditions (Table 7–4).

Differential Diagnosis

Other psychiatric illnesses. Although the medical conditions that mimic anxiety disorder are usually easily ruled out, psychiatric conditions that involve pathological anxiety can make the differential diagnosis of panic disorder difficult. By far the most problematic is the differentiation of primary anxiety disorder from depression.

Patients with depression often manifest signs of anxiety and may even have frank panic attacks. Although the differentiation of anxiety from depression can at times strain even the most experienced clinician, several points are helpful. Patients with panic disorder generally do not demonstrate the full range of vegetative symptoms seen in depression. Thus, anxious patients usually have trouble falling asleep rather than experiencing early-morning awakening, and they do not lose their appetite. Diurnal mood fluctuation is uncommon in anxiety disorder. Perhaps of greatest importance is the fact that most anxious patients do not lose the capacity to enjoy things or to be cheered up as endogenously depressed patients do.

TABLE 7–4. Psychiatric and medical differential diagnosis of panic disorders

Psychiatric

Generalized anxiety disorder	Depersonalization disorder
Depressive disorders	Somatoform disorders
Schizophrenia	Character disorders

Medical

Hyperthyroidism	Pheochromocytoma
Hypothyroidism	Hypoglycemia
Hyperparathyroidism	True vertigo
Mitral valve prolapse	Drug withdrawal
Cardiac arrhythmias	Alcohol withdrawal
Coronary insufficiency	

The order of developing symptoms also differentiates depression from anxiety. In cases of panic disorder, anxiety symptoms usually precede any seriously altered mood. Patients can generally recall having anxiety attacks first, then becoming gradually more disgusted with life, and then feeling depressed. In depression, patients usually experience dysphoria first, with anxiety symptoms coming later. However, panic disorder can be complicated by secondary major depression and vice versa.

A few other psychiatric conditions often need to be differentiated from panic disorder. Patients with somatization disorder complain of various physical ailments and discomforts, none of which are substantiated by physical or laboratory findings. Unlike panic disorder patients, somatizing patients present with physical problems that do not usually occur in episodic attacks but are virtually constant.

Patients with depersonalization disorder have episodes of derealization/depersonalization without the other symptoms of a panic attack. However, panic attacks not infrequently involve depersonalization and derealization as prominent symptoms.

Although patients with panic disorder

often fear they will lose their minds or go crazy, psychotic illness is not an outcome of anxiety disorder. Reassuring the patient on this point is often the first step in a successful treatment.

Undoubtedly some patients with anxiety disorders abuse alcohol and drugs such as sedatives in attempts at self-medication (Quitkin and Babkin 1982). In one study, after successful detoxification, a group of alcoholic patients with a history of panic disorder were treated with medication to block spontaneous panic attacks (Quitkin and Babkin 1982). These patients did not resume alcohol consumption once their panic attacks were eliminated.

Hyperthyroidism and hypothyroidism. Both hyperthyroidism and hypothyroidism can present with anxiety unaccompanied by other signs or symptoms. For this reason, it is imperative that all patients complaining of anxiety undergo routine thyroid function tests, including the evaluation of the level of thyroid-stimulating hormone. It should be remembered, however, that thyroid disease can act as one of the predisposing triggers to panic disorder, so that even when the apparently primary thyroid disease is corrected, panic attacks may continue until specifically treated.

Cardiac disease. The relationship of mitral valve prolapse to panic disorder has attracted a great deal of attention over the years. This usually benign condition has been shown by several investigators to occur more frequently in patients with panic disorder than in healthy control subjects. However, screening of patients known to have mitral valve prolapse reveals no greater frequency of panic disorder than is found in the overall population.

Other medical illnesses. Hyperparathyroidism occasionally presents as anxiety symptoms, warranting a serum calcium level determination before definitive diagnosis is made.

Various cardiac conditions can initially present as anxiety symptoms, although, in most cases, the patient's prominent complaints are of chest pain, skipped beats, or palpitations. Ischemic heart disease and arrhythmias, especially paroxysmal atrial tachycardia, should be ruled out by electrocardiography.

Pheochromocytoma is a rare, usually benign tumor of the adrenal medulla that secretes catecholamines in episodic bursts. During an active phase, the patient characteristically experiences flushing, tremulousness, and anxiety. Blood pressure is usually elevated during the active phase of catecholamine secretion but not at other times. Therefore, merely finding a normal blood pressure does not rule out a pheochromocytoma. If this condition is suspected, urine is collected for 24 hours so that a diagnosis can be attempted through determination of catecholamine metabolite concentration.

Disease of the vestibular nerve can cause episodic bouts of vertigo, lightheadedness, nausea, and anxiety that mimic panic attacks. Rather than merely feeling dizzy, patients with disease of the vestibular nerve often experience true vertigo in which the room seems to spin in one direction during each attack. Otolaryngology consultation is warranted when this condition is suspected.

Treatment

Pharmacotherapy

Antidepressants. When initiating a drug regimen for a patient with panic disorder, it is crucial that the patient understand that the drug will block the panic attacks but may not necessarily decrease the amount of intervening anticipatory anxiety and avoidance, at least initially.

For patients with severe anxiety, it can be helpful to initially prescribe a concomitant benzodiazepine, which can be gradually tapered and discontinued after several weeks of antidepressant treatment. It is also important to be aware that some patients with panic disorder display an initial hypersensitivity to antidepressants, whether TCAs or serotonin reuptake inhibitors, during which they complain of jitteriness, agitation, a "speedy" feeling, and insomnia. Although this effect is usually transient, it is unfortunately one of the primary reasons that patients choose to discontinue medication early in treatment. For this reason, it is strongly recommended that patients with panic disorder be started on lower doses of antidepressants than would be given to depressed patients.

The central feature in the treatment of panic disorder is the pharmacological blockade of the spontaneous panic attacks. Several classes of medication have been shown to be effective in accomplishing this goal; a summary of the pharmacological treatment of panic disorder is presented in Table 7–5.

TABLE 7–5.   Pharmacological treatment of panic disorder

Selective serotonin reuptake inhibitors (SSRIs)

  General indications: first-line, alone or in combination with benzodiazepines if needed; also first choice with comorbid obsessive-compulsive disorder, generalized anxiety disorder, depression, and social phobia

  Start at very low doses and increase; response seen with low to moderate doses

  Sertraline, paroxetine: U.S. Food and Drug Administration–approved

  Fluvoxamine, fluoxetine, citalopram: appear similarly efficacious

Tricyclic antidepressants

  General indication: established efficacy, second line if SSRIs fail or are not tolerated

  Imipramine: well studied

  Clomipramine: high efficacy but not easily tolerated

  Desipramine: if patient has low tolerance to anticholinergic side effects

  Nortriptyline: if patient is elderly or prone to orthostatic hypotension

Monoamine oxidase inhibitors

  General indications: poor response or tolerance of other antidepressants; comorbid atypical depression or social phobia without good SSRI response

  Phenelzine: most studied

  Tranylcypromine: less sedation

High-potency benzodiazepines

  General indications: poor response or tolerance of antidepressants; prominent anticipatory anxiety or phobic avoidance; initial treatment phase until antidepressant begins to work

  Clonazepam: longer-acting, less frequent dosing, less withdrawal, first choice

  Alprazolam: well studied

Other medications

  Other antidepressants: venlafaxine and nefazodone are less studied but seem efficacious

  Other options: particularly as augmentation in patients who are refractory or intolerant of all above medications, not well tested to date:

  Pindolol: effective augmentation in one controlled trial

  Valproate: studied in open trials only

  Inositol: studied in open trials only

  Clonidine: in open trials, initial response later tended to fade

The first medications to be widely studied in the treatment of panic disorder were the TCAs, especially imipramine (Mavissakalian and Michelson 1986a, 1986b; McNair and Kahn 1981; Sheehan et al. 1980; Zitrin et al. 1980, 1983). Other TCAs, such as desipramine, have also been found to be effective, although they have not been studied as extensively as imipramine. Nortriptyline has not been systematically studied, but clinical experience indicates that it is also efficacious and is often better tolerated than other TCAs. The presence of depressed mood is not a predictor or requirement for these drugs to be effective in blocking panic attacks. In recent years, the SSRIs have been shown to be efficacious in treating panic, and because of their several advantages over TCAs, they have become the first-line treatment for panic. TCAs are now reserved, for the most part, for treatment of patients who do not have a good response to, or who do not tolerate, serotonin reuptake inhibitors and related medications.

Results of a number of open and controlled treatment trials have now shown that the potent serotonin reuptake inhibitors are highly effective in the treatment of panic. Given their greater safety and ease of administration in comparison with TCAs, they have become the first-line treatment in panic disorder, either alone or in combination with a benzodiazepine when needed. As a first-line treatment, they also offer the advantage of being effective for several of the common comorbid disorders, such as depression, social phobia, GAD, and OCD.

Although only paroxetine and sertraline are approved by the U.S. Food and Drug Administration (FDA) for this indication, there is no particular reason to think that SSRIs do not all have comparable efficacy in panic. Several controlled trials have documented the efficacy of flu-

voxamine at doses up to 150 mg/day (Den Boer 1988; Hoehn-Saric et al. 1993a). Paroxetine has also been demonstrated to be effective in controlled trials, at doses of 20–60 mg daily according to one study (Oehrberg et al. 1995). In another study, however, only the 40-mg daily dose reached statistically significant superiority over placebo during a 10-week period, whereas the 10-mg and 20-mg doses did not, a finding that highlights the importance of trying higher doses if response to lower doses is inadequate (Ballenger et al. 2000). Not surprisingly, another paroxetine study documented that it was as efficacious as clomipramine in treating panic disorder but better tolerated (Lecrubier et al. 1997). Both medications retained their efficacy during a blinded maintenance period of 9 months, leading to further improvement and highlighting the importance of longer-term treatment (Lecrubier and Judge 1997).

The SSRI sertraline has also been found to be efficacious in treating panic disorder in large controlled trials using doses of 50–200 mg/day (Pohl et al. 1998). Not only did sertraline markedly decrease the number of panic attacks, it also led to significant improvement in life quality and had a low dropout rate (Pohl et al. 1998).

Another SSRI, citalopram, has been shown to be efficacious in treating panic disorder. In an acute 8-week controlled trial, the middle dose of 20–30 mg/day conferred the most advantageous risk–benefit ratio compared with the higher and lower doses used (Wade et al. 1997). In a 1-year controlled maintenance extension of that study, the lowest dose of 10–15 mg/day was not superior to placebo, whereas the middle dose of 20–30 mg/day again showed the best response (Lepola et al. 1998).

Fluoxetine is similarly efficacious in treating panic. Fluoxetine, especially at a daily dosage of 20 mg rather than 10 mg, was shown to be superior to placebo in the acute treatment of panic disorder (D. Michelson et al. 1998). Over a 6-month maintenance-treatment period, the initial responders to acute fluoxetine treatment demonstrated significant further improvement if randomized to fluoxetine and significant worsening if randomized to placebo (D. Michelson et al. 1999).

Clomipramine, used at doses of 25–200 mg/day titrated to patients' individual responses, appears at least as efficacious—and better tolerated at lower versus higher doses—in treating panic attacks and, to a lesser degree, avoidance (Caillard et al. 1999). Clomipramine is generally less well tolerated than the SSRIs (Lecrubier et al. 1997) and therefore is not routinely used as a first-line treatment in panic.

Like the TCAs, SSRIs can cause uncomfortable overstimulation in patients with panic disorder if started at the usual doses. It is therefore suggested that treatment be started very cautiously, at 5–10 mg/day for fluoxetine, paroxetine, and citalopram and at 25 mg/day for sertraline and fluvoxamine. The dosage can then be gradually increased to an average dose by weekly adjustments. A moderate or lower daily dose is usually adequate for most patients, as described in the trials above, and high doses are generally not needed and are less well tolerated.

MAOIs are as effective as the TCAs and the SSRIs in treating panic. Both phenelzine and tranylcypromine successfully treat panic, although phenelzine has been studied more extensively. MAOIs are an option to consider for patients who fail to tolerate or to respond well to other antidepressants. In patients with concomitant atypical depression or social phobia, MAOIs may be an appropriate earlier choice for treatment if SSRIs do not confer adequate results.

Full remission of panic attacks with antidepressants usually requires 4–12 weeks of treatment. Subsequently, the duration of required treatment to prevent relapse is a function of the natural course of panic disorder. The disorder can probably best be characterized as chronic, with an exacerbating and remitting course. Therefore, complete agreement has not been reached regarding the recommended course of treatment. In a naturalistic follow-up study, Noyes et al. (1989) found that most patients with panic disorder initially treated with TCAs had a relatively good prognosis when followed over a few years, whether they had continued (60% of the sample) or stopped (40% of the sample) taking medication. In a controlled and prospective study with somewhat less optimistic results, a very high relapse rate for panic was found when imipramine therapy was discontinued after 6 months of acute treatment. However, half-dose imipramine at around 80 mg/day was successful in preventing relapse during 1 year of maintenance treatment (Mavissakalian and Perel 1992). Thus, a reasonable recommendation for treating patients with panic disorder is to keep them on full-dose medication for at least 6 months to prevent early relapse. Afterward, doses can be tapered to the half-dose level and patients can be followed to ensure that clinical improvement is maintained. Subsequently, the clinician may attempt gradual dosage decreases every few months, as long as the improvement is maintained, to reach a minimal dose at which the patient is relatively symptom free. Some patients may eventually be able to discontinue drug therapy. Other patients may require more chronic maintenance treatment, especially in light of the morbidity and mortality risk that may be associated with the disorder.

Benzodiazepines. Although clinicians prefer to use antidepressants for the first-line treatment of panic, high-potency benzodiazepines are also highly effective in treating the condition. In a large, multicenter treatment study, 82% of patients treated acutely with alprazolam showed at least moderate improvement in panic, compared with 43% of patients taking placebo. Onset of response was rapid, in that significant improvement occurred in the first couple weeks of treatment, and the mean final dosage was 5.7 mg/day (Ballenger et al. 1988). Clonazepam appears equally promising in the acute treatment of panic according to a large multicenter trial (Rosenbaum et al. 1997). In the acute treatment of panic attacks, the lowest dose of 0.5 mg/day was least efficacious, but doses of 1.0 mg/day or higher (2, 3, and 4 mg/day) were equally efficacious and the lower doses of 1–2 mg/day were better tolerated. Long-term efficacy, possible tolerance and dependency, and difficulties in discontinuing the medication are the main areas of concern in the selection of benzodiazepine treatment. Results of naturalistic follow-up studies of long-term benzodiazepine treatment appear generally optimistic, in that most patients maintain their therapeutic gains without requiring an increase in benzodiazepine dose over time (Nagy et al. 1989).

Benzodiazepines have fewer initial side effects than TCAs and serotonin reuptake inhibitors. However, the general treatment principle is that anxiolytics should be reserved until the different classes of antidepressants have failed, because anxiolytics do pose some risk for tolerance, dependence, and withdrawal. For patients with severe acute distress and disability who may require immediate relief, it may be indicated to start with a benzodiazepine and then replace it with an antidepressant.

Clonazepam should generally be the first choice, because it is longer acting and thus has the advantage of less-frequent twice-daily or even once-daily dosing and less risk of withdrawal symptoms compared with alprazolam. Clonazepam should generally be started at 0.5 mg twice daily and is increased only if needed, usually to a maximum dose of 4 mg/day. Alprazolam is usually started at 0.5 mg four times daily and is gradually increased to an average dose of 4 mg/day, with a range of 2–10 mg/day according to the individual patient. A treatment duration of at least 6 months is recommended, as with the antidepressants. Discontinuation must be gradual to prevent withdrawal: 15% of the total dose weekly is generally a safe regimen, but an even slower rate may be required to prevent the recurrence of panic. It has been convincingly shown that the introduction of cognitive-behavioral therapy (CBT) greatly increases the likelihood that patients with panic disorder will be able to successfully reduce and eventually discontinue benzodiazepine dosages (Otto et al. 1993; Spiegel et al. 1994).

Although benzodiazepines are generally safe, with side effects limited mainly to sedation, there is a concern that some patients may develop tolerance or even become addicted to these medications. However, available data indicate that most patients are able to stop taking them without serious sequelae and that the problem of tolerance and dependence is overestimated.

Other medications. Venlafaxine, found to be efficacious in one controlled study (Pollack et al. 1996), definitely merits further study and consideration when SSRIs do not work well. Nefazodone, a serotonin reuptake inhibitor and serotonin type 2 (5-HT$_2$) antagonist, appears promising in the treatment of panic. Ten of 14 patients (70%) treated openly for 8 weeks with doses of 200–600 mg/day significantly improved (DeMartinis et al. 1996).

Nefazodone was again shown to have some efficacy in treating panic disorder in another small open trial (Papp et al. 2000). If these findings are replicated in a larger, controlled study, this medication may hold some benefits in terms of initial anxiogenic response and long-term sexual side effects compared with SSRIs. Panic attacks also receded in four patients who were treated openly with the combined serotonin and norepinephrine reuptake inhibitor (SNRI) venlafaxine at low doses of 50–75 mg/day (Geracioti 1995).

Buspirone, a $5-HT_{1A}$ agonist nonbenzodiazepine antianxiety agent, has not been found to be effective in treating panic. Similarly, there is no evidence that β-adrenergic–blocking drugs, such as propranolol, are effective in blocking spontaneous panic attacks. However, if panic attacks occur in a specific social context, such as public speaking, a trial of a β-blocker would be indicated.

Clonidine, which inhibits locus coeruleus discharge, would seem for theoretical reasons to be a good antipanic drug. Although two-thirds of patients in a small series responded initially, the therapeutic effect tends to be lost in a matter of weeks, despite continuation of dose (Liebowitz et al. 1981). A later study confirmed a similar pattern of loss of response during a 10-week trial (Uhde et al. 1989). This loss of response, plus a number of bothersome side effects, makes clonidine a poor initial choice for treatment of panic disorder. However, one controlled study found clonidine to be efficacious for both panic disorder and GAD (Hoehn-Saric et al. 1981).

When response to SSRIs and other antidepressants is inadequate, one augmentation strategy, shown to be effective in a small, blinded trial, may be to add pindolol at 2.5 mg three times a day (Hirschmann et al. 2000).

Valproate may also have some benefi-cial effects in the treatment of panic attacks (Keck et al. 1993). In one open trial, all of 12 patients were moderately to markedly improved after 6 weeks of treatment, and 11 continued the medication and maintained their gains after 6 months (Woodman and Noyes 1994). Controlled trials however have not been reported. A fairly large controlled trial of another mood stabilizer, gabapentin, at flexible doses of 600–3,600 mg/day showed it to be no better than placebo in treating panic disorder (Pande et al. 2000), although a post hoc analysis revealed some efficacy for gabapentin in the more severely symptomatic patients, suggesting that an augmentation study in refractory panic might be worthwhile.

In a placebo-controlled 4-week trial, inositol, an intracellular second-messenger precursor, was found to be effective in treating panic disorder at a dosage of 12 g/day (Benjamin et al. 1995). This finding has not yet been replicated.

Psychotherapy

Psychodynamic psychotherapy. Even after medication has blocked the actual panic attacks, a subgroup of panic disorder patients remain wary of independence and assertiveness. In addition to supportive and behavioral treatment, traditional psychodynamic psychotherapy might be helpful for some of these patients. Significant unconscious conflict over separations during childhood sometimes appears to operate in patients with panic disorder, leading to a reemergence of anxiety symptoms in adult life each time a new separation is imagined or threatened. Furthermore, it has been found that comorbid personality disorder is the major predictor of continued social maladjustment in patients otherwise treated for panic disorder (Noyes et al. 1990), which suggests that psychodynamic therapy may be an important additional treatment for at least some patients with panic disorder.

Unfortunately, few systematic studies document the efficacy of psychodynamic psychotherapy in panic disorder. Psychodynamically oriented clinicians tend to agree that psychological factors do not appear to be significant in a proportion of patients with panic disorder, and they emphasize the importance of conducting a psychodynamic assessment to determine whether a particular patient may benefit from a psychodynamic treatment component (Gabbard 2000).

Supportive psychotherapy. Despite adequate treatment of panic attacks with medication, phobic avoidance may remain. Supportive psychotherapy and education about the illness are necessary in order for the patient to confront the phobic situation. Patients who fail to respond may then need additional psychotherapy, dynamic or behavioral. Encouragement from other patients with similar conditions is often quite helpful.

Cognitive-behavioral therapy. Treatments involving cognitive and behavioral approaches have long focused on phobic avoidance, but more recently, techniques have been developed and shown to be effective for panic attacks per se. In the past few years, interest in cognitive and behavioral therapy for panic has surged, and these approaches have become firmly established in the treatment of this disorder.

The major behavioral techniques used for the treatment of panic attacks are breathing retraining, to control both acute and chronic hyperventilation; exposure to somatic cues, usually involving a hierarchy of exposure to feared sensations through imaginal and behavioral exercises; and relaxation training. Cognitive treatment of panic involves cognitive restructuring designed to provide a more benign interpretation for the uncomfortable affects and physical sensations associated with panic. These cognitive-behavioral techniques can be administered in various combinations. The extreme cognitive view is that panic attacks consist of normal physical sensations (e.g., palpitations, slight dizziness) to which patients with panic disorder grossly overreact with catastrophic cognitions. A more moderate view is that although panic patients do have extreme physical sensations such as bursts of tachycardia, they can still help themselves to a significant degree by changing their interpretation of these events from "I am going to die of a heart attack" to "There go my heart symptoms again."

Several studies have shown that these various cognitive-behavioral techniques are undoubtedly quite successful in the treatment of panic disorder (Barlow et al. 1989; Beck et al. 1992; L. Michelson et al. 1990; Salkovskis et al. 1986). Group-format cognitive-behavioral treatment for panic has also been shown to be highly successful (Telch et al. 1993). After the initiation of medication treatment for initial symptom control, the introduction of CBT seems greatly to increase the likelihood that a patient will be successful in gradually reducing and eventually discontinuing medication (Otto et al. 1993). Preliminary findings on long-term outcome of panic treated with cognitive-behavioral techniques appear to be favorable, especially in the case of combined cognitive restructuring and exposure (Craske et al. 1991).

Treatment of the agoraphobic component of panic disorder. It is generally accepted that some form of treatment involving exposure of agoraphobic patients to the feared situations is necessary for overall improvement. Some studies have not found imipramine to have a significant effect on agoraphobia when given alone or with antiexposure instructions (I.M. Marks et al. 1983; Telch et al. 1985), whereas others have shown imipramine alone to decrease phobic avoidance at combined plasma levels of 110–140 ng/mL. Most studies concur that the combination of medication and behavioral treatment (exposure) is superior to either modality alone for treating phobic avoidance (de Beurs et al. 1995; Mavissakalian and Michelson 1986a; Telch et al. 1985; Zitrin et al. 1980).

In summary, antidepressants in combination with cognitive-behavioral treatment should generally be instituted. Combination therapy appears to be superior to either treatment alone. In a large controlled study of alprazolam plus exposure in patients with panic and agoraphobia, the improvement in attacks, anxiety, and avoidance were found to be largely independent of each other, and only early improvement in avoidance predicted global improvement after treatment (Basoglu et al. 1994).

Generalized Anxiety Disorder

GAD is the main diagnostic category for prominent and chronic anxiety in the absence of panic disorder (Table 7–6). The essential feature of this syndrome, according to DSM-IV, is persistent anxiety lasting at least 6 months. The symptoms of this type of anxiety fall within two broad categories: 1) apprehensive expectation and worry and 2) physical symptoms. Patients with GAD are constantly worried over trivial matters, fearful, and anticipating the worst. Muscle tension, restlessness or a "keyed up" feeling, difficulty concentrating, insomnia, irritability, and fatigue are typical signs of generalized anxiety that also—as a result

of a number of studies that attempted to single out the physical symptoms that are the most distinctive and characteristic of GAD—constitute the DSM-IV symptom criteria for GAD. Motor tension and hypervigilance better differentiate GAD from other anxiety states than does autonomic hyperactivity (Marten et al. 1993; Starcevic et al. 1994).

The diagnosis of GAD is made when a patient experiences at least 6 months of chronic anxiety and excessive worry. At least three of six physical symptoms must also be present. Finally, this chronic anxiety must not be secondary to another Axis I disorder or a specific organic factor such as medical illness or substance use.

Epidemiology and Comorbidity

The National Comorbidity Survey assessed DSM-III-R–diagnosed GAD and found it to have a current (past-year) prevalence of 3.1% and a lifetime prevalence of 5.1% in the 15- to 45-year age group, to be twice as common in women as in men, and to have a very high lifetime comorbidity (90%) with a wide spectrum of other psychiatric disorders. Even so, the prevalence and comorbidity patterns of current GAD supported its conceptualization as a distinct disorder. More recent studies using DSM-IV criteria (Carter et al. 2001) have confirmed a similar epidemiology for GAD, with a 1-year prevalence of 1.5% for threshold GAD and of 3.6% for subthreshold GAD. Higher rates of the disorder were found in women (2.7%) and in the elderly (2.2%). A high degree of comorbidity was again confirmed: 59% for major depression and 56% for other anxiety disorders.

Biological Theories

Although the neurobiology of generalized anxiety is among the least investigated in the anxiety disorders, advances are now

---

TABLE 7–6.   DSM-IV-TR diagnostic criteria for generalized anxiety disorder

A. Excessive anxiety and worry (apprehensive expectation), occurring more days than not for at least 6 months, about a number of events or activities (such as work or school performance).

B. The person finds it difficult to control the worry.

C. The anxiety and worry are associated with three (or more) of the following six symptoms (with at least some symptoms present for more days than not for the past 6 months).
    Note: Only one item is required in children.
    (1) restlessness or feeling keyed up or on edge
    (2) being easily fatigued
    (3) difficulty concentrating or mind going blank
    (4) irritability
    (5) muscle tension
    (6) sleep disturbance (difficulty falling or staying asleep, or restless unsatisfying sleep)

D. The focus of the anxiety and worry is not confined to features of an Axis I disorder, e.g., the anxiety or worry is not about having a panic attack (as in panic disorder), being embarrassed in public (as in social phobia), being contaminated (as in obsessive-compulsive disorder), being away from home or close relatives (as in separation anxiety disorder), gaining weight (as in anorexia nervosa), having multiple physical complaints (as in somatization disorder), or having a serious illness (as in hypochondriasis), and the anxiety and worry do not occur exclusively during posttraumatic stress disorder.

E. The anxiety, worry, or physical symptoms cause clinically significant distress or impairment in social, occupational, or other important areas of functioning.

F. The disturbance is not due to the direct physiological effects of a substance (e.g., a drug of abuse, a medication) or a general medical condition (e.g., hyperthyroidism) and does not occur exclusively during a mood disorder, a psychotic disorder, or a pervasive developmental disorder.

---

being made. Recent work has focused on brain circuits underlying the neurobiology of fear in animal models and in humans, and on how inherited and acquired vulnerabilities in these circuits might underlie a variety of anxiety disorders. It is speculated that alterations in the structure and function of the amygdala, which are central to fear-related behaviors, may be associated with generalized anxiety. This was supported in a magnetic resonance imaging (MRI) volumetric study comparing children and adolescents with GAD with healthy comparison subjects matched for other general characteristics. GAD children had larger right and total amygdalar volumes, whereas other brain regions were comparable in size between the two groups (DeBellis et al. 2000). The frontal cortex and medial temporal lobe are involved in controlling fear and anxiety, and there is evidence for heightened cortical activity and decreased basal ganglia activity in GAD, possibly accounting for the observed arousal and hypervigilance (Buchsbaum et al. 1987; Wu et al. 1991).

Cognitive Theories

With regard to the origins of generalized anxiety, it has been proposed that insecure attachment relationships, ambivalence toward caregivers, and parental overprotection and lack of emotional warmth may all contribute to later development of anxiety. Regarding mechanisms that may perpetuate GAD, three are summarized. First, worry is used as a strategy for avoiding intense negative affects. Second, worry about unlikely and future threat removes the need to deal with more proximal and realistic threats and limits the capacity to find solutions to more immediate conflicts. Finally, individuals with GAD engage in a certain degree of magical thinking and believe that their worry helps to prevent feared outcomes, thus leading to a negative reinforcement of the process of worrying. In terms of the etiology of GAD, cognitive theory speculates a relationship either to early cognitive schemas—derived from negative experiences—of the world as a dangerous place (Barlow 1988) or to insecure, anxious early attachments to important caregivers (Cassidy 1995).

Course and Prognosis

In contrast with panic disorder, no single, overwhelming event prompts the patient with GAD to seek help. Such patients seem only over time to develop the recognition that their experience of chronic tension, hyperactivity, worry, and anxiety is excessive. GAD appears to be a more chronic condition than panic disorder with fewer periods of spontaneous remission (Raskin et al. 1982; Woodman et al. 1999). Of subjects with GAD followed over a 5-year period, only 18%–35% were found to be in full remission (Woodman et al. 1999; Yonkers et al. 1996). GAD patients with an earlier onset of anxiety symptoms in the first two decades of life appear to be more impaired overall, to have more severe anxiety that may not be precipitated by specific stressful events, and to have histories of more childhood fears, disturbed family environments, and greater social maladjustment (Hoehn-Saric et al. 1993b). Breslau and Davis (1985) showed that if GAD persists for 6 months, as required under the DSM-III-R definition and in the DSM-IV criteria, the comorbidity of depressive disorder will be very high, and the probability of remission over time is lower with comorbid depression (Yonkers et al. 1996). Contrary to panic disorder, which de-

clines with old age, GAD appears to account for many of the anxiety states that arise in late life, often comorbidly with medical illnesses (Flint 1994).

Treatment

Pharmacotherapy

The pharmacological treatment of GAD is summarized in Table 7–7. In past years, benzodiazepines have been the first-line treatment of GAD, and they continue to be a first-line option today, despite certain concerns over their chronic use and new medication choices such as buspirone, SSRIs, and SNRIs. Several controlled studies clearly show that chronically anxious patients respond well to benzodiazepines, and all benzodiazepines are probably similarly efficacious in treating GAD (Rickels et al. 1983; Ruiz 1983). There is some evidence that benzodiazepines may be more effective in treating the physical symptoms of anxiety, whereas antidepressants, whether TCAs or SSRIs, may be more effective in treating the psychic symptoms. Available data indicate that the concern about benzodiazepine abuse in chronically anxious populations is overestimated; in reality, most patients continue to derive clinical benefits without developing abuse or dependence (Romach et al. 1995).

Buspirone, a $5-HT_{1A}$ agonist nonbenzodiazepine antianxiety agent, may have similar efficacy to the benzodiazepines in treating GAD. Its advantages are a different side-effect profile without sedation and the absence of tolerance and withdrawal. Its disadvantage is a slower rate of onset (Rickels et al. 1988), which can lead to early patient noncompliance. Treatment with buspirone is usually started at 5 mg three times a day, and the dose can be increased until a maximum dose of 60 mg/day is reached. A twice-daily regimen is probably as efficacious as a three-times-

TABLE 7–7. Pharmacological treatment of generalized anxiety disorder

Venlafaxine extended release

General indications: first-line treatment; U.S. Food and Drug Administration–approved, proven efficacy in large controlled trials; generally well tolerated; once-daily dosing; recommended starting dose is 75 mg/day, which may be adequate for a number of patients

Selective serotonin reuptake inhibitors (SSRIs)

General indications: first-line treatment; proven efficacy for paroxetine in large controlled trials; generally well tolerated; once-daily dosing; recommended starting dose is 20 mg/day, which may be adequate for many patients; SSRIs other than paroxetine have not been extensively tested but are probably efficacious

Benzodiazepines

General indications: well-known efficacy and widely used; all appear similarly efficacious; issues with dependence and withdrawal in certain patients; may be more effective for physical rather than cognitive symptoms of generalized anxiety disorder

Buspirone

General indications: proven efficacy; well tolerated; a trial is generally indicated in all patients; compared with benzodiazepines, requires longer to take effect and is not associated with a "high"; may have less efficacy and be associated with less compliance in the presence of very recent benzodiazepine use

Tricyclic antidepressants

General indications: shown efficacy in few trials; more side effects than benzodiazepines, buspirone, and newer antidepressants; delayed action in comparison with benzodiazepines; may be more effective for cognitive rather than physical symptoms of anxiety

Imipramine: shown efficacy

Trazodone: shown efficacy

Other medications

Nefazodone: one open trial

Mirtazapine: one open trial with comorbid major depression

Clonidine: tends to lose initial response

Propranolol: may be a useful adjuvant in patients with pronounced palpitations and tremor

a-day regimen and easier to comply with.

DeMartinis et al. (2000) retrospectively analyzed a large dataset with respect to history of benzodiazepine use prior to a controlled clinical trial. They found that clinical response to buspirone was similar to benzodiazepine response in patients who had never used or remotely used benzodiazepines, but patients who had used benzodiazepines within 1 month of starting the trial had a higher attrition rate and less clinical improvement if they were randomized to buspirone rather than to a benzodiazepine. There is recent evidence, from a controlled trial (Rickels et al. 2000), that in long-term benzodiazepine users, a successful strategy may be to initiate treatment with buspirone or an antidepressant 1 month before undertaking a gradual 4- to 6-week taper of the benzodiazepine. Other independent predictors of successful benzodiazepine taper were lower initial doses and less severe and chronic anxiety symptoms.

Over the past few years, newer antidepressants have become established as first-line treatments for GAD; they tend to be well tolerated, require only once-daily dosing, and do not risk abuse and dependence. Three large controlled trials to date have established the efficacy of extended-release venlafaxine, an SNRI, in treating GAD. An approximately 70% response rate was found, with benefits appearing as early as the first 2 weeks of treatment (Gelenberg et al. 2000). The trials did not demonstrate differences between the doses of venlafaxine, suggesting it can be started at 75 mg/day for GAD and subsequently increased if clinical improvement is not adequate and side effects permit.

In addition to venlafaxine, the SSRI paroxetine has recently been found to be efficacious in treating GAD in several controlled studies at dosages of 20–50 mg/day (Pollack et al. 2001). About two-thirds of patients who did not respond to the initial 20-mg dose responded to higher paroxetine doses of 30 mg, 40 mg, or 50 mg daily (McCafferty et al. 2001). Although SSRIs other than paroxetine have not been tested in GAD to date, it is likely that they also would be efficacious. Finally, nefazodone was successful in treating GAD in one open trial (Hedges et al. 1996) and mirtazapine was successful in treating GAD in an open trial with comorbid major depression (Goodnick et al. 1999).

Several older studies have shown TCAs to be effective in treating chronically anxious patients independent of the presence of depressive symptoms, although TCA use has largely fallen out of favor recently in light of the newer, better-tolerated antidepressants.

β-Adrenergic–blocking drugs such as propranolol may only be rarely indicated as an adjuvant in patients who experience significant palpitations or tremor. One controlled study found clonidine to be efficacious for both panic disorder and GAD (Hoehn-Saric et al. 1981).

Psychotherapy

Research into the psychotherapy of GAD has not been as extensive as for other anxiety disorders. Still, a number of studies exist that clearly show various psychotherapies to be helpful in treating GAD.

Given the previously described cognitive profile of GAD, several aspects of the disorder can serve as the foci of psychotherapeutic interventions. These include the heightened tendency to perceive threat, the expectation of low-likelihood catastrophic outcomes, poor problem solving especially in the face of ambivalence or ambiguity, the central feature of worry, and the physical symptoms of anxiety. A variety of treatments have been developed for GAD, including cognitive restructuring, behavioral anxiety management such as relaxation and rebreathing techniques, exposure therapy with or without a cognitive component, and psychodynamic treatment.

CBT is superior to general nondirective or supportive therapy in treating GAD (Chambless and Gillis 1993) and possibly superior to behavior therapy alone (Borkovec and Costello 1993). Cognitive therapy alone may have an edge over behavioral therapy alone according to some studies (Butler et al. 1991), but not others (Ost and Breitholtz 2000).

Finally, there are minimal data on the use of combined psychotherapy and medication in the treatment of GAD. In one study comparing CBT and benzodiazepine alone, and combined, with placebo (Power et al. 1990), CBT alone or with medication tended to emerge as superior. It appears however that the CBT component of the study was more intensive than the medication treatment, and further studies are clearly needed in this area.

Phobic Disorders: Social Phobia and Specific Phobias

A *phobia* is defined as a persistent and irrational fear of a specific object, activity, or situation that results in a compelling desire to avoid the dreaded object, activity, or situation (i.e., phobic stimulus). The fear is recognized by the individual as excessive or unreasonable in proportion to the actual dangerousness of the object, activity, or situation. Irrational fears and avoidance behavior are seen in a number of psychiatric disorders. However, in DSM-IV-TR the diagnosis of phobic disorder is made only when single or multiple phobias are the predominant aspect of the clinical picture and a source of significant distress to the individual and are not the result of another mental disorder (Tables 7–8, 7–9, and 7–10).

TABLE 7–8. DSM-IV-TR diagnostic criteria for agoraphobia without history of panic disorder

A. The presence of agoraphobia related to fear of developing panic-like symptoms (e.g., dizziness or diarrhea).
B. Criteria have never been met for panic disorder.
C. The disturbance is not due to the direct physiological effects of a substance (e.g., a drug of abuse, a medication) or a general medical condition.
D. If an associated general medical condition is present, the fear described in Criterion A is clearly in excess of that usually associated with the condition.

In the National Comorbidity Survey (Kessler et al. 1994; Magee et al. 1996), which employed DSM-III-R criteria, specific phobias had a lifetime prevalence of 11.3%. Social phobia had a lifetime occurrence of 13.3%, a 1-year incidence of 7.9%, and a 1-month incidence of 4.5%, and was somewhat more common in women than in men (lifetime 15.5% in women vs. 11.1% in men). Agoraphobia had a lifetime prevalence of 6.7% and a 1-month incidence of 2.3%. Median ages at illness onset were 15 years for specific phobias, 16 years for social phobia, and 29 years for agoraphobia. The phobias were highly comorbid with each other, and despite significant functional impairment, only a minority of the individuals interviewed had sought professional help.

Agoraphobia in the absence of panic disorder was traditionally thought to be rare, and thus, for the purposes of this chapter, agoraphobia is discussed under panic disorder. Therefore, in this section we discuss two major phobic disorders, social phobia and specific phobias.

Social Phobia

Clinical Description

In social phobia, the individuals' central fear is that they will act in such a way that they will humiliate or embarrass themselves in front of others. Typical social phobias relate to speaking, eating, or writing in public; using public lavatories; and attending parties or interviews. In addition, a common fear of socially phobic individuals is that other people will detect and ridicule their anxiety in social situations. Social phobia is described as generalized if the social fear encompasses most social situations as opposed to being present in circumscribed ones. Generalized social phobia is overall a more serious and impairing condition. Generalized social phobia can be reliably diagnosed as a subtype; afflicted patients have an earlier age at onset, are more often single, and have more interactional fears and greater comorbidity with atypical depression and alcoholism (Mannuzza et al. 1995). Individuals who have only limited social fears may be functioning well overall and may be relatively asymptomatic unless confronted with the necessity of entering their phobic situation. When faced with this necessity, they are often subject to intense anticipatory anxiety.

As in specific phobias, the anxiety in social phobia is stimulus-bound. When

TABLE 7–9.   DSM-IV-TR diagnostic criteria for social phobia

A. A marked and persistent fear of one or more social or performance situations in which the person is exposed to unfamiliar people or to possible scrutiny by others. The individual fears that he or she will act in a way (or show anxiety symptoms) that will be humiliating or embarrassing.   **Note:** In children, there must be evidence of the capacity for age-appropriate social relationships with familiar people and the anxiety must occur in peer settings, not just in interactions with adults.

B. Exposure to the feared social situation almost invariably provokes anxiety, which may take the form of a situationally bound or situationally predisposed panic attack.   **Note:** In children, the anxiety may be expressed by crying, tantrums, freezing, or shrinking from social situations with unfamiliar people.

C. The person recognizes that the fear is excessive or unreasonable.   **Note:** In children, this feature may be absent.

D. The feared social or performance situations are avoided or else are endured with intense anxiety or distress.

E. The avoidance, anxious anticipation, or distress in the feared social or performance situation(s) interferes significantly with the person's normal routine, occupational (academic) functioning, or social activities or relationships, or there is marked distress about having the phobia.

F. In individuals under age 18 years, the duration is at least 6 months.

G. The fear or avoidance is not due to the direct physiological effects of a substance (e.g., a drug of abuse, a medication) or a general medical condition and is not better accounted for by another mental disorder (e.g., panic disorder with or without agoraphobia, separation anxiety disorder, body dysmorphic disorder, a pervasive developmental disorder, or schizoid personality disorder).

H. If a general medical condition or another mental disorder is present, the fear in Criterion A is unrelated to it, e.g., the fear is not of Stuttering, trembling in Parkinson's disease, or exhibiting abnormal eating behavior in anorexia nervosa or bulimia nervosa.

Specify if:

   Generalized: if the fears include most social situations (also consider the additional diagnosis of avoidant personality disorder)

forced or surprised into the phobic situation, the individual experiences profound anxiety accompanied by various somatic symptoms. Interestingly, different anxiety disorders tend to be characterized by their own constellation of most prominent somatic symptoms. For example, palpitations and chest pain or pressure are more common in panic attacks, whereas sweating, blushing, and dry mouth are more common in social anxiety (Amies et al. 1983; Reich et al. 1988). Actual panic attacks may also occur in individuals with social phobia in response to feared social situations. Blushing is the cardinal physical symptom in social phobia, whereas commonly encountered cognitive constel-

lations include tendencies for self-focused attention, negative self-evaluation regarding social performance, difficulty gauging nonverbal aspects of one's behavior, discounting of social competence in positive interactions, and a positive bias toward appraising others' social performance (Alden and Wallace 1995).

Epidemiology and Comorbidity

The National Comorbidity Survey identified a 13.3% lifetime and 7.9% 1-year prevalence (Magee et al. 1996). Of those, about one-third reported exclusively public-speaking fears, whereas the rest were characterized by at least one other social

---

TABLE 7–10. DSM-IV-TR diagnostic criteria for specific phobia

---

A. Marked and persistent fear that is excessive or unreasonable, cued by the presence or anticipation of a specific object or situation (e.g., flying, heights, animals, receiving an injection, seeing blood).

B. Exposure to the phobic stimulus almost invariably provokes an immediate anxiety response, which may take the form of a situationally bound or situationally predisposed panic attack. **Note:** In children, the anxiety may be expressed by crying, tantrums, freezing, or clinging.

C. The person recognizes that the fear is excessive or unreasonable. **Note:** In children, this feature may be absent.

D. The phobic situation(s) is avoided or else is endured with intense anxiety or distress.

E. The avoidance, anxious anticipation, or distress in the feared situation(s) interferes significantly with the person's normal routine, occupational (or academic) functioning, or social activities or relationships, or there is marked distress about having the phobia.

F. In individuals under age 18 years, the duration is at least 6 months.

G. The anxiety, panic attacks, or phobic avoidance associated with the specific object or situation are not better accounted for by another mental disorder, such as obsessive-compulsive disorder (e.g., fear of dirt in someone with an obsession about contamination), posttraumatic stress disorder (e.g., avoidance of stimuli associated with a severe stressor), separation anxiety disorder (e.g., avoidance of school), social phobia (e.g., avoidance of social situations because of fear of embarrassment), panic disorder with agoraphobia, or agoraphobia without history of panic disorder.

Specify type:

Animal Type

Natural Environment Type (e.g., heights, storms, water)

Blood-Injection-Injury Type

Situational Type (e.g., airplanes, elevators, enclosed places)

Other Type (e.g., fear of choking, vomiting, or contracting an illness; in children, fear of loud sounds or costumed characters)

---

fear. About one-third had multiple fears qualifying for the generalized type of social phobia, which was found to be more persistent, impairing, and comorbid than the specific public speaking type. However, the two types did not differ in age at onset, family history, and certain sociodemographic variables (Kessler et al. 1998). In a large epidemiological survey of social phobia, Schneier et al. (1992) found that 70% of those afflicted were women. Mean age at onset was 15 years, and there was substantial associated morbidity, including greater financial dependency and increased suicidal ideation. Epidemiological studies have consistently found significant comorbidity between lifetime social phobia and various mood disorders, with an approx-

imately three- to sixfold higher risk for dysthymia, depression, and bipolar disorder (Kessler et al. 1999b). Social phobia almost always predates the mood disorder, and is a predictor not only of higher likelihood of future mood disorder, but also of more severity and chronicity.

Social phobia can be associated with a variety of personality disorders, in particular avoidant personality disorder (Dyck et al. 2001). In epidemiologically identified probands with social phobia alone, avoidant personality disorder alone, or both, a similarly elevated familial risk of social phobia has been found, suggesting that the Axis I and II disorders may represent dimensions of social anxiety rather than discrete conditions (Tillfors et al.

2001). Indeed, a recent review of the literature comparing generalized social phobia, avoidant personality disorder, and shyness concluded that all three may exist on a continuum (Rettew 2000).

Social phobia, in and of itself, is a highly disabling disorder whose effect on functioning and quality of life has probably been greatly underestimated and hidden in past years. Recent studies (M.B. Stein and Kean 2000) show that persons with social phobia are impaired on a broad spectrum of measures, ranging from dropping out of school to significant disability in whatever their main activity is. They describe dissatisfaction for many aspects of their lives and the quality of their lives is rated as quite low. Importantly, comorbid depression seems to contribute only modestly to these outcomes. Even in preadolescent children, pervasive and serious functional impairment can already be found (Beidel et al. 1999).

Etiology

Psychosocial theories. A number of mechanisms are proposed by learning theories as contributors to the pathogenesis of social phobia (Ost 1987; Stemberger et al. 1995). These include direct exposure to socially related traumatic events, vicarious learning through observing others engaged in such traumatic situations, and information transfer, things that one hears in various contexts regarding social interactions. There is a significant familial component to social phobia, part of which is thought to be heritable (see "Genetics" under "Biological Theories" subsection below) and part acquired. Parents, whether socially anxious themselves or not, might rear socially anxious children through various mechanisms such as lack of adequate exposure to social situations and development of social skills, overprotectiveness, controlling and critical behavior, modeling

of socially anxious behaviors, and fearful information conveyed about social situations (Hudson and Rapee 2000).

Parental social phobia is a strong risk factor for social phobia among adolescent offspring, as is parental depression, any other anxiety disorder, any alcohol use disorder, and parental overprotection or rejection; overall family functioning was not predictive (Lieb et al. 2000).

Biological theories. *Genetics.* A strong familial risk for social phobia has been identified, which is believed to be partly heritable and partly environmental. First-degree relatives of probands with generalized social phobia have an approximately 10-fold higher risk for generalized social phobia or avoidant personality disorder (M.B. Stein et al. 1998a). One twin study has not supported a genetic component to social and specific phobia, in contrast to panic disorder, GAD, and PTSD, suggesting environmental causation (Skre et al. 1993). However, in another study of phobias in twins, Kendler et al. (1992b) determined that the familial aggregation of phobias was mostly accounted for by genetic factors, with a modest heritability of 30%–40% depending on the particular phobia. Environmental factors also played a significant role in the development of phobic disorders. An adolescent female twin study estimated the heritability of social phobia to be 28%, with strong evidence for shared genetic vulnerability between social phobia and major depression.

Neurochemistry. Neurochemical studies of social phobia have not been as systematic or as consistently replicated as those in panic disorder, but to date they have implicated a number of neurotransmitter systems, including noradrenergic, GABAergic, dopaminergic, and serotonergic. In one study, patients with social phobia exhibited a blunted GH response to clonidine challenge, suggesting an underlying norad-renergic dysfunction similar to that in patients with panic disorder (Tancer et al. 1993); however, this finding was not repli-cated in a subsequent study (Tancer et al. 1994). Patients with social phobia also show evidence of altered autonomic responsivity, such as an exaggerated response to the Val-salva maneuver, in comparison with healthy control subjects (M.B. Stein et al. 1994). GABA–benzodiazepine receptor involve-ment in social phobia is unclear. One study found that the benzodiazepine antagonist flumazenil did not induce a greater surge in anxiety in social phobia patients compared with control subjects (Coupland et al. 2000). However, another study showed sig-nificantly decreased peripheral benzodiaz-epine receptor density in patients with gen-eralized social phobia compared with a healthy control group (M.R. Johnson et al. 1998).

Despite the now-documented efficacy of serotonin reuptake inhibitors in treat-ing social phobia, little is directly known about serotonergic involvement in the disorder. Subjects in one study demon-strated increased cortisol response to fen-fluramine suggestive of altered seroto-nergic sensitivity (Tancer et al. 1994). However, social phobia patients in other studies showed no signs of altered seroto-nin reuptake sites in platelets (M.B. Stein et al. 1995b) and no abnormalities in the prolactin response to m-CPP (Hollander et al. 1998). Although two studies found normal basal functioning of the HPA axis in patients with social phobia, as mea-sured by basal cortisol levels and the dex-amethasone suppression test (Uhde et al. 1994), HPA studies of these patients un-der conditions of social stress might be more telling. Finally, social phobia was associated with a significant 20% decrease in dopamine transporter site density in the striatum by SPECT (Tiihonen et al. 1997b) and, similarly, with lowered

dopamine D_2 receptor binding potential (Schneier et al. 2000).

Course and Prognosis

Social phobia has its onset mainly in ado-lescence and early adulthood, earlier than agoraphobia, and the course of illness is very chronic. Mean age at onset in two clinical series was 19 years (Amies et al. 1983; I.M. Marks and Gelder 1966). Onset of symptoms is sometimes acute (e.g., following a humiliating social expe-rience) but is more usually insidious over months or years and without a clear-cut precipitant.

Social phobia is clearly a chronic and potentially highly impairing condition. It has been found that more than half of patients report significant impairment in some area(s) of their lives, independent of the degree of social support (Schneier et al. 1994; M.B. Stein and Kean 2000). Pre-dictors of good outcome in social phobia are onset after age 11 years, absence of psychiatric comorbidity, and higher edu-cational status (Davidson et al. 1993a). In a recent very large retrospective survey of individuals ages 15–64 years with lifetime social phobia, approximately half of the sample had recovered from their illness at the time of the survey, with a median ill-ness duration of 25 years. Significant pre-dictors of recovery were childhood social context (e.g., no siblings and small-town rearing), onset after age 7 years, fewer symptoms, and either absence of comor-bid health problems or depression or occurrence of these conditions before the onset of social phobia (DeWit et al. 1999).

Diagnosis and Differential Diagnosis

Avoidance of social situations may be seen as part of avoidant, schizoid, and paranoid personality disorders, agoraphobia, OCD, depressive disorders, schizophrenia, and paranoid disorders. Persons with paranoid disorders fear that something unpleasant will be done to them by others. In avoidant personality disorder, the central fear is also of rejection, ridicule, or humiliation by others, but usually there is broader interpersonal impairment.

Some agoraphobic patients say that they are afraid they will embarrass themselves by losing control if they panic while in a social situation. Patients with psychotic vulnerabilities and massive social isolation or poor interpersonal skills may occasionally be mistaken as having social phobia if seen when they are in nonpsychotic or prepsychotic phases of illness. Social withdrawal seen in depressive disorders is usually associated with a lack of interest or pleasure in the company of others rather than a fear of scrutiny. In contrast, individuals with social phobia generally express the wish to be able to interact appropriately with others and anticipate pleasure in this eventuality.

Treatment

Pharmacotherapy. The pharmacological treatment of social phobia is summarized in Table 7–11. In performance-type social phobia, studies have shown β-blocker efficacy, particularly when these agents are used acutely before a performance (Brantigan et al. 1982; Hartley et al. 1983; I.M. James et al. 1977, 1983; Liden and Gottfries 1974; Neftel et al. 1982). Although a variety of β-blockers have been used in studies and are probably efficacious for performance anxiety, the most common ones used are propranolol 20 mg or atenolol 50 mg, taken about 45 minutes before a performance. It also seems that β-blockers are more effective in controlling stage fright, with minimal or no side effects, than are benzodiazepines, which may decrease subjective anxiety but not optimize performance and may have an adverse effect on "sharpness."

Until recently, the MAOIs were the most proven effective medications in treating generalized social phobia. Liebowitz et al. (1992) conducted a controlled study comparing phenelzine, atenolol, and placebo in the treatment of patients with DSM-III–diagnosed social phobia. About two-thirds of the patients had a marked response to phenelzine at dosages of 45–90 mg/day, whereas atenolol was not superior to placebo. Tranylcypromine in dosages of 40–60 mg/day was also associated with significant improvement in about 80% of patients with DSM-III–diagnosed social phobia treated openly for 1 year (Versiani et al. 1988). Another study (Gelernter et al. 1991) compared cognitive-behavioral group treatment with phenelzine, alprazolam, and placebo. Although all groups improved significantly with treatment, phenelzine tended to be superior in regard to absolute clinical response and decreased impairment. Despite their proven efficacy in social phobia, MAOIs are no longer a first-line treatment, because of their dietary and medication restrictions, potential for hypertensive crises, and frequently poorly tolerated side effects.

Traditionally, benzodiazepines have held promise and have been used to treat generalized social phobia, despite the usual concerns about their use. Several open trials reported positive results, and in one controlled study, clonazepam at doses of 0.5–3.0 mg/day (mean dosage, 2.4 mg/day) was found to be superior to placebo, with a response rate of 78% and improvement in social anxiety, avoidance, performance, and negative self-evaluation (Davidson et al. 1993b). Alprazolam was also found to be superior to placebo and to have results comparable with those of phenelzine and CBT. However, the alpra-

---

TABLE 7–11. Pharmacological treatment of social phobia

Selective serotonin reuptake inhibitors (SSRIs)

General indications: first-line treatment; shown efficacy; well tolerated; once-daily dosing; effective for comorbid depression, panic, generalized anxiety disorder, or obsessive-compulsive disorder

Paroxetine: best studied in large controlled trials; U.S. Food and Drug Administration–approved; average dosage 40 mg/day

Fluvoxamine: smaller controlled trials, average dosage 200 mg/day

Sertraline: one controlled trial, 50–200 mg/day

Fluoxetine: open trials

Citalopram: open trials

Monoamine oxidase inhibitors

General indications: demonstrated high effectiveness; may be difficult to tolerate and require dietary restrictions; effective for several comorbid conditions including atypical depression, social phobia, and panic; well worth trying in otherwise refractory patients

Phenelzine: most studied

Tranylcypromine: also effective

Benzodiazepines

General indications: clinically widely used and reportedly efficacious in open trials; generally well tolerated; concerns about dependence and withdrawal in certain patients

Clonazepam: long-acting; efficacy demonstrated in controlled trial

Gabapentin

General indication: found effective in controlled trial, mean dose 2,900 mg/day, consider as augmentation or second-line treatment if inadequate response to or intolerance of SSRIs

β-Blockers

General indications: highly effective for performance anxiety, taken on an as-needed basis about 1 hour before event; for the most part, not helpful in patients with generalized social phobia

Propranolol, atenolol

Other medications

Buspirone: well tolerated, effective in open but not in controlled trial

Nefazodone: effective in open trial

Venlafaxine: effective in open trial

Bupropion: effective in open trial

Reversible monoamine oxidase inhibitors: moclobemide modestly effective to ineffective, not marketed in the United States.

---

zolam group had the highest relapse rate 2 months after treatment discontinuation (Gelernter et al. 1991). Given its longer half-life, clonazepam is a better choice than alprazolam. The benzodiazepines would not be considered a first-line treatment for social phobia.

In recent years, the SSRIs have become the first-line treatment for the disorder. SSRIs are generally well tolerated, are easy to dispense and monitor, and are used in standard doses comparable with those used in depression. Paroxetine is now FDA approved for treating social phobia, its efficacy having been demonstrated in two controlled trials (Baldwin et al. 1999; M.B. Stein et al. 1998c). About one-half to two-thirds of patients with social phobia responded to acute treatment with paroxetine, at average doses of about 40 mg/day. In one controlled trial, fluvoxamine at 150 mg/day for 12 weeks resulted in substantial improvement in 46% of patients, compared with 7% improvement in the placebo group (van Vliet et al. 1994), and this success was subsequently replicated in a larger study with a comparable mean dose of 200 mg/day and a response rate of 43% (M.B. Stein et al. 1999). Of 20 patients treated openly with sertraline for at least 8 weeks, 80% showed some improvement of their social phobia (Van Ameringen et al. 1994), and the efficacy of sertraline was duplicated in a placebo-controlled study at dosages of 50–200 mg/day (Katzelnick et al. 1995). A very recent large 20-week trial of sertraline versus placebo confirmed its efficacy, with flexible dosing up to 200 mg/day and a 53% response rate (Van Ameringen et al. 2001). Similar response rates were found in an open trial of fluoxetine (Van Ameringen et al. 1993) and an open trial of citalopram (Bouwer and Stein 1998).

In addition, other medications seem to hold some promise in treating social phobia. Buspirone, a $5-HT_{1A}$ agonist, initially appeared promising in an open trial (Schneier et al. 1993), but findings from a subsequent controlled trial were negative (van Vliet et al. 1997). It is conceivable that doses higher than the 30 mg/day employed in the controlled trial may have been more beneficial. An open trial of nefazodone was positive (Van Ameringen et al. 1999), and nefazodone may be a good option in patients who cannot tolerate SSRIs. Similarly, a small open trial of venlafaxine—interestingly, in patients who had not responded to SSRIs—reported positive results (Altamura et al. 1999). Bupropion is the least-studied antidepressant to date, but even it may have some efficacy in social phobia (Emmanuel et al. 1991). Finally, the anticonvulsant gabapentin represents another medication class that has been studied in a controlled setting and therefore merits serious con-

sideration as a second-line agent for patients in whom SSRIs are ineffective or not tolerated. Although gabapentin has not been directly compared with SSRIs, alone or as augmentation, to date, a placebo-controlled trial in patients with social phobia found gabapentin to be superior to placebo at a mean dose of about 2,900 mg/day, with a response rate approaching 40% (Pande et al. 1999).

Cognitive and behavioral therapies. Three major cognitive-behavioral techniques are used in the treatment of social phobia: exposure, cognitive restructuring, and social skills training. Exposure treatment involves imaginal or in vivo exposure to specific feared performance and social situations. Although patients with very high levels of social anxiety may need to start out with imaginal exposure until a certain degree of habituation is attained, therapeutic results are not gained until in vivo exposure to the real-life feared situations is done. Social skills training employs modeling, rehearsal, role-playing, and assigned practice to help individuals learn appropriate behaviors and decrease their anxiety in social situations, with an expectation that this will lead to more positive responses from others. This type of training is not necessary for all individuals with social phobia and is more applicable to those who have actual deficits in social interacting above and beyond their anxiety or avoidance of social situations. Cognitive restructuring focuses on poor self-concepts, the fear of negative evaluation by others, and the attribution of positive outcomes to chance or circumstance and negative outcomes to one's own shortcomings. Treatment consists of a variety of homework exercises focused on identifying negative thoughts, evaluating their accuracy, and reframing them in a more realistic way.

Studies show that exposure, cognitive restructuring, and social skills training may all be of significant benefit in patients with social phobia. In addition, these techniques appear superior to nonspecific supportive therapy, as shown in a randomized controlled study comparing supportive therapy with initial individual cognitive therapy followed by group social skills training (Cottraux et al. 2000). The success of CBT appears to be mediated, at least in part, by a decrease in self-focused attention (Woody et al. 1997). Heimberg et al. (1990a) compared cognitive-behavioral group treatment with a credible psychoeducational-supportive control intervention in patients with DSM-III–diagnosed social phobia; both groups got better, but the cognitive-behavioral group showed more improvement, especially in patients' self-appraisal. Finally, it has been suggested that cognitive aspects may be of greater importance in social phobia than in other anxiety or phobic conditions, and therefore cognitive restructuring may be a necessary component to maximize treatment gains. Mattick et al. (1989) reported that combination treatment was superior to either exposure or cognitive restructuring alone in social phobia; cognitive restructuring alone was inferior to exposure alone in decreasing avoidant behavior, but exposure alone did not change self-perception and attitude.

Although long-term outcome is more difficult to assess, studies suggest that CBT leads to long-lasting gains (Turner et al. 1995) and therefore may be of particular significance in this disorder, which tends to have a chronic, often lifetime, course. At this point, it appears that in vivo exposure is a critical component of the treatment, and that the introduction of cognitive restructuring at some point in the treatment contributes to further gains and to their long-term maintenance.

Social phobia is a disorder that often starts in the early years, and it is encouraging to know that in prepubertal children, both behavioral therapy consisting of social skills training and anxiety reduction techniques (Beidel et al. 2000) and CBT alone or with the parents (Spence et al. 2000) have been found to be highly effective in controlled trials.

Other psychotherapies. In recent years, the successful use of medication and/or behavioral treatments has resulted in psychodynamic therapy for phobias falling out of favor to some degree (Gabbard 2000). However, in those patients in whom underlying conflicts associated with phobic anxiety and avoidance can be identified by the clinician and lend themselves to insightful exploration, psychodynamic therapy may be of benefit. Furthermore, a psychodynamic approach may be valuable in elucidating and resolving the secondary interpersonal ramifications that phobic patients and their partners often become caught up in and that could serve as resistances to the successful implementation of medication or behavioral treatments (Gabbard 2000).

Specific Phobias

Specific phobias are circumscribed fears of specific objects, situations, or activities. The syndrome has three components: an anticipatory anxiety brought on by the possibility of confrontation with the phobic stimulus, the central fear itself, and the avoidance behavior by which the individual minimizes anxiety. These fears are excessive, unreasonable, and enduring, so that although most individuals with specific phobias will readily acknowledge that they know there is really nothing to be afraid of, reassuring them of this does not diminish their fear.

In DSM-IV, for the first time, types of specific phobias were adopted: natural environment (e.g., storms); animal (e.g., insects); blood-injury-injection; situational (e.g., cars, elevators, bridges); and other (e.g., choking, vomiting). The validity of such distinctions is supported by data showing that these types tend to differ with respect to age at onset, mode of onset, familial aggregation, and physiological responses to the phobic stimulus (Curtis and Thyer 1983; Fyer et al. 1990; Himle et al. 1991; Ost 1987). A comparable structure has been found in child and adolescent specific phobia, clustering into three subtypes (Muris et al. 1999).

The general population prevalence of specific phobias is around 10%, and women are affected more than twice as often as men (Magee et al. 1996). In a community study of adolescents, the prevalence of specific phobias was found to be 3.5%, higher in girls than boys, and with significant comorbidity with depressive and somatoform disorders in about one-third of the sample (Essau et al. 2000). Most commonly, individuals never seek treatment for this disorder.

Etiology

Psychodynamic theory. With the 1909 publication of the case of Little Hans, Freud started to develop a psychological theory of phobic symptom formation (Freud 1909/1955). Little Hans was a 5-year-old boy who developed a phobia of horses. Through an analysis of the boy's conversations with his parents over a period of months, Freud hypothesized that Little Hans's sexual feelings for his mother, aggressive feelings toward his father, and the guilty fear of retribution and castration by his father generated anxiety as a signal of oedipal conflict. The conflict became displaced and projected onto an avoidable object, horses, which

Little Hans consequently feared would bite him. According to Freud, such a phobic symptom had two advantages. First, it avoided the ambivalence inherent in Little Hans's original conflict, because he not only hated but also loved his father. Second, it allowed his ego to cease generating anxiety as long as he could avoid the sight of horses. The cost of this compromise was that Little Hans had become housebound. Psychodynamic work with phobias, then, focuses on the symbolic meanings that the phobic object carries for any individual and the conflicts that it serves to avoid.

Behavioral theories.   In learning theory, phobic anxiety is thought to be a conditioned response acquired through association of the phobic object (i.e., the conditioned stimulus) with a noxious experience (i.e., the unconditioned stimulus). Initially, the noxious experience (e.g., an electric shock) produces an unconditioned response of pain, discomfort, and fear. If the individual frequently receives an electric shock when in contact with the phobic object, then by contiguous conditioning the appearance of the phobic object alone may come to elicit an anxiety response (i.e., conditioned response). Avoidance of the phobic object prevents or reduces this conditioned anxiety and is therefore perpetuated through drive reduction. This classical learning theory model of phobias has received much reinforcement from the relative success of behavioral (i.e., deconditioning) techniques in the treatment of many patients with specific phobias. However, it has also been criticized on the grounds that it is not consistent with a number of empirically observed aspects of phobic behavior in humans.

Models regarding the etiology of specific phobias have been elaborated and critiqued by Fyer (1998). She posited that, in order to satisfactorily explain specific phobia, a modified conditioning model would be needed, on four counts. First, many phobic patients do not recall an initial aversive event, suggesting that if such an event had occurred it must be encoded by amygdala-based emotional memory but not by hippocampus-based episodic memory, either because it occurred before age 3 or was encoded under highly stressful conditions. Second, it turns out that a very small number of objects account for most human phobias, suggesting that there may be an evolutionarily wired biological preparedness toward specific stimuli which would be easily conditioned but difficult to extinguish. Third, only a minority of individuals exposed to a certain stimulus develop a phobic reaction, suggesting that additional factors such as genetic vulnerabilities or previous experiences play a role. Fourth, most phobias are resistant to extinction in the absence of specific interventions, despite belief and evidence that there is nothing to fear.

Another model of specific phobias is the nonassociative learning model (Fyer 1998), which is in a sense the converse of the conditioned model above. It proposes that each species has certain innate fears that are part of normal development and that essentially what goes wrong in specific phobia is a failure to habituate over time to these intrinsic developmental fears. This could be due to various processes such as stressful life events, constitutional vulnerabilities or unsafe environments.

Biological theories. Some interesting recent hypotheses about the origin of phobias have resulted from integration of ethological, biological, and learning theory approaches. Fyer et al. (1990) found high familial transmission for specific phobias, with a roughly threefold risk for first-

degree relatives of affected subjects; there was no increased risk for other comorbid phobic or anxiety disorders. However, one twin study did not support a genetic component to specific phobias, suggesting environmental causation (Skre et al. 1993). In a large study of phobias in twins, Kendler et al. (1992b) determined that the familial aggregation of phobias was mostly accounted for by genetic factors, with a modest heritability of 30% to 40% depending on the particular phobia. Environmental factors also played a significant role in the development of phobic disorders.

The neurobiology of specific phobias has barely been studied. Two studies examining response to CO_2 inhalation in subjects with specific phobia have found no differences from healthy subjects and no hypersensitivity as is found in panic disorder (Verburg et al. 1994). Brain-imaging studies in specific phobia have been few and inconclusive. One showed no findings during exposure to the phobic stimulus (Mountz et al. 1989), whereas two other studies showed activation of the visual associative cortex (Fredrikson et al. 1993) and the somatosensory cortex (Rauch et al. 1995) suggesting that visual and tactile imagery is one component of the phobic response; findings regarding limbic activation appear equivocal.

Course and Prognosis

Animal phobias usually begin in childhood, whereas situational phobias tend to start later in life. I.M. Marks (1969) found the mean age at onset for animal phobias to be 4.4 years, whereas patients with situational phobias had a mean age at onset of 22.7 years. Although systematic prospective studies are limited, it appears that specific phobias follow a chronic course unless treated. A recent study followed up specific phobia 10–16 years after an initial treatment, and found that even among responders with complete initial recovery, about half were clinically symptomatic at follow-up, and none of the patients who had not improved with the initial treatment were any better at follow-up; the study suggests that specific phobias may be resistant to treatment or often do not receive treatment (Lipsitz et al. 1999b).

Treatment

Exposure. The treatment of choice for specific phobias is exposure. The challenge lies in persuading the patient that exposure is worth trying and will be beneficial. Exposure treatments may be divided into two groups, depending on whether exposure to the phobic object is "in vivo" or "imaginal." In vivo exposure involves the patient in real-life contact with the phobic stimulus. Imaginal techniques confront the phobic stimulus through the therapist's descriptions and the patient's imagination.

In both the in vivo and the imaginal techniques, the method of exposure can be graded or ungraded. Graded exposure uses a hierarchy of anxiety-provoking events, varying from least to most stressful. The patient begins at the least-stressful level and gradually progresses up the hierarchy. Ungraded exposure begins with the patients confronting the most stressful items in the hierarchy.

Studies thus far have not conclusively shown any one exposure technique to be superior to other techniques or to be specifically indicated for particular phobic subtypes. In those patients whose phobic symptoms include panic attacks, antipanic medication may also be indicated.

Pharmacotherapy. Medications have not been shown to be effective in treating specific phobias. TCAs, benzodiazepines,

and β-blockers generally do not appear useful for specific phobias, at least on the basis of the limited number of studies conducted to date. A report of positive results for paroxetine was recently published, however. In this very small controlled trial, 11 patients were randomized to receive either placebo or paroxetine dosages up to 20 mg/day for 4 weeks (Benjamin et al. 2000). The authors reported that 1 of 6 patients responded to placebo and 3 of 5 to paroxetine. Further trials of serotonergic agents may be warranted.

Obsessive-Compulsive Disorder

The essential features of OCD are obsessions or compulsions. The DSM-IV-TR definition and criteria for OCD are presented in Table 7–12.

The various presentations of OCD are based on symptom clusters. One group includes patients with obsessions about dirt and contamination, patients whose rituals center on compulsive washing and avoidance of contaminated objects. A second group includes patients who engage in pathological counting and compulsive checking. A third group includes purely obsessional patients with no compulsions. Primary obsessional slowness is evident in another group of patients in whom slowness is the predominant symptom; patients may spend many hours every day getting washed, dressed, and eating breakfast, and life goes on at an extremely slow speed. Some patients with OCD, called hoarders, are unable to throw anything out for fear they might someday need something they discarded.

Even though obsessions are typically experienced as ego-dystonic, patients with OCD have a wide range of insight. Although most patients have some degree

---

TABLE 7–12. DSM-IV-TR diagnostic criteria for obsessive-compulsive disorder

---

A. Either obsessions or compulsions:

Obsessions as defined by (1), (2), (3), and (4):

(1) recurrent and persistent thoughts, impulses, or images that are experienced, at some time during the disturbance, as intrusive and inappropriate and that cause marked anxiety or distress

(2) the thoughts, impulses, or images are not simply excessive worries about real-life problems

(3) the person attempts to ignore or suppress such thoughts, impulses, or images, or to neutralize them with some other thought or action

(4) the person recognizes that the obsessional thoughts, impulses, or images are a product of his or her own mind (not imposed from without as in thought insertion)

Compulsions as defined by (1) and (2):

(1) repetitive behaviors (e.g., hand washing, ordering, checking) or mental acts (e.g., praying, counting, repeating words silently) that the person feels driven to perform in response to an obsession, or according to rules that must be applied rigidly

(2) the behaviors or mental acts are aimed at preventing or reducing distress or preventing some dreaded event or situation; however, these behaviors or mental acts either are not connected in a realistic way with what they are designed to neutralize or prevent or are clearly excessive

B. At some point during the course of the disorder, the person has recognized that the obsessions or compulsions are excessive or unreasonable. **Note:** This does not apply to children.

C. The obsessions or compulsions cause marked distress, are time consuming (take more than 1 hour a day), or significantly interfere with the person's normal routine, occupational (or academic) functioning, or usual social activities or relationships.

D. If another Axis I disorder is present, the content of the obsessions or compulsions is not restricted to it (e.g., preoccupation with food in the presence of an eating disorder; hair pulling in the presence of trichotillomania; concern with appearance in the presence of body dysmorphic disorder; preoccupation with drugs in the presence of a substance use disorder; preoccupation with having a serious illness in the presence of hypochondriasis; preoccupation with sexual urges or fantasies in the presence of a paraphilia; or guilty ruminations in the presence of major depressive disorder).

E. The disturbance is not due to the direct physiological effects of a substance (e.g., a drug of abuse, a medication) or a general medical condition.

Specify if:

With Poor Insight: if, for most of the time during the current episode, the person does not recognize that the obsessions and compulsions are excessive or unreasonable

---

of insight, about 5% are convinced that their obsessions and compulsions are reasonable (Foa et al. 1995). On the basis on this finding, DSM-IV specified a poor-insight type of OCD. DSM-IV has also made explicit the fact that compulsions can be either behavioral or mental. Mental rituals are encountered in the great majority of patients with OCD and, like behavioral compulsions, are intended to reduce anxiety or prevent harm. Although more than 90% of patients have features of both obsessions and compulsions, 28% are bothered mainly by obsessions, 20% by compulsions, and 50% by both (Foa et al. 1995).

Clinical Description

Onset

OCD usually begins in adolescence or early adulthood but can begin before that time; 31% of first episodes occur between ages 10 and 15 years and 75% develop by age 30 years. In most cases, no particular stress or event precipitates the onset of OCD symptoms, and after an insidious onset there is a chronic and often progressive course. However, some patients describe a sudden onset of symptoms. This is particularly true of patients with a neurological basis for their illness. There is evidence of OCD onset associated with the 1920s encephalitis epidemic, abnormal birth events (Capstick and Seldrup 1977), head injury (McKeon et al. 1984), and seizures (Kehl and Marks 1986). Of interest are more recent reports of new onset of OCD during pregnancy (Neziroglu et al. 1992).

Symptoms

Obsessions. An obsession is an intrusive, unwanted mental event usually evoking anxiety or discomfort. Obsessions may be thoughts, ideas, images, ruminations, convictions, fears, or impulses and often involve content of an aggressive, sexual, religious, disgusting, or nonsensical nature. Obsessional convictions are often characterized by an element of magical thinking, such as "step on the crack, break your mother's back." Obsessional ruminations may involve prolonged, excessive, and inconclusive thinking about metaphysical questions. Obsessional fears often involve dirt or contamination and differ from phobias in that they are present in the absence of the phobic stimulus. Other common obsessional fears have to do with harm coming to oneself or to others as a consequence of one's misdoings, such as one's home catching on fire because the stove was not checked or running over a pedestrian because of careless driving. Obsessional impulses may be aggressive or sexual, such as intrusive impulses of stabbing one's spouse or raping one's child.

Attributing these obsessions to an internal source, the patient resists or controls them to a variable degree, and sig-

nificant impairment in functioning can result. Resistance is the struggle against an impulse or intrusive thought, and control is the patient's actual success in diverting his or her thinking. Obsessions are usually accompanied by compulsions but may also occur as the main or only symptom.

Another hallmark of obsessive thinking involves lack of certainty or persistent doubting. In contrast to manic or psychotic patients, who manifest premature certainty, OCD patients are unable to achieve a sense of certainty between incoming sensory information and internal beliefs.

Compulsions. A compulsive ritual is a behavior that usually reduces discomfort but is carried out in a pressured or rigid fashion. Such behavior may include rituals involving washing, checking, repeating, avoiding, striving for completeness, and being meticulous. In the DSM-IV field trial, washing and checking were the two most common groups of compulsions. Although slowness results from most rituals, it is the major feature of the rare and disabling syndrome of primary obsessional slowness. It may take several hours for the obsessionally slow individual to get dressed or get out of the house. Mental compulsions are also quite common and should be inquired about directly, because they could go undetected if the clinician asks only about behavioral rituals. Such patients, for example, may replay over and over in their minds past conversations with others to make sure they did not somehow incriminate themselves.

One study examined the distribution and grouping of obsessive-compulsive symptoms in about 300 patients with OCD and found that a total of four symptom dimensions accounted for more than 60% of variance: obsessions and checking, symmetry and ordering, cleanliness and washing, and hoarding (Leckman et al. 1997).

Character Traits

Psychoanalytic theorists have suggested that a continuum exists between compulsive personality and OCD. Janet (1908) stated that all obsessional patients have a premorbid personality causally related to the disorder. Freud (1913/1958) noted an association between obsessional neurosis (i.e., OCD) symptoms and personality traits such as obstinacy, parsimony, punctuality, and orderliness.

However, phenomenological and epidemiological evidence suggests that OCD is frequently distinct from obsessive-compulsive personality disorder (OCPD). In more recent, standardized evaluations, only a minority of patients with OCD had DSM-III-R–diagnosed OCPD, whereas other personality disorders, such as avoidant or dependent personality disorder, were more common (Thomsen and Mikkelsen 1993). In addition, personality disorders may be more common in the presence of OCD of a longer duration, which suggests that they could be secondary to the Axis I disorder, and criteria for personality disorders may no longer be met after successful treatment of the OCD (Baer and Jenike 1992; Baer et al. 1990). A recent study suggested that a familial spectrum of OCD and OCPD may exist (Samuels et al. 2000).

Epidemiology

OCD was previously considered one of the rarest mental disorders. Current data from the ECA study (described earlier in this chapter) suggest that OCD is quite common, with a 1-month prevalence of 1.3%, a 6-month prevalence of 1.5%, and a lifetime rate of 2.5% (Regier et al. 1988).

A slightly higher 1-month prevalence was found for women (1.5%) compared with men (1.1%), which was accounted for in the age range of 25–64 years, but this difference was not significant (Regier et al. 1988). However, in childhood-onset OCD, about 70% of patients are male (Hollingsworth et al. 1980; Swedo et al. 1989c). This difference seems to be accounted for by the earlier age at onset in males, and it may also suggest partly differing etiologies or vulnerabilities in the two sexes.

Twin and family studies have found a greater degree of concordance for OCD (defined broadly to include obsessional features) among monozygotic twins than among dizygotic twins (Carey and Gottesman 1981), which suggests that some predisposition to obsessional behavior is inherited. There have been no studies of OCD in adopted children or monozygotic twins raised apart. Studies of first-degree relatives of patients with OCD show a higher-than-expected incidence of various psychiatric symptoms and disorders, including obsessive-compulsive symptoms, anxiety disorders, and depression (Black et al. 1992; Carey and Gottesman 1981; Rapoport et al. 1981). Findings from family studies suggest a genetic link between OCD and Tourette's disorder (Nee et al. 1982). A recent large family study reported that OCD was about fourfold more common in relatives of OCD probands than in control relatives, and this finding was more robust for obsessions. Interestingly, age at onset of OCD in probands was very strongly related to familiality; no OCD was detected in relatives of probands with onset after age 18 years (Nestadt et al. 2000b). This study suggests, as does a similar study of panic disorder, that there may exist a more strongly familial subtype of OCD with an earlier onset.

Etiology

Psychodynamic Theory

Psychodynamic theory views OCD as residing on a continuum with obsessive-

compulsive character pathology and suggests that OCD develops when defense
mechanisms fail to contain the obsessional
character's anxiety. In this model, obsessive-compulsive pathology involves fixation and subsequent regression from the
oedipal to the earlier anal developmental
phase. The fixation is presumably due to
excessive investment in anal eroticism, resulting from excessive frustrations or grat-
ifications in the anal phase.

Obsessive-compulsive patients are
thought to use the defense mechanisms of
isolation, undoing, reaction formation,
and displacement to control unacceptable
sexual and aggressive impulses. The defense mechanisms are unconscious and
thus not readily apparent to the patient.

Cognitive and Behavioral Theories

Certain types of cognitions and cognitive
processes are highly characteristic of OCD
and presumably contribute, if not to the
genesis, to the maintenance of the disorder. In particular, negative beliefs about
responsibility, especially responsibility
surrounding intrusive cognitions, may be
a key factor that influences obsessive behavior. Individuals with OCD also appear
to have memory biases toward disturbing
themes—for example, better memory for
contaminated objects in comparison with
control subjects with comparable memory. Individuals with OCD who check
have been found to have not memory impairments—which presumably could account for the increased checking—but
rather decreased confidence in their memory. Deficits in selective attention have
been reported in people with OCD, and it
has been proposed that such deficits may
relate to their diminished ability to selectively ignore intrusive cognitive stimuli.
Deficits in spatial working memory, spatial
recognition, and motor initiation and execution have also been found in OCD. In
contrast to findings in adults, neuropsy-

chological deficits have not been found in
children with OCD, suggesting that OCD
symptoms may not interfere with cognition earlier in the illness.

Biological Theories

The association of OCD with a variety of
neurological conditions or more subtle
neurological findings has been known for
some time. Such findings include the
onset of OCD following head trauma
(McKeon et al. 1984) or von Economo's
disease (Schilder 1938); a high incidence
of neurological premorbid illnesses in
OCD (Grimshaw 1964); an association of
OCD with birth trauma (Capstick and
Seldrup 1977); abnormalities on EEG
(Pacella et al. 1944), auditory evoked
potentials (Ciesielski et al. 1981; Towey
et al. 1990), and ventricular–brain ratio
(VBR) on computed tomography scan
(Behar et al. 1984); an association with
diabetes insipidus (Barton 1965); and the
presence of significantly more neurological
soft signs in patients with OCD compared
with healthy control subjects (Hollander
et al. 1990). Basal ganglia abnormalities
were particularly suspected in the pathogenesis of OCD, given that OCD is closely
associated with Tourette's disorder (Nee
et al. 1982; Pauls et al. 1986), in which
basal ganglia dysfunction results in abnormal involuntary movements, as well as
with Sydenham's chorea, another disorder of the basal ganglia (Barton 1965;
Swedo et al. 1989b). Neuropsychological
findings in OCD are also of some interest,
although not always consistent; they have
suggested abnormalities in memory, memory confidence, trial-and-error learning,
and processing speed (Christensen et al.
1992; Galderisi et al. 1996; McNally and
Kohlbeck 1993; Otto 1992; Rubenstein
et al. 1993).

Advances in neuroimaging techniques
have permitted a more sophisticated and
elaborate elucidation of the functional

anatomy underpinning OCD. In particular, orbitofrontal–limbic–basal ganglia circuits have been implicated in numerous studies. It has been suggested that the severity of obsessive urges correlates with orbitofrontal and basal ganglia activity, whereas the accompanying anxiety is reflected by activity in the hippocampus and cingulate cortex (McGuire et al. 1994). With functional MRI, it has been possible to demonstrate that during the behavioral provocation of symptoms in patients with OCD, significant increases in relative blood flow occur in "real time" in the caudate, cingulate cortex, and orbitofrontal cortex relative to the resting state (Adler et al. 2000; Breiter et al. 1996; Rauch et al. 1994). In addition, higher-resolution MRI techniques have revealed volume abnormalities in a variety of brain regions in OCD subjects, including reduced orbitofrontal and amygdalar volumes (Szeszko et al. 1999), smaller basal ganglia (Rosenberg et al. 1997), and enlarged thalamus (Gilbert et al. 2000).

Of great interest are an increasing number of studies that demonstrate not only functional but also structural brain changes after various treatments for OCD. After treatment of OCD with serotonin reuptake inhibitors or with behavior therapy, hyperactivity decreases in the caudate, in the orbitofrontal lobes, and in the cingulate cortex in those patients who have good treatment responses (Baxter et al. 1992; Benkelfat et al. 1990; Perani et al. 1995; Swedo et al. 1992a). Also after successful behavioral treatment, the correlations in brain activity between the orbital gyri and the caudate nucleus decrease significantly, suggesting a decoupling of malfunctioning brain circuits (J.M. Schwartz et al. 1996). In children with OCD, MRI scanning revealed a decrease in initially abnormally large thalamic volumes with successful response to paroxetine treatment (Gilbert et al. 2000). This finding was not replicated in children who responded to CBT (Rosenberg et al. 2000b). Magnetic resonance spectroscopy has also revealed a decrease in initially elevated caudate glutamate concentration in children with OCD after successful paroxetine treatment (Rosenberg et al. 2000a).

Course and Prognosis

About 24%–33% of patients have a fluctuating course, 11%–14% have a phasic course with periods of complete remission, and 54%–61% have a constant or progressive course. Although prognosis of OCD has traditionally been considered to be poor, new developments in behavioral and pharmacological treatments have considerably improved this prognosis. The disorder usually has a major impact on daily functioning, with some patients spending many waking hours consumed with their obsessions and rituals. Patients are often socially isolated, marry at an older age, and have high celibacy rates. Depression and anxiety are common complications of OCD.

Recently, a major follow-up study reported on the course of OCD in patients followed over a 40-year period in Sweden, from approximately the 1950s to the 1990s (Skoog and Skoog 1999). Findings were more optimistic than one might have expected, with improvement noted in 83% of individuals. Of those, about half were fully or almost fully recovered. Importantly, predictors of worse outcome were earlier age at onset, a more chronic course at baseline, poorer social functioning at baseline, having both obsessions and compulsions, and magical symptoms.

In terms of acute treatment, the presence of hoarding obsessions and compulsions is associated with poorer response to medication treatment (Mataix-Cols et al. 1999).

Diagnosis

Although a variety of biological and neuro-psychiatric markers have been associated with OCD, the diagnosis rests solely on the psychiatric examination and history. DSM-IV defines OCD as the presence of either obsessions or compulsions that cause marked distress, are time consuming, or interfere with social or occupational functioning. Although all other Axis I disorders are allowed to be comorbidly present, the OCD symptoms must not be merely secondary to another disorder (e.g., thoughts about food in the presence of an eating disorder, guilty thoughts in the presence of major depression). The diagnosis is usually clear-cut, but occasionally it can be more difficult to distinguish OCD from depression, psychosis, phobias, or severe OCPD.

Differential Diagnosis

In some cases, the course of OCD may more closely resemble that of schizophrenia, with chronic debilitation, decline, and profound impairment in social and occupational functioning. Sometimes it is difficult to distinguish between an obsession (i.e., contamination) and a delusion (i.e., being poisoned). An obsession is typically ego-dystonic, resisted, and recognized as having an internal origin. A delusion is not resisted and is believed to be external. However, OCD patients may lack insight, and in 12% of cases obsessions may become delusions. Yet longitudinal studies show that OCD patients are not at increased risk of developing schizophrenia.

Individuals with OCD frequently have complicating depressions, and these individuals may be difficult to distinguish from depressed individuals who have complicating obsessive symptoms. Depressive ruminations, in contrast to pure obsessions, are often focused on a past incident rather than on a current or future event and are rarely resisted.

A close connection exists between OCD and phobic and anxiety disorders. Patients with OCD who are compulsive cleaners appear very similar to phobic individuals and are often mislabeled "germ phobics." Both have avoidant behavior, both show intense subjective and autonomic responses to focal stimuli, and both are said to respond to similar behavioral interventions. Both have excessive fear, although disgust is prominent in OCD patients and not in phobic patients. Also, patients with OCD can never entirely avoid the obsession, whereas phobic patients have more focal, external stimuli that they can successfully avoid.

Patients with OCD who experience high levels of anxiety may describe panic-like episodes, but these are secondary to obsessions and do not arise spontaneously. Unlike panic disorder patients, in OCD patients there is no precipitation of anxiety attack with lactate infusions (Gorman et al. 1985).

Treatment

Pharmacotherapy

Advances in the pharmacotherapy of OCD have been quite dramatic and have generated a great deal of excitement and optimism for successful treatment of this disorder. What was previously thought to be a rare, psychodynamically laden, and difficult-to-treat illness now appears to have a strong biological component and to respond well to potent serotonin reuptake inhibitors. The pharmacological treatment approach to OCD is summarized in Table 7–13.

Serotonin reuptake inhibitors. The most extensively studied medication for the treatment of OCD is clomipramine, a potent serotonin reuptake inhibitor with weak norepinephrine reuptake blockade.

TABLE 7–13. Pharmacological treatment of obsessive-compulsive disorder (OCD)

Serotonin reuptake inhibitors

General indications: first-line treatments; moderate to high doses

Fluoxetine, fluvoxamine, sertraline: efficacy shown in large controlled trials

Paroxetine, citalopram: less studied, similar efficacy

Clomipramine: efficacy shown in multiple controlled trials; may have small superiority over SSRIs; however, typically not used until at least two SSRIs have failed secondary to side-effect profile; can be used in low doses in combination with SSRIs in more refractory patients—clomipramine + desmethylclomipramine levels must be closely followed for toxicity

Augmentation strategies

General indications: partial response to SSRIs; presence of other target symptoms

Pimozide: comorbid tic disorders or schizotypal personality

Haloperidol: comorbid tic disorders or schizotypal personality

Risperidone: effective augmentation in controlled trial, regardless of tics or schizotypy

Olanzapine: effective in open trials

Pindolol: effective in controlled trial

Clonazepam: effective in controlled trial; comorbid very high anxiety

Buspirone: one positive trial, three negative

Lithium: ineffective in controlled trial

Trazodone: ineffective in controlled trial

Monoamine oxidase inhibitors: hardly any evidence; ? phenelzine in symmetry obsessions

Other medications

Intravenous clomipramine: efficacy in controlled trial of oral clomipramine–refractory patients

Plasma exchange and intravenous immunoglobulin: effective in children with streptococcus-related OCD

A series of well-controlled double-blind studies have indisputably documented the efficacy of clomipramine in reducing OCD symptoms (Ananth et al. 1981; As-berg et al. 1982). The largest of these was a multicenter trial in which clomipramine was compared with placebo in more than 500 patients with OCD. At an average dose of 200–250 mg/day of clomipramine, the average reduction in OCD symptoms was about 40%, and about 60% of all patients were clinically much or very much improved. Patients should typically be started on 25 mg of clomipramine taken at bedtime, and the dose should then be gradually increased by 25 mg every 4 days or by 50 mg every week, until a maximum dose of 250 mg is reached. Some patients are unable to tolerate the highest dose and may be stabilized on 150 or 200 mg. Improvement with clomipramine is relatively slow, with maximal response occurring after 5–12 weeks of treatment. Controlled studies have also demonstrated that clomipramine is effective in treating OCD when other antidepressants, such as amitriptyline, nortriptyline, desipramine, and the MAOI clorgyline have no therapeutic effect (Ananth et al. 1981; Leonard et al. 1989; Zohar and Insel 1987). This finding strongly suggests that improvement in OCD symptoms is mediated through the blockade of serotonin reuptake.

Studies with the SSRIs have further supported this hypothesis in that these agents have turned out to be essentially as efficacious as clomipramine. Numerous large, controlled trials emerged in the 1990s that definitively documented the efficacy of all SSRIs for this disorder. Fluoxetine at dosages of 20–60 mg/day was shown to be superior to placebo in treating OCD, with greater efficacy at higher doses (Montgomery et al. 1993; Tollefson et al. 1994). Similarly, fluoxetine has been shown to be safe and efficacious in treating OCD in children (Riddle et al. 1992).

Fluvoxamine was also found to have a significant antiobsessional effect in several controlled studies (Goodman et al. 1989,

1990b; Jenike et al. 1990a; Perse et al. 1987), with efficacy comparable to that of clomipramine (Freeman et al. 1994; Koran et al. 1996). Goodman and his group (1990b) showed that fluvoxamine is superior to desipramine in treating OCD. In their study, 52% of patients demonstrated marked clinical improvement independent of initial depression. The required daily dose is titrated up to a maximum of 300 mg. The efficacy of fluvoxamine for OCD has also been demonstrated in adolescent patients, at dosages of 100–300 mg/day (Apter et al. 1994). The efficacy of fluvoxamine in the treatment of pediatric OCD (ages 8–17 years) was further confirmed in a multicenter trial that used doses of 50–200 mg/day. Forty-two percent of the subjects were responders (defined as a 25% symptomatic improvement), and the medication was well tolerated; asthenia and insomnia were the most common side effects (Riddle et al. 2001).

Sertraline is another serotonin reuptake inhibitor whose efficacy in OCD has been established. Although an initial placebo-controlled study revealed no beneficial effect (Jenike et al. 1990b), subsequent studies have shown sertraline to be superior to placebo at daily doses ranging from 50 to 200 mg (Chouinard 1992; Greist et al. 1995a). Similarly, sertraline has been found to be effective in treating childhood OCD (ages 6–17 years) in a large multicenter trial that used doses up to 200 mg/day (March et al. 1998b).

Although paroxetine and citalopram have not been as extensively studied as other SSRIs in the treatment of adult OCD (Koponen et al. 1997; Montgomery et al. 2001; Mundo et al. 1997; D.J. Stein et al. 2001; Zohar and Judge 1996), they appear to be as efficacious and are widely used at dosages of 20–60 mg/day. There is also limited evidence that citalopram may be helpful in refractory OCD (Bejerot and

Bodlund 1998; Marazziti et al. 2001; Pallanti et al. 1999). In open trials of pediatric subjects with OCD, both paroxetine (Rosenberg et al. 1999) and citalopram (Thomsen 1997) have been found to be effective and safe.

Three meta-analytic studies retrospectively analyzed treatment data from OCD trials; results supported a small but significant superiority for clomipramine over the SSRIs (Greist et al. 1995b; Piccinelli et al. 1995). However, the clinical applicability of this finding may be limited, because in clinical practice, actual or expected tolerability of different medications often takes precedence over small differences in efficacy. For most patients, the SSRIs are better tolerated than clomipramine and have therefore become the well-established first line of treatment for OCD. If patients do not have a good response to an adequate trial of at least two SSRIs, clomipramine augmentation or monotherapy should be undertaken.

Augmentation strategies. It is useful to remember that approximately 40%–60% of patients with OCD improve by about 30%–60% with a first-line drug. Thus, various combination and augmentation strategies are often needed to attain a satisfactory response. The most commonly used augmenting agents, unfortunately not always with strong scientific findings supporting their effectiveness, are buspirone, lithium, tryptophan, trazodone, clonazepam, risperidone, olanzapine, pindolol, desipramine, inositol, and the MAOIs. With more rigorous testing in recent years, many of these augmentation strategies no longer look as promising as was initially thought. Still, given the relatively limited treatment options, these strategies are well worth undertaking sequentially, beginning with the most compelling ones.

Although a small study initially reported similar efficacy for clomipramine alone versus buspirone alone in treating OCD (Pato et al. 1991), three other studies failed to show a significant benefit for buspirone augmentation in clomipramine-treated (Pigott et al. 1992b), fluoxetine-treated (Grady et al. 1993), or fluvoxamine-treated (McDougle et al. 1993b) patients, whereas one study described clinical improvement in 10 of 20 OCD patients who underwent buspirone augmentation of fluoxetine treatment (Jenike et al. 1991a). If buspirone is tried, higher doses of 30–60 mg/day should be aimed for. A controlled study of lithium augmentation of clomipramine did not detect any benefit (Pigott et al. 1991). A controlled study of trazodone monotherapy in OCD likewise found no benefit in comparison with placebo (Pigott et al. 1992a). A controlled crossover study showed clonazepam to be effective in 40% of subjects with OCD who had failed to respond to clomipramine trials (Hewlett et al. 1992a), and clonazepam may also be helpful with the very high anxiety levels frequently associated with OCD (Hewlett et al. 1990). Evidence in support of MAOIs is very weak despite a positive report (Vallejo et al. 1992), possibly with the exception of some benefit for symmetry obsessions from phenelzine (Jenike et al. 1997). A controlled trial of lithium augmentation was negative (McDougle et al. 1991a), as were controlled trials of trazodone monotherapy (Pigott et al. 1992a) and desipramine augmentation of SSRI treatment (Barr et al. 1997). In a small open trial, 10 patients with OCD who had not responded to serotonin reuptake inhibitor trials were treated with inositol augmentation, at 18 mg/day, for 6 weeks; only 3 patients reported clinically significant improvement, leaving inositol also as an option of unclear efficacy (Seedat and Stein 1999).

Antipsychotics are a major medication class that can be successfully used to augment partial response to serotonin reuptake inhibitors in OCD. McDougle et al. (1990) first reported that about 50% of patients with OCD improved noticeably when pimozide was added to fluvoxamine therapy; comorbid tic disorders or schizotypal personality predicted a good response to treatment (Goodman et al. 1990a). OCD patients with comorbid tic disorders may actually be less responsive to SSRI monotherapy (McDougle et al. 1993a), and they appear to respond well to haloperidol augmentation (McDougle et al. 1994).

In more recent years, atypical antipsychotics have received increasing attention as a major augmentation strategy for OCD, regardless of comorbid tics or schizotypy, and the effectiveness of this strategy is now supported by controlled trials. After promising open-trial findings with risperidone (Pfanner et al. 2000), a controlled 6-week trial of risperidone in patients refractory to a serotonin reuptake inhibitor found significant improvement in half of the patients (McDougle et al. 2000); this response was not associated with whether tics or schizotypy were present. Four pediatric patients with refractory OCD were also described as responsive to risperidone augmentation (Fitzgerald et al. 1999). Olanzapine appears to be as promising as risperidone. In a 3-month open augmentation trial with olanzapine in OCD patients unresponsive to fluvoxamine, almost half showed notable improvement (Bogetto et al. 2000). Similarly, benefits were noted in the majority of subjects who had partially responded to an SSRI and were augmented openly with olanzapine for 8 weeks (Weiss et al. 1999). In a probably more refractory sample of nine OCD patients who had failed to respond in more than three serotonin reuptake inhibitor trials, three showed at least a 30% improvement with 8-week open olanzapine augmentation at doses of 2.5–10.0 mg/day (Koran et al. 2000).

Other than the antipsychotics, pindolol is the only additional medication that has been proven to be a useful augmentation agent in a controlled study (Dannon et al. 2000). Fourteen patients with treatment-refractory OCD who had not responded to three SSRI trials received paroxetine augmentation with pindolol or placebo for 6 weeks. In comparison with placebo, pindolol at 2.5 mg three times daily was significantly superior in reducing OCD symptoms.

The combination of clomipramine with an SSRI is another strategy commonly used in the treatment of patients with refractory OCD. Although clomipramine is generally well tolerated, lower doses of clomipramine should be used and blood levels monitored to avoid toxicity (because clomipramine levels can become markedly elevated). In one small randomized trial in patients with refractory OCD, citalopram combined with clomipramine led to significantly greater improvement than did citalopram alone (Pallanti et al. 1999).

When oral medications fail to be successful enough in highly refractory patients, other options can be considered, such as cognitive-behavioral techniques (which are described later on) and several other biological interventions. Intravenously administered clomipramine was found to be more effective than intravenous placebo in a trial of 54 patients with OCD refractory to oral clomipramine; 58% of the patients were responders, and the treatment was safely tolerated (Fallon et al. 1998). Plasma exchange and intravenous immunoglobulin have been found to be effective in lessening symptom severity in children with streptococcal infection–triggered OCD (Perlmutter et al. 1999). In extreme cases of refractory, severely impaired OCD patients, neurosurgery can

be considered. Jenike et al. (1991b), in a thorough retrospective analysis, estimated that cingulotomy resulted in notable improvement in at least 25%–30% of patients. This response rate was confirmed in a 2-year prospective cingulotomy study (Baer et al. 1995). A comparable response rate of 38% was reported in another study at follow-up 10 years after the sterotactic surgery (Hay et al. 1993). Most recently, transcranial magnetic stimulation has been used in OCD and appears to show some promise; however, this technique requires much further study (Greenberg et al. 1997).

Although there are no definitive predictors of medication treatment response, several factors appear to be predictive of a poorer prognosis, including earlier age at onset, longer duration of illness, higher frequency of compulsions, presence of washing rituals, a chronic course, prior hospitalizations, and comorbid avoidant, borderline, and schizotypal as well as multiple personality disorders (Ackerman et al. 1994; Baer and Jenike 1992; Baer et al. 1992; Ravizza et al. 1995). A recent review of 274 patients with OCD found no differences between responsive and nonresponsive subjects in age, gender, age at onset, duration of illness, or symptom subtypes. Responders had a higher incidence of family history of tics, sudden onset of OCD, and an episodic course of illness. Nonresponders had more severe symptoms, poorer insight into their OCD, and comorbid eating disorder (Hollander et al. 2001).

OCD tends to be a chronic illness, and many patients may require ongoing drug treatment to stay well. In a double-blind discontinuation study of OCD patients who had done well on clomipramine for about 1 year, 90% experienced substantial worsening within 7 weeks (Pato et al. 1988). The same relapse rate of 90% was found in a group of adolescent OCD patients when chronic clomipramine was blindly substituted with 8 weeks of desipramine (Leonard et al. 1991). At follow-up several years later, most of the patients remained symptomatic and required continued pharmacotherapy, with a substantial minority of 20% remaining refractory to multiple treatment regimens (Leonard et al. 1993).

Behavioral Therapy

Behavioral treatments of OCD involve two separate components: 1) exposure procedures, which aim to decrease the anxiety associated with obsessions, and 2) response prevention techniques, which aim to decrease the frequency of rituals or obsessive thoughts. Exposure techniques include systematic desensitization with brief imaginal exposure and flooding (in which prolonged exposure to the real-life ritual-evoking stimuli causes profound discomfort). The ultimate goal of exposure techniques is to decrease the discomfort associated with the eliciting stimuli through habituation. In exposure therapy, the patient is assigned homework exercises, performance of which may require assistance either from the therapist (via home visits) or from family members. Response prevention requires patients to face feared stimuli (e.g., dirt, chemicals) without resorting to excessive hand washing or to tolerate doubt (e.g., "Is the door really locked?") without succumbing to excessive checking. Initial work may involve delaying performance of the ritual, but ultimately the patient works to fully resist the compulsions. The psychoeducation and support of family members can be pivotal to the success of the behavioral therapy, because family dysfunction is prevalent, and the majority of parents or spouses accommodate to or are involved in the patients' rituals, possibly as a way to reduce the anxiety or anger that pa-

tients may direct at their family members (Calvocoressi et al. 1995; Shafran et al. 1996).

It is generally agreed that combined behavioral techniques (e.g., exposure with response prevention) yield the greatest improvement. When the combined techniques of in vivo exposure and response prevention were used, up to 75% of ritualizing patients willing and able to undergo the arduous treatment were reported to show significant improvement (I.M. Marks et al. 1975). The addition of imaginal exposure to in vivo exposure/response prevention was reported to help maintain treatment gains, perhaps by moderating obsessive fears of future catastrophes (Steketee et al. 1982).

Cognitive Therapy

Another modality that has more recently been advocated in the treatment of OCD is cognitive therapy, which centers on cognitive reformulation of themes related to the perception of danger, estimation of catastrophe, expectations about anxiety and its consequences, excessive responsibility, thought–action fusion, and illogical inferences (Freeston et al. 1996; O'Connor and Robillard 1996; Rachman et al. 1995; vanOppen and Arntz 1994). A review of 15 open and controlled cognitive trials in patients with OCD showed little evidence of improvement overall when cognitive therapy was added to the existing pharmacological and behavioral techniques (I.A. James and Blackburn 1995). However, one controlled study found cognitive therapy's effectiveness to be similar to that of exposure and response prevention in treating OCD (vanOppen et al. 1995).

Combination Therapy

Combination therapy is commonly used and recommended in the treatment of

OCD. Unless symptoms are mild or subjects highly motivated to begin with CBT
techniques, a common approach used in
clinical practice is to start out with medication, attain a degree of improvement
that will allow better utilization of CBT,
and then possibly attempt some degree of
medication taper once CBT has been mastered and observed to be effective. In a
recent study testing this commonly used
paradigm, it appeared to be quite effective
(Simpson et al. 1999). Patients who remained symptomatic with a 12-week
course of an SSRI received a course of
exposure and ritual prevention and demonstrated a 50% decrease in their OCD
symptoms (Simpson et al. 1999). Another study that compared behavioral or
cognitive monotherapy with initial SSRI
treatment subsequently complemented
with such therapies showed no differences
among the treatments. These findings were
interpreted as suggesting that psychotherapy alone may be sufficient, at least in this
group of subjects (van Balkom et al. 1998).
Finally, a meta-analytic comparison study
of OCD treatments, after controlling for a
number of confounding variables, found
that clomipramine, SSRIs, and exposure
with response prevention had comparable
results (Kobak et al. 1998).

Other Psychotherapies

Patients with OCD frequently present
with symptoms that appear laden with
unconscious symbolism and dynamic
meaning. However, OCD has generally
proven refractory to psychoanalytically
oriented, as well as to loosely structured,
nondirective exploratory psychotherapies.
In contrast to its lack of efficacy in
treating chronic OCD, dynamic psychotherapy may be helpful for patients with
acute and limited symptoms who are otherwise psychologically minded and motivated to explore their conflicts, as well as
in dealing with obsessive character traits
of perfectionism, doubting, procrastina-
tion, and indecisiveness (Salzman 1985).
However, controlled clinical data are not
yet available to support these clinical impressions.

Posttraumatic Stress Disorder

PTSD was first introduced in DSM-III, its
inclusion spurred in part by the increasing
recognition of posttraumatic conditions
in veterans of the Vietnam War. The current DSM-IV-TR criteria for PTSD are
presented in Table 7–14.

Not all investigators agree that PTSD
belongs with the anxiety disorders. In the
past decade, attention has increasingly
been focused on the concept of "trauma-
spectrum" disorders, which can include
admixtures of posttraumatic stress, dissociative, somatoform, and conversion
symptoms, and the classification approach
to trauma-related conditions is a subject
of ongoing debate.

In acknowledgment of the spectrum
of disorders stemming from severe stress,
DSM-IV added acute stress disorder (ASD)
to the anxiety disorders. Acute stress disorder is similar to PTSD with regard to
the precipitating traumatic event and to
symptomatology but is time limited, occurring up to 1 month after the event.
ASD is a highly reliable predictor of developing PTSD down the road; it may well
be that the two should not be defined as
discrete disorders. The DSM-IV-TR diagnostic criteria for ASD are presented in
Table 7–15.

TABLE 7–14.   DSM-IV-TR diagnostic criteria for posttraumatic stress disorder

A. The person has been exposed to a traumatic event in which both of the following were present:
   (1) the person experienced, witnessed, or was confronted with an event or events that involved actual or threatened death or serious injury, or a threat to the physical integrity of self or others
   (2) the person's response involved intense fear, helplessness, or horror.   **Note:** In children, this may be expressed instead by disorganized or agitated behavior

B. The traumatic event is persistently reexperienced in one (or more) of the following ways:
   (1) recurrent and intrusive distressing recollections of the event, including images, thoughts, or perceptions.   **Note:** In young children, repetitive play may occur in which themes or aspects of the trauma are expressed.
   (2) recurrent distressing dreams of the event.   **Note:** In children, there may be frightening dreams without recognizable content.
   (3) acting or feeling as if the traumatic event were recurring (includes a sense of reliving the experience, illusions, hallucinations, and dissociative flashback episodes, including those that occur on awakening or when intoxicated).   **Note:** In young children, trauma-specific reenactment may occur.
   (4) intense psychological distress at exposure to internal or external cues that symbolize or resemble an aspect of the traumatic event
   (5) physiological reactivity on exposure to internal or external cues that symbolize or resemble an aspect of the traumatic event

C. Persistent avoidance of stimuli associated with the trauma and numbing of general responsiveness (not present before the trauma), as indicated by three (or more) of the following:
   (1) efforts to avoid thoughts, feelings, or conversations associated with the trauma
   (2) efforts to avoid activities, places, or people that arouse recollections of the trauma
   (3) inability to recall an important aspect of the trauma
   (4) markedly diminished interest or participation in significant activities
   (5) feeling of detachment or estrangement from others
   (6) restricted range of affect (e.g., unable to have loving feelings)
   (7) sense of a foreshortened future (e.g., does not expect to have a career, marriage, children, or a normal life span)

D. Persistent symptoms of increased arousal (not present before the trauma), as indicated by two (or more) of the following:
   (1) difficulty falling or staying asleep
   (2) irritability or outbursts of anger
   (3) difficulty concentrating
   (4) hypervigilance
   (5) exaggerated startle response

E. Duration of the disturbance (symptoms in Criteria B, C, and D) is more than 1 month.

F. The disturbance causes clinically significant distress or impairment in social, occupational, or other important areas of functioning.

Specify if:
   Acute: if duration of symptoms is less than 3 months
   Chronic: if duration of symptoms is 3 months or more
Specify if:
   With Delayed Onset: if onset of symptoms is at least 6 months after the stressor

TABLE 7–15.   DSM-IV-TR diagnostic criteria for acute stress disorder

A. The person has been exposed to a traumatic event in which both of the following were present:
   (1) the person experienced, witnessed, or was confronted with an event or events that involved actual or threatened death or serious injury, or a threat to the physical integrity of self or others
   (2) the person's response involved intense fear, helplessness, or horror
B. Either while experiencing or after experiencing the distressing event, the individual has three (or more) of the following dissociative symptoms:
   (1) a subjective sense of numbing, detachment, or absence of emotional responsiveness
   (2) a reduction in awareness of his or her surroundings (e.g., "being in a daze")
   (3) derealization
   (4) depersonalization
   (5) dissociative amnesia (i.e., inability to recall an important aspect of the trauma)
C. The traumatic event is persistently reexperienced in at least one of the following ways: recurrent images, thoughts, dreams, illusions, flashback episodes, or a sense of reliving the experience; or distress on exposure to reminders of the traumatic event.
D. Marked avoidance of stimuli that arouse recollections of the trauma (e.g., thoughts, feelings, conversations, activities, places, people).
E. Marked symptoms of anxiety or increased arousal (e.g., difficulty sleeping, irritability, poor concentration, hypervigilance, exaggerated startle response, motor restlessness).
F. The disturbance causes clinically significant distress or impairment in social, occupational, or other important areas of functioning or impairs the individual's ability to pursue some necessary task, such as obtaining necessary assistance or mobilizing personal resources by telling family members about the traumatic experience.
G. The disturbance lasts for a minimum of 2 days and a maximum of 4 weeks and occurs within 4 weeks of the traumatic event.
H. The disturbance is not due to the direct physiological effects of a substance (e.g., a drug of abuse, a medication) or a general medical condition, is not better accounted for by brief psychotic disorder, and is not merely an exacerbation of a preexisting Axis I or Axis II disorder.

Epidemiology

Although there are marked individual differences in how people react to stress, when stressors become extreme, such as in concentration camp situations or in extended combat, the rate of morbidity rapidly increases (Krystal 1968).

In a large, random community survey of young adults, the lifetime prevalence of PTSD was 9.2% (Breslau et al. 1991). The prevalence was higher in women (11.3%) than in men (6%). In the more recent National Comorbidity Survey, the lifetime prevalence of PTSD was similarly found to be 7.8% and was again more common in women. The most common stressors were combat exposure in men and sexual assault in women (Kessler et al. 1995). PTSD prevalence is higher in women, a gender difference that has been consistent across several studies. It appears that women are more likely to develop PTSD than are men with comparable exposure to traumatic events, especially if exposure occurs before age 15 years (Breslau et al. 1997b).

A high rate of comorbid disorders is found in PTSD. In the survey by Breslau et al. (1991), a high comorbidity risk was found for OCD, agoraphobia, panic, and depression, whereas the association with drug or alcohol abuse was weaker. Epidemiological analyses suggest that in trauma survivors, the vulnerabilities for PTSD and depression are not separate; rather, the risk for depression is highly elevated in just those trauma survivors who manifest PTSD (Breslau et al. 2000). On the other hand, a prospective study of a large sample of trauma survivors found depression and PTSD to be independent sequelae of trauma (Shalev et al. 1998b). Regardless of causality, it is clear that PTSD in women increases the risk for a new onset of both depression and alcohol use disorder (Breslau et al. 1997a).

Etiology

The Role of the Stressor

The severity of the stressor in PTSD differs in magnitude from that found in adjustment disorder, which is usually less severe and within the range of common life experience, although the relationship between the severity of the stressor and the type of subsequent symptomatology is not always predictable. In effect, it has generally been underemphasized that in the average community setting, events such as sudden loss of a spouse are a much more frequent cause of PTSD than are assault and violence (Breslau et al. 1998).

Nevertheless, events such as sexual assault or armed robbery, which are interpersonal insults to integrity, self-esteem, and security, are particularly likely to lead to PTSD. The ECA study found that in men who had served in Vietnam, 4% of those who were in combat but were not wounded had PTSD, whereas 20% of combat veterans who had been wounded developed PTSD. In even more horrendous conditions, such as those endured by U.S. prisoners of war of the Japanese in World War II, extremely high PTSD incidence rates have been reported: 84% lifetime and 59% decades after (Engdahl et al. 1997). Variable PTSD rates have been found in individuals subjected to major noninterpersonal trauma; for example, reported rates in severely injured accident

victims range from a very low 2% (Schnyder et al. 2001) to 32% (Koren et al. 1999). In those sustaining severe traumatic brain injury, a 27% PTSD incidence has been reported (Bryant et al. 2000a). Childhood interpersonal trauma can often result in PTSD, as is widely known clinically and documented by numerous studies. In an inner-city child psychiatry clinic, more than half of the traumatized children had syndromal or subsyndromal PTSD, with experiencing physical abuse or witnessing domestic violence being the strongest contributors (Silva et al. 2000). In a large community sample followed prospectively into young adulthood, about one-third of the children who had suffered substantiated sexual abuse, physical abuse, or neglect had PTSD (Widom 1999). On average, it is estimated that approximately one-fourth of all individuals who experience major trauma develop PTSD (Breslau et al. 1991). In addition, as described by McFarlane, a definite dose–response relationship exists between the impact of the trauma and PTSD. Still, it is rare even for overwhelming trauma to lead to PTSD in more than half of the exposed populations, clearly suggesting that other etiological factors also play a role (McFarlane 1990). A discussion of such predictors follows.

Risk Factors and Predictors

There is general agreement in the literature that a variety of premorbid risk factors predispose to the development of PTSD. Although the disorder can certainly develop in people without significant preexisting psychopathology, a number of biological and psychological variables have been identified that render individuals more vulnerable to the development of PTSD.

It has been suggested that the greater the amount of previous trauma experienced by an individual, the more likely he or she is to develop symptoms after a stressful life event. In addition, individuals with previous traumatic experiences may be more likely to become exposed to future traumas, because they can be prone to reenact the original trauma behaviorally (van der Kolk 1989). In a study of Vietnam veterans, individuals with PTSD had higher rates of childhood physical abuse than veterans without PTSD, as well as a significantly higher rate of total traumatic events before entrance into the military (Bremner et al. 1993a).

McFarlane (1989) found that the severity of exposure to disaster was the major determinant of early posttraumatic morbidity, whereas preexisting psychological disorders better predicted the persistence of posttraumatic symptoms over time. A number of psychiatric conditions in probands and in their relatives appear to predispose these individuals to develop PTSD. In the ECA sample, a history of childhood conduct problems before age 15 years was predictive of PTSD. An epidemiological survey identified (albeit retrospectively) different risk factors for being exposed to trauma versus developing PTSD after traumatic exposure (Breslau et al. 1991). Risk factors for exposure to trauma were male sex, childhood conduct problems, extraversion, and family history of substance abuse or psychiatric problems. Risk factors for developing PTSD after traumatic exposure were disrupted parental attachments, anxiety, depression, and a family history of anxiety. Having an Axis II disorder also was found to increase the risk for chronic PTSD (Ursano et al. 1999a). Having a past history of PTSD increases the risk for both acute and chronic PTSD (Ursano et al. 1999b). Compared with nonchronic PTSD, chronic PTSD (PTSD of more than 1 year's duration) has been specifically associated with higher rates of comorbid anxiety and depressive disorders and a family history of antisocial behavior (Breslau and Davis 1992).

Interestingly, parental PTSD is a risk factor for PTSD in offspring, even in the absence of elevated trauma (Yehuda et al. 1998b). Findings with regard to gender are conflicting, in that female gender was found to be associated with chronic PTSD in one study (Breslau and Davis 1992) but with only acute PTSD in another (Ursano et al. 1999a). An additional factor that has been associated with a higher likelihood of developing PTSD is lower premorbid intelligence (Macklin et al. 1998). Neurological compromise, with increased neurological soft signs and a childhood history of neurodevelopmental problems and lower intelligence, is associated with PTSD and could possibly be a predisposing risk factor (Gurvits et al. 2000).

Early predictors of PTSD after a traumatic event have also received great attention, and their potential significance for early intervention and prevention is obvious. As previously stated, the occurrence of ASD in the first month after trauma is a very strong predictor of later PTSD. ASD diagnosis combined with a resting heart rate greater than 90 has a surprisingly high sensitivity, 88%, and specificity, 85%, in predicting development of PTSD (Bryant et al. 2000b). Similarly, high heart rate and decreased cortisol in the acute aftermath of trauma strongly correlate with later PTSD (Yehuda et al. 1998a). Even elevated heart rate, on its own, shortly after trauma is a significant predictor of later PTSD (Shalev et al. 1998a). The importance of the very early reaction to a traumatic event in predicting PTSD cannot be underestimated: early PTSD-type symptoms within 1 week of a traffic accident predict PTSD 1 year later (Koren et al. 1999).

In recent years, increased attention has been given to dissociative phenomena and to their relationship with posttraumatic symptoms (Spiegel and Cardena 1990). Greater dissociation around the time of the traumatic event is a strong predictor of subsequent development of PTSD (Marmar et al. 1994; Shalev et al. 1996). Individuals with peritraumatic dissociation are 4–5 times more likely than those without such phenomena to develop both acute and chronic PTSD (Ursano et al. 1999b). It may be that early peritraumatic dissociation can serve as a "marker" to identify individuals who will be at high risk of developing PTSD in the future.

Cognitive and Behavioral Theories

A cognitive model proposed to explain the persistence of PTSD symptoms postulates that PTSD becomes persistent when individuals process their trauma in a way that leads to a sense of serious and current threat. Such threat processing consists of excessively negative appraisals of the trauma or its consequences and a disruption in autobiographical memory involving poor contextualization and strong associative memory (Ehlers and Clark 2000).

Behavioral theory suggests that a disturbance of conditioned responses occurs in PTSD. Autonomic responses to both innocuous and aversive stimuli are elevated, with larger responses to unpaired cues and reduced extinction of conditioned responses (Peri et al. 2000). It is proposed that individuals with PTSD have higher sympathetic system arousal at the time of conditioning and therefore are more conditionable than trauma-exposed individuals without PTSD (Orr et al. 2000). Individuals with PTSD also generalize fear-related conditioned responses across stimuli, having been sensitized by stress (Grillon and Morgan 1999).

Recent studies have also revealed a number of disturbances in cognitive processes associated with PTSD. For example, the high incidence of PTSD after severe traumatic brain injury involving loss of consciousness but few traumatic memories suggests that trauma can mediate PTSD in part at an implicit level (Bryant et al. 2000a). Impairments in explicit memory have been associated with PTSD (Bremner et al. 1993b; Jenkins et al. 1998) and may be related to hippocampal toxicity resulting from stress-mediated elevations in norepinephrine (Bremner et al. 1995). In addition, subjects with PTSD may exhibit recall deficits not for trauma-related words, but rather for positive and neutral words, suggesting that avoidance of the encoding of disturbing information does not occur in PTSD (McNally et al. 1998). This appears consistent with the intrusive nature of traumatic memories clinically encountered in the disorder. Indeed, there appears to be an attentional bias toward traumatic stimuli in PTSD (Bryant and Harvey 1997), whereas generalized attentional disturbances have not been found (Golier et al. 1997).

Biological Theories

Noradrenergic system. The neurobiological response to acute stress and trauma involves the release of various stress hormones that allow the organism to respond adaptively to stress. These releases include heightened secretion of catecholamines and cortisol. When PTSD develops under severe or repeated trauma, the stress response becomes dysregulated and chronic autonomic hyperactivity sets in, manifesting itself in the "positive" symptoms of PTSD—that is, the hyperarousal and intrusive recollections. A wide range of data support this hypothesis. The noradrenergic system, originating in the locus coeruleus, regulates arousal (Southwick et al. 1999). In patients with PTSD, heightened physiological responses to stressful stimuli, such as blood pressure, heart rate, respiration, galvanic skin response, and electromyographic activity, have been consistently documented (Kolb 1987; Pitman et al. 1987). Long-standing increases in the urinary catecholamines norepinephrine and epinephrine have been found in patients with PTSD (Kosten et al. 1987; Spivak et al. 1999), as well as elevated plasma norepinephrine (Spivak et al. 1999). Agents that stimulate the arousal system, such as lactate (Rainey et al. 1987) and yohimbine (Southwick et al. 1993, 1997), induce flashbacks and increases in core PTSD symptoms. Clinical improvement in intrusive recollections and hyperarousal during open treatment with adrenergic-blocking agents, such as clonidine or propranolol, also suggests adrenergic hyperactivity (Kolb et al. 1984). A decrease in the number and sensitivity of α_2-adrenergic receptors, possibly as a consequence of chronic noradrenergic hyperactivity, has been reported in PTSD (Perry et al. 1987). Downregulation of the α_2-adrenergic receptor is also supported by one case report of a PTSD patient with a blunted GH response to clonidine, which normalized after behavioral treatment (Hansenne et al. 1991).

Endogenous opioid system. Whereas affective numbing was understood, in the past, primarily as a psychological defense against overwhelming emotional pain, more recent research has suggested a biological component to the "negative" symptoms of PTSD. van der Kolk et al. (1984) proposed that animal models of inescapable shock may parallel the development of PTSD in humans. Animals that are prevented from escaping from severe stress develop a syndrome of learned helplessness (Maier and Seligman 1976) that resembles the symptoms of constricted affect, withdrawal, amotivation, and decline in functioning associated with PTSD.

Animals exposed to prolonged or repeated inescapable stress develop analgesia, which appears to be mediated by release of endogenous opiates and which is blocked by the opiate antagonist naloxone (Kelly 1982; Maier et al. 1980). Similarly, it is suggested that in humans who have experienced prolonged or repeated trauma, endogenous opiates are readily released with any stimulus that is reminiscent of the original trauma, leading to analgesia and psychic numbing (van der Kolk et al. 1984). Pitman et al. (1990) compared pain intensity in response to thermal stimuli in Vietnam veterans with PTSD and veterans without PTSD who were watching a war videotape. PTSD patients, but not control subjects, had a 30% analgesic effect (i.e., decreased pain intensity) when pretreated with a placebo injection; this analgesia was eliminated with naloxone pretreatment. On the basis of such findings, the concept of trauma addiction has been proposed (van der Kolk et al. 1984). After a transient opioid burst on reexposure to traumatic stimuli, accompanied by a subjective sense of calm and control, opiate withdrawal may set in. This withdrawal may then contribute to the hyperarousal symptoms of PTSD, leading the individual into a vicious cycle of traumatic reexposures to gain transient symptomatic relief.

Serotonergic system. The serotonergic system has also been implicated in the symptomatology of PTSD. The septohippocampal brain system contains serotonergic pathways and mediates behavioral inhibition and constraint. The role of serotonergic deficit in impulsive aggression has been studied extensively. In animals, repeated inescapable shock can lead to serotonin depletion. Thus, the irritability and outbursts seen in patients with PTSD may be related to serotonergic deficit. The partial serotonin agonist m-CPP induces an increase in PTSD symptoms suggestive of serotonergic sensitization

(Southwick et al. 1997). Decreased plasma serotonin levels have been found in PTSD patients (Spivak et al. 1999). A blunted prolactin response to fenfluramine challenge is similarly supportive of central serotonergic dysregulation in PTSD (Davis et al. 1999). Moreover, the efficacy of SSRIs in PTSD is indirectly supportive of dysregulated serotonergic modulation in PTSD.

Hypothalamic-pituitary-adrenal axis. A number of findings in PTSD have implicated a chronic dysregulation of HPA axis functioning that is highly characteristic of this disorder and distinct from that seen in other psychiatric disorders such as depression. The findings include elevated CSF corticotropin-releasing hormone (D.G. Baker et al. 1999; Bremner et al. 1997a), low urinary cortisol concentrations (J.W. Mason et al. 1986) and an elevated urinary norepinephrine–cortisol ratio (J.W. Mason et al. 1988), a blunted ACTH response to CRF (Smith et al. 1989), enhanced suppression of cortisol in response to dexamethasone administration, and a decrease in lymphocyte glucocorticoid receptor number. All of these findings are consistent with a model of a highly sensitized HPA axis that is hyperresponsive to stress and the effects of cortisol (Yehuda et al. 1993, 1995a).

Brain circuitry and neuroimaging findings. A number of neuroimaging findings, both structural and functional, in PTSD studies over the past several years have begun to delineate a model suggestive of limbic sensitization and diminished cortical inhibition in PTSD, with specific dysfunction in the brain areas involved in memory, emotion, and visuospatial processing (Bremner et al. 1999a). Functional deficits in verbal memory have been correlated with decreased hippocampal volume on MRI in combat-related PTSD (Brem-

ner et al. 1995). Similarly, a decrease in hippocampal volume has been found in a study of adult survivors of childhood abuse (Bremner et al. 1997b). PET imaging with PTSD symptom provocation via audiotaped traumatic scripts has revealed activation of the right limbic and paralimbic systems and of the visual cortex (Rauch et al. 1996). Finally, PET imaging conducted during auditory exposure to traumatic scripts has shown that abuse memories are associated with decreased blood flow in the medial prefrontal cortex, hippocampus, and visual association cortex (Bremner et al. 1999a).

Genetics. A large study of Vietnam veteran twins found that genetic factors accounted for 13%–34% of the variance in liability to the various PTSD symptom clusters, whereas no etiological role was found for shared environment (True et al. 1993). Molecular genetic studies of PTSD are sparse. An initial study found an association between PTSD and a polymorphism of the dopamine D_2 receptor (Comings et al. 1996); however, this finding was not replicated in a later study (Gelernter et al. 1999).

Course and Prognosis

Scrignar (1984) divided the clinical course of PTSD into three stages. Stage I involves the response to trauma. Nonsusceptible persons may experience an adrenergic surge of symptoms immediately after the trauma but do not dwell on the incident. Predisposed persons have higher levels of anxiety and dissociation at baseline, an exaggerated response to the trauma, and an obsessive preoccupation with the trauma after the trauma has occurred. If symptoms persist beyond 4–6 weeks, the patient enters stage II, or acute PTSD. Feelings of helplessness and loss of control, symptoms of increased autonomic arousal, reliving of the trauma, and somatic symptoms may occur. The patient's life becomes centered around the trauma, with subsequent changes in lifestyle, personality, and social functioning. Phobic avoidance, startle responses, and angry outbursts may occur. In stage III, chronic PTSD develops, with disability, demoralization, and despondency. The patient's emphasis changes from preoccupation with the actual trauma to preoccupation with the physical disability resulting from the trauma. Somatic symptoms, chronic anxiety, and depression are common complications at this time, as are substance abuse, disturbed family relations, and unemployment. Some patients may focus on compensation and lawsuits.

It was reported in one study that the rate of full remission from chronic PTSD over a 5-year prospectively studied period was only 18%, highlighting the frequent chronicity of the illness. Histories of alcohol abuse and childhood trauma were associated with less remission (Zlotnick et al. 1999).

Diagnosis

The diagnosis of PTSD is usually not difficult if there is a clear history of exposure to a traumatic event, followed by symptoms of intense anxiety lasting at least 1 month, along with arousal and stimulation of the autonomic nervous system, numbing of responsiveness, and avoidance or reexperiencing of the traumatic event. However, a wide variety of anxiety, depressive, somatic, and behavioral symptoms for which the relationship between their onset and the traumatic event is less clear-cut may easily lead to misdiagnosis.

Differential Diagnosis

Following acute physical traumas, head trauma, or concussion, an organic mental disorder must be ruled out, because this diagnosis has important treatment implications. Mild concussions may leave no immediate apparent neurological signs but may have residual long-term effects on mood and concentration. A careful evaluation of the nature of the head trauma, including a review of medical records and witnesses' observations, followed by mental status evaluation and neurological examination, and, if indicated, laboratory examinations, is essential in a diagnostic workup. Malnutrition may occur during prolonged stressful periods and may also lead to organic brain syndromes.

Organic mental disorders that could mimic PTSD include organic personality syndrome, delirium, amnestic syndrome, organic hallucinosis, and organic intoxication and withdrawal states. In addition, patients with PTSD may cope with their disorder through excessive use of alcohol, drugs, caffeine, or tobacco and thus may present with a combination of organic and psychological factors. In such cases, each concomitant disorder should be diagnosed.

There is much overlap between PTSD and major mood disorders. Symptoms such as psychic numbing, irritability, sleep disturbance, fatigue, anhedonia, impairments in family and social relationships, anger, concern with physical health, and pessimistic outlook may occur in both disorders. Major depression is a frequent complication of PTSD; when it occurs, major depression must be treated aggressively, because comorbidity carries an increased risk of suicide.

After a traumatic event, patients may be aversively conditioned to the surroundings of the trauma and may develop a phobia of objects, surroundings, or situations that remind them of the trauma itself. Phobic patients experience anxiety in the feared situation, whereas avoidance is accompanied by anxiety reduction that reinforces the avoidant behavior. In PTSD, the phobia may be symptomatically similar to specific phobia, but the nature of the precipitant and the symptom cluster of PTSD distinguish this condition from simple phobia.

The symptoms of GAD, such as motor tension, autonomic hyperactivity, apprehensive expectation, and vigilance and scanning, are also present in PTSD. However, the onset and course of the illness differ: GAD has an insidious or gradual onset and a course that fluctuates with environmental stressors, whereas PTSD has an acute onset often followed by a chronic course.

Patients with PTSD may also experience panic attacks. In some patients, panic attacks predate the PTSD or do not occur exclusively in the context of stimuli reminiscent of the traumatic event. In other patients, however, panic attacks develop after the PTSD and are cued solely by traumatic stimuli.

Adjustment disorder differs from PTSD in that the stressor in adjustment disorder is usually less severe and within the range of common experience and the characteristic symptoms of PTSD, such as reexperiencing the trauma, are absent. The prognosis of full recovery in adjustment disorder is usually excellent.

Both factitious disorder and malingering involve conscious deception and feigning of illness, although the motivation for each condition differs. Factitious disorder may present with physical or psychological symptoms, the feigning of symptoms is under voluntary control, and the motivation is to assume the "patient" role. Chronic factitious disorder with physical symptoms (i.e., Munchausen syndrome) involves frequent doctor visits and surgical interventions. PTSD differs from this disorder by absence of fabricated symptoms, acute onset after a trauma, and absence of a bizarre pretraumatic medical history.

Malingering involves the conscious fabrication of an illness for the purpose of achieving a definite goal such as obtaining money or compensation. Malingerers often reveal an inconsistent history, unexpected symptom clusters, a history of antisocial behavior and substance abuse, and a chaotic lifestyle, and there is often a discrepancy between history, claimed distress, and objective data.

Treatment

Pharmacotherapy

A variety of different psychopharmacological agents have been used in the treatment of PTSD by clinicians and reported in the literature as case reports, open clinical trials, and controlled studies. A summary of the pharmacological treatment of PTSD is presented in Table 7–16. In the past few years, SSRIs and other serotonergic agents have emerged as the first-line pharmacological treatment of PTSD.

Adrenergic blockers. Kolb et al. (1984) treated 12 Vietnam veterans with PTSD in an open trial of the β-blocker propranolol over a 6-month period. Dosage ranged from 120 to 160 mg/day. Eleven patients reported a positive change in self-assessment at the end of the 6-month period, with less explosiveness, fewer nightmares, improved sleep, and a decrease in intrusive thoughts, hyperalertness, and startle response. Another open pilot study by this group (Kolb et al. 1984) using clonidine, an noradrenergic α_2 agonist, was conducted in nine Vietnam veterans with PTSD. Daily dosages of 0.2–0.4 mg of clonidine were administered over a 6-month period. Eight patients reported reduced explosiveness and improvement in their capacity to control their emotions, and a majority reported improvements in sleep and nightmares; lowered startle response, hyperalertness,

TABLE 7–16.   Pharmacotherapy of posttraumatic stress disorder (PTSD)

Selective serotonin reuptake inhibitors (SSRIs)
   General indications: first-line treatment; well tolerated; once-daily dosing; documented efficacy
   Sertraline: U.S. Food and Drug Administration–approved, large controlled trials
   Fluoxetine: large controlled trials
   Fluvoxamine, paroxetine: open trials, similar efficacy
   Nefazodone: next first-line option if poor response to or intolerance of SSRIs; several open
      trials, one in treatment-refractory patients; no controlled trials
Other antidepressants
   Tricyclics: overall modest results when tested in double-blind fashion
   Monoamine oxidase inhibitors: may be superior to tricyclics, especially for intrusive symptoms
Augmentation
   General indications: when response to first-line options not adequate; additional treatment of
      specific PTSD symptoms or comorbid disorders
   Clonidine: some efficacy in open treatment
   Lithium: improvement in intrusive symptoms and irritability in open trial
   Carbamazepine: decreased intrusive symptoms, anger, impulsivity in open treatment
   Valproate: decreased hyperarousal and intrusion, not numbing, in open treatment
   Lamotrigine: very small controlled trial, some efficacy
   Buspirone: efficacy in an open trial
   Triiodothyronine: improvement in small open trial, possibly antidepressant response
   Cyproheptadine: case reports of decreased nightmares
   Bupropion: no change in PTSD, improvement in depression
   Trazodone, benzodiazepines, diphenhydramine: sleep disturbance
   Nefazodone

and intrusive thinking; and psychosocial improvement.

Tricyclic antidepressants.   Until about a decade ago, most reports on the pharmacotherapy of PTSD involved the use of TCAs. A retrospective study examining 25 patients with PTSD treated with a variety of different antidepressants, including TCAs and MAOIs, reported good or moderate results in 67% of the patients treated. Response was not clearly related to the presence of somatization symptoms, depression, or panic attacks. Antidepressants appeared to be more useful than major tranquilizers. Although antidepressants improved intrusion-type symptoms, their most prominent impact was decreased insomnia and an overall sedative effect.

Burstein (1984), in administering

imipramine at daily doses of 50–350 mg to 10 patients with recent-onset PTSD, observed significant improvement in intrusive recollections, sleep and dream disturbance, and flashbacks. Similar improvement in intrusive symptomatology was reported with an open trial of desipramine (Kauffman et al. 1987). A positive effect of imipramine on posttraumatic night terrors was reported by J.R. Marshall (1975).

Although controlled studies of TCAs in PTSD were subsequently conducted, they were unable to replicate the earlier trials' success in decreasing posttraumatic symptoms. In a 4-week, double-blind crossover study of desipramine and placebo in 18 veterans with PTSD, only depressive symptoms improved; anxiety, intrusive symptoms, and avoidance did not change with desipramine therapy (Reist et al. 1989). Davidson et al. (1990) conducted a 4- to 8-week double-blind comparison of amitriptyline and placebo in 46 veterans with PTSD. Although depression and anxiety decreased with amitriptyline therapy, the decrease in intrusive and avoidant symptoms was apparent only in the subgroup of patients who completed 8 weeks of amitriptyline therapy and was marginal. At the end of the study, roughly two-thirds of patients in both treatment groups still met the criteria for PTSD.

Monoamine oxidase inhibitors. An early study of MAOIs described five patients with "traumatic war neurosis" in whom phenelzine, at doses of 45–75 mg/day, improved traumatic dreams, flashbacks, startle reactions, and violent outbursts (Hogben and Cornfield 1981). Panic attacks were also described in all of the patients in this study. Positive effects of phenelzine on intrusive posttraumatic symptoms have been reported in subsequent small open trials (Davidson et al. 1987; van der Kolk 1983).

An 8-week randomized double-blind trial subsequently compared phenelzine (71 mg), imipramine (240 mg), and placebo in 34 veterans with PTSD (Frank et al. 1988). Both antidepressants resulted in some overall improvement in patients' posttraumatic symptoms, and phenelzine tended to be superior to imipramine. The most marked improvement was the decrease in intrusive symptoms in patients receiving phenelzine, with an average reduction of 60% on the intrusion scale measure.

Serotonin reuptake inhibitors. In the past few years SSRIs have become the medications of choice for this disorder. Several initial open trials of fluoxetine reported marked improvement in PTSD symptoms at a wide range of doses (Da-

vidson et al. 1991; McDougle et al. 1991b; Shay 1992). Subsequently, in a double-blind trial comparing fluoxetine and placebo, fluoxetine led to a significant reduction of PTSD symptomatology, especially for arousal and numbing symptoms (van der Kolk et al. 1994). An initial open trial of sertraline (Brady et al. 1995) also claimed benefit for PTSD. Sertraline is now FDA approved for the treatment of PTSD, in the wake of two large controlled trials that recently documented its efficacy. In a 12-week, multicenter, placebo-controlled trial, sertraline at doses of 50–200 mg/day resulted in significant benefits that began to appear by week 2. The response rate was over 50%, and improvement in both numbing and arousal symptoms, although not in reexperiencing, was significantly greater than with placebo (Brady et al. 2000). Comparable results were reported in another large sertraline study with very similar design (Davidson et al. 2001), with a 60% response rate by conservative intent-to-treat analysis. Open trials of other SSRIs, such as fluvoxamine (De Boer et al. 1992) and paroxetine (R.D. Marshall et al. 1998), suggest that these medications have similar efficacy in PTSD, despite the lack of controlled trials.

Mood stabilizers and anticonvulsants. In a small open trial of lithium treatment of PTSD, van der Kolk (1983) reported improvement in intrusive recollections and irritability in more than half of the patients treated. However, there have been no controlled trials. In an open trial of carbamazepine in 10 patients with PTSD, Lipper et al. (1986) reported moderate to great improvement in intrusive symptoms in 7 patients. Wolf et al. (1988) reported decreased impulsivity and angry outbursts in 10 veterans who were also treated with carbamazepine; all patients had normal EEGs. Valproate was initially reported to decrease irritability and angry outbursts in two veterans with PTSD (Szymanski and Olympia 1991). More recently, in an open trial of 16 patients treated with valproate for 8 weeks, a significant decrease in symptoms of hyperarousal and intrusion, but not of numbing, was reported (Clark et al. 1999b). In a very small, placebo-controlled trial of lamotrigine at dosages up to 500 mg/day, more patients appeared to respond to lamotrigine than to placebo (Hertzberg et al. 1999), a finding that warrants additional studies with larger samples.

Other medications.   Several open trials have described benefits with nefazodone treatment. A 12-week study using a mean dose of 430 mg/day showed improvement in all three symptom clusters in patients with previously treatment-refractory PTSD (Zisook et al. 2000). An 8-week open trial reported similar improvements in patients with chronic PTSD (Davis et al. 2000), whereas another report found a 60% response rate in treatment completers (Davidson et al. 1998), and yet another described improvement in all 10 patients treated (Hertzberg et al. 1998). Thus, nefazodone appears very promising in treating PTSD and a controlled trial is warranted.

Psychotherapy

It is generally agreed that some form of psychotherapy is necessary in the treatment of posttraumatic pathology. Crisis intervention shortly after the traumatic event is effective in reducing immediate distress, possibly preventing chronic or delayed responses, and, if the pathological response is still tentative, may allow for briefer intervention.

Brief dynamic psychotherapy has been advocated both as an immediate treatment procedure and as a way of preventing chronic disorder. The therapist must

establish a working alliance that allows the patient to work through his or her reactions.

The literature has suggested that persons with disrupted early attachments or abuse, who have been traumatized earlier in their lives, are more likely to develop PTSD than are those with stable backgrounds. The occurrence of psychic trauma in a person's past may psychologically and biologically predispose him or her to respond excessively and maladaptively to intense experiences and affects (Herman et al. 1989; Krystal 1968; van der Kolk 1987b). Therefore, attempting to modify preexisting conflicts, developmental difficulties, and defensive styles that render the person especially vulnerable to traumatization by particular experiences is central to the treatment of traumatic syndromes.

The "phase oriented" treatment model suggested by Horowitz (1976) strikes a balance between initial supportive interventions to minimize the traumatic state and increasingly aggressive "working through" interventions at later stages of treatment. Establishment of a safe and communicative relationship, reappraisal of the traumatic event, revision of the patient's inner model of self and world, and planning for termination with a reexperiencing of loss are all important therapeutic issues in the treatment of PTSD. Herman et al. (1989) emphasized the importance of validating the patient's traumatic experiences as a precondition for reparation of damaged self-identity.

Embry (1990) outlined seven major parameters for effective psychotherapy in war veterans with chronic PTSD: 1) initial rapport building, 2) limit setting and supportive confrontation, 3) affective modeling, 4) defocusing on stress and focusing on current life events, 5) sensitivity to transference–countertransference issues, 6) understanding of secondary gain, and

7) therapist's maintenance of a positive treatment attitude.

Group psychotherapy can also serve as an important adjunctive treatment, or as the central treatment mode, in traumatized patients (van der Kolk 1987a). Because of past experiences, such patients are often mistrustful and reluctant to depend on authority figures, whereas the identification, support, and hopefulness of peer settings can facilitate therapeutic change.

Cognitive and Behavioral Therapies

A variety of cognitive and behavioral techniques have gained increasing popularity and validation in the treatment of PTSD. People involved in traumatic events such as accidents frequently develop phobias or phobic anxiety related to or associated with these situations. When a phobia or phobic anxiety is associated with PTSD, systematic desensitization or graded exposure has been found to be effective. This is based on the principle that when patients are gradually exposed to a phobic or anxiety-provoking stimulus, they will become habituated or deconditioned to the stimulus. Variations of this treatment include using imaginal techniques (i.e., imaginal desensitization) and exposure to real-life situations (i.e., in vivo desensitization). Prolonged exposure (i.e., flooding), if tolerated by a patient, can also be useful and has been reported to be successful in the treatment of Vietnam veterans (Fairbank and Keane 1982).

Relaxation techniques produce the beneficial physiological result of reducing motor tension and lowering the activity of the autonomic nervous system, effects that may be particularly efficacious in PTSD. Progressive muscle relaxation involves contracting and relaxing various muscle groups to induce the relaxation response. This technique is useful for symptoms of autonomic arousal such as somatic symptoms, anxiety, and insomnia. Hypnosis has also been used, with success, to induce the relaxation response in PTSD.

Cognitive therapy and thought stopping, in which a phrase and momentary pain are paired with thoughts or images of the trauma, have been used to treat unwanted mental activity in PTSD. A recent randomized trial compared imaginal exposure and cognitive therapy in 72 patients with chronic PTSD (Tarrier et al. 1999). Both treatments resulted in comparable significant improvement, although not complete remission, of symptoms. Another controlled study in 87 patients with chronic PTSD compared exposure therapy, cognitive restructuring, their combination, and simple relaxation techniques (I. Marks et al. 1998). Both the behavioral and the cognitive treatment resulted in marked improvement, with gains maintained after 6 months; in contrast, their combination was of no additional benefit, and relaxation yielded only modest improvement. In another study, exposure therapy, stress inoculation training, their combination, and a waiting-list control condition were compared in women with chronic PTSD who had experienced an assault (Foa et al. 1999). The three active treatments produced comparable improvement, and the gains were maintained through 1-year follow-up. In another study that attempted to boost the effects of individual exposure therapy by adding family behavioral interventions, the latter rendered no additional benefit (Glynn et al. 1999).

Another approach, affect management, also appears to be beneficial. In a randomized study of adult women with PTSD and a history of childhood sexual abuse who were already receiving individual psychotherapy and pharmacotherapy, those who underwent a 3-month course of group affect-management treatment demonstrated significantly fewer PTSD and dissociative symptoms after the treatment (Zlotnick et al. 1997).

Other Treatments

Eye movement desensitization and reprocessing (EMDR) is a relatively new technique that has been applied to the treatment of trauma-related pathology in the past decade. There continues to be controversy in the literature regarding EMDR's efficacy as well as the underlying mechanisms of its action. In a 5-year follow-up study of a small group of veterans who had initially shown modest benefits from treatment with EMDR, all benefit was found to have disappeared at follow-up (Macklin et al. 2000). Although EMDR has been found to be superior to relaxation in treating PTSD (Carlson et al. 1998), relaxation is not considered one of the first-line treatments for this disorder. A recent randomized study comparing EMDR with CBT found that CBT was significantly more effective and that its superiority was even more apparent at 3-month follow-up (Devilly and Spence 1999).

Transcranial magnetic stimulation was found to have some transient efficacy in decreasing core PTSD symptoms in 10 patients treated openly, and thus may warrant more investigation in PTSD (Grisaru et al. 1998).

Conclusions

In this chapter we endeavored to present a comprehensive discussion of panic disorder, GAD, the phobic disorders, OCD, and PTSD. A review of history, differing theoretical models, and new developments in epidemiology, classification, pathophysiology, and treatment, has been presented. An explosion of research has led to dramatic developments in the understanding and alleviation of various forms of anxiety and has made the anxiety disorders an exciting field of modern psychiatry.

References

Ackerman DL, Greenland S, Bystritsky A, et al: Predictors of treatment response in obsessive-compulsive disorder: multivariate analyses from a multicenter trial of clomipramine. J Clin Psychopharmacol 14:247–254, 1994

Adler CM, McDonough-Ryan P, Sax KW, et al: fMRI of neuronal activation with symptom provocation in unmedicated patients with obsessive compulsive disorder. J Psychiatr Res 34:317–324, 2000

Alden LE, Wallace ST: Social phobia and social appraisal in successful and unsuccessful social interactions. Behav Res Ther 33: 497–505, 1995

Altamura AC, Pioli R, Vitto M, et al: Venlafaxine in social phobia: a study in selective serotonin reuptake inhibitor non-responders. Int Clin Psychopharmacol 14:239–245, 1999

American Psychiatric Association: Diagnostic and Statistical Manual of Mental Disorders, 4th Edition. Washington, DC, American Psychiatric Association, 1994

American Psychiatric Association: Diagnostic and Statistical Manual of Mental Disorders, 4th Edition, Text Revision. Washington, DC, American Psychiatric Association, 2000

Amies PL, Gelder MG, Shaw PM: Social phobia: a comparative clinical study. Br J Psychiatry 142:174–179, 1983

Ananth J, Pecknold JC, Van Den Steen N, et al: Double-blind comparative study of clomipramine and amitriptyline in obsessive neurosis. Prog Neuropsychopharmacol Biol Psychiatry 5:257–262, 1981

Apter A, Ratzoni G, King RA, et al: Fluvoxamine open-label treatment of adolescent inpatients with obsessive-compulsive disorder or depression. J Am Acad Child Adolesc Psychiatry 33:342–8, 1994

Asberg M, Thoren P, Bertilsson L: Clomipramine treatment of obsessive-compulsive disorder: biochemical and clinical aspects. Psychopharmacol Bull 18:13–21, 1982

Baer L, Jenike MA: Personality disorders in obsessive-compulsive disorder. Psychiatr Clin North Am 15:803–812, 1992

Baer L, Jenike MA, Ricciardi JN, et al: Standardized assessment of personality disorders in obsessive-compulsive disorder. Arch Gen Psychiatry 47:826–830, 1990

Baer L, Jenike MA, Black DW, et al: Effect of Axis II diagnoses on treatment outcome with clomipramine in 55 patients with obsessive-compulsive disorder. Arch Gen Psychiatry 49:862–862, 1992

Baer L, Rauch SL, Ballantine HT, et al: Cingulotomy for intractable obsessive-compulsive disorder: prospective long-term follow-up of 18 patients. Arch Gen Psychiatry 52:384–392, 1995

Baker DG, West SA, Nicholson WE, et al: Serial CSF corticotropin-releasing hormone levels and adrenocortical activity in combat veterans with posttraumatic stress disorder. Am J Psychiatry 156:585–588, 1999

Baldwin D, Bobes J, Stein DJ, et al: Paroxetine in social phobia/social anxiety disorder: a randomized, double-blind, placebo-controlled study. Br J Psychiatry 175:120–126, 1999

Ballenger JC, Burrows GD, DuPont RL Jr, et al: Alprazolam in panic disorder and agoraphobia: results from a multicenter trial, I: efficacy in short-term treatment. Arch Gen Psychiatry 45:413–422, 1988

Ballenger JC, Wheadon DE, Steiner M, et al: Double-blind, fixed-dose, placebo-controlled study of paroxetine in the treatment of panic disorder. Am J Psychiatry 155:36–42, 2000

Barlow DH: Anxiety and Its Disorders: The Nature and Treatment of Anxiety and Panic. New York, Guilford, 1988

Barlow DH, Craske MG, Cerny JA, et al: Behavioral treatment of panic disorder. Behav Ther 20:261–282, 1989

Barr LC, Goodman WK, Anand A, et al: Addition of desipramine to serotonin reuptake inhibitors in treatment-resistant obsessive-compulsive disorder. Am J Psychiatry 154:1293–1295, 1997

Barton R: Diabetes insipidus and obsessional neurosis: a syndrome. Lancet 1:133–135, 1965

Basoglu M, Marks IM, Kilic C, et al: Relationship of panic, anticipatory anxiety, agoraphobia and global improvement in panic disorder with agoraphobia treated with alprazolam and exposure. Br J Psychiatry 164:647–652, 1994

Baxter LR Jr, Schwartz JM, Bergman KS, et al: Caudate glucose metabolic rate changes with both drug and behavior therapy for obsessive-compulsive disorder. Arch Gen Psychiatry 49:681–689, 1992

Beck AT, Sokol L, Clark DA, et al: A crossover study of focused cognitive therapy for panic disorder. Am J Psychiatry 149:778–783, 1992

Behar D, Rapoport JL, Berg CJ, et al: Computerized tomography and neuropsychological test measures in adolescents with obsessive-compulsive disorder. Am J Psychiatry 141:363–369, 1984

Beidel DC, Turner SM, Morris TL: Psychopathology of childhood social phobia. J Am Acad Child Adolesc Psychiatry 38:643–650, 1999

Beidel DC, Turner SM, Morris TL: Behavioral treatment of childhood social phobia. J Consult Clin Psychol 68:1072–1080, 2000

Bejerot S, Bodlund O: Response to high doses of citalopram in treatment-resistant obsessive-compulsive disorder. Acta Psychiatr Scand 98:423–424, 1998

Benjamin J, Levine J, Fux M, et al: Double-blind, placebo-controlled, crossover trial of inositol treatment for panic disorder. Am J Psychiatry 152:1084–1086, 1995

Benjamin J, Ben-Zion IZ, Karbofsky E, et al: Double-blind, placebo-controlled study of paroxetine for specific phobia. Psychopharmacology (Berl) 149:194–196, 2000

Benkelfat C, Nordahl TE, Semple WE, et al: Local cerebral glucose metabolic rates in obsessive-compulsive disorder: patients treated with clomipramine. Arch Gen Psychiatry 47:840–848, 1990

Black DW, Noyes R, Goldstein RB, et al: A family study of obsessive-compulsive disorder. Arch Gen Psychiatry 49:362–368, 1992

Bogetto F, Bellino S, Vaschetto P, et al: Olanzapine augmentation of fluvoxamine-refractory obsessive-compulsive disorder (OCD): a 12-week open trial. Psychiatry Res 96:91–98, 2000

Borkovec TD, Costello E: Efficacy of applied relaxation and cognitive-behavioral therapy in the treatment of generalized anxiety disorder. J Consult Clin Psychol 61:611–619, 1993

Bouwer C, Stein DJ: Use of the selective serotonin reuptake inhibitor citalopram in the treatment of generalized social phobia. J Affect Disord 49:79–82, 1998

Bowlby J: Attachment and Loss, Vol 2: Separation: Anxiety and Anger. New York, Basic Books, 1973

Brady KT, Sonne SC, Roberts JM: Sertraline treatment of comorbid posttraumatic stress disorder and alcohol dependence. J Clin Psychiatry 56:502–505, 1995

Brady K[T], Pearlstein T, Asnis GM, et al: Efficacy and safety of sertraline treatment of posttraumatic stress disorder: a randomized controlled trial. JAMA 283:1837–1844, 2000

Brantigan CO, Brantigan TA, Joseph N: Effect of beta blockade and beta stimulation on stage fright. Am J Med 72:88–94, 1982

Breiter HC, Rauch SL, Kwong KK, et al: Functional magnetic resonance imaging of symptom provocation in obsessive-compulsive disorder. Arch Gen Psychiatry 53:595–606, 1996

Bremner JD, Southwick SM, Johnson DR, et al: Childhood physical abuse and combat-related posttraumatic stress disorder in Vietnam veterans. Am J Psychiatry 150:235–239, 1993a

Bremner JD, Scott TM, Delaney RC, et al: Deficits in short-term memory in posttraumatic stress disorder. Am J Psychiatry 150:1015–1019, 1993b

Bremner JD, Randall P, Scott TM, et al: MRI-based measurement of hippocampal volume in patients with combat-related posttraumatic stress disorder. Am J Psychiatry 152:973–981, 1995

Bremner JD, Licinio J, Darnell A, et al: Elevated CSF corticotropin-releasing factor concentrations in posttraumatic stress disorder. Am J Psychiatry 154:624–629, 1997a

Bremner JD, Randall P, Vermetten E, et al: Magnetic resonance imaging-based measurement of hippocampal volume in posttraumatic stress disorder related to childhood physical and sexual abuse: a preliminary report. Biol Psychiatry 41:23–32, 1997b

Bremner JD, Staib LH, Kaloupek D, et al: Neural correlates of exposure to traumatic pictures and sound in Vietnam combat veterans with and without posttraumatic stress disorder: a positron emission tomography study. Biol Psychiatry 45:806–816, 1999a

Bremner JD, Innis RB, White T, et al: SPECT [I-123] iomazenil measurement of the benzodiazepine receptor in panic disorder. Biol Psychiatry 47:96–106, 2000

Breslau N, Davis GC: DSM-III generalized anxiety disorder: an empirical investigation of more stringent criteria. Psychiatry Res 15:231–238, 1985

Breslau N, Davis GC: Posttraumatic stress disorder in an urban population of young adults: risk factors for chronicity. Am J Psychiatry 149:671–675, 1992

Breslau N, Davis GC, Andreski P, et al: Traumatic events and posttraumatic stress disorder in an urban population of young adults. Arch Gen Psychiatry 48:216–222, 1991

Breslau N, Davis GC, Peterson EL, et al: Psychiatric sequelae of posttraumatic stress disorder in women. Arch Gen Psychiatry 54:81–87, 1997a

Breslau N, Davis GC, Andreski P, et al: Sex differences in posttraumatic stress disorder. Arch Gen Psychiatry 54:1044–1048, 1997b

Breslau N, Kessler RC, Chilcoat HD, et al: Trauma and posttraumatic stress disorder in the community: the 1996 Detroit Area Survey of Trauma. Arch Gen Psychiatry 55:626–632, 1998

Breslau N, Davis GC, Peterson EL, et al: A second look at comorbidity in victims of trauma: the posttraumatic stress disorder–major depression connection. Biol Psychiatry 48:902–909, 2000

Bryant RA, Harvey AG: Attentional bias in posttraumatic stress disorder. J Trauma Stress 10:635–644, 1997

Bryant RA, Marosszeky JE, Crooks J, et al: Posttraumatic stress disorder after severe traumatic brain injury. Am J Psychiatry 157:629–631, 2000a

Bryant RA, Harvey AG, Guthrie RM, et al: A prospective study of psychophysiological arousal, acute stress disorder, and posttraumatic stress disorder. J Abnorm Psychol 109:341–344, 2000b

Buchsbaum MS, Wu J, Haier R, et al: Positron emission tomography assessment of effects of benzodiazepines on regional glucose metabolic rate in patients with anxiety disorder. Life Sci 40:2393–2400, 1987

Burstein A: Treatment of post-traumatic stress disorder with imipramine. Psychosomatics 25:681–687, 1984

Butler G, Fennell M, Robson P, et al: Comparison of behavior therapy and cognitive behavior therapy in the treatment of generalized anxiety disorder. J Consult Clin Psychol 59:167–175, 1991

Caillard V, Rouillon F, Viel JF, et al: Comparative effects of low and high doses of clomipramine and placebo in panic disorder: a double-blind, controlled study. French University Antidepressant Group. Acta Psychiatr Scand 99:51–58, 1999

Calvocoressi L, Lewis B, Harris M, et al: Family accommodation in obsessive-compulsive disorder. Am J Psychiatry 152:441–443, 1995

Capstick N, Seldrup V: Obsessional states: a study in the relationship between abnormalities occurring at birth and subsequent development of obsessional symptoms. Acta Psychiatr Scand 56:427–439, 1977

Carey G, Gottesman II: Twin and family studies of anxiety, phobic, and obsessive disorders, in Anxiety: New Research and Changing Concepts. Edited by Klein DF, Rabkin J. New York, Raven, 1981, pp 117–136

Carlson JG, Chemtob CM, Rusnak K, et al: Eye movement desensitization and reprocessing (EMDR) treatment for combat-related posttraumatic stress disorder. J Trauma Stress 11:3–24, 1998

Carter RM, Wittchen HU, Pfister H, et al: One-year prevalence of subthreshold and threshold DSM-IV generalized anxiety disorder in a nationally representative sample. Depress Anxiety 13:78–88, 2001

Cassidy J: Attachment and generalized anxiety disorder, in Rochester Symposium on Developmental Psychopathology, Vol 6: Emotion, Cognition and Representation. Edited by Cicchetti D, Toth S. New York, University of Rochester Press, 1995

Chambless DL, Gillis MM: Cognitive therapy of anxiety disorders. J Consult Clin Psychol 61:248–260, 1993

Charney DS, Heninger GR: Abnormal regulation of noradrenergic function in panic disorders: effects of clonidine in healthy subjects and patients with agoraphobia and panic disorder. Arch Gen Psychiatry 43:1042–1054, 1986

Charney DS, Heninger GR, Breier A: Noradrenergic function in panic anxiety: effects of yohimbine in healthy subjects and patients with agoraphobia and panic disorder. Arch Gen Psychiatry 41:751–763, 1984

Chouinard G: Sertraline in the treatment of obsessive compulsive disorder: two double-blind, placebo-controlled studies. Int Clin Psychopharmacol 7 (suppl 2):37–41, 1992

Christensen KJ, Kim SW, Dysken MW, et al: Neuropsychological performance in obsessive-compulsive disorder. Biol Psychiatry 31:4–18, 1992

Ciesielski KT, Beech HR, Gordon PK: Some electrophysiological observations in obsessional states. Br J Psychiatry 138:479–484, 1981

Clark RD, Canive JM, Calais LA, et al: Divalproex in posttraumatic stress disorder: an open-label clinical trial. J Trauma Stress 12:395–401, 1999b

Comings DE, Muhleman D, Gysin R: Dopamine D2 receptor (DRD2) gene and susceptibility to posttraumatic stress disorder: a study and replication. Biol Psychiatry 40:368–372, 1996

Cooper AM: Will neurobiology influence psychoanalysis? Am J Psychiatry 142:1395–1402, 1985

Coplan JD, Lydiard RB: Brain circuits in panic disorder. Biol Psychiatry 44:1264–1276, 1998

Coplan JD, Pine D, Papp L, et al: Uncoupling of the noradrenergic-hypothalamic-pituitary-adrenal axis in panic disorder patients. Neuropsychopharmacology 13:65–73, 1995

Coplan JD, Papp LA, Pine D, et al: Clinical improvement with fluoxetine therapy and noradrenergic function in patients with panic disorder. Arch Gen Psychiatry 54:643–648, 1997

Cottraux J, Note I, Albuisson E, et al: Cognitive behavior therapy versus supportive therapy in social phobia: a randomized controlled trial. Psychother Psychosom 69:137–146, 2000

Coupland NJ, Bell C, Potokar J, et al: Flumazenil challenge in social phobia. Anxiety 111:27–30, 2000

Craske MG, Brown TA, Barlow DH: Behavioral treatment of panic disorder: a two-year follow-up. Behav Ther 22:289–304, 1991

Crowe RR, Noyes R, Pauls DL, et al: A family study of panic disorder. Arch Gen Psychiatry 40:1065–1069, 1983

Crowe RR, Wang Z, Noyes R, et al: Candidate gene study of eight GABAA receptor subunits in panic disorder. Am J Psychiatry 154:1096–1100, 1997

Curtis GC, Thyer B: Fainting on exposure to phobic stimuli. Am J Psychiatry 140:771–774, 1983

Curtis GC, Abelson JL, Gold PW: Adrenocorticotropic hormone and cortisol responses to corticotropin-releasing hormone: changes in panic disorder and effects of alprazolam treatment. Biol Psychiatry 41:76–85, 1997

Dannon PN, Sasson Y, Hirschmann S, et al: Pindolol augmentation in treatment-resistant obsessive compulsive disorder: a double-blind placebo controlled trial. Eur Neuropsychopharmacol 10:165–169, 2000

Davidson J[R], Walker JI, Kilts C: A pilot study of phenelzine in the treatment of post-traumatic stress disorder. Br J Psychiatry 150:252–255, 1987

Davidson J[R], Kudler H, Smith R, et al: Treatment of posttraumatic stress disorder with amitriptyline and placebo. Arch Gen Psychiatry 47:259–266, 1990

Davidson J[R], Roth S, Newman E: Fluoxetine in post-traumatic stress disorder. J Trauma Stress 4:419–423, 1991

Davidson JR, Hughes DL, George LK, et al: The epidemiology of social phobia: findings from the Duke Epidemiological Catchment Area Study. Psychol Med 23:709–718, 1993a

Davidson JR, Potts N, Richichi E, et al: Treatment of social phobia with clonazepam and placebo. J Clin Psychopharmacol 13:423–428, 1993b

Davidson JR, Weisler RH, Malik ML, et al: Treatment of posttraumatic stress disorder with nefazodone. Int Clin Psychopharmacol 13:111–113, 1998

Davidson JR, Rothbaum BO, van der Kolk BA, et al: Multicenter, double-blind comparison of sertraline and placebo in the treatment of posttraumatic stress disorder. Arch Gen Psychiatry 58:485–492, 2001

Davis LL, Clark DM, Kramer GL, et al: D-fenfluramine challenge in posttraumatic stress disorder. Biol Psychiatry 45:928–930, 1999

Davis LL, Nugent AL, Murray J, et al: Nefazodone treatment for chronic posttraumatic stress disorder: an open trial. J Clin Psychopharmacol 20:159–164, 2000

DeBellis MD, Casey BJ, Dahl RE, et al: A pilot study of amygdala volumes in pediatric generalized anxiety disorder. Biol Psychiatry 48:51–57, 2000

de Beurs E, van Balkom AJ, Lange A, et al: Treatment of panic disorder with agoraphobia: comparison of fluvoxamine, placebo and psychological panic management combined with exposure and of exposure in vivo alone. Am J Psychiatry 152:683–691, 1995

De Boer M, Op den Velde W, Falger PJ, et al: Fluvoxamine treatment for chronic PTSD: a pilot study. Psychother Psychosom 57:158–163, 1992

Deckert J, Catalano M, Heils A, et al: Functional promoter polymorphism of the human serotonin transporter: lack of association with panic disorder. Psychiatr Genet 7:45–47, 1997

Deckert J, Nothen MM, Franke P, et al: Systematic mutation screening and association study of the A1 and A2a adenosine receptor genes in panic disorder suggest a contribution of the A2a gene to the development of the disease. Mol Psychiatry 3:81–85, 1998

Deckert J, Catalano M, Syagailo YV, et al: Excess of high activity monoamine oxidase A gene promoter alleles in female patients with panic disorder. Hum Mol Genet 81:228–234, 1999

DeMartinis N, Schweizer E, Rickels K: An open-label trial of nefazodone in high comorbidity panic disorder. J Clin Psychiatry 57:245–248, 1996

DeMartinis N, Rynn M, Rickels K, et al: Prior benzodiazepine use and buspirone response in the treatment of generalized anxiety disorder. J Clin Psychiatry 61:91–94, 2000

Den Boer JA: Serotonergic Mechanisms in Anxiety Disorders: An Inquiry into Serotonin Function in Panic Disorder. The Hague, The Netherlands, Cip-Gegevens Koninklijke Bibliotheek, 1988

Devilly GJ, Spence SH: The relative efficacy and treatment distress of EMDR and a cognitive-behavior trauma treatment protocol in the amelioration of posttraumatic stress disorder. J Anxiety Disord 13:131–157, 1999

DeWit DJ, Ogborne A, Offord DR, et al: Antecedents of the risk of recovery from DSM-III-R social phobia. Psychol Med 29:569–582, 1999

Dimsdale JE, Moss J: Plasma catecholamines in stress and exercise. JAMA 243:340–342, 1980

Dyck IR, Phillips KA, Warshaw MG, et al: Patterns of personality pathology in patients with generalized anxiety disorder, panic disorder with and without agoraphobia, and social phobia. J Personal Disord 15:60–71, 2001

Ehlers A, Clark DM: A cognitive model of posttraumatic stress disorder. Behav Res Ther 38:319–345, 2000

Elam M, Yoat TP, Svensson TH: Hypercapnia and hypoxia: chemoreceptor-mediated control of locus coeruleus neurons and splanchnic, sympathetic nerves. Brain Res 222:373–381, 1981

Embry CK: Psychotherapeutic interventions in chronic posttraumatic stress disorder, in Posttraumatic Stress Disorder: Etiology, Phenomenology, and Treatment. Edited by Wolf ME, Mosnaim AD. Washington, DC, American Psychiatric Press, 1990, pp 226–236

Emmanuel NP, Lydiard BR, Ballenger JC: Treatment of social phobia with bupropion. J Clin Psychopharmacol 11:276–277, 1991

Engdahl B, Dikel TN, Eberly R, et al: Posttraumatic stress disorder in a community group of former prisoners of war: a normative response to severe trauma. Am J Psychiatry 154:1576–1581, 1997

Essau CA, Conradt J, Petermann F: Frequency, comorbidity, and psychosocial impairment of specific phobia in adolescents. J Clin Child Psychol 29:221–231, 2000

Fairbank TA, Keane TM: Flooding for combat-related stress disorders: assessment of anxiety reduction across traumatic memories. Behav Ther 13:499–510, 1982

Fallon BA, Liebowitz MR, Campeas R, et al: Intravenous clomipramine for obsessive-compulsive disorder refractory to oral clomipramine: a placebo-controlled study. Arch Gen Psychiatry 55:918–924, 1998

Faravelli C, Pallanti S: Recent life events and panic disorder. Am J Psychiatry 146:622–626, 1989

Fitzgerald KD, Stewart CM, Tawile V, et al: Risperidone augmentation of serotonin reuptake inhibitor treatment of pediatric obsessive compulsive disorder. J Child Adolesc Psychopharmacol 9:115–123, 1999

Flescher J: A dualistic viewpoint on anxiety. J Am Psychoanal Assoc 3:415–446, 1955

Flint AJ: Epidemiology and comorbidity of anxiety disorders in the elderly. Am J Psychiatry 151:640–649, 1994

Foa EB, Kozak MJ, Goodman WK, et al: DSM-IV field trial: obsessive-compulsive disorder. Am J Psychiatry 152:90–96, 1995

Foa EB, Dancu CV, Hembree EA, et al: A comparison of exposure therapy, stress inoculation therapy, and their combination for reducing posttraumatic stress disorder in female assault victims. J Consult Clin Psychol 67:194–200, 1999

Frank JB, Kosten TR, Giller EL Jr, et al: A randomized clinical trial of phenelzine and imipramine for posttraumatic stress disorder. Am J Psychiatry 145:1289–1291, 1988

Fredrikson M, Wik G, Greitz T, et al: Regional cerebral blood flow during experimental phobic fear. Psychophysiology 30:126–130, 1993

Freeman CP, Trimble MR, Deakin JF, et al: Fluvoxamine versus clomipramine in the treatment of obsessive compulsive disorder: a multicenter, randomized, double-blinded, parallel group comparison. J Clin Psychiatry 55:301–305, 1994

Freeston MH, Rheaume J, Ladouceur R: Correcting faulty appraisals of obsessional thoughts. Behav Res Ther 34:433–446, 1996

Freud S: On the grounds for detaching a particular syndrome from neurasthenia under the description anxiety neurosis (1895 [1894]), in The Standard Edition of the Complete Psychological Works of Sigmund Freud, Vol 3. Translated and edited by Strachey J. London, England, Hogarth, 1962b, pp 85–117

Freud S: Analysis of a phobia in a five-year-old boy (1909), in The Standard Edition of the Complete Psychological Works of Sigmund Freud, Vol 10. Translated and edited by Strachey J. London, England, Hogarth, 1955, pp 1–149

Freud S: The disposition to obsessional neurosis: a contribution to the problem of choice of neurosis (1913), in The Standard Edition of the Complete Psychological Works of Sigmund Freud, Vol 12. Translated and edited by Strachey J. London, England, Hogarth, 1958, pp 311–326

Freud S: Inhibitions, symptoms and anxiety (1926), in The Standard Edition of the Complete Psychological Works of Sigmund Freud, Vol 20. Translated and edited by Strachey J. London, England, Hogarth Press, 1959, pp 75–175

Fyer AJ: Current approaches to etiology and pathophysiology of specific phobia. Biol Psychiatry 44:1295–1304, 1998

Fyer AJ, Mannuzza S, Gallops MS, et al: Familial transmission of simple phobias and fears: a preliminary report. Arch Gen Psychiatry 47:252–256, 1990

Gabbard GO: Psychodynamic Psychiatry in Clinical Practice, 3rd Edition. Washington, DC, American Psychiatric Publishing, 2000

Galderisi S, Mucci A, Catapano F, et al: Neuropsychological slowness in obsessive-compulsive patients. Is it confined to tests involving the fronto-subcortical systems? Br J Psychiatry 167:394–398, 1996

Gelernter CS, Uhde TW, Cimbolic P, et al: Cognitive-behavioral and pharmacological treatments of social phobia: a controlled study. Arch Gen Psychiatry 48:938–945, 1991

Gelernter J. Southwick S, Goodson S, et al: No association between D2 dopamine receptor (DRD2) "A" system alleles or DRD2 haplotypes and posttraumatic stress disorder. Biol Psychiatry 45:620–625, 1999

Geracioti TD: Venlafaxine treatment of panic disorder: a case series. J Clin Psychiatry 56:408–410, 1995

Gilbert AR, Moore GJ, Keshavan MS, et al: Decrease in thalamic volumes of pediatric patients with obsessive-compulsive disorder who are taking paroxetine. Arch Gen Psychiatry 57:449–456, 2000

Glynn SM, Eth S, Randolph ET, et al: A test of behavioral family therapy to augment exposure for combat-related posttraumatic stress disorder. J Consult Clin Psychol 67: 243–251, 1999

Goddard AW, Mason GF, Almai A, et al: Reductions in occipital cortex GABA levels in panic disorder detected with 1H-magnetic resonance spectroscopy. Arch Gen Psychiatry 58:556–561, 2001

Goldstein RB, Wickramaratne PJ, Horwath E, et al: Familial aggregation and phenomenology of "early" onset (at or before age 20 years) panic disorder. Arch Gen Psychiatry 54:271–278, 1997

Golier J, Yehuda R, Cornblatt B, et al: Sustained attention in combat-related posttraumatic stress disorder. Integr Physiol Behav Sci 32:52–61, 1997

Goodman WK, Price LH, Rasmussen SA, et al: Efficacy of fluvoxamine in obsessive-compulsive disorder: a double-blind comparison with placebo. Arch Gen Psychiatry 46:36–44, 1989

Goodman WK, McDougle CJ, Price LH, et al: Beyond the serotonin hypothesis: a role for dopamine in some forms of obsessive compulsive disorder? J Clin Psychiatry 51 (suppl):36–43, 1990a

Goodman WK, Price LH, Delgado PL, et al: Specificity of serotonin reuptake inhibitors in the treatment of obsessive-compulsive disorder: comparison of fluvoxamine and desipramine. Arch Gen Psychiatry 47: 577–585, 1990b

Goodnick PJ, Ruiz A, DeVane CL, et al: Mirtazapine in major depression with comorbid generalized anxiety disorder. J Clin Psychiatry 60:446–448, 1999

Gorman JM, Askanazi J, Liebowitz MR, et al: Response to hyperventilation in a group of patients with panic disorder. Am J Psychiatry 141:857–861, 1984

Gorman JM, Liebowitz MR, Fyer AJ, et al: Lactate infusions in obsessive-compulsive disorder. Am J Psychiatry 142:864–866, 1985

Gorman JM, Battista D, Goetz RR, et al: A comparison of sodium bicarbonate and sodium lactate infusion in the induction of panic attacks. Arch Gen Psychiatry 46: 145–150, 1989a

Gorman JM, Kent JM, Sullivan GM, et al: Neuroanatomical hypothesis of panic disorder, revised. Am J Psychiatry 157:493–505, 2000

Grady TA, Pigott TA, L'Heureux F, et al: Double-blind study of adjuvant buspirone for fluoxetine-treated patients with obsessive-compulsive disorder. Am J Psychiatry 150:819–821, 1993

Greenberg BD, George MS, Martin JD, et al: Effect of prefrontal repetitive transcranial magnetic stimulation in obsessive-compulsive disorder: a preliminary study. Am J Psychiatry 154:867–869, 1997

Greist J, Chouinard G, DuBoff E, et al: Double-blind parallel comparison of three dosages of sertraline and placebo in outpatients with obsessive-compulsive disorder. Arch Gen Psychiatry 52:289–295, 1995a

Greist JH, Jefferson JW, Kobak KA, et al: Efficacy and tolerability of serotonin transport inhibitors in obsessive-compulsive disorder. A meta-analysis. Arch Gen Psychiatry 52:53–60, 1995b

Grillon C, Morgan CA: Fear-potentiated startle conditioning to explicit and contextual cues in Gulf War veterans with posttraumatic stress disorder. J Abnorm Psychol 108:134–142, 1999

Grimshaw L: Obsessional disorder and neurological illness. J Neurol Neurosurg Psychiatry 27:229–231, 1964

Grisaru N, Amir M, Cohen H, et al: Effect of transcranial magnetic stimulation in posttraumatic stress disorder: a preliminary study. Biol Psychiatry 44:52–55, 1998

Gurvits TV, Gilbertson MW, Lasko NB, et al: Neurologic soft signs in chronic posttraumatic stress disorder. Arch Gen Psychiatry 57:181–186, 2000

Hansenne M, Pitchot W, Ansseau M: The clonidine test in posttraumatic stress disorder (letter). Am J Psychiatry 148:810–811, 1991

Hartley LR, Ungapen S, Davie I, et al: The effect of beta adrenergic blocking drugs on speakers' performance and memory. Br J Psychiatry 142:512–517, 1983

Hay P, Sachdev P, Cumming S, et al: Treatment of obsessive-compulsive disorder by psychosurgery. Acta Psychiatr Scand 87:197–207, 1993

Hedges DW, Reimherr FW, Strong RE, et al: An open trial of nefazodone in adult patients with generalized anxiety disorder. Psychopharmacol Bull 32:671–676, 1996

Heimberg RG, Dodge CS, Hope DA, et al: Cognitive behavioral group treatment for social phobia: comparison with a credible placebo control. Cognitive Therapy and Research 14:1–23, 1990a

Herman JL, Perry JC, van der Kolk BA: Childhood trauma in borderline personality disorder. Am J Psychiatry 146:490–495, 1989

Hertzberg MA, Feldman ME, Beckham JC, et al: Open trial of nefazodone for combat-related posttraumatic stress disorder. J Clin Psychiatry 59:460–464, 1998

Hertzberg MA, Butterfield MI, Feldman ME, et al: A preliminary study of lamotrigine for the treatment of posttraumatic stress disorder. Biol Psychiatry 45:1226–1229, 1999

Hewlett WA, Vinogradov S, Agras WS: Clonazepam treatment of obsessions and compulsions. J Clin Psychiatry 51:158–161, 1990

Hewlett WA, Vinogradov S, Agras WS: Clomipramine, clonazepam, and clonidine treatment of obsessive-compulsive disorder. J Clin Psychopharmacol 12:420–430, 1992a

Himle JA, Crystal D, Curtis GC, et al: Mode of onset of simple phobia subtypes: further evidence of heterogeneity. Psychiatry Res 36:37–43, 1991

Hirschmann S, Dannon PN, Iancu I, et al: Pindolol augmentation in patients with treatment-resistant panic disorder: a double-blind, placebo-controlled trial. J Clin Psychopharmacol 20:556–559, 2000

Hoehn-Saric R, Merchant AF, Keyser ML, et al: Effects of clonidine on anxiety disorders. Arch Gen Psychiatry 38:1278–1282, 1981

Hoehn-Saric R, McLeod DR, Hipsley PA: Effect of fluvoxamine on panic disorder. J Clin Psychopharmacol 13:321–326, 1993a

Hoehn-Saric R, Hazlett RL, McLeod DR: Generalized anxiety disorder with early and late onset of anxiety symptoms. Compr Psychiatry 34:291–298, 1993b

Hogben GL, Cornfield RB: Treatment of traumatic war neurosis with phenelzine. Arch Gen Psychiatry 38:440–445, 1981

Hollander E, Liebowitz MR, Gorman JM, et al: Cortisol and sodium lactate-induced panic. Arch Gen Psychiatry 46:135–140, 1989

Hollander E, Schiffman E, Cohen B, et al: Signs of central nervous system dysfunction in obsessive-compulsive disorder. Arch Gen Psychiatry 47:27–32, 1990

Hollander E, Kwon J, Weiller F, et al: Serotonergic function in social phobia: comparison to normal control and obsessive-compulsive disorder subjects. Psychiatry Res 79:213–217, 1998

Hollander E, Bienstock C, Pallanti S, et al: The International Treatment Refractory OCD Consortium: preliminary findings. Presented at the 5th International OCD Conference, Sardinia, Italy, March 29–April 1, 2001

Hollingsworth CE, Tanguay PE, Grossman L, et al: Long-term outcome of obsessive-compulsive disorder in childhood. Journal of the American Academy of Child Psychiatry 19:134–144, 1980

Horesh N, Amir M, Kedem P, et al: Life events in childhood, adolescence and adulthood and the relationship to panic disorder. Acta Psychiatr Scand 96:373–378, 1997

Horowitz MJ: Stress-Response Syndromes. New York, Jason Aronson, 1976

Horwath E, Johnson J, Hornig CD: Epidemiology of panic disorder in African Americans. Am J Psychiatry 150:465–469, 1993

Hudson J, Rapee R: The origins of social phobia. Behav Modif 24:102–129, 2000

Ishiguro H, Arinami T, Yamada K, et al: An association study between a transcriptional polymorphism in the serotonin transporter gene and panic disorder in a Japanese population. Psychiatry Clin Neurosci 51:333–335, 1997

James IA, Blackburn IM: Cognitive therapy with obsessive-compulsive disorder. Br J Psychiatry 166:444–450, 1995

James IM, Griffith DNW, Pearson RM, et al: Effect of oxprenolol on stage-fright in musicians. Lancet 2:952–954, 1977

James IM, Borgoyne W, Savage IT: Effect of pindolol on stress-related disturbances of musical performance: preliminary communication. J R Soc Med 76:194–196, 1983

Janet P: Les Obsessions et la Psychasthenie, 2nd Edition. Paris, France, Bailliere, 1908

Jenike MA, Hyman S, Baer L, et al: A controlled trial of fluvoxamine in obsessive-compulsive disorder: implications for a serotonergic theory. Am J Psychiatry 147:1209–1215, 1990a

Jenike MA, Baer L, Summergrad P, et al: Sertraline in obsessive-compulsive disorder: a double-blind comparison with placebo. Am J Psychiatry 147:923–928, 1990b

Jenike MA, Baer L, Buttolph L, et al: Buspirone augmentation of fluoxetine in patients with obsessive-compulsive disorder. J Clin Psychiatry 52:13–14, 1991a

Jenike MA, Baer L, Ballantine HT, et al: Cingulotomy for refractory obsessive-compulsive disorder: a long-term follow-up of 33 patients. Arch Gen Psychiatry 48:548–555, 1991b

Jenike MA, Baer L, Minichiello WE, et al: Placebo-controlled trial of fluoxetine and phenelzine for obsessive-compulsive disorder. Am J Psychiatry 154:1261–1264, 1997

Jenkins MA, Langlasi PJ, Delis D, et al: Learning and memory in rape victims with posttraumatic stress disorder. Am J Psychiatry 155:278–279, 1998

Johnson MR, Marazziti D, Brawman MO, et al: Abnormal benzodiazepine receptor density associated with generalized social phobia. Biol Psychiatry 43:306–309, 1998

Katschnig H, Amering M, Stolk JM, et al: Long-term follow-up after a drug trial for panic disorder. Br J Psychiatry 167:487–494, 1995

Katzelnick DJ, Kobak KA, Greist JH, et al: Sertraline for social phobia: a double-blind, placebo-controlled crossover study. Am J Psychiatry 152:1368–1371, 1995

Kauffman CD, Reist C, Djenderedjian A, et al: Biological markers of affective disorders and posttraumatic stress disorder: a pilot study with desipramine. J Clin Psychiatry 48:366–367, 1987

Keck PE, Taylor VE, Tugrul KC, et al: Valproate treatment of panic disorder and lactate-induced panic attacks. Biol Psychiatry 33:542–546, 1993

Kehl PA, Marks IM: Neurological factors in obsessive-compulsive disorder: two case reports and a review of the literature. Br J Psychiatry 149:315–319, 1986

Kelly DD: The role of endorphins in stress-induced analgesia. Ann N Y Acad Sci 398:260–271, 1982

Kendler KS, Neale MC, Kessler RC, et al: The genetic epidemiology of phobias in women: the interrelationship of agoraphobia, social phobia, situational phobia, and simple phobia. Arch Gen Psychiatry 49:273–281, 1992b

Kendler KS, Neale MC, Kessler RC, et al: Panic disorder in women: a population-based twin study. Psychol Med 23:397–406, 1993

Kennedy JL, Bradwejn J, Koszycki D, et al: Investigation of cholecystokinin system genes in panic disorder. Mol Psychiatry 4:284–285, 1999

Kessler RC, McGonagle KA, Zhao S, et al: Lifetime and 12-month prevalence of DSM-III-R psychiatric disorders in the United States. Results from the National Comorbidity Survey. Arch Gen Psychiatry 51:8–19, 1994

Kessler RC, Sonnega A, Bromet E, et al: Post-traumatic stress disorder in the National Comorbidity Survey. Arch Gen Psychiatry 52:1048–1060, 1995

Kessler RC, Stein MB, Berglund P: Social phobia subtypes in the National Comorbidity Survey. Am J Psychiatry 155:613–619, 1998

Kessler RC, Stang P, Wittchen HU, et al: Lifetime co-morbidities between social phobia and mood disorders in the US National Comorbidity Survey. Psychol Med 29: 555–567, 1999b

Klein DF: Anxiety reconceptualized, in Anxiety: New Research and Changing Concepts. Edited by Klein DF, Rabkin JG. New York, Raven Press, 1981, pp 235–263

Klein M: A contribution to the theory of anxiety and guilt. Int J Psychoanal 29:114–123, 1948

Knowles JA, Fyer AJ, Vieland VJ, et al: Results of a genome-wide genetic screen for panic disorder. Am J Med Genet 28:139–147, 1998

Kobak KA, Greist JH, Jefferson JW, et al: Behavioral versus pharmacological treatments of obsessive compulsive disorder: a meta-analysis. Psychopharmacology (Berl) 136:205–216, 1998

Kolb LC: A neuropsychological hypothesis explaining posttraumatic stress disorders. Am J Psychiatry 144:989–995, 1987

Kolb LC, Burris BC, Griffiths S: Propranolol and clonidine in treatment of the chronic post-traumatic stress disorders of war, in Post-Traumatic Stress Disorder: Psychological and Biological Sequelae. Edited by van der Kolk BA. Washington, DC, American Psychiatric Press, 1984, pp 97–105

Koponen H, Lepola U, Leinonen E, et al: Citalopram in the treatment of obsessive-compulsive disorder: an open pilot study. Acta Psychiatr Scand 96:343–346, 1997

Koran LM, McElroy SL, Davidson JR, et al: Fluvoxamine versus clomipramine for obsessive-compulsive disorder: a double-blind comparison. J Clin Psychopharmacol 16:121–129, 1996

Koran LM, Ringold AL, Elliott MA: Olanzapine augmentation for treatment-resistant obsessive-compulsive disorder. J Clin Psychiatry 61:514–517, 2000

Koren D, Arnon I, Klein E: Acute stress response and posttraumatic stress disorder in traffic accident victims: a one-year prospective, follow-up study. Am J Psychiatry 156:367–373, 1999

Kosten TR, Mason JW, Giller EL, et al: Sustained urine norepinephrine and epinephrine elevation in PTSD. Psychoneuroendocrinology 12:13–20, 1987

Krystal H: Massive Psychic Trauma. New York, International Universities Press, 1968

Leckman JF, Grice DE, Boardman J, et al: Symptoms of obsessive compulsive disorder. Am J Psychiatry 154:911–917, 1997

Lecrubier Y, Judge R: Long-term evaluation of paroxetine, clomipramine and placebo in panic disorder. Collaborative Paroxetine Panic Study Investigators. Acta Psychiatr Scand 95:153–160, 1997

Lecrubier Y, Bakker A, Dunbar G, et al: A comparison of paroxetine, clomipramine and placebo in the treatment of panic disorder. Collaborative Paroxetine Panic Study Investigators. Acta Psychiatr Scand 95:145–152, 1997

Leonard HL, Swedo SE, Rapoport JL, et al: Treatment of obsessive-compulsive disorder with clomipramine and desipramine in children and adolescents: a double-blind crossover comparison. Arch Gen Psychiatry 46:1088–1092, 1989

Leonard HL, Swedo SE, Lenane MC, et al: A double-blind desipramine substitution during long-term clomipramine treatment in children and adolescents with obsessive-compulsive disorder. Arch Gen Psychiatry 48:922–927, 1991

Leonard HL, Swedo SE, Lenane MC, et al: A 2- to 7-year follow-up study of 54 obsessive compulsive children and adolescents. Arch Gen Psychiatry 50:429–439, 1993

Lepola UM, Wade AG, Leinonen EV, et al: A controlled, prospective, 1-year trial of citalopram in the treatment of panic disorder. J Clin Psychiatry 59:528–534, 1998

Liden S, Gottfries CG: Beta-blocking agents in the treatment of catecholamine-induced symptoms in musicians (letter). Lancet 2(7879):529, 1974

Lieb R, Wittchen HU, Hofler M, et al: Parental psychopathology, parenting styles, and the risk of social phobia in offspring: a prospective-longitudinal community study. Arch Gen Psychiatry 57:859–866, 2000

Liebowitz MR, Fyer AJ, McGrath P, et al: Clonidine treatment of panic disorder. Psychopharmacol Bull 17:122–123, 1981

Liebowitz MR, Gorman JM, Fyer AJ, et al: Lactate provocation of panic attacks, II: biochemical and physiological findings. Arch Gen Psychiatry 42:709–719, 1985a

Liebowitz MR, Schneier F, Campeas R, et al: Phenelzine vs atenolol in social phobia: a placebo-controlled comparison. Arch Gen Psychiatry 49:290–300, 1992

Lipper S, Davidson JRT, Grady TA, et al: Preliminary study of carbamazepine in posttraumatic stress disorder. Psychosomatics 27:849–854, 1986

Lipsitz JD, Mannuzza S, Klein DF, et al: Specific phobia 10–16 years after treatment. Depress Anxiety 10:105–111, 1999b

Lundh LG, Czyzykow S, Ost LG: Explicit and implicit memory bias in panic disorder with agoraphobia. Behav Res Ther 35: 1003–1014, 1997

Macklin ML, Metzger LJ, Litz BT, et al: Lower precombat intelligence is a risk factor for posttraumatic stress disorder. J Consult Clin Psychol 66:323–326, 1998

Macklin ML, Metzger LJ, Lasko NB, et al: Five-year follow-up study of eye movement desensitization and reprocessing therapy for combat-related posttraumatic stress disorder. Compr Psychiatry 41:24–27, 2000

Magee WJ, Eaton WW, Wittchen HU, et al: Agoraphobia, simple phobia, and social phobia in the National Comorbidity Survey. Arch Gen Psychiatry 53:159–168, 1996

Maier SF, Seligman ME: Learned helplessness: theory and evidence. J Exp Psychol 105: 3–46, 1976

Maier SF, Dovies S, Gran JW: Opiate antagonists and long-term analgesic reaction induced by inescapable shock in rats. J Comp Physiol Psychol 94:1172–1183, 1980

Malizia AL, Cunningham VJ, Bell CJ, et al: Decreased brain GABA(A)-benzodiazepine receptor binding in panic disorder: preliminary results from a quantitative PET study. Arch Gen Psychiatry 55:715–720, 1998

Mannuzza S, Schneier FR, Chapman TF, et al: Generalized social phobia. Reliability and validity. Arch Gen Psychiatry 52:230–237, 1995

Marazziti D, Dell'Osso L, Gemignani A, et al: Citalopram in refractory obsessive-compulsive disorder: an open study. Int Clin Psychopharmacol 16:215–219, 2001

March JS, Biederman J, Wolkow R, et al: Sertraline in children and adolescents with obsessive-compulsive disorder: a multicenter randomized controlled trial. JAMA 280:1752–1756, 1998b

Marks IM: Fears and Phobias. New York, Academic Press, 1969

Marks IM, Gelder MG: Different ages on onset in varieties of phobia. Am J Psychiatry 123:218–221, 1966

Marks IM, Hodgson R, Rachman S: Treatment of chronic obsessive-compulsive neurosis by in vivo exposure: a two-year follow-up and issues in treatment. Br J Psychiatry 127:349–364, 1975

Marks IM, Gray S, Cohen D, et al: Imipramine and brief therapist-aided exposure in agoraphobics having self-exposure homework. Arch Gen Psychiatry 40:153–162, 1983

Marks I, Lovell K, Noshirvani H, et al: Treatment of posttraumatic stress disorder by exposure and/or cognitive restructuring: a controlled study. Arch Gen Psychiatry 55: 317–325, 1998

Marmar CR, Weiss DS, Schlenger WE, et al: Peritraumatic dissociation and posttraumatic stress in male Vietnam theater veterans. Am J Psychiatry 151:902–907, 1994

Marshall JR: The treatment of night terrors associated with posttraumatic syndrome. Am J Psychiatry 132:293–295, 1975

Marshall RD, Schneier FR, Fallon BA, et al: An open trial of paroxetine in patients with noncombat-related, chronic posttraumatic stress disorder. J Clin Psychopharmacol 18:10–18, 1998

Marten PA, Brown TA, Barlow DH, et al: Evaluation of the ratings comprising the associated symptom criterion of DSM-III-R generalized anxiety disorder. J Nerv Ment Dis 181:676–682, 1993

Mason JW, Giller EL, Kosten TR, et al: Urinary free-cortisol levels in posttraumatic stress disorder patients. J Nerv Ment Dis 174:145–149, 1986

Mason JW, Giller EL, Kosten TR, et al: Elevation of urinary norepinephrine/cortisol ratio in posttraumatic stress disorder. J Nerv Ment Dis 176:498–502, 1988

Mataix-Cols D, Rauch SL, Manzo PA, et al: Use of factor-analyzed symptom dimensions to predict outcome with serotonin reuptake inhibitors and placebo in the treatment of obsessive-compulsive disorder. Am J Psychiatry 156:1409–1416, 1999

Mattick RP, Peters L, Clarke JC: Exposure and cognitive restructuring for social phobia: a controlled study. Behav Ther 20:3–23, 1989

Mavissakalian M, Michelson L: Agoraphobia: relative and combined effectiveness of therapist-assisted in vivo exposure and imipramine. J Clin Psychiatry 47:117–122, 1986a

Mavissakalian M, Michelson L: Two-year follow-up of exposure and imipramine treatment of agoraphobia. Am J Psychiatry 143:1106–1112, 1986b

Mavissakalian M, Perel JM: Clinical experiments in maintenance and discontinuation of imipramine therapy in panic disorder with agoraphobia. Arch Gen Psychiatry 49:318–323, 1992

McCafferty JP, Bellew KM, Zaninelli RM: Paroxetine treatment of GAD: an analysis of response by dose. Poster presented at the 154th annual meeting of the American Psychiatric Association, New Orleans, LA, May 2001

McDougle CJ, Goodman WK, Price LH, et al: Neuroleptic addition in fluvoxamine-refractory obsessive-compulsive disorder. Am J Psychiatry 147:652–654, 1990

McDougle CJ, Price LH, Goodman WK, et al: A controlled trial of lithium augmentation in fluvoxamine-refractory obsessive-compulsive disorder: lack of efficacy. J Clin Psychopharmacol 11:175–181, 1991a

McDougle CJ, Southwick SM, Charney DS, et al: An open trial of fluoxetine in the treatment of posttraumatic stress disorder. J Clin Psychopharmacol 11:325–327, 1991b

McDougle CJ, Goodman WK, Leckman JF, et al: The efficacy of fluvoxamine in obsessive-compulsive disorder: effects of comorbid chronic tic disorder. J Clin Psychopharmacol 13:354–358, 1993a

McDougle CJ, Goodman WK, Leckman JF, et al: Limited therapeutic effect of addition of buspirone in fluvoxamine-refractory obsessive-compulsive disorder. Am J Psychiatry 150:647–649, 1993b

McDougle CJ, Goodman WK, Leckman JF, et al: Haloperidol addition in fluvoxamine-refractory obsessive-compulsive disorder. A double-blind, placebo-controlled study in patients with and without tics. Arch Gen Psychiatry 51:302–308, 1994

McDougle CJ, Epperson CN, Pelton GH, et al: A double-blind, placebo-controlled study of risperidone addition in serotonin reuptake inhibitor-refractory obsessive-compulsive disorder. Arch Gen Psychiatry 57:794–801, 2000

McFarlane AC: The aetiology of post-traumatic morbidity: predisposing, precipitating and perpetuating factors. Br J Psychiatry 154:221–228, 1989

McFarlane AC: Vulnerability to posttraumatic stress disorder, in Posttraumatic Stress Disorder: Etiology, Phenomenology, and Treatment. Edited by Wolf ME, Mosnaim AD. Washington, DC, American Psychiatric Press, 1990, pp 2–20

McGuire PK, Bench CJ, Frith CD, et al: Functional anatomy of obsessive-compulsive phenomena. Br J Psychiatry 164:459–468, 1994

McKeon J, McGuffin P, Robinson P: Obsessive-compulsive neurosis following head injury: a report of four cases. Br J Psychiatry 144:190–192, 1984

McNair DM, Kahn RJ: Imipramine compared with a benzodiazepine for agoraphobia, in Anxiety: New Research and Changing Concepts. Edited by Klein DF, Rabkin JG. New York, Raven, 1981, pp 69–80

McNally RJ, Kohlbeck PA: Reality monitoring in obsessive-compulsive disorder. Behav Res Ther 31:24–53, 1993

McNally RJ, Hornig CD, Otto MW, et al: Selective encoding of threat in panic disorder: application of a dual priming paradigm. Behav Res Ther 35:543–549, 1997

McNally RJ, Metzger LJ, Lasko NB, et al: Directed forgetting of trauma cues in adult survivors of childhood sexual abuse with and without posttraumatic stress disorder. J Abnorm Psychol 107:596–601, 1998

Michels R, Frances A, Shear MK: Psychodynamic models of anxiety, in Anxiety and the Anxiety Disorders. Edited by Tuma AH, Maser JD. Hillsdale, NJ, Lawrence Erlbaum, 1985, pp 595–618

Michelson D, Lydiard RB, Pollack MH, et al: Outcome assessment and clinical improvement in panic disorder: evidence from a randomized controlled trial of fluoxetine and placebo. The Fluoxetine Panic Disorder Study Group. Am J Psychiatry 155:1570–1577, 1998

Michelson D, Pollack M, Lydiard RB, et al: Continuing treatment of panic disorder after acute response: randomized, placebo-controlled trial with fluoxetine. The Fluoxetine Panic Disorder Study Group. Br J Psychiatry 174:213–218, 1999

Michelson L, Marchione K, Greenwald M, et al: Panic disorder: cognitive-behavioral treatment. Behav Res Ther 28:141–151, 1990

Miller HE, Deakin JF, Anderson IM: Effect of acute tryptophan depletion on CO2-induced anxiety in patients with panic disorder and normal volunteers. Br J Psychiatry 176:182–188, 2000

Montgomery SA, McIntyre A, Osterheider M, et al: A double-blind, placebo-controlled study of fluoxetine in patients with DSM-III-R obsessive-compulsive disorder. The Lilly European OCD Study Group. Eur Neuropsychopharmacol 3:143–152, 1993

Montgomery SA, Kasper S, Stein DJ, et al: Citalopram 20 mg, 40 mg, and 60 mg are all effective and well tolerated compared with placebo in obsessive-compulsive disorder. Int Clin Psychopharmacol 16:75–86, 2001

Mountz JM, Modll JG, Wilson MW, et al: Positron emission tomographic evaluation of cerebral blood flow during state anxiety in simple phobia. Arch Gen Psychiatry 46:501–504, 1989

Mundo E, Bianchi L, Bellodi L: Efficacy of fluvoxamine, paroxetine, and citalopram in the treatment of obsessive-compulsive disorder: a single-blind study. J Clin Psychopharmacol 17:267–271, 1997

Muris P, Schmidt H, Meckelbach H: Ther structure of specific phobia symptoms among children and adolescents. Behav Res Ther 37:863–868, 1999

Nagy LM, Krystal JH, Woods SW, et al: Clinical and medication outcome after short-term alprazolam and behavioral group treatment in panic disorder: 2.5-year naturalistic follow-up study. Arch Gen Psychiatry 46:993–999, 1989

Nee LE, Caine ED, Polinsky RJ, et al: Gilles de la Tourette syndrome: clinical and family study of 50 cases. Ann Neurol 7:41–49, 1982

Neftel KA, Adler RH, Kappell K, et al: Stage fright in musicians: a model illustrating the effect of beta blockers. Psychosom Med 44:461–469, 1982

Nemiah JC: A psychoanalytic view of phobias. Am J Psychoanal 41:115–120, 1981

Nemiah JC: The psychodynamic view of anxiety: an historical approach, in Handbook of Anxiety, Vol 1. Edited by Roth M, Noyes R, Burrows GD. Amsterdam, The Netherlands, Elsevier, 1988, pp 277–303

Nestadt G, Samuels J, Riddle M, et al: A family study of obsessive-compulsive disorder. Arch Gen Psychiatry 57:358–363, 2000b

Neziroglu F, Anemone R, Yaryura-Tobias JA: Onset of obsessive-compulsive disorder in pregnancy. Am J Psychiatry 149:947–950, 1992

Noyes R Jr, Garvey MJ, Cook BL: Follow-up study of patients with panic disorder and agoraphobia with panic attacks treated with tricyclic antidepressants. J Affect Disord 16:249–257, 1989

Noyes R Jr, Reich JH, Christiansen J, et al: Outcome of panic disorder: relationship to diagnostic subtypes and comorbidity. Arch Gen Psychiatry 47:809–818, 1990

Noyes R Jr, Reich JH, Suelzer M, et al: Personality traits associated with panic disorder: change associated with treatment. Compr Psychiatry 32:283–294, 1991

Noyes R Jr, Clancy J, Woodman C, et al: Environmental factors related to the outcome of panic disorder: a seven-year follow-up study. J Nerv Ment Dis 181:529–538, 1993

Nutt DJ: Altered central a2-adrenoreceptor sensitivity in panic disorder. Arch Gen Psychiatry 46:165–169, 1989

Nutt DJ, Glue P, Lawson C, et al: Flumazenil provocation of panic attacks: evidence for altered benzodiazepine receptor sensitivity in panic disorder. Arch Gen Psychiatry 47:917–925, 1990

O'Connor K, Robillard S: Inference processes in obsessive-compulsive disorder: some clinical observations. Behav Res Ther 33:887–896, 1996

Oehrberg S, Christiansen PE, Behnke K, et al: Paroxetine in the treatment of panic disorder. A randomised, double-blind, placebo-controlled study. Br J Psychiatry 167:374–379, 1995

O'Rourke D, Fahy TJ, Brophy J, et al: The Galway study of panic disorder, III: outcome at 5 to 6 years. Br J Psychiatry 168:462–469, 1996

Orr SP, Metzger LJ, Lasko NB, et al: De novo conditioning in trauma-exposed individuals with and without posttraumatic stress disorder. J Abnorm Psychol 109:290–298, 2000

Ost LG: Age of onset of different phobias. J Abnorm Psychol 96:223–229, 1987

Ost LG, Breitholtz E: Applied relaxation versus cognitive therapy in the treatment of generalized anxiety disorder. Behav Res Ther 38:777–790, 2000

Otto MW: Normal and abnormal information processing: a neuropsychological perspective on obsessive-compulsive disorder. Psychiatr Clin North Am 15:825–848, 1992

Otto MW, Pollack MH, Sachs GS, et al: Discontinuation of benzodiazepine treatment: efficacy of cognitive-behavioral therapy for patients with panic disorder. Am J Psychiatry 150:1485–1490, 1993

Pacella BL, Polatin P, Nagler SH: Clinical and EEG studies in obsessive-compulsive states. Am J Psychiatry 100:830–838, 1944

Pallanti S, Quercioli L, Paiva RS, et al: Citalopram for treatment-resistant obsessive-compulsive disorder. Eur Psychiatry 14:101–106, 1999

Pande AC, Davidson JRT, Jefferson JW, et al: Treatment of social phobia with gabapentin: a placebo-controlled study. J Clin Psychopharmacol 19:341–348, 1999

Pande AC, Pollack MH, Crockatt J, et al: Placebo-controlled study of gabapentin treatment of panic disorder. J Clin Psychopharmacol 20:467–471, 2000

Papp LA, Coplan JD, Marinez JM, et al: Efficacy of open-label nefazodone treatment in patients with panic disorder. J Clin Psychopharmacol 20:544–546, 2000

Pato MT, Zohar-Kadouch R, Zohar J, et al: Return of symptoms after discontinuation of clomipramine in patients with obsessive-compulsive disorder. Am J Psychiatry 145:1521–1525, 1988

Pato MT, Pigott TA, Hill JL, et al: Controlled comparison of buspirone and clomipramine in obsessive-compulsive disorder. Am J Psychiatry 148:127–129, 1991

Pauls DL, Towbin KE, Leckman JF, et al: Gilles de la Tourette's and obsessive-compulsive disorder: evidence supporting a genetic relationship. Arch Gen Psychiatry 43:1180–1182, 1986

Perani D, Colombo C, Bressi S, et al: [18F] FDG PET study in obsessive-compulsive disorder. A clinical/metabolic correlation study after treatment. Br J Psychiatry 166:244–250, 1995

Peri T, Ben Shakhar G, Orr SP, et al: Psychophysiologic assessment of aversive conditioning in posttraumatic stress disorder. Biol Psychiatry 47:512–519, 2000

Perlmutter SJ, Leitman SF, Garvey MA, et al: Therapeutic plasma exchange and intravenous immunoglobulin for obsessive-compulsive disorder and tic disorders in childhood. Lancet 354:1153–1158, 1999

Perry BD, Giller EL Jr, Southwick SM: Altered plasma alpha2-adrenergic binding sites in posttraumatic stress disorder (letter). Am J Psychiatry 144:1511–1512, 1987

Perse TL, Greist JH, Jefferson JW, et al: Fluvoxamine treatment of obsessive-compulsive disorder. Am J Psychiatry 144:1543–1548, 1987

Pfanner C, Marazziti D, Dell'Osso L, et al: Risperidone augmentation in refractory obsessive-compulsive disorder: an open-label study. Int Clin Psychopharmacol 15:297–301, 2000

Piccinelli M, Pini S, Bellantuono C, et al: Efficacy of drug treatment in obsessive-compulsive disorder. A meta-analytic review. Br J Psychiatry 166:424–443, 1995

Pigott TA, Pato MT, L'Heureux F, et al: A controlled comparison of adjuvant lithium carbonate or thyroid hormone in clomipramine-treated patients with obsessive-compulsive disorder. J Clin Psychopharmacol 11:242–248, 1991

Pigott TA, L'Heureux F, Rubenstein CS, et al: A double-blind, placebo controlled study of trazodone in patients with obsessive-compulsive disorder. J Clin Psychopharmacol 12:156–162, 1992a

Pigott TA, L'Heureux F, Hill JL, et al: A double-blind study of adjuvant buspirone hydrochloride in clomipramine-treated patients with obsessive-compulsive disorder. J Clin Psychopharmacol 12:11–18, 1992b

Pitman RK, Orr SP, Forgue DF, et al: Psychophysiologic assessment of post-traumatic stress disorder imagery in Vietnam combat veterans. Arch Gen Psychiatry 44:970–975, 1987

Pitman RK, van der Kolk BA, Orr SP, et al: Naloxone-reversible analgesic response to combat-related stimuli in posttraumatic stress disorder: a pilot study. Arch Gen Psychiatry 47:541–544, 1990

Pitts FN, McClure JN: Lactate metabolism in anxiety neurosis. N Engl J Med 277:1329–1336, 1967

Pohl RB, Wolkow RM, Clary CM: Sertraline in the treatment of panic disorder: a double-blind multicenter trial. Am J Psychiatry 155:1189–1195, 1998

Pollack MH, Worthington JJ 3rd, Otto MW, et al: Venlafaxine for panic disorder: results of a double-blind, placebo-controlled study. Psychopharmacol Bull 32:667–670, 1996

Pollack MH, Zaninelli R, Goddard A, et al: Paroxetine in the treatment of generalized anxiety disorder: results of a placebo-controlled, flexible-dosage trial. J Clin Psychiatry 62:350–357, 2001

Power KG, Simpson RJ, Swanson V, et al: A controlled comparison of cognitive-behaviour therapy, diazepam, and placebo, alone and in combination, for the treatment of generalized anxiety disorder. J Anxiety Disord 4:267–292, 1990

Quitkin F, Babkin J: Hidden psychiatric diagnosis in the alcoholic, in Alcoholism and Clinical Psychiatry. Edited by Soloman J. New York, Plenum, 1982, pp 129–140

Rachman S, Thordarson DS, Shafran R, et al: Perceived responsibility: structure and significance. Behav Res Ther 33:779–784, 1995

Rainey JM Jr, Aleem A, Ortiz A, et al: Laboratory procedure for the inducement of flashbacks. Am J Psychiatry 144:1317–1319, 1987

Rapoport JL, Elkins R, Langer DH, et al: Childhood obsessive-compulsive disorder. Am J Psychiatry 138:1545–1554, 1981

Raskin M, Peeke HVS, Dickman W, et al: Panic and generalized anxiety disorders: developmental antecedents and precipitants. Arch Gen Psychiatry 39:687–689, 1982

Rauch SL, Jenike MA, Alpert NM, et al: Regional cerebral blood flow measured during symptom provocation in obsessive-compulsive disorder using oxygen 15-labeled carbon dioxide and positron emission tomography. Arch Gen Psychiatry 51:62–70, 1994

Rauch SL, Savage CR, Alpert NM, et al: A positron emission tomographic study of simple phobic symptom provocation. Arch Gen Psychiatry 52:20–28, 1995

Rauch SL, van der Kolk BA, Fisler RE, et al: A symptom provocation study of posttraumatic stress disorder using positron emission tomography and script-driven imagery. Arch Gen Psychiatry 53:380–387, 1996

Ravizza L, Barzega G, Bellino S, et al: Predictors of drug treatment response in obsessive-compulsive disorder. J Clin Psychiatry 56:368–373, 1995

Regier DA, Boyd JH, Burke JD Jr, et al: One-month prevalence of mental disorders in the United States, based on five Epidemiologic Catchment Area sites. Arch Gen Psychiatry 45:977–986, 1988

Reich J, Noyes R, Yates W: Anxiety symptoms distinguishing social phobia from panic and generalized anxiety disorders. J Nerv Ment Dis 176:510–513, 1988

Reist C, Kauffmann CD, Haier RJ, et al: A controlled trial of desipramine in 18 men with posttraumatic stress disorder. Am J Psychiatry 146:513–516, 1989

Rettew DC: Avoidant personality disorder, generalized social phobia, and shyness: putting the personality back into personality disorders. Harv Rev Psychiatry 8:283–297, 2000

Rickels K, Csanalosi I, Greisman P, et al: A controlled clinical trial of alprazolam for the treatment of anxiety. Am J Psychiatry 140:82–85, 1983

Rickels K, Schweizer E, Csanalosi I, et al: Long-term treatment of anxiety and risk of withdrawal: prospective comparison of clorazepate and buspirone. Arch Gen Psychiatry 45:444–450, 1988

Rickels K, DeMartinis N, Garcia-Espana F, et al: Imipramine and buspirone in treatment of patients with generalized anxiety disorder who are discontinuing long-term benzodiazepine therapy. Am J Psychiatry 157:1973–1979, 2000

Riddle MA, Scahill L, King RA, et al: Double-blind, crossover trial of fluoxetine and placebo in children and adolescents with obsessive-compulsive disorder. J Am Acad Child Adolesc Psychiatry 31:1062–1069, 1992

Riddle MA, Reeve EA, Yaryura-Tobias JA, et al: Fluvoxamine for children and adolescents with obsessive-compulsive disorder: a randomized, controlled, multicenter trial. J Am Acad Child Adolesc Psychiatry 40:222–229, 2001

Romach M, Busto U, Somer G, et al: Clinical aspects of chronic use of alprazolam and lorazepam. Am J Psychiatry 152:1161–1167, 1995

Rosenbaum JF, Moroz G, Bowden CL: Clonazepam in the treatment of panic disorder with or without agoraphobia: a dose–response study of efficacy, safety, and discontinuance. Clonazepam Panic Disorder Dose–Response Study Group. J Clin Psychopharmacol 17:390–400, 1997

Rosenberg DR, Keshavan MS, O'Hearn KM, et al: Frontostriatal measurement in treatment-naïve children with obsessive-compulsive disorder. Arch Gen Psychiatry 54:824–830, 1997

Rosenberg DR, Stewart CM, Fitzgerald KD, et al: Paroxetine open-label treatment of pediatric outpatients with obsessive-compulsive disorder. J Am Acad Child Adolesc Psychiatry 38:1180–1185, 1999

Rosenberg DR, MacMaster FP, Keshavan MS, et al: Decrease in caudate glutamatergic concentrations in pediatric obsessive-compulsive disorder patients taking paroxetine. J Am Acad Child Adolesc Psychiatry 39:1096–1103, 2000a

Rosenberg DR, Benazon NR, Gilbert A, et al: Thalamic volume in pediatric obsessive-compulsive disorder patients before and after cognitive behavioral therapy. Biol Psychiatry 48:294–300, 2000b

Roy-Byrne PP, Cowley DS, Greenblatt DJ, et al: Reduced benzodiazepine sensitivity in panic disorder. Arch Gen Psychiatry 47:534–538, 1990

Rubenstein CS, Peynircioglu ZF, Chambless DL, et al: Memory in sub-clinical obsessive-compulsive checkers. Behav Res Ther 31:759–765, 1993

Ruiz AT: A double-blind study of alprazolam and lorazepam in the treatment of anxiety. J Clin Psychiatry 44:60–62, 1983

Salkovskis PM, Jones DRO, Clark DM: Respiratory control in the treatment of panic attacks: replication and extension with concurrent measurement of behaviour and pCO2. Br J Psychiatry 148:526–532, 1986

Salzman L: Comments on the psychological treatment of obsessive-compulsive patients, in Obsessive-Compulsive Disorder: Psychological and Pharmacological Treatment. Edited by Mavissakalian M, Turner SM, Michelson L. New York, Plenum, 1985, pp 155–165

Samuels J, Nestadt G, Bienvenu OJ, et al: Personality disorders and normal personality dimensions in obsessive-compulsive disorder. Br J Psychiatry 177:457–462, 2000

Schilder P: The organic background of obsessions and compulsions. Am J Psychiatry 94:1397–1416, 1938

Schneier FR, Johnson J, Hornig CD, et al: Social phobia: comorbidity and morbidity in an epidemiologic sample. Arch Gen Psychiatry 49:282–288, 1992

Schneier FR, Saoud JB, Campeas R, et al: Buspirone in social phobia. J Clin Psychopharmacol 13:251–256, 1993

Schneier FR, Heckelman LR, Garfinkel R, et al: Functional impairment in social phobia. J Clin Psychiatry 55:322–331, 1994

Schneier F, Liebowitz MR, Abi-Dargham A, et al: Low dopamine D2 binding potential in social phobia. Am J Psychiatry 157:457–459, 2000

Schnyder U, Moergeli H, Klaghofer R, et al: Incidence and prediction of posttraumatic stress disorder symptoms in severely injured accident victims. Am J Psychiatry 158:595–599, 2001

Schwartz JM, Stoessel PW, Baxter LR, et al: Systematic changes in cerebral glucose metabolic rate after successful behavior modification treatment in obsessive-compulsive disorder. Arch Gen Psychiatry 53:109–113, 1996

Scrignar CB: Post-Traumatic Stress Disorder: Diagnosis, Treatment, and Legal Issues. New York, Praeger, 1984

Seedat S, Stein DJ: Inositol augmentation of serotonin reuptake inhibitors in treatment-refractory obsessive-compulsive disorder: an open trial. Int Clin Psychopharmacol 14:353–356, 1999

Shafran R, Ralph J, Tallis F: Obsessive-compulsive symptoms and the family. Bull Menninger Clin 59:472–479, 1996

Shalev AY, Peri T, Canetti L, et al: Predictors of PTSD in injured trauma survivors: a prospective study. Am J Psychiatry 153:2219–2225, 1996

Shalev AY, Sahar T, Freedman S, et al: A prospective study of heart rate response following trauma and the subsequent development of posttraumatic stress disorder. Arch Gen Psychiatry 55:553–559, 1998a

Shalev AY, Freedman S, Peri T, et al: Prospective study of posttraumatic stress disorder and depression following trauma. Am J Psychiatry 155:630–637, 1998b

Shay J: Fluoxetine reduces explosiveness and elevates mood of Vietnam combat vets with PTSD. J Trauma Stress 5:97–101, 1992

Shear MK, Cooper AM, Klerman GL, et al: A psychodynamic model of panic disorder. Am J Psychiatry 150:859–866, 1993

Sheehan DV, Ballenger J, Jacobsen G: Treatment of endogenous anxiety with phobic, hysterical, and hypochondriacal symptoms. Arch Gen Psychiatry 37:51–59, 1980

Silva RR, Alpert M, Munoz DM, et al: Stress and vulnerability to posttraumatic stress disorder in children and adolescents. Am J Psychiatry 157:1229–1235, 2000

Simpson HB, Gorfinkle KS, Liebowitz MR: Cognitive-behavioral therapy as an adjunct to serotonin reuptake inhibitors in obsessive-compulsive disorder: an open trial. J Clin Psychiatry 60:584–590, 1999

Skoog G, Skoog I: A 40-year follow-up of patients with obsessive-compulsive disorder. Arch Gen Psychiatry 56:121–127, 1999

Skre I, Onstad S, Torgensen S, et al: A twin study of DSM-III-R anxiety disorders. Acta Psychiatr Scand 88:85–92, 1993

Smith MA, Davidson J, Ritchie JC, et al: The corticotropin releasing hormone test in patients with posttraumatic stress disorder. Biol Psychiatry 26:349–355, 1989

Southwick SM, Krystal JH, Morgan CA, et al: Abnormal noradrenergic function in posttraumatic stress disorder. Arch Gen Psychiatry 50:266–274, 1993

Southwick SM, Krystal JH, Bremner JD, et al: Noradrenergic and serotonergic function in posttraumatic stress disorder. Arch Gen Psychiatry 54:749–758, 1997

Southwick SM, Bremner JD, Rasmusson A, et al: Role of norepinephrine in the pathophysiology and treatment of posttraumatic stress disorder. Biol Psychiatry 46:1192–1204, 1999

Spence SH, Donovan C, Brechman TM: The treatment of childhood social phobia: the effectiveness of a social skills training-based, cognitive-behavioural intervention, with and without parental involvement. J Child Psychol Psychiatry 41:713–762, 2000

Spiegel D, Cardena E: Dissociative mechanisms in posttraumatic stress disorder, in Posttraumatic Stress Disorder: Etiology, Phenomenology, and Treatment. Edited by Wolf ME, Mosnaim AD. Washington, DC, American Psychiatric Press, 1990, pp 22–34

Spiegel DA, Bruce TJ, Gregg SF, et al: Does cognitive behavior therapy assist slow-taper alprazolam discontinuation in panic disorder? Am J Psychiatry 151:876–881, 1994

Spivak B, Vered Y, Graff E, et al: Low platelet-poor plasma concentrations of serotonin in patients with combat-related posttraumatic stress disorder. Biol Psychiatry 45:840–845, 1999

Starcevic V, Fallon S, Uhlenhuth EH: The frequency and severity of generalized anxiety disorder symptoms. Toward a less cumbersome conceptualization. J Nerv Ment Dis 182:80–84, 1994

Stein DJ, Spadaccine E, Hollander E: Meta-analysis of pharmacotherapy trials for obsessive-compulsive disorder. Int Clin Psychopharmacol 10:11–18, 1995

Stein DJ, Montgomery SA, Kasper S, et al: Predictors of response to pharmacotherapy with citalopram in obsessive-compulsive disorder. Int Clin Psychopharmacol 16:357–361, 2001

Stein MB, Kean YM: Disability and quality of life in social phobia: epidemiologic findings. Am J Psychiatry 157:1606–1613, 2000

Stein MB, Asmundson G, Chartier M: Autonomic responsivity in generalized social phobia. J Affect Disord 31:211–221, 1994

Stein MB, Delaney SM, Chartier M, et al: 3H paroxetine binding to platelets of patients with social phobia: comparison to patients with panic disorder and healthy volunteers. Biol Psychiatry 37:224–228, 1995b

Stein MB, Walker JR, Anderson G, et al: Childhood physical and sexual abuse in patients with anxiety disorders and in a community sample. Am J Psychiatry 153:275–277, 1996

Stein MB, Chartier MJ, Hazen AL, et al: A direct-interview family study of generalized social phobia. Am J Psychiatry 155:90–97, 1998a

Stein MB, Liebowitz MR, Lydiard B, et al: Paroxetine treatment of generalized social phobia (social anxiety disorder): a randomized controlled trial. JAMA 280:708–713, 1998c

Stein MB, Fyer AJ, Davidson JRT, et al: Fluvoxamine treatment of social phobia (social anxiety disorder): a double-blind, placebo-controlled study. Am J Psychiatry 156:756–760, 1999

Steketee GS, Foa EB, Grayson JB: Recent advances in the behavioral treatment of obsessive-compulsives. Arch Gen Psychiatry 39:1365–1371, 1982

Stemberger RT, Turner SM, Beidel DC, et al: Social phobia: an analysis of possible developmental factors. J Abnorm Psychol 104:526–531, 1995

Strohle A, Kellner M, Holsboer F, et al: Behavioral, neuroendocrine, and cardiovascular response to flumazenil: no evidence for an altered benzodiazepine receptor sensitivity in panic disorder. Biol Psychiatry 45:321–326, 1999

Swedo SE, Rapoport JL, Cheslow DL, et al: Increased incidence of obsessive-compulsive symptoms in patients with Sydenham's chorea. Am J Psychiatry 146:246–249, 1989b

Swedo SE, Rapoport JL, Leonard H, et al: Obsessive-compulsive disorder in children and adolescents: clinical phenomenology of 70 consecutive cases. Arch Gen Psychiatry 46:335–341, 1989c

Swedo SE, Pietrini P, Leonard HL, et al: Cerebral glucose metabolism in childhood-onset obsessive-compulsive disorder: revisualization during pharmacotherapy. Arch Gen Psychiatry 49:690–694, 1992a

Szegedi A, Wetzel H, Leal M, et al: Combination treatment with clomipramine and fluvoxamine: drug monitoring, safety, and tolerability data. J Clin Psychiatry 57:257–264, 1996

Szeszko PR, Robinson D, Alvir JM, et al: Orbital frontal and amygdala volume reductions in obsessive-compulsive disorder. Arch Gen Psychiatry 56:913–919, 1999

Szymanski HV, Olympia J: Divalproex in posttraumatic stress disorder (letter). Am J Psychiatry 148:1086–1087, 1991

Tancer ME, Stein MB, Uhde TW: Growth hormone response to intravenous clonidine in social phobia: comparison to patients with panic disorder and healthy volunteers. Biol Psychiatry 34:591–595, 1993

Tancer ME, Mailman RB, Stein MB, et al: Neuroendocrine responsivity to monoaminergic system probes in generalized social phobia. Anxiety 1:216–223, 1994

Tarrier N, Pilgrim H, Sommerfield C, et al: A randomized trial of cognitive therapy and imaginal exposure in the treatment of chronic posttraumatic stress disorder. J Consult Clin Psychol 67:13–18, 1999

Telch MJ, Agras WG, Taylor CM, et al: Combined pharmacological and behavioral treatment for agoraphobia. Behav Res Ther 23:325–335, 1985

Telch MJ, Lucas JA, Schmidt NB, et al: Group cognitive-behavioral treatment of panic disorder. Behav Res Ther 31:279–287, 1993

Thomsen PH: Child and adolescent obsessive-compulsive disorder treated with citalopram: findings from an open trial of 23 cases. J Child Adolesc Psychopharmacol 7:157–166, 1997

Thomsen PH, Mikkelsen HU: Development of personality disorders in children and adolescents with obsessive-compulsive disorder: a 6- to 22-year follow-up study. Acta Psychiatr Scand 87:456–462, 1993

Tiihonen J, Kuikka J, Bergstrom K, et al: Dopamine reuptake site densities in patients with social phobia. Am J Psychiatry 154:239–242, 1997b

Tillfors M, Furmark T, Ekselius L, et al: Social phobia and avoidant personality disorder as related to parental history of social anxiety: a general population study. Behav Res Ther 39:289–298, 2001

Tollefson GD, Rampey AH, Potvin JH, et al: A multicenter investigation of fixed-dose fluoxetine in the treatment of obsessive-compulsive disorder. Arch Gen Psychiatry 51:559–567, 1994

Torgersen S: Genetic factors in anxiety disorders. Arch Gen Psychiatry 40:1085–1089, 1983

Towey J, Bruder G, Hollander E, et al: Endogenous event-related potentials in obsessive-compulsive disorder. Biol Psychiatry 28:92–98, 1990

True WR, Rice J, Eisen SA, et al: A twin study of genetic and environmental contributions to liability for posttraumatic stress symptoms. Arch Gen Psychiatry 50:257–264, 1993

Turner SM, Beidel DC, Cooley-Quille MR: Two-year follow-up of social phobias treated with Social Effectiveness Therapy. Behav Res Ther 33:553–555, 1995

Tweed JL, Schoenbach VJ, George LK, et al: The effects of childhood parental death and divorce on six-month history of anxiety disorders. Br J Psychiatry 154:823–828, 1989

Uhde TW, Stein MB, Vittone BJ, et al: Behavioral and physiologic effects of short-term and long-term administration of clonidine in panic disorder. Arch Gen Psychiatry 46:170–177, 1989

Uhde TW, Tancer ME, Gelernter CS, et al: Normal urinary free cortisol and post-dexamethasone cortisol in social phobia: comparison to normal volunteers. J Affect Disord 30:155–161, 1994

Ursano RJ, Fullerton CS, Epstein RS, et al: Acute and chronic posttraumatic stress disorder in motor vehicle accident victims. Am J Psychiatry 156:589–595, 1999a

Ursano RJ, Fullerton CS, Epstein RS, et al: Peritraumatic dissociation and posttraumatic stress disorder following motor vehicle accidents. Am J Psychiatry 156:1808–1810, 1999b

Vallejo J, Olivares J, Marcos T, et al: Clomipramine versus phenelzine in obsessive-compulsive disorder: a controlled clinical trial. Br J Psychiatry 161:665–670, 1992

Van Ameringen M, Mancini C, Streiner DL: Fluoxetine efficacy in social phobia. J Clin Psychiatry 54:27–32, 1993

Van Ameringen M, Mancini C, Streiner D: Sertraline in social phobia. J Affect Disord 31:141–145, 1994

Van Ameringen M, Mancini C, Oakman JM: Nefazodone in social phobia. J Clin Psychiatry 60:96–100, 1999

Van Ameringen MA, Lane RM, Walker JR, et al: Sertraline treatment of generalized social phobia: a 20-week, double-blind, placebo-controlled study. Am J Psychiatry 158:275–281, 2001

van Balkom AJ, de Haan E, van Oppen P, et al: Cognitive and behavioral therapies alone versus in combination with fluvoxamine in the treatment of obsessive compulsive disorder. J Nerv Ment Dis 186:492–499, 1998

van der Kolk BA: Psychopharmacological issues in posttraumatic stress disorder. Hosp Community Psychiatry 34:683–691, 1983

van der Kolk BA: The role of the group in the origin and resolution of the trauma response, in Psychological Trauma. Edited by van der Kolk BA. Washington, DC, American Psychiatric Press, 1987a, pp 153–171

van der Kolk BA: The separation cry and the trauma response: developmental issues in the psychobiology of attachment and separation, in Psychological Trauma. Edited by van der Kolk BA. Washington, DC, American Psychiatric Press, 1987b, pp 31–62

van der Kolk BA: The compulsion to repeat the trauma: reenactment, revictimization, and masochism. Psychiatr Clin North Am 12:389–411, 1989

van der Kolk BA, Boyd H, Krystal J, et al: Posttraumatic stress disorder as a biologically based disorder: implications of the animal model of inescapable shock, in Post-Traumatic Stress Disorder: Psychological and Biological Sequelae. Edited by van der Kolk BA. Washington, DC, American Psychiatric Press, 1984, pp 123–134

van der Kolk BA, Dreyfuss D, Michaels M, et al: Fluoxetine in posttraumatic stress disorder. J Clin Psychiatry 55:517–522, 1994

vanOppen P, Arntz A: Cognitive therapy for obsessive-compulsive disorder. Behav Res Ther 32:79–87, 1994

vanOppen P, deHaan E, vanBalkom AJ, et al: Cognitive therapy and exposure in vivo in the treatment of obsessive compulsive disorder. Behav Res Ther 33:379–390, 1995

van Vliet IM, den Boer JA, Westenberg HG: Psychopharmacological treatment of social phobia: a double blind placebo controlled study with fluvoxamine. Psychopharmacology (Berl) 115:128–134, 1994

van Vliet IM, den Boer JA, Westenberg HGM, et al: Clinical effects of buspirone in social phobia: a double-blind placebo-controlled study. J Clin Psychiatry 58:164–168, 1997

Verburg C, Griez C, Meijer J: A 35% carbon dioxide challenge in simple phobias. Acta Psychiatr Scand 90:420–423, 1994

Versiani M, Mundim FD, Nardi AE, et al: Tranylcypromine in social phobia. J Clin Psychopharmacol 8:279–283, 1988

Wade AG, Lepola U, Koponen HJ, et al: The effect of citalopram in panic disorder. Br J Psychiatry 170:549–553, 1997

Wang Z, Valdes J, Noyes R, et al: Possible association of a cholecystokinin promoter polymorphism (CCK-36CT) with panic disorder. Am J Med Genet 81:228–234, 1998

Weiss EL, Potenza MN, McDougle CJ, et al: Olanzapine addition in obsessive-compulsive disorder refractory to selective serotonin reuptake inhibitors: an open-label case series. J Clin Psychiatry 60:524–527, 1999

Weissman MM, Leckman JF, Merikangas KR, et al: Depression and anxiety disorders in parents and children. Arch Gen Psychiatry 41:845–852, 1984

Weissman MM, Wickramaratne P, Adams PB, et al: The relationship between panic disorder and major depression: a new family study. Arch Gen Psychiatry 50:767–780, 1993

Widom CS: Posttraumatic stress disorder in abused and neglected children grown up. Am J Psychiatry 156:1223–1229, 1999

Wilkinson DJ, Thompson JM, Lambert GW, et al: Sympathetic activity in patients with panic disorder at rest, under laboratory mental stress, and during panic attacks. Arch Gen Psychiatry 55:511–520, 1998

Wolf ME, Alavi A, Mosnaim AD: Posttraumatic stress disorder in Vietnam veterans, clinical and EEG findings: possible therapeutic effects of carbamazepine. Biol Psychiatry 23:642–644, 1988

Woodman CL, Noyes R: Panic disorder: treatment with valproate. J Clin Psychiatry 55:134–136, 1994

Woodman CL, Noyes R, Black DW, et al: A 5-year follow-up study of generalized anxiety disorder and panic disorder. J Nerv Ment Dis 187:3–9, 1999

Woody SR, Chambless DL, Glass CR: Self-focused attention in the treatment of social phobia. Behav Res Ther 35:117–129, 1997

Wu JC, Buchsbaum MS, Hershey TG, et al: PET in generalized anxiety disorder. Biol Psychiatry 29:1181–1199, 1991

Yehuda R, Southwick SM, Krystal JH, et al: Enhanced suppression of cortisol following dexamethasone administration in posttraumatic stress disorder. Am J Psychiatry 150:83–86, 1993

Yehuda R, Boisoneau D, Lowy MT, et al: Dose-response changes in plasma cortisol and lymphocyte glucocorticoid receptors following dexamethasone administration in combat veterans with and without posttraumatic stress disorder. Arch Gen Psychiatry 52:583–593, 1995a

Yehuda R, McFarlane AC, Shalev AY: Predicting the development of posttraumatic stress disorder from the acute response to a traumatic event. Biol Psychiatry 44:1305–1313, 1998a

Yehuda R, Schmeidler J, Wainberg M, et al: Vulnerability to posttraumatic stress disorder in adult offspring of Holocaust survivors. Am J Psychiatry 155:1163–1171, 1998b

Yonkers KA, Warshaw MG, Massion AO, et al: Phenomenology and course of generalised anxiety disorder. Br J Psychiatry 168:308–313, 1996

Zisook S, Chentsova-Dutton YE, Smith-Vaniz A, et al: Nefazodone in patients with treatment-refractory posttraumatic stress disorder. J Clin Psychiatry 61:203–208, 2000

Zitrin CM, Klein DF, Woerner MG: Treatment of agoraphobia with group exposure in vivo and imipramine. Arch Gen Psychiatry 37:63–72, 1980

Zitrin CM, Klein DF, Woerner MG, et al: Treatment of phobias, I: comparison of imipramine hydrochloride and placebo. Arch Gen Psychiatry 40:125–138, 1983

Zlotnick C, Shea TM, Rosen K, et al: An affect-management group for women with posttraumatic stress disorder and histories of childhood sexual abuse. J Trauma Stress 10:425–436, 1997

Zlotnick C, Warshaw M, Shea MT, et al: Chronicity in posttraumatic stress disorder (PTSD) and predictors of course of comorbid PTSD in patients with anxiety disorders. J Trauma Stress 12:89–100, 1999

Zohar J, Insel TR: Obsessive-compulsive disorder: psychobiological approaches to diagnosis, treatment, and pathophysiology. Biol Psychiatry 22:667–687, 1987

Zohar J, Judge R: Paroxetine versus clomipramine in the treatment of obsessive-compulsive disorder. OCD Paroxetine Study Investigators. Br J Psychiatry 169: 468–474, 1996

CHAPTER 8

Somatoform Disorders

Sean H. Yutzy, M.D.

In DSM-IV-TR, the disorders included under the somatoform rubric are *somatization disorder, undifferentiated somatoform disorder, conversion disorder, pain disorder, hypochondriasis, body dysmorphic disorder,* and the residual category *somatoform disorder not otherwise specified (NOS)*. The grouping is based on the clinical utility of a shared diagnostic concern rather than assumptions regarding a shared etiology or mechanism: the exclusion of occult "physical" or "organic" pathology underlying the symptoms. In DSM-IV-TR terminology, such etiologies are referred to as "general medical conditions" or the "direct effects of a substance." General medical conditions include all conditions not included in the mental disorders section of ICD-10 (World Health Organization 1992b). As examples, all infectious and parasitic, endocrine, nutritional, metabolic, immunity, and congenital disorders affecting virtually any organ system (including the nervous system) in the body are considered general medical conditions. This terminology was adopted to avoid the implication that *mental* (i.e., psychiatric) conditions do not have *organic* causes and to underscore the view that psychiatric disorders are also *medical* conditions.

The utility of grouping disorders on the basis of a shared clinical concern was endorsed by the symptom-driven *Diagnostic and Statistical Manual of Mental Disorders, Fourth Edition, Primary Care Version* (DSM-IV–PC; American Psychiatric Association 1995), which included "unexplained physical symptoms" as the basis of 1 of its 10 algorithms. Likewise, the ICD-10 *Diagnostic and Management Guidelines for Mental Disorders in Primary Care* (World Health Organization 1996) was organized with a diagnostic category for "unexplained somatic complaint."

It is assumed that the specific disorders in the somatoform grouping are heterogeneous. In somatization, undifferentiated somatoform, conversion, and pain disorders, the focus is on the symptoms themselves. In hypochondriasis and body dysmorphic disorder, the emphasis is on preoccupations: in hypochondriasis, with the interpretation and possible implications of bodily symptoms; in body dysmorphic disorder, with an imagined or exaggerated defect in appearance. Because of their emphasis on preoccupations, hypochondriasis and body dysmorphic disorder more closely resemble obsessive-compulsive or even psychotic disorders than they do the symptom-centered somatoform disorders (Hollander et al. 1992; Phillips et al. 1995).

The *somatoform* concept, with a

history dating only to the introduction of DSM-III in 1980 (American Psychiatric Association 1980), must not be equated with two concepts of long tradition: *psychosomatic illness* and *somatization*. Theoretically, in psychosomatic illnesses, structural or physiological changes result from psychological factors. In the somatoform disorders, however, such changes generally are not evident. The "classic" psychosomatic illnesses described by Alexander (1950) included bronchial asthma, ulcerative colitis, thyrotoxicosis, essential hypertension, rheumatoid arthritis, neurodermatitis, and peptic ulcer. In DSM-IV-TR, these illnesses are considered general medical conditions.

Given the heterogeneity of the somatoform disorder class, extensive discussion of the class, in general, is not particularly useful. The specific somatoform disorders are best discussed individually. Thus, with the exception of pain disorder, we review the somatoform disorders included in DSM-IV-TR. For convenience, the disorders are discussed in the order in which they appear in DSM-IV-TR.

Somatization Disorder

Definition and Clinical Description

The core features of somatization disorder are recurrent multiple physical complaints that are not fully explained by physical factors and that result in medical attention or significant impairment.

Somatization disorder is the most pervasive somatoform disorder. By definition, somatization disorder is a polysymptomatic disorder affecting multiple body systems. Symptoms of other specific somatoform disorders (e.g., conversion disorder and pain disorder) are included in the diagnostic criteria for somatization disorder. Undifferentiated somatoform disor-

der, in essence, represents a syndrome similar to somatization disorder but with a less extensive symptomatology. From a hierarchical perspective, none of these disorders is diagnosed if symptoms occur exclusively during the course of somatization disorder.

Somatization disorder has been the most rigorously studied somatoform disorder and is the best validated in terms of diagnostic reliability, stability over time, prediction of medical utilization, and even heritability. Yet its validity as a discrete syndrome has been challenged (Bass and Murphy 1990). Vaillant (1984), noting that most of the research on this disorder has emanated from four academic centers in the midwestern United States, went so far as to state that the diagnosis "lies in the eyes of the beholder" (p. 543).

Diagnosis

The DSM-IV-TR criteria for somatization disorder are the product of a long and inconsistent approach to a syndrome characterized by multiple unexplained physical complaints (Martin 1988).

A comprehensive reassessment of the extant literature and preexisting data sets was coordinated by the American Psychiatric Association. On the basis of this review, Cloninger and Yutzy (1993) suggested a diagnostic strategy that simplified the criteria for somatization disorder and appeared useful in routine practice. Data from a sample of 500 psychiatric outpatients were reanalyzed, leading to the development of an empirically derived algorithm for the diagnosis of somatization disorder. This algorithm required four pain symptoms, two nonpain gastrointestinal symptoms, one nonpain sexual or reproductive symptom, and one pseudoneurological (conversion or dissociative) symptom. This approach was adopted for DSM-IV (American Psychiatric Association 1994) (Table 8–1).

TABLE 8–1. DSM-IV-TR diagnostic criteria for somatization disorder

A. A history of many physical complaints beginning before age 30 years that occur over a period of several years and result in treatment being sought or significant impairment in social, occupational, or other important areas of functioning.

B. Each of the following criteria must have been met, with individual symptoms occurring at any time during the course of the disturbance:

    (1) *four pain symptoms:* a history of pain related to at least four different sites or functions (e.g., head, abdomen, back, joints, extremities, chest, rectum, during menstruation, during sexual intercourse, or during urination)

    (2) *two gastrointestinal symptoms:* a history of at least two gastrointestinal symptoms other than pain (e.g., nausea, bloating, vomiting other than during pregnancy, diarrhea, or intolerance of several different foods)

    (3) *one sexual symptom:* a history of at least one sexual or reproductive symptom other than pain (e.g., sexual indifference, erectile or ejaculatory dysfunction, irregular menses, excessive menstrual bleeding, vomiting throughout pregnancy)

    (4) *one pseudoneurological symptom:* a history of at least one symptom or deficit suggesting a neurological condition not limited to pain (conversion symptoms such as impaired coordination or balance, paralysis or localized weakness, difficulty swallowing or lump in throat, aphonia, urinary retention, hallucinations, loss of touch or pain sensation, double vision, blindness, deafness, seizures; dissociative symptoms such as amnesia; or loss of consciousness other than fainting)

C. Either (1) or (2):

    (1) after appropriate investigation, each of the symptoms in Criterion B cannot be fully explained by a known general medical condition or the direct effects of a substance (e.g., a drug of abuse, a medication)

    (2) when there is a related general medical condition, the physical complaints or resulting social or occupational impairment are in excess of what would be expected from the history, physical examination, or laboratory findings

D. The symptoms are not intentionally produced or feigned (as in factitious disorder or malingering).

The new criteria were tested in a multicenter field trial designed to examine their concordance with previous diagnostic criteria. This study (Yutzy et al. 1995) found excellent agreement with the newly proposed diagnostic strategy and these earlier criteria in DSM-III and DSM-III-R. These findings supported the DSM-IV diagnostic strategy for somatization disorder.

Differential Diagnosis

The symptom picture encountered in somatization disorder is frequently nonspecific and can overlap with a multitude of medical disorders. According to Cloninger (1994), three features are useful in discriminating between somatization dis-

order and physical illness: 1) involvement of multiple organ systems, 2) early onset and chronic course without development of physical signs of structural abnormalities, and 3) absence of characteristic laboratory abnormalities of the suggested physical disorder. These features should be considered in cases for which careful analysis leaves the etiology unclear. The clinician also should be aware that several medical disorders may be confused with somatization disorder. Patients with multiple sclerosis and systemic lupus erythematosus (SLE) may have vague functional and sensory disturbances with unclear physical signs. Patients with acute intermittent porphyria (AIP) may have a history of episodic pain and various neurological disturbances, and patients with hemochromatosis often have vague and diffuse pains, which may be confused with patients who have somatization disorder.

According to Cloninger (1994), three psychiatric disorders must be carefully considered in the differential diagnosis of somatization disorder: anxiety disorders (in particular, panic disorder), mood disorders, and schizophrenia. The most troublesome distinction is between anxiety disorders and somatization disorder. Individuals with generalized anxiety disorder may have a multitude of physical complaints that are also frequently found in patients with somatization disorder. Individuals with anxiety disorders also may have disease concerns and hypochondriacal complaints common to somatization disorder. Similarly, patients with somatization disorder often report panic (anxiety) attacks. Although the usual parameters of age at onset and course may be helpful in differentiating between an anxiety disorder and somatization disorder, the presence of certain traits, symptoms, and social factors can be of assistance. In particular, the presence of histrionic personality traits, conversion and dissociative symptoms, sexual and menstrual problems, and social impairment supports a diagnosis of somatization disorder (Cloninger 1994). In addition, gender should be considered because men are much more likely to have anxiety disorders than somatization disorder. Precise diagnosis, although difficult, is clinically important because the medical management of somatization disorder differs from that of anxiety disorders.

Patients with mood disorders, especially depression, may have somatic complaints. Commonly, the chief complaint may be headache, gastrointestinal disturbance, or unexplained pain. However, such symptoms resolve with successful treatment of the mood disorder, whereas in somatization disorder, the physical complaints continue. Patients with somatization disorder frequently complain of depression and often fulfill the criteria for major depression (DeSouza et al. 1988). It is not clear, however, whether these complaints truly reflect the clinical state or are simply a reflection of overreporting.

Patients with schizophrenia may have unexplained somatic complaints. Careful evaluation often identifies delusions, hallucinations, and/or a formal thought disorder. Rarely will the somatic symptoms be extensive enough to meet the criteria for somatization disorder. It should be noted that occasionally a patient with extensive somatic symptomatology and no evidence of psychosis subsequently will develop clinical symptoms of schizophrenia (Goodwin and Guze 1996).

Individuals with antisocial, borderline, and/or histrionic personality disorder may have an associated somatization disorder (Cloninger et al. 1997; Hudziak et al. 1996; Stern et al. 1993). Antisocial personality disorder has been shown to cluster both within individuals and within families (Cloninger and Guze 1970; Cloninger et al. 1975) and may have a common etiology in many cases.

Patients with somatization disorder often complain of psychological or interpersonal problems in addition to somatic symptoms. Wetzel et al. (1994) summarized these as "psychoform symptoms." In this study, Minnesota Multiphasic Personality Inventory (MMPI; Hathaway and McKinley 1943) profiles of somatization disorder patients mimicked multiple psychiatric disorders.

Commonly, individuals with somatization disorder are inconsistent historians, and obtaining the medical records often will be necessary to definitively establish the diagnosis.

Natural History

Somatization disorder is a chronic illness with fluctuations in the frequency and diversity of symptoms, but it rarely, if ever, totally remits (Guze and Perley 1963; Guze et al. 1986). The most active symptomatic phase is usually early adulthood, but aging does not lead to total remission (Goodwin and Guze 1996). Pribor et al. (1994) found that patients with somatization disorder age 55 years and older did not differ from younger patients in terms of the number of somatization symptoms or the use of health care services. Longitudinal prospective studies have confirmed that 80%–90% of the patients diagnosed with somatization disorder maintain consistent clinical syndrome and retain the same diagnosis over many years (Cloninger et al. 1986; Guze et al. 1986; Perley and Guze 1962).

According to Goodwin and Guze (1996), the most frequent and important complications of somatization disorder are repeated surgical operations, drug dependence, suicide attempts, and marital separation or divorce. These authors suggested that the first two complications are preventable if the disorder is recognized and the patient's symptoms are managed appropriately. Generally, because of awareness that somatization disorder is an alternative explanation for various pains and other symptoms, invasive techniques can be withheld or postponed when objective indications are absent or equivocal. There is no evidence of excess mortality in patients with somatization disorder.

Avoidance of prescribing habit-forming or addictive substances for persistent or recurrent complaints of pain should be paramount in the mind of the treating physician. Suicide attempts are common, but completed suicide is not (Martin et al. 1985; G.E. Murphy and Wetzel 1982). It is unclear whether marital or occupational dysfunction can be minimized through psychotherapy.

Epidemiology

The lifetime risk, prevalence, and incidence of somatization disorder are unclear. The lifetime risk for somatization disorder was estimated at about 2% in women when age at onset and method of assessment were taken into account (Cloninger et al. 1975). This risk is similar to the previously noted 2% prevalence rate identified by Woodruff et al. (1971). Cloninger et al. (1984), using complete lifetime medical records, found a 3% frequency of somatization disorder in 859 Swedish women in the general population. However, the ECA study (L.N. Robins et al. 1984), using nonphysician interviewers, found a lifetime risk of somatization disorder of only 0.2%–0.3% for women. However, the prevalence of somatization disorder may be underestimated in studies relying on interviews by nonphysicians. In a study by L.N. Robins et al. (1981), nonphysicians, when compared with psychiatrists, showed high (i.e., 97%–99%) diagnostic specificity for somatization disorder. However, diagnostic sensitivity for nonphysicians was low (55% for Feighner-defined hysteria and 41% for DSM-III-defined somatization disorder). The diagnostic criteria for somatization disorder require judgments as to whether symptoms are fully explained medically. Patients with somatization disorder often attribute symptoms to various physical disorders. Nonphysicians rarely have the expertise to evaluate such statements critically and may tend to accept them. To properly assess somatic complaints relative to objective findings and the known course of disease may require that the interviewer have an adequate medical background (Cloninger 1994).

Additionally, patients may be less inclined to describe physical complaints to non-physicians. All of these factors may lead to the underdiagnosis of somatization disorder, which may account for the low prevalence of somatization disorder in large-scale population surveys that use nonphysician interviewers.

Somatization disorder is diagnosed predominantly in women and rarely in men. Some have suggested that this sex difference may be artifactual because somatization disorder criteria are biased against making the diagnosis in men because of the inapplicability of pregnancy and menstrual complaints. Also, men tend to report fewer symptoms than do women.

Etiology

The etiology of somatization disorder is unknown, but it is clearly a familial disorder. In several studies, approximately 20% of the female first-degree relatives of patients with somatization disorder also met criteria (Cloninger and Guze 1970; Guze et al. 1986; Woerner and Guze 1968). Guze et al. (1986) further demonstrated the familial nature of somatization disorder in a "blind" family study and documented an association between somatization disorder and antisocial personality in male and female relatives.

A relationship between somatization disorder and certain personality disorders has been posited. Hudziak et al. (1996) and Cloninger et al. (1997) identified similarities and even overlap between somatization disorder and borderline personality disorder, as did Stern et al. (1993) with personality disorders broadly. These studies support the interpretation that somatization disorder is more of a personality (Axis II) disorder than an Axis I disorder, considering its early onset, nonremitting nature, and pervasiveness, which in some

cases results in chronic dysfunctional states.

Treatment

Somatization disorder is difficult to treat, and there appears to be no single superior treatment approach (G.E. Murphy 1982). Primary care physicians generally can manage patients with somatization disorder adequately, but the expertise of at least a consulting psychiatrist has been shown to be useful. In a prospective, randomized controlled study, Smith et al. (1986) found a reduction in health care costs for patients with somatization disorder who received a psychiatric consultation as opposed to those who did not receive a consultation. Reduced expenditures were largely the result of decreased rates of hospitalization. These gains were accomplished with no decrement in medical status or in patient satisfaction, suggesting that many of the evaluations and treatments otherwise provided to patients with somatization disorder are unnecessary. Smith et al. (1986) suggested that treatment include regularly scheduled visits with an appropriate physician. The frequency of visits should be determined on the basis of support for the patient, not in response to the frequency or severity of complaints.

Scallet et al. (1976) reviewed the earlier psychiatric literature on treatment of hysteria and reported the success rates of various approaches. Although most of the studies were uncontrolled and otherwise methodologically flawed, one study conducted by Luff and Garrod (1935) noted a 51% improvement rate at 3-year follow-up in patients treated with an "eclectic approach." As summarized by Scallet et al. (1976), this treatment involved "re-education, reassurance and suggestion" (p. 348). These techniques also were described by Carter (1949) as being effective in the treatment of acute conversion.

An eclectic approach comports well with the general principles of treatment recommended by Quill (1985), Cloninger (1994), and Smith et al. (1986). Three important suggestions emerge from review of these reports: 1) establish a firm therapeutic alliance with the patient, 2) educate the patient about the manifestations of somatization disorder, and 3) provide consistent reassurance. Implementation of these principles, as described in more detail in the following paragraphs, may greatly facilitate clinical management of somatization disorder and prevent potentially serious complications, including the effects of unnecessary diagnostic and therapeutic procedures. The superiority of more specific treatment approaches has not been documented by controlled trials (Kellner 1989).

First, a firm therapeutic alliance must be established. The basis of any satisfactory treatment relationship is a firm therapeutic alliance; it is particularly important in the treatment of patients with somatization disorder, but it is often difficult to attain. Generally, multiple physicians already have been consulted in an attempt to discover a physical explanation for the symptoms offered. The patient usually has received the message (overtly or covertly) that the difficulty is "mental," "psychological," or "psychiatric," and the physician is not particularly interested in continuing to provide care to him or her. That message promotes a pattern of "doctor shopping," which may lead to unnecessary diagnostic procedures and treatments. To prevent harm, a therapeutic alliance is essential. The first step in establishing such an alliance is for the physician to acknowledge the patient's pain and suffering. This acknowledgment communicates to the patient that the physician is caring, compassionate, and interested in providing assistance. The physician should

then conduct an exhaustive review of the patient's medical history, including careful examination of medical records. Such a review generally will strengthen the incipient therapeutic bond, demonstrating the physician's willingness to take the time and effort to gain an understanding of the patient. In addition, this step is crucial in ruling out medical disorders that can include nonspecific motor and sensory abnormalities or transient or equivocal signs (e.g., multiple sclerosis, SLE, AIP, hemochromatosis). Also, a thorough medical knowledge of the patient initially will allow better ongoing assessment of symptomatology. After the diagnosis of somatization disorder is firmly established, elaborate diagnostic evaluations should be conducted based on objective evidence and not just subjective complaints. However, the clinician must always remain cognizant that patients with somatization disorder are not immune to developing physical illness.

Education is the second general principle. Cloninger (1994) favors informing the patient of the diagnosis and describing the various facets of somatization disorder in a positive light. The patient should be advised that he or she is not "crazy" but has a medically recognized illness. The condition will not lead to chronic mental or physical deterioration (or death). The clinician should be careful to strike a balance between painting a positive picture of the disorder and conducting a realistic discussion of prognosis, goals, and treatment.

The third principle is consistent reassurance. Patients with somatization disorder often become concerned that the physician is not performing a sufficiently thorough evaluation and may threaten to seek care from a different physician. Such challenges should be directly addressed with reassurance that the possibility of an undiscovered physical illness is being appropriately assessed on a continuing basis and that changing physicians would place decisions in the hands of someone unaware of the complexities of the patient's case. The patient should be reassured that there is no evidence of a physical cause for the complaint but that there may be a link with "stress." A thorough review of complaints commonly identifies a temporal association of symptoms with interpersonal, social, or occupational problems. Discussion of such associations may help the patient gain insight that the problems may precipitate somatic or psychological symptoms. In patients for whom introspection is difficult, modification of behavior by using simple behavioral management techniques may be useful.

Pharmacotherapy in the management of patients with somatization disorder must be tempered with the knowledge that these patients may take medicines inconsistently and unpredictably, may develop drug dependence, and may overdose in suicide gestures or attempts.

The clinician should develop a relationship with the patient's family. This facilitates attaining a better appreciation of the patient's social structure, which may be crucial to understanding and managing the patient's often chaotic personal lifestyle. When appropriate, the clinician must place firm limits on excessive demands, manipulations, and attention seeking (G.E. Murphy 1982; G.E. Murphy and Guze 1960).

Undifferentiated Somatoform Disorder

Definition and Clinical Description

The essential aspect of undifferentiated somatoform disorder is the presence of one or more clinically significant medically unexplained somatic symptoms with a duration of 6 months or more that are not better accounted for by another mental disorder (Table 8–2).

TABLE 8–2. DSM-IV-TR diagnostic criteria for undifferentiated somatoform disorder

A. One or more physical complaints (e.g., fatigue, loss of appetite, gastrointestinal or urinary complaints).
B. Either (1) or (2):
  (1) after appropriate investigation, the symptoms cannot be fully explained by a known general medical condition or the direct effects of a substance (e.g., a drug of abuse, a medication)
  (2) when there is a related general medical condition, the physical complaints or resulting social or occupational impairment is in excess of what would be expected from the history, physical examination, or laboratory findings
C. The symptoms cause clinically significant distress or impairment in social, occupational, or other important areas of functioning.
D. The duration of the disturbance is at least 6 months.
E. The disturbance is not better accounted for by another mental disorder (e.g., another somatoform disorder, sexual dysfunction, mood disorder, anxiety disorder, sleep disorder, or psychotic disorder).
F. The symptom is not intentionally produced or feigned (as in factitious disorder or malingering).

Diagnosis

History

The diagnostic category of undifferentiated somatoform disorder did not exist prior to DSM-III-R. At that time, it was added to cover those syndromes that in DSM-III simply would have been included under "atypical somatoform disorder." It is not clear whether the category *undifferentiated somatoform disorder* has been well adopted by clinicians, but several studies support its existence.

DSM-IV Criteria

After some debate, minor changes in the category *undifferentiated somatoform disorder* were made in DSM-IV. The only changes involved substituting the standard "general medical condition" for DSM-III-R's "organic pathology." A threshold for diagnosis also was added, requiring clinically significant distress or impairment. Instead of excluding the diagnosis on the basis of "occurrence exclusively during the course of another mental disorder," exclusion in DSM-IV was on the basis of "not better accounted for by another mental disorder."

Differential Diagnosis

Principal considerations in the differential diagnosis include the question of whether, with follow-up, criteria for somatization disorder will be met. Patients with somatization disorder are typically inconsistent historians. During one evaluation, they may report many symptoms and fulfill criteria for the full syndrome, whereas during another, they may report fewer symptoms, perhaps only fulfilling criteria for an abridged syndrome (Martin et al. 1979). Another consideration is whether the somatic symptoms qualifying a patient for the diagnosis of undifferentiated somatoform disorder are the manifestation of a depressive or an anxiety disorder. Indeed, high rates of major depression and anxiety disorders have been found in somatizing patients attending family medicine clinics (Kirmayer et al. 1993).

Epidemiology

Some investigators have argued that undifferentiated somatoform disorder is the most common somatoform disorder. Esco-bar et al. (1991) used a construct requiring six somatic symptoms for women and four for men and reported that in the United States 11% of non-Hispanic whites and Hispanics, as well as 15% of blacks, fulfilled the criteria. In Puerto Rico, 20% met the criteria. A preponderance of women was evident in all groups except the Puerto Rican sample.

Etiology

If undifferentiated somatoform disorder is simply an abridged form of somatization disorder, etiological theories reviewed under that diagnosis should also apply to undifferentiated somatoform disorder.

Treatment

Existing data have been derived from studies fraught with methodological problems, including the use of diverse groups with only a certain number of chronic somatic complaints in common. Several studies suggested that improvement is accelerated with psychotherapy of a supportive, rather than a nondirective, type. However, a substantial proportion of patients improve or recover with no formal psychotherapy.

Conversion Disorder

Definition and Clinical Description

The essential features of conversion disorder are the nonintentionally produced symptoms or deficits affecting voluntary motor or sensory function that suggest but are not fully explained by a neurological or general medical condition, by the direct effects of a substance, or by a culturally sanctioned behavior or experience. Specific symptoms mentioned as examples in DSM-IV-TR include motor symptoms such as impaired coordination or balance, paralysis or localized weakness, difficulty swallowing or lump in throat (e.g., "globus hystericus"), aphonia, and urinary retention; sensory symptoms, including hallucinations, loss of touch or pain sensation, double vision, blindness, and deafness; and seizures or convulsions with voluntary motor or sensory components. Single episodes usually involve one symptom, but longitudinally, other conversion symptoms will be evident as well. Psychological factors generally appear to be involved in that symptoms often occur in the context of a conflictual situation that may in some way be resolved with the development of the symptom.

Diagnosis

History

Some of the major early contributions to the study of conversion disorder were by neurologists, including Charcot (Torack 1978) and Breuer and Freud (1893 1895/1955) in the late nineteenth century and early twentieth century.

Acute hysteria has been used to refer to such states. Unfortunately, conversion disorder or *conversion hysteria* was used by some clinicians synonymously with *hysteria*, a term replaced by somatization disorder in DSM-III. Generally, hysteria was used to describe a more pervasive, chronic, and polysymptomatic disorder. Although conversion symptoms are perhaps the most dramatic symptoms of somatization disorder, the disorder is characterized by multiple unexplained symptoms in many organ systems. In conversion disorder, a single symptom, traditionally of a pseudoneurological type (i.e., suggesting neurological disease), suffices. Such inconsistency in the use of terms has resulted in a great deal of confusion, both in research and in clinical practice.

Adding to this confusion was a change introduced in DSM-III and retained in

DSM-III-R, wherein the concept of conversion was expanded to include disorders characterized by symptoms involving any "loss of, or alteration in, physical functioning suggesting a physical disorder" (American Psychiatric Association 1987, p. 259) as long as the mechanism of conversion was evident; that is, the symptom was "an expression of a psychological conflict or need" (American Psychiatric Association 1987, p. 257). Thus, symptoms involving the autonomic or endocrine systems, such as vomiting (supposedly representing revulsion and disgust) and pseudocyesis (as a manifestation of unconscious conflict about, or the need for, pregnancy), were included as examples of conversion symptoms.

DSM-IV-TR Criteria

As defined in DSM-IV-TR, nonintentional "symptoms or deficits affecting voluntary motor or sensory function" (American Psychiatric Association 2000, p. 498) are central to conversion disorder (see Table 8–3). The majority of such symptoms will suggest a neurological condition (i.e., are pseudoneurological), but other general medical conditions may be suggested as well. Pseudoneurological symptoms remain the classic symptomatology. By definition, symptoms limited to pain or disturbance in sexual functioning are not included.

In conversion disorder, as in the other somatoform disorders, the symptom cannot be fully explained by a known physical disorder. This criterion is perhaps the most imperative diagnostic consideration. In addition, the symptom is defined as not fully explained by a culturally sanctioned behavior or experience. Symptoms such as seizurelike episodes occurring in conjunction with certain religious ceremonies and culturally expected responses, in times past, such as women swooning in response to excitement would qualify as examples.

TABLE 8–3. DSM-IV-TR diagnostic criteria for conversion disorder

A. One or more symptoms or deficits affecting voluntary motor or sensory function that suggest a neurological or other general medical condition.

B. Psychological factors are judged to be associated with the symptom or deficit because the initiation or exacerbation of the symptom or deficit is preceded by conflicts or other stressors.

C. The symptom or deficit is not intentionally produced or feigned (as in factitious disorder or malingering).

D. The symptom or deficit cannot, after appropriate investigation, be fully explained by a general medical condition, or by the direct effects of a substance, or as a culturally sanctioned behavior or experience.

E. The symptom or deficit causes clinically significant distress or impairment in social, occupational, or other important areas of functioning or warrants medical evaluation.

F. The symptom or deficit is not limited to pain or sexual dysfunction, does not occur exclusively during the course of somatization disorder, and is not better accounted for by another mental disorder.

Specify type of symptom or deficit:
With Motor Symptom or Deficit
With Sensory Symptom or Deficit
With Seizures or Convulsions
With Mixed Presentation

DSM-IV-TR specifies that the symptoms in conversion disorder are not intentionally produced, thus distinguishing conversion symptoms from those of a factitious disorder or malingering. Although this judgment is difficult to make, it is an important one because the recommended management and expected outcome of factitious disorder and malingering are markedly different.

Clinical judgment also is required in determining whether psychological factors are etiologically related to the symp-

tom. Inclusion of this criterion is perhaps a holdover from the initial conceptualization of conversion symptoms as representing the conversion of unconscious psychic conflict into a physical symptom. As reviewed by Cloninger (1987), such determination is virtually impossible except in cases in which there is a temporal relationship between a psychosocial stressor and the symptom or in cases in which similar situations led to conversion symptoms in the past.

Differential Diagnosis

Conversion symptoms suggest physical illness, and nonpsychiatrists are generally seen initially. Neurologists are frequently consulted by primary care physicians for such symptoms because most suggest neurological disease. It has been estimated that 1% of the patients admitted to the hospital for neurological problems have conversion symptoms (Marsden 1986).

One major problem with conversion symptoms is that they suggest neurological or general medical conditions, and conversion (mis)diagnosis may be applied when the true illness is present. Some older studies found that significant proportions of patients initially diagnosed with conversion symptoms had neurological illnesses on follow-up. Slater and Glithero (1965) found a misdiagnosis rate of 50% during a 7- to 11-year follow-up; Gatfield and Guze (1962) reported 21%; but more recently, Mace and Trimble (1996) observed a rate of 15%. The trend toward less misdiagnosis may reflect an increasing sophistication in neurological diagnosis. Although Slater and Glithero's study often has been used to challenge the validity of hysteria (now somatization disorder), its importance lies in underscoring the need to remain tentative in making a diagnosis of conversion disorder.

Symptoms of various neurological illnesses may seem to be inconsistent with known neurophysiology or neuropathology and may suggest conversion. Diseases to be considered include multiple sclerosis (consider blindness secondary to optic neuritis with initially normal fundi), myasthenia gravis, periodic paralysis, myoglobinuric myopathy, polymyositis, other acquired myopathies (all of which may include marked weakness in the presence of normal deep tendon reflexes), and Guillain-Barré syndrome, in which early weakness of the arms and legs may be inconsistent (Cloninger 1994). As reviewed by Ford and Folks (1985), more than 13% of actual neurological cases are diagnosed as "functional" before the elucidation of a neurological illness. Initial evidence of some neurological disease is predictive of a subsequent neurological explanation (Mace and Trimble 1996).

Complicating diagnosis is the fact that physical illness and conversion (or other apparent psychiatric overlay) are not mutually exclusive. Patients who have incapacitating and frightening physical illnesses may appear to exaggerate their symptoms. Patients with actual neurological illness also may have "pseudosymptoms." For example, patients with actual seizures often have pseudoseizures (Desai et al. 1982).

Considering these observations, physicians should resist an incautious diagnosis of conversion disorder when faced with difficult-to-interpret symptoms. The occurrence of apparent conversion symptoms mandates a thorough evaluation for possible underlying physical explanation. This evaluation may include physical and psychiatric examination, X rays, and blood and urine tests as the symptoms and signs would indicate.

Longitudinal studies indicate the most reliable predictor that a patient with apparent conversion symptoms will not later be shown to have a physical disorder is a

history of conversion or other unexplained symptoms (Cloninger 1994). Patients with somatization disorder will manifest multiple symptoms in multiple organ systems, including the voluntary motor and sensory nervous systems. Thus, apparent conversion symptoms in the context of somatization disorder should indicate that an underlying physical disorder is unlikely. Although conversion symptoms may occur at any age, vulnerability for conversion symptoms is first manifested most often in late adolescence or early adulthood (Cloninger 1994). Conversion symptoms first occurring in middle age or later should increase suspicion of an occult physical illness.

An association between conversion symptoms affecting voluntary motor and sensory functioning and dissociative symptoms affecting memory and identity should be noted. Traditionally, such symptoms have been attributed to similar psychological mechanisms. The two types of symptoms often occur in the same individual, sometimes during the same episode of illness (consider the example of the patient with conversion disorder discussed at the beginning of this section). Thus, patients with conversion disorder should be screened for dissociative symptoms, and patients with dissociative disorder should be evaluated for conversion symptoms.

Natural History

Onset is generally from late childhood to early adulthood. Conversion disorder is rare before age 10 years (Maloney 1980) and seldom first presents after age 35 years, but it has been reported to begin as late as the ninth decade (Weddington 1979). When onset is in middle or late age, the possibility of a neurological or other medical condition is increased.

Onset of conversion disorder is generally acute, but it may be characterized by gradually increasing symptomatology. The typical course of individual conversion symptoms is generally short; half (Folks et al. 1984) to nearly all (Carter 1949) patients show a disappearance of symptoms by the time of hospital discharge. However, 20%–25% will relapse within 1 year. Factors traditionally associated with good prognosis include acute onset, presence of clearly identifiable stress at the time of onset, short interval between onset and institution of treatment, and good intelligence (Toone 1990).

In general, individual conversion symptoms are self-limited and do not lead to physical changes or disabilities. Occasionally, physical sequelae such as atrophy may occur, but this is rare. Morbidity in terms of marital and occupational impairment appears to be less than that in somatization disorder (Kent et al. 1995; Tomasson et al. 1991). In a long-term follow-up study (up to 44 years) of a small number ($N = 28$) of individuals with conversion disorder, excess mortality by unnatural causes was observed (Coryell and House 1984). None of the deaths in this study was by suicide.

Epidemiology

Conclusions regarding the epidemiology of conversion disorder are compromised by methodological differences in diagnostic boundaries as well as by ascertainment procedures from study to study. Vastly different estimates have been reported. Lifetime prevalence rates of treated conversion symptoms in general populations have ranged from 11/100,000 to 500/100,000 (Ford and Folks 1985; Toone 1990). A marked excess of women compared with men develop conversion symptoms. More than 25% of healthy postpartum and medically ill women report having had conversion symptoms some-

time during their lives (Cloninger 1994).

Approximately 5%–24% of psychiatric outpatients, 5%–14% of general hospital patients, and 1%–3% of outpatient psychiatric referrals have a history of conversion symptoms (Cloninger 1994; Ford 1983; Toone 1990). Conversion is associated with lower socioeconomic status, lower education, lack of psychological sophistication, and rural setting (Folks et al. 1984; Guze and Perley 1963; Lazare 1981; Stefansson et al. 1976; Weinstein et al. 1969). Consistent with this finding, much higher rates (nearly 10%) of outpatient psychiatric referrals in developing countries are for conversion symptoms. As countries develop, there may be a declining incidence over time, which may relate to increasing levels of education and sophistication (Stefanis et al. 1976).

Conversion disorder appears to be diagnosed more often in women than in men, with ratios varying from 2:1 (Ljundberg 1957; Stefansson et al. 1976) to 10:1 (Raskin et al. 1966). In part, this variance may relate to referral patterns, but it also appears that indeed a predominance of women compared with men develop conversion symptoms.

Etiology

An etiological hypothesis is implicit in the term *conversion*. The term conversion, in fact, is derived from the hypothesized conversion of psychological conflict into a somatic symptom. Several psychological factors have been implicated in the pathogenesis, or at least pathophysiology, of conversion disorder. However, as the following discussion will show, such etiological relationships are difficult to establish.

In *primary gain*, anxiety is theoretically reduced by keeping an internal conflict or need out of awareness by symbolic expression of an unconscious wish as a conversion symptom. However, individuals with active conversion symptoms often continue to show marked anxiety, especially on psychological tests (Lader and Sartorius 1968; Meares and Horvath 1972). Symbolism is infrequently evident, and its evaluation involves highly inferential and unreliable judgments (Raskin et al. 1966). Interpretation of symbolism in persons with occult medical disorder has been noted to contribute to misdiagnosis. *Secondary gain*, whereby conversion symptoms allow avoidance of noxious activities or the obtaining of otherwise unavailable support, also may occur in persons who have medical conditions, who often take advantage of such benefits (Raskin et al. 1966; Watson and Buranen 1979).

Individuals with conversion disorder may show a lack of concern, in keeping with the nature or implications of the symptom (the so-called *la belle indifference*). However, such indifference to symptoms is not invariably present in conversion disorder (Lewis and Berman 1965; Sharma and Chaturvedi 1995), and it also can be seen in individuals with general medical conditions (Raskin et al. 1966), sometimes as denial or stoicism (Pincus 1982). Conversion symptoms may be revealed in a dramatic or histrionic fashion. A minority of individuals with conversion disorder fulfill criteria for histrionic personality disorder. A dramatic presentation of conversion disorder can be seen in distressed individuals with medical conditions. Even symptoms based on underlying medical conditions often respond to suggestion, at least temporarily (Gatfield and Guze 1962). Patients with conversion disorder may have a history of disturbed sexuality (Lewis 1974), with many (one-third) reporting a history of sexual abuse, especially incestuous. (Thus, two-thirds do *not* report such a history.) Individuals with conversion disorder are often reported to be the youngest, or else the youngest of a sex, in sibling order, although these are not consistent findings (Stephens and Kamp 1962; Ziegler et al. 1960).

Treatment

Generally, the initial aim in treating conversion disorder is the removal of the symptom. The pressure behind accomplishing this goal depends on the distress and disability associated with the symptom (Merskey 1989). If the patient is not in particular discomfort and the need to regain function is not great, direct attention may not be necessary. In any situation, direct confrontation is not recommended. Such a communication may cause a patient to feel even more isolated. A conservative approach of reassurance and relaxation is effective. Reassurance need not come from a psychiatrist but can be performed effectively by the primary physician. Once physical illness is excluded, prognosis for conversion symptoms is good. Folks et al. (1984), for example, found that half of 50 general hospital patients with conversion symptoms showed complete remission by the time of discharge.

If symptoms do not resolve with a conservative approach and there is an immediate need for symptom resolution, several techniques, including narcoanalysis (e.g., amobarbital interview), hypnosis, and behavior therapy, may be tried (Merskey 1989). It does appear that prompt resolution of conversion symptoms is important in that the duration of conversion symptoms is associated with greater risk of recurrence and chronic disability (Cloninger 1994).

In narcoanalysis, amobarbital or another sedative-hypnotic medication such as lorazepam is given to the patient intravenously to the point of drowsiness. Sometimes this is followed by administration of a stimulant medication such as methamphetamine. The patient is then encouraged to discuss stressors and conflicts. This technique may be effective in the short term, leading to at least temporary symptom relief and expansion of the information known about the patient. This technique has not been shown to be especially effective with more chronic conversion symptoms. In hypnotic therapy, symptoms may be removed during a hypnotic state, with the suggestion that the symptoms will gradually improve posthypnotically. Information about stressors and conflicts may be explored as well. Behavior therapy, including relaxation training and even aversion therapy, has been proposed and reported by some investigators to be effective.

It is evident that it may not be the particular technique that is associated with symptom relief but the influence of suggestion. Various rituals such as exorcism and other religious ceremonies undoubtedly have led to immediate "cures." Suggestion seems to play a big part in cases of mass hysteria, in which individuals exposed to a "toxin" develop similar symptoms that do not appear to have any organic basis. Often, the epidemic can be contained if affected individuals are segregated. Simple announcements that no toxin was present and that reported "symptomatology" is linked to mass hysteria have been effective.

Anecdotal reports exist of positive response to somatic treatments such as phenothiazines, lithium, and even electroconvulsive therapy (ECT). Of course, in some cases, such a response again may be attributable to suggestion. In others, it may be that symptom removal occurred because of resolution of another psychiatric disorder, especially a mood disorder.

Thus far, the discussion on treatment of conversion disorder has centered on acute treatment primarily for symptom removal. Longer-term approaches would include strategies that were previously described for somatization disorder. These involve a pragmatic, conservative approach that entails support for and exploration of various areas of conflict, particularly interpersonal relationships. Ford (1995) suggested a treatment strategy based on "three Ps," whereby predisposing factors, precipitating stressors, and perpetuating factors are each identified and addressed. A certain degree of insight may be attained, at least in terms of appreciating relationships between various conflicts and stressors and the development of symptoms. More ambitious goals have been adopted by some in terms of long-term, intensive insight-oriented psychotherapy, especially of a psychodynamic nature. Reports of such approaches date from Freud's work with Anna O. Three studies involving a series of patients treated with psychoanalytic psychotherapy have reported success (Merskey 1989).

Hypochondriasis

Definition and Clinical Description

The essential feature in hypochondriasis is preoccupation not with symptoms themselves but rather with the fear or idea of having a serious disease, based on the misinterpretation of bodily signs and sensations. The preoccupation persists despite evidence to the contrary and reassurance from physicians. Some degree of preoccupation with disease is apparently quite common. As reviewed by Kellner (1987), 10%–20% of "normal" and 45% of "neurotic" persons have intermittent, unfounded worries about illness, with 9% of patients doubting reassurances given by physicians. In another review, Kellner (1985) estimated that 50% of all patients attending physicians' offices either "suffer…from primary hypochondriacal syndromes or have 'minor somatic disorders with hypochondriacal overlay'" (p. 822). How these estimates relate to hypochondriasis as a disorder is difficult to assess, because they do not appear to distinguish between preoccupation with symptoms (as is present in somatization disorder) and preoccupation with the implications of the symptoms (as is the case in hypochondriasis).

Diagnosis

History

Clinical descriptions of a syndrome designated *hypochondriasis* and characterized by preoccupation with bodily function can be found in the writings of the Hippocratic era (Stoudemire 1988). The Greeks attributed the syndrome to disturbances of viscera below the xiphoid cartilage, hence the term *hypochondria*. Even into the nineteenth century, the term *hypochondriasis*, unlike the topographically nonspecific concept of more recent usage, was used specifically for somatic complaints below the diaphragm (Cloninger et al. 1984). As reviewed by M.R. Murphy (1990), Gillespie, in 1928, encapsulated a concept of hypochondriasis that is essentially identical to modern concepts, emphasizing preoccupation with a disease conviction "far in excess of what is justified," implying "an indifference to the opinion of the environment, including irresponsiveness to persuasion" (p. 28). Gillespie considered hypochondriasis a discrete disease entity.

Throughout the modern period, there has been controversy over whether hypochondriasis represents an independent, discrete disease entity, as proposed by Gillespie. Kenyon (1976), in an often quoted but perhaps methodologically flawed study (see M.R. Murphy 1990), concluded that hypochondriasis was virtu-

ally always secondary to another psychiatric disorder, usually depression. Barsky and various colleagues (Barsky and Klerman 1983; Barsky et al. 1986, 1993) extensively studied patients with hypochondriacal complaints using a set of operational criteria derived from DSM-III. These authors concluded that of the many patients with such complaints, few will meet criteria for the full diagnosis. However, they noted no bimodality, suggesting that hypochondriasis represents a continuum rather than a discrete entity.

DSM-IV-TR Criteria

Specific criteria for the diagnosis of hypochondriasis are included in Table 8–4.

Differential Diagnosis

The first step in evaluating patients with hypochondriasis is to assess the possibility of physical disease. The list of serious diseases associated with the type of complaints seen in hypochondriacal patients is extensive, yet certain general categories emerge (Kellner 1985, 1987). These include neurological diseases, such as myasthenia gravis and multiple sclerosis; endocrine diseases; systemic diseases, such as SLE, that affect several organ systems; and occult malignancies.

If after appropriate assessment the probability of physical illness appears low, the condition should be considered relative to other psychiatric disorders (i.e., whether the hypochondriacal symptoms represent a primary disorder or are secondary to another psychiatric illness). As previously mentioned, one useful criterion is whether the belief is of delusional proportions. Patients with hypochondriasis as a primary disorder, although extremely preoccupied, are generally able to acknowledge the possibility that their concerns are unfounded. Delusional patients, on the other hand, are not. Hypo-

TABLE 8–4. DSM-IV-TR diagnostic criteria for hypochondriasis

A. Preoccupation with fears of having, or the idea that one has, a serious disease based on the person's misinterpretation of bodily symptoms.
B. The preoccupation persists despite appropriate medical evaluation and reassurance.
C. The belief in Criterion A is not of delusional intensity (as in delusional disorder, somatic type) and is not restricted to a circumscribed concern about appearance (as in body dysmorphic disorder).
D. The preoccupation causes clinically significant distress or impairment in social, occupational, or other important areas of functioning.
E. The duration of the disturbance is at least 6 months.
F. The preoccupation is not better accounted for by generalized anxiety disorder, obsessive-compulsive disorder, panic disorder, a major depressive episode, separation anxiety, or another somatoform disorder.

Specify if:

With Poor Insight: if, for most of the time during the current episode, the person does not recognize that the concern about having a serious illness is excessive or unreasonable

chondriasis, with poor insight, would lie somewhere in between, with the patient not recognizing that the concern is unwarranted for most of the episode. Somatic delusions of serious illness are seen in some cases of major depressive disorder and in schizophrenia. A useful discriminator is the presence of other psychiatric symptoms. A patient with hypochondriacal concerns secondary to depression should show other symptoms of depression such as sleep and appetite disturbance, feelings of worthlessness, and self-reproach, although elderly patients particularly may deny sadness or other expressions of depressed mood. Generally, schizophrenic patients will have bizarre delusions of illness (e.g., "I have congenital Hodgkin's caused by a snail hormone imbalance") and will show other signs of schizophrenia such as looseness of associations, peculiarities of thought and behavior, hallucinations, and other delusions. A confounding feature is the fact that hypochondriacal patients often will develop anxiety or depression in association with their hypochondriacal concerns. In general, characterizing the chronology of the episode will separate such patients from those with hypochondriasis.

Treatment trials also may have diagnostic significance. Depressed patients who are hypochondriacal may respond to antidepressant medication or ECT (often necessary in reversing a depressive state of sufficient severity to lead to such profound symptoms), with resolution of the hypochondriacal as well as the depressive symptoms. In schizophrenic patients, a disease-related delusion may show improvement with neuroleptic treatment. Although, if questioned carefully, the patient still may report a somatic delusion, preoccupation with the delusion will have diminished.

Natural History

Traditionally, limited data suggested that approximately one-fourth of the patients with a diagnosis of hypochondriasis do poorly, two-thirds show a chronic but fluctuating course, and one-tenth recover. However, such predictions may not reflect advances in psychopharmacology. It also must be remembered that such findings pertain to the full syndrome. A much more variable course is seen in patients who have some hypochondriacal concerns.

Epidemiology

Estimates of the frequency of hypochondriacal symptoms warranting a diagnosis are somewhat compromised in that DSM-III-R did not provide threshold criteria, other than requiring a duration of more than 6 months. The ECA study (L.N. Robins et al. 1984) did not assess for hypochondriasis. One study reported prevalence figures ranging from 3% to 13% in different cultures (Kenyon 1965), but it is not clear whether this range represented the full syndrome or just hypochondriacal symptoms. As previously mentioned, many patients have such symptoms as part of other psychiatric disorders, particularly depressive and anxiety disorders, whereas others develop transient hypochondriacal symptoms in response to stress, particularly serious physical illness.

Etiology

In considering hypochondriasis as an aspect of depression or anxiety disorders, it has been posited that these conditions create a state of hypervigilance to insult, including overperception of physical problems (Barsky and Klerman 1983).

More recently, hypochondriasis has been included by some authors in a posited "obsessive-compulsive spectrum disorder," which includes, in addition to obsessive-compulsive disorder, body dysmorphic disorder, anorexia nervosa, Tourette's disorder, and certain impulsive disorders (e.g., trichotillomania and pathological gambling; Hollander et al. 1992). This clustering is based, in part, on the phenomenological similarity of repetitive thoughts and behaviors that are difficult or impossible to delay or inhibit (Martin and Yutzy 1997).

Treatment

Patients referred early for psychiatric evaluation and treatment of hypochondriasis appear to have a better prognosis than do patients continuing with only medical evaluations and treatments (Kellner 1983). Psychiatric referral should be performed with sensitivity. Perhaps the best guideline to follow is for the referring physician to stress that the patient's distress is serious and that psychiatric evaluation will be a supplement to, not a replacement for, continued medical care.

Hypochondriacal symptoms secondary to depressive and anxiety disorders may improve with successful treatment of the primary disorder. However, until recently, hypochondriasis as a primary condition was not considered to be responsive to known psychopharmacological medications. Early results of placebo-controlled, double-blind studies are pending, but anecdotal case reports, open-label trials, and review of preliminary data reveal some promise for the selective serotonin reuptake inhibitors (SSRIs; Fallon et al. 1996). Interestingly, these medications have been shown to be effective in obsessive-compulsive disorder, and preliminary data are promising for their use in other obsessive-compulsive spectrum disorders, including body dysmorphic disorder and anorexia nervosa.

Investigators have tried many psychotherapeutic approaches in treating hypochondriasis. These may be summarized as supportive, rational, ventilative, and educative (Kellner 1987). However, no evidence shows the superiority of any one of these methods over the others. An approach suggested by Stoudemire (1988)—one that includes consistent treatment, generally by the same primary physician, with supportive, regularly scheduled office visits not based on the evaluation of symptoms—should be considered. Hospitalization, medical tests, and medications with addictive potential are to be avoided if possible. Focus during the office visits gradually should be shifted from symptoms to social or interpersonal problems. Psychotherapeutic approaches may be enhanced greatly by the promising potential of effective pharmacotherapy. Thus, there is increasing hope for attaining the overriding goal in treating hypochondriacal patients: preventing adoption of the sick role and chronic invalidism (Kellner 1987).

Body Dysmorphic Disorder

Definition and Clinical Description

The essential feature of body dysmorphic disorder is a preoccupation with some imagined defect in appearance or markedly excessive concern with a minor physical anomaly (Table 8–5). Such preoccupation persists even after reassurance. Common complaints include a diversity of imagined flaws of the face or head, such as various defects in the hair (too much or too little), skin, shape of the face, or facial features. However, any body part may be the focus, including genitals, breasts, buttocks, extremities, shoulders, and even overall body size. De Leon et al. (1989) stated that the nose, ears, face, and sexual organs are most often involved. It is not surprising, then, that patients with body dysmorphic disorder are found most commonly among persons seeking cosmetic surgery.

Diagnosis

History

The syndrome, generally under the rubric of dysmorphophobia, has a long history in the European and Japanese literature, with much less attention in the United States literature (Phillips and Hollander 1996). Because the symptoms are not really of a typical phobic nature with avoidance behavior, the condition was renamed *body dysmorphic disorder* in DSM-III-R. Debate continues as to whether body dys-

TABLE 8–5. DSM-IV-TR diagnostic criteria for body dysmorphic disorder

A. Preoccupation with an imagined defect in appearance. If a slight physical anomaly is present, the person's concern is markedly excessive.
B. The preoccupation causes clinically significant distress or impairment in social, occupational, or other important areas of functioning.
C. The preoccupation is not better accounted for by another mental disorder (e.g., dissatisfaction with body shape and size in anorexia nervosa).

morphic disorder is a discrete disorder. It is variously argued that it represents a variant of one of the major disorders, including social phobia, mood disorder, obsessive-compulsive disorder, hypochondriasis, and psychosis (particularly delusional disorder), or just the extreme of the continuum of normal concern with appearance. ICD-9 did not include the disorder. ICD-10 lists it as a type of hypochondriacal disorder. Since inclusion of body dysmorphic disorder in DSM-III-R, increased study has occurred so that the disorder is now more clearly characterized.

DSM-IV-TR Criteria

In DSM-IV-TR, the wording of the criterion "preoccupation with an imagined defect in appearance" (Table 8–5) represents a slight change from that in DSM-III-R, in which the phrase "in a normal-appearing person" was included. Because a person with some defect may have a preoccupation with a different imagined or exaggerated defect, this phrase was dropped.

As in other somatoform disorders, diagnosis requires that the preoccupation causes clinically significant distress or impairment to exclude those individuals with trivial symptoms. As is explained in the following discussion, body dysmorphic disorder is not diagnosed if the preoccupation is better accounted for by another mental disorder. On the other hand, DSM-IV-TR dropped exclusion on the basis of the preoccupation being delusional, which was included in DSM-III-R and in ICD-10.

Differential Diagnosis

By definition, body dysmorphic disorder is not diagnosed when the body preoccupation is better accounted for by another mental disorder. Anorexia nervosa, in which there is dissatisfaction with body shape and size, is specifically mentioned in the criteria as an example of such an exclusion. In DSM-III-R, transsexualism (gender identity disorder in DSM-IV-TR) also was mentioned as such a disorder. Although not specifically mentioned in DSM-IV, if a preoccupation is limited to discomfort or a sense of inappropriateness of one's primary and secondary sex characteristics, coupled with a strong and persistent cross-gender identification, body dysmorphic disorder would not be diagnosed. Diagnostic problems may develop when a patient has the mood-congruent ruminations of major depression (e.g., preoccupation with a perceived unattractive appearance in association with poor self-esteem). However, such concerns generally lack the focus on a particular body part that is seen in body dysmorphic disorder. Somatic obsessions and even grooming or cleaning rituals in obsessive-compulsive disorder may suggest body dysmorphic disorder; however, in such cases, other obsessions and compulsions are seen as well. In body dysmorphic disorder, the preoccupations are limited to concerns with appearance. Preoccupations in body dysmorphic disorder may reach delusional proportions, and patients with this disorder may show ideas of ref-

erence regarding defects in their appearance, which may lead to consideration of the diagnosis of schizophrenia. However, bizarre delusions and hallucinations are not seen in patients with body dysmorphic disorder. From the other perspective, schizophrenic patients with somatic delusions generally do not focus on a specific defect in appearance.

Unlike the diagnostic guideline for hypochondriasis, if the preoccupation is of psychotic proportions, a diagnosis of body dysmorphic disorder still can be made. De Leon et al. (1989) point out the difficulties in determining whether a dysmorphophobic concern is delusional or not. They suggest that cases be classified as "primary dysmorphophobia" without attempting to distinguish between delusional and nondelusional concerns, as long as schizophrenia, major depression, and organic mental disorders are excluded. This point of view was adopted in DSM-IV (Phillips and Hollander 1996). In body dysmorphic disorder, it appears that a continuum exists between preoccupations and delusions, and thus it is difficult, if not impossible, to draw a discrete boundary between body dysmorphic disorder and delusional disorder, somatic type. Furthermore, individual patients seem to move along this continuum. Thus, it was decided to allow both diagnoses if a dysmorphic preoccupation was delusional.

Patients with body dysmorphic disorder often isolate themselves, and social phobia may be suspected. However, in social phobia alone the person may feel self-conscious but will not focus on a specific imagined defect. Persons with histrionic personality disorder may be vain and excessively concerned with appearance. However, in this disorder, the focus is on maintaining a good or even an exceptional appearance rather than preoccupation with a defect.

Natural History

Onset of body dysmorphic disorder peaks in adolescence or early adulthood (Phillips 1991). The disorder is generally a chronic condition, with a waxing and waning of intensity but rarely full remission (Phillips et al. 1993). Over a lifetime, multiple preoccupations are typical. (In their study, Phillips et al. 1993 found an average of four.) In some people, the same preoccupation remains unchanged; in others, preoccupations with newly perceived defects are added to the original ones. In some individuals, symptoms remit only to be replaced by others.

Body dysmorphic disorder is highly incapacitating. Almost all persons with this disorder show marked impairment in social and occupational activities. About 75% will never marry, and among those who do, most will divorce (Phillips 1995). Perhaps a third will become housebound. Most attribute their limitations to embarrassment concerning their "defect." The extent to which patients with body dysmorphic disorder receive surgery or medical treatments is unknown. Superimposed depressive episodes are common, as are suicidal ideation and suicide attempts. The actual suicide risk is unknown.

Epidemiology

The lifetime risk of body dysmorphic disorder in the general population is unknown. Although body dysmorphic disorder is seldom encountered in psychiatric settings, Andreasen and Bardach (1977) estimated that 2% of the patients seeking corrective cosmetic surgery have this disorder. Generally, patients with body dysmorphic disorder are seen psychiatrically only after referral from plastic surgery, dermatology, and otorhinolaryngology clinics (De Leon et al. 1989). The male-to-female ratio is about 1:1 (Phillips 1995).

Etiology

Traditionally, little emphasis was devoted to etiological possibilities other than suggested relationships to underlying mood disorders, schizophrenia, obsessive-compulsive disorder, or social phobia. More recently, body dysmorphic disorder has been included with a posited obsessive-compulsive spectrum disorder and with delusional disorders for which a variety of biological pathologies have been proffered (Phillips et al. 1995). The latter association is reflected in DSM-IV-TR's allowing both disorders to be diagnosed in the same patient for the same symptoms.

Treatment

Simply recognizing that a complaint derives from body dysmorphic disorder may have therapeutic benefit by interrupting an unending procession of repeated evaluations by physicians and eliminating the possibility of needless surgery. Surgery actually has been recommended as a treatment for this disorder, but there is no clear evidence that it is helpful. There is a long history of anecdotal reports suggesting the value of diverse treatments, including behavior therapy, dynamic psychotherapy, and pharmacotherapy. Recommended medications include neuroleptics and antidepressants (De Leon et al. 1989). Response to neuroleptic treatment has been suggested as a diagnostic test to distinguish body dysmorphic disorder from delusional disorder, somatic type (Riding and Munro 1975). Delusional syndromes, in general, may respond to neuroleptics, whereas in body dysmorphic disorder, even when the bodily preoccupations are psychotic, there is less likelihood of success. Pimozide has been singled out as a neuroleptic having specific effectiveness for somatic delusions, but this drug does not appear to be any more effective than other neuroleptics in treating body dysmorphic disorder.

In earlier reports, it was not clear if reported response to antidepressant drugs or ECT was due to amelioration of dysmorphic symptoms per se or to improvement in depressive symptoms. Several studies have suggested that SSRIs, including fluoxetine, fluvoxamine, and clomipramine, have been effective in treating the disorder (Hollander et al. 1993; Phillips et al. 1993). Patients showing a partial response to the SSRI may benefit further from augmentation with buspirone. Improvement with SSRIs seems to be a primary effect in that response was not predicted on the basis of coexisting major depression or obsessive-compulsive disorder. Also of note are observations that patients with somatic delusions may respond to SSRIs.

Somatoform Disorder Not Otherwise Specified

Definition and Clinical Description

Somatoform disorder NOS is the true residual category for the somatoform disorders. By definition, conditions included under this category are characterized by somatoform symptoms that do not meet the criteria for any of the specified somatoform disorders. DSM-IV-TR gives several examples, but syndromes potentially included under this category are not limited to those examples. Unlike undifferentiated somatoform disorder, no minimum duration is required. In fact, some disorders may be relegated to NOS because they do not meet the time requirements for a specified somatoform disorder.

Diagnosis

DSM-IV-TR Criteria

The basic DSM-IV-TR requirement for a diagnosis of somatoform disorder NOS is

that a disorder with somatoform symptoms does not meet criteria for a specified somatoform disorder. The first example listed in DSM-IV-TR is pseudocyesis. In DSM-III and DSM-III-R, pseudocyesis was included as a conversion disorder under criteria broadened to include any alteration or loss of physical functioning, suggesting a physical disorder that was an expression of psychological conflict or need. After contraction of conversion disorder to voluntary motor and sensory dysfunction in DSM-IV, pseudocyesis was excluded and relegated to the NOS category. Oddly enough, pseudocyesis lends itself to a quite specific definition (see Table 8–6). However, given its rarity, pseudocyesis is not listed as a specified somatoform disorder.

Two other examples given are syndromes that resemble specified somatoform syndromes, somatization disorder, undifferentiated somatoform disorder, or hypochondriasis but have a duration less than the required 6 months. An additional example is a condition described as involving complaints such as fatigue or body weakness not due to another mental disorder, again with a duration of less than 6 months. Such a syndrome would resemble neurasthenia, a syndrome with a long historical tradition. Included in DSM-II (American Psychiatric Association 1968), ICD-9, and ICD-10, neurasthenia was considered for inclusion as a specified DSM-IV somatoform disorder. After careful review, neurasthenia was not adopted because it was difficult to delineate from depressive, anxiety, and other somatoform disorders, and there was a lack of systematic study supporting it. Finally, there was concern that neurasthenia would become a wastebasket category, the availability of which might promote premature closure of the diagnostic process so that other mental disorders, as well as other general medical disorders, would be overlooked.

TABLE 8–6. DSM-IV-TR diagnostic criteria for somatoform disorder not otherwise specified

This category includes disorders with somatoform symptoms that do not meet the criteria for any specific somatoform disorder. Examples include

1. Pseudocyesis: a false belief of being pregnant that is associated with objective signs of pregnancy, which may include abdominal enlargement (although the umbilicus does not become everted), reduced menstrual flow, amenorrhea, subjective sensation of fetal movement, nausea, breast engorgement and secretions, and labor pains at the expected date of delivery. Endocrine changes may be present, but the syndrome cannot be explained by a general medical condition that causes endocrine changes (e.g., a hormone-secreting tumor).
2. A disorder involving nonpsychotic hypochondriacal symptoms of less than 6 months' duration.
3. A disorder involving unexplained physical complaints (e.g., fatigue or body weakness) of less than 6 months' duration that are not due to another mental disorder.

Differential Diagnosis

As mentioned in the preceding discussion, DSM-IV-TR lists several syndromes that, if not for their short duration, would qualify for a diagnosis as the specified somatoform disorder that they resemble.

Epidemiology, Etiology, and Treatment

Discussion of epidemiology, etiology, and treatment for a residual category such as somatoform disorder NOS would not be meaningful because it represents a grouping of diverse disorders. Conditions that would warrant diagnosis of a specified somatoform disorder except for their insufficient duration (less than 6 months) are probably best considered to be in the spectrum of the resembled disorder. Thus, the epidemiological, etiological, and treatment considerations pertaining to the specified disorder should be reviewed because these may apply, at least in part, to the shorter-duration syndromes.

In a comprehensive review of pseudocyesis, Small (1986) stated: "Of all that has been written on the subject [of pseudocyesis], therapy is least discussed." In another report, Whelan and Stewart (1990) emphasized two principles in treating pseudocyesis. First, the patient is to be clearly, yet "empathically" advised that she (or the rare he) is not pregnant. If such simple advice is not effective, objective procedures such as ultrasound are recommended to demonstrate to the patient that there is no visible evidence of a fetus. Alternatively, menses are to be induced. Remarkably, such straightforward approaches are often effective (Cohen 1982). According to Whelan and Stewart (1990), the second principle, which goes hand in hand with the first, is that the patient's expectations, fears, and fantasies should be explored to discover the reason that the false pregnancy was "needed." They also advised providing a face-saving resolution to the patient's lack of pregnancy, such as allowing the patient to take the position that a "miscarriage" has occurred. However, systematic data on the effectiveness of these and other approaches are lacking. Whatever the therapy, relapses are common. According to Ford (1995), there are limited data on the prognosis for women with pseudocyesis. Concomitant disorders such as major depression should be treated in the usual manner.

Conclusions

Syndromes now subsumed under the rubric "somatoform disorders" have had a tortuous course in the evolution of psychiatric nosology and therapy. Yet, they are extremely important because they are disorders that must be differentiated from conditions with identifiable, and often treatable, physical bases.

Developments in the past decade are encouraging. Coordinated effort has been made to establish a common, globally used nomenclature. Somatoform disorders as delineated in DSM-IV-TR are compatible with, although not identical to, counterparts in ICD-10. A common and more explicitly defined nosology is conducive to empirical research that is truly comparable from one investigation to the next. Initial observations on the pharmacological treatment of several of the disorders, namely hypochondriasis and body dysmorphic disorder, are promising and not only may add to our therapeutic armamentarium but also may suggest avenues for improved pathophysiological as well as etiological understanding of these two somatoform disorders.

Ultimately, it may prove possible to obtain a better understanding of the somatoform disorders, a group of complex, incapacitating disorders. Better understanding should facilitate more effective treatments. Already, there has been some preliminary discussion regarding the development of practice guidelines for somatoform disorders. Consideration of guidelines would have been highly unlikely even a few years ago.

References

Alexander F: Psychosomatic Medicine: Its Principles and Applications. New York, WW Norton, 1950

American Psychiatric Association: Diagnostic and Statistical Manual of Mental Disorders, 2nd Edition. Washington, DC, American Psychiatric Association, 1968

American Psychiatric Association: Diagnostic and Statistical Manual of Mental Disorders, 3rd Edition. Washington, DC, American Psychiatric Association, 1980

American Psychiatric Association: Diagnostic and Statistical Manual of Mental Disorders, 3rd Edition, Revised. Washington, DC, American Psychiatric Association, 1987

American Psychiatric Association: Diagnostic and Statistical Manual of Mental Disorders, 4th Edition. Washington, DC, American Psychiatric Association, 1994

American Psychiatric Association: Diagnostic and Statistical Manual of Mental Disorders, 4th Edition, Primary Care Version. Washington, DC, American Psychiatric Association, 1995

American Psychiatric Association: Diagnostic and Statistical Manual of Mental Disorders, 4th Edition, Text Revision. Washington, DC, American Psychiatric Association, 2000

Andreasen NC, Bardach J: Dysmorphophobia: symptom or disease? Am J Psychiatry 134:673–676, 1977

Barsky AJ, Klerman GL: Overview: hypochondriasis, bodily complaints, and somatic styles. Am J Psychiatry 140:273–283, 1983

Barsky AJ, Wyshak G, Klerman GL: Hypochondriasis: an evaluation of the DSM-III criteria in medical outpatients. Arch Gen Psychiatry 43:493–500, 1986

Barsky AJ, Cleary PD, Sarnie MK, et al: The course of transient hypochondriasis. Am J Psychiatry 150:484–488, 1993

Bass CM, Murphy MR: Somatization disorder: critique of the concept and suggestions for future research, in Somatization: Physical Symptoms and Psychological Illness. Edited by Bass C. Oxford, England, Blackwell Scientific, 1990, pp 301–332

Breuer J, Freud S: Studies on hysteria (1893–1895), in the Standard Edition of the Complete Psychological Works of Sigmund Freud, Vol 2. Translated and edited by Strachey J. London, England, Hogarth, 1955, pp 1–311

Carter AB: The prognosis of certain hysterical symptoms. BMJ 1:1076–1079, 1949

Cloninger CR: Diagnosis of somatoform disorders: a critique of DSM-III, in Diagnosis and Classification in Psychiatry: A Critical Appraisal of DSM-III. Edited by Tischler GL. New York, Cambridge University Press, 1987, pp 243–259

Cloninger CR: Somatoform and dissociative disorders, in The Medical Basis of Psychiatry, 2nd Edition. Edited by Winokur G, Clayton P. Philadelphia, PA, WB Saunders, 1994, pp 169–192

Cloninger CR, Guze SB: Psychiatric illness and female criminality: the role of sociopathy and hysteria in the antisocial woman. Am J Psychiatry 127:303–311, 1970

Cloninger CR, Yutzy S: Somatoform and dissociative disorders: a summary of changes for DSM-IV, in Current Psychiatric Therapy. Edited by Dunner DL. Philadelphia, PA, WB Saunders, 1993, pp 310–313

Cloninger CR, Reich T, Guze SB: The multifactorial model of disease transmission, III: familial relationship between sociopathy and hysteria (Briquet's syndrome). Br J Psychiatry 127:23–32, 1975

Cloninger CR, Sigvardsson S, von Knorring AL, et al: An adoption study of somatoform disorders, II: identification of two discrete somatoform disorders. Arch Gen Psychiatry 41:863–871, 1984

Cloninger CR, Martin RL, Guze SB, et al: A prospective follow-up and family study of somatization in men and women. Am J Psychiatry 143:873–878, 1986

Cloninger CR, Bayon C, Przybeck TR: Epidemiology and Axis I comorbidity of antisocial personality, in Handbook of Antisocial Behavior. Edited by Stoff DM, Breiling J, Maser JD. New York, Wiley, 1997, pp 12–21

Cohen LM: A current perspective of pseudocyesis. Am J Psychiatry 139:1140–1144, 1982

Coryell W, House D: The validity of broadly defined hysteria and DSM-III conversion disorder: outcome, family history, and mortality. J Clin Psychiatry 45:252–256, 1984

De Leon J, Bott A, Simpson GM: Dysmorphophobia: body dysmorphic disorder or delusional disorder, somatic subtype? Compr Psychiatry 30:457–472, 1989

Desai BT, Porter RJ, Penry K: Psychogenic seizures: a study of 42 attacks in six patients, with intensive monitoring. Arch Neurol 39:202–209, 1982

DeSouza C, Othmer E, Gabrielli W Jr, et al: Major depression and somatization disorder: the overlooked differential diagnosis. Psychiatr Ann 18:340–348, 1988

Escobar JI, Swartz M, Rubio-Stipec M, et al: Medically unexplained symptoms: distribution, risk factors, and comorbidity, in Current Concepts of Somatization: Research and Clinical Perspectives. Edited by Kirmayer LJ, Robbins JM. Washington, DC, American Psychiatric Press, 1991, pp 63–78

Fallon BA, Schneir FR, Narshall R, et al: The pharmacotherapy of hypochondriasis. Psychopharmacol Bull 32:607–611, 1996

Folks DG, Ford CV, Regan WM: Conversion symptoms in a general hospital. Psychosomatics 25:285–295, 1984

Ford CV: The Somatizing Disorders: Illness as a Way of Life. New York, Elsevier, 1983

Ford CV: Conversion disorder and somatoform disorder not otherwise specified, in Treatment of Psychiatric Disorders, 2nd Edition. Edited by Gabbard GO. Washington, DC, American Psychiatric Press, 1995, pp 1737–1753

Ford CV, Folks DG: Conversion disorders: an overview. Psychosomatics 26:371–383, 1985

Gatfield PD, Guze SB: Prognosis and differential diagnosis of conversion reactions (a follow-up study). Diseases of the Nervous System 23:623–631, 1962

Goodwin DW, Guze SB: Psychiatric Diagnosis, 5th Edition. New York, Oxford University Press, 1996

Guze SB, Perley MJ: Observations on the natural history of hysteria. Am J Psychiatry 119:960–965, 1963

Guze SB, Cloninger CR, Martin RL, et al: A follow-up and family study of Briquet's syndrome. Br J Psychiatry 149:17–23, 1986

Hathaway SR, McKinley JC: Minnesota Multiphasic Personality Schedule. Minneapolis, MN, University of Minnesota Press, 1943

Hollander E, Neville D, Frenkel M, et al: Body dysmorphic disorder: diagnostic issues and related disorders. Psychosomatics 33:156–165, 1992

Hollander E, Cohen LJ, Simeon D: Body dysmorphic disorder. Psychiatr Ann 23:359–364, 1993

Hudziak JJ, Boffeli TJ, Kreisman JJ, et al: Clinical study of the relation of borderline personality disorder to Briquet's syndrome (hysteria), somatization disorder, antisocial personality disorder, and substance abuse disorders. Am J Psychiatry 153:1598–1606, 1996

Kellner R: The prognosis of treated hypochondriasis: a clinical study. Acta Psychiatr Scand 67:69–79, 1983

Kellner R: Functional somatic symptoms and hypochondriasis: a survey of empirical studies. Arch Gen Psychiatry 42:821–833, 1985

Kellner R: Hypochondriasis and somatization. JAMA 258:2718–2722, 1987

Kellner R: Somatization disorder, in Treatments of Psychiatric Disorders: A Task Force Report of the American Psychiatric Association, Vol 3. Washington, DC, American Psychiatric Association, 1989, pp 2166–2171

Kent D, Tomasson K, Coryell W: Course and outcome of conversion and somatization disorders: a four-year follow-up. Psychosomatics 36:138–144, 1995

Kenyon FE: Hypochondriasis: a survey of some historical, clinical, and social aspects. Br J Psychiatry 138:117–133, 1965

Kenyon FE: Hypochondriacal states. Br J Psychiatry 129:1–14, 1976

Kirmayer LJ, Robbins JM, Dworkind M, et al: Somatization and the recognition of depression and anxiety in primary care. Am J Psychiatry 150:734–741, 1993

Lader M, Sartorius N: Anxiety in patients with hysterical conversion symptoms. J Neurol Neurosurg Psychiatry 31:490–495, 1968

Lazare A: Conversion symptoms. N Engl J Med 305:745–748, 1981

Lewis WC: Hysteria: the consultant's dilemma: twentieth century demonology, pejorative epithet, or useful diagnosis? Arch Gen Psychiatry 30:145–151, 1974

Lewis WC, Berman M: Studies of conversion hysteria, I: operational study of diagnosis. Arch Gen Psychiatry 13:275–282, 1965

Ljundberg L: Hysteria: clinical, prognostic and genetic study. Acta Psychiatr Scand Suppl 32:1–162, 1957

Luff MC, Garrod M: The after-results of psychotherapy in 500 adult cases. BMJ 2:54–59, 1935

Mace CJ, Trimble MR: Ten-year prognosis of conversion disorder. Br J Psychiatry 169:282–288, 1996

Maloney MJ: Diagnosing hysterical conversion disorders in children. J Pediatr 97:1016–1020, 1980

Marsden CD: Hysteria: a neurologist's view. Psychol Med 16:277–288, 1986

Martin RL: Problems in the diagnosis of somatization disorder: effects on research and clinical practice. Psychiatr Ann 18:357–362, 1988

Martin RL, Yutzy SH: Somatoform disorders, in Psychiatry. Edited by Tasman A, Kay J, Lieberman JA. Philadelphia, PA, WB Saunders, 1997, pp 1119–1155

Martin RL, Cloninger CR, Guze SB: The evaluation of diagnostic concordance in follow-up studies, II: a blind prospective follow-up of female criminals. J Psychiatr Res 15:107–125, 1979

Martin RL, Cloninger CR, Guze SB, et al: Mortality in a follow-up of 500 psychiatric outpatients, II: cause-specific mortality. Arch Gen Psychiatry 42:58–66, 1985

Meares R, Horvath T: "Acute" and "chronic" hysteria. Br J Psychiatry 121:653–657, 1972

Merskey H: Conversion disorder, in Treatments of Psychiatric Disorders: A Task Force Report of the American Psychiatric Association, Vol 3. Washington, DC, American Psychiatric Association, 1989, pp 2152–2159

Murphy GE: The clinical management of hysteria. JAMA 247:2559–2564, 1982

Murphy GE, Guze SB: Setting limits. Am J Psychother 14:30–47, 1960

Murphy GE, Wetzel RD: Family history of suicidal behavior among suicide attempters. J Nerv Ment Dis 170:86–90, 1982

Murphy MR: Classification of the somatoform disorders, in Somatization: Physical Symptoms and Psychological Illness. Edited by Bass C. Oxford, England, Blackwell Scientific, 1990, pp 10–39

Perley M, Guze SB: Hysteria: the stability and usefulness of clinical criteria: a quantitative study based upon a 6–8 year follow-up of 39 patients. N Engl J Med 266:421–426, 1962

Phillips KA: Body dysmorphic disorder: the distress of imagined ugliness. Am J Psychiatry 148:1138–1149, 1991

Phillips KA: Body dysmorphic disorder: clinical features and drug treatment. CNS Drugs 3:30–40, 1995

Phillips KA, Hollander E: Body dysmorphic disorder, in DSM-IV Sourcebook, Vol 2. Edited by Widiger TA, Frances AJ, Pincus HA, et al. Washington, DC, American Psychiatric Press, 1996, pp 949–960

Phillips KA, McElroy SL, Keck PE Jr, et al: Body dysmorphic disorder: 30 cases of imagined ugliness. Am J Psychiatry 150:302–308, 1993

Phillips KA, Kim JM, Hudson JI: Body image disturbance in body dysmorphic disorder and eating disorders: obsessions or delusions? Psychiatr Clin North Am 18:317–334, 1995

Pincus J: Hysteria presenting to a neurologist, in Hysteria. Edited by Roy A. London, England, Wiley, 1982, pp 131–144

Pribor EF, Smith DS, Yutzy SH: Somatization disorder in the elderly. Am J Geriatr Psychiatry 2:109–117, 1994

Quill TE: Somatization disorder: one of medicine's blind spots. JAMA 254:3075–3079, 1985

Raskin M, Talbott JA, Meyerson AT: Diagnosis of conversion reactions: predictive value of psychiatric criteria. JAMA 197:530–534, 1966

Riding J, Munro A: Pimozide in the treatment of monosymptomatic hypochondriacal psychosis. Acta Psychiatr Scand 52:23–30, 1975

Robins LN, Helzer JE, Croughan J, et al: National Institute of Mental Health Diagnostic Interview Schedule: its history, characteristics, and validity. Arch Gen Psychiatry 38:381–389, 1981

Robins LN, Helzer JE, Weissman MM, et al: Lifetime prevalence of specific psychiatric disorders in three sites. Arch Gen Psychiatry 41:949–958, 1984

Scallet A, Cloninger CR, Othmer E: The management of chronic hysteria: a review and double-blind trial of electrosleep and other relaxation methods. Diseases of the Nervous System 37:347–353, 1976

Sharma P, Chaturvedi SK: Conversion disorder revisited. Acta Psychiatr Scand 92:301–304, 1995

Slater ETO, Glithero C: A follow-up of patients diagnosed as suffering from "hysteria." J Psychosom Res 9:9–13, 1965

Small GW: Pseudocyesis: an overview. Can J Psychiatry 31:452–457, 1986

Smith GR Jr, Monson RA, Ray DC: Psychiatric consultation in somatization disorder: a randomized controlled study. N Engl J Med 314:1407–1413, 1986

Stefanis C, Markidis M, Christodoulou G: Observations on the evolution of the hysterical symptomatology. Br J Psychiatry 128:269–275, 1976

Stefansson JH, Messina JA, Meyerowitz S: Hysterical neurosis, conversion type: clinical and epidemiological considerations. Acta Psychiatr Scand 59:119–138, 1976

Stephens JH, Kamp M: On some aspects of hysteria: a clinical study. J Nerv Ment Dis 134:305–315, 1962

Stern J, Murphy M, Bass C: Personality disorders in patients with somatization disorder: a controlled study. Br J Psychiatry 163:785–789, 1993

Stoudemire GA: Somatoform disorders, factitious disorders, and malingering, in American Psychiatric Press Textbook of Psychiatry. Edited by Talbott JA, Hales RE, Yudofsky SC. Washington, DC, American Psychiatric Press, 1988, pp 533–556

Tomasson K, Kent D, Coryell W: Somatization and conversion disorders: comorbidity and demographics at presentation. Acta Psychiatr Scand 84:288–293, 1991

Toone BK: Disorders of hysterical conversion, in Physical Symptoms and Psychological Illness. Edited by Bass C. London, England, Blackwell Scientific, 1990, pp 207–234

Torack RM: Historical overview of dementia, in The Pathologic Physiology of Dementia. Edited by Torack RA. New York, Springer-Verlag, 1978, pp 1–16

Vaillant GE: The disadvantages of DSM-III outweigh its advantages. Am J Psychiatry 141:542–545, 1984

Watson CG, Buranen C: The frequency and identification of false positive conversion reactions. J Nerv Ment Dis 167:243–247, 1979

Weddington WW: Conversion reaction in an 82-year-old man. J Nerv Ment Dis 167:368–369, 1979

Weinstein EA, Eck RA, Lyerly OG: Conversion hysteria in Appalachia. Psychiatry 32:334–341, 1969

Wetzel RD, Guze SB, Cloninger CR, et al: Briquet's syndrome (hysteria) is both a somatoform and a "psychoform" illness: an MMPI study. Psychosom Med 56:564–569, 1994

Whelan CI, Stewart DE: Pseudocyesis: a review and report of six cases. Int J Psychiatry Med 20:97–108, 1990

Woerner PI, Guze SB: A family and marital study of hysteria. Br J Psychiatry 114:161–168, 1968

Woodruff RA, Clayton PJ, Guze SB: Hysteria: studies of diagnosis, outcome, and prevalence. JAMA 215:425–428, 1971

World Health Organization: International Statistical Classification of Diseases and Related Health Problems, 10th Revision. Geneva, Switzerland, World Health Organization, 1992b

World Health Organization: Diagnostic and Management Guidelines for Mental Disorders in Primary Care: ICD-10 Chapter V Primary Care Version. Gottingen, Germany, Hogrefe & Huber, 1996

Yutzy SH, Cloninger CR, Guze SB, et al: The DSM-IV field trial: somatization disorder: testing a new proposal. Am J Psychiatry 152:97–101, 1995

Ziegler FJ, Imboden JB, Meyer E: Contemporary conversion reactions: a clinical study. Am J Psychiatry 116:901–910, 1960

CHAPTER 9

Factitious Disorders and Malingering

Martin H. Leamon, M.D.

Marc D. Feldman, M.D.

Charles L. Scott, M.D.

Factitious Disorder

Introduction

Factitious disorder is characterized by a person intentionally fabricating or inducing signs or symptoms of other illnesses solely to become identified as "ill" or as a "patient." Such patients have been described in medical writing throughout history (Feldman et al. 1994; Gavin 1843) and throughout the world (Bappal et al. 2001; Cizza et al. 1996; Linde 1996; Mizuta et al. 2000; Seersholm et al. 1991). The concept became firmly established in modern medical thinking in 1951 when Asher (1951) described what has since been classified a subtype of factitious disorders, Munchausen syndrome. In many patients, factitious disorders remain undiagnosed, and even when recognized, they often go untreated (Toth and Baggaley 1991). Yet, factitious disorders cause significant morbidity and mortality (Baker and Major 1994; Folks 1995; Higgins 1990), consume an astonishing amount of medical resources (Feldman 1994a;

Frumkin and Victoroff 1990; Higgins 1990; Powell and Boast 1993a; Schwarz et al. 1993), and cause significant emotional distress in the patients themselves, in their caregivers, and in their close relationships (Feldman and Smith 1996). Over the past decade, the literature about factitious disorders has expanded, with the publication of lay and professional books on the topic (Feldman and Eisendrath 1996; Feldman et al. 1994) and the establishment of a factitious disorders Web site (http://munchausen.com; Feldman 2003).

Classification

DSM-IV-TR (American Psychiatric Association 2000) requires three criteria for the diagnosis of factitious disorder (Table 9–1). The first, the intentional production or feigning of physical or psychological signs or symptoms, distinguishes factitious disorder from the somatoform disorders, in which physical symptoms are viewed as unconsciously produced. The second and third criteria, that the motivation for the behavior is to assume the sick

TABLE 9–1. DSM-IV-TR diagnostic criteria for factitious disorder

A. Intentional production or feigning of physical or psychological signs or symptoms.
B. The motivation for the behavior is to assume the sick role.
C. External incentives for the behavior (such as economic gain, avoiding legal responsibility, or improving physical well-being, as in Malingering) are absent.

Code based on type:

300.16 With Predominantly Psychological Signs and Symptoms: if psychological signs and symptoms predominate in the clinical presentation

300.19 With Predominantly Physical Signs and Symptoms: if physical signs and symptoms predominate in the clinical presentation

300.19 With Combined Psychological and Physical Signs and Symptoms: if both psychological and physical signs and symptoms are present but neither predominates in the clinical presentation

role and that external incentives for the behavior are absent, distinguish factitious disorder from malingering.

DSM-IV-TR classifies the disorder on the basis of the predominant type of factitious symptom presented—physical or psychological. Individual case histories (Bauer and Boegner 1996; Craddock and Brown 1993; Miner and Feldman 1998) suggest that this categorization may be somewhat arbitrary because the same patient may have different presentations across time. Rogers et al. (1989) also raised epistemological objections to this subtyping, arguing, in part, that factitious disorder with predominantly psychological signs and symptoms confers a psychiatric disorder to someone who, by definition, is merely pretending to have one. The fourth subtype is factitious disorder not otherwise specified. This code should be used

for disorders with factitious symptoms that do not meet criteria for one of the other subtypes. An example is factitious disorder by proxy (discussed in the "Factitious Disorder by Proxy" section later in this chapter).

Other authors have used different typologies. Nadelson (1979) distinguished between factitious disorders of the Munchausen and the non-Munchausen type. This typology may have prognostic and treatment implications. *Munchausen syndrome*, a term coined by Asher (1951), accounts for about 10% of patients with factitious disorders (Eisendrath 1994). In this special type of factitious disorder, multiple hospitalizations with dramatic and often life-threatening presentations, wandering from hospital to hospital (peregrination), and pathological lying (*pseudologia fantastica*, the telling of dramatic tales that merge truth and falsehood and that the listener initially finds intriguing) are prominent. Asher, using the anglicized spelling, drew the term from Rudolf Erich Raspe's 1784 book, *Baron Münchhausen's Narrative of His Marvelous Travels and Campaigns in Russia* (Carswell 1950), a whimsical account of the adventures of a real-life German cavalry officer in the Russian army, Baron Karl Friedrich Hieronymous von Münchhausen (1720–1797).

Other expressions concerning patients of this type have been quite colorful but often with derogatory overtones: *peregrinating problem patients* (Chapman 1957) and, for a subset of plastic surgery patients, *the SHAFT syndrome* (Kasdan et al. 1998).

The vast majority of factitious disorder patients are of the non-Munchausen type. Characterized by several authors (Carney 1980; Ford 1986; Freyberger et al. 1994; Guziec et al. 1994; Plassmann 1994b; Reich and Gottfried 1983), these patients are mostly young women with conforming lifestyles and more family support and involvement than Munchausen patients. These patients have been described as passive and immature, and a significant proportion have health-related jobs or training. Most are not wanderers, have single-system complaints, and generate fewer hospitalizations than do Munchausen patients, but the overall severity and morbidity of their illness may be just as great (Sutherland and Rodin 1990).

Others (Eisendrath 1996; Overholser 1990) have classified patients with factitious disorders according to the manner in which illness is simulated and by the type of simulated illness. Patients may simply report invented symptoms and false medical histories (Feldman 2000), or they may exaggerate symptoms. They may manipulate diagnostic instruments to give false readings (Aduan et al. 1979; Ludwigs et al. 1994) or tamper with laboratory specimens. Finally, they may purposefully cause actual tissue damage or biochemical abnormalities in their bodies, either inducing new injury or exacerbating existing conditions.

Classification by type of simulated illness is most useful to the clinician who begins to suspect factitious illness and who then looks for evidence to support the suspicion. Wallach (1994) and Nordmeyer (1994) give thorough descriptions of presentations of factitious illness in the different organ systems and some suggestions for their detection. Almost any conceivable condition can be simulated, depending on the knowledge, motivation, creativity, and covert skill of the patient. An exhaustive list of the medical disorders that have been feigned or produced by patients with factitious disorder would approximate the index of a pathology textbook (Feldman et al. 2001).

Diagnosis

Many factors can suggest a diagnosis of factitious disorder (Freyberger et al. 1994;

Popli et al. 1992). There can be discrepancies between objective findings (Ziv et al. 1998), or objective findings might be inconsistent with clinical history or symptoms. The illness course could be markedly atypical, or the condition can fail to respond as expected to usual therapies. A patient may be unusually acquiescent to invasive diagnostic studies or may be unusually quarrelsome and argumentative with staff, particularly when it comes to trying to obtain old records to confirm history. A patient who describes a flamboyant, fascinating life with connections to well-known people may nevertheless have no visitors or callers.

These indicators notwithstanding, verification of the DSM-IV-TR diagnostic criteria can be problematic. The first criterion requires that the patient be feigning or intentionally producing illness. The physician becomes a detective, working against the patient's overt desires, trying to discover the ruse. This role shift destabilizes the relationship (Paar 1994). The dilemma is especially complex when patients have combinations of feigned and actual illness (Nordmeyer 1994; Sutherland and Rodin 1990) or develop an actual illness in the attempt to simulate one. Additionally, some general medical conditions may be difficult to diagnose initially, leading to an erroneous clinical impression of fabricated symptoms (Baddley et al. 1998; Koo et al. 1996). Other illnesses, such as multiple sclerosis or systemic lupus erythematosus, may have fluctuating courses, or in themselves produce inconsistent findings (Liebson et al. 1996).

The DSM-IV-TR criteria also require that the feigning be intentional. Psychoses (Gielder 1994), mood disorders (Roy and Roy 1995), and dissociative disorders (Goodwin 1988; Toth and Baggaley 1991) need to be ruled out as alternative etiologies. The hunt for intentionality raises ethical and legal issues of informed consent, right to privacy, and malpractice (Frumkin and Victoroff 1990; Houck 1992; Markantonakis and Lee 1988; Powell and Boast 1993a). Almost by definition, patients with factitious disorders deny their simulations. Rather than being proved irrefutably, intentionality is more likely to be inferred through a process of diagnostic and treatment procedures that "confirm the absence" of any naturally occurring disease process that can account for the observed physical problem (Dixon and Abbey 1995; Feldman et al. 2001).

Furthermore, the patient's specific motivation must be "to assume the sick role" (American Psychiatric Association 2000). Yet such patients often are unaware of their motivations, despite being aware of their role in producing their illness (Bhugra 1988; Eisendrath 1996). Patients can be extremely resistant to psychological inquiry or may prematurely leave the hospital (Bauer and Boegner 1996), rendering psychological motivational assessment incomplete (Baker and Major 1994; Churchill et al. 1994; Harrington et al. 1990; Topazian and Binder 1994). Motivations may be multiple and mixed (Rogers et al. 1989), with clear secondary gains coexisting with less conscious or more subtle ones (Khan et al. 2000; Lawrie et al. 1993). Nonetheless, thorough attempts must be made to investigate and clarify the motivational factors operative in the patients (e.g., Feldman and Russell 1991; Feldman et al. 1994).

The notion of the sick role (Parsons 1951) is complex. Some authors see it as a nonpathological mode of functioning that the factitious disorder patient adopts for pathological reasons. Others see the sick role of the factitious disorder patient as inherently pathological (Plassmann 1994b; Spivak et al. 1994).

Another factor complicating the diagnosis is the high prevalence of comorbid disorders (Sutherland and Rodin 1990). Substance use disorders (Bauer and Boegner 1996; Burge and Lacey 1993; Kent 1994; McDaniel et al. 1992; Popli et al. 1992), personality disorders (particularly borderline and antisocial) (Bauer and Boegner 1996; Nadelson 1979; Overholser 1990), malingering (Gorman and Winograd 1988; Harrington et al. 1990), dissociative disorders (Goodwin 1988; Toth and Baggaley 1991), eating disorders (Burge and Lacey 1993; Mizuta et al. 2000), suicidality, and mood disorders (Gielder 1994; Paar 1994; Roy and Roy 1995; Sutherland and Rodin 1990) may coexist. The comorbidities can overwhelm the diagnostic picture, and the diagnosis can be ignored altogether (Roy and Roy 1995; Toth and Baggaley 1991).

There are no diagnostic tests for factitious disorders. Psychological testing may reflect comorbid conditions (Babe et al. 1992) or, in cases of factitious disorder with predominantly psychological signs and symptoms, may give "fake bad" or invalid results (Zimmerman et al. 1991). Such results are not pathognomonic (Liebson et al. 1996).

Epidemiology

Data on the epidemiology of factitious disorder are difficult to gather and vary considerably. Sutherland and Rodin (1990) diagnosed factitious disorder in 0.8% of all psychiatric consultation-liaison service referrals of medical or surgical inpatients. Bhugra (1988) found 0.5% of psychiatric admissions to have Munchausen syndrome. Bauer and Boegner (1996) diagnosed factitious disorders in 0.3% of neurological admissions. Others (Eisendrath 1996) have reported rates between approximately 2% and 10%, with the higher rates in case series of fevers of unknown origin. Most reported cases have been in patients in their 20s to 40s, but it has been reported in children, adolescents, and geriatric patients (Joseph-Di Caprio and Remafedi 1997; Libow 2000; Pfefferbaum et al. 1999; Zimmerman et al. 1991).

Etiology

Psychodynamic explanations for these paradoxical disorders have been provided by several authors. Many have noted the apparent prevalence of histories of early childhood physical or sexual abuse, with disturbed parental relationships and emotional deprivation. Histories of early illness or extended hospitalizations also have been noted. Nadelson (1979) conceptualized factitious disorder as a manifestation of borderline character pathology rather than as an isolated clinical syndrome. Plassmann (1994b, 1994c) viewed the disorders as a "symptom of a psychic problem complex." Early traumas are dealt with narcissistically and through dissociation, denial, and a type of projection. The patient's body, or part of the body, becomes perceived as an external object or as a fused, symbiotic combination of self and object, which then comes to represent negative affects (hate, fear, pain), the associated negative object concepts, and negative self-concepts. In the face of early deprivation and assaults, the "body self" is split off to preserve the "psychic self" (Hirsch 1994). Eventually, the patient acts out or involves the medical system in a type of countertransference identification. Other intrapsychic, cognitive, social learning, and behavioral theories have been advanced as well (Barsky et al. 1992; Ford 1996b; Schwartz et al. 1994; Spivak et al. 1994).

Neuropathological foundations for the disorders also have been suggested, on the basis of neuroimaging (Babe et al. 1992; Fenelon et al. 1991; Lawrie et al. 1993; Mountz et al. 1996) and neuropsychological testing (Pankratz and Lezak 1987), but no consistent findings have yet been reported.

Although many cases of factitious disorder are chronic (Sutherland and Rodin 1990; Zimmerman et al. 1991), the stressor of recurrent object loss, or fear of loss, occurs over and over in the literature as an antecedent of a factitious episode (Ballard and Stoudemire 1992; Carney 1980; Linde 1996; Songer 1995).

Treatment

Once the diagnosis is suspected, it is essential to examine the treatment system for countertransference reactions. Plassmann (1994b) saw the patient's ability to induce a countertransference identification in the physician as a core of the disorder, and several authors (Amirault 1995; Freyberger et al. 1994; Kalivas 1996) viewed the physician's countertransference feelings as partially diagnostic for the disorder. The risk of nontherapeutic countertransference reactions usually calls for obtaining additional psychiatric consultation that then often involves working with the entire treatment team of physicians, nurses, ethics and risk management committees, and others (Eisendrath and Feder 1996). As Feldman and Feldman (1995) described, countertransference can lead to adverse consequences, such as therapeutic nihilism (Bhugra 1988; Toth and Baggaley 1991), anger and aversion (Lewis 1993; Powell and Boast 1993a), breaches of confidentiality (Markantonakis and Lee 1988; Powell and Boast 1993a), overidentification with the patient, or activation of rescue fantasies (Willenberg 1994).

Erroneous diagnosis of a factitious disorder can result in its own trauma and may be perpetuated in medical records (Feldman et al. 1994; Guziec et al. 1994). Teasell and Shapiro (1994), however, argued against the necessity of a completely accurate diagnosis of factitious disorder once the contribution of general medical illness has been factored out. The patient then must be informed of a change in treatment plan, and an attempt must be made to enlist him or her in that plan. Treatment begins at this point, and it is best done indirectly, with minimal expectation that the patient "confess" or acknowledge the deception. It is a delicate process, with patients frequently leaving the hospital against medical advice or otherwise leaving treatment (Baile et al. 1992; Baker and Major 1994; Songer 1995). Guziec et al. (1994) aptly likened this process to making a psychodynamic interpretation. Eisendrath (1989) described techniques for reducing confrontation, such as using inexact interpretations, therapeutic double binds, and other strategic and face-saving techniques to allow the patient tacitly to relinquish the factitious signs and symptoms. Using a systems approach to reframe the doctor–patient relationship can place the patient's factitious behavior in a more comprehensible context and may help avoid countertherapeutic oppositional positions (van der Feltz-Cornelis 2002).

Some authors recommend inpatient psychiatric hospitalization (Aduan et al. 1979; Plassmann 1994a; Powell and Boast 1993b). However, many (e.g., Ballard and Stoudemire 1992; Guziec et al. 1994; Spivak et al. 1994; Teasell and Shapiro 1994) describe treatment being initiated in the general medical inpatient setting where the factitious disorder has been diagnosed and continuing in the psychiatric outpatient setting.

No comparative studies of different therapeutic approaches have been done, but several different techniques have been described. Regardless of modality, treatment must be collaborative and involve some level of communication among all of the patient's treatment providers (Eisendrath and Feder 1996; Feldman and Duval 1997; Higgins 1990). The psycho-dynamic approach to treatment (Plassmann 1994a; Spivak et al. 1994) generally focuses not on the factitious behaviors themselves but on the underlying dynamic issues. Strategic-behavioral approaches also have been used (Schwarz et al. 1993; Solyom and Solyom 1990; Teasell and Shapiro 1994), implementing standard behavioral techniques as well as the therapeutic double bind, in which the only way out is to abandon the target factitious behaviors. Pharmacotherapy, when used, targets specific symptoms, such as depression or transient psychosis, or comorbid disorders. Some patients cease factitious behaviors on their own as a result of unanticipated life change (e.g., marriage or involvement in a church group that provides the requisite attention and support). Perceiving an "addictive" quality to their factitious behaviors, others have creatively evolved personal "12-step" programs that have helped them end the deceptions. Medicolegal issues must be considered, both in the malpractice and in the workers' compensation arenas (Houck 1992; Janofsky 1994).

Insufficient studies have been done to address conclusively the prognostic factors in factitious disorder, but children, patients with major depression, and those without personality disorders may have better prognoses (Folks 1995; Libow 2000). The literature on this disorder is certainly ample, and it implies that the factitious disorder patient, although requiring considerable therapeutic skill, may be approached with a cautious hope for improvement (Mayo and Haggerty 1984).

Factitious Disorder by Proxy

Introduction

In 1977, the British pediatrician Roy Meadow described another scenario involving factitious illness (R. Meadow 1977). He presented his observations on a number of cases, each of which involved a mother who had intentionally induced illness in her infant rather than in herself. Concealing the deception, the mother then presented the child for medical care, resulting in extensive, often invasive, evaluations and examinations of the child. Despite displaying an outward appearance of being concerned and caring, the mother continued to fabricate illness in her child. Meadow coined the term *Munchausen syndrome by proxy* (MSBP) to describe such scenarios. The children in these situations may be subject to considerable and prolonged morbidity, with a mortality of 6%–10% (Rosenberg 1987; Schreier and Libow 1993b).

Over the past decade, there has been a continued expansion of the medical literature about this type of fabricated illness, with the publication of lay and professional books on the topic (Adshead and Brooke 2001; Allison and Roberts 1998; Brownlee 1996; Feldman and Eisendrath 1996; Firstman and Talan 1997; Levin and Sheridan 1995; Schreier and Libow 1993a, 1996).

Classification

DSM-IV-TR provides research criteria for factitious disorder by proxy (American Psychiatric Association 2000). The criteria are similar to those for factitious disorder, with the addition of the "by proxy" specification (see Table 9–2). Much of the literature, however, retains the use of the eponym MSBP, and there is considerable debate about how best to use the terms *factitious disorder by proxy* and *MSBP* (Fisher and Mitchell 1995; R. Meadow 1995; Morley 1995; Schreier 2002a). The debate is not merely academic but may have serious legal implications as well (see Schreier 2002b).

TABLE 9–2. DSM-IV-TR research criteria for factitious disorder by proxy

A. Intentional production or feigning of physical or psychological signs or symptoms in another person who is under the individual's care.
B. The motivation for the perpetrator's behavior is to assume the sick role by proxy.
C. External incentives for the behavior (such as economic gain) are absent.
D. The behavior is not better accounted for by another mental disorder.

DSM-IV-TR uses factitious disorder by proxy to describe *a mental disorder in an individual.* Because factitious disorder by proxy is a research diagnosis, an individual meeting factitious disorder by proxy criteria would actually be given a diagnosis of factitious disorder not otherwise specified. The proxy, if psychiatrically diagnosed, would receive diagnoses other than factitious disorder, depending on the circumstances and the proxy's psychiatric symptoms (American Psychiatric Association 2000).

R. Meadow (1995) used MSBP to refer to *a particular form of child abuse* characterized by a particular behavior and attitude on the part of the mother. MSBP is something a mother commits, not a disorder she has (S.R. Meadow 1995). Bools (1996) viewed the attempt to label the perpetrator of child abuse with any new diagnosis as "(pseudo) psychiatric" and reserved either term to describe a situation of child abuse. Other authors similarly use the terms to refer to situations of abuse (Blix and Brack 1988; Donald and Jureidini 1996; Fisher and Mitchell 1995; Rosenberg 1996). In contrast to DSM-IV-TR, ICD-10 also classifies factitious disorder by proxy not as a disorder but as a form of child abuse (World Health Organization 1992).

Schreier and Libow (1993a) applied

the term *MSBP* to describe a disorder in the fabricator who has a specific and particular primary motivation, which is "the mother's intense need to be in a relationship with doctors and/or hospitals. The child is used to gain and maintain this contact" (p. 13). This motivation is a true perversion in the analytical sense of the term (Schreier 1992). Schreier's (1996) later writing included perpetrators who fabricate with a proxy in order to build "a highly manipulative relationship with a powerful transferential figure," specifically "professionals who occupy positions of power in society," not just physicians.

Another authority, Ford (1996a), argued that the fabricator should receive no syndrome-related diagnosis for the factitious behavior out of concern that diagnosis may provide a legal defense for behavior he views as predominantly criminal. Uniquely, however, he would use the diagnosis of factitious disorder not otherwise specified to apply to the proxy-victim.

In 2002, a multidisciplinary task force of the American Professional Society on the Abuse of Children issued revised definitions (Ayoub et al. 2002). Factitious disorder by proxy is the DSM-IV-TR disorder of factitious disorder not otherwise specified and applies to the fabricator-perpetrator. Pediatric condition falsification (PCF) is a form of child maltreatment or abuse and applies to the child proxy. Munchausen by proxy is then an overarching term used to describe the combination of PCF, factitious disorder by proxy, and the involvement of others (family, health care providers, etc.).

Although the overwhelming majority of cases involve mother as perpetrator and child as proxy (McClure et al. 1996), instances have been described in which the proxies were able-bodied adults or hospital and nursing home patients and the perpetrators were fathers, other relatives, baby-sitters, partners, health care professionals, or paraprofessionals (Chantada et al. 1994; Repper 1995; Sigal et al. 1986; Yorker 1996a).

For the purposes of this chapter, we use the terms *factitious disorder by proxy* and *MSBP* (Rappaport and Hochstadt 1993) interchangeably, rely primarily on the DSM-IV-TR research criteria, and use the paradigm of the mother perpetrator and the child proxy-victim.

Diagnosis

Certain clusters of warning signs (Table 9–3) can suggest a diagnosis of factitious disorder by proxy.

TABLE 9–3. Warning signs for factitious disorder by proxy

The episodes of illness begin only when the child is, or has recently been, with the parent.

The parent has taken the child to numerous caregivers, resulting in multiple diagnostic evaluations but neither cure nor definitive diagnosis.

The other parent (usually the father) is notably uninvolved despite the ostensive health crises.

The parent is proved to have provided false information to health care professionals or others.

The parent is not reassured by normal test results and continually advocates for painful or risky diagnostic tests for the child.

The child persistently fails to tolerate or respond to usual medical therapies.

Signs and symptoms abate or do not occur when the child is separated from the parent.

Another child in the family has had unexplained illness or childhood death.

The parent has a personal history of factitious disorder.

Source. Data from Bools et al. 1992; Jani et al. 1992; Jureidini 1993; Libow 1995; R. Meadow 1982; Schreier and Libow 1996.

A proposed diagnostic indicator, described by Szajnberg et al. (1996), is a particular type of countertransference: "the clinician has a recurrent, uncanny, ego-dystonic, and uncomfortable sense of *disbelief* that this parent has perpetrated his or her child's symptoms and illness" (p. 230).

Verification of the DSM-IV-TR diagnosis is a process fraught with the same type of difficulties mentioned in the discussion of factitious disorder earlier in this chapter. The mother's principal motivation must be determined (Kahan and Yorker 1991; Morley 1995; Schreier 1996), and any motivation other than attaining the sick role by proxy must be ruled out (Bools 1996; R. Meadow 1995). Also required is the determination that the mother is intentionally fabricating or inducing the child's illness. Because child abuse is a crime, proving the fabrication becomes a forensic process rather than a clinical medical investigation (Yorker 1996b). Various techniques have been used, including covert video surveillance in the hospital (Byard and Burnell 1994; Lacey et al. 1993; Samuels et al. 1992), searching rooms and belongings (Ford 1996a; Ostfeld and Feldman 1996), and special handling of laboratory specimens (Kahan and Yorker 1991). Some of these techniques raise obvious legal and ethical issues that must be resolved before they are implemented (Evans 1995; Ford 1996a; Samuels et al. 1992). Once the deceptions are exposed, the intentionality usually is readily inferred (McClure et al. 1996; Samuels et al. 1992; Sigal et al. 1990).

The ability of the mother with factitious disorder by proxy to deceive and to appear to be a caring, concerned parent can be astounding. In one case in which the mother confessed to poisoning her children, the mother was "so convincing in her performance that local authorities were reported as digging up pipes in the street looking for contamination," presumably of the water supply (Coombe 1995, p. 195). Video surveillance has clearly shown how the caring presentation is a performance; when the mother thinks she is unobserved, she gives the child minimal attention (Samuels et al. 1992) or is abusive.

The cautions against making a false-positive diagnosis of factitious disorder apply to factitious disorder by proxy as well (R. Meadow 1995; Schreier and Libow 1994). Added to these risks is that of making false criminal accusations with adverse results on the involved family (Rand and Feldman 1999; Schreier and Libow 1993b).

Once factitious disorder by proxy has been diagnosed, it is important to assess the entire family. Other children also may be proxies, other family members may be participating in the factitious behavior, and the proxy himself or herself may be actively cooperating with the fabrications (Alexander et al. 1990; Kosmach et al. 1996; Rand 1996; Smith and Ardern 1989).

Epidemiology

The prevalence of factitious disorder by proxy is unknown, but one study estimated 2.8 cases per 100,000 children age 1 year or younger or 0.5 cases per 100,000 children age 16 years or younger (McClure et al. 1996). Among select populations (Chantada et al. 1994; Jani et al. 1992; Schreier and Libow 1993b), the rates may be substantially higher. The child typically is 2–5 years old at diagnosis (Donald and Jureidini 1996; Yorker and Kahan 1990). Length of time from onset of symptoms in the child to diagnosis can vary widely, from months (Rosenberg 1987) to years (Libow 1995). In most cases, multiple methods such as smothering, poisoning, and fabricated history of seizures or fever have been used to fabricate a variety of illnesses in the child (Bools et al. 1992). Behavioral conditions and psychiatric disorders also may be feigned (Schreier 2000).

No consistent profile of mothers has been shown on psychological testing (Rand 1996). In contrast to factitious disorder, the most common comorbid psychiatric disorder in factitious disorder by proxy is a personality disorder (Schreier 1992), and substance use disorders are less commonly reported.

Etiology

Although perpetrators rarely make themselves available for psychiatric or psychological study, most authors postulate that the maternal pathology arises from childhood roots, characterized by "quietly traumatic" emotional neglect and abandonment (Schreier and Libow 1993a; Sigal et al. 1988). Schreier and Libow (1993a) and Parnell and Day (1998) have written extensively on the etiological hypotheses of factitious disorder, and the reader is referred to their texts.

Treatment and Prognosis

Mothers with factitious disorder by proxy are regarded as very difficult to treat (Schreier and Libow 1994). Some of the difficulty stems from the mother's massive use of denial and projective identification (Coombe 1995; Feldman 1994b; Schreier 1992). Another source stems from the process by which treatment is usually initiated. Because of the necessity to protect the proxy, the indirect approach used in treating factitious disorder that permits some continued factitious behavior is not possible. The first stage of treatment in factitious disorder by proxy usually begins with the involvement of child protection authorities, the initiation

of legal proceedings against the parent, and the removal of the child from the home.

Treatment of factitious disorder by proxy requires coordinated multidisciplinary, multiagency involvement (Coombe 1995; Lyons-Ruth et al. 1991; Parnell and Day 1998; Smith and Ardern 1989). Individual treatment is long-term psychotherapy (group, individual, or combined) (Coombe 1995; Lyons-Ruth et al. 1991). As with the treatment of factitious disorder, the factitious behavior is rarely the primary focus. Pharmacotherapy is used only to treat comorbid conditions.

Treatment results in unselected patient samples have been distinctly unfavorable; thus, the overall prognosis is guarded, with a high likelihood of continued factitious disorder by proxy behavior (Bools et al. 1993, 1994; Davis et al. 1998; Libow 1995; R. Meadow 1993; see also Berg and Jones 1999). Management is usually coordinated and directed through the legal system, and protection of the child is the priority (Brady 1994; Kahan and Yorker 1991; Ostfeld and Feldman 1996).

Malingering

Classification

In DSM-IV-TR, malingering is classified under "Other Conditions That May Be a Focus of Clinical Attention" and is not considered to be a mental disorder or a psychiatric illness. Malingering is defined as the "intentional production of false or grossly exaggerated physical or psychological symptoms, motivated by external incentives" (American Psychiatric Association 2000, p. 739). The term *malingering by proxy* also has been suggested (Bools 1996) for those cases in which illness is fabricated in a child for secondary gain; for example, for the purpose of obtaining social assistance benefits money (Cassar et al. 1996).

Other disorders to consider in the differential diagnosis of malingering include factitious disorder, conversion disorder, and somatoform disorders. Although all three of these diagnoses may involve physical symptoms, none involve the production of symptoms for external incentives. In addition, individuals who confabulate should be distinguished from malingerers because they are unintentionally filling in information that they believed to have happened, when, in fact, it did not happen at all (Newmark et al. 1999; Resnick 2000).

Diagnostic confusion between malingering and other mental disorders, particularly factitious disorders, can be traced to Asher's (1951) original description of Munchausen syndrome. He attributed several possible motives for Munchausen syndrome, including "a desire to escape from the police" and "a desire to get free board and lodgings for the night" (p. 339), motives that would now clearly classify feigned illness behavior as malingering. There are many examples of patients with factitious disorder who also malinger (see "Diagnosis" subsection of "Factitious Disorder" section earlier in this chapter).

Diagnosis

Malingering is "so easy to define but so difficult to diagnose" (Resnick 1997). The individual may present inconsistencies in what he or she actually reports. A malingerer's observed behavior may differ significantly from the symptoms he or she reports. Malingerers may behave in a dramatically different way depending on who they believe is observing them. Psychological test data may be inconsistent with the history provided by malingerers. Finally, malingerers often report symptoms that are inconsistent with how genuine symptoms normally manifest. The better clini-

cians understand characteristics of a true illness, the more likely they will be able to detect feigned symptoms (Resnick 2000).

A care provider's natural inclination is to accept the person's reported symptoms at face value. Rosenhan (2001) conducted a famous study that showed clinicians' tendency to blindly accept reported mental health symptoms. In this study, eight non–mentally ill individuals presented to a psychiatric hospital alleging that they were hearing very atypical voices. Based on this one reported symptom, every person was admitted to the hospital and given schizophrenia diagnoses, even though each person ceased reporting any symptom after admission.

Table 9–4 provides a suggested clinical decision model for the assessment of malingered psychosis (Resnick 1997). In determining whether reported hallucinations or delusions are fabricated or exaggerated, the factors outlined in Table 9–5 also may prove helpful (Resnick 1997). Note that a bona fide diagnosis of a past psychotic disorder does not necessarily exclude a presentation of manufactured psychotic symptoms (Tyrer et al. 2001).

When evaluating possible malingering, the clinician should consider obtaining additional information from collateral sources and psychological testing to verify the person's reported symptoms. Psychological testing may include structured interviews to evaluate psychotic symptoms (Rogers 1992), various personality inventories, and neuropsychological testing to assess cognitive deficits (Liebson et al. 1996). Witztum et al. (1996) described several military inductees who received erroneous diagnoses of malingering; diagnoses of severe psychiatric disorders were missed because of assessment problems. Those authors also noted, as did DuAlba and Scott (1993), the important role of cross-cultural issues in the assessment of malingering.

TABLE 9–4. Clinical decision model for the assessment of malingering

The evaluee's presentation meets the following criteria:

A. Understandable motive to malinger.
B. Marked variability of presentation as observed in at least one of the following:
  1. Marked discrepancies in interview and noninterview behavior.
  2. Gross inconsistencies in reported psychotic symptoms.
  3. Blatant contradictions between reported prior episodes and documented psychiatric history.
C. Improbable psychiatric symptoms as evidenced by one or more of the following:
  1. Reporting elaborate psychotic symptoms that lack common paranoid, grandiose, or religious themes.
  2. Sudden emergence of purported psychotic symptoms to explain antisocial behavior.
  3. Atypical hallucinations or delusions (see Table 9–5).
D. Confirmation of malingered psychosis by either
  1. Admission of malingering following confrontation.
  2. Presence of strong corroborative information, such as psychometric data or history of malingering.

TABLE 9–5. Threshold model for the assessment of hallucinations and delusions

Malingering should be suspected if any combination of the following are observed:
Hallucinations
  Continuous rather than intermittent hallucinations
  Vague or inaudible hallucinations
  Hallucinations not associated with delusions
  Stilted language reported in hallucinations
  Inability to state strategies to diminish voices
  Self-report that all command hallucinations were obeyed
  Visual hallucinations in black and white
Delusions
  Abrupt onset or termination
  Eagerness to call attention to delusions
  Conduct markedly inconsistent with delusions
  Bizarre content without disordered thinking

Epidemiology

Malingering is not a rare event. In a study of malingered mental illness in a metropolitan emergency department, 13% of patients were strongly suspected or considered to be malingering (Yates et al. 1996). Rogers et al. (1993) estimated that approximately half of the individuals evaluated for personal injury claims were feigning all or part of their cognitive deficits.

Treatment

When a determination of malingering is made, the clinician is faced with the dilemma of how to "treat" a nondisorder. Depending on the situation, the clinician may elect to confront the individual with the assessment. Pankratz and Erickson (1990) emphasized the importance of permitting the malingering individual to save face. Possible verbal interventions include statements such as "You haven't told me the whole truth" or "The type of symptoms that you are reporting are not consistent with any known mental illness" (Inbau and Reid 1967). The clinician should be prepared for some individuals to react defensively and to refuse to accept this assessment, even when faced with strong evidence that they are faking their symptoms. Finally, many of Houck's (1992) warnings about the medicolegal pitfalls in the assessment and treatment of a factitious disorder also apply to the assessment and disposition of the malingerer.

References

Adshead G, Brooke D (eds): Munchausen's Syndrome By Proxy: Current Issues in Assessment, Treatment and Research. London, England, Imperial College Press, 2001

Aduan RP, Fauci AS, Dale DC, et al: Factitious fever and self-induced infection: a report of 32 cases and review of the literature. Ann Intern Med 90:230–242, 1979

Alexander R, Smith W, Stevenson R: Serial Munchausen syndrome by proxy. Pediatrics 86:581–585, 1990

Allison DB, Roberts MS: Disordered Mother or Disordered Diagnosis? Munchausen By Proxy Syndrome. Hillsdale, NJ, Analytic Press, 1998

American Psychiatric Association: Diagnostic and Statistical Manual of Mental Disorders, 4th Edition, Text Revision. Washington, DC, American Psychiatric Association, 2000

Amirault C: Pseudologica fantastica and other tall tales: the contagious literature of Munchausen syndrome. Lit Med 14:169–190, 1995

Asher R: Munchausen's syndrome. Lancet 1:339–341, 1951

Ayoub CC, Alexander R, Beck D, et al: Position paper: definitional issues in Munchausen by proxy. Child Maltreatment 7:105–111, 2002

Babe KS Jr, Peterson AM, Loosen PT, et al: The pathogenesis of Munchausen syndrome: a review and case report. Gen Hosp Psychiatry 14:273–276, 1992

Baddley J, Daberkow D, Hilton C: Insulinoma masquerading as factitious hypoglycemia. South Med J 91:1067–1069, 1998

Baile WF Jr, Kuehn CV, Straker D: Factitious cancer. Psychosomatics 33:100–105, 1992

Baker CE, Major E: Munchausen's syndrome: a case presenting as asthma requiring ventilation. Anaesthesia 49:1050–1051, 1994

Ballard RS, Stoudemire A: Factitious apraxia. Int J Psychiatry Med 22:275–280, 1992

Bappal B, George M, Nair R, et al: Factitious hypoglycemia: a tale from the Arab world. Pediatrics 107:180–181, 2001

Barsky AJMD, Wyshak G, Klerman GL: Psychiatric comorbidity in DSM-III-R hypochondriasis. Arch Gen Psychiatry 49:101–108, 1992

Bauer M, Boegner F: Neurological syndromes in factitious disorder. J Nerv Ment Dis 184:281–288, 1996

Berg B, Jones D: Outcome of psychiatric intervention in factitious illness by proxy (Munchausen's syndrome by proxy). Arch Dis Child 81:465–472, 1999

Bhugra D: Psychiatric Munchausen's syndrome: literature review with case reports. Acta Psychiatr Scand 77:497–503, 1988

Blix S, Brack G: The effects of a suspected case of Munchausen's syndrome by proxy on a pediatric nursing staff. Gen Hosp Psychiatry 10:402–409, 1988

Bools C: Factitious illness by proxy: Munchausen syndrome by proxy. Br J Psychiatry 169:268–275, 1996

Bools CN, Neale BA, Meadow SR: Co-morbidity associated with fabricated illness (Munchausen syndrome by proxy). Arch Dis Child 67:77–79, 1992

Bools CN, Neale BA, Meadow SR: Follow up of victims of fabricated illness (Munchausen syndrome by proxy). Arch Dis Child 69:625–630, 1993

Bools C, Neale B, Meadow R: Munchausen syndrome by proxy: a study of psychopathology. Child Abuse Negl 18:773–788, 1994

Brady MM: Munchausen syndrome by proxy: how should we weigh our options? Law and Psychology Review 18:361–375, 1994

Brownlee S: Mother love betrayed: children are tools for parents with a rare psychiatric disorder. U.S. News and World Report 120:29, 1996

Burge CK, Lacey JH: A case of Munchausen's syndrome in anorexia nervosa. Int J Eat Disord 14:379–381, 1993

Byard RW, Burnell RH: Covert video surveillance in Munchausen syndrome by proxy: ethical compromise or essential technique? Med J Aust 160:352–356, 1994

Carney MW: Artefactual illness to attract medical attention. Br J Psychiatry 136:542–547, 1980

Carswell J: The Romantic Rogue; Being the Singular Life and Adventures of Rudolph Eric Raspe, Creator of Baron Munchausen. New York, Dutton, 1950

Cassar J, Hales E, Longhurst J, et al: Can disability benefits make children sicker? J Am Acad Child Adolesc Psychiatry 35: 700–701, 1996

Chantada G, Casak S, Plata JD, et al: Children with fever of unknown origin in Argentina: an analysis of 113 cases. Pediatr Infect Dis J 13:260–263, 1994

Chapman JS: Peregrinating problem patients; Munchausen's syndrome. JAMA 165: 927–933, 1957

Churchill DR, De Cock KM, Miller RF: Feigned HIV infection/AIDS: malingering and Munchausen's syndrome. Genitourinary Medicine 70:314–316, 1994

Cizza G, Nieman L, Doppman J, et al: Factitious Cushing syndrome. J Clin Endocrinol Metab 81:3573–3577, 1996

Coombe P: The inpatient psychotherapy of a mother and child at the Cassel Hospital: a case of Munchausen's syndrome by proxy. British Journal of Psychotherapy 12:195–207, 1995

Craddock N, Brown N: Munchausen syndrome presenting as mental handicap. Mental Handicap Research 6:184–190, 1993

Davis P, McClure R, Rolfe K, et al: Procedures, placement, and risks of further abuse after Munchausen syndrome by proxy, non-accidental poisoning, and non-accidental suffocation. Arch Dis Child 78:217–221, 1998

Dixon D, Abbey S: Cupid's arrow: an unusual presentation of factitious disorder. Psychosomatics 36:502–504, 1995

Donald T, Jureidini J: Munchausen syndrome by proxy: child abuse in the medical system. Arch Pediatr Adolesc Med 150:753–758, 1996

DuAlba L, Scott RL: Somatization and malingering for workers' compensation applicants: a cross-cultural MMPI study. J Clin Psychol 49:913–917, 1993

Eisendrath SJ: Factitious physical disorders: treatment without confrontation. Psychosomatics 30:383–387, 1989

Eisendrath SJ: Factitious physical disorders. West J Med 160:177–179, 1994

Eisendrath SJ: Current overview of factitious physical disorders, in The Spectrum of Factitious Disorders. Edited by Feldman MD, Eisendrath SJ. Washington, DC, American Psychiatric Press, 1996, pp 21–36

Eisendrath SJ, Feder A: Management of factitious disorders, in The Spectrum of Factitious Disorders. Edited by Feldman MD, Eisendrath SJ. Washington, DC, American Psychiatric Press, 1996, pp 195–213

Evans D: The investigation of life-threatening child abuse and Munchausen syndrome by proxy. J Med Ethics 21:9–13, 1995

Feldman MD: The costs of factitious disorders. Psychosomatics 35:506–507, 1994a

Feldman MD: Denial in Munchausen syndrome by proxy: the consulting psychiatrist's dilemma. Int J Psychiatry Med 24: 121–128, 1994b

Feldman M: Munchausen by Internet: detecting factitious illness and crisis on the Internet. South Med J 93:669–672, 2000

Feldman MD: Factitious Disorders, Munchausen, and Munchausen by Proxy Web page. Available at http://munchausen.com. Accessed April 23, 2003

Feldman M, Duval N: Factitious quadriplegia: a rare new case and literature review. Psychosomatics 38:76–80, 1997

Feldman MD, Eisendrath SJ (eds): The Spectrum of Factitious Disorders. Washington, DC, American Psychiatric Press, 1996

Feldman MD, Feldman JM: Tangled in the web: countertransference in the therapy of factitious disorders. Int J Psychiatry Med 25:389–399, 1995

Feldman MD, Russell JL: Factitious cyclic hypersomnia: a new variant of factitious disorder. South Med J 84:379–381, 1991

Feldman MD, Smith R: Personal and interpersonal toll of factitious disorders, in The Spectrum of Factitious Disorders. Edited by Feldman MD, Eisendrath SJ. Washington, DC, American Psychiatric Press, 1996, pp 175–194

Feldman MD, Ford CV, Reinhold T: Patient or Pretender: Inside the Strange World of Factitious Disorders. New York, Wiley, 1994

Feldman MD, Hamilton JC, Deemer HN: A critical analysis of factitious disorders, in Somatoform and Factitious Disorders. Edited by Phillips KA. Washington, DC, American Psychiatric Publishing, 2001, pp 129–166

Fenelon G, Mahieux F, Roullet E, et al: Munchausen's syndrome and abnormalities on magnetic resonance imaging of the brain. BMJ 302:996–997, 1991

Firstman R, Talan J: The Death of Innocents. New York, Bantam Books, 1997

Fisher GC, Mitchell I: Is Munchausen syndrome by proxy really a syndrome? Arch Dis Child 72:530–534, 1995

Folks DG: Munchausen's syndrome and other factitious disorders. Neurol Clin 13:267–281, 1995

Ford CV: The somatizing disorders. Psychosomatics 27:327–331, 335–337, 1986

Ford CV: Ethical and legal issues in factitious disorders: an overview, in The Spectrum of Factitious Disorders. Edited by Feldman MD, Eisendrath SJ. Washington, DC, American Psychiatric Press, 1996a, pp 51–63

Ford CV: Lies! Lies!! Lies!!! The Psychology of Deceit. Washington, DC, American Psychiatric Press, 1996b

Freyberger H, Nordmeyer JP, Freyberger HJ, et al: Patients suffering from factitious disorders in the clinico-psychosomatic consultation liaison service: psychodynamic processes, psychotherapeutic initial care and clinico-interdisciplinary cooperation. Psychother Psychosom 62:108–122, 1994

Frumkin LR, Victoroff JI: Chronic factitious disorder with symptoms of AIDS. Am J Med 88:694–696, 1990

Gavin H: On Feigned and Factitious Diseases, Chiefly of Soldiers and Seamen, on the Means Used to Simulate or Produce Them, and on the Best Mode of Discovering Imposters: Being the Prize Essay in the Class of Military Surgery, in the University of Edinburgh, Session, 1835-6, With Additions. London, England, John Churchill Princes Street Soho, 1843

Gielder U: Factitious disease in the field of dermatology. Psychother Psychosom 62: 48–55, 1994

Goodwin J: Munchausen's syndrome as a dissociative disorder. Dissociation: Progress in the Dissociative Disorders 1:54–60, 1988

Gorman WF, Winograd M: Crossing the border from Munchausen to malingering. J Fla Med Assoc 75:147–150, 1988

Guziec J, Lazarus A, Harding JJ: Case of a 29-year-old nurse with factitious disorder: the utility of psychiatric intervention on a general medical floor. Gen Hosp Psychiatry 16:47–53, 1994

Harrington WZ, Jackimczyk KC, Seligson RA: Thiopental-facilitated interview in respiratory Munchausen's syndrome. Ann Emerg Med 19:941–942, 1990

Higgins PM: Temporary Munchausen syndrome. Br J Psychiatry 157:613–616, 1990

Hirsch M: The body as a transitional object. Psychother Psychosom 62:78–81, 1994

Houck CA: Medicolegal aspects of factitious disorder. Psychiatric Medicine 10:105–116, 1992

Inbau FE, Reid JE: Criminal Interrogation and Confessions. Baltimore, MD, Williams & Wilkins, 1967

Jani S, White M, Rosenberg LA, et al: Munchausen syndrome by proxy. Int J Psychiatry Med 22:343–349, 1992

Janofsky JS: The Munchausen syndrome in civil forensic psychiatry. Bulletin of the American Academy of Psychiatry and the Law 22:489–497, 1994

Joseph-Di Caprio J, Remafedi GJ: Adolescents with factitious HIV disease. J Adolesc Health 21:102–106, 1997

Jureidini J: Obstetric factitious disorder and Munchausen syndrome by proxy. J Nerv Ment Dis 181:135–137, 1993

Kahan B, Yorker BC: Munchausen syndrome by proxy: clinical review and legal issues. Behav Sci Law 9:73–83, 1991

Kalivas J: Malingering versus factitious disorder (letter). Am J Psychiatry 153:1108, 1996

Kasdan ML, Soergel TM, Johnson AL, et al: Expanded profile of the SHAFT syndrome. J Hand Surg [Am] 23:26–31, 1998

Kent JD: Munchausen's syndrome and substance abuse. J Subst Abuse Treat 11:247–251, 1994

Khan I, Fayaz I, Ridgley J, et al: Factitious clock drawing and constructional apraxia. J Neurol Neurosurg Psychiatry 68:106–107, 2000

Koo J, Gambla C, Fried R: Pseudopsychodermatologic disease. Dermatol Clin 14:525–530, 1996

Kosmach B, Tarbell S, Reyes J, et al: "Munchausen by proxy" syndrome in a small bowel transplant recipient. Transplant Proc 28:2790–2791, 1996

Lacey SR, Cooper C, Runyan DK, et al: Munchausen syndrome by proxy: patterns of presentation to pediatric surgeons. J Pediatr Surg 28:827–832, 1993

Lawrie SM, Goodwin G, Masterton G: Munchausen's syndrome and organic brain disorder. Br J Psychiatry 162:545–549, 1993

Levin AV, Sheridan MS (eds): Munchausen Syndrome by Proxy: Issues in Diagnosis and Treatment. New York, Lexington Books, 1995

Lewis EJ: Kidney-related Munchausen's syndrome and the Red Baron. N Engl J Med 328:60–61, 1993

Libow JA: Munchausen by proxy victims in adulthood: a first look. Child Abuse Negl 19:1131–1142, 1995

Libow J: Child and adolescent illness falsification. Pediatrics 105:336–342, 2000

Liebson E, White R, Albert M: Cognitive inconsistencies in abnormal illness behavior and neurological disease. J Nerv Ment Dis 184:122–125, 1996

Linde P: A bewitching case of factitious disorder in Zimbabwe. Gen Hosp Psychiatry 18:440–443, 1996

Ludwigs U, Ruiz H, Isaksson H, et al: Factitious disorder presenting with acute cardiovascular symptoms. J Intern Med 236:685–690, 1994

Lyons-Ruth K, Kaufman M, Masters N, et al: Issues in the identification and long-term management of Munchausen by proxy syndrome within a clinical infant service. Infant Mental Health Journal 12:309–320, 1991

Markantonakis A, Lee AS: Psychiatric Munchausen's syndrome: a college register (letter). Br J Psychiatry 152:867, 1988

Mayo JP Jr, Haggerty JJ Jr: Long-term psychotherapy of Munchausen syndrome. Am J Psychother 38:571–578, 1984

McClure RJ, Davis PM, Meadow SR, et al: Epidemiology of Munchausen syndrome by proxy, non-accidental poisoning, and non-accidental suffocation. Arch Dis Child 75:57–61, 1996

McDaniel JS, Desoutter L, Firestone S, et al: Factitious disorder resulting in bilateral mastectomies. Gen Hosp Psychiatry 14:355–356, 1992

Meadow R: Munchausen syndrome by proxy: the hinterland of child abuse. Lancet 2(8033):343–345, 1977

Meadow R: Munchausen syndrome by proxy. Arch Dis Child 57:92–98, 1982

Meadow R: False allegations of abuse and Munchausen syndrome by proxy. Arch Dis Child 68:444–447, 1993

Meadow R: What is, and what is not, 'Munchausen syndrome by proxy'? Arch Dis Child 72:534–538, 1995

Meadow SR: Munchausen syndrome by proxy. Med Leg J 63:89–104, 1995

Miner I, Feldman M: Factitious deafblindness: an imperceptible variant of factitious disorder. Gen Hosp Psychiatry 20:48–51, 1998

Mizuta I, Fukunaga T, Sato H, et al: A case report of comorbid eating disorder and factitious disorder. Psychiatry Clin Neurosci 54:603–606, 2000

Morley CJ: Practical concerns about the diagnosis of Munchausen syndrome by proxy. Arch Dis Child 72:528–529, 1995

Mountz JM, Parker PE, Liu HG, et al: Tc-99m HMPAO brain SPECT scanning in Munchausen syndrome. J Psychiatry Neurosci 21:49–52, 1996

Nadelson T: The Munchausen spectrum: borderline character features. Gen Hosp Psychiatry 1:11–17, 1979

Newmark N, Adityanjee, Kay J: Pseudologia fantastica and factitious disorder: review of the literature and a case report. Compr Psychiatry 40:89–95, 1999

Nordmeyer JP: An internist's view of patients with factitious disorders and factitious clinical symptomatology. Psychother Psychosom 62:30–40, 1994

Ostfeld BM, Feldman MD: Factitious disorder by proxy: clinical features, detection, and management, in The Spectrum of Factitious Disorders. Edited by Feldman MD, Eisendrath SJ. Washington, DC, American Psychiatric Press, 1996, pp 83–108

Overholser JC: Differential diagnosis of malingering and factitious disorder with physical symptoms. Special Issue: Malingering and Deception: An Update. Behav Sci Law 8:55–65, 1990

Paar GH: Factitious disorders in the field of surgery. Psychother Psychosom 62:41–47, 1994

Pankratz L, Erickson RC: Two views of malingering. Clinical Neuropsychologist 4:379–389, 1990

Pankratz L, Lezak MD: Cerebral dysfunction in the Munchausen syndrome. Hillside Journal of Clinical Psychiatry 9:195–206, 1987

Parnell TF, Day DO: Munchausen by Proxy Syndrome: Misunderstood Child Abuse. Thousand Oaks, CA, Sage, 1998

Parsons T: The Social System. Glencoe, IL, Free Press, 1951

Pfefferbaum B, Allen J, Lindsey E, et al: Fabricated trauma exposure: an analysis of cognitive, behavioral, and emotional factors. Psychiatry 62:293–302, 1999

Plassmann R: Inpatient and outpatient long-term psychotherapy of patients suffering from factitious disorder. Psychother Psychosom 62:96–107, 1994a

Plassmann R: Munchausen syndromes and factitious diseases. Psychother Psychosom 62:7–26, 1994b

Plassmann R: Structural disturbances in the body self. Psychother Psychosom 62:91–95, 1994c

Popli AP, Masand PS, Dewan MJ: Factitious disorders with psychological symptoms. J Clin Psychiatry 53:315–318, 1992

Powell R, Boast N: The million dollar man: resource implications for chronic Munchausen's syndrome. Br J Psychiatry 162:253–256, 1993a

Powell R, Boast N: Resource implications of Munchausen's syndrome (letter). Br J Psychiatry 162:848, 1993b

Rand DC: Comprehensive psychosocial assessment in factitious disorder by proxy, in The Spectrum of Factitious Disorders. Edited by Feldman MD, Eisendrath SJ. Washington, DC, American Psychiatric Press, 1996, pp 109–133

Rand DC, Feldman MD: Misdiagnosis of Munchausen syndrome by proxy: a literature review and four new cases (review). Harv Rev Psychiatry 7:94–101, 1999

Rappaport SR, Hochstadt NJ: Munchausen syndrome by proxy (MSBP): an intergenerational perspective. Journal of Mental Health Counseling 15:278–289, 1993

Reich P, Gottfried LA: Factitious disorders in a teaching hospital. Ann Intern Med 99:240–247, 1983

Repper J: Munchausen syndrome by proxy in health care workers. J Adv Nurs 21:299–304, 1995

Resnick PJ: Malingered psychosis, in Clinical Assessment of Malingering and Deception, 2nd Edition. Edited by Rogers R. New York, Guilford, 1997, pp 47–67

Resnick PJ: The clinical assessment of malingered mental illness, in Annual Board Review Course Syllabus. Bloomfield, CT, American Academy of Psychiatry and the Law, 2000, pp 842–866

Rogers R: Structured Interview of Reported Symptoms. Odessa, FL, Psychological Assessment Resources, 1992

Rogers R, Bagby RM, Rector N: Diagnostic legitimacy of factitious disorder with psychological symptoms. Am J Psychiatry 146:1312–1314, 1989

Rogers R, Harrell EH, Liff CD: Feigning neuropsychological impairment: a critical review of methodological and clinical considerations. Clin Psychol Rev 13:255–274, 1993

Rosenberg DA: Web of deceit: a literature review of Munchausen syndrome by proxy. Child Abuse Negl 11:547–563, 1987

Rosenberg D: Child neglect and Munchausen syndrome by proxy. Washington, DC, National Criminal Justice Reference Service, 1996

Rosenhan DL: On being sane in insane places, in Down to Earth Sociology: Introductory Readings, 11th Edition. Edited by Henslin JA. New York, Free Press, 2001, pp 278–289

Roy M, Roy A: Factitious hypoglycemia: an 11-year follow-up. Psychosomatics 36:64–65, 1995

Samuels MP, McClaughlin W, Jacobson RR, et al: Fourteen cases of imposed upper airway obstruction. Arch Dis Child 67:162–170, 1992

Schreier HA: The perversion of mothering: Munchausen syndrome by proxy. Bull Menninger Clin 56:421–437, 1992

Schreier HA: Repeated false allegations of sexual abuse presenting to sheriffs: when is it Munchausen by proxy? Child Abuse Negl 20:985–991, 1996

Schreier H: Factitious disorder by proxy in which the presenting problem is behavioral or psychiatric. J Am Acad Child Adolesc Psychiatry 39:668–670, 2000

Schreier H: Munchausen by proxy defined. Pediatrics 110:985–988, 2002a

Schreier H: On the importance of motivation in Munchausen by proxy: the case of Kathy Bush. Child Abuse and Neglect 26:537–549, 2002b

Schreier HA, Libow JA: Hurting for Love: Munchausen by Proxy Syndrome. New York, Guilford, 1993a

Schreier HA, Libow JA: Munchausen syndrome by proxy: diagnosis and prevalence. Am J Orthopsychiatry 63:318–321, 1993b

Schreier HA, Libow JA: Munchausen by proxy syndrome: a clinical fable for our times. J Am Acad Child Adolesc Psychiatry 33:904–905, 1994

Schreier HA, Libow JA: Munchausen by proxy: the deadly game. Saturday Evening Post 268:40–41, 1996

Schwartz SM, Gramling SE, Mancini T: The influence of life stress, personality, and learning history on illness behavior. J Behav Ther Exp Psychiatry 25:135–142, 1994

Schwarz K, Harding R, Harrington D, et al: Hospital management of a patient with intractable factitious disorder. Psychosomatics 34:265–267, 1993

Seersholm NJ, Frolich S, Jensen NH, et al: Factitious disorder: an iatrogenic disease? Ugeskr Laeger 153:2133–2135, 1991

Sigal MD, Altmark D, Carmel I: Munchausen syndrome by adult proxy: a perpetrator abusing two adults. J Nerv Ment Dis 174:696–698, 1986

Sigal M, Carmel I, Altmark D, et al: Munchausen syndrome by proxy: a psychodynamic analysis. Med Law 7:49–56, 1988

Sigal M, Gelkopf M, Levertov G: Medical and legal aspects of the Munchausen by proxy perpetrator. Med Law 9:739–749, 1990

Smith NJ, Ardern MH: "More in sickness than in health": a case study of Munchausen by proxy in the elderly. Journal of Family Therapy 11:321–334, 1989

Solyom C, Solyom L: A treatment program for functional paraplegia/Munchausen syndrome. J Behav Ther Exp Psychiatry 21:225–230, 1990

Songer DA: Factitious AIDS: a case reported and literature review. Psychosomatics 36:406–411, 1995

Spivak H, Rodin G, Sutherland A: The psychology of factitious disorders: a reconsideration. Psychosomatics 35:25–34, 1994

Sutherland AJ, Rodin GM: Factitious disorders in a general hospital setting: clinical features and a review of the literature. Psychosomatics 31:392–399, 1990

Szajnberg NM, Moilanen I, Kanerva A, et al: Munchausen-by-proxy syndrome: countertransference as a diagnostic tool. Bull Menninger Clin 60:229–237, 1996

Teasell RW, Shapiro AP: Strategic-behavioral intervention in the treatment of chronic non-organic motor disorders. Am J Phys Med Rehabil 73:44–50, 1994

Topazian M, Binder HJ: Factitious diarrhea detected by measurement of stool osmolality. N Engl J Med 330:1418–1419, 1994

Toth EL, Baggaley A: Coexistence of Munchausen's syndrome and multiple personality disorder: detailed report of a case and theoretical discussion. Psychiatry 54:176–186, 1991

Tyrer P, Babidge N, Emmanuel J, et al: Instrumental psychosis: the good soldier Svejk syndrome. J R Soc Med 94:22–25, 2001 van der Feltz-Cornelis CM: The impact of factitious disorder on the physician–patient relationship: an epistemological model. Medicine, Health Care and Philosophy 5: 253–261, 2002

Wallach J: Laboratory diagnosis of factitious disorders. Arch Intern Med 154:1690–1696, 1994

Willenberg H: Countertransference in factitious disorder. Psychother Psychosom 62:129–134, 1994

Witztum E, Grinshpoon A, Margolin J, et al.: The erroneous diagnosis of malingering in a military setting. Mil Med 161:225–229, 1996

World Health Organization: The ICD-10 Classification of Mental and Behavioral Disorders. Geneva, Switzerland, World Health Organization, 1992

Yates BD, Nordquist CR, Schultz-Ross RA: Feigned psychiatric symptoms in the emergency room. Psychiatr Serv 47:998–1000, 1996

Yorker BC: Hospital epidemics of factitious disorder by proxy, in The Spectrum of Factitious Disorders. Edited by Feldman MD, Eisendrath SJ. Washington, DC, American Psychiatric Press, 1996a, pp 157–174

Yorker BC: Legal issues in factitious disorder by proxy, in The Spectrum of Factitious Disorders. Edited by Feldman MD, Eisendrath SJ. Washington, DC, American Psychiatric Press, 1996b, pp 135–156

Yorker BC, Kahan BB: Munchausen's syndrome by proxy as a form of child abuse. Arch Psychiatr Nurs 4:313–318, 1990

Zimmerman JG, Hussian RA, Tintner R, et al: Factitious disorder in a geriatric patient. Clin Gerontol 11:3–11, 1991

Ziv I, Djaldetti R, Zoldan Y, et al: Diagnosis of "non-organic" limb paresis by a novel objective motor assessment: the quantitative Hoover's test. J Neurol 245:797–802, 1998

CHAPTER 10

Dissociative Disorders

José R. Maldonado, M.D.

David Spiegel, M.D.

The dissociative disorders involve a disturbance in the integrated organization of identity, memory, perception, or consciousness. Events normally experienced on a smooth continuum are isolated from the other mental processes with which they would ordinarily be associated. This isolation results in a variety of dissociative disorders depending on the primary cognitive process affected. When memories are poorly integrated, the resulting disorder is *dissociative amnesia*. Fragmentation of identity results in *dissociative fugue* or *dissociative identity disorder* (DID; formerly multiple personality disorder). Disordered perception yields *depersonalization disorder*. Dissociation of aspects of consciousness produces *acute stress disorder* and various dissociative trance and possession states.

These dissociative disorders are a disturbance more in the organization or structure of mental contents than in the contents themselves. Memories in dissociative amnesia are not so much distorted or bizarre as they are segregated from one another. The identity temporarily lost in dissociative fugue, or the aspects of the self that are fragmented in DID, are two-dimensional aspects of an overall personality structure. In this sense, it has been said that patients with DID suffer not from having more than

one personality, but rather from having less than one personality. The problem is the failure of integration rather than the contents of the fragments. In summary, all types of dissociative disorders have in common a lack of immediate access to the entire personality structure or mental content in one form or another.

The dissociative disorders have a long history in classical psychopathology but until recently have been largely ignored. Nonetheless, the phenomena are sufficiently persistent and interesting that they have elicited growing attention from both professionals and the public. The dissociative disorders remain an area of psychopathology for which the best treatment is psychotherapy (Maldonado et al. 2000). As mental disorders, they have much to teach us about the way humans adapt to traumatic stress and about information processing in the brain.

Models and Mechanisms of Dissociation

Dissociation and Information Processing

Modern information processing–based theories, including connectionist and parallel distributed processing (PDP) models

(Rumelhart and McClelland 1986), take a bottom-up rather than a top-down approach to cognitive organization. Traditional models emphasize a superordinate organization in which broad categories of information structure the processing of specific examples. In the PDP models, subunits or neural nets process information through computation of co-occurring input stimuli. The activation patterns in these neural nets allow for category recognition. The output of one set of nets becomes the input to another, thereby gradually building up integrated and complex patterns of activation and inhibition. Such bottom-up processing models have the advantage of accounting for the processing of vast amounts of information and for the human ability to recognize patterns on the basis of approximate information. However, such models make the classification and integration of information problematic. In PDP models, it is theoretically likely that failures in integration of mental contents will occur. Indeed, attempts have been made to model psychopathology based on difficulties in neural net information processing, for example, in schizophrenia and bipolar disorder (Hoffman 1987), as well as in dissociative disorders (D. Li and Spiegel 1992). The idea is that when a net runs into difficulty in balancing the processing of input information (a model for traumatic input), it is more likely to have difficulty achieving a unified and balanced output. Such neural nets tend to fall into a "dissociated" situation in which they move in one direction or another but cannot reach an optimal balanced solution, and therefore they are unable to process smoothly all of the incoming information.

Dissociation and Memory Systems

Modern research on memory shows that there are at least two broad categories of memory, variously described as *explicit* and *implicit* (Schacter 1992; Squire 1992) or *episodic* and *semantic* (Tulving 1983). These two memory systems serve different functions. *Explicit* (or *episodic*) *memory* involves recall of personal experience identified with the self (e.g., "I was at the ball game last week"). *Implicit* (or *semantic*) *memory* involves the execution of routine operations, such as riding a bicycle or typing. Such operations may be carried out with a high degree of proficiency with little conscious awareness of either their current execution or the learning episodes on which the skill is based. Indeed, these two types of memory may well have different anatomical localizations: the limbic system, especially the hippocampal formation, and mammillary bodies for episodic memory; and the basal ganglia and cortex for procedural (or semantic) memory (Mishkin and Appenzeller 1987; Squire 1992).

Indeed, the distinction between these two types of memory may account for certain dissociative phenomena (D. Spiegel et al. 1993). The automaticity observed in certain dissociative disorders may be a reflection of the separation of self-identification in certain kinds of explicit memory from routine activity in implicit or semantic memory. It is thus not at all foreign to our mental processing to act in an automatic way devoid of explicit self-identification. Were it necessary for us to retrieve explicit memories of how and when we learned all of the activities we are required to perform, it is highly unlikely that we would be able to function with anything like the degree of efficiency we have.

Meares (1999) suggested that traumatic memories are represented in a way that is qualitatively different from nontraumatic memories. His argument depends on a concept of self that is double, involving mental life and the individual's own reflection on it. If trauma is seen as causing an uncoupling, or dedoubling, of consciousness, then the traumatic diminishment of the subject–object distinction in psychic life will have several effects. First, it will change the form of conscious awareness to a state that is focused on the present and on immediate stimuli. Second, the memory system in which the traumatic events are recorded will be non-episodic, thus lacking the reflective component, making it unconscious. Third, the traumatized–traumatizer dyad will be represented not as two persons in a relationship, but more as a nearly fused unit. This fused representation will not be integrated into the system of self as the stream of consciousness but is more likely to remain relatively sequestered. Finally, in an "uncoupled" state, the interpretation of the "meaning" of the traumatic event is impaired, and its construction will be determined by affect.

Dissociation and Trauma

An important development in the modern understanding of dissociative disorders is the exploration of the link between trauma and dissociation (D. Spiegel and Cardeña 1991). Trauma can be understood as the experience of being made into an object or a thing, the victim of someone else's rage or of nature's indifference. It is the ultimate experience of helplessness and loss of control over one's own body. There is growing clinical and some empirical evidence that dissociation may occur especially as a defense during trauma—an attempt to maintain mental control at the very moment when physical control has been lost (Bremner and Brett 1997; Butler et al. 1996; Eriksson and Lundin 1996; Kluft 1984a, 1984c; Koopman et al. 1995, 1996; Putnam 1985; D. Spiegel 1984; D. Spiegel et al. 1988).

An accumulating literature suggests a connection between a history of physical and sexual abuse in childhood and the development of dissociative symptoms (Anderson et al. 1993; L. Brown et al. 1999; Chu et al. 1999; Coons 1994; Coons and Milstein 1986; Ellason et al. 1996; Farley and Keaney 1997; Irwin 1999; Kaplan et al. 1995; Kluft 1984c, 1985a; Mulder et al. 1998; Roesler and McKenzie 1994; Sar et al. 1996; Saxe et al. 1993; Scroppo et al. 1998; D. Spiegel 1984). Similarly, evidence is accumulating that dissociative symptoms are more prevalent in patients with Axis II disorders such as borderline personality disorder when there has been a history of childhood abuse (Brenner 1996a, 1996b; Brodsky et al. 1995; Chu and Dill 1990; Darves-Bornoz 1997; Herman et al. 1989; Zweig-Frank et al. 1994). When Mulder et al. (1998) examined the relation between childhood sexual abuse, childhood physical abuse, current psychiatric illness, and measures of dissociation in an adult population, they found that 6.3% of the abused population had three or more frequently occurring dissociative symptoms. Among these individuals, the rate of childhood sexual abuse was two and one-half times as high, the rate of physical abuse was five times as high, and the rate of current psychiatric disorder was four times as high as the respective rates for the other subjects.

In the following discussions, we review the diagnosis and treatment of the dissociative disorders as defined in DSM-IV-TR.

Dissociative Amnesia

The hallmark of dissociative amnesia is the inability to recall important personal information, usually of a traumatic or stressful nature, which cannot be explained by ordinary forgetfulness (American Psychiatric Association 2000) (Table 10–1). Dissociative amnesia is considered the most common of all dissociative disorders (Putnam 1985). Amnesia is a symptom commonly found in several other dissociative and anxiety disorders, including acute stress disorder, PTSD, somatization disorder, dissociative fugue, and DID (American Psychiatric Association 2000). A higher incidence of dissociative amnesia has been described in the context of war and natural and other disasters (Maldonado et al. 2000). There appears to be a direct relation between the severity of the exposure to trauma and the incidence of amnesia (G.R. Brown and Anderson 1991; Chu and Dill 1990; Kirshner 1973; Putnam 1985, 1993; Sargant and Slater 1941).

Dissociative amnesia is the classical functional disorder of memory and involves difficulty in retrieving discrete components of episodic memory. It does not, however, involve a difficulty in memory storage, as in Wernicke-Korsakoff syndrome. Because the amnesia involves primarily difficulties in retrieval rather than encoding or storage, the memory deficits usually are reversible. Once the amnesia has cleared, normal memory function is resumed (Schacter et al. 1982). Dissociative amnesia has three primary characteristics:

1. The memory loss is episodic. The first-person recollection of certain events is lost, rather than knowledge of procedures.
2. The memory loss is for a discrete period of time, ranging from minutes to years. It is not vagueness or inefficient retrieval of memories, but rather a dense unavailability of memories that previously had been clearly available. Unlike in the amnestic disorders, there is usually no difficulty in learning *new* episodic information. Thus, the amne-

TABLE 10–1. DSM-IV-TR diagnostic criteria for dissociative amnesia

A. The predominant disturbance is one or more episodes of inability to recall important personal information, usually of a traumatic or stressful nature, that is too extensive to be explained by ordinary forgetfulness.
B. The disturbance does not occur exclusively during the course of dissociative identity disorder, dissociative fugue, posttraumatic stress disorder, acute stress disorder, or somatization disorder and is not due to the direct physiological effects of a substance (e.g., a drug of abuse, a medication) or a neurological or other general medical condition (e.g., amnestic disorder due to head trauma).
C. The symptoms cause clinically significant distress or impairment in social, occupational, or other important areas of functioning.

sia is typically of the retrograde rather than the anterograde variety (Loewenstein 1991a), with one or more discrete periods of past information becoming unavailable.
3. The memory loss generally involves events of a traumatic or stressful nature.

Dissociative amnesia is most common in the third and fourth decades of life (Abeles and Schilder 1935; Coons and Milstein 1986). It usually involves one episode, but multiple periods of lost memory are not uncommon (Coons and Milstein 1986). Comorbidity with conversion disorder, bulimia, alcohol abuse, and depression is common, and Axis II diagnoses of histrionic, dependent, and borderline personality disorders occur in a substantial minority of such patients (Coons and Milstein 1986).

Dissociative amnesia usually involves discrete boundaries around the period of time unavailable to consciousness. Individuals with such a disorder lose their ability to recall what happened during a specific period. They demonstrate not vagueness or spotty memory but rather a loss of any episodic memory for a finite period. Such individuals initially may not be aware of the memory loss—that is, they may not remember that they do not remember.

Dissociative amnesia most frequently occurs after an episode of trauma, and the onset may be sudden or gradual. Some individuals do experience episodes of selective amnesia, usually for specific traumatic incidents, which may be more interwoven with periods of intact memory. In these cases, the amnesia is for a type of material remembered rather than for a discrete period of time. Despite the fact that certain information is kept out of consciousness in dissociative amnesia, such information may exert an influence on consciousness.

Individuals with dissociative amnesia generally do not have disturbances of identity, except to the extent that their identity is influenced by the warded-off memory. It is not uncommon for such individuals to develop depressive symptoms as well, especially when the amnesia is in the wake of a traumatic episode.

Treatment

To date, no controlled studies have addressed the treatment of dissociative amnesia. No established pharmacological treatments are available, except for the use of benzodiazepines or barbiturates for drug-assisted interviews (Maldonado et al. 2000). Most cases of dissociative amnesia revert spontaneously, especially when the individuals are removed from stressful or threatening situations, when they feel physically and psychologically safe, and/or when they are exposed to cues from the

past (i.e., family members) (W. Brown 1918; Kardiner and Spiegel 1947; Loewenstein 1991b; Maldonado et al. 2000; Reither and Stoudemire 1988). When a safe environment is not enough to restore normal memory functioning, the amnesia sometimes can be breached through use of techniques such as pharmacologically mediated interviews (i.e., barbiturates and benzodiazepines) (Baron and Nagy 1988; Naples and Hackett 1978; J.C. Perry and Jacobs 1982; Wettstein and Fauman 1979).

On the other hand, most patients with dissociative disorder are highly hypnotizable on formal testing and therefore are easily able to make use of hypnotic techniques such as age regression (H. Spiegel and Spiegel 1978/1987). Patients are hypnotized and instructed to experience a time before the onset of the amnesia as though it were the present. Then the patients are reoriented in hypnosis to experience events during the amnesic period. Hypnosis can enable such patients to reorient temporally and therefore to achieve access to otherwise dissociated memories. If the warded-off memory has traumatic content, patients may abreact (i.e., express strong emotion) as these memories are elicited, and they will need psychotherapeutic help in integrating these memories and the associated affect into consciousness.

One technique that can help bring such memories into consciousness while modulating the affective response to them is the screen technique (D. Spiegel 1981). In this approach, patients are taught, by using hypnosis, to relive the traumatic event as if they were watching it on an imaginary movie or television screen. This technique is often helpful for individuals who are unable to relive the event as if it were occurring in the present tense, either because that process is too emotionally taxing or because they are not sufficiently

hypnotizable to be able to engage in hypnotic age regression. The screen technique
also can be used to provide dissociation
between the psychological and the somatic aspects of the memory retrieval.
Individuals can be put into self-hypnosis
and instructed to get their bodies into a
state of floating comfort and safety. They
are reminded that no matter what they
see on the screen, their bodies will be safe
and comfortable. This allows them to
remember the trauma without re-experi-
encing the somatic memories that often
accompany flashbacks and spontaneous
abreactions. This technique may also be
used by a skillful clinician to help patients
remember what they may have done during the trauma to maintain or regain control.

Dissociative Fugue

Dissociative fugue combines failure of
integration of certain aspects of personal
memory with loss of customary identity
and automatisms of motor behavior (Table
10–2). Patients appear "normal," usually
showing no signs of psychopathology or
cognitive deficit. Fugue involves one or
more episodes of sudden, unexpected,
purposeful travel away from home, coupled with an inability to recall portions or
all of one's past, and a loss of identity or
the assumption of a new identity. In contrast to patients who have DID, if patients
with dissociative fugue develop a new
identity, the old and new identities do not
alternate. The onset is usually sudden, and
it frequently occurs after a traumatic experience or bereavement. A single episode
is not uncommon, and spontaneous remission of symptoms can occur without treatment.

It was thought that the assumption of
a new identity, as in the classical case of
the Reverend Ansel Bourne (James 1890/

1950), was typical of dissociative fugue.
However, Reither and Stoudemire (1988),
in their review of the literature, documented that in most cases, there is loss of
personal identity but no clear assumption
of a new identity.

Many cases of dissociative fugue remit
spontaneously. But again, hypnosis can be
useful in accessing dissociated material
(H. Spiegel and Spiegel 1978/1987). As
mentioned previously, hypnosis can be
useful in accessing dissociated material
(H. Spiegel and Spiegel 1978/1987). In
those cases in which no spontaneous resolution occurs, hypnosis may be helpful in
accessing otherwise unavailable components of memory and identity. The approach used is similar to that for dissociative amnesia. Hypnotic age regression can
be used as the framework for accessing
information previously unavailable. Demonstrating to patients that such information can be made available to consciousness enhances their sense of control over
the material and facilitates the therapeutic working-through of its emotion-laden
aspects.

Patients with dissociative fugue may
be helped with a psychotherapeutic approach that facilitates conscious integration of dissociated memories and motivations for behavior previously experienced
as automatic and unwilled. It is often
helpful to address current psychosocial
stressors, such as marital conflict, with the
involved individuals. To the extent that
current psychosocial stress triggers fugue,
resolution of that stress can help resolve
the fugue state and reduce the likelihood
of recurrence.

In the past, sodium amobarbital or
another short-acting sedative was used to
reverse dissociative amnesia or fugue.
However, such techniques offer no advantage over hypnosis and are not especially
effective (J.C. Perry and Jacobs 1982).
There is at least one case report of the use

TABLE 10–2. DSM-IV-TR diagnostic criteria for dissociative fugue

A. The predominant disturbance is sudden, unexpected travel away from home or one's customary place of work, with inability to recall one's past.
B. Confusion about personal identity or assumption of a new identity (partial or complete).
C. The disturbance does not occur exclusively during the course of dissociative identity disorder and is not due to the direct physiological effects of a substance (e.g., a drug of abuse, a medication) or a general medical condition (e.g., temporal lobe epilepsy).
D. The symptoms cause clinically significant distress or impairment in social, occupational, or other important areas of functioning.

TABLE 10–3. DSM-IV-TR diagnostic criteria for depersonalization disorder

A. Persistent or recurrent experiences of feeling detached from, and as if one is an outside observer of, one's mental processes or body (e.g., feeling like one is in a dream).
B. During the depersonalization experience, reality testing remains intact.
C. The depersonalization causes clinically significant distress or impairment in social, occupational, or other important areas of functioning.
D. The depersonalization experience does not occur exclusively during the course of another mental disorder, such as schizophrenia, panic disorder, acute stress disorder, or another dissociative disorder, and is not due to the direct physiological effects of a substance (e.g., a drug of abuse, a medication) or a general medical condition (e.g., temporal lobe epilepsy).

of a locator beacon attached to a patient with dissociative fugue, which has proven effective in the curtailment of dissociative fugue episodes (Macleod 1999).

Depersonalization Disorder

The essential feature of depersonalization disorder is the occurrence of persistent feelings of unreality, detachment, or estrangement from oneself or one's body, usually with the feeling that one is an outside observer of one's own mental processes (Steinberg 1991). Thus, depersonalization disorder is primarily a disturbance in the integration of perceptual experience (Table 10–3). Individuals who have depersonalization disorder are distressed by it. Different from those with delusional disorders and other psychotic processes, those with depersonalization disorder have intact reality testing. Patients are aware of some distortion in their perceptual experience and therefore are

not delusional. The symptom is often transient and may co-occur with a variety of other symptoms, especially anxiety, panic, or phobic symptoms. Indeed, the content of the anxiety may involve fears of "going crazy." Derealization frequently co-occurs with depersonalization disorder, in which affected individuals notice an altered perception of their surroundings, resulting in the world seeming unreal or dreamlike. Affected individuals often will ruminate about this alteration and be preoccupied with their own somatic and mental functioning.

Depersonalization as a symptom is seen in several psychiatric and neurological disorders (Pies 1991; Putnam 1985). Unlike other dissociative disorders, the presence of which excludes other mental disorders such as schizophrenia and substance abuse, depersonalization disorder frequently co-occurs with such disorders. It is often a symptom of anxiety disorders and PTSD. In fact, about 69% of patients

with panic disorder experience depersonalization or derealization during their
panic attacks (Ball et al. 1997). Episodes
of depersonalization also may occur as a
symptom of alcohol and drug abuse, as
a side effect of prescription medication,
and during stress and sensory deprivation.
Depersonalization is considered a disorder
when it is a persistent and predominant
symptom. The phenomenology of the
disorder involves both the initial symptoms themselves and the reactive anxiety
caused by them.

Treatment

Depersonalization is most often transient
and may remit without formal treatment.
Recurrent or persistent depersonalization
should be thought of both as a symptom in
and of itself and as a component of other
syndromes requiring treatment, such as
anxiety disorders and schizophrenia.

The symptom itself may respond to
self-hypnosis training. Often, hypnotic induction will induce transient depersonalization symptoms in patients. This is a
useful exercise, because by having a structure for inducing the depersonalization
symptoms, one provides patients with a
context for understanding and controlling
them. The symptoms are presented as a
spontaneous form of hypnotic dissociation that can be modified. Individuals for
whom this approach is effective can be
taught to induce a pleasant sense of floating lightness or heaviness in place of the
anxiety-related somatic detachment. Often, the use of an imaginary screen to picture problems in a way that detaches
them from the typical somatic response
is also helpful (H. Spiegel and Spiegel
1978/1987).

Other treatment modalities used (Maldonado et al. 2000) include behavioral
techniques, such as paradoxical intention
(Blue 1979), record keeping, and positive

reward (Dollinger 1983); flooding (Sookman and Solyom 1978); psychotherapy,
especially psychodynamic (Noyes and
Kletti 1977; Schilder 1939; Shilony and
Grossman 1993; Torch 1987); and psychoeducation (Fewtrell 1986; Torch 1987).
Some have suggested the use of psychotropic medications, including psychostimulants (Cattell and Cattell 1974; Davison
1964; Shorvon 1946), antidepressants
(Fichtner et al. 1992; Hollander et al.
1989, 1990; Noyes et al. 1987; Walsh
1975), antipsychotics (Ambrosino 1973;
Nuller 1982), anticonvulsants (Stein and
Uhde 1989), and benzodiazepines (Ballenger et al. 1988; Nuller 1982; Spier
et al. 1986; Stein and Uhde 1989). Finally, others have suggested the use of
electroconvulsive therapy (ECT; Ambrosino 1973; Davison 1964; Roth 1959;
Shorvon 1946). Appropriate treatment of
comorbid disorders is an important part of
treatment. Use of antianxiety medications for generalized anxiety or phobic disorders and antipsychotic medications for
schizophrenia should help in these conditions.

Dissociative Identity Disorder (Multiple Personality Disorder)

Prevalence

There are no convincing studies of the absolute prevalence of DID. The initial systematic report on the epidemiology of
DID estimated a prevalence in the general
population of 0.01% (Coons 1984). The
estimated prevalence is approximately 3%
of psychiatric inpatients (Ross 1991; Ross
et al. 1991b). Studies conducted in the
general population suggest a prevalence
higher than that initially reported by
Coons (1984) but lower (about 1%) than
the prevalence described in psychiatric

settings and specialized treatment units (Ross 1991; Vanderlinden et al. 1991). Loewenstein (1994) reported that the prevalence of DID in North America is about 1%, compared with a prevalence of 10% for all dissociative disorders as a group. Loewenstein's findings were replicated by Rifkin et al. (1998), who studied 100 randomly selected women, ages 16–50 years, who had been admitted to an acute psychiatric hospital. One percent of the subjects were found to have DID.

The number of reported DID cases has risen considerably in recent years. Factors that account for this increase include a more general awareness of the diagnosis among mental health professionals; the availability, starting with DSM-III, of specific diagnostic criteria (Table 10–4); and reduced misdiagnosis of DID as schizophrenia or borderline personality disorder. Although the increase in reported cases is best documented in North America, a recent study showed similar phenomenology and link to trauma history in Europe (Boon and Draijer 1993a, 1993b; Gast et al. 2001; Nijenhuis et al. 1998). In fact, there are reports of DID in almost all societies and races, making it a true cross-cultural diagnosis (Coons et al. 1991). Case reports have described DID or related disorders among Asians (Putnam 1989; Yap 1960), blacks (Coons and Milstein 1986; R. Solomon 1983; Stern 1984), Europeans (Boon and Draijer 1993a, 1993b; Freyberger et al. 1998; Nijenhuis et al. 1998; Spitzer et al. 1999; van der Hart 1993), Hispanics (Allison 1974; Ronquillo 1991; R. Solomon 1983), and inhabitants of Australia and New Zealand (L. Brown et al. 1999; Gelb 1993; Middleton and Butler 1998; Price and Hess 1979), Canada (Horen et al. 1995; Ross et al. 1989, 1991a, 1991b; Vincent and Pickering 1988), the Caribbean (Wittkower 1970), India (Adityanjee et al. 1989; Varma et al. 1981), Japan (Berger et al. 1994), the

Netherlands (Boon and Draijer 1993b; Draijer and Langeland 1999; Friedl and Draijer 2000; Nijenhuis et al. 1997; Sno and Schalken 1999; van der Hart and Nijenhuis 1993; Vanderlinden et al. 1991; van Dyck 1993), Norway (Boe et al. 1993), Sweden (Eriksson and Lundin 1996), Switzerland (Modestin et al. 1996), and Turkey (Akyuz et al. 1999; Chodoff 1997; Sar et al. 1996; Tutkun et al. 1998; Yargic et al. 1998).

TABLE 10–4. DSM-IV-TR diagnostic criteria for dissociative identity disorder

A. The presence of two or more distinct identities or personality states (each with its own relatively enduring pattern of perceiving, relating to, and thinking about the environment and self).

B. At least two of these identities or personality states recurrently take control of the person's behavior.

C. Inability to recall important personal information that is too extensive to be explained by ordinary forgetfulness.

D. The disturbance is not due to the direct physiological effects of a substance (e.g., blackouts or chaotic behavior during alcohol intoxication) or a general medical condition (e.g., complex partial seizures).

Note: In children, the symptoms are not attributable to imaginary playmates or other fantasy play.

Other authors attribute the increase in reported cases to hypnotic suggestion and misdiagnosis (Brenner 1994, 1996a; Frankel 1990; Ganaway 1989, 1995; Mayer-Gross et al. 1969; McHugh 1995a, 1995b; Piper 1994; Spanos et al. 1985, 1986). Proponents of this point of view argue that individuals with DID are as a group highly hypnotizable and therefore quite suggestible and that a few specialist clinicians usually make the vast majority of diagnoses. However, it has been observed that the symptomatology of patients diagnosed by specialists in dissociation does not differ from that assessed by psychiatrists, psychologists, and physicians in more general practices, who diagnose one or two cases a year.

In a study (Chu et al. 1999) of female patients admitted to a unit specializing in the treatment of trauma-related disorders, participants reporting any type of childhood abuse had elevated levels of dissociative symptoms that were significantly higher than those in subjects not reporting abuse. Higher dissociative symptom levels were correlated with early age at onset of physical and sexual abuse and with more frequent sexual abuse. A substantial proportion of participants with all types of abuse reported partial or complete amnesia for abuse memories. For physical and sexual abuse, early age at onset was correlated with greater levels of amnesia. Participants who reported recovering memories of abuse generally recalled these experiences while at home, alone, or with family or friends. Although some participants were in treatment at the time, very few were in therapy sessions during their first memory recovery. Suggestion was generally denied as a factor in memory recovery, and most participants were able to find strong corroboration of their recovered memories.

If such patients were so suggestible and subject to directive influence by diagnosticians, then it is surprising that their presenting symptoms persisted for an average of 6.5 years before the diagnosis was made (Putnam et al. 1986). Rather, it would seem likely that such patients would accept a suggestion that they have another disorder, such as schizophrenia or borderline personality disorder, because they encounter many clinicians who are unaware of or not familiar with DID. Because these patients are indeed highly hypnotizable and therefore suggestible

(Frischholz 1985), care must be taken in the manner in which the illness is presented to them. However, it is unlikely that the increased number of cases currently reported is accounted for by suggestion alone. Rather, a reduction in previous misdiagnoses and an increase in recognition of the prevalence and sequelae of physical and sexual abuse in childhood (Braun 1990; Bryer et al. 1987; Coons et al. 1988; Finkelhor 1984; Frischholz 1985; Goodwin 1982; Herman et al. 1989; Kluft 1984c, 1991; Pribor and Dinwiddie 1992; Putnam 1988; Putnam et al. 1986; Ross 1989; Russell 1986; D. Spiegel 1984; Terr 1991) are also likely explanations. There have been reports of "definite independent confirmation of the histories of abuse" (Coons 1994; Martinez-Taboas 1996) confirming not only the association between dissociative disorders and trauma but also the occurrence of amnesia in response to traumatic experiences. Furthermore, a recent study among Dutch psychiatrists (Sno and Schalken 1999) reported that 40% have made the diagnosis of DID at least once. The diagnosis was made statistically significantly more frequently by female psychiatrists, by psychiatrists age 50 years or younger, and by psychiatrists certified after 1982. No correlation was observed with the psychiatrist's primary theoretical orientation or the type or topography of work facility. The mean age of the selected patients was 33.2, and the female-to-male ratio was 9:1. Similar to their American counterparts, most Dutch DID patients were seen once a week in an outpatient setting, and individual psychotherapy and adjunctive anxiolytic or antidepressant medications were the most widely endorsed treatment modalities. Different from more typical American practice, hypnosis was rarely used. This study suggested that the diagnosis of DID should not be dismissed as a local (American) eccentricity and minimized the roles of suggestibility, hypnosis, and culture.

Course

Although DID is being diagnosed in childhood with increasing frequency (Kluft 1984a; 1984b), it typically emerges between adolescence and the third decade of life. DID rarely presents as a new disorder after an individual reaches age 40 years; however, there is often considerable delay between initial symptom presentation and diagnosis (American Psychiatric Association 2000; Putnam et al. 1986). The female:male sex ratio of DID is 5:4 in children and adolescents and 9:1 in adults (Hocke and Schmidtke 1998; Sno and Schalken 1999).

Untreated, DID is a chronic and recurrent disorder. It rarely remits spontaneously, but the symptoms may not be evident for some time (Kluft 1985b). DID has been called "a pathology of hiddenness" (Gutheil, as quoted in Kluft 1988, p. 575). The dissociation itself hampers self-monitoring and accurate reporting of symptoms. Many patients with the disorder are not fully aware of the extent of the dissociative symptomatology. They may be reluctant to bring up symptoms because of having encountered frequent skepticism. Furthermore, because most patients with DID report histories of sexual and physical abuse (Braun and Sachs 1985; Coons and Milstein 1992; Coons et al. 1988; Kluft 1985a, 1988, 1991; Putnam 1988; Putnam et al. 1986; Ross 1989; Ross et al. 1990; Schultz et al. 1989; D. Spiegel 1984), the shame associated with that experience, as well as fear of retribution, may inhibit reporting of symptoms.

Comorbidity

The major comorbid psychiatric illnesses of DID are the depressive disorders (Put-

nam et al. 1986; Ross and Norton 1989; Ross et al. 1989; Yargic et al. 1998), substance use disorders (Anderson et al. 1993; Coons 1984; Dunn et al. 1995; Ellason et al. 1996; Putnam et al. 1986; Rivera 1991), and borderline personality disorder (Anderson et al. 1993; Brodsky et al. 1995; Horevitz and Braun 1984; Shearer 1994; Yargic et al. 1998). Sexual (Brenner 1996b; van der Kolk et al. 1994), eating (Berger et al. 1994; Valdiserri and Kihlstrom 1995; van der Kolk et al. 1994), somatoform (Spitzer et al. 1999; Yargic et al. 1998), and sleep disorders (Putnam et al. 1986) occur less commonly. Patients with DID frequently engage in self-mutilative behavior (Bliss 1980, 1984; Coons 1984; Gainer and Torem 1993; Greaves 1980; Putnam et al. 1986; Ross and Norton 1989; Zweig-Frank et al. 1994), impulsiveness, and overvaluing and devaluing of relationships that make approximately a third of DID patients fit the criteria for borderline personality disorder as well. Such individuals also show higher levels of depression (Horevitz and Braun 1984). Conversely, research shows dissociative symptoms in many patients with borderline personality disorder, especially those who report histories of physical and sexual abuse (Chu and Dill 1990; Ogata et al. 1990).

Comorbidity is complex in that patients with concurrent diagnoses of DID and borderline personality disorder (approximately one-third) also are more likely to meet the criteria for major depressive disorder. In addition, they frequently meet the criteria for PTSD, with intrusive flashbacks, recurring dreams of physical and sexual abuse, avoidance and loss of pleasure of usually pleasurable activities, and symptoms of hyperarousal, especially when exposed to reminders of childhood trauma (Kluft 1991; Putnam 1993; D. Spiegel 1990b; van der Kolk and Fisler 1995; van der Kolk et al. 1994, 1996).

In addition, these patients are often misdiagnosed as having schizophrenia (Coons 1984; Ellason and Ross 1995; Kluft 1987; Putnam et al. 1986; Ross and Norton 1988; Ross et al. 1990; Steinberg et al. 1994). This diagnostic confusion is understandable given that the first-rank criterion for schizophrenia is that the patient has an apparent delusion (e.g., that his or her body is occupied by more than one person). These patients frequently have auditory hallucinations in which one personality state speaks to or comments on the activities of another (Bliss 1986; Bliss et al. 1983; Coons 1984; Kluft 1987; Peterson 1995; Putnam et al. 1986; Ross et al. 1990). When these patients receive misdiagnoses of schizophrenia, they are frequently given neuroleptics, with poor therapeutic response.

Individuals with DID report an average of 15 somatic or conversion symptoms (Anderson et al. 1993; Bowman 1993; Bowman and Markand 1996; Kaplan et al. 1995; Ross et al. 1989, 1990) and other psychosomatic symptoms such as migraine headaches (D. Spiegel 1987) and complex partial seizures (Schenk and Bear 1981).

Psychological Testing

The diagnosis of DID can be facilitated through psychological testing (Scroppo et al. 1998). Form level on the Rorschach Test usually is within the normal range, but emotionally dramatic responses are common, often involving mutilation, especially on the color cards (such responses are often seen in patients with histrionic personality disorder as well). Good form level is useful in distinguishing DID patients from schizophrenic patients, who have poor form level. Leavitt and Labott (1998) replicated these findings. Their results indicated that Rorschach signs for the Labott, Barach, and Wagner Rorschach markers

were significantly better than chance at classifying patients as having DID or as not having DID. The Labott system, which performed the best, was able to accurately classify 92% of the sample. The fact that two relatively rare sets of signs (DID and Rorschach) converged in the same small sector of the psychiatric population represents evidence of linkage that is clinically meaningful and not explainable on the basis of artificial creation. That the Rorschach signs operate independent of external bias, yet correspond to the diagnoses obtained through psychiatric evaluation in an inpatient setting, argues for the validity of the DID diagnosis. Also, unlike individuals with schizophrenia, those with DID score far higher than healthy individuals on standard measures of hypnotizability, whereas schizophrenic patients tend to show lower than normal or the absence of high hypnotizability (Lavoie and Sabourin 1980; Lavoie et al. 1973; Pettinati 1982; Pettinati et al. 1990; D. Spiegel and Fink 1979; D. Spiegel et al. 1982; van der Hart and Spiegel 1993). Thus, there is comparatively little overlap in the hypnotizability scores of schizophrenic patients and those of DID patients.

More recently, scales of trait dissociation have been developed (Bernstein and Putnam 1986; Ross 1989), and patients with DID score extremely high on these scales in contrast to healthy populations and other patient groups (Ross et al. 1990; Steinberg et al. 1990). These include the DES (Bernstein and Putnam 1986; Carlson et al. 1993), the Somatoform Dissociation Questionnaires (SDQ-20 and SDQ-5; Nijenhuis et al. 1996, 1997, respectively), the Clinician-Administered Dissociative States Scale (Bremner et al. 1998), the Structured Clinical Interview for DSM-IV Dissociative Disorders—Revised (Steinberg 2000), and the Adolescent Dissociative Experiences Scale (Armstrong et al. 1997).

Treatment

Psychotherapy

Therapeutic direction. It is possible to help patients with DID gain control in several ways over the dissociative process underlying their symptoms. The fundamental psychotherapeutic stance should involve meeting patients halfway in the sense of acknowledging that they experience themselves as fragmented, yet the reality is that the fundamental problem is a failure of integration of disparate memories and aspects of the self. Therefore, the goal in therapy is to facilitate integration of disparate elements. This can be done in a variety of ways.

TABLE 10–5. "Rules of engagement" in the treatment of dissociative identity disorder

---

1. Free access to all pertinent records
2. Review of all available and pertinent records
3. Freedom to discuss all past and current pertinent information with previous therapists
4. Complete organic/neurological workup
5. Contract for safety
6. Increased communication and cooperation among alters
7. "No secrets" policy
8. Establishment of hierarchical pattern of communication
9. Establishment of hierarchical pattern of responsibility
10. Limited exploration followed by therapeutic condensation of memories
11. "All details are not needed" policy
12. Rules regarding contact during hospitalizations and continued therapy after discharge
13. Videotaping
14. Ultimate goal: "full integration"
15. "One day you will make me obsolete" principle

Secrets are frequently a problem with DID patients, who attempt to use the therapist to reinforce a dissociative strategy that withholds relevant information from certain personality states. Such patients often like to confide plans or stories to the therapist with the idea that the information is to be kept from other parts of the self, for example, traumatic memories or plans for self-destructive activities. Clear limit setting and commitment on the part of the therapist to helping all portions of a patient's personality structure learn about warded-off information are important. It is wise to clarify explicitly that the therapist will not become involved in secret collusion. Furthermore, when important agreements are negotiated, such as a commitment on the part of the patient to seek medical help before acting on a thought to harm self or others, it is useful to discuss with the patient that this is an "all-points bulletin," that is, one that requires attention from all the relevant personality states. The excuse that certain personality states were "not aware" of the agreement should not be accepted.

Maldonado (2000) described a series of "Rules of Engagement" (see Table 10–5) to be used in the treatment of DID. These rules were designed to facilitate the therapist–patient contract by establishing clear lines of communication, delineating therapeutic boundaries, eliminating splitting, and enhancing control over dissociative experiences. The rules call for free access to all pertinent old records and permission to discuss all past and current pertinent information with previous therapists; cooperation in the completion of a full organic/neurological workup; a contract for safety; the establishment of a hierarchical pattern of communication and a hierarchical pattern of responsibility; agreement for a limited exploration followed by therapeutic condensation of memories—that is, an "all details are not needed" policy rather than an endless fishing exploration; a "no secrets" policy; an increased level of communication and cooperation between patient and therapist and between alters; detailed rules regarding therapist–patient contact during hospitalization and continued therapy after discharge; need for videotaping; and, finally, clear understanding of the ultimate treatment goal: "full integration."

Hypnosis. Hypnosis can be helpful in therapy as well as in diagnosis (Braun 1984; Kluft 1982, 1985b, 1992, 1999; Maldonado and Spiegel 1995, 1998; Maldonado et al. 2000; Smith 1993; H. Spiegel and Spiegel 1978/1987). The capacity to elicit such symptoms on command provides the first hint of the ability to control these symptoms. Most of these patients have the experience of being unable to stop dissociative symptoms but are often intrigued by the possibility of starting them. This carries with it the potential for changing or stopping the symptoms as well.

Hypnosis can be helpful in facilitating access to dissociated personalities. The personalities may simply occur spontaneously during hypnotic induction. An alternative strategy is to hypnotize the patient and use age regression to help the patient reorient to a time when a different personality state was manifest. An instruction later to change times back to the present tense usually elicits a return to the other personality state. This then becomes an alternative means of teaching the patient control over the dissociation. Alternatively, entering the state of hypnosis may make it possible to simply "call up" different identities or personality states.

Memory retrieval. Because loss of memory in DID is complex and chronic, its retrieval is likewise a more extended and integral part of the psychotherapeutic process. The therapy becomes an integrating experience of information sharing among disparate personality elements. In conceptualizing DID as a chronic PTSD, the psychotherapeutic strategy involves a focus on working through traumatic memories in addition to controlling the dissociation.

Controlled access to memories greatly facilitates psychotherapy. As in the treatment of dissociative amnesia, a variety of strategies can be used to help DID patients break down amnesic barriers. Use of hypnosis to go to that place in imagination and ask one or more such parts of the self to interact can be helpful.

Once these memories of earlier traumatic experience have been brought into consciousness, it is crucial to help the patient work through the painful affect, inappropriate self-blame, and other reactions to these memories. A model of grief work is helpful, enabling the patient to acknowledge and bear the import of such memories (Lindemann 1944; D. Spiegel 1981). It may be useful to have the patient visualize the memories rather than relive them as a way of making their intensity more manageable. It also can be useful to have the patient divide the memories onto two sides of an imaginary screen; for example, on one side, picturing something an abuser did to him or her and on the other side, picturing how the patient tried to protect himself or herself from the abuse. Such techniques can help make the traumatic memories more bearable by placing them in a broader perspective, one in which the trauma victim also can identify adaptive aspects of his or her response to the trauma.

This technique and similar approaches can help these individuals work through traumatic memories, enabling them to bear the memories in consciousness and therefore reducing the need for dissociation as a means of keeping such memories out of consciousness. Although these techniques can be helpful and often result in reduced fragmentation and integration (Kluft 1985b, 1986, 1992; Maldonado and Spiegel 1995, 1998; D. Spiegel 1984, 1986a), several complications can occur in the psychotherapy of these patients as well.

The information retrieved from memory in these ways should be reviewed, traumatic memories put into perspective, and emotional expression encouraged and worked through, with the goal of sharing the information as widely as possible among various parts of the patient's personality structure. Instructing other alter personalities to "listen" while a given alter is talking, and reviewing previously dissociated material uncovered, can be helpful. The therapist conveys his or her desire to disseminate the information, without accepting responsibility for transmitting it across all personality boundaries.

Given the intensity of the material that often emerges involving memories of sexual and physical abuse, and the sudden shifts in mental state accompanied by amnesia, the therapist is called on to take a clear and structured role in managing the psychotherapy. Appropriate limits must be set about self-destructive or threatening behavior and agreements made regarding physical safety and treatment compliance, and other matters must be presented to the patient in such a way that dissociative ignorance is not an acceptable explanation for failure to live up to agreements.

Traumatic transference. Transference applies with special meaning in patients who have been physically and sexually abused. These patients have had presumed caregivers who acted instead in an exploitative and sometimes sadistic fashion. These patients thus expect the same

from their therapists. Although their reality testing is good enough that they can perceive genuine caring, they expect therapists either to exploit them, with the patients viewing the working through of traumatic memories as a reinflicting of the trauma and the therapists' taking sadistic pleasure in the patients' suffering, or to be excessively passive, with the patients identifying the therapists with some uncaring family figure who knew abuse was occurring but did little or nothing to stop it. It is important in managing the therapy to keep these issues in mind and make them frequent topics of discussion. Attention to these issues can diffuse, but not eliminate, such traumatic transference distortions of the therapeutic relationship (Maldonado and Spiegel 1995, 1998; D. Spiegel 1988).

Integration. The ultimate goal of psychotherapy for patients with DID is integration of the disparate states. There can be considerable resistance to this process. Early in therapy, the patient views the dissociation as tremendous protection: "I knew my father could get some of me, but he couldn't get all of me." Indeed, he or she may experience efforts of integration as an attempt on the part of the therapist to "kill" personalities. These fears must be worked through and the patient shown how to control the degree of integration, giving the patient a sense of gradually being able to control his or her dissociative processes in the service of working through traumatic memories. The process of the psychotherapy, in emphasizing control, must alter rather than reinforce the content, which involves reexperiencing of helplessness, a symbolic reenactment of trauma (D. Spiegel 1986b).

As previously mentioned, a patient with DID often fears integration as an attempt to kill alter personalities and make the patient more vulnerable to mistreat-

ment by depriving him or her of the dissociative defense. At the same time, this defense represents an internalization of the
abusive person or persons in the patient's
memory. Setting aside the defense also
means acknowledging and bearing the discomfort of helplessness at having been
victimized and working through the irrational self-blame that gave the patient a
fantasy of control over events that he or
she was in fact helpless to control. Yet difficult as it is, ultimately, the goal of psychotherapy is mastery over the dissociative process, controlled access to dissociative states, integration of warded-off
painful memories and material, and a
more integrated continuum of identity,
memory, and consciousness (Maldonado
and Spiegel 1995, 1998; D. Spiegel 1988).
Although there have been no controlled
trials of psychotherapy outcome in patients with this disorder, case series reports indicate a positive outcome in most
cases (Kluft 1984c, 1986, 1991).

Cognitive-Behavioral Approaches

Fine (1999) summarized the tactical-
integration model for the treatment of
dissociative disorders. This model consists
of structured cognitive-behavioral–based
treatments that foster symptom relief,
followed by integration of the personalities and/or ego states into one mainstream
of consciousness. This approach promotes
proficiency in control over posttraumatic
and dissociative symptoms, is collaborative and exploratory, and conveys a consistent message of empowerment to the
patient.

Psychopharmacology

To date, no good evidence shows that
medication of any type has a direct therapeutic effect on the dissociative process
manifested by patients with DID (Loewenstein 1991b; Markowitz and Gill

1996; Putnam 1989). In fact, most dissociative symptoms seem relatively resistant
to pharmacological intervention (Loewenstein 1991a, 1991b). Thus, pharmacological treatment has been limited to the control of signs and symptoms afflicting
patients with DID or comorbid conditions
rather than the treatment of dissociation
per se.

Whereas in the past, short-acting barbiturates such as sodium amobarbital were
used intravenously to reverse functional
amnesias, this technique is no longer used,
largely because of poor results (J.C. Perry
and Jacobs 1982).

Benzodiazepines have at times been
used to facilitate recall through controlling secondary anxiety associated with
retrieval of traumatic memories. However, these effects may be nonspecific at
best. Furthermore, sudden mental state
transitions induced by medications may
increase rather than decrease amnesic barriers, as the recent concern about triazolam, a short-acting benzodiazepine hypnotic, indicates. Thus, inducing state
changes pharmacologically could in theory
add to difficulty in retrieval. The only systematic study on the use of benzodiazepines in patients with DID was conducted by Loewenstein et al. (1988). In
their study, they used clonazepam successfully to control PTSD-like symptoms
in a small sample ($n = 5$) of DID patients,
achieving improvement in sleep continuity and a decrease in frequency of flashbacks and nightmares.

Antidepressants are the most useful
class of psychotropic agents for patients
with DID. Such patients frequently have
dysthymic disorder or major depression as
well, and when these disorders are present, especially with somatic signs and suicidal ideation, antidepressant medication
can be helpful. At least two studies report
on the successful use of antidepressant
medications (Barkin et al. 1986; Kluft

1984a, 1985a). The use of antidepressants should be limited to the treatment of DID patients who experience symptoms of major depression (Barkin et al. 1986). The newer selective serotonin reuptake inhibitors (SSRIs) are effective at reducing comorbid depressive symptoms and have the advantage of far less lethality in overdose compared with tricyclic antidepressants (TCIs) and monoamine oxidase inhibitors (MAOIs). Medication compliance is a problem with such patients because dissociated personality states may interfere with the taking of medication by the patients' "hiding" or hoarding of pills, or patients may overdose.

Antipsychotics are rarely useful in reducing dissociative symptoms. They are used occasionally for containing impulsive behavior, with varying effect. More often, they are used with little benefit when DID patients have been given misdiagnoses of schizophrenia (Kluft 1987). In addition to the risks of side effects such as tardive dyskinesia, the neuroleptics may reduce the range of affect, thereby making patients with DID look spuriously as though they were schizophrenic. In fact, most DID researchers have reported an extremely high incidence of adverse side effects with the use of neuroleptic medications (Barkin et al. 1986; Kluft 1984a, 1988; Putnam 1989; Ross 1989).

Anticonvulsants have been used to treat seizure disorders (Mesulam 1981; Schenk and Bear 1981), which have a high rate of comorbidity with DID, mood disorders (Fichtner et al. 1990), and the impulsiveness associated with personality disorders. These agents have been used to reduce impulsive behavior but are rarely definitively helpful. The high incidence of serious side effects (Devinsky et al. 1989) and abuse or overdose potential also should be kept in mind.

Case reports have suggested that β-blockers may be useful in the treatment of hyperarousal, anxiety, poor impulse control, disorganized thinking, and rapid or uncontrolled switching in patients with DID (Braun 1990). However, little information is available about the actual success rate, comorbid diagnoses, or prevalence of adverse drug reactions.

DeBattista et al. (1998) reported on four cases of DID associated with severe self-destructive behavior and comorbid major depression treated with ECT. In three of the patients, ECT appeared to be helpful in treating the comorbid depression without adversely affecting the DID.

Legal Aspects of Memory Work and Hypnosis Recall

Maldonado (2000) summarized and adapted the guidelines provided by the American Medical Association (AMA; Orne et al. 1985) and the American Society of Clinical Hypnosis (ASCH; Hammond et al. 1995) for the use of hypnosis as a method of memory enhancement. The guidelines suggest that when hypnosis or any other memory enhancement method is being used for forensic purposes or in the context of working out traumatic memories, especially those related to childhood physical and/or sexual abuse, the steps shown in Table 10–6 should be applied.

Dissociative Trance Disorder

Cultural Context

Dissociative phenomena are ubiquitous around the world, occurring in virtually every culture (Castillo 1994a, 1994b; Kirmayer 1993; Lewis-Fernandez 1993). These phenomena seem to be more prevalent in the less heavily industrialized Second and Third World countries, although they can be found everywhere. For this

TABLE 10–6. Guidelines for the use of hypnosis in memory work

1. Before hypnosis use, perform a thorough evaluation of the patient.
2. Explore the patient's expectations about treatment in general and hypnosis use in particular.
3. Obtain the patient's permission to consult with his or her attorney.
4. Clarify your role (i.e., therapist vs. forensic consultant) before initiating any assessment and/or treatment. Make sure the patient clearly understands your role in the case.
5. Obtain written informed consent regarding the nature of hypnotic retrieval (explain to the subject and his or her attorney about the nature of hypnotically retrieved memories) and possible side effects of memory work.
6. Clarify the patient's expectation regarding hypnotically enhanced or recovered memories.
7. Maintain neutrality throughout every interaction with the patient.
8. Make a videotape recording of the interview and hypnotic session.
9. Thoroughly document any and all prehypnosis memories.
10. Objectively measure hypnotizability.
11. Carefully document your discussion of hypnosis and memory, issues of accuracy of memory, informed consent, and the maintenance of a stance of neutrality and nonleading approach.
12. Use an expert as a hypnosis consultant.
13. Conduct the interview in a neutral tone; avoid leading or suggestive questions.
14. Demonstrate a balance between supportiveness and empathy, while assisting the patient to critically evaluate the elicited material.
15. Do not encourage patients to institute litigation or to confront alleged perpetrators based solely on information retrieved under hypnosis.
16. Carefully debrief the subject at the end of each session.
17. Carefully document and produce a report containing
     Detailed prehypnotic memories
     Hypnotizability score
     Hypnotic techniques used
     Any significant behavior
     Any confirmed or new memories and details

reason, some scholars have argued against the inclusion of possession or trance disorder as a DSM diagnostic category (Noll 1993). There are descriptions of mediums or possession episodes in different cultures, but they all may serve a similar purpose. There are shamans among Hispanics (Alonso 1988; Pineros et al. 1998) and in Brazil (Shapiro 1992), China (Gaw et al. 1998; Kua et al. 1993), India (Moore 1993; Nuckolls 1991), Iran (Safa 1988), Israel (Bilu and Beit-Hallahmi 1989; Shirali et al. 1986), Japan (Eguchi 1991; Etsuko 1991), Madagascar (Lambek 1988; Sharp 1990, 1994), Malaysia (McLellan 1991; Ong 1988), New Guinea (Schieffelin 1996), Samoa (Mageo 1996),

Singapore (Kua et al. 1986), South Africa (Heap and Ramphele 1991), South Asia (Castillo 1994a, 1994b), Thailand (Trangkasombat et al. 1995, 1998), Zambia (Pullela 1986), and Zanzibar (Tantam 1993). Other dissociative syndromes include demonic possession in Brazil (Heap and Ramphele 1991), Chilopa ritual sacrifices in Malawi (Machleidt and Peltzer 1991), and Zar possession in Northern Sudan (Boddy 1988) and Ethiopia (Witztum et al. 1996).

Most scholars agree that the most common clinical features of trance states are amnesia, emotional disturbances, and loss of identity (D. Li and Spiegel 1992) (Table 10–7). In a study comparing the

A. Either (1) or (2):

   (1) trance, i.e., temporary marked alter-
        ation in the state of consciousness or
        loss of customary sense of personal
        identity without replacement by an
        alternate identity, associated with at
        least one of the following:

        (a) narrowing of awareness of imme-
             diate surroundings, or unusually
             narrow and selective focusing on
             environmental stimuli

        (b) stereotyped behaviors or move-
             ments that are experienced as
             being beyond one's control

   (2) possession trance, a single or episodic
        alteration in the state of consciousness
        characterized by the replacement of
        customary sense of personal identity
        by a new identity. This is attributed to
        the influence of a spirit, power, deity,
        or other person, as evidenced by one
        (or more) of the following:

        (a) stereotyped and culturally deter-
             mined behaviors or movements
             that are experienced as being con-
             trolled by the possessing agent

        (b) full or partial amnesia for the
             event

B. The trance or possession trance state is not
    accepted as a normal part of a collective
    cultural or religious practice.

C. The trance or possession trance state caus-
    es clinically significant distress or impair-
    ment in social, occupational, or other
    important areas of functioning.

D. The trance or possession trance state does
    not occur exclusively during the course of
    a psychotic disorder (including mood dis-
    order with psychotic features and brief
    psychotic disorder) or dissociative iden-
    tity disorder and is not due to the direct
    physiological effects of a substance or a
    general medical condition.

characteristic features of the possession
trance in three different ethnic groups of
Chinese, Malayans, and Indians, Kua et al.

(1986) found a set of similarities, including alteration in the level of consciousness,
amnesia for the period of the trance, stereotyped behavior characteristic of a deity, duration of less than 1 hour, fatigue at
the termination of the trance, normal behavior in the interval between trances, onset before age 25 years, low social class
status, poor educational level, and prior
witnessing of a trance.

Dissociative symptoms are widely understood as an idiom of distress. The major purposes served by possession and
trance states include the need to gain
power, prestige, and status and the desire
to express aggressive and sexual impulses
(Shirali et al. 1986), especially given the
cultural overdetermination of women's
selfhood (Boddy 1988). Dissociative
trance disorders, especially possession disorder, are probably more common than is
usually thought. Ferracuti et al. (1996) reported on 10 patients undergoing exor-
cisms for devil trance possession state.
Subjects were studied with the Dissociative Disorders Diagnostic Schedule and
the Rorschach Test. Subjects were found
to have many traits in common with patients with DID. Despite claiming possession by a demon and various paranormal
phenomena, most of them managed to
maintain normal social functioning. Thus,
in this sample of subjects reporting demonic possession, dissociative trance disorder appeared to be a distinct clinical
manifestation of a dissociative continuum,
sharing some features with dissociative
disorders in general and DID in particular.

Ataque de nervios is a common, self-
labeled Hispanic folk diagnosis that describes episodic, dramatic outbursts of
negative emotion in response to a stressor,
sometimes involving destructive behavior.
A study among 70 Hispanic outpatients
conducted by Schechter et al. (2000)
found that significantly more subjects
with an anxiety or a mood disorder plus

ataque de nervios reported a history of physical abuse, sexual abuse, and/or a substance-abusing caregiver than did those with psychiatric disorder but no *ataque de nervios*. As in the case of dissociative disorders, in some Hispanic individuals, *ataque de nervios* may represent a culturally sanctioned expression of extreme affect dysregulation associated with antecedent childhood trauma.

In a case–control study of 32 girls ages 9–14 years afflicted with an outbreak of spirit possession in the south of Thailand, Trangkasombat et al. (1998) found that the children with spirit possession were firstborn and came from small families (e.g., one to three children); had experienced more psychosocial stressors and significantly higher rates of psychiatric disorders; and had been exposed to more spirit possession ceremonies than the control children.

Similarly, Gaw et al. (1998) described the clinical characteristics of 20 hospitalized psychiatric patients in the Hebei Province of China who believed that they were possessed. The mean age was 37 years; most patients were women from rural areas with little education; and most reported significant events preceding the episode of possession, including interpersonal conflicts, subjectively meaningful circumstances, illness, and death of an individual or dreaming of a deceased individual. In most instances, the initial experience of possession typically came on acutely and often became a chronic relapsing event. Almost all subjects manifested the loss of control over their actions, change in their usual pattern of behavior, loss of awareness of surroundings, loss of personal identity, inability to distinguish reality from fantasy, change in tone of voice, and loss of perceived sensitivity to pain.

Some even suggest that possession can be interpreted as historical discourse, usu-

ally containing tales of tradition (Mageo 1996), or even as an alternative method of healing—not too different from Western psychotherapy (C. Li et al. 1992; Machleidt and Peltzer 1991; Mulhern 1991; Tantam 1993)—thus performing a wider social function. In fact, "when the embodiment of an alternative identity is exercised in the cross-cultural complex of spirit possession, it provides a conduit through which subjective suffering can be transcended and through which the past, present, and future can be expressed" (Mulhern 1991).

The trance and possession categories of dissociative trance disorder constitute by far the most common kinds of dissociative disorders around the world. Several studies of dissociative disorders in India, for example, reported that dissociative trance and possession are the most prevalent dissociative disorders (i.e., approximately 3.5% of psychiatric admissions; Adityanjee et al. 1989; Saxena and Prasad 1989). On the other hand, DID, which is relatively more common in the United States, is virtually never diagnosed in India. Cultural and biological factors may account for the different content and form of dissociative symptoms.

These dissociative episodes usually are understood as an idiom of distress, yet they are not viewed as normal. That is, they are not a generally accepted part of cultural and religious practice that may often involve normal trance phenomena, such as trance dancing in the Balinese Hindu culture. Trance dancers in that culture are remarkable for being the only portion of this socially stable society able to elevate their social status. This elevation of social status is done through developing an ability to enter trance states. They are able within the social ceremony to induce an altered state of consciousness in which they dance over hot coals, hold a sword at their throat, or in other ways show exceptional powers of concentration and physical prowess. This form of trance is considered socially normal and even exalted. By contrast, trance and possession disorder is viewed by the local community as a common but aberrant form of behavior that requires intervention. Although trance and possession disorder is clearly an idiom of distress (e.g., discomfort in a new family environment), most individuals use an array of alternative strategies for coping with such distress. Thus, cultural informants make it clear that individuals with trance and possession trance disorders are acting abnormally, if recognizably.

Classification

Dissociative trance disorder has been divided into two broad categories: dissociative trance and possession trance.

Dissociative Trance

Dissociative trance phenomena are characterized by a sudden alteration in consciousness that is not accompanied by distinct alternative identities. In this form, the dissociative symptom involves consciousness rather than identity. Also, in dissociative trance, the activities performed are rather simple, usually involving sudden collapse, immobilization, dizziness, shrieking, screaming, or crying. Memory is rarely affected, and amnesia, if any, is fragmented.

Dissociative trance phenomena frequently involve sudden, extreme changes in sensory and motor control. Classic examples include *ataque de nervios*, which is prevalent throughout Latin America. This condition, for example, is estimated to have a lifetime prevalence rate of 12% in Puerto Rico (Lewis-Fernandez 1993). Typically, the individual suddenly begins to shake convulsively, hyperventilate, scream, and show agitation and aggressive

movements. These behaviors may be followed by collapse and loss of consciousness. Afterward, such individuals report being exhausted and may have some amnesia for the event (Lewis-Fernandez 1993).

Falling out occurs frequently among African Americans in the southern United States. Affected individuals may collapse suddenly, unable to see or speak even though they are conscious. These persons may be confused afterward but usually are not amnesic to the episode (Lewis-Fernandez 1993).

In the Malay version of trance disorder, *latah*, affected individuals may have a sudden vision of a spirit that is threatening them. These persons scream or cry, strike out physically, and may need restraints. They may report amnesia, but they do not clearly take on the identity of the offending spirit (Lewis-Fernandez 1993).

Possession Trance

In contrast to dissociative trance, possession trance involves the assumption of a distinct alternate identity, usually that of a deity, an ancestor, or a spirit. The person in this trance often engages in rather complex activities, which may take the form of expressing otherwise forbidden thoughts or needs, negotiating for change in family or social status, or engaging in aggressive behavior. Possession usually involves amnesia for a large portion of the episode during which the alternate identity was in control of the person's behavior.

In Indian possession syndrome, the affected individual suddenly begins speaking in an altered voice with an altered identity, usually that of a deity recognizable to others. Through this voice, a person may refer to himself or herself in the third person. The affected person's "spirit" may negotiate for changes in the family environment or become agitated or aggressive. Possession syndrome typically occurs in a recently married woman who finds herself uncomfortable or unwelcome in her mother-in-law's home. Such individuals usually are unable to directly express their discomfort.

Treatment

Treatment of these disorders varies from culture to culture. Most syndromes occur within the context of acute social stress and thus serve the purpose of recruiting help from the family and other support systems or removing the subject from the immediate danger or threat. Ceremonies to remove or appease the invading spirit are commonly used (Pineros et al. 1998). The role of psychiatry should be focused on ruling out any possible organic cause for the symptoms shown, treating comorbid psychiatric conditions (if any are present), avoiding excess medication, understanding the social context and role of the syndrome, and facilitating a favorable outcome.

Conclusions

The dissociative disorders constitute a challenging component of psychiatric illness. The failure of integration of memory, identity, perception, and consciousness seen in these disorders results in symptomatology that illustrates fundamental problems in the organization of mental processes. Dissociative phenomena often occur during and after physical trauma but also may represent transient or chronic defensive patterns. Dissociative disorders are generally treatable and constitute a domain in which psychotherapy is a primary modality, although pharmacological treatment of comorbid conditions such as depression can be quite helpful. The dissociative disorders are ubiquitous around the world, although they take a variety of forms. They repre-

sent a fascinating window into the processing of identity, memory, perception, and consciousness, and they pose a variety of diagnostic, therapeutic, and research challenges.

References

Abeles M, Schilder P: Psychogenic loss of personal identity: amnesia. Archives of Neurology and Psychiatry 34:587–604, 1935

Adityanjee, Raju GSP, Khandelwal SK: Current status of multiple personality disorder in India. Am J Psychiatry 146:1607–1610, 1989

Akyuz G, Dogan O, Sar V, et al: Frequency of dissociative identity disorder in the general population in Turkey. Compr Psychiatry 40:151–159, 1999

Allison RB: A new treatment approach for multiple personalities. Am J Clin Hypn 17:15–32, 1974

Alonso L: Mental illness complicated by the santeria belief in spirit possession. Hosp Community Psychiatry 39:1188–1191, 1988

Ambrosino SV: Phobic anxiety-depersonalization syndrome. New York State Journal of Medicine 73:419–425, 1973

American Psychiatric Association: Diagnostic and Statistical Manual of Mental Disorders, 4th Edition, Text Revision. Washington, DC, American Psychiatric Association, 2000

Anderson G, Yasenik L, Ross CA: Dissociative experiences and disorders among women who identify themselves as sexual abuse survivors. Child Abuse Negl 17:677–686, 1993

Armstrong JG, Putnam FW, Carlson EB, et al: Development and validation of a measure of adolescent dissociation: the Adolescent Dissociative Experiences Scale. J Nerv Ment Dis 185:491–497, 1997

Ball S, Robinson A, Shekhar A, et al: Dissociative symptoms in panic disorder. J Nerv Ment Dis 185:755–760, 1997

Ballenger JC, Burrows GD, Dupont RL, et al: Alprazolam in panic disorder and agoraphobia: results from a multicenter trial, I: efficacy in short term treatment. Arch Gen Psychiatry 45:413–422, 1988

Barkin R, Braun BG, Kluft RP: The dilemma of drug therapy for multiple personality disorder, in Treatment of Multiple Personality Disorder. Edited by Braun BG. Washington, DC, American Psychiatric Press, 1986, pp 107–132

Baron DA, Nagy R: The amobarbital interview in a general hospital setting, friend or foe: a case report. Gen Hosp Psychiatry 10: 220–222, 1988

Berger D, Saito S, Ono Y, et al: Dissociation and child abuse histories in an eating disorder cohort in Japan. Acta Psychiatr Scand 90:274–280, 1994

Bernstein EM, Putnam FW: Development, reliability, and validity of a dissociation scale. J Nerv Ment Dis 174:727–735, 1986

Bilu Y, Beit-Hallahmi B: Dybbuk-possession as a hysterical symptom: psychodynamic and socio-cultural factors. Isr J Psychiatry Relat Sci 26:138–149, 1989

Bliss EL: Multiple personalities: a report of 14 cases with implications for schizophrenia and hysteria. Arch Gen Psychiatry 37: 1388–1397, 1980

Bliss EL: A symptom profile of patients with multiple personalities, including MMPI results. J Nerv Ment Dis 172:197–202, 1984

Bliss EL: Multiple Personality, Allied Disorders, and Hypnosis. New York, Oxford University Press, 1986

Bliss EL, Larson EM, Nakashima SR: Auditory hallucinations and schizophrenia. J Nerv Ment Dis 171:30–33, 1983

Blue FR: Use of directive therapy in the treatment of depersonalization neurosis. Psychol Rep 49:904–906, 1979

Boddy J: Spirits and selves in Northern Sudan: the cultural therapeutics of possession and trance. American Ethnologist 15:4–27, 1988

Boe T, Haslerud J, Knudsen H: Multiple personality: a phenomenon also in Norway? Tidsskr Nor Laegeforen 113:3230–3232, 1993

Boon S, Draijer N: Multiple personality disorder in the Netherlands: a clinical investigation of 71 patients. Am J Psychiatry 150:489–494, 1993a

Boon S, Draijer N: Multiple Personality Disorder in the Netherlands: A Study on Reliability and Validity of the Diagnosis. Amsterdam, The Netherlands, Swets & Zeitlinger, 1993b

Bowman ES: Etiology and clinical course of pseudoseizures: relationship to trauma, depression, and dissociation. Psychosomatics 34:333–342, 1993

Bowman ES, Markand ON: Psychodynamics and psychiatric diagnoses of pseudoseizure subjects. Am J Psychiatry 153:57–63, 1996

Braun BG: Uses of hypnosis with multiple personality. Psychiatr Ann 14:34–36, 39–40, 1984

Braun BG: Multiple personality disorder: an overview. Am J Occup Ther 44:971–976, 1990

Braun BG, Sachs RG: The development of multiple personality disorder: predisposing, precipitating, and perpetuating factors, in Childhood Antecedents of Multiple Personality Disorder. Edited by Kluft RP. Washington, DC, American Psychiatric Press, 1985, pp 37–64

Bremner JD, Brett E: Trauma-related dissociative states and long-term psychopathology in posttraumatic stress disorder. J Trauma Stress 10:37–49, 1997

Bremner JD, Krystal JH, Putnam FW, et al: Measurement of dissociative states with the Clinician-Administered Dissociative States Scale (CADSS). J Trauma Stress 11:125–136, 1998

Brenner I: The dissociative character: a reconsideration of "multiple personality." J Am Psychoanal Assoc 42:819–846, 1994

Brenner I: The characterological basis of multiple personality. Am J Psychother 50:154–166, 1996a

Brenner I: On trauma, perversion, and "multiple personality." J Am Psychoanal Assoc 44:785–814, 1996b

Brodsky BS, Cloitre M, Dulit RA: Relationship of dissociation to self-mutilation and childhood abuse in borderline personality disorder. Am J Psychiatry 152:1788–1792, 1995

Brown GR, Anderson B: Psychiatric morbidity in adult inpatients with childhood histories of sexual and physical abuse. Am J Psychiatry 148:55–61, 1991

Brown L, Russell J, Thornton C, et al: Dissociation, abuse and the eating disorders: evidence from an Australian population. Aust N Z J Psychiatry 33:521–528, 1999

Brown W: The treatment of cases of shell shock in an advanced neurological centre. Lancet 2:197–200, 1918

Bryer JB, Nelson BA, Miller JB, et al: Childhood sexual and physical abuse as factors in adult psychiatric illness. Am J Psychiatry 144:1426–1430, 1987

Butler LD, Duran EFD, Jasiukatis P, et al: Hypnotizability and traumatic experience: a diathesis-stress model of dissociative symptomatology. Am J Psychiatry 153:42–63, 1996

Carlson EB, Putnam FW, Ross CA, et al: Validity of the Dissociative Experiences Scale in screening for multiple personality disorder: a multicenter study. Am J Psychiatry 150:1030–1036, 1993

Castillo RJ: Spirit possession in South Asia, dissociation or hysteria? I: theoretical background. Cult Med Psychiatry 18:1–21, 1994a

Castillo RJ: Spirit possession in South Asia, dissociation or hysteria? II: case histories. Cult Med Psychiatry 18:141–162, 1994b

Cattell JP, Cattell JS: Depersonalization: psychological and social perspectives, in American Handbook of Psychiatry. Edited by Arieti S. New York, Basic Books, 1974, pp 767–799

Chodoff P: Turkish dissociative identity disorder (letter). Am J Psychiatry 154:1179, 1997

Chu JA, Dill DL: Dissociative symptoms in relation to childhood physical and sexual abuse. Am J Psychiatry 147:887–892, 1990

Chu JA, Frey LM, Ganzel BL, et al: Memories of childhood abuse: dissociation, amnesia, and corroboration. Am J Psychiatry 156:749–755, 1999

Coons PM: The differential diagnosis of multiple personality: a comprehensive review. Psychiatr Clin North Am 7:51–65, 1984

Coons PM: Confirmation of childhood abuse in child and adolescent cases of multiple personality disorder and dissociative disorder not otherwise specified. J Nerv Ment Dis 182:461–464, 1994

Coons PM, Milstein V: Psychosexual disturbances in multiple personality: characteristics, etiology, and treatment. J Clin Psychiatry 47:106–110, 1986

Coons PM, Milstein V: Psychogenic amnesia: a clinical investigation of 25 cases. Dissociation 5:73–79, 1992

Coons PM, Bowman ES, Milstein V: Multiple personality disorder: a clinical investigation of 50 cases. J Nerv Ment Dis 17:519–527, 1988

Coons PM, Bowman ES, Kluft RP, et al: The cross-cultural occurrence of MPD: additional cases from a recent survey. Dissociation 4:124–128, 1991

Darves-Bornoz JM: Rape-related psychotraumatic syndromes. Eur J Obstet Gynecol Reprod Biol 71:59–65, 1997

Davison K: Episodic depersonalization: observations on 7 patients. Br J Psychiatry 110:505–513, 1964

DeBattista C, Solvason HB, Spiegel D: ECT in dissociative identity disorder and comorbid depression. J ECT 14:275–279, 1998

Devinsky O, Putnam F, Grafman J, et al: Dissociative states and epilepsy. Neurology 39:835–840, 1989

Dollinger S: A case report of dissociative neurosis (depersonalization disorder) in an adolescent treated with family therapy and behavior modification. J Consult Clin Psychol 51:479–484, 1983

Draijer N, Langeland W: Childhood trauma and perceived parental dysfunction in the etiology of dissociative symptoms in psychiatric inpatients. Am J Psychiatry 156: 379–385, 1999

Dunn GE, Ryan JJ, Paolo AM, et al: Comorbidity of dissociative disorders among patients with substance use disorders. Psychiatr Serv 46:153–156, 1995

Eguchi S: Between folk concepts of illness and psychiatric diagnosis: kitsune-tsuki (fox possession) in a mountain village of western Japan. Cult Med Psychiatry 15:421–451, 1991

Ellason JW, Ross CA: Positive and negative symptoms in dissociative identity disorder and schizophrenia: a comparative analysis. J Nerv Ment Dis 183:236–241, 1995

Ellason JW, Ross CA, Sainton K, et al: Axis I and II comorbidity and childhood trauma history in chemical dependency. Bull Menninger Clin 60:39–51, 1996

Eriksson NG, Lundin T: Early traumatic stress reactions among Swedish survivors of the Estonia disaster. Br J Psychiatry 169:713–716, 1996

Etsuko M: The interpretations of fox possession: illness as metaphor. Cult Med Psychiatry 15:453–477, 1991

Farley M, Keaney JC: Physical symptoms, somatization, and dissociation in women survivors of childhood sexual assault. Women Health 25:33–45, 1997

Ferracuti S, Sacco R, Lazzari R: Dissociative trance disorder: clinical and Rorschach findings in ten persons reporting demon possession and treated by exorcism. J Pers Assess 66:525–539, 1996

Fewtrell W: Depersonalization: a description and suggested strategies. British Journal of Guidance and Counseling 14:263–269, 1986

Fichtner CG, Kuhlman DT, Gruenfeld MJ, et al: Decreased episodic violence and increased control of dissociation in a carbamazepine-treated case of multiple personality. Biol Psychiatry 27:1045–1052, 1990

Fichtner CG, Horevitz RP, Braun BG: Fluoxetine in depersonalization disorder. Am J Psychiatry 149:1750–1751, 1992

Fine CG: The tactical-integration model for the treatment of dissociative identity disorder and allied dissociative disorders. Am J Psychother 53:361–376, 1999

Finkelhor D: Child Sexual Abuse: New Theory and Research. New York, Free Press, 1984

Frankel FH: Hypnotizability and dissociation. Am J Psychiatry 147:823–829, 1990

Freyberger HJ, Spitzer C, Stieglitz RD, et al: Questionnaire on dissociative symptoms: German adaptation, reliability and validity of the American Dissociative Experience Scale (DES). Psychother Psychosom Med Psychol 48:223–229, 1998

Friedl MC, Draijer N: Dissociative disorders in Dutch psychiatric inpatients. Am J Psychiatry 157:1012–1013, 2000

Frischholz EJ: The relationship among dissociation, hypnosis, and child abuse in the development of multiple personality disorder, in Childhood Antecedents of Multiple Personality Disorder. Edited by Kluft RP. Washington, DC, American Psychiatric Press, 1985, pp 99–126

Gainer MJ, Torem MS: Ego-state therapy for self-injurious behavior. Am J Clin Hypn 35:257–266, 1993

Ganaway GK: Historical versus narrative truth: clarifying the role of exogenous trauma in the etiology of MPD and its variants. Dissociation 2:205–220, 1989

Ganaway GK: Hypnosis, childhood trauma, and dissociative identity disorder: toward an integrative theory. Int J Clin Exp Hypn 43:127–144, 1995

Gast U, Rodewald F, Nickel V, et al: Prevalence of dissociative disorders among psychiatric inpatients in a German university clinic. J Nerv Ment Dis 189:249–257, 2001

Gaw AC, Ding Q, Levine RE, et al: The clinical characteristics of possession disorder among 20 Chinese patients in the Hebei province of China. Psychiatr Serv 49:360–365, 1998

Gelb JL: Multiple personality disorder and satanic ritual abuse. Aust N Z J Psychiatry 27:701–708, 1993

Goodwin J: Sexual Abuse: Incest Victims and Their Families. Boston, MA, Wright/PSG, 1982

Greaves GB: Multiple personality: 165 years after Mary Reynolds. J Nerv Ment Dis 168:577–596, 1980

Hammond DC, Garver RB, Mutter CB, et al: Clinical Hypnosis and Memory: Guidelines for Clinicians and for Forensic Hypnosis. Bloomingdale, IL, American Society of Clinical Hypnosis Press, 1995

Heap M, Ramphele M: The quest for wholeness: health care strategies among the residents of council-built hostels in Cape Town. Soc Sci Med 32:117–126, 1991

Herman JL, Perry JC, van der Kolk BA: Childhood trauma in borderline personality disorder. Am J Psychiatry 146:490–495, 1989

Hocke V, Schmidtke A: "Multiple personality disorder" in childhood and adolescence. Z Kinder Jugendpsychiatr Psychother 26:273–284, 1998

Hoffman RE: Computer simulations of neural information processing and the schizophrenia-mania dichotomy. Arch Gen Psychiatry 44:178–188, 1987

Hollander E, Fairbanks J, Decaria C, et al: Pharmacological dissection of panic and depersonalization (letter). Am J Psychiatry 146:402, 1989

Hollander E, Liebowitz MR, Decaria C, et al: Treatment of depersonalization with serotonin reuptake blockers. J Clin Psychopharmacol 10:200–203, 1990

Horen SA, Leichner PP, Lawson JS: Prevalence of dissociative symptoms and disorders in an adult psychiatric inpatient population in Canada. Can J Psychiatry 40:185–191, 1995

Horevitz RP, Braun BG: Are multiple personalities borderline? An analysis of 33 cases. Psychiatr Clin North Am 7:69–87, 1984

Irwin HJ: Pathological and nonpathological dissociation: the relevance of childhood trauma. J Psychol 133:157–164, 1999

James W: The Principles of Psychology (1890). New York, Dover, 1950

Kaplan ML, Asnis GM, Lipschitz DS, et al: Suicidal behavior and abuse in psychiatric outpatients. Compr Psychiatry 36:229–235, 1995

Kardiner A, Spiegel H: War, Stress and Neurotic Illness. New York, Hoeber, 1947

Kirmayer LJ: Pacing the void: social and cultural dimensions of dissociation, in Dissociation: Culture, Mind, and Body. Edited by Spiegel D. Washington, DC, American Psychiatric Press, 1993, pp 91–122

Kirshner LA: Dissociative reactions: an historical review and clinical study. Acta Psychiatr Scand 49:698–711, 1973

Kluft RP: Varieties of hypnotic intervention in the treatment of multiple personality. Am J Clin Hypn 24:230–240, 1982

Kluft RP: An introduction to multiple personality disorder. Psychiatric Annals 14:19–24, 1984a

Kluft RP: Multiple personality in childhood. Psychiatr Clin North Am 7:121–134, 1984b

Kluft RP: Treatment of multiple personality disorder: a study of 33 cases. Psychiatr Clin North Am 7:9–29, 1984c

Kluft RP: The natural history of multiple personality disorder, in Childhood Antecedents of Multiple Personality. Edited by Kluft RP. Washington, DC, American Psychiatric Press, 1985a, pp 197–238

Kluft RP: Using hypnotic inquiry protocols to monitor treatment progress and stability in multiple personality disorder. Am J Clin Hypn 28:63–75, 1985b

Kluft RP: Personality unification in multiple personality disorder: a follow-up study, in Treatment of Multiple Personality Disorder. Edited by Braun BG. Washington, DC, American Psychiatric Press, 1986, pp 29–60

Kluft RP: First-rank symptoms as a diagnostic clue to multiple personality disorder. Am J Psychiatry 144:293–298, 1987

Kluft RP: The dissociative disorders, in American Psychiatric Press Textbook of Psychiatry. Edited by Talbott JA, Hales RE, Yudofsky SC. Washington, DC, American Psychiatric Press, 1988, pp 557–585

Kluft RP: Multiple personality disorder, in American Psychiatric Press Review of Psychiatry, Vol 10. Edited by Tasman A, Goldfinger SM. Washington, DC, American Psychiatric Press, 1991, pp 161–188

Kluft RP: The use of hypnosis with dissociative disorders. Psychiatr Med 10:31–46, 1992

Kluft RP: An overview of the psychotherapy of dissociative identity disorder. Am J Psychother 53:289–319, 1999

Koopman C, Classen C, Cardeña E, et al: When disaster strikes, acute stress disorder may follow. J Trauma Stress 8:29–46, 1995

Koopman C, Classen C, Spiegel D: Dissociative responses in the immediate aftermath of the Oakland/Berkeley firestorm. J Trauma Stress 9:521–540, 1996

Kua EH, Sim LP, Chee KT: A cross-cultural study of the possession-trance in Singapore. Aust N Z J Psychiatry 20:361–364, 1986

Kua EH, Chew PH, Ko SM: Spirit possession and healing among Chinese psychiatric patients. Acta Psychiatr Scand 88:447–450, 1993

Lambek M: Spirit possession/spirit succession: aspects of social continuity among Malagasy speakers in Mayotte. American Ethnologist 15:710–731, 1988

Lavoie G, Sabourin M: Hypnosis and schizophrenia: a review of experimental and clinical studies, in Handbook of Hypnosis and Psychosomatic Medicine. Edited by Burrows GD, Dennerstein L. New York, Elsevier, 1980

Lavoie G, Sabourin M, Langlois J: Hypnotic susceptibility, amnesia, and IQ in chronic schizophrenia. Int J Clin Exp Hypn 21:157–168, 1973

Leavitt F, Labott SM: Rorschach indicators of dissociative identity disorders: clinical utility and theoretical implications. J Clin Psychol 54:803–810, 1998

Lewis-Fernandez R: Culture and dissociation: a comparison of ataque de nervios among Puerto Ricans and "possession syndrome" in India, in Dissociation: Culture, Mind, and Body. Edited by Spiegel D. Washington, DC, American Psychiatric Press, 1993, pp 123–167

Li C, Sun Y, Fang M: Trance states, altered states of consciousness, and related issues. Chinese Mental Health Journal 6:167–170, 1992

Li D, Spiegel D: A neural network model of dissociative disorders. Psychiatr Ann 22:144–147, 1992

Lindemann E: Symptomatology and management of acute grief. Am J Psychiatry 101:141–148, 1944

Loewenstein RJ: An official mental status examination for complex chronic dissociative symptoms and multiple personality disorder. Psychiatr Clin North Am 14:567–604, 1991a

Loewenstein RJ: Psychogenic amnesia and psychogenic fugue: a comprehensive review, in American Psychiatric Press Review of Psychiatry, Vol 10. Edited by Tasman A, Goldfinger SM. Washington, DC, American Psychiatric Press, 1991b, pp 189–222

Loewenstein RJ: Diagnosis, epidemiology, clinical course, treatment, and cost effectiveness of treatment of dissociative disorders and MPD: report submitted to the Clinton Administration Task Force on Health Care Financing Reform. Dissociation 7:3–11, 1994

Loewenstein RJ, Hornstein N, Farber B: Open trial of clonazepam in the treatment of posttraumatic stress symptoms in MPD. Dissociation 1:3–12, 1988

Machleidt W, Peltzer K: The Chilopa ceremony: a sacrificial ritual for mentally (spiritually) ill patients in a traditional healing centre in Malawi. Psychiatria Danubina 3:205–227, 1991

Macleod AD: Posttraumatic stress disorder, dissociative fugue and a locator beacon. Aust N Z J Psychiatry 33:102–104, 1999

Mageo JM: Spirit girls and marines: possession and ethnopsychiatry as historical discourse in Samoa. American Ethnologist 23:61–82, 1996

Maldonado JR: Diagnosis and treatment of dissociative disorders, in Manual for the Course: Advanced Hypnosis: The Use of Hypnosis in Medicine and Psychiatry. Annual meeting of the American Psychiatric Association, Chicago, IL, May 13–18, 2000

Maldonado JR, Spiegel D: Using hypnosis, in Treating Women Molested in Childhood. Edited by Classen C. San Francisco, CA, Jossey-Bass, 1995, pp 163–186

Maldonado JR, Spiegel D: Trauma, dissociation, and hypnotizability, in Trauma, Memory, and Dissociation. Edited by Marmar CR, Bremmer JD. Washington, DC, American Psychiatric Press, 1998, pp 57–106

Maldonado JR, Butler LD, Spiegel D: Treatment of dissociative disorders, in Treatments That Work. Edited by Nathan P, Gorman JM. New York, Oxford University Press, 2000, pp 463–493

Markowitz JS, Gill HS: Pharmacotherapy of dissociative identity disorder. Ann Pharmacother 30:1498–1499, 1996

Martinez-Taboas A: Repressed memories: some clinical data contributing toward its elucidation. Am J Psychother 50:217–230, 1996

Mayer-Gross W, Slater E, Roth M: Clinical Psychiatry, 3rd Edition. London, England, Bailliere, Tindal & Cassell, 1969

McHugh PR: Dissociative identity disorder as a socially constructed artifact. Journal of Practical Psychiatry and Behavioral Health 1:158–166, 1995a

McHugh PR: Witches, multiple personalities, and other psychiatric artifacts. Nat Med 1:110–114, 1995b

McLellan S: Deviant spirits in West Malaysian factories. Anthropologica 33:145–160, 1991

Meares R: The "adualistic" representation of trauma: on malignant internalization. Am J Psychother 53:392–402, 1999

Mesulam MM: Dissociative states with abnormal temporal lobe EEG: multiple personality and the illusion of possession. Arch Neurol 38:178–181, 1981

Middleton W, Butler J: Dissociative identity disorder: an Australian series. Aust N Z J Psychiatry 32:794–804, 1998

Mishkin M, Appenzeller T: The anatomy of memory. Sci Am 256:80–89, 1987

Modestin J, Ebner G, Junghan M, et al: Dissociative experiences and dissociative disorders in acute psychiatric inpatients. Compr Psychiatry 37:355–361, 1996

Moore EP: Gender, power, and legal pluralism: Rajasthan, India. American Ethnologist 20:522–542, 1993

Mulder RT, Beautrais AL, Joyce PR, et al: Relationship between dissociation, childhood sexual abuse, childhood physical abuse, and mental illness in a general population sample. Am J Psychiatry 155:806–811, 1998

Mulhern S: Patients reporting ritual abuse in childhood (letter and comment). Child Abuse Negl 15:609–613, 1991

Naples M, Hackett T: The Amytal interview: history and current uses. Psychosomatics 19:98–105, 1978

Nijenhuis ER, Spinhoven P, van Dyck R, et al: The development and psychometric characteristics of the Somatoform Dissociation Questionnaire (SDQ-20). J Nerv Ment Dis 184:688–694, 1996

Nijenhuis ER, Spinhoven P, van Dyck, et al: The development of the Somatoform Dissociation Questionnaire (SDQ-5) as a screening instrument for dissociative disorders. Acta Psychiatr Scand 96:311–318, 1997

Nijenhuis ER, Spinhoven P, van Dyck R, et al: Degree of somatoform and psychological dissociation in dissociative disorder is correlated with reported trauma. J Trauma Stress 11:711–730, 1998

Noll R: Exorcism and possession: the clash of worldviews and the hubris of psychiatry. Dissociation 6(special issue):250–253, 1993

Noyes R, Kletti R: Depersonalization in response to life-threatening danger. Compr Psychiatry 18:375–384, 1977

Noyes R, Kupperman S, Olson SB: Desipramine: a possible treatment for depersonalization. Can J Psychiatry 32:782–784, 1987

Nuckolls CW: Deciding how to decide: possession-mediumship in Jalari divination. Med Anthropol 13(special issue):57–82, 1991

Nuller YL: Depersonalization: symptoms, meaning, therapy. Acta Psychiatr Scand 66:451–458, 1982

Ogata SN, Silk KR, Goodrich S, et al: Childhood sexual and physical abuse in adult patients with borderline personality disorder. Am J Psychiatry 147:1008–1013, 1990

Ong A: The production of possession: spirits and the multinational corporation in Malaysia. American Ethnologist 15:28–42, 1988

Orne MT, Axelrad AD, Diamond BL, et al: Scientific status of refreshing recollection by the use of hypnosis. JAMA 253:1918–1923, 1985

Perry JC, Jacobs D: Overview: clinical applications of the Amytal interview in psychiatric emergency settings. Am J Psychiatry 139:552–559, 1982

Peterson G: Auditory hallucinations and dissociative identity disorder. Am J Psychiatry 152:1403–1404, 1995

Pettinati HM: Measuring hypnotizability in psychotic patients. Int J Clin Exp Hypn 30:404–416, 1982

Pettinati HM, Kogan LG, Evans FJ, et al: Hypnotizability of psychiatric inpatients according to two different scales. Am J Psychiatry 147:69–75, 1990

Pies R: Depersonalization's many faces. Psychiatric Times 8:27–28, 1991

Pineros M, Rosselli D, Calderon C: An epidemic of collective conversion and dissociation disorder in an indigenous group of Colombia: its relation to cultural change. Soc Sci Med 46:1425–1428, 1998

Piper A Jr: Multiple personality disorder. Br J Psychiatry 164:600–612, 1994

Pribor EF, Dinwiddie SH: Psychiatric correlates of incest in childhood. Am J Psychiatry 149:52–56, 1992

Price J, Hess NC: Behaviour therapy as precipitant and treatment in a case of dual personality. Aust N Z J Psychiatry 13:63–66, 1979

Pullela S: An outbreak of epidemic hysteria: an illustrative case study. Irish Journal of Psychiatry 7:9–11, 1986

Putnam FW: Dissociation as a response to extreme trauma, in Childhood Antecedents of Multiple Personality. Edited by Kluft RP. Washington, DC, American Psychiatric Press, 1985, pp 65–97

Putnam FW: The disturbance of "self" in victims of childhood sexual abuse, in Incest-Related Syndromes of Adult Psychopathology. Edited by Kluft RP. Washington, DC, American Psychiatric Press, 1988, pp 113–132

Putnam FW: Diagnosis and Treatment of Multiple Personality Disorder. New York, Guilford, 1989

Putnam FW: Dissociative disorders in children: behavioral profiles and problems. Child Abuse Negl 17:39–45, 1993

Putnam FW, Guroff JJ, Silberman EK, et al: The clinical phenomenology of multiple personality disorder: review of 100 recent cases. J Clin Psychiatry 47:285–293, 1986

Reither AM, Stoudemire A: Psychogenic fugue states: a review. South Med J 81:568–571, 1988

Rifkin A, Ghisalbert D, Dimatou S, et al: Dissociative identity disorder in psychiatric inpatients. Am J Psychiatry 155:844–845, 1998

Rivera M: Multiple personality disorder and the social systems: 185 cases. Dissociation 4:79–82, 1991

Roesler TA, McKenzie N: Effects of childhood trauma on psychological functioning in adults sexually abused as children. J Nerv Ment Dis 182:145–150, 1994

Ronquillo EB: The influence of "espiritismo" on a case of multiple personality disorder. Dissociation 4:39–45, 1991

Ross CA: Multiple Personality Disorder: Diagnosis, Clinical Features, and Treatment. New York, Wiley, 1989

Ross CA: Epidemiology of multiple personality disorder and dissociation. Psychiatr Clin North Am 14:503–518, 1991

Ross CA, Norton GR: Multiple personality disorder patients with a prior diagnosis of schizophrenia. Dissociation 1:39–42, 1988

Ross CA, Norton GR: Suicide and parasuicide in multiple personality disorder. Psychiatry 52:365–371, 1989

Ross CA, Norton GR, Wozney K: Multiple personality disorder: an analysis of 236 cases. Can J Psychiatry 34:413–418, 1989

Ross CA, Miller SD, Reagor P, et al: Structured interview data on 102 cases of multiple personality disorder from four centers. Am J Psychiatry 147:596–601, 1990

Ross CA, Joshi S, Currie R: Dissociative experiences in the general population: a factor analysis. Hosp Community Psychiatry 42: 297–301, 1991a

Ross CA, Anderson G, Fleischer WP, et al: The frequency of multiple personality disorder among psychiatric inpatients. Am J Psychiatry 148:1717–1720, 1991b

Roth M: The phobic-anxiety-depersonalization syndrome. Proceedings of the Royal Society of Medicine 52:587–595, 1959

Rumelhart DE, McClelland JL: Parallel Distributed Processing: Explorations in the Microstructure of Cognition, Vols 1 and 2. Cambridge, MA, MIT Press, 1986

Russell DEH: The Secret Trauma: Incest in the Lives of Girls and Women. New York, Basic Books, 1986

Safa K: Reading Saedi's Ahl-e Hava: pattern and significance in spirit possession beliefs on the southern coasts of Iran. Cult Med Psychiatry 12:85–111, 1988

Sar V, Yargic LI, Tutkun H: Structured interview data on 35 cases of dissociative identity disorder in Turkey. Am J Psychiatry 153:1329–1333, 1996

Sargant W, Slater E: Amnestic syndromes in war. Proceedings of the Royal Society of Medicine 34:757–764, 1941

Saxe GN, van der Kolk BA, Berkowitz R, et al: Dissociative disorders in psychiatric inpatients. Am J Psychiatry 150:1037–1042, 1993

Saxena S, Prasad KVSR: DSM-III subclassification of dissociative disorders applied to psychiatric outpatients in India. Am J Psychiatry 146:261–262, 1989

Schacter DL: Understanding implicit memory: a cognitive neuroscience approach. Am Psychol 47:559–569, 1992

Schacter DL, Wang PL, Tulving E, et al: Functional retrograde amnesia: a quantitative case study. Neuropsychologia 20: 523–532, 1982

Schechter DS, Marshall R, Salman E, et al: Ataque de nervios and history of childhood trauma. J Trauma Stress 13:529–534, 2000

Schenk L, Bear D: Multiple personality and related dissociative phenomena in patients with temporal lobe epilepsy. Am J Psychiatry 138:1311–1316, 1981

Schieffelin EL: Evil spirit sickness, the Christian disease: the innovation of a new syndrome of mental derangement and redemption in Papua, New Guinea. Cult Med Psychiatry 20:1–39, 1996

Schilder P: The treatment of depersonalization. Bulletin of the New York Academy of Science 15:258–272, 1939

Schultz R, Braun BG, Kluft RP: Multiple personality disorder: phenomenology of selected variables in comparison to major depression. Dissociation 2:45–51, 1989

Scroppo JC, Drob SL, Weinberger JL, et al: Identifying dissociative identity disorder: a self-report and projective study. J Abnorm Psychol 107:272–284, 1998

Shapiro DJ: Symbolic fluids: the world of spirit mediums in Brazilian possession groups. Dissertation Abstracts International 53: 867–868, 1992

Sharp LA: Possessed and dispossessed youth: spirit possession of school children in northwest Madagascar. Cult Med Psychiatry 14:339–364, 1990

Sharp LA: Exorcists, psychiatrists, and the problems of possession in northwest Madagascar. Soc Sci Med 38:525–542, 1994

Shearer SL: Dissociative phenomena in women with borderline personality disorder. Am J Psychiatry 151:1324–1328, 1994

Shilony E, Grossman FK: Depersonalization as a defense mechanism in survivors of trauma. J Trauma Stress 6:119–128, 1993

Shirali P, Kishwar A, Bharti SP: Life stress, demographic variables and personality (TAT) in eleven cases of possession (trance medium) in Shimla Tehsil. Personality Study and Group Behaviour 6: 73–81, 1986

Shorvon HJ: The depersonalization syndrome. Proceedings of the Royal Society of Medicine 39:779–785, 1946

Smith WH: Incorporating hypnosis into the psychotherapy of patients with multiple personality disorder. Bull Menninger Clin 57:344–354, 1993

Sno HN, Schalken HF: Dissociative identity disorder: diagnosis and treatment in the Netherlands. European Psychiatry: the Journal of the Association of European Psychiatrists 14:270–277, 1999

Solomon R: The use of the MMPI with multiple personality patients. Psychol Rep 53:1004–1006, 1983

Sookman D, Solyom L: Severe depersonalization treated with behavior therapy. Am J Psychiatry 135:1543–1545, 1978

Spanos NP, Weekes JR, Bertrand LD: Multiple personality: a social psychological perspective. J Abnorm Psychol 94:362–376, 1985

Spanos NP, Weekes JR, Menary E, et al: Hypnotic interview and age regression procedures in elicitation of multiple personality symptoms: a simulation study. Psychiatry 49:298–311, 1986

Spiegel D: Vietnam grief work using hypnosis. Am J Clin Hypn 24:33–40, 1981

Spiegel D: Multiple personality as a posttraumatic stress disorder. Psychiatr Clin North Am 7:101–110, 1984

Spiegel D: Dissociating damage. Am J Clin Hypn 29:123–131, 1986a

Spiegel D: Dissociation, double binds, and posttraumatic stress in multiple personality disorder, in Treatment of Multiple Personality Disorder. Edited by Braun BG. Washington, DC, American Psychiatric Press, 1986b, pp 61–77

Spiegel D: Chronic pain masks depression, multiple personality disorder. Hosp Community Psychiatry 38:933–935, 1987

Spiegel D: Dissociation and hypnosis in posttraumatic stress disorders. J Trauma Stress 1:17–33, 1988

Spiegel D: Trauma, dissociation, and hypnosis, in Incest-Related Syndromes of Adult Psychopathology. Edited by Kluft RL. Washington, DC, American Psychiatric Press, 1990b, pp 247–261

Spiegel D, Cardeña E: Disintegrated experience: the dissociative disorders revisited. J Abnorm Psychol 100:366–378, 1991

Spiegel D, Fink R: Hysterical psychosis and hypnotizability. Am J Psychiatry 136:777–781, 1979

Spiegel D, Detrick D, Frischholz E: Hypnotizability and psychopathology. Am J Psychiatry 139:431–437, 1982

Spiegel D, Hunt T, Dondershine HE: Dissociation and hypnotizability in posttraumatic stress disorder. Am J Psychiatry 145:301–305, 1988

Spiegel D, Frischholz EJ, Spira J: Functional disorders of memory, in American Psychiatric Press Review of Psychiatry, Vol 12. Edited by Oldham JM, Riba MB, Tasman A. Washington, DC, American Psychiatric Press, 1993, pp 747–782

Spiegel H, Spiegel D: Trance and Treatment: Clinical Uses of Hypnosis (1978). Washington, DC, American Psychiatric Press, 1987

Spier SA, Tesar GE, Rosenbaum JF, et al: Treatment of panic disorder and agoraphobia with clonazepam. J Clin Psychiatry 47:238–242, 1986

Spitzer C, Spelsberg B, Grabe HJ, et al: Dissociative experiences and psychopathology in conversion disorders. J Psychosom Res 46:291–294, 1999

Squire LR: Memory and the hippocampus: a synthesis from findings with rats, monkeys, and humans. Psychol Rev 99:195–231, 1992

Stein MB, Uhde TW: Depersonalization disorder: effects of caffeine and response to pharmacotherapy. Biol Psychiatry 26:315–320, 1989

Steinberg M: The spectrum of depersonalization: assessment and treatment, in American Psychiatric Press Review of Psychiatry, Vol 10. Edited by Tasman A, Goldfinger SM. Washington, DC, American Psychiatric Press, 1991, pp 223–247

Steinberg M, Rounsaville B, Cicchetti DV: The Structured Clinical Interview for DSM-III-R Dissociative Disorders: preliminary report on a new diagnostic instrument. Am J Psychiatry 147:76–82, 1990

Steinberg M, Cicchetti D, Buchanan J, et al: Distinguishing between multiple personality disorder (dissociative identity disorder) and schizophrenia using the Structured Clinical Interview for DSM-IV Dissociative Disorders. J Nerv Ment Dis 182:495–502, 1994

Steinberg M: Advances in the clinical assessment of dissociation: the SCID-D-R. Bull Menninger Clin 64:146–163, 2000

Stern CR: The etiology of multiple personalities. Psychiatr Clin North Am 7:149–160, 1984

Tantam D: An exorcism in Zanzibar: insights into groups from another culture. Group Analysis 26:251–260, 1993

Terr LC: Childhood traumas: an outline and overview. Am J Psychiatry 148:10–20, 1991

Trangkasombat U, Su-Umpan U, Churujikul V, et al: Epidemic dissociation among school children in southern Thailand. Dissociation 8:130–141, 1995

Trangkasombat U, Su-Umpan U, Churujiporn V, et al: Risk factors for spirit possession among school girls in southern Thailand. J Med Assoc Thai 81:541–546, 1998

Torch EM: The psychotherapeutic treatment of depersonalization disorder. Hillside Journal of Clinical Psychiatry 9:133–143, 1987

Tulving E: Elements of Episodic Memory. Oxford, England, Clarendon Press, 1983

Tutkun H, Sar V, Yargic LI, et al: Frequency of dissociative disorders among psychiatric inpatients in a Turkish university clinic. Am J Psychiatry 155:800–805, 1998

Valdiserri S, Kihlstrom JF: Abnormal eating and dissociative experiences. Int J Eat Disord 17:373–380, 1995

van der Hart O: Multiple personality disorder in Europe: impressions. Dissociation 6:102–118, 1993

van der Hart O, Nijenhuis E: Dissociative disorders, especially multiple personality disorder. Ned Tijdschr Geneeskd 137:1865–1868, 1993

van der Hart O, Spiegel D: Hypnotic assessment and treatment of trauma-induced psychoses: the early psychotherapy of Breukink and modern views. Int J Clin Exp Hypn 41:191–209, 1993

van der Kolk BA, Fisler R: Dissociation and the fragmentary nature of traumatic memories: overview and exploratory study. J Trauma Stress 8:505–525, 1995

van der Kolk BA, Hostetler A, Herron N, et al: Trauma and the development of borderline personality disorder. Psychiatr Clin North Am 17:715–730, 1994

van der Kolk BA, Pelcovitz D, Roth S, et al: Dissociation, somatization, and affect dysregulation: the complexity of adaptation of trauma. Am J Psychiatry 153 (suppl 7):83–93, 1996

Vanderlinden J, Van Dyck R, Vandereycken W, et al: Dissociative experiences in the general population of the Netherlands and Belgium: a study with the Dissociative Questionnaire (DIS-Q). Dissociation 4:180–184, 1991

van Dyck R: Dissociation, hypnosis and multiple personality disorders. Ned Tijdschr Geneeskd 137:1863–1864, 1993

Varma VK, Bouri M, Wig NN: Multiple personality in India: comparison with hysterical possession state. Am J Psychother 35:113–120, 1981

Vincent M, Pickering MR: Multiple personality disorder in childhood. Can J Psychiatry 33:524–529, 1988

Walsh RN: Depersonalization: definition and treatment (letter). Am J Psychiatry 132:873–874, 1975

Wettstein RM, Fauman BJ: The amobarbital interview. JACEP 8:272–274, 1979

Wittkower ED: Transcultural psychiatry in the Caribbean: past, present and future. Am J Psychiatry 127:162–166, 1970

Witztum E, Grisaru N, Budowski D: The "Zar" possession syndrome among Ethiopian immigrants to Israel: cultural and clinical aspects. Br J Med Psychol 69:207–225, 1996

Yap PM: The possession syndrome: a comparison of Hong Kong and French findings. Journal of Mental Science 106:114–137, 1960

Yargic LI, Sar V, Tutkun H, et al: Comparison of dissociative identity disorder with other diagnostic groups using a structured interview in Turkey. Compr Psychiatry 39: 345–351, 1998

Zweig-Frank H, Paris J, Guzder J: Psychological risk factors for dissociation and self-mutilation in female patients with borderline personality disorder. Can J Psychiatry 39:259–264, 1994

CHAPTER 11

Sexual and Gender Identity Disorders

Judith V. Becker, Ph.D.

Bradley R. Johnson, M.D.

Clinicians see patients who have a variety of sexual disorders or dysfunctions. A woman who is sexually assaulted may no longer experience sexual desire. A man who is recently widowed may experience difficulty in achieving erections when he begins to date. A woman with multiple sclerosis may no longer have orgasms. A man who is taking antihypertensive medication may have difficulty obtaining an erection. Recently postmenopausal women may find intercourse painful. Patients given antidepressants or antipsychotic medication may report impairment in sexual functioning. An adolescent may request a consultation because his cross-dressing troubles him. An adult man who has been fantasizing about sex with prepubertal children may seek treatment because he is fearful that he will act on his fantasies. Adolescents or adults may compulsively view pornographic images on the Internet or visit sexual chat rooms to the point that it interferes with life functions. Consequently, it is important for clinicians to become educated about the categories of sexual disorders and become adept at taking sexual histories and using the various modalities and interventions.

Gender Identity Disorders

Gender and Sexual Differentiation

The genetic sex of an individual is determined at conception, but development from that point on is influenced by many factors. For the first few weeks of gestation, the gonads are undifferentiated. If the Y chromosome is present in the embryo, the gonads will differentiate into testes. A substance referred to as the H-Y antigen is responsible for this transformation. If the Y chromosome or H-Y antigen is not present in the developing embryo, the gonads will develop into ovaries.

Like the gonads, the internal and external genital structures are initially undifferentiated in the fetus. If the gonads differentiate into testes, fetal androgen (i.e., testosterone) is secreted, and these structures develop into male genitalia (epididymis, vas deferens, ejaculatory ducts, penis, and scrotum). In the absence of fetal androgen, these structures develop into female genitalia (fallopian tubes, uterus, clitoris, and vagina). It is important to note that the development of genitalia in utero depends on the presence or absence of fetal androgen, from whatever source. Thus, if fetal androgen is present in a genetically determined female (e.g., adrenal hyperplasia), male genitalia will develop, even in the presence of ovaries, and the child will be born with either ambiguous or male genitals. Likewise, if fetal androgen is missing (e.g., enzyme deficiency) or the androgen receptors are defective (e.g., testicular feminization), female genitalia will develop even though the individual has the Y chromosome and testes.

Psychosexual development also is thought to be influenced by a complex interaction of factors, both pre- and postnatal. Before discussing these factors, however, it is important to break down psychosexual behavior into several components. *Gender identity* is an individual's perception and self-awareness of being male or female. *Gender role* is the behavior that an individual engages in that identifies him or her to others as being male or female (e.g., wearing dresses and makeup). *Sexual orientation* is the erotic attraction that an individual feels (e.g., arousal to men, women, children, nonsexual objects).

Prenatal hormones play a role in the differentiation of the mammalian brain. However, their exact effect on psychosexual development in humans has not been established. Gender identity appears to develop in the early years of life and generally is established by age 3 years. Gender identity seems to depend on the sex in which an individual is reared, regardless of biological factors.

Gender identity, once it is firmly established, is extremely resistant to change. For example, if a genetic female is reared as a boy (e.g., as a result of exposure to fetal androgens) but suddenly develops breasts and other female secondary sex characteristics during puberty, his gender identity will remain male, and he will want to cor-

rect the changes. Biological factors that have not yet been discovered may influence the development of gender identity, and in some instances, it has been suggested that biological factors may override sex assignment at birth (Ehrhardt and Meyer-Bahlburg 1981). According to a learning theory model, gender identity begins to develop when the child imitates or identifies with same-sex models. The child is then reinforced for this identification and for engaging in "appropriate" sex-role behaviors. In psychoanalytic theory, gender identity develops as part of overall identity formation in the phase of separation and individuation and is very much dependent on the quality of the mother–infant dyad.

Criteria for Diagnosing Gender Identity Disorder

Gender identity disorders are characterized by strong and persistent cross-gender identification (not merely a desire for any perceived cultural advantages of being the other sex) as well as a persistent discomfort with one's sex or sense of inappropriateness in the gender role of that sex (Table 11–1).

Gender Identity Disorder of Adulthood

Up to this point, the essential features of the principal diagnostic categories in the subclass *transsexualism* were a persistent sense of discomfort and inappropriateness about one's anatomical sex and a persistent wish to be rid of one's genitals and to live as a member of the other sex.

The term *transsexualism* was eliminated in DSM-IV (American Psychiatric Association 1994). A single diagnostic term, *gender identity disorder*, exists for the childhood form and for the adult and adolescent form. The elimination of the term *transsexualism* alters the sense that it exists as a single disorder and presents it

---

TABLE 11–1. DSM-IV-TR diagnostic criteria for gender identity disorder

---

A. A strong and persistent cross-gender identification (not merely a desire for any perceived cultural advantages of being the other sex).

In children, the disturbance is manifested by four (or more) of the following:

(1) repeatedly stated desire to be, or insistence that he or she is, the other sex

(2) in boys, preference for cross-dressing or simulating female attire; in girls, insistence on wearing only stereotypical masculine clothing

(3) strong and persistent preferences for cross-sex roles in make-believe play or persistent fantasies of being the other sex

(4) intense desire to participate in the stereotypical games and pastimes of the other sex

(5) strong preference for playmates of the other sex

In adolescents and adults, the disturbance is manifested by symptoms such as a stated desire to be the other sex, frequent passing as the other sex, desire to live or be treated as the other sex, or the conviction that he or she has the typical feelings and reactions of the other sex.

B. Persistent discomfort with his or her sex or sense of inappropriateness in the gender role of that sex.

In children, the disturbance is manifested by any of the following: in boys, assertion that his penis or testes are disgusting or will disappear or assertion that it would be better not to have a penis, or aversion toward rough-and-tumble play and rejection of male stereotypical toys, games, and activities; in girls, rejection of urinating in a sitting position, assertion that she has or will grow a penis, or assertion that she does not want to grow breasts or menstruate, or marked aversion toward normative feminine clothing.

In adolescents and adults, the disturbance is manifested by symptoms such as preoccupation with getting rid of primary and secondary sex characteristics (e.g., request for hormones, surgery, or other procedures to physically alter sexual characteristics to simulate the other sex) or belief that he or she was born the wrong sex.

C. The disturbance is not concurrent with a physical intersex condition.

D. The disturbance causes clinically significant distress or impairment in social, occupational, or other important areas of functioning.

Code based on current age:

302.6 Gender Identity Disorder in Children

302.85 Gender Identity Disorder in Adolescents or Adults

Specify if (for sexually mature individuals):

Sexually Attracted to Males

Sexually Attracted to Females

Sexually Attracted to Both

Sexually Attracted to Neither

---

conceptually as a spectrum of disorders.

The term *gender dysphoria* has been used to characterize a person's sense of discomfort or unease about his or her status as male or female (Zucker and Green 1997). Gender dysphoria has been classified as primary or secondary as it relates to transsexualism (Person and Ovesey 1974). *Primary transsexuals* have a life-long, profound disturbance of core gender identity. *Secondary transsexuals* also can have a long history of gender identity confusion; however, in these individuals, the identity disturbance follows other cross-gender behavior such as transvestism or effeminate homosexuality.

Epidemiology

Gender identity disorder of adulthood is rare, with estimates of 30,000 cases worldwide (Lothstein 1980). Approximately 1 per 30,000 adult males and 1 per 100,000 females seek sex-reassignment surgery (American Psychiatric Association 2000). Transsexual individuals most commonly request *sex reassignment*; that is, change in their physical appearance (usually by hormonal and surgical means) to correspond with their self-perceived gender. It is important to conduct a thorough evaluation before recommending sex reassignment.

Three to four times as many males as females apply for sex reassignment, but approximately equal numbers of males and females are reassigned (J.K. Meyer 1982). Virtually all of the women who apply have a sexual orientation toward women. Male transsexuals are predominantly homosexual in orientation, but approximately 25% are sexually attracted to women. Some of these "heterosexual" transsexuals enter into "lesbian" relationships after they are reassigned as females. Many male and female transsexuals also have been described as being hyposexual or asexual.

Comorbidity

Among those adults who are diagnosed as having gender identity disorder, there is a high degree of concomitant psychiatric disorder, most commonly borderline, antisocial, or narcissistic personality disorder; substance abuse; and suicidal or self-destructive behavior (J.K. Meyer 1982).

Etiology

There are no well-established or exhaustive explanations for the development of gender identity disorder. As noted earlier in this chapter, gender identity appears to be established and influenced by psychosocial factors during the first few years of life. However, many authors have argued that biological factors, if not causative,

may predispose an individual to a gender identity disorder. It is important to realize, however, that researchers still have been unable to identify a biological anomaly or variant associated specifically with gender identity disorder.

As mentioned earlier in this section, prenatal sex hormones probably have little causal effect on gender identity and possibly sexual orientation. However, studies of females with congenital adrenal hyperplasia caused by high levels of androgens prenatally (Collaer and Hines 1995) suggest there may be a relation between such disorders and gender identity problems. This type of example leads us to realize that further research in this area needs to be done.

Some researchers have found decreased levels of testosterone in male transsexuals and abnormally high levels of testosterone in female transsexuals, but the findings have been inconsistent, and the studies from which they were obtained were not well controlled. Tests for H-Y antigen have been found to be negative in male transsexuals and positive in female transsexuals in a high percentage of cases; however, there has been a consistent failure to replicate these findings (Hoenig 1985).

Although no correlation has been made with specific temporal lobe abnormalities, there have been case reports of individuals who developed gender identity disorder following onset of temporal lobe seizures, which reverted with the use of anticonvulsive medication. Studies of electroencephalograms (EEGs) in male and female transsexuals have detected abnormalities in 30%–70%; however, only one of the studies used control groups, and the effect of medications, especially estrogen, was not taken into account (Hoenig 1985).

Family studies have been difficult to carry out given the low incidence of gender identity disorders. To date, no clear increase in familial incidence has been documented. Learning theory models suggest that gender dysphoria arises from absent or inconsistent reinforcement for identification with same-sex models. Psychoanalytic theory argues that early deprivation of the male child by his mother leads to a symbiotic merger with the mother and lack of full individuation as a separate person. Clinical studies (Green 1987; Stoller 1968, 1975a, 1975b, 1979) describe that boys with gender identity disorder often have an overly close relationship with their mother and a distant, ambivalent relationship with their father. Stoller (1968) argued that the boy who is excessively close to his mother, in absence of the father, may have difficulty in separating himself from the female body and feminine behavior.

Diagnosis and Evaluation

Individuals who request sex reassignment require careful and patient evaluation by a psychiatrist or psychologist with experience in the management of gender identity disorders. Patients with other primary psychiatric diagnoses may present as transsexuals. Psychotic patients may have delusions centered around their genitalia. When the psychosis is treated, the cross-gender wishes usually resolve. Individuals with severe personality disorders, especially borderline, can have transient wishes to change gender as part of their overall identity diffusion during times of stress. Effeminate homosexuals may desire to change sex in order to be more attractive to men; usually this desire fluctuates with time. Adolescents sometimes become gender dysphoric because of developing homosexual feelings that need to be resolved. For each of these patients, psychotherapy is indicated to deal with the appropriate issues leading to their request for sex reassignment.

Unfortunately, individuals requesting sex reassignment often hide the truth in an effort to obtain hormonal and surgical change. Therefore, it is imperative to contact significant others in the patient's life to confirm the pervasive and nonremitting nature of the gender identity disturbance.

Treatment

Because most gender dysphoric individuals have adamant requests for sex reassignment, it is extremely difficult to engage these patients in treatment with anything other than surgical sex reassignment as the goal. These patients see psychotherapy as a means of discouraging them from surgery. However, because surgery is irreversible, it is important to engage these patients in psychotherapy, even if surgery is indicated. The therapist should be careful to base the goals of therapy on what is desired by the patient.

Supportive psychotherapy can serve various purposes in transsexual individuals. First, there have been reports, albeit few, of reversal of patients' gender identity disorders. Second, a trial of psychotherapy is often useful in cases in which the diagnosis is not clear. Third, dealing with patients' fears of homosexuality may sometimes change their wishes for surgical reassignments. Fourth, psychotherapy plays an important role in patients' adjustment to the process of sex reassignment. Finally, therapy is often helpful in the postsurgical adjustment of patients with gender identity disorder.

Psychoanalysis generally is not indicated in the treatment of transsexuals secondary to occasional poor ego functioning (J.K. Meyer 1982). Dynamic psychotherapy may be used but must involve parameters applied to borderline patients (i.e., structured therapy, limit setting, ego support, and short-term goals).

Behavior therapy has been used with success in ego-dystonic male transsexuals in several cases (Barlow et al. 1979). The treatment can be helpful to those who wish to alter their effeminate behaviors, including female patterns of behavior. These behaviors are then changed with videotapes and modeling of masculine behaviors in which the patients are trained to engage.

Green and Fleming (1990) reviewed the literature published during 1979 through 1989 on both male-to-female and female-to-male postoperative transsexuals. Only 11 follow-up studies were located in the literature. These authors concluded that preoperative factors that were indicative of a favorable outcome included an absence of psychosis, as well as mental and emotional stability shown prior to the surgery; a successful adaptation to the desired gender for at least 1 year; an understanding of the consequences and limitations of the surgery; and the seeking of preoperative psychotherapy. Data from this report indicated that outcomes were considered satisfactory for 97% of the female-to-male transsexuals and for 87% of the male-to-female transsexuals.

Smith et al. (2001) conducted a prospective follow-up study with 20 treated adolescent transsexuals to evaluate early sex reassignment and with 21 nontreated and 6 delayed-treatment adolescents to evaluate the decisions not to allow them to start sex reassignment, especially at an early age. The treated group who received sex-reassignment surgery did not continue to have gender dysphoria, and they were thought to be psychologically and socially functioning quite well 1–4 years postoperatively.

Sex reassignment is a long process that must be carefully monitored. Patients with other primary psychiatric diagnoses and secondary transsexuals should be screened out and given other appropriate treatment. If the patient is considered ap-propriate for sex reassignment, psychotherapy should be started to prepare the patient for the cross-gender role. The patient should then go out into the world and live in the cross-gender role before surgical reassignment. Males should cross-dress, have electrolysis, and practice female behaviors. They can even change their identity to female on official documents and at work. Females should cut their hair, bind or conceal their breasts, and similarly take on the identity of a man. After 1–2 years, if these measures have been successful and the patient still wishes reassignment, hormone treatment is begun. After 1–2 years of hormone therapy, the patient may be considered for surgical reassignment if such a procedure is still desired. In the male-to-female patient, this consists of bilateral orchiectomy, penile amputation, and creation of an artificial vagina. Female-to-male patients undergo bilateral mastectomy and optional hysterectomy with removal of ovaries. Efforts to create an artificial penis have met with mixed results thus far. Psychotherapy after surgery is indicated to help the patient adjust to the surgical changes and discuss sexual functioning and satisfaction.

Gender Identity Disorder of Childhood

Because of the difficulty and turmoil involved in treating late-adolescent and adult patients who have gender identity disorder, researchers and clinicians began to evaluate and treat children with gender identity problems. Strictly speaking, this disorder is seen in a child who perceives himself or herself as being of the opposite sex.

However, it is often difficult to separate gender identity from gender role behavior in children. Boys with normal gender identity may play with "girl" dolls.

Many girls in our culture are "tomboys" and like rough and contact games. However, in this gender identity syndrome, there is a repeated pattern of opposite-gender role behavior accompanied by a disturbance in the child's perception of "being" a boy or a girl. The exact incidence of gender identity disorder in children is not known, but, like adult gender dysphoria, it is a rare disorder.

Etiology

As with adult gender dysphoria, the etiology of childhood gender identity disorder is unclear. The theories outlined earlier in this chapter for adults who have gender identity disorder also apply to children. Additional factors that have been suggested are parents' indifference to or encouragement of opposite-sex behavior; regular cross-dressing as a young boy by a female; lack of male playmates during a boy's first years of socialization; excessive maternal protection, with inhibition of rough-and-tumble play; or absence of or rejection by an older male early in life (Green 1974). Gender identity disorder in children has been posited as being the result of child and family pathology (Zucker and Bradley 1995).

Course

Retrospective studies of transsexuals (Green 1974) have shown a high incidence of childhood cross-gender behavior. Follow-up studies of children with gender identity disorder have found a high incidence of continued manifestations in adulthood, with a higher incidence of homosexual or bisexual behavior and fantasies than those in a control group (Green 1985).

Treatment

Treatment of gender identity disorder in the child is offered in an attempt to help the child avoid peer ostracism and humiliation, be comfortable with his or her own sex, and avoid the possible development of adult gender dysphoria. An eclectic approach to treatment has been advocated that involves developing a close, trusting relationship between a male therapist and the boy; stopping parental encouragement of feminine behaviors; interrupting the excessively close relationship between mother and son; enhancing the role of father and son; and reinforcing male behaviors (Green 1974).

Sexual Dysfunctions

Male and Female Physiology

Human sexual functioning requires a complex interaction of the nervous, vascular, and endocrine systems to produce arousal and orgasm. Sexual arousal in men occurs in the presence of visual stimuli (e.g., a naked partner), fantasies, or physical stimulation of the genitals or other areas of the body (e.g., the nipples). This stimulation leads to involuntary discharge in the parasympathetic nerves that control the diameter and valves of the penile blood vessels. Blood flow increases into the corpora cavernosa, two cylinders of specialized tissue in the penis that distend with blood to produce an erection. Continued stimulation leads to emission of semen and ejaculation, which are controlled through sympathetic fibers and the pudendal nerve. Dopaminergic systems in the central nervous system facilitate arousal and ejaculation, whereas serotonergic systems inhibit these functions. In addition, androgens must be present to expedite sexual arousal (and to some extent erection and ejaculation).

In women, as in men, arousal depends on fantasies, visual stimuli, and physical stimulation; in general, the latter is more important for women, whereas visual cues are more important for men. Again, this stimulation leads to parasympathetic nervous discharge that increases blood flow to the female genitalia, resulting in lubrication of the vagina and some enlargement of the clitoris. Continued stimulation of the clitoris either directly or through intercourse results in orgasm. Estrogens and progestins play a role in female sexual functioning; however, androgens are important in the maintenance of sexual arousal in women. As in men, dopaminergic systems facilitate female sexual arousal and orgasm, whereas serotonergic systems inhibit these functions.

It is readily apparent that normal sexual functioning and processes require intact neural and vascular connections to the genitals along with normal endocrine functioning. Any illness that interferes with these systems can lead to sexual dysfunction: neurological diseases (e.g., multiple sclerosis, lumbar or sacral spinal cord trauma, herniated disks), thrombosis of the arteries or veins of the penis, diabetes mellitus (which causes both neurological and vascular damage), endocrine disorders (e.g., hyperprolactinemia), liver disease (which leads to a buildup of estrogens), and so forth. Similarly, drugs that affect these systems also can impair sexual functioning (Table 11–2).

The sexual response cycle of men and women consists of four stages: appetitive, excitement, orgasm, and resolution (Masters and Johnson 1970). Sexual dysfunctions occur when there are disruptions of any of the four stages of sexual response because of anatomical, physiological, or psychological factors. Sexual orientation is not a determining factor, and sexual dysfunctions may be lifelong or may develop after a period of normal sexual functioning. Sexual dysfunctions may be further characterized as to whether they are present in all sexual activities or are situational.

TABLE 11–2. Some commonly used medications that may interfere with sexual functioning

Abused drugs
  Alcohol
  Opiates
  Cocaine
Antihypertensives
  Diuretics (thiazides, spironolactone)
  Methyldopa
  Clonidine
  β-Blockers
  Reserpine
  Guanethidine
Antipsychotics
  Thioridazine (retarded ejaculation)
  Thiothixine
  Chlorpromazine
  Perphenazine
  Fluphenazine
  Risperidone
  Olanzapine
Antidepressants
  Tricyclics
  Monoamine oxidase inhibitors
  Serotonin reuptake inhibitors
  Trazodone (priapism)
  Nefazodone (rare)
  Venlafaxine
  Mirtazapine (rare)
Others
  Cimetidine
  Steroids
  Estrogens

Epidemiology

The exact prevalence of sexual dysfunctions is difficult to determine. Frank et al. (1978) surveyed 100 well-educated, happily married couples. Forty percent of the men reported having experienced erectile or ejaculatory dysfunctions at some point during their lives. Sixty-three percent of the women reported arousal or orgasmic dysfunctions at some point. In addition, 50% of the men and 77% of the women reported other sexual difficulties, including lack of interest or inability to relax.

Simons and Cary (2001) recently reviewed the published literature since the publication of the Spector and Carey (1990) review. They reported prevalence figures for community samples of 0%–3% for male orgasmic disorder, 0%–5% for male erectile disorder, 0%–3% for male hypoactive sexual desire disorder, and 4%–5% for premature ejaculation. For female orgasmic disorder, the rates were 7%–10%.

A comprehensive survey conducted on a representative sample of the United States population between ages 19 and 59 suggested the following prevalence estimates: 3% for male dyspareunia, 15% for female dyspareunia, 10% for male orgasm problems, 25% for female orgasm problems, 33% for female hypoactive sexual desire, 27% for premature ejaculation, 20% for female arousal problems, and 10% for male erectile difficulties (American Psychiatric Association 2000).

Etiology

Kaplan (1974) argued for a multicausal theory of sexual dysfunctions on several levels (intrapsychic, interpersonal, and behavioral) and listed four factors as playing a role in the development of these disorders (Table 11–3).

TABLE 11–3. Multicausal theory of sexual dysfunctions

---

1. Misinformation or ignorance regarding sexual and social interaction
2. Unconscious guilt and anxiety concerning sex
3. Performance anxiety, as the most common cause of erectile and orgasmic dysfunctions
4. Partners' failure to communicate to each other their sexual feelings and those behaviors in which they want to engage

---

Other factors that may lead to the development of a sexual dysfunction include an unacknowledged homosexual orientation and attempts to function sexually with a person of the opposite sex. Many sexual problems are related to sexual trauma. For example, a history of incest, child sexual abuse, or rape may place an individual at risk for developing sexual problems (Becker et al. 1986). Many sexual dysfunctions occur secondary to major psychiatric disorders such as schizophrenia, depression, and severe personality disorders (Fagan et al. 1988). As previously discussed, physical, neurological, and physiological problems can lead to sexual dysfunction.

The side effects of various forms of medications also may cause sexual dysfunctions. A multicenter, prospective, descriptive clinical study was conducted with 344 patients who were taking selective serotonin reuptake inhibitors (SSRIs). Of the 344 patients, 200 reported some form of sexual dysfunction. The adverse effects varied by type of SSRI. Paroxetine was more likely to interfere with erection than were fluoxetine, fluvoxamine, or sertraline. Sexual dysfunctions included loss of libido, delayed orgasm or ejaculation, anorgasmia, and erectile dysfunction. Although the male patients showed a higher incidence of sexual dysfunction, the women's dysfunctions were more intense. The dysfunction remitted within 6 months in only 5.8% of the patients (Montejo-Gonzalez et al 1997).

Interestingly, no DSM category describes a primary disorder of increased sexual desire, but this has been reported in a few cases with the use of SSRIs (Greil et al. 2001).

Differential Diagnosis

Patients with a sexual dysfunction should be medically evaluated by a gynecologist or urologist to rule out treatable organic etiologies. These organic factors may be

local diseases of the genitals, vascular illnesses, neurological diseases, endocrine
disorders, or systemic illnesses. Patients
always should be asked about medications, including over-the-counter medicines and illegal drugs.

Psychophysiological procedures have
been developed to assess patients' erections. During rapid eye movement (REM)
sleep, men experience penile erections
defined as nocturnal penile tumescence
(NPT). Although NPT measures can be
equivocal, they help in evaluating a patient with erectile problems for organic
factors. Other assessment procedures include Doppler flow studies and penile
blood pressure measurement, arteriography and papaverine injections of the corpora cavernosa to assess vascular competence, and nerve root stimulation to assess
neurological impairment.

Descriptions and Treatments of Sexual Dysfunctions

Sexual Desire Disorders

Hypoactive sexual desire disorder.
Hypoactive sexual desire disorder (also
known as inhibited sexual desire) is characterized by the following DSM-IV-TR
criteria:

A. Persistently or recurrently deficient
   sexual fantasies and desire for sexual
   activity.
B. The disturbance also causes marked
   distress or interpersonal difficulty.
C. The diagnosis is made if the dysfunction does not occur exclusively during
   the course of another Axis I disorder
   (e.g., major depression) and is not due
   to the direct effects of a substance (alcohol or illegal drugs or prescription
   drugs) or a general medical condition.

It is also important to determine
whether hypoactive sexual desire is the

primary problem or the consequence of
another underlying sexual problem. It is
also important to differentiate this disorder, in which there is an absence of sexual
desire and fantasies, from sexual aversion,
in which there is avoidance of sexual activity because of extreme anxiety. It is important to assess whether the desire disorder
is substance induced (i.e., drugs or medications). Assessment of individuals with
hypoactive sexual desire disorder requires
medical workup, psychological evaluation,
and assessment of the relationship.

Hypoactive sexual desire disorder has
been the most difficult of all the dysfunctions to treat. Testosterone has been used
(in both men and women) to treat inhibited sexual desire with mixed results. Recently, Segraves et al. (2001) reported on
the use of bupropion sustained release in
the treatment of hypoactive sexual desire
disorder in nondepressed women.

The most effective treatments involve
a combination of cognitive therapy to deal
with maladaptive beliefs and marital therapy. When the problem is secondary to
prescription medication, one could consider waiting for the patient to accommodate to the drug, lowering the dose, giving
drug holidays, changing to another drug
within the same therapeutic class, changing to a new therapeutic class, or adding a
pharmacological antidote (although none
is currently approved by the U.S. Food
and Drug Administration for this purpose)
(Finger 2001).

Sexual aversion disorder.   Sexual aversion disorder is characterized by the following DSM-IV-TR criteria:

A. A persistent or recurrent extreme
   aversion to, and avoidance of, all (or
   almost all) genital sexual contact with
   a partner.
B. The disturbance causes marked distress or interpersonal difficulty.

C. The sexual dysfunction is not better accounted for by another Axis I disorder.

The major goal of treatment is to reduce the patient's fear and avoidance of sex. This goal can be accomplished via systematic desensitization, in which the patient is gradually exposed in imagination and then in vivo to the actual sexual situations that generate anxiety.

Sexual Arousal Disorders

Male erectile disorder. Male erectile disorder is characterized by the following DSM-IV-TR criteria:

A. Persistent or recurrent inability to attain, or to maintain until completion of the sexual activity, an adequate erection.
B. The disturbance causes marked distress or interpersonal difficulty.
C. The erectile difficulty is not better accounted for by another Axis I disorder.

Feldman et al. (1994) reported that 35% of men between ages 40 and 70 have severe or complete erectile dysfunction, as do 50% of men older than 70. Until recently, the most frequently used interventions have been behavioral.

A successful treatment for arousal and erectile disorders in patients with partners has been the use of behavioral assignments to gradually decrease performance anxiety. Sarwer and Durlak (1997) reported on 365 married couples who received treatment over a 7-week period. Sessions were provided once a week for approximately 4 hours. The treatment success rate for the total sample was 65%.

Vasoactive injections into the corpora cavernosa can be used to treat erectile disorders. These injections can produce erections that last up to several hours. Most injections consist of a combination of papaverine (a smooth-muscle relaxant) and phentolamine (an α-adrenergic blocker), although other agents (e.g., prostaglandin E_1) also can be used (Mahmoud et al. 1992). Success rates for this treatment are high (about 85%), with improvements in erectile capacity, sexual satisfaction, and frequency of intercourse (Althof et al. 1991).

Oral medications such as yohimbine, an α-adrenergic antagonist, also have been used to treat erectile dysfunction. Full or partial improvement has been reported in about 34%–38% of patients taking these agents compared with those taking a placebo, although the benefits can require several weeks to take effect (Sonda et al. 1990; Susset et al. 1989). Dopamine agonists such as bromocriptine also have been found to be effective in preliminary trials (Lal et al. 1991).

Sildenafil is now widely used in the treatment of erectile disorders by releasing nitric oxide into the corpus cavernosum. This activates the enzyme guanylate cyclase, which results in increased levels of cyclic guanosine monophosphate (cGMP), producing smooth-muscle relaxation in the corpus cavernosum and allowing the inflow of blood during sexual stimulation. Salerian et al. (2000) recently reported on the treatment of 61 men and 31 women who had psychotropic-induced sexual dysfunction. Ninety-one percent of the men reported improvement in erectile functioning. Seidman et al. (2001) also recently reported not only that sildenafil was efficacious for erectile dysfunction but also that the improvement in erectile dysfunction due to sildenafil was associated with marked improvement in the depressive symptoms often seen in this population.

For men with pure organic or combination organic–psychogenic impotence who do not respond to other treatment measures, penile prostheses can be implanted.

Female sexual arousal disorder.
Female sexual arousal disorder is characterized by the following DSM-IV-TR criteria:

A. Persistent or recurrent inability to attain, or to maintain until completion of the sexual activity, an adequate lubrication-swelling response of sexual excitement.
B. The disturbance causes marked distress or interpersonal difficulty.
C. The sexual dysfunction is not better accounted for by another Axis I disorder (except another sexual dysfunction) and is not due to the direct physiological effects of a substance (e.g., a drug of abuse, a medication) or a general medical condition.

Treatment of impairment of sexual arousal in women often involves the reduction of anxiety associated with sexual activity. Thus, behavioral techniques such as those involving sensate focus are most often effective (Kaplan 1974). Although not yet approved by the Food and Drug Administration for use in women, treatment with sildenafil improved sexual arousal in 77% of the women in one study (Salerian et al. 2000).

Orgasmic Disorders

Female orgasmic disorder. Female orgasmic disorder is characterized by the following DSM-IV-TR criteria:

A. Persistent or recurrent delay in, or absence of, orgasm following a normal sexual excitement phase. Women exhibit wide variability in the type or intensity of stimulation that triggers orgasm. The diagnosis of female orgasmic disorder should be based on the clinician's judgment that the woman's orgasmic capacity is less than would be reasonable for her age, sexual experience, and the adequacy of sexual stimulation she receives.
B. The disturbance causes marked distress or interpersonal difficulty.
C. The orgasmic dysfunction is not better accounted for by another Axis I disorder and is not due exclusively to the direct physiological effects of a substance or a general medical condition.

The most likely way for a woman with general anorgasmia (i.e., never having had an orgasm) to become orgasmic is through a program of directed masturbation (LoPiccolo and Stock 1986). Use of sexual fantasies combined with stimulation is also taught. Once the woman is able to have an orgasm through self-stimulation, she then teaches her sexual partner (using sensate focus exercises) the type of genital stimulation she requires to have an orgasm.

The most frequent complaint of women experiencing an orgasmic problem is that they are not orgasmic through penile–vaginal intercourse. When becoming orgasmic through intercourse is a patient's treatment goal, the clinician should ensure that she and her partner are aware that adequate stimulation both before and during intercourse is necessary. In addition, the clinician may suggest various sexual positions that allow stimulation of the clitoris by the patient or her partner during intercourse. For women who are fearful of "letting go" during intercourse, systematic desensitization is often helpful. The therapist may wish to explore with the patient psychodynamic reasons, religious concerns, or personal beliefs regarding intercourse and sexual pleasure.

Recently, there have been reports of improved orgasmic responding in women who have been prescribed sildenafil. Berman et al. (2001) reported that 67% of the women in their study reported an increased ability to have an orgasm, as did 67% of the women in the Salerian et al. (2000) study.

Male orgasmic disorder. Male orgasmic disorder is characterized by the following DSM-IV-TR criteria:

A. Persistent or recurrent delay in, or absence of, orgasm following a normal sexual excitement phase during sexual activity that the clinician, taking into account the person's age, judges to be adequate in focus, intensity, and duration.

B. The disturbance causes marked distress or interpersonal difficulty.

C. The orgasmic difficulty is not better accounted for by another Axis I disorder.

The treatment of male orgasmic disorder is similar to that used for female orgasmic disorder. The patient should be told that when he masturbates, he should masturbate as quickly as possible to ejaculation while fantasizing that his penis is inside his partner's vagina and ejaculating. A second technique is to teach the patient and his partner sensate focus exercises.

Salerian et al. (2000) reported that 77% of those men who had psychotropically induced sexual dysfunctions improved in orgasmic functioning after taking sildenafil.

Premature ejaculation. Premature ejaculation is characterized by the following DSM-IV-TR criteria:

A. Persistent or recurrent ejaculation with minimal sexual stimulation before, on, or shortly after penetration and before the person wishes it. The clinician must take into account factors that affect duration of the excitement phase, such as age, novelty of the sexual partner or situation, and recent frequency of sexual activity.

B. The disturbance causes marked distress or interpersonal difficulty.

C. The premature ejaculation is not due exclusively to the direct effects of a substance.

Premature ejaculation is the most prevalent of all male sexual problems. The treatment of premature ejaculation can involve training the individual to tolerate high levels of excitement without ejaculating and reducing anxiety associated with sexual arousal. One successful intervention is the start–stop technique (Semans 1956).

A second procedure, the "squeeze" technique (Masters and Johnson 1970), can be done in conjunction with the start–stop technique.

Metz and Pryor (2000) distinguished several subtypes of biogenic and psychogenic premature ejaculation. Biogenic types include neurological constitution, physical illness, physical injury, and pharmacological side effects. Medical conditions that can contribute to premature ejaculation include arteriosclerosis, benign prostatic hyperplasia, cardiovascular disease, diabetes, injury to the sympathetic nervous system, pelvic injuries, prostate cancer, prostatitis, urethritis, urinary incontinence, polycythemia, and polyneuritis (Baum and Spieler 2001). Psychogenic types consist of psychological constitution (chronic psychological disorders), psychological distress, and psychosexual skills deficit.

Somatic treatments for premature ejaculation have included intracavernous injection of papaverine and phentolamine (Fein 1990) and oral medications such as clomipramine (Colpi et al. 1991). However, Baum and Spieler (2001) discussed newer medical interventions for premature ejaculation, including the use of SSRIs (can decrease libido and delay orgasm), topical creams such as SS-cream (can cause mild penile burning or pain) or anesthetic creams (can cause penile numbness), and Chloraseptic mouthwash (can retard sexual stimulation).

Sexual Pain Disorders

Dyspareunia. Dyspareunia is characterized by the following DSM-IV-TR criteria:

A. Recurrent or persistent genital pain associated with intercourse in either a male or a female.
B. The disturbance causes marked distress or interpersonal difficulty.
C. The disturbance is not caused exclusively by vaginismus or lack of lubrication and is not better accounted for by another Axis I disorder.

It is imperative that a comprehensive physical and gynecological or urological examination be conducted. In the absence of organic pathology, the patient's fear and anxiety underlying sexual functioning should be investigated. Systematic desensitization has been found to be successful in the treatment of this disorder in some women. Graziottin (2001) reported that a diagnosis integrating medical and psychosexual factors is the first step in the effective treatment of dyspareunia and that intervention involves physiopathologically oriented treatment of the organic factors and therapy targeted toward the individual's and/or the couple's psychosexual issues.

Vaginismus. Vaginismus is characterized by the following DSM-IV-TR criteria:

A. Recurrent or persistent involuntary spasm of the musculature of the outer

third of the vagina that interferes with sexual intercourse.
B. The disturbance causes marked distress or interpersonal difficulty.
C. The disturbance is not better accounted for by another Axis I disorder.

Vaginismus can be diagnosed with certainty only through a gynecological examination. Some women who are anxious about sex may experience muscular tightening and some pain during penetration, but these women do not have vaginismus. It is important to rule out other Axis I disorders (e.g., somatization disorder), substance-induced disorders, or a general medical condition.

Systematic desensitization has been the most effective treatment method for vaginismus. A useful procedure involves the systematic insertion of dilators of graduated sizes, either in the physician's office or in the privacy of the patient's home. Some clinicians have the patient or her partner gradually insert a tampon or fingers until penile penetration can be effected (Kaplan 1974). The clinician may suggest that the patient gently stroke her genitals, including her clitoris, during the insertion procedure. Additionally, penile penetration should be effected with the partner lying on his back and the patient controlling the actual insertion and subsequent movement during intercourse. Follow-up studies have reported maintenance of treatment gains over time for most women (Scholl 1988).

Sexual Dysfunction Due to a General Medical Condition

The diagnosis of sexual dysfunction due to a general medical condition is made if there is evidence from the history, physical examination, or laboratory findings of a general medical condition judged to be etiologically related to the sexual dysfunction.

Substance-Induced Sexual Dysfunction

The diagnosis of substance-induced sexual dysfunction is made if there is a clinically significant sexual dysfunction that results in marked distress or interpersonal difficulty. Depending on the substance involved, the dysfunction may involve impaired desire, arousal, or orgasm or sexual pain. Individuals who abuse drugs have a high rate (up to 60%) of sexual dysfunctions (Cocores et al. 1988; Schiavi 1990).

Paraphilias

The paraphilias (Table 11–4) are characterized by the experiencing, over a period of at least 6 months, of recurrent, intense sexually arousing fantasies, sexual urges, or behaviors generally involving nonhuman objects or nonconsenting partners. Examples of paraphilias are fetishism (i.e., sexual arousal to nonliving objects, female undergarments), transvestic fetishism (i.e., sexual urges and fantasies involving cross-dressing), and pedophilia (i.e., sexual urges and fantasies involving prepubescent children). Sexual sadism involves urges toward, and sexually arousing fantasies of, acts (real, not simulated) in which the psychological and/or physical suffering (including humiliation) of the victim is sexually exciting to the perpetrator. In sexual masochism, an individual derives sexual excitement from being humiliated, beaten, bound, or otherwise made to suffer.

Other paraphilias that involve nonconsenting partners are exhibitionism (i.e., exposure of genitals to an unsuspecting stranger), voyeurism (i.e., observing an unsuspecting person naked, in the process of disrobing, or engaging in sexual activity), and frottage (i.e., sexual arousal caused by rubbing up against a stranger). Some individuals are aroused by sexual

TABLE 11–4.   Paraphilias

Exhibitionism
Fetishism
Frotteurism
Pedophilia
Sexual masochism
Sexual sadism
Transvestic fetishism
Voyeurism
Paraphilia not otherwise specified
Sexual disorder not otherwise specified

contact with corpses (necrophilia), urine (urophilia), feces (coprophilia), or enemas (klismaphilia).

In diagnosing all of the paraphilias, a further criterion is that the person has acted on the urges or is markedly distressed by them.

Epidemiology

The paraphilias rarely cause personal distress, and individuals with these disorders usually come for treatment because of pressure from their partners or the authorities. Thus, there are few data on the prevalence or course of many of these disorders. Two large studies of incarcerated sex offenders found that the offenders had committed only a small number of sexually deviant acts (Gebhard et al. 1965). In contrast, studies of nonincarcerated pedophiles have found a high number of paraphilic acts: 23.2–281.7 acts per offender (Abel et al. 1985).

The vast majority of individuals with these disorders are male. For example, among reported cases of sexual abuse, more than 90% of the offenders are men (Finkelhor 1986). Faller (1989) reported that 5%–15% of sexual abuse perpetrators are women. It also has been traditionally held that persons with paraphilias engage in only one type of deviant sexual behavior. However, studies have suggested that these individuals often have multiple paraphilias (Abel et al. 1985). It is important to note that more than 50% of these individuals develop the onset of their paraphilic arousal before age 18 years.

Etiology

Various theories have been put forth to explain the development of paraphilias. As with the gender identity disorders, biological factors have been postulated. In animals, destruction of parts of the limbic system causes hypersexual behavior (Klüver-Bucy syndrome), and temporal lobe diseases such as psychomotor seizures or temporal lobe tumors have been implicated in some persons with paraphilias. It also has been suggested that abnormal levels of androgens may contribute to inappropriate sexual arousal. Most studies, however, have dealt only with violent sex offenders and have yielded inconclusive results (Bradford and McLean 1984).

According to learning theory, sexual arousal develops when an individual engages in a sexual behavior that is subsequently reinforced through sexual fantasies and masturbation. It is thought that there are certain vulnerable periods (e.g., puberty) when the development of sexual arousal can occur.

Another theoretical model of the development of paraphilias is based on cognitive distortions. Distortions in thinking, or thinking errors, provide a way for an individual to give himself or herself permission to engage in inappropriate or deviant sexual behaviors. Examples of such faulty beliefs include the following: it is all right to have sex with a child as long as the child agrees; watching a woman through a window as she undresses does not cause her any harm; and if a child stares at my penis, he or she likes what he or she is seeing and wants to be sexual (Abel et al. 1984).

Diagnosis

It is important to distinguish between paraphilias such as fetishism and transvestism and normal variations of sexual behavior. Only when these activities are the exclusive or preferred means of achieving sexual excitement and orgasm, or when the sexual behavior is not consensual, is the paraphilia diagnosed. Obviously, nonconsensual sexual activities such as sexual contact with children or exhibitionism never can be appropriate; children never can give consent for sexual activity with an adult.

In evaluating an individual for paraphilic behavior, a careful psychiatric evaluation must be done to exclude the aforementioned possible causes of this behavior. A detailed sexual history should be taken, noting the onset and course of paraphilic and appropriate sexual fantasies and behavior and the present degree of control over the deviant behavior. In addition, the individual should be evaluated for faulty beliefs about his or her sexual behavior (i.e., cognitive distortions), social and assertive skills with appropriate adult partners, sexual dysfunctions, and sexual knowledge.

Phallometric assessments (i.e., measurements of penile erection) have been used to objectively assess sexual arousal in individuals who have engaged in paraphilic behavior. Phallometric assessments of sexual age and gender preferences have excellent discriminant validity with extrafamilial child molesters (Freund and Blanchard 1989). However, exclusively incestuous offenders are less likely to show inappropriate sexual age preferences in phallometric assessment as compared with extrafamilial child molesters (Barbaree and Marshall 1989).

Recently, there has been an effort to examine other methods to assess deviant sexual interest. The Abel Assessment for

Sexual Interest is an instrument that measures the subject's viewing time of specially designed photographs of clothed models, assuming that the length of viewing time may correlate to the measure of sexual interest. Measuring sexual interest may not be the same as sexual arousal; thus, both the Abel Assessment for Sexual Interest and plethysmography may have their separate uses.

Treatment

Biological treatments traditionally have been reserved for individuals with pedophilia or exhibitionism, although occasionally, individuals with other paraphilias receive treatment with medications. In view of the important role androgens play in maintaining sexual arousal, treatments have focused on blocking or decreasing the level of circulating androgens. Surgical castration has been used widely in Europe with incarcerated sex offenders. However, studies have suggested that surgical castration is not an effective means of eliminating deviant sexual behavior and that almost one-third of castrated men can still engage in intercourse. Many view surgical castration not only as highly intrusive but also as cruel and unusual punishment. The results from this procedure are variable, unpredictable, and irreversible (Heim 1981).

Antiandrogenic medications have been used widely throughout the world since the late 1960s to treat sex offenders. The most extensively used and studied are the progestin derivatives medroxyprogesterone acetate (MPA) and cyproterone acetate (CPA). They act to decrease libido and thus break the individual's pattern of compulsive deviant sexual behavior. MPA and CPA thus work best in those paraphilic persons with a high sexual drive and less well in those with a low sexual drive or an antisocial personality (Cooper 1986). The use of antiandrogenic medications often is referred to as *chemical castration*. Although the legal issues raised concerning surgical castration are similar to those concerning chemical castration, the use of these medications is at least reversible and less invasive.

Another promising focus of research has been on the use of other forms of pharmacological treatment. Fluoxetine has been used successfully in the treatment of patients with voyeurism (Emmanuel et al. 1991), exhibitionism, pedophilia, and frottage (Perilstein et al. 1991) and in persons who have committed rape (Kafka 1991).

Stein et al. (1992) discussed the use of serotonergic medications (i.e., fluoxetine, clomipramine, fluvoxamine, or fenfluramine) in the treatment of sexual obsessions, addictions, and paraphilias. Stein et al. (1992) hypothesized that compulsivity and impulsivity may occur on a neurobiological spectrum on which obsessions and compulsions are at the compulsive end of the spectrum and paraphilias are at the impulsive end.

Kafka (2000) summarized the existing data on the current knowledge regarding the use of SSRIs in the treatment of both paraphilias and paraphilia-related disorders. The SSRIs can be prescribed in the typical antidepressant doses, although in our experience, higher doses, as often are necessary in the treatment of obsessions, are sometimes necessary. It is important to realize, however, that more research is needed regarding the use of SSRIs for this purpose because the knowledge is based mostly on case reports and open clinical trials. There are no current published double-blind, placebo-controlled studies of their use in the sex offender population or with men or women who have paraphilias.

Kafka and Hennen (2000) described an open trial of psychostimulants added to SSRIs when treating paraphilias in men.

They concluded that methylphenidate sustained release can be cautiously and effectively combined with SSRIs in ameliorating paraphilias in some selected cases. Coleman et al. (2000) published results of a retrospective study that concluded that nefazodone may decrease the frequency of sexual obsessions without the undesired sexual side effects sometimes seen with SSRIs.

Krueger and Kaplan (2001) described the successful treatment of paraphilias with depot leuprolide. This new class of antiandrogen medication has fewer side effects than MPA does. The authors reported that treatment resulted in a significant suppression of deviant sexual interests and behavior as measured by self-report. However, of the 12 patients receiving the therapy, 3 who were receiving long-term treatment developed bone mineralization.

A variety of behavior therapies have been used to treat paraphilias. Various aversive conditioning methods (e.g., noxious odors) and covert sensitization have been used to decrease deviant sexual behavior. (In the latter approach, the individual pairs his or her inappropriate sexual fantasies with aversive, anxiety-provoking scenes, under the guidance of a therapist.) Satiation is a technique in which the individual uses his or her deviant fantasies postorgasm in a repetitive manner to the point of satiating himself or herself with the deviant stimuli, in essence making the fantasies and behavior boring (Marshall and Barbaree 1978).

Skills training and cognitive restructuring to change the individual's maladaptive beliefs are also used in behavioral treatments. Marshall et al. (1991), in an extremely comprehensive review of the literature of treatment outcome studies for a variety of sex offenders, concluded that treatment programs that use comprehensive cognitive-behavioral interventions, as well as those that use antiandrogens in combination with psychological treatment, are the most effective. Recent outcome studies of sex offender programs have yielded generally optimistic results regarding recidivism outcome (Freeman-Longo and Knopp 1992; Marshall and Pithers 1994).

Hanson (2000) conducted a meta-analytic review of the effectiveness of psychological treatment for sex offenders. Forty-two studies were reviewed (a combined sample of 9,316 participants). Treatment was associated with a reduction in both sexual and general recidivism.

References

Abel GG, Becker JV, Cunningham-Rathner J: Complications, consent, and cognitions in sex between children and adults. Int J Law Psychiatry 7:89–103, 1984

Abel GG, Mittelman MS, Becker JV: Sexual offenders: results of assessment and recommendations for treatment, in Clinical Criminology. Edited by Ben-Aron HH, Hucker SI, Webster CD. Toronto, ON, Canada, MM Graphics, 1985, pp 191–205

Althof SE, Turner LA, Levine SB, et al: Sexual, psychological, and marital impact of self-injection of papaverine and phentolamine: a long-term prospective study. J Sex Marital Ther 17:101–112, 1991

American Psychiatric Association: Diagnostic and Statistical Manual of Mental Disorders, 4th Edition. Washington, DC, American Psychiatric Association, 1994

American Psychiatric Association: Diagnostic and Statistical Manual of Mental Disorders, 4th Edition, Text Revision. Washington, DC, American Psychiatric Association, 2000

Barbaree HE, Marshall WL: Erectile responses among heterosexual child molesters, father-daughter incest offenders, and matched non-offenders: five distinct age preference profiles. Canadian Journal of Behavioral Sciences 21:70–82, 1989

Barlow DH, Abel GG, Blanchard EB: Gender identity change in transsexuals: follow-up and replications. Arch Gen Psychiatry 36: 1001–1007, 1979

Baum N, Spieler B: Medical management of premature ejaculation. Medical Aspects of Human Sexuality 1:15–25, 2001

Becker JV, Skinner LJ, Abel GG, et al: Level of postassault sexual functioning in rape and incest victims. Arch Sex Behav 15:37–49, 1986

Berman JR, Berman LA, Lin H, et al: Effect of sildenafil on subjective and physiologic parameters of the female sexual response in women with sexual arousal disorder: J Sex Marital Ther 27:411–420, 2001

Bradford JMW, McLean D: Sexual offenders, violence, and testosterone: a clinical study. Can J Psychiatry 29:335–343, 1984

Cocores JA, Miller NS, Pottash AC, et al: Sexual dysfunction in abusers of cocaine and alcohol. Am J Drug Alcohol Abuse 14:169–173, 1988

Coleman E, Gratzer T, Nesvacil L, et al: Nefazodone and the treatment of nonparaphilic compulsive sexual behavior: a retrospective study (abstract). J Clin Psychiatry 61:282–284, 2000

Collaer ML, Hines M: Human behavioral sex differences: a role for gonadal hormones during early development? Psychol Bull 118:55–107, 1995

Colpi GM, Fanciullacci F, Aydos K, et al: Effectiveness mechanism of clomipramine by neurophysiological tests in subjects with true premature ejaculation. Andrologia 23:45–47, 1991

Cooper AJ: Progestogens in the treatment of male sex offenders: a review. Can J Psychiatry 31:73–79, 1986

Ehrhardt AA, Meyer-Bahlburg HFL: Effects of prenatal sex hormones on gender-related behavior. Science 211:1312–1318, 1981

Emmanuel NP, Lydiard RB, Ballenger JC: Fluoxetine treatment of voyeurism (letter). Am J Psychiatry 148:950, 1991

Fagan PJ, Schmidt CW Jr, Wise TN, et al: Sexual dysfunction and dual psychiatric diagnoses. Compr Psychiatry 29:278–284, 1988

Faller KC: Characteristics of a clinical sample of sexually abused children: how boy and girl victims differ. Child Abuse Negl 13: 281–291, 1989

Fein RL: Intracavernous medication for treatment of premature ejaculation. Urology 35:301–303, 1990

Feldman HA, Goldstein I, Hatzichristou DG, et al: Impotence and its medical and psychosocial correlates: results of the Massachusetts Male Ageing Study. J Urol 15: 54–61, 1994

Finger WW: Antidepressants and sexual dysfunction: managing common treatment pitfalls. Medical Aspects of Human Sexuality 1:12–18, 2001

Finkelhor D: Source Book on Child Sex Abuse. Beverly Hills, CA, Sage, 1986

Frank E, Anderson C, Rubenstein D: Frequency of sexual dysfunctions in normal couples. N Engl J Med 299:111–115, 1978

Freeman-Longo RE, Knopp FH: State-of-the-art sex offender treatment: outcome and issues. Annals of Sex Research 5:141–160, 1992

Freund K, Blanchard R: Phallometric diagnosis of pedophilia. J Consult Clin Psychol 57:100–105, 1989

Gebhard PH, Gagnon JH, Pomeroy WB, et al: Sex Offenders. New York, Harper & Row, 1965

Graziottin A: Clinical approaches to dyspareunia. J Sex Marital Ther 27:489–501, 2001

Green R: Sexual Identity Conflict in Children and Adults. New York, Basic Books, 1974

Green R: Gender identity in childhood and later sexual orientation: follow-up of 78 males. Am J Psychiatry 142:339–341, 1985

Green R: "The Sissy Boys Syndrome" and the Development of Homosexuality. New Haven, CT, Yale University Press, 1987

Green R, Fleming DT: Transsexual surgery follow-up: status in the 1990s, in Annual Review of Sex Research, Vol 1. Edited by Bancroft J, Davis CM, Weinstein D. Lake Mills, IA, Society for the Scientific Study of Sex, 1990, pp 163–174

Greil W, Horvath A, Sassim N, et al: Disinhibition of libido: an adverse effect of SSRI? J Affect Disord 62:225–228, 2001

Hanson RK: The 2000 ATSA report on the effectiveness of treatment for sex offenders. Sex Abuse Vol 12, 2000

Heim N: Sexual behavior of castrated sex offenders. Arch Sex Behav 10:11–19, 1981

Hoenig J: Etiology of transsexualism, in Gender Dysphoria: Development, Research, Management. Edited by Steiner BW. New York, Plenum, 1985, pp 33–73

Kafka MP: Successful treatment of paraphilic coercive disorder (a rapist) with fluoxetine hydrochloride. Br J Psychiatry 158: 844–847, 1991

Kafka MP: Psychopharmacologic treatments for nonparaphilic compulsive sexual behaviors. CNS Spectrums 5:49–59, 2000

Kafka MP, Hennen J: Psychostimulant augmentation during treatment with selective serotonin reuptake inhibitors in men with paraphilias and paraphilia-related disorders: a case series. J Clin Psychiatry 61:664–670, 2000

Kaplan HS: The New Sex Therapy: Active Treatment of Sexual Dysfunctions. New York, Brunner/Mazel, 1974

Krueger RB, Kaplan MS: Depot-leuprolide acetate for treatment of paraphilias: a report of twelve cases: Arch Sex Behav 30:409–422, 2001

Lal S, Kiely ME, Thavundayil JX, et al: Effect of bromocriptine in patients with apomorphine-responsive erectile impotence: an open study. J Psychiatry Neurosci 16: 262–266, 1991

LoPiccolo J, Stock WE: Treatment of sexual dysfunction. J Consult Clin Psychol 54: 158–167, 1986

Lothstein L: The postsurgical transsexual: empirical and theoretical considerations. Arch Sex Behav 9:547–564, 1980

Mahmoud KZ, el Dakhli MR, Fahmi IM, et al: Comparative value of prostaglandin E_1 and papaverine in treatment of erectile failure: double-blind crossover study among Egyptian patients. J Urol 147:623–626, 1992

Marshall WL, Barbaree HE: The reduction of deviant arousal: satiation treatment for sexual aggressors. Criminal Justice and Behavior 5:294–303, 1978

Marshall WL, Pithers W: A reconsideration of treatment outcome with sex offenders. Criminal Justice and Behavior 21:6–27, 1994

Marshall WL, Jones R, Ward T, et al: Treatment outcome with sex offenders. Clin Psychol Rev 11:465–485, 1991

Masters WH, Johnson VE: Human Sexual Inadequacy. Boston, MA, Little, Brown, 1970

Metz ME, Pryor JL: Premature ejaculation: a psychophysiological approach for assessment and management. J Sex Marital Ther 26:293–320, 2000

Meyer JK: The theory of gender identity disorders. J Am Psychoanal Assoc 30:381–418, 1982

Montejo-Gonzalez AL, Llorca G, Izquierdo JA, et al: SSRI-induced sexual dysfunction: fluoxetine, paroxetine, sertraline, and fluvoxamine in a prospective, multicenter, and descriptive clinical study of 344 patients. J Sex Marital Ther 23:176–194, 1997

Perilstein RD, Lipper S, Friedman LJ: Three cases of paraphilias responsive to fluoxetine treatment. J Clin Psychiatry 52:169–170, 1991

Person E, Ovesey L: The transsexual syndrome in males, II: secondary transsexualism. Am J Psychother 28:174–193, 1974

Salerian AJ, Vittone BJ, Geyer SP, et al: Sildenafil for psychotropic-induced sexual dysfunction in 31 women and 61 men. J Sex Marital Ther 26:133–140, 2000

Sarwer DB, Durlak JA: A field trial of the effectiveness of behavioral treatment for sexual dysfunction. J Sex Marital Ther 23: 87–102, 1997

Schiavi RC: Chronic alcoholism and male sexual dysfunction. J Sex Marital Ther 16: 23–33, 1990

Scholl GM: Prognostic variables in treating vaginismus. Obstet Gynecol 72:231–235, 1988

Segraves RT, Croft H, Kavoussi R, et al: Bupropion sustained release (SR) for the treatment of hypoactive sexual desire (HSDD) in nondepressed women. J Sex Marital Ther 27:303–316, 2001

Seidman SN, Roose SP, Menza MA, et al: Treatment of erectile dysfunction in men with depressive symptoms: results of a placebo-controlled trial with sildenafil citrate. Am J Psychiatry 158:1623–1630, 2001

Semans JH: Premature ejaculation: a new approach. South Med J 9:353–357, 1956

Simons JS, Carey M: Prevalence of sexual dysfunctions: results from a decade of research. Arch Sex Behav 30:177–219, 2001

Smith Y, Ban Goozen S, Cohen-Kettenis PT: Adolescents with gender identity disorder who were accepted or rejected for sex reassignment surgery: a prospective follow-up study. J Am Acad Child Adolesc Psychiatry 40:472–481, 2001

Sonda LP, Mazo R, Chancellor MB: The role of yohimbine for the treatment of erectile impotence. J Sex Marital Ther 16:15–21, 1990

Spector IP, Carey MP: Incidence and prevalence of the sexual dysfunctions: a critical review of the empirical literature. Arch Sex Behav 19:389–408, 1990

Stein DJ, Hollander E, Anthony DT, et al: Serotonergic medications for sexual obsessions, sexual addictions and paraphilias. J Clin Psychiatry 53:267–271, 1992

Stoller RJ: Sex and Gender, Vol 1: The Development of Masculinity and Femininity. New York, Science House, 1968

Stoller RJ: Perversion: The Erotic Form of Hatred. New York, Pantheon, 1975a

Stoller RJ: Sex and Gender, Vol 2: The Transsexual Experiment. London, England, Hogarth Press, 1975b

Stoller RJ: Fathers of transsexual children. J Am Psychoanal Assoc 27:837–866, 1979

Susset JG, Tessier CD, Wincze J, et al: Effect of yohimbine hydrochloride on erectile impotence: a double-blind study. J Urol 141:1360–1363, 1989

Zucker KJ, Bradley SJ: Gender Identity Disorder and Psychosexual Problems in Children and Adolescents. New York, Guilford, 1995

Zucker KJ, Green R: Gender identity and psychosexual disorders, in Textbook of Child and Adolescent Psychiatry, 2nd Edition. Edited by Wiener JM. Washington, DC, American Psychiatric Press, 1997, pp 657–676

CHAPTER 12

Adjustment Disorders

James J. Strain, M.D.

Jeffrey Newcorn, M.D.

Adjustment disorder—a subthreshold diagnosis—has undergone a major evolution since DSM-I (American Psychiatric Association 1952) (Table 12–1). DSM-IV-TR (American Psychiatric Association 2000) has updated the "Associated Features and Disorders" section to clarify comorbidity with other disorders. For example,

> Adjustment disorders are associated with suicide attempts, suicide, excessive substance use, and somatic complaints. Adjustment disorder has been reported in individuals with preexisting mental disorders in selected samples, such as children and adolescents and in general medical and surgical patients. The presence of an adjustment disorder may complicate the course of illness in individuals who have a general medical condition (e.g., decreased compliance with the recommended medical regimen or increased length of hospital stay). (pp. 680–681)

With regard to specific culture, age, and gender issues, it is necessary to take these attributes into account in making the clinical judgment of whether the individual's response to the stressor is maladaptive or in excess of that which nor-

mally would be expected. Women are given the diagnosis of adjustment disorder twice as often as men. However, in children and adolescents, the gender assignment of adjustment disorder is equivalent.

The section on prevalence has been altered to include rates in children, adolescents, and the elderly (2%–8% in community samples). "Adjustment Disorder has been diagnosed in up to 12% of general hospital inpatients who are referred for a mental health consultation, in 10%–30% of those in mental health outpatient settings, and in as many as 50% in special populations that have experienced a specific stressor (e.g., following cardiac surgery)" (American Psychiatric Association 2000, p. 681). Those populations with increased stressors (e.g., from poverty) are at higher risk for adjustment disorder.

In the "Course" section, information about progression to other disorders has been added. Adjustment disorder may progress to more severe mental disorders in children and adolescents more frequently than in adults. However, this increased risk may be secondary to the co-occurrence of other mental disorders or the fact that the subthreshold presenta-

This work was funded by The Malcolm Gibbs Foundation, Inc., New York, New York.

TABLE 12–1. Diagnostic categories of adjustment disorder

DSM-I (1952): Transient Situational Personality Disorder

  Gross stress reaction

  Adult situational reaction

  Adjustment reaction of infancy

  Adjustment reaction of childhood

  Adjustment reaction of adolescence

  Adjustment reaction of late life

  Other transient situational personality disturbance

DSM-II (1968): Transient Situational Disturbance

  Adjustment reaction of infancy

  Adjustment reaction of childhood

  Adjustment reaction of adolescence

  Adjustment reaction of adult life

  Adjustment reaction of late life

DSM-III (1980): Adjustment Disorder

  Adjustment disorder with depressed mood

  Adjustment disorder with anxious mood

  Adjustment disorder with mixed emotional features

  Adjustment disorder with disturbance of conduct

  Adjustment disorder with mixed disturbance of emotions and conduct

  Adjustment disorder with work (or academic) inhibition

  Adjustment disorder with withdrawal

  Adjustment disorder with atypical features

DSM-III-R (1987): Adjustment Disorder

  Adjustment disorder with depressed mood

  Adjustment disorder with anxious mood

  Adjustment disorder with mixed emotional features

  Adjustment disorder with disturbance of conduct

  Adjustment disorder with mixed disturbance of emotions and conduct

  Adjustment disorder with work (or academic) inhibition

  Adjustment disorder with withdrawal

  Adjustment disorder with physical complaints

  Adjustment disorder not otherwise specified

DSM-IV (1994) and DSM-IV-TR (2000): Adjustment Disorder

  Adjustment disorder with depressed mood

  Adjustment disorder with anxiety

  Adjustment disorder with mixed anxiety and depressed mood

  Adjustment disorder with disturbance of conduct

  Adjustment disorder with mixed disturbance of emotions and conduct

  Adjustment disorder unspecified

tion was an early phase of a more pernicious mental disorder.

As a subthreshold diagnosis, the adjustment disorder diagnosis can be used with another Axis I diagnosis if the symptoms of that diagnosis meet criteria for a major diagnosis (e.g., major depressive disorder) even if a stressor had precipitated that major depressive disorder. The not otherwise specified disorders do not require a stressor. Posttraumatic stress disorder (PTSD) and acute stress disorder require extreme stressors and the presence of a specifically defined array of symptoms. If the symptoms extant are secondary to the direct physiological effects of a general medical condition and/or its treatment, adjustment disorder should not be diagnosed.

Adjustment disorder occupies an important place in the psychiatric lexicon spectrum: 1) normal behavior, 2) problem-level diagnoses (V codes), 3) adjustment disorders, 4) categories of disorders classified as not otherwise specified, and 5) major mental disorders.

Adjustment disorder is a stress-related phenomenon in which the stressor has precipitated maladaptation and symptoms (within 3 months of the occurrence of the stressor) that are time limited until the stressor is removed or a new state of adaptation takes place (Table 12–2). As the diagnosis of adjustment disorder has evolved, other stress-related disorders (e.g., PTSD) have become recognized. An acute stress disorder was designated in DSM-IV (American Psychiatric Association 1994)—encompassing, for example, those stress reactions that follow a disaster or cataclysmic personal event (Spiegel 1994).

The diagnosis of adjustment disorder also requires a careful assessment of the timing of the stressor to the adverse psychological sequelae, and until DSM-IV, a time limit was imposed on how long

TABLE 12–2. DSM-IV-TR diagnostic criteria for adjustment disorders

A. The development of emotional or behavioral symptoms in response to an identifiable stressor(s) occurring within 3 months of the onset of the stressor(s).

B. These symptoms or behaviors are clinically significant as evidenced by either of the following:
   (1) marked distress that is in excess of what would be expected from exposure to the stressor
   (2) significant impairment in social or occupational (academic) functioning

C. The stress-related disturbance does not meet the criteria for another specific Axis I disorder and is not merely an exacerbation of a preexisting Axis I or Axis II disorder.

D. The symptoms do not represent bereavement.

E. Once the stressor (or its consequences) has terminated, the symptoms do not persist for more than an additional 6 months.

Specify if:
   Acute: if the disturbance lasts less than 6 months
   Chronic: if the disturbance lasts for 6 months or longer

Adjustment disorders are coded based on the subtype, which is selected according to the predominant symptoms. The specific stressor(s) can be specified on Axis IV.

   309.0 With Depressed Mood
   309.24 With Anxiety
   309.28 With Mixed Anxiety and Depressed Mood
   309.3 With Disturbance of Conduct
   309.4 With Mixed Disturbance of Emotions and Conduct
   309.9 Unspecified

this diagnosis could be used. Adjustment disorder was a transitory diagnosis that could not exceed 6 months, after which if the patient remained symptomatic, it was necessary to invoke another diagnosis.

Definition and History

Wise (1988) summarized the historical evolution of the adjustment disorders since 1945. The diagnostic concept included the notion of a transient situational disturbance, initially codified by developmental epochs (Table 12–1). It evolved to embody a disorder of adjustment characterized by mood, behavior, or work (or academic) inhibition (DSM-III [American Psychiatric Association 1980]). Finally, it was defined to include physical complaints as well as other mood and behavioral disturbances (DSM-III-R [American Psychiatric Association 1987]).

As a result of the review of the literature and the Western Psychiatric Institute and Clinic data reanalysis supported by a MacArthur grant, the American Psychiatric Association (APA) Task Force on Psychological System Interface Disorders recommended that specific changes be included in DSM-IV and now DSM-IV-TR:

1. Enhance the clarity of the language.
2. Describe the time of the reaction to reflect duration: acute (less than 6 months) or chronic (6 months or longer).
3. Allow for the continuation of the stressor for an indefinite period.
4. Eliminate the subtypes of mixed emotional features, work (or academic) inhibition, withdrawal, and physical complaints.

Although it might be argued that the adjustment disorders could be placed in an innovative category of "stress response syndromes" or, for that matter, in several diverse locations within the DSM classification (Strain et al. 1993), the literature does not offer data to support such an alternative placement. In addition, research findings show that adjustment disorder is a valid diagnosis (Kovacs et al. 1994, 1995).

Kovacs et al. (1994) examined pro-

spectively the course of adjustment disorder among 30 subjects aged 8–13 years to determine whether long-term negative outcomes of those with adjustment disorder are referable to the disorder itself or to comorbid conditions and compared them with control subjects without adjustment disorder. Those with adjustment disorder recovered rapidly and had similar rates of new psychiatric disorders as those without adjustment disorder.

The criterion and predictive validity of the diagnosis of adjustment disorder in 92 children who had new-onset type 1 diabetes mellitus were examined. DSM-III criteria plus four clinically significant signs or symptoms were used, and the time frame was extended to 6 months after the diagnosis of diabetes. Thirty-three percent of the cohort developed adjustment disorder (mean = 29 days after the medical diagnosis), and the average episode length was 3 months, with a recovery rate of 100%. The 5-year cumulative probability of a new psychiatric disorder was 0.48 in comparison to 0.16 for the non–adjustment disorder subjects. The findings support the criterion validity of the adjustment disorder diagnosis.

Construct validity also was observed in a retrospective data study comparing outpatients with single-episode major depression, recurrent major depression, dysthymia, depression not otherwise specified, and adjustment disorder with depressed mood with or without mixed anxiety (Jones et al. 1999). The Medical Outcomes Study 36-item Short Form Health Status Survey (SF-36) was completed before and 6 months after treatment. The diagnostic categories were significantly different at baseline but did not differ with regard to outcome at follow-up. Females were significantly more likely to be given the diagnosis of major depression or dysthymia than adjustment disorder. Females also were more likely than males to score lower on the Mental Component Summary scales of the

SF-36 at admission. Patients with adjustment disorder scored higher on all SF-36 scales, as did the other diagnostic groups at baseline and again at follow-up. No significant difference was seen among diagnostic groups with regard to treatment outcome. The authors concluded that the results support the construct validity of the adjustment disorder diagnostic category (Jones et al. 1999).

In reviewing the diagnosis of adjustment disorder for DSM-IV, two issues emerged as fundamental. First, the effect of the imprecision of this diagnosis on reliability and validity because of the lack of behavioral or operational criteria must be determined. One study (Aoki et al. 1995), however, found three psychological tests—Zung's Self-Rating Anxiety Scale (Zung 1971), Zung's Self-Rating Depression Scale (Zung 1965), and Profile of Mood States (McNair et al. 1971)—to be useful tools for adjustment disorder diagnosis among physical rehabilitation patients. Although Aoki et al. (1995) succeeded in reliably differentiating patients with adjustment disorder from healthy patients, they did not distinguish them from patients with major depression or PTSD.

Second, the classification of syndromes that do not fulfill the criteria for a major mental illness but indicate serious (or incipient) symptomatology that requires intervention and/or treatment, by default, may be viewed as "subthreshold" and afforded a subthreshold interest by health care workers and third-party payers. Thus, the construct of adjustment disorder is designed as a means for classifying psychiatric conditions having a symptom profile that is as yet insufficient to meet the more specifically operationalized criteria for the major syndromes but that is 1) clinically significant and deemed to be in excess of a normal reaction to the stressor in question (taking culture into account), 2) associated with impaired vocational or interpersonal functioning, and 3) not solely the result of a psychosocial problem (V code) requiring medical attention (e.g., noncompliance, phase of life problem).

In contrast to other DSM-IV-TR disorders, adjustment disorder includes no specific profile (or checklist) of symptoms that collectively constitutes a psychiatric (medical) syndrome or disorder. The V codes, a problem level of diagnoses, understandably are devoid of a symptom-based diagnostic schema. The imprecision of the diagnostic criteria for adjustment disorder is immediately apparent in DSM-IV-TR's description of this disorder as a maladaptive reaction to an identifiable psychosocial or physical stressor, or stressors, that occurs within 3 months after onset of the stressor. It is assumed that the disturbance will remit soon after the stressor ceases or, if the stressor persists, when a new level of adaptation is achieved (American Psychiatric Association 2000). Difficulties are inherent within each of these diagnostic conceptual elements.

The patient's functional status evaluation (Axis V) is not linked via an algorithm to the adjustment disorder construct in DSM-IV-TR. Fabrega et al. (1987) contend that both subjective symptoms and decrement in social function can be considered maladaptive and that the severity of either of these is subject to great individual variation. Using data from Axis V and their "Axis VI"—an additional and more specific functional status axis on their Initial Evaluation Form (Mezzich et al. 1981)[1]—these

---

[1]The functional status measure, involving seven levels of impairment, is used to assess "current functioning" of patients in three dimensions: "at work or at school, with family, and with other persons or groups" (Fabrega et al. 1987, p. 569).

authors could not conclude that the level of psychopathology correlates with impaired functioning.

Second, no criteria or "guidelines" are offered in DSM-IV-TR to quantify stressors for adjustment disorder or to assess their effect or meaning for a particular individual at a given time. The measurement of the severity of the stressor and its temporal and causal relationship to demonstrable symptoms are often uncertain and at times impossible to discern.

The time course and chronicity of both stressors and symptoms need further exploration. The modifications introduced in DSM-IV, which differentiate between acute and chronic forms of adjustment disorder, solved the problem of a 6-month limitation in DSM-III-R's criteria. This change was validated by Despland et al. (1995), who observed that 16% of the patients with adjustment disorder required treatment for longer than 1 year, with the mean length exceeding the prior limitation of 6 months.

Serious symptomatology (e.g., suicidal behavior) that is not regarded as part of a major mental disorder needs treatment and a "diagnosis" under which it can be placed. De Leo et al. (1986a, 1986b) reported on adjustment disorder and suicidality. Recent life events, which would constitute an acute stress, were commonly found to correlate with suicidal behavior in a group that included those with adjustment disorder (Isometsa et al. 1996). Spalletta et al. (1996) observed that assessment of suicidal behavior is an important tool in differentiating major depression, dysthymia, and adjustment disorder. Furthermore, patients with adjustment disorder were observed to be among the most common recipients of a deliberate self-harm diagnosis, with the majority involving self-poisoning (Vlachos et al. 1994). Thus, deliberate self-harm is more common in these patients (Vlachos et al.

1994), whereas the percentage of suicidal behavior was found to be higher in depressed patients (Spalletta et al. 1996). Clearly, what is regarded as a subthreshold diagnosis—adjustment disorder—does not necessarily imply the presence of subthreshold symptomatology.

DSM-III-R had been described as "medical illness and age unfair" (i.e., it did not sufficiently take into account the issues of age and/or medical illness) (L. George, personal communication, June 1981; Strain 1981). DSM-IV was developed to overcome some of these deficiencies. Eventually, to enhance reliability and validity, there needs to be a psychiatric taxonomy that considers developmental epochs (e.g., children and youth, adults, young elderly, and old elderly) and medical illness with its symptomatology. For example, with regard to the latter issue, Endicott (1984) has described replacing vegetative with ideational symptoms when evaluating depressed patients with medical illness. Rapp and Vrana (1989) confirmed Endicott's proposed changes in the diagnostic criteria for depression in medically ill elderly persons and observed a maintenance of specificity and sensitivity, respectively, when substituting ideational for vegetative symptoms. Recent studies found patients with adjustment disorder to be significantly younger compared with patients who have a major psychiatric diagnosis (Despland et al. 1995; Mok and Walter 1995). Zarb's (1996) study suggested that cognitively impaired elderly, when evaluated with individual items of the Geriatric Depression Scale (Yesavage et al. 1982–1983), had adjustment disorder rather than major depression. In addition, Despland et al. (1995) reported that the patients with adjustment disorder (with depressive or mixed symptoms) included more women than men, thus resulting in a sex ratio resembling that for major depression or dysthymia.

Epidemiology

Andreasen and Wasek (1980) reported that 5% of an inpatient and outpatient sample were labeled as having adjustment disorder. Fabrega et al. (1987) observed that 2.3% of a sample of patients at a walk-in clinic (diagnostic and evaluation center) met criteria for adjustment disorder, with no other diagnoses on Axis I or Axis II; 20% had the diagnosis of adjustment disorder when patients with other Axis I diagnoses (i.e., Axis I comorbidities) also were included. In general hospital psychiatric consultation populations, adjustment disorder was diagnosed in 21.5% (Popkin et al. 1990), 18.5% (Foster and Oxman 1994), and 11.5% (Snyder and Strain 1989).

Strain et al. (1998b) examined the consultation-liaison data from seven university teaching hospitals in the United States, Canada, and Australia. The sites had all used a common clinical database to examine 1,039 consecutive referrals. Adjustment disorder was diagnosed in 125 patients (12.0%); it was the sole diagnosis in 81 (7.8%) and comorbid with other Axis I and II diagnoses in 44 (4.2%). It had been considered as a "rule-out" diagnosis in an additional 110 (10.6%). Adjustment disorder with depressed mood, anxious mood, or mixed emotions were the most common subcategories. Adjustment disorder was diagnosed comorbidly most frequently with personality disorder and organic mental disorder. Patients with adjustment disorder were referred significantly more often for problems of anxiety, coping, and depression; had less past psychiatric illness; and were rated as functioning better than those patients with major mental disorders—all consistent with the construct of adjustment disorder as a maladaptation to a psychosocial stressor. Interventions were similar to those for other Axis I and II diagnoses, including the prescription of antidepressant medications. Patients with adjustment disorder required a similar amount of clinical time and resident supervision when compared with patients with other Axis I and II disorders.

Oxman et al. (1994) observed that 50.7% of elderly patients (age 55 years or older) receiving elective surgery for coronary artery disease developed adjustment disorder related to the stress of surgery. Thirty percent had symptomatic and functional impairment 6 months after surgery. Kellermann et al. (1999) reported that 27% of elderly patients examined 5–9 days after a cerebrovascular accident fulfilled the criteria for adjustment disorder. Spiegel (1996) observed that half of all cancer patients have a psychiatric disorder, usually an adjustment disorder with depression. Because patients treated for their mental states had longer survival times (although this finding is currently being questioned based on random controlled trials now under way and those already reported), treatment of depression in cancer patients should be considered integral to their medical treatment. Adjustment disorder is frequently diagnosed in patients with head and neck surgery (16.8%) (Kugaya et al. 2000), patients with HIV (dementia and adjustment disorder, 73%) (Pozzi et al. 1999), cancer patients from a multicenter survey of consultation-liaison psychiatry in oncology (27%) (Grassi et al. 2000), dermatology patients (29% of the 9% who had psychiatric diagnoses) (Pulimood et al. 1996), and suicide attempters (22%) examined in an emergency department (Schnyder and Valach 1997). Other studies include the diagnosis of adjustment disorder in more than 60% of burned inpatients (Perez-Jimenez et al. 1994), 20% of patients in early stages of multiple sclerosis (Sullivan et al. 1995), and 40% of poststroke patients (Shima et al. 1994).

Andreasen and Wasek (1980), using a chart review, stated that more adolescents than adults with adjustment disorder experienced acting out and behavioral symptoms, but adults had significantly more depressive symptomatology (87.2% vs. 63.8%). Anxiety symptoms were frequent at all ages.

Fabrega et al. (1987) and Mezzich et al. (1981) evaluated 64 symptoms present in three cohorts: subjects with specific diagnoses, those with adjustment disorder, and those who were not ill. Vegetative, substance use, and characterological symptoms were greatest in the specific-diagnosis group, intermediate in the adjustment disorder group, and least in the group with no illness. The symptoms of mood and affect, general appearance, behavior, disturbance in speech and thought pattern, and cognitive functioning had a similar distribution. The adjustment disorder group was significantly different from the no-illness group with regard to more "depressed mood" and "low self-esteem" ($P < 0.0001$). The adjustment disorder and no-illness groups both had minimal pathology of thought content and perception. Twenty-nine percent of the adjustment disorder group, compared with 9% of the no-illness group, had a positive response on the suicide indicators. The three cohorts did not differ on the frequency of Axis III disorders.

An example of associated features in adjustment disorder was provided by Andreasen and Wasek (1980), who observed that in their adjustment disorder cohorts, 21.6% of the adolescents' and 11.8% of the adults' fathers had problems with alcohol. Greenberg et al. (1995) observed more substance abuse in adults with diagnosed adjustment disorder compared with those with other diagnoses. Breslow et al. (1996) examined patients with adjustment disorder and patients with

other psychiatric diagnoses and found that alcohol or substance use/abuse did not help to differentiate between diagnostic groups.

Runeson et al. (1996) observed from psychological autopsy methods that the median interval between first suicidal communication and suicide was very short in the patients with adjustment disorder (<1 month) compared with patients who have major depression (3 months), borderline personality disorder (30 months), or schizophrenia (47 months).

Etiology

Stress has been described as the etiological agent for adjustment disorder. However, diverse variables and modifiers are involved regarding who will experience an adjustment disorder following stress. Cohen (1981) argued that 1) acute stresses are different from chronic ones in both psychological and physiological terms, 2) the meaning of the stress is affected by "modifiers" (e.g., ego strengths, support systems, prior mastery), and 3) the manifest and latent meanings of the stressor(s) must be differentiated (e.g., loss of job may be a relief or a catastrophe).

Axis IV of DSM-III was included to allow the clinician to assess for the presence of stress in the multiaxial diagnoses of psychiatric disorders, but it has been confounded by low reliability (Rey et al. 1988; Spitzer and Forman 1979; Zimmerman et al. 1987). Almost 100% presence of stressors on Axis IV was reported by Despland et al. (1995) for adjustment disorder with depressed mood, whereas 83% was reported for major depression, 80% for dysthymia, and only 67% for nonspecific depression, supporting the importance of stressors in the adjustment disorder diagnosis.

From the examination of several studies, it has been difficult to establish a significant temporal link between the onset of an identified stressor and the occurrence of depressive illness (Akiskal et al. 1978; Andreasen and Winokur 1979; Benjaminsen 1981; Garvey et al. 1984; Hirschfeld 1981; Paykel and Tanner 1976; Winokur 1985).

Andreasen and Wasek (1980) described the differences between the types of stressors found in adolescents and those found in adults: 59% and 35%, respectively, of the precipitants had been present for a year or more and 9% and 39% for 3 months or less. Fabrega et al. (1987) reported that their adjustment disorder group had greater registration of stressors compared with the specific-diagnosis and the non-illness cohorts. There was a significant difference in the amount of stressors reported relevant to the clinical request for evaluation: the group with adjustment disorder, compared with the specific-diagnosis and the nonillness patients, was overrepresented in the "higher stress category." Popkin et al. (1990) reported that in 68.6% of the cases in their consultation cohort, the medical illness itself was judged to be the primary psychosocial stressor. Snyder and Strain (1989) observed that stressors as assessed on Axis IV were significantly higher ($P = 0.0001$) for consultation patients with adjustment disorder than for patients with other diagnostic disorders. Illescas-Rico et al. (2002) report the increased incidence of anxiety and depression during bone marrow transplant.

Clinical Features

In DSM-IV-TR, adjustment disorder was reduced to six types that again are classified according to their clinical features: with depressed mood, with anxiety, with mixed anxiety and depressed mood, with disturbance of conduct, with mixed disturbance of emotions and conduct, and unspecified (Table 12–3).

Treatment

Treatment of adjustment disorder rests primarily on psychotherapeutic measures that enable reduction of the stressor, enhanced coping with the stressor that cannot be reduced or removed, and establishment of a support system to maximize adaptation (Angelino and Treisman 2001). The first goal is to note significant dysfunction secondary to a stressor and help the patient to moderate this imbalance. Many stressors may be avoided or minimized. Other stressors may elicit an overreaction on the part of the patient (e.g., abandonment by a lover). The patient may attempt suicide or become reclusive, damaging his or her source of income. In this situation, the therapist attempts to help the patient put his or her rage and other feelings into words rather than into destructive actions. The role of verbalization cannot be overestimated in an attempt to reduce the pressure of the stressor and enhance coping.

Counseling, psychotherapy, crisis intervention, family therapy, and group treatment may be used to encourage the verbalization of fears, anxiety, rage, helplessness, and hopelessness related to the stressors imposed on a patient. The goals of treatment in each case are to expose the concerns and conflicts that the patient is experiencing, identify means to reduce the stressors, enhance the patient's coping skills, and help the patient gain perspective on the adversity and establish relationships (i.e., a support network) to assist in the management of the stressors and the self. Cognitive-behavioral therapy was successfully used in young military recruits (Nardi et al. 1994).

Although the primary treatment for

TABLE 12–3. Types of DSM-IV-TR adjustment disorder

Adjustment disorder with depressed mood	The predominant symptoms are those of a minor depression. For example, the symptoms might be depressed mood, tearfulness, and hopelessness.
Adjustment disorder with anxiety	This type of adjustment disorder is diagnosed when anxiety symptoms are predominant, such as nervousness, worry, and jitteriness. The differential diagnosis would include anxiety disorders.
Adjustment disorder with mixed anxiety and depressed mood	This category should be used when the predominant symptoms are a combination of depression and anxiety or other emotions. An example would be an adolescent who, after moving away from home and parental supervision, reacts with ambivalence, depression, anger, and signs of increased dependence.
Adjustment disorder with disturbance of conduct	The symptomatic manifestations are those of behavioral misconduct that violated societal norms or the rights of others. Examples are fighting, truancy, vandalism, and reckless driving.
Adjustment disorder with mixed disturbance of emotions and conduct	This diagnosis is made when the disturbance combines affective and behavioral features of adjustment disorder with mixed emotional features and adjustment disorder with disturbance of conduct.
Adjustment disorder unspecified	This is a residual diagnosis within the diagnostic category. This diagnosis can be used when a maladaptive reaction that is not classified under other adjustment disorders occurs in response to stress. An example would be a patient who, when given a diagnosis of cancer, denies the diagnosis of malignancy and is noncompliant with treatment recommendations.

adjustment disorder is talking, small doses of antidepressants and anxiolytics may be appropriate. Minimal data are available on pharmacological treatment of adjustment disorder, and randomized controlled pharmacological trials are rare. Formal psychotherapy appears to be the current treatment of choice (Uhlenhuth et al. 1995), although psychotherapy combined with benzodiazepines also is used, especially for patients with severe life stress(es) and a significant anxious component (Shaner 2000; Uhlenhuth et al. 1995). Tricyclic antidepressants or buspirone was recommended in place of benzodiazepines for patients with current or past heavy alcohol use because of the greater risk of dependence in these patients (Uhlenhuth et al. 1995). Tianeptine, alprazolam, and mianserin were found to be equally effective in symptom improvement in patients with adjustment disorder with anxiety (Ans-

seau et al. 1996). In a randomized double-blind study, trazodone was more effective than clorazepate in cancer patients for the relief of anxious and depressed symptoms (Razavi et al. 1999). Similar findings were observed in HIV-positive patients with adjustment disorder (DeWit et al. 1999).

It is important to note that there are no randomized controlled trials employing SSRIs, mixed SSRI atypicals (nefazodone and venlafaxine), buspirone, or mirtazapine. These newer antidepressant medications have fewer side effects and may offer symptom relief of dysphoric moods with minimal adverse reactions and interactions. The difficulty in obtaining an adjustment disorder study cohort with reliable and valid diagnoses may impede the conduct of a controlled clinical trial comparing these newer antidepressant agents against placebo and psychotherapy.

A significant aspect of treatment is for the clinician to keep alert to the fact that the diagnosis of adjustment disorder may indicate a patient who is in the early phase of a major mental disorder that has not yet evolved to full-blown symptoms. Therefore, if a patient continues to worsen, becomes more symptomatic, and does not respond to treatment, it is critical to review the patient's symptoms and the diagnosis for the presence of a major mental disorder.

Course and Prognosis

With regard to the long-term outcome of adjustment disorder, Andreasen and Hoenk (1982) suggested that the prognosis is good for adults but that in adolescents, many major psychiatric illnesses eventually occur. At 5-year follow-up, 71% of the adults were completely well, 8% had an intervening problem, and 21% developed a major depressive disorder or alcoholism. In adolescents at 5-year follow-up, only 44% were without a psychiatric diagnosis; 13% had an intervening psychiatric illness, and 43% went on to develop major psychiatric morbidity (e.g., schizophrenia, schizoaffective disorder, major depression, bipolar disorder, substance abuse, personality disorders). In contrast to the predictors for major pathology in adults, the chronicity of the illness and the presence of behavioral symptoms in the adolescents were the strongest predictors for major pathology at the 5-year follow-up.

As was reported by Chess and Thomas (1984), it is important to note that adjustment disorder with disturbance of conduct, regardless of age, has a more guarded outcome.

Despland et al. (1997) observed 52 patients with adjustment disorder at the end of treatment or after 3 years of treatment. Results showed the occurrence of psychiatric comorbidity (31%), suicide attempts (14%), development of a more serious psychiatric disorder (29%), and an unfavorable clinical state (23%). Jones et al. (2002) described decreased readmission rates for adjustment disorders with depressed moods in comparison with other mood disorders. Finally, Krzyhanovskaya and Canterbury (2001) discussed suicidal behavior in patients with adjustment disorders.

Conclusions

The issues of diagnostic rigor and clinical utility seem at odds for the adjustment disorders. Clinicians need a diagnosis in which they can place subthreshold symptomatology, and field studies need to use reliable and valid instruments (e.g., depression or anxiety rating scales, stress assessments, length of disability, treatment outcome, family patterns). Identification of the time course, remission or evolution to another diagnosis, and evaluation of stressors (characteristics, duration, and nature of adaptation to stress) would enhance the understanding of the concept of a stress-response illness.

Studies with adequate symptom checklists rated independently from the establishment of the diagnosis would be helpful in clarifying the threshold between major and minor depression and anxiety, as well as help guide an entry level threshold for adjustment disorder. Although the upper threshold of adjustment disorder is established by the criteria for the major syndromes, the lower threshold between adjustment disorder and problems of living/normality is bereft of operational criteria that would define an entry "boundary."

Regardless of their position on the diagnostic tree, subthreshold syndromes can encompass significant psychopathology that must be not only recognized but also treated (e.g., suicidal ideation or behavior). Cross-sectionally, adjustment disorder may appear to be the incipient phase of an emerging major syndrome. Consequently, adjustment disorder, despite its problems with reliability and validity, serves an important diagnostic function in the practice of psychiatry. Problem- and subthreshold-level diagnoses are critical to the function of any medical discipline. Because this disorder may be the initial phase, or a mild form, of a dysfunction that is not yet fully developed, the relation between the incipient and the developed and between the subthreshold and the defined must be described.

Combined with the remaining problem of the certainty of the diagnosis, the question prevails: Should drugs be used in the treatment of adjustment disorders? It is better to be cautious and delay psychotropic drug administration rather than subject the patient to the risk of unfavorable other drug–psychotropic drug interaction(s). The condition may resolve, or it may evolve into a major psychiatric illness that needs to be treated accordingly, which could include pharmacological agents.

References

Akiskal HS, Bitar AH, Puzantian VR, et al: The nosological status of neurotic depression: a prospective three- to four-year follow-up examination in light of the primary-secondary and unipolar-bipolar dichotomies. Arch Gen Psychiatry 35:756–766, 1978

American Psychiatric Association: Diagnostic and Statistical Manual: Mental Disorders. Washington, DC, American Psychiatric Association, 1952

American Psychiatric Association: Diagnostic and Statistical Manual of Mental Disorders, 3rd Edition. Washington, DC, American Psychiatric Association, 1980

American Psychiatric Association: Diagnostic and Statistical Manual of Mental Disorders, 3rd Edition, Revised. Washington, DC, American Psychiatric Association, 1987

American Psychiatric Association: Diagnostic and Statistical Manual of Mental Disorders, 4th Edition. Washington, DC, American Psychiatric Association, 1994

American Psychiatric Association: Diagnostic and Statistical Manual of Mental Disorders, 4th Edition, Text Revision. Washington, DC, American Psychiatric Association, 2000

Andreasen NC, Hoenk PR: The predictive value of adjustment disorders: a follow-up study. Am J Psychiatry 139:584–590, 1982

Andreasen NC, Wasek P: Adjustment disorders in adolescents and adults. Arch Gen Psychiatry 37:1166–1170, 1980

Andreasen NC, Winokur G: Secondary depression: familial, clinical, and research perspectives. Am J Psychiatry 136:62–66, 1979

Angelino AF, Treisman GJ: Major depression and demoralization in cancer patients: diagnostic and treatment considerations. Support Care Cancer 9:344–349, 2001

Ansseau M, Bataille M, Briole G, et al: Controlled comparison of tianeptine, alprazolam and mianserin in the treatment of adjustment disorders with anxiety and depression. Human Psychopharmacology Clinical and Experimental 11:293–298, 1996

Aoki T, Hosaka T, Ishida A: Psychiatric evaluation of physical rehabilitation patients. Gen Hosp Psychiatry 17:440–443, 1995

Benjaminsen S: Stressful life events preceding the onset of neurotic depression. Psychol Med 11:369–378, 1981

Breslow RE, Klinger BI, Erickson BJ: Acute intoxication and substance abuse among patients presenting to a psychiatric emergency service. Gen Hosp Psychiatry 18:183–191, 1996

Chess S, Thomas A: Origins and Evolution of Behavior Disorders: From Infancy to Early Adult Life. New York, Brunner/Mazel, 1984

Cohen F: Stress and bodily illness. Psychiatr Clin North Am 4:269–286, 1981

De Leo D, Pellegrini C, Serraiotto L: Adjustment disorders and suicidality. Psychol Rep 59:355–358, 1986a

De Leo D, Pellegrini C, Serraiotto L, et al: Assessment of severity of suicide attempts: a trial with the dexamethasone suppression test and two rating scales. Psychopathology 19:186–191, 1986b

Despland JN, Monod L, Ferrero F: Clinical relevance of adjustment disorder in DSM-III-R and DSM-IV. Compr Psychiatry 36:456–460, 1995

Despland JN, Monod L, Ferrero F: Etude clinique du trouble de l'adaptation selon le DSM-III-R. Schweizer Archiv fuer Neurologie und Psychiatrie 148:19–24, 1997

DeWit S, Cremers L, Hirsch D, et al: Efficacy and safety of trazodone versus clorazepate in the treatment of HIV-positive subjects with adjustment disorders: a pilot study. J Int Med Res 27:223–232, 1999

Endicott J: Measurement of depression in patients with cancer. Cancer 53:2243–2249, 1984

Fabrega H Jr, Mezzich JE, Mezzich AC: Adjustment disorder as a marginal or transitional illness category in DSM-III. Arch Gen Psychiatry 44:567–572, 1987

Foster P, Oxman T: A descriptive study of adjustment disorder diagnoses in general hospital patients. Irish Journal of Psychological Medicine 11:153–157, 1994

Garvey MJ, Tollefson GD, Mungas D, et al: Is the distinction between situational and nonsituational primary depression valid? Compr Psychiatry 25:372–375, 1984

Grassi L, Gritti P, Rigatelli M, et al: Psychosocial problems secondary to cancer: an Italian multicenter survey of consultation-liaison psychiatry in oncology. Italian Consultation-Liaison Group. Eur J Cancer 36:579–585, 2000

Greenberg WM, Rosenfeld DN, Ortega EA: Adjustment disorder as an admission diagnosis. Am J Psychiatry 152:459–461, 1995

Hirschfeld RMA: Situational depression: validity of the concept. Br J Psychiatry 139:297–305, 1981

Illescas-Rico R, Amaya-Ayala F, Jiminez-Lopez JL, et al: Increased incidence of anxiety and depression during bone marrow transplantation. Arch Med Res 33:144–147, 2002

Isometsa E, Heikkinen M, Henriksson M, et al: Suicide in non-major depressions. J Affect Disord 36:117–127, 1996

Jones R, Yates WR, Williams S, et al: Outcome for adjustment disorder with depressed mood: comparison with other mood disorders. J Affect Disord 55:55–61, 1999

Jones R, Yates WR, Zhou HH: Readmission rates for adjustment disorders: comparison with other mood disorders. J Affect Disord 71:199–203, 2002

Kellermann M, Fekete I, Gesztelyi R, et al: Screening for depressive symptoms in the acute phase of stroke. Gen Hosp Psychiatry 21:116–121, 1999

Kovacs M, Gatsonis C, Pollock M, et al: A controlled prospective study of DSM-III adjustment disorder in childhood: short term prognosis and long-term predictive validity. Arch Gen Psychiatry 51:535–541, 1994

Kovacs M, Ho V, Pollock MH: Criterion and predictive validity of the diagnosis of adjustment disorder: a prospective study of youths with new-onset insulin-dependent diabetes mellitus. Am J Psychiatry 152:523–528, 1995

Krzyhanovskaya L, Canterbury R: Suicidal behavior in patients with adjustment disorder. Journal of Crisis Intervention and Suicide 22:125–131, 2001

Kugaya A, Akechi T, Okuyama T, et al: Prevalence, predictive factors, and screening for psychological distress in patients with newly diagnosed head and neck cancers. Cancer 88:2817–2823, 2000

McNair DM, Lorr M, Doppelman LF (eds): Manual for the Profile of Mood States. San Diego, CA, Educational & Industrial Testing Service, 1971

Mezzich JE, Dow JT, Rich CL, et al: Developing an efficient clinical information system for a comprehensive psychiatric institute, II: initial evaluation form. Behavioral Research Methods and Instrumentation 13:464–478, 1981

Mok H, Walter C: Brief psychiatric hospitalization: preliminary experience with an urban short-stay unit. Can J Psychiatry 40: 415–417, 1995

Nardi C, Lichtenberg P, Kaplan Z: Adjustment disorder of conscripts as a military phobia. Mil Med 159:612–616, 1994

Oxman TE, Barrett JE, Freeman DH, et al: Frequency and correlates of adjustment disorder relates to cardiac surgery in older patients. Psychosomatics 35:557–568, 1994

Paykel ES, Tanner J: Life events, depressive relapse and maintenance treatment. Psychol Med 6:481–485, 1976

Perez-Jimenez JP, Gomez-Bajo GJ, Lopez-Catillo JJ, et al: Psychiatric consultation and post-traumatic stress disorder in burned patients. Burns 20:532–536, 1994

Popkin MK, Callies AL, Colón EA, et al: Adjustment disorders in medically ill patients referred for consultation in a university hospital. Psychosomatics 31:410–414, 1990

Pozzi G, Del Borgo C, Del Forna A, et al: Psychological discomfort and mental illness in patients with AIDS: implications for home care. AIDS Patient Care STDS 13: 555–564, 1999

Pulimood S, Rajagopalan B, Rajagopalan M, et al: Psychiatric morbidity among dermatology inpatients. Natl Med J India 9:208–210, 1996

Rapp SR, Vrana S: Substituting nonsomatic for somatic symptoms in the diagnosis of depression in elderly male medical patients. Am J Psychiatry 146:1197–1200, 1989

Razavi D, Kormoss N, Collard A, et al: Comparative study of the efficacy and safety of trazodone versus clorazepate in the treatment of adjustment disorders in cancer patients: a pilot study. J Int Med Res 27: 264–272, 1999

Rey JM, Stewart GW, Plapp JM, et al: DSM-III Axis IV revisited. Am J Psychiatry 145: 286–292, 1988

Runeson BS, Beskow J, Waern M: The suicidal process in suicides among young people. Acta Psychiatr Scand 93:35–42, 1996

Schnyder U, Valach L: Suicide attempters in a psychiatric emergency room population. Gen Hosp Psychiatry 19:119–129, 1997

Shaner R: Benzodiazepines in psychiatric emergency settings. Psychiatr Ann 30:268–275, 2000

Shima S, Kitagawa Y, Kitamura T, et al: Post-stroke depression. Gen Hosp Psychiatry 16:286–289, 1994

Snyder S, Strain JJ: Differentiation of major depression and adjustment disorder with depressed mood in the medical setting. Gen Hosp Psychiatry 12:159–165, 1989

Spalletta G, Troisi A, Saracco M, et al: Symptom profile: Axis II comorbidity and suicidal behaviour in young males with DSM-III-R depressive illnesses. J Affect Disord 39:141–148, 1996

Spiegel D: DSM-IV Options Book. Washington, DC, American Psychiatric Association, 1994

Spiegel D: Cancer and depression. Br J Psychiatry 168 (suppl 30):109–116, 1996

Spitzer RL, Forman JBW: DSM-III field trials, II: initial experience with the multiaxial system. Am J Psychiatry 136:818–820, 1979

Strain JJ: Diagnostic considerations in the medical setting. Psychiatr Clin North Am 4:287–300, 1981

Strain JJ, Newcorn J, Wolf D, et al: Considering changes in adjustment disorder. Hosp Community Psychiatry 44:13–15, 1993

Strain JJ, Smith GC, Hammer JS, et al: Adjustment disorder: a multisite study of its utilization and interventions in the consultation-liaison psychiatry setting. Gen Hosp Psychiatry 20:139–149, 1998b

Sullivan MJ, Winshenker B, Mikail S: Screening for major depression in the early stages of multiple sclerosis. Can J Neurol Sci 22: 228–231, 1995

Uhlenhuth EH, Balter MB, Ban TA, et al: International study of expert judgment on therapeutic use of benzodiazepines and other psychotherapeutic medications, III: clinical features affecting experts' therapeutic recommendations in anxiety disorders. Psychopharmacol Bull 31:289–296, 1995

Vlachos IO, Bouras N, Watson JP, et al: Deliberate self-harm referrals. European Journal of Psychiatry 8:25–28, 1994

Winokur G: The validity of neurotic-reactive depression: new data and reappraisal. Arch Gen Psychiatry 42:1116–1122, 1985

Wise MG: Adjustment disorders and impulse disorders not otherwise classified, in American Psychiatric Press Textbook of Psychiatry. Edited by Talbot JA, Hales RE, Yudofsky SC. Washington, DC, American Psychiatric Press, 1988, pp 605–620

Yesavage JA, Brink TL, Rose TL, et al: Development and validation of geriatric depression screening scale: a preliminary report. J Psychiatry Res 17:37–49, 1982–1983

Zarb J: Correlates of depression in cognitively impaired hospitalized elderly referred for neuropsychological assessment. J Clin Exp Neuropsychol 18:713–723, 1996

Zimmerman M, Pfohl B, Coryell W, et al: The prognostic validity of DSM-III Axis IV in depressed inpatients. Am J Psychiatry 144:102–106, 1987

Zung W: A self-rating depression scale. Arch Gen Psychiatry 12:63–70, 1965

Zung W: A rating instrument for anxiety disorders. Psychosomatics 12:371–379, 1971

CHAPTER 13

Impulse-Control Disorders Not Elsewhere Classified

Charles L. Scott, M.D.

Donald M. Hilty, M.D.

Michael Brook, B.S.

The DSM-IV-TR (American Psychiatric Association 2000) category "impulse-control disorders not elsewhere classified" includes five separate diagnoses whose single unifying theme is clinically significant impulsive behavior that is not better accounted for by another DSM-IV-TR diagnosis (Frances et al. 1995). The five diagnoses described in this section are intermittent explosive disorder, kleptomania, pyromania, pathological gambling, and trichotillomania. The diagnosis of impulse-control disorder not otherwise specified describes those individuals who have an impulse-control disorder that does not meet criteria for any of the specific impulse-control disorders or other DSM-IV-TR diagnoses.

When considering a diagnosis of an impulse-control disorder, the clinician must carefully review the established criteria for each of the diagnoses. Numerous other psychiatric disorders have impulsive behavior as one component. The possible diagnostic range for impulsive behavior includes antisocial and borderline personality disorders, conduct disorder, atten-tion-deficit/hyperactivity disorder, oppositional defiant disorder, delirium, dementia, substance-related disorders, schizophrenia and other psychotic disorders, and mood disorders. The clinician should consider alternative motivations such as vengeance or monetary gain that may account for the impulsive-appearing behavior, particularly when considering the diagnoses of intermittent explosive disorder, kleptomania, and pyromania.

Intermittent Explosive Disorder

Definition and Diagnostic Criteria

The classification of individuals who have episodic violent behavior has undergone considerable change in the literature. In 1956, Menninger and Mayman introduced the term *episodic dyscontrol*, and Menninger (1963), in his book *The Vital Balance*, mentioned a disorganized episodic violence type of seizure disorders and brain-damage syndromes.

In 1970, Mark and Ervin described a "dyscontrol syndrome" that was thought to represent behavioral manifestations of disordered brain physiology, particularly in the limbic system. That same year, Monroe (1970) reinforced the idea that subtle brain dysfunction could cause episodic violent behavior and also used the term *episodic dyscontrol*.

Eventually, terms began appearing in formal classification systems. The diagnostic term *intermittent explosive disorder* first appeared in ICD-9-CM (World Health Organization 1978). This was the first time that an official diagnostic nomenclature had categorized episodic violence as a disorder separate from personality. Intermittent explosive disorder with different diagnostic criteria appeared in DSM-III (American Psychiatric Association 1980) and then in DSM-III-R (American Psychiatric Association 1987). In DSM-IV-TR (Table 13–1), the requirement that impulsivity be absent between episodes has been eliminated and additional exclusionary diagnoses have been added.

Two DSM-IV-TR diagnoses are currently available to the clinician who wishes to diagnose primarily episodic violent behavior: *intermittent explosive disorder* and *personality change due to a general medical condition, aggressive type*. Intermittent explosive disorder has numerous exclusion criteria, whereas personality change due to a general medical condition requires the presence of a specific organic factor that is judged to be causally related to the violence, including a medication (Shaw and Fletcher 2000). Most individuals with episodic violent behavior do not meet the diagnostic criteria for either disorder but have another psychiatric disorder such as schizophrenia, paranoid disorder, mania, substance abuse, drug withdrawal, delirium, a personality disorder (especially borderline or anti-

TABLE 13–1. DSM-IV-TR diagnostic criteria for intermittent explosive disorder

A. Several discrete episodes of failure to resist aggressive impulses that result in serious assaultive acts or destruction of property.
B. The degree of aggressiveness expressed during the episodes is grossly out of proportion to any precipitating psychosocial stressors.
C. The aggressive episodes are not better accounted for by another mental disorder (e.g., antisocial personality disorder, borderline personality disorder, a psychotic disorder, a manic episode, conduct disorder, or attention-deficit/hyperactivity disorder) and are not due to the direct physiological effects of a substance (e.g., a drug of abuse, a medication) or a general medical condition (e.g., head trauma, Alzheimer's disease).

social), mental retardation, a conduct disorder, or organic brain disease (Tardiff 1992).

Epidemiology

According to a review of the literature published between 1937 and 1991, episodic violent behavior is quite common in the general population, but strictly diagnosed intermittent explosive disorder is quite rare because of the exclusionary criteria (American Psychiatric Association 1994b). Males account for 80% of the persons who have episodic violence (American Psychiatric Association 1994b). Fava (1997) correctly noted that patients diagnosed with intermittent explosive disorder are complex and heterogeneous in terms of symptoms and etiologies.

One study examined the characteristics of 842 individuals reported to have episodic violent behavior (American Psychiatric Association 1994b). When all 842 cases were carefully reviewed and compared against DSM-III-R criteria for intermittent explosive disorder, only 17 patients were found to have possible intermittent explosive disorder. Mattes (1990) reported 4 of 51 (8%) patients diagnosed with intermittent explosive disorder who were free of any evidence of organicity.

Patients with episodic violent behavior frequently have abnormal neurological examination results (65%), abnormal neuropsychological test results (58%), abnormal electroencephalogram (EEG) results (55%), a history of attention-deficit/hyperactivity disorder (45%), or a history of learning disability (38%). Despite evidence of central nervous system (CNS) dysfunction, it is often impossible to establish a clear cause-and-effect relationship between the CNS dysfunction and episodic violent behavior.

Etiology

Episodic violent behavior occurs in patients because of biological (e.g., neuronal discharges), psychological (e.g., motivational), and social reasons (Lesch and Merschdorf 2000). A continuum exists between "faulty learning" and "faulty equipment" (Monroe 1970). Individuals with episodic violence have abnormalities in serotonergic and noradrenergic function (Eichelman 1992; Kruesi et al. 1992; Tardiff 1992; Virkkunen et al. 1996), as well as increased testosterone, dopamine, and arginine vasopressin levels (Kavoussi et al. 1997). Reduced γ-aminobutyric acid (GABA) and acetylcholine function also have been associated with agitation (Lindenmayer 2000). A review by Chernasky and Hollander (1997) of the neurobiology and neurophysiology of aggression and impulsivity indicated that it was unclear whether all of these findings pertain to those with intermittent explosive disorder.

Experimental paradigms of punishment, extinction, and novelty provide a method for studying the neurobiology of behavioral inhibition (Stein et al. 1993). For example, decrease in serotonergic transmission leads to an inability to adopt passive or waiting attitudes or to accept situations that necessitate or create inhibitory tendencies (Soubrie 1986). Animal studies of impulse control typically have used one of three models: delay of reward, differential reinforcement, or autoshaping (behaviors naturally engaged without reinforcement) (Monterosso and Ainslie 1999). Models of self-control also may be of utility, including control of attention, control of emotions, and choice bundling (bundling a current choice with a series of future choices) (Monterosso and Ainslie 1999).

Associated Diagnoses

Because relatively few patients have intermittent explosive disorder, associated diagnoses have not been thoroughly evaluated. There may be significant overlap with other disorders with agitation (e.g., dementia, cerebrovascular accident) impulse-control dysregulation (e.g., kleptomania), antisocial personality disorder, or borderline personality disorder.

Evaluation

The evaluation of the patient with potential intermittent explosive disorder includes a review of the chief complaint, history of the present illness, psychiatric and substance use history, family history, personal and developmental history, medical history (e.g., history of seizures), mental status, and results of physical examination. Information from the patient, relatives, therapist, primary care physician, prior evaluations of violence, and police and criminal records may be of utility. The onset, course, and severity of the violent behavior, as well as other types of reckless behavior (e.g., suicidal behavior, reckless driving, destruction of property, reckless spending, and reckless sexual behavior), are assessed. It may be helpful to quantify the behavior with the Overt Aggression Scale (Yudofsky et al. 1986) or Overt Agitation Severity Scale (Yudofsky et al. 1997). Visual evoked potential studies and special diagnostic techniques (e.g., electroencephalographic activation with chloralose) may prove useful in evaluation of these patients (Bars et al. 2001; Monroe 1970).

Treatment

Although information on the management and treatment of aggressive behavior is available, no information exists on the treatment of rigorously diagnosed intermittent explosive disorder. Studies of aggressive behavior consist primarily of anecdotal case reports or open drug trials; few studies are placebo controlled. Research in this area is also complicated by the ethical dilemma of randomizing potentially violent patients to placebo treatment, although this is critical because the rates of response are most likely lower than those for other disorders (e.g., depression).

The treatment of a patient who becomes acutely violent, regardless of the underlying etiology, commonly involves physical restraint, seclusion, and sedation. Neuroleptics and benzodiazepines, such as haloperidol and lorazepam (or a combination of the two), are often appropriate and effective interventions to control an acutely violent individual (Wise et al. 2002). A task force of professionals from more than 40 disciplines recently reviewed the literature with regard to practice parameters for intravenous sedation for adult patients in the intensive care setting (Shapiro et al. 1995). Evidence for use of haloperidol was convinc-

ingly justifiable on scientific evidence alone, whereas use of lorazepam was reasonably justifiable by available scientific evidence and strongly supported by expert critical care opinion. However, intravenous haloperidol may induce arrhythmia such that a pretreatment check of the QTc interval and monitoring are recommended (Lawrence and Nasraway 1997).

The development of a treatment plan for a patient who has long-standing, episodic aggressive behavior is complicated and involves the assessment and amelioration (when possible) of multiple factors: temperament, sensory cues, neuroanatomy, neurochemical and neuroendocrine function, stress, and social conditions (Eichelman 1992). Long-term psychotherapy is effective in diminishing violent behavior in some individuals (Eichelman 1992; Tardiff 1992).

No drug is currently specifically approved by the U.S. Food and Drug Administration (FDA) for the treatment of intermittent explosive disorder or other forms of aggression. However, numerous pharmacological agents have been reported to be effective in diminishing violent behavior in some individuals, largely in anecdotal reports: neuroleptics, benzodiazepines, lithium, β-blockers (especially propranolol), anticonvulsants (especially carbamazepine), serotonin-modulating drugs (tryptophan, trazodone, buspirone, clomipramine, selective serotonin reuptake inhibitors [SSRIs]), polycyclic antidepressants, monoamine oxidase inhibitors (MAOIs), and psychostimulants (Eichelman 1992; Tardiff 1992). Medications with few long-term side effects are advantageous because the duration of the disorder is currently unknown but may be persistent like other aggressive disorders.

Lithium and other mood stabilizers may be useful in the treatment of aggression not associated with a manic episode.

Campbell et al. (1984) treated children who had conduct disorder with lithium and reported decreases in aggressive behavior, especially when the behavior contained strong affective components. In a double-blind, placebo-controlled study, Sheard et al. (1976) found that lithium reduced aggression in prisoners who did not have mood disorders. Fava (1997) noted that lithium appears to be effective in the treatment of aggression in prison inmates without epilepsy, mentally retarded and disabled patients, children with conduct disorder, and patients with bipolar disorder. On the basis of the hypothetical relationship between seizures and aggressive behavior, carbamazepine was used in the early 1970s to treat patients with rage outbursts, especially patients who had seizure foci located in the temporal lobe or limbic structures (Mattes 1986). Carbamazepine reduces aggressive behavior in patients with intermittent explosive disorder and without overt epilepsy (Mattes 1990); the average dose was 860 mg, and the mean serum level was 8.6 μg/mL. Other studies have suggested the benefit of carbamazepine for developmentally disabled individuals with agitation (Folks et al. 1982) and for persons with dementia (Gleason and Schneider 1990), as well as valproate for those with borderline personality disorder (Stein et al. 1995a) and dementia (Lott et al. 1995; Narayan and Nelson 1997).

Antipsychotic medication has been used for acute and long-term violence of many etiologies, although the side effect risk has prompted reevaluation of that practice. Atypical antipsychotics have a better profile than typical antipsychotics. In a 12-week, double-blind, placebo-controlled trial, risperidone was better than haloperidol and placebo for behavioral disturbance associated with dementia (De Deyn et al. 1999).

Elliott (1977) was among the first to use propranolol to treat the aggressive behavior seen in brain-injured patients. Numerous other studies showed the relative benefit of β-blockers in patients with and without overt brain injury (Mattes 1990; Sheard 1988; Williams et al. 1982; Yudofsky et al. 1981). More recent research has suggested that compounds that modulate serotonin transmission, such as buspirone, serotonin reuptake inhibitors, trazodone, and clomipramine, may benefit some patients. This also appears true in disorders of pathological aggression (Fava 1997).

Course and Prognosis

Few patients are under study for intermittent explosive disorder in terms of its epidemiology, diagnosis, treatment, and course. Accordingly, more data need to be collected in each of these areas.

Kleptomania

Definition and Diagnostic Criteria

In DSM-IV-TR, kleptomania is defined as the recurrent failure to resist impulses to steal objects that are not needed for personal use or for their monetary gain (Table 13–2). The individual with kleptomania experiences an increasing sense of tension immediately before the theft, followed by a sense of pleasure, gratification, or relief at the time of committing the theft. The stealing is not in response to psychotic symptoms, such as a delusion or hallucination, and is not committed to express anger or vengeance. In addition, the individual is not given the diagnosis of kleptomania if the stealing is better accounted for by conduct disorder, a manic episode, or antisocial personality disorder (American Psychiatric Association 2000).

Kleptomania should be distinguished

TABLE 13–2. DSM-IV-TR diagnostic
criteria for kleptomania

A. Recurrent failure to resist impulses to
   steal objects that are not needed for personal use or for their monetary value.
B. Increasing sense of tension immediately
   before committing the theft.
C. Pleasure, gratification, or relief at the time
   of committing the theft.
D. The stealing is not committed to express
   anger or vengeance and is not in response
   to a delusion or a hallucination.
E. The stealing is not better accounted for by
   conduct disorder, a manic episode, or
   antisocial personality disorder.

from other behaviors such as stealing and
compulsive buying. Stealing involves the
planned taking of objects for secondary
gain or profit (Christenson et al. 1994;
Yates 1986). In contrast, compulsive buying involves the purchase rather than the
theft of items. Although compulsive buying is not a recognized DSM-IV-TR diagnosis, proposed criteria include maladaptive preoccupations or impulses with
buying or shopping that cause marked distress; are time-consuming; significantly
interfere with social, occupational, or financial functioning; and do not occur exclusively during periods of hypomania or
mania (McElroy et al. 1994).

   In their study of 20 persons with kleptomania, McElroy et al. (1991b) found
that some individuals with kleptomania
atoned for stealing by donating stolen
goods to charity, returning to victimized
stores to pay for stolen items or to buy
unneeded items, or calling stores to alert
clerks of their stealing.

Epidemiology

Kleptomania has been described as a rare
diagnosis. Prevalence estimates among
identified shoplifters range between 4%
(Singer 1978) and 8% (Bradford and Bal-

maceda 1983). Because many persons
with kleptomania are never caught, the
actual prevalence may be higher (McElroy
et al. 1995). Although some authors have
suggested that kleptomania is more common in men (Gibbens 1962), most case
reports and studies indicate that kleptomania occurs primarily in women.

Etiology

Numerous theories have been proposed
in an effort to understand the stealing behavior of individuals with kleptomania.
Explanations have included a need for
stimulation to help treat underlying depression (Fishbain 1987) and a desire to
emotionally compensate for an actual or
anticipated loss (Cupchik and Atcheson
1983). Psychoanalytic theory proposes
that stealing gratifies id impulses (Fenichel 1945) and compensates for issues
related to childhood neglect (Abraham
1949).

   Human and animal research suggests
that serotonergic neurotransmission is
important in the development of impulse-control disorders (Virkkunen et al.
1989) and therefore may play a role in
the etiology of kleptomania. Finally, various neurological conditions have been
described as precipitating the onset of
kleptomania-type behavior. These include dementia (Khan and Martin 1977),
intracranial lesions or masses (Chiswick
1976), and normal-pressure hydrocephalus (McIntyre and Emsley 1990).

Associated Diagnoses

Substantial comorbid psychopathology
has been described in studies of individuals with kleptomania. Associated disorders that have been reported include
mood disorders, anxiety disorders, eating
disorders (Wiedemann 1998), other
impulse-control disorders, obsessive-
compulsive disorder (OCD), and alcohol

and substance abuse disorders (Hudson and Pope 1990; McElroy et al. 1991a).

In a study of 37 individuals who had a DSM-IV (American Psychiatric Association 1994a) diagnosis of kleptomania, more than 80% reported current psychiatric problems, 54% reported family psychiatric illness, and nearly half were receiving psychiatric treatment at the time of the study. The most common diagnoses were depressive disorders, anxiety disorders, and sleeping disorders. More than 30% had attempted suicide, and more than 20% had a history of alcohol misuse or abuse (Sarasalo et al. 1996).

Evaluation

The practitioner must consider whether the stealing behavior represents a choice to commit an antisocial act with potential secondary gain rather than the taking of items not needed for personal use. Because many patients with kleptomania do not report their stealing behavior to mental health evaluators, specific questions must be asked. Such questions involve the onset, frequency, duration, and magnitude of stealing behavior as well as any previous treatment. In addition, the clinician should evaluate for a comorbid psychiatric disorder, including depression, mania, alcohol or substance abuse, anxiety disorder, eating disorder, personality disorder, or other impulse-control disorder, as well as a family history of mental illness. The evaluator also should screen for any possible head injury or organic disorder, with particular attention in elderly individuals referred for new-onset stealing behavior (Moak 1988).

Treatment

Various treatment approaches have been described for kleptomania. Nonpharmacological treatments that have been used include systematic desensitization (Mar-

zagao 1972), "assertive training" (Wolpe 1958), aversive conditioning (Keutzer 1972), covert sensitization (Gauthier and Pellerin 1982; Glover 1985), self-imposed banning by shoppers (Goldman 1991), adjunctive sexual counseling for those with disturbed sexual relationships (Turnbull 1987), and Shoplifters Anonymous. Pharmacotherapy also has been used to help decrease impulsive urges to steal.

A few published case reports suggest that SSRIs, such as paroxetine (Kraus 1999), fluvoxamine (Chong and Low 1996), and fluoxetine (McElroy et al. 1989), may be useful in decreasing the frequency of stealing behavior in individuals with kleptomania. The use of antidepressants may be particularly helpful in individuals with kleptomania with a comorbid depressive disorder. Therapeutic efficacy has also been reported with lithium, valproate, amitriptyline, imipramine, nortriptyline, trazodone, and electroconvulsive therapy (ECT) in adults with kleptomania (McElroy et al. 1995).

Course and Prognosis

Kleptomania appears to be a disorder that has a pattern established early in life (Goldman 1991), with most patients having an onset of symptoms before age 21. In most patients, the symptoms are long-standing, lasting more than 10 years (Sarasalo et al. 1996).

Pyromania

Definition and Diagnostic Criteria

In DSM-IV-TR, pyromania is defined as deliberate and purposeful fire setting on more than one occasion. The DSM-IV-TR criteria describe a period of tension or arousal preceding the act, fascination with

TABLE 13–3. DSM-IV-TR diagnostic
criteria for pyromania

A. Deliberate and purposeful fire setting on
   more than one occasion.
B. Tension or affective arousal before the act.
C. Fascination with, interest in, curiosity
   about, or attraction to fire and its situational contexts (e.g., paraphernalia, uses,
   consequences).
D. Pleasure, gratification, or relief when
   setting fires, or when witnessing or participating in their aftermath.
E. The fire setting is not done for monetary
   gain, as an expression of sociopolitical
   ideology, to conceal criminal activity, to
   express anger or vengeance, to improve
   one's living circumstances, in response to
   a delusion or hallucination, or as a result
   of impaired judgment (e.g., in dementia,
   mental retardation, substance intoxication).
F. The fire setting is not better accounted
   for by conduct disorder, a manic episode,
   or antisocial personality disorder.

fire and its consequences, followed by
pleasure, gratification, or relief (Table 13–
3). DSM-IV-TR outlines circumstances in
which the diagnosis of pyromania should
not be given, including when the individual is intoxicated or is acting under the
influence of a hallucination or delusion.

Individuals who commit acts of arson
should be distinguished from those who
meet diagnostic criteria for pyromania.
Arson is commonly defined as the willful
and malicious setting of a fire. Numerous
motives for fire setting, independent of
pyromania, exist and include anger or re-
venge toward an individual or agency, insurance fraud, vandalism, crime conceal-
ment, or a failed suicide attempt.

Epidemiology

Studies indicate that pyromania is diagnosed in 0%–4% of examined arsonists
when DSM-III or DSM-IV criteria are

used (Koson and Dvoskin 1982; Rasanen
et al. 1995; Ritchie and Huff 1999).
Although pyromania is rare, acts of arson
are common in the United States. In
1997, more than 80,000 acts of arson
were reported to the Federal Bureau of
Investigation (1998). However, pyromania is rarely diagnosed when established
criteria are applied to arsonists. Although
Lewis and Yarnell (1951) diagnosed 39%
of their sample of 1,500 arsonists with
pyromania, this significant percentage was
achieved by a poorly defined classification
system.

Fire setting is also relatively common
among the mentally ill. Geller and Bertsch
(1985) found that 26% of nongeriatric
state hospital psychiatric inpatients had
engaged in some form of fire-setting
behavior, and 18% had actually set fires
(Geller et al. 1992a, 1992b).

Etiology

The vast majority of the literature related
to fire setting addresses factors associated
with arsonists, individuals who usually do
not qualify for a diagnosis of pyromania.
Family backgrounds of fire setters have
indicated higher than expected rates of
mental illness, antisocial personality disorder, and alcoholism.

Biological factors associated with arson
also have been examined. In their study of
individuals who had committed arson,
Lewis and Yarnell (1951) found that these
individuals had a higher-than-expected
frequency of long-standing physical abnormalities. In one study, more than 18% of
the arsonists were noted to have EEG abnormalities (Hill et al. 1982). Reactive hypoglycemia and decreased cerebrospinal
fluid concentrations of 3-methoxy-4-hy-
droxyphenylglycol (MHPG) and 5-
hydroxyindoleacetic acid (5-HIAA) also
have been found in arsonists and violent
offenders (Virkkunen et al. 1994).

Associated Diagnoses

Although most arsonists will not meet the DSM criteria for pyromania, many will have a psychiatric diagnosis. In his study of 153 adult arsonists, Rix (1994) found that 54% of the arsonists met criteria for a personality disorder. The most common personality disorder was antisocial personality disorder, although borderline, avoidant, dependent, and paranoid types were nearly as common. In addition, intoxication with alcohol, drugs, or both was frequently noted. Research indicates that between one-third and two-thirds of fire setters are intoxicated at the time of their act (Ritchie and Huff 1999; Rix 1994). Other diagnoses overrepresented among fire setters when compared with the general population include schizophrenia (Lewis and Yarnell 1951; Ritchie and Huff 1999), mania (Ritchie and Huff 1999), and mental retardation (Hill et al. 1982; Rix 1994).

Evaluation

When evaluating a fire setter for the diagnosis of pyromania, the clinician must carefully determine whether the individual meets the established diagnostic criteria for this disorder. Additional important areas to review include the person's motive; location of the fire; means of starting the fire; history and progression of fire-setting behavior; age at first offense; aggression toward other inanimate objects; presence or absence of a co-conspirator; intent to harm persons, property, or both; history of violence; history of "watching" other fires or spending time in fire stations; history of setting off fire alarms; actions during the fire; behaviors after setting the fire; self-injurious behavior using fire; history of smoking; access to flammables; and a family history of arson. An EEG is appropriate for those individuals with symptoms consistent with a seizure disorder.

In some situations, fire setting represents a suicide attempt, and further inquiry regarding suicidal intent is recommended. Careful attention also must be given to the presence of intoxication, personality disorders, mental retardation, mood disorders, and psychosis. In particular, psychotic arsonists almost always act alone (Molnar et al. 1984), and their targets are frequently outsiders of the community rather than individuals they know (Virkkunen 1974). Virkkunen (1974) also found that hallucinations and delusions were the principal motivation for the fire-setting behavior in one-third of schizophrenic arsonists.

Treatment

Limited studies have been conducted on effective treatment strategies for pyromania. Traditional psychoanalytic approaches have not proven effective, and no research supports the theory that pyromania is caused by unresolved psychosexual conflicts. Other treatment modalities that have been implemented include behavior therapy with aversive conditioning (McGrath and Marshall 1979), positive reinforcement (Bumpass et al. 1983), social skills training (Jackson et al. 1987), and implementation of a relapse prevention plan (Stewart 1993). Because no single approach has been proven effective for all fire setters, treatment should be individualized with a combination of interventions as appropriate.

Course and Prognosis

Virtually all research examining the course and prognosis of individuals who set fires deals with fire setters whose symptoms do not meet criteria for pyromania. A study of 243 male arsonists found that repeat fire setters differed from those with only one episode by being younger, having more extensive criminal histories, being less likely to set fires for psychotic reasons, and being more likely to have a personality disorder (Rice and Harris 1991). A 20-year follow-up of 67 arsonists found a conviction rate for arson of approximately 4%. Those who reoffended were solitary offenders with chronic problems of social adjustment (Soothill and Pope 1973).

Mentally disordered fire setters have been shown to have a higher rate of recurrence than do non–mentally disordered fire setters (Barnett et al. 1997). Furthermore, Barnett et al. (1999) found that 9% of the arsonists who had been found not guilty by reason of insanity received a conviction of arson in a 10-year follow-up period. When examining a group of 50 patients who had engaged in at least one fire-setting behavior in their lifetime, Geller et al. (1992a, 1992b) determined that 28% of these had fire-setting behavior, and 16% actually set a fire in the 7-year follow-up period.

Pathological Gambling

Definition and Diagnostic Criteria

According to DSM-IV-TR (Table 13–4), pathological gambling is characterized by a continuous or periodic inability to control gambling behavior, a preoccupation with gambling and with obtaining gambling funds, irrational thinking, and a continuation of the behavior despite adverse consequences and/or desire to quit. Pathological gambling is a disorder that results in a high degree of emotional and physical suffering to gamblers and those around them. Approximately 60% of pathological gamblers engage in criminal activities, such as forgery and fraud, to maintain their addiction (Blaszczynski and Silove 1996). Stress-related medical conditions such as hypertension, peptic ulcer disease,

TABLE 13–4.   DSM-IV-TR diagnostic criteria for pathological gambling

A. Persistent and recurrent maladaptive gambling behavior as indicated by five (or more) of the following:
   (1) is preoccupied with gambling (e.g., preoccupied with reliving past gambling experiences, handicapping or planning the next venture, or thinking of ways to get money with which to gamble)
   (2) needs to gamble with increasing amounts of money in order to achieve the desired excitement
   (3) has repeated unsuccessful efforts to control, cut back, or stop gambling
   (4) is restless or irritable when attempting to cut down or stop gambling
   (5) gambles as a way of escaping from problems or of relieving a dysphoric mood (e.g., feelings of helplessness, guilt, anxiety, depression)
   (6) after losing money gambling, often returns another day to get even ("chasing" one's losses)
   (7) lies to family members, therapist, or others to conceal the extent of involvement with gambling
   (8) has committed illegal acts such as forgery, fraud, theft, or embezzlement to finance gambling
   (9) has jeopardized or lost a significant relationship, job, or educational or career opportunity because of gambling
   (10) relies on others to provide money to relieve a desperate financial situation caused by gambling
B. The gambling behavior is not better accounted for by a manic episode.

and migraine headaches are also common among pathological gamblers. Twenty percent of the individuals seeking treatment for pathological gambling have a history of a suicide attempt (American Psychiatric Association 2000).

Studies of pathological gamblers classified two broad subtypes: antisocial-impulsive (also known as action subtype) and obsessive-dependent (escape subtype). Although both subtypes have characteristics common to many pathological gamblers (such as neuroticism, low self-esteem, and manipulativeness), important differences exist. Action gamblers are predominantly male and achieve a euphoric state through gambling. Such individuals tend to be domineering, controlling, and manipulative; have an above-average IQ; and view themselves as friendly, sociable, gregarious, and generous. They are often energetic, assertive, persuasive, and confident in their interpersonal interactions. Action gamblers are reluctant to recognize that they have a gambling problem and generally are resistant to treatment. In contrast, escape gamblers are represented nearly equally by men and women. These individuals tend to be nurturing, responsible, and active in their family life prior to the onset of pathological gambling. In their interpersonal relationships, they are passive-avoidant, unassertive, and in need of empowerment. Escape gamblers often have a history of physical, sexual, or emotional abuse and use gambling as a means to escape their problems. These individuals describe feelings of temporary elation and release from physical and emotional pain while gambling. They may seek professional help for assistance with their gambling, relationship issues, or both. Escape gamblers are more malleable to treatment, with a better prognosis when compared with action gamblers (Blaszczynski et al. 1997; Committee on the Social and Economic Impact of Pathological Gambling 1999).

Epidemiology

Studies have placed the prevalence of pathological gambling in the adult population at 1%–4%. The likelihood that an individual would have a gambling addiction at some point in his or her life was estimated as 1.6%. Groups with a higher prevalence of pathological gambling included adolescents (6.1%) and adults of low socioeconomic status (17.2%). Men compose approximately 75% of the total pathological gambling population, and women make up the remaining 25%, with most women falling within the escape subtype (Committee on the Social and Economic Impact of Pathological Gambling 1999; Lepage et al. 2000).

Etiology

Anderson and Brown (1987) proposed that gamblers have low autonomic arousal that they seek to augment by gambling. Consequently, pathological gamblers become addicted to their own arousal because of its self-reinforcing physical and psychological effects. Follow-up studies suggest that increased arousal and risk taking described in pathological gamblers may be linked to noradrenergic system dysfunction (Roy et al. 1988). Although abnormalities in the endorphin system also have been suggested as a possible contributor to increased arousal in pathological gamblers, studies examining this link have not noted significant differences in plasma β-endorphin levels between pathological gamblers and nongamblers (Blaszczynski et al. 1986). Abnormalities in the dopaminergic reward pathways of pathological gamblers have been shown to account for the addictive symptoms of the disorder (Bergh et al. 1997; Comings 1998), and serotonergic system dysfunction has been linked to the impulsive and compulsive traits (DeCaria et al. 1998). Blanco et al. (1996) reported lower platelet monoamine oxidase activity (a peripheral marker of serotonin function) among pathological gamblers as compared with nongamblers.

An increased prevalence of pathological gambling has been described in family members of individuals diagnosed with the disorder when compared with individuals who gamble recreationally. In their study of 3,359 twins, Eisen et al. (1998) showed that 56% of three or more and 62% of four or more DSM-III-R criteria for pathological gambling endorsed by the participants in their study could be accounted for by familial factors, such as genetic predisposition and environmental influences. Comings et al. (1999) identified a repeat polymorphism of the 48th base pair of the D_4 dopamine receptor gene (DRD4) as a potential genetic abnormality in pathological gamblers.

Associated Diagnoses

A significant relationship exists between pathological gambling and substance abuse, with more than 60% of pathological gamblers meeting criteria for a substance abuse disorder at least once in their lifetime. The incidence of pathological gambling is 8–10 times greater among those with alcohol dependence than in the general population (Crockford and el-Guebaly 1998; Lejoyeux et al. 2000). One study examining the overlap of alcoholism and pathological gambling suggested a common genetic vulnerability for these two disorders (Slutske et al. 2000). Depressive disorders co-occur in approximately 18% of pathological gamblers, a rate similar to that found among substance-dependent populations (Crockford and el-Guebaly 1998).

Personality disorders have been reported to have moderate comorbidity with pathological gambling. In a study of 82 inpatient pathological gamblers, more than 90% met criteria for a personality disorder, primarily narcissistic, histrionic, or borderline (Blaszczynski and Steel 1998; Steel and Blaszczynski 1998). Although possible comorbidity with antisocial per-

sonality disorder has been alluded to in the literature, research shows that the antisocial behavior conducted by individuals with pathological gambling typically occurs after their gambling becomes problematic rather than as a result of a separate antisocial personality disorder (Blaszczynski and Silove 1996).

Evaluation

The evaluator's primary task is to carefully determine whether the individual meets the diagnostic criteria for pathological gambling and to assess the extent of comorbid conditions. In addition to the DSM-IV-TR criteria, the South Oaks Gambling Screen (Lesieur and Blume 1987) may be useful in assessing the severity of the gambling behavior. Potential comorbid diagnoses to consider include alcohol and substance abuse, personality disorders, depression, and bipolar mania. Pathological gambling is not diagnosed if the gambling behavior is the result of a manic episode. The examiner's challenge is to distinguish between the elation sometimes induced by gambling behavior and the euphoria secondary to mania.

Because of the high suicide risk among pathological gamblers, a brief inpatient stay may be warranted.

Collateral contacts are helpful in evaluating the extent of the individual's involvement in and the veracity of his or her accounts of gambling behavior. Useful sources of information include significant others, family members, credit reports, credit card statements, banking statements, and employers.

Treatment

Behavioral and cognitive-behavioral approaches have been identified as highly successful in achieving abstinence from gambling in the short term (i.e., 1 month or less). For example, behavioral models that emphasize desensitization and aversion have been successful in achieving short-term abstinence in 30% of treated patients (Committee on the Social and Economic Impact of Pathological Gambling 1999; Symes and Nicki 1997). Sylvain et al. (1997) described a multimodal cognitive-behavioral approach, which combined cognitive restructuring, problem solving, social skills training, and active relapse prevention and was shown to alleviate pathological symptomatology in 86% of participating gamblers, most of whom were able to maintain abstinence as indicated at the 6- and 12-month follow-up assessment.

Several pharmacological agents have been prescribed with varied rates of success, particularly in the presence of a comorbid psychiatric disorder. Lithium carbonate has helped decrease gambling behavior in pathological gamblers with bipolar disorder (Moskowitz 1980). SSRIs have been shown to assist particularly in alleviating impulsive and compulsive aspects of gambling behavior. Hollander et al. (2000) reported complete cessation of gambling for 8 weeks in 7 of 10 pathological gamblers in response to 220 mg/day of fluvoxamine therapy. Studies note that comorbid diagnosis of depression may further warrant treatment with an antidepressant that affects serotonergic activity. Concerns have been raised about the possibility that SSRIs may induce underlying mania in some patients with mood disorders. Screening for comorbid mood disorders should diminish the possibility of a manic episode following SSRI treatment of pathological gambling. Opioid antagonists have been shown to block the excitement or pleasure of addictive behavior and have been suggested as a possible treatment for pathological gambling. In particular, naltrexone has shown promising results for curbing intense cravings that often accompany pathological gambling behavior (Kim 1998).

Relapse prevention strategies such as self-help and group therapies are important in achieving successful and lasting abstinence (Hodgins and el-Guebaly 2000). Gamblers Anonymous is one popular self-help group and is modeled on the 12-Step approach used by Alcoholics Anonymous. Surveys show that people are more likely to turn to Gamblers Anonymous for help than any other form of intervention; however, follow up studies indicate that 82% of "graduates" relapse within 1 year of completing the program (Committee on the Social and Economic Impact of Pathological Gambling 1999).

Course and Prognosis

A commonly identified course of pathological gambling consists of three progressive stages: 1) the winning phase, 2) the losing phase, and 3) the desperation phase. During the winning stage, pathological gamblers regard gambling as a social activity and are often able to attain substantial profits. This self-reinforcing dynamic facilitates feelings of grandiosity, with the increase in finances directed toward gambling. In the losing stage, gamblers begin to "chase" their losses by placing increasingly larger bets. Gamblers fantasize about winning and attempt to conceal their addiction by lying to family and friends, borrowing money from various resources, and taking out loans. Once the desperation phase is reached, the gambler experiences feelings of hopelessness as losses continue to mount and personal relationships crumble. Gamblers no longer see their gambling as a choice. They often become aloof and emotionally callous and may engage in antisocial behaviors such as stealing, swindling, or forgery to continue gambling. The risk of suicide is highest at this stage (Lesieur and

Custer 1984). Pathological gamblers commonly experience all three phases before seeking help.

The prognosis for pathological gambling appears to be affected by age at onset and type of gambling behavior. In general, the earlier the gambling behavior commences, the greater the likelihood of it becoming pathological. In comparing action with escape gamblers, action gamblers tend to begin gambling at an early age (often in adolescence) and gradually progress through the stages of the disease. In contrast, escape gamblers usually begin gambling later in life (often after 30) but experience the onset of pathological symptoms earlier in the course of their gambling career (Committee on the Social and Economic Impact of Pathological Gambling 1999).

Trichotillomania

Definition and Diagnostic Criteria

Trichotillomania is a term created by Hallopeau in 1889 to describe a compulsion to pull out one's own hair (Krishnan et al. 1985). DSM-IV-TR diagnostic criteria include recurrent pulling out of one's hair, tension before pulling, and pleasure or gratification when pulling (Table 13–5). A significant number of individuals considered to have trichotillomania, however, do not fulfill Criteria B and C (Christenson and Crow 1996). Trichotillomania produces irregular, nonscarring focal patches of hair loss that are linear, rectangular, or oval. Hair loss usually occurs in the scalp region but can involve eyebrows, eyelashes, or pubic hair. These areas of hair loss are more likely to be found on the opposite side of the body from the dominant hand. In addition to the current impulse-control disorder classification, trichotillo-

mania has been conceptualized as an affective or anxiety (e.g., OCD) spectrum disorder (Christenson et al. 1991b; Jenike 1989; McElroy et al. 1992; Swedo and Leonard 1992). Krishnan et al. (1985) noted that trichotillomania also can be present as a major symptom in mental retardation, schizophrenia, and borderline personality disorder.

TABLE 13–5.   DSM-IV-TR diagnostic criteria for trichotillomania

A. Recurrent pulling out of one's hair resulting in noticeable hair loss.
B. An increasing sense of tension immediately before pulling out the hair or when attempting to resist the behavior.
C. Pleasure, gratification, or relief when pulling out the hair.
D. The disturbance is not better accounted for by another mental disorder and is not due to a general medical condition (e.g., a dermatological condition).
E. The disturbance causes clinically significant distress or impairment in social, occupational, or other important areas of functioning.

Epidemiology

In a questionnaire survey of 2,579 first-year college students, Christenson et al. (1991b) found a prevalence of between 0.6% and 1.5% for males and between 0.6% and 3.4% for females. This suggested that trichotillomania may not be as rare as previously suspected and that males may be affected as frequently as females. Most patients who seek treatment are female (Christenson et al. 1991a; Swedo et al. 1989).

The dermatological literature most commonly reports pathological hair pulling in preadolescent children. Stroud (1983), a dermatologist, found that 10% of 59 patients who came to his office with hair loss in 1982 had trichotillomania.

Oranje et al. (1986) found that the female-to-male ratio was 2.5:1 and also that 25% of the children with trichotillomania had associated onychophagy, trichophagy, or automutilation.

Christenson et al. (1991a) described the phenomenology of trichotillomania in a report of 60 adult hair pullers. The mean age at onset was 13 years, and 93% of the subjects were female. Hair pulling can last from a few minutes to a few hours (Swedo et al. 1991; Winchel et al. 1992a). Hair was pulled primarily from the scalp (67%); however, subjects also pulled eyelashes (22%), eyebrows (8%), facial hair (2%), and pubic hair (2%). All subjects believed that their hair pulling was an excessive or unusual behavior, and 95% reported a diurnal variation, with the worst hair pulling in the evening. Interestingly, it has been reported that the symptoms of trichotillomania may worsen the week before menstruation (Keuthen et al. 1997). After pulling, 48% of patients also initiate oral behaviors (e.g., running the hair across their lips, eating the hair) (Christenson et al. 1991a). Accordingly, dental erosion and trichophagy may occur, as well as skin infections.

Etiology

A number of biological etiologies have been proposed for trichotillomania. Christenson et al. (1992) reported that 8% of 161 patients knew a first-degree relative who had pulled hair, and in other family studies, between 4% and 5% of relatives reported current or past hair-pulling behavior (Diefenbach et al. 2000). A neuroethological theory views trichotillomania and OCD as pathology of the neurobiological mechanisms responsible for grooming behavior. Neurotransmitter dysregulation is supported by phenomenological similarities of trichotillomania symptoms to those of other disorders, studies of neurotransmitter and other neuroendocrine function, and treatment studies with SSRIs. Some reports in the literature suggest that trichotillomania may be a type of OCD (Jenike 1989; Swedo et al. 1989). Stanley et al. (1992, 1993), however, reported several differences between OCD and trichotillomania, including the facts that hair pulling usually is associated with pleasure, patients with trichotillomania have few associated obsessive-compulsive symptoms, and patients with OCD differ from patients with trichotillomania in terms of anxiety, depression, and personality characteristics. Regional cerebral blood flow studies indicate that women with trichotillomania have increased activity of the cerebellar and right superior parietal area, compared with increased frontal cortex activity in women with OCD (Christenson and Crow 1996; Swedo et al. 1991). One way to understand these findings is a dimension from primarily impulsive (i.e., risk seeking) to primarily compulsive (i.e., harm avoidance) (Hollander et al. 1996). Trichotillomania may be closer to the impulsive end, whereas obsessive-compulsive disorder may be closer to the compulsive end.

Many psychosocial theories have been described for trichotillomania. From a psychoanalytic perspective, hair can represent beauty, virility, sexual conflicts, physical prowess, and sexuality; haircutting or plucking can signify castration (Krishnan et al. 1985). Hair pulling may result from poor object relations or represent a means of working through real or perceived threats of object loss (Greenberg and Sarner 1965; Krishnan et al. 1985). Behavior theories include tension reduction (i.e., negative reinforcement), modeling, and response covariation (e.g., thumb sucking and hair pulling co-occur, and with treatment of the former, the latter resolves). For children, the syndrome usually develops during a time of psychosocial stress (e.g., a disturbed mother–child relationship, hospitalization, or family stress) (Oranje et al. 1986) but may persist even though the stressor(s) may no longer be present.

Associated Diagnoses

Psychiatric disorders are commonly comorbid with trichotillomania (e.g., mood [65%], anxiety [57%], personality disorders [25%–55%]) (Christenson et al. 1991b; Diefenbach et al. 2000; Soriano et al. 1996; Swedo et al. 1993; Winchel et al. 1992a).

Evaluation

The clinical interview requires a substantial collection of historical information, including quantitative and qualitative pulling of one's hair from the scalp, eyelashes, eyebrows, facial hair, and other regions; tension before pulling; and pleasure or gratification when pulling. A relation, if any, to psychosocial stressors, menstruation, and other triggers should be explored. Family history of hair pulling should be noted. Screening for symptoms of obsessive-compulsive, depressive, other anxiety, and tic disorders may identify comorbid psychiatric conditions. Medical disorders (e.g., dermatological) are prudent to evaluate in collaboration with primary and other specialty physicians as indicated.

Self-monitoring, self-report, and clinical interview instruments are available for use in the diagnosis of trichotillomania. A daily diary of hair pulling and saving pulled hairs may be useful but can be limited by trichophagy, pulling without awareness, and nonadherence for various reasons. The Massachusetts General Hospital Hairpulling Scale is the only self-report questionnaire with established psychometric properties (Keuthen et al. 1995; O'Sullivan et al. 1995). Several

clinical rating scales for trichotillomania have been developed, including the Yale-Brown Obsessive-Compulsive Scale modified for trichotillomania (Y-BOCS TM; Stanley et al. 1992) and the Psychiatric Institute Trichotillomania Scale (PITS; Winchel et al. 1992b). The Y-BOCS TM substitutes "thoughts of hair-pulling" for obsessions and "hair-pulling" for compulsions. The PITS is more specific to trichotillomania and can be administered more quickly.

Physical examination and procedures may substantiate the diagnosis of trichotillomania. Adult patients generally do not have changes in fingernails or toenails (except possibly signs of nail biting) usually associated with dermatological conditions. Hair regrowth follows the application of collodion to the area of hair loss for 1 week. In children, careful parental observation of the child includes looking for hair among the child's playthings. The child also may practice onychophagy (i.e., nail biting). If the child complains of gastrointestinal symptoms such as abdominal pain, diarrhea, and/or constipation, or decreased appetite, examination of the oral cavity for evidence of trichophagy (i.e., eating hair) and X-ray examination of the stomach for a trichobezoar (i.e., hairball) are warranted. In addition, a skin biopsy may provide evidence for the diagnosis by ruling out other conditions. Finally, longitudinal photographs may facilitate changes in the course or responses to treatment.

Treatment

Patients who receive both behavioral and medication treatment show a greater reduction in hair-pulling scores than do those receiving either treatment alone (Keuthen et al. 1998). A review of the literature finds several controlled medication trials, many open case series, and a multitude of case reports for the acute treatment of trichotillomania. Swedo et al. (1989) found that clomipramine was significantly more effective than desipramine in a double-blind crossover treatment of 20 patients with trichotillomania. Rothbaum and Ninan (1992) found that clomipramine was superior to placebo, but in a repeat trial, the difference was not significant (Ninan et al. 2000). Recently, Neudecker et al. (2001) reported that paroxetine was superior to placebo. Christenson et al. (1991d), in another placebo-controlled, double-blind crossover study, reported that fluoxetine was no better than placebo for 21 patients with chronic hair pulling. Streichenwein and Thornby (1995), in a placebo-controlled, double-blind crossover trial, found that fluoxetine was not effective in 23 chronic hair pullers.

Open trials indicate favorable response to fluoxetine (Winchel et al. 1992a), fluvoxamine (Stanley et al. 1997), venlafaxine (Ninan et al. 1998), lithium carbonate (Christenson et al. 1991c), and haloperidol (Van Ameringen et al. 1999). Augmentation of SSRIs also has been successful with haloperidol (Van Ameringen et al. 1999), pimozide (Stein and Hollander 1992), and risperidone (Epperson et al. 1999; Stein et al. 1997). Isolated case reports of successful treatment of trichotillomania in adults have been published regarding the following drugs: buspirone, citalopram, amitriptyline, a monoamine oxidase inhibitor, chlorpromazine in a patient with comorbid schizophrenia, and olanzapine augmentation of an SSRI. For children and adolescents, paroxetine and fluoxetine use has been reported. A steroid topical cream also has been used in combination with clomipramine when hair pulling is cued by itch (Black and Blum 1992). Another topical cream has been used to increase physical sensitivity (Ristvedt and Christenson 1996).

Psychosocial treatments are now beginning to be evaluated in controlled trials. In a study of 23 patients, Ninan et al. (2000) showed that cognitive-behavioral treatment had a dramatic effect in reducing symptoms of trichotillomania and was significantly more effective than clomipramine or placebo. Neudecker et al. (2001) reported that multimodal behavior therapy, weekly for 45 treatments, was superior to placebo in a study of 20 patients. Multimodal behavior therapy consisted of behavioral, functional, and motivation analysis and training in symptom-centered techniques. Other potential treatments include habit reversal training, hypnosis, and individual behavior modification techniques (e.g., biofeedback, aversion therapy, extinction, response prevention).

Course and Prognosis

According to Stroud (1983), most cases of trichotillomania in young children resolve spontaneously because it usually represents a transient behavior in response to a psychosocial stressor or a habit without the presence of an obvious precipitant. If hair loss persists, psychiatric consultation is indicated, and inquiry into areas of parent–child relationships or other areas of potential conflict may illuminate the problem. Psychiatric evaluation is indicated when trichotillomania occurs in adolescents and adults. Trichotillomania in adults typically follows a chronic course, frequently involves multiple hair sites, and is associated with high rates of psychiatric comorbidity (Christenson et al. 1991a).

The long-term response of symptoms to pharmacotherapy and behavior therapy is variable. At 4-year follow-up, a 40% reduction of symptoms was maintained with clomipramine (Swedo et al. 1993). Keuthen et al. (1998) completed a naturalistic survey study of 63 patients who had received behavioral treatment (90%), medication (73%), or both (41%). At 6-year follow-up, 52% of the subjects rated themselves as treatment responders, and 51% were still in active treatment, with 62% receiving therapy or medication and 25% receiving both; subjects receiving both showed a greater reduction in hair-pulling scores than did those receiving either treatment alone. In a longitudinal study evaluating hair pulling, sickness impact, and self-esteem in a more structured fashion, Keuthen et al. (2001) noted that responders maintained their symptomatic improvement but did not continue to improve. Interestingly, self-esteem continued to be problematic even in subjects with reduced hair-pulling and sickness impact scores.

References

Abraham K: Manifestation of the female castration complex, in Selected Papers on Psychoanalysis, Vol 1. Translated by Bryan D, Strachey A. New York, Basic Books, 1949, pp 338–369

American Psychiatric Association: Diagnostic and Statistical Manual of Mental Disorders, 3rd Edition. Washington, DC, American Psychiatric Association, 1980

American Psychiatric Association: Diagnostic and Statistical Manual of Mental Disorders, 3rd Edition, Revised. Washington, DC, American Psychiatric Association, 1987

American Psychiatric Association: Diagnostic and Statistical Manual of Mental Disorders, 4th Edition. Washington, DC, American Psychiatric Association, 1994a

American Psychiatric Association: DSM-IV Sourcebook, Vol 2. Washington, DC, American Psychiatric Association, 1994b

American Psychiatric Association: Diagnostic and Statistical Manual of Mental Disorders, 4th Edition, Text Revision. Washington, DC, American Psychiatric Association, 2000

Anderson G, Brown RIF: Some applications of reversal theory to the explanation of gambling and gambling addictions. Journal of Gambling Behavior 3:179–189, 1987

Barnett W, Richter P, Sigmund D, et al: Recidivism and concomitant criminality in pathological firesetters. J Forensic Sci 42:879–883, 1997

Barnett W, Richter P, Renneberg B: Repeated arson: data from criminal records. Forensic Sci Int 101:49–54, 1999

Bars DR, Heyrend FL, Simpson CD, et al: Use of visual evoked-potential studies and EEG data to classify aggressive, explosive behavior of youths. Psychiatr Serv 52:81–86, 2001

Bergh C, Eklund P, Sodersten P, et al: Altered dopamine action in pathological gambling. Psychol Med 27:473–475, 1997

Black DW, Blum N: Trichotillomania treated with clomipramine and a topical steroid (letter). Am J Psychiatry 149:842–843, 1992

Blanco C, Orensanz-Munoz L, Blanco-Jerez C, et al: Pathological gambling and platelet MAO activity: a psychobiological study. Am J Psychiatry 153:119–121, 1996

Blaszczynski A, Silove D: Pathological gambling: forensic issues. Aust N Z J Psychiatry 30:358–369, 1996

Blaszczynski A, Steel Z: Personality disorders among pathological gamblers. Journal of Gambling Studies 14:51–71, 1998

Blaszczynski AP, Winter SW, Simon W, et al: Plasma endorphin levels in pathological gambling. Journal of Gambling Behavior 2:3–14, 1986

Blaszczynski A, Steel Z, McConaghy N: Impulsivity in pathological gambling: the antisocial impulsivist. Addiction 92:75–87, 1997

Bradford J, Balmaceda R: Shoplifting: is there a specific psychiatric syndrome? Can J Psychiatry 28:248–253, 1983

Bumpass ER, Fagelman FD, Brix RJ: Intervention with children who set fires. Am J Psychother 37:328–345, 1983

Campbell M, Perry R, Green WH, et al: Use of lithium in children and adolescents. Psychosomatics 25:95–101, 105–106, 1984

Chernasky S, Hollander E: The neuropsychiatric aspects of impulsivity and aggression, in The American Psychiatric Press Textbook of Neuropsychiatry, 3rd edition. Edited by Yudofsky SC, Hales RE. Washington, DC, American Psychiatric Press, 1997, pp 488–492

Chiswick D: Shoplifting, depression and an unusual intracranial lesion (case report). Med Sci Law 16:266–268, 1976

Chong SA, Low BL: Treatment of kleptomania with fluvoxamine. Acta Psychiatr Scand 93:314–315, 1996

Christenson GA, Crow SJ: The characterization and treatment of trichotillomania. J Clin Psychiatry 57:42–49, 1996

Christenson GA, Mackenzie TB, Mitchell JE: Characteristics of 60 adult chronic hair pullers. Am J Psychiatry 148:365–370, 1991a

Christenson GA, Pyle RL, Mitchell JE: Estimated lifetime prevalence of trichotillomania in college students. J Clin Psychiatry 52:415–417, 1991b

Christenson GA, Popkin MK, Mackenzie TB, et al: Lithium treatment of chronic hair pulling. J Clin Psychiatry 52:116–120, 1991c

Christenson GA, Mackenzie TB, Mitchell JE, et al: A placebo-controlled, double-blind crossover study of fluoxetine in trichotillomania. Am J Psychiatry 148:1566–1571, 1991d

Christenson GA, Mackenzie TB, Reeve EA: Familial trichotillomania (letter). Am J Psychiatry 149:283, 1992

Christenson GA, Faber RJ, de Zwaan M, et al: Compulsive buying: descriptive characteristics and psychiatric comorbidity. J Clin Psychiatry 55:5–11, 1994

Comings DE: The molecular genetics of pathological gambling. CNS Spectrums 3:20–37, 1998

Comings DE, Gonzalez N, Wu S, et al: Studies of the 48 repeat polymorphism of the DRD4 gene in impulsive, compulsive, addictive behaviors; Tourette syndrome; ADHD; pathological gambling; and substance abuse. Am J Med Genet 88:358–368, 1999

Committee on the Social and Economic Impact of Pathological Gambling (CSEIPG), Committee on Law and Justice, Commission on Behavioral and Social Sciences and Education, National Research Council: Pathological Gambling: A Critical Review. Washington, DC, National Academy Press, 1999

Crockford DN, el-Guebaly N: Psychiatric comorbidity in pathological gambling: a critical review. Can J Psychiatry 43:43–50, 1998

Cupchik W, Atcheson JD: Shoplifting: an occasional crime of the moral majority. Bull Am Acad Psychiatry Law 11:343–352, 1983

DeCaria CM, Begaz T, Hollander E: Serotonergic and noradrenergic function in pathological gambling. CNS Spectrums 3:38–47, 1998

De Deyn PP, Rabheru K, Rasmussen A, et al: A randomized trial of risperidone, placebo, and haloperidol for behavioral symptoms of dementia. Neurology 53:946–955, 1999

Diefenbach GJ, Reitman D, Williamson DA: Trichotillomania: a challenge to research and practice. Clin Psychol Rev 20:289–309, 2000

Eichelman B: Aggressive behavior: from laboratory to clinic. Quo vadit? Arch Gen Psychiatry 49:488–492, 1992

Eisen SA, Lin N, Lyons MJ, et al: Familial influences on gambling behavior: an analysis of 3359 twin pairs. Addiction 93:1375–1384, 1998

Elliott FA: Propranolol for the control of belligerent behavior following acute brain damage. Ann Neurol 1:489–491, 1977

Epperson CN, Fasula D, Wasylink S, et al: Risperidone addition in serotonin reuptake inhibitor-resistant trichotillomania: three cases. J Child Adolesc Psychopharmacol 9:43–49, 1999

Fava M: Psychopharmacologic treatment of pathologic aggression, in The Psychiatric Clinics of North America. Edited by Fava M. Philadelphia, PA, WB Saunders, 1997, p 444

Federal Bureau of Investigation: Crime in the United States: Uniform Crime Reports for the United States. Washington, DC, U.S. Department of Justice, 1998

Fenichel O: The Psychoanalytic Theory of Neurosis. New York, WW Norton, 1945

Fishbain DA: Kleptomania as risk-taking behavior in response to depression. Am J Psychother 41:598–603, 1987

Folks DG, King LD, Dowdy SB, et al: Carbamazepine treatment of selected affectively disordered inpatients. Am J Psychiatry 139:115–117, 1982

Frances A, First MB, Pincus HA: Impulse control disorders not elsewhere classified, in DSM-IV Guidebook. Washington, DC, American Psychiatric Press, 1995, pp 343–352

Gauthier J, Pellerin D: Management of compulsive shoplifting through covert sensitization. J Behav Ther Exp Psychiatry 13:73–75, 1982

Geller JL, Bertsch G: Firesetting behavior in the histories of a state hospital population. Am J Psychiatry 142:464–468, 1985

Geller JL, Fisher WH, Moynihan K: Adult lifetime prevalence of fire setting behaviors in a state hospital population. Psychiatr Q 63:129–142, 1992a

Geller JL, Fisher WH, Bertsch G: Who repeats? A follow-up study of state hospital patients' firesetting behavior. Psychiatr Q 63:143–156, 1992b

Gibbens TCN: Shoplifting. Med Leg J 30:6–19, 1962

Gleason RP, Schneider LS: Carbamazepine treatment of agitation in Alzheimer's outpatients refractory to neuroleptics. J Clin Psychiatry 51:115–118, 1990

Glover J: A case of kleptomania treated by covert sensitization. Br J Clin Psychol 24:213–214, 1985

Goldman MJ: Kleptomania: making sense of the nonsensical. Am J Psychiatry 148:986–996, 1991

Greenberg HR, Sarner CA: Trichotillomania: symptom and syndrome. Arch Gen Psychiatry 12:482–489, 1965

Hill RW, Langevin R, Paitich D, et al: Is arson an aggressive act or a property offense? A controlled study of psychiatric referrals. Can J Psychiatry 27:648–654, 1982

Hodgins DC, el-Guebaly N: Natural and treatment-assisted recovery from gambling problems: a comparison of resolved and active gamblers. Addiction 95:777–789, 2000

Hollander E, Kwon JH, Stein DJ, et al: Obsessive-compulsive spectrum disorders: overview and quality of life issues. J Clin Psychiatry 57(suppl 8):3–6, 1996

Hollander E, DeCaria CM, Finkell JN, et al: A randomized double-blind fluvoxamine/placebo crossover trial in pathologic gambling. Biol Psychiatry 47:813–817, 2000

Hudson JI, Pope HG Jr: Affective spectrum disorder: does antidepressant response identify a family of disorders with a common pathophysiology? Am J Psychiatry 147:552–564, 1990

Jackson HF, Glass C, Hope S: A functional analysis of recidivistic arson. Br J Clin Psychol 26:175–185, 1987

Jenike MA: Obsessive-compulsive and related disorders (editorial). N Engl J Med 321:539–541, 1989

Kavoussi R, Armstead P, Coccaro E: The neurobiology of impulsive aggression, in The Psychiatric Clinics of North America. Edited by Fava M. Philadelphia, PA, WB Saunders, 1997, pp 395–403

Keuthen NJ, O'Sullivan RL, Ricciardi JN, et al: The Massachusetts General Hospital (MGH) Hairpulling Scale, 1: development and factor analyses. Psychother Psychosom 64:141–145, 1995

Keuthen NJ, O'Sullivan RL, Hayday CF, et al: The relationship of menstrual cycle and pregnancy to compulsive hair-pulling. Psychother Psychosom 66:33–37, 1997

Keuthen NJ, O'Sullivan RL, Goodchild P, et al: Retrospective review of treatment outcome for 63 patients with trichotillomania. Am J Psychiatry 155:560–561, 1998

Keuthen NJ, Fraim C, Deckersbach T, et al: Longitudinal follow-up of naturalistic treatment outcome in patients with trichotillomania. J Clin Psychiatry 62:101–107, 2001

Keutzer CS: Kleptomania: a direct approach to treatment. Br J Med Psychol 45:159–163, 1972

Khan K, Martin ICA: Kleptomania as a presenting feature of cortical atrophy. Acta Psychiatr Scand 56:168–172, 1977

Kim SW: Opioid antagonists in the treatment of impulse-control disorders. J Clin Psychiatry 59:159–164, 1998

Koson DF, Dvoskin J: Arson: a diagnostic study. Bull Am Acad Psychiatry Law 10: 39–49, 1982

Kraus JE: Treatment of kleptomania with paroxetine. J Clin Psychiatry 60:793, 1999

Krishnan KRR, Davidson JRT, Guajardo C: Trichotillomania: a review. Compr Psychiatry 26:123–128, 1985

Kruesi MJP, Hibbs ED, Zahn TP, et al: A 2-year prospective follow-up study of children and adolescents with disruptive behavior disorders: prediction by cerebrospinal fluid 5-hydroxyindoleacetic acid, homovanillic acid, and autonomic measures? Arch Gen Psychiatry 49:429–435, 1992

Lawrence K, Nasraway S: Conduction disturbances associated with administration of butyrophenone antipsychotics in the critically ill: a review of the literature. Pharmacotherapy 17:531–537, 1997

Lejoyeux M, McLoghlin M, Ades J: Epidemiology of behavioral dependence: literature review and results of original studies. European Psychiatry 15:129–134, 2000

Lepage C, Ladouceur R, Jacques C: Prevalence of problem gambling among community service users. Community Ment Health J 36:597–601, 2000

Lesch KP, Merschdorf U: Impulsivity, aggression, and serotonin: a molecular psychobiological perspective. Behav Sci Law 18: 581–604, 2000

Lesieur HR, Blume SB: The South Oaks Gambling Screen (SOGS): a new instrument for the identification of pathological gamblers. Am J Psychiatry 144:1184–1188, 1987

Lesieur HR, Custer RL: Pathological gambling: roots, phases and treatments. Annals of the American Academy of Political and Social Science 74:146–156, 1984

Lewis NDC, Yarnell H: Pathological Firesetting (Pyromania) (Nervous and Mental Disease Monogr 82). New York, Coolidge Foundation, 1951

Lindenmayer J-P: The pathophysiology of agitation. J Clin Psychiatry 61(suppl 14):5–10, 2000

Lott AD, McElroy SL, Keys MA: Valproate in the treatment of behavioral agitation in elderly patients with dementia. J Neuropsychiatry Clin Neurosci 7:314–319, 1995

Mark V, Ervin F: Violence and the Brain. New York, Harper & Row, 1970

Marzagao LR: Systematic desensitization treatment of kleptomania. J Behav Ther Exp Psychiatry 3:327–328, 1972

Mattes JA: Psychopharmacology of temper outbursts: a review. J Nerv Ment Dis 174: 464–470, 1986

Mattes JA: Comparative effectiveness of carbamazepine and propranolol for rage outbursts. J Neuropsychiatry Clin Neurosci 2:159–164, 1990

McElroy SL, Keck PE, Pope HG, et al: Pharmacological treatment of kleptomania and bulimia nervosa. J Clin Psychopharmacol 9:358–360, 1989

McElroy SL, Hudson JI, Pope HG Jr, et al: Kleptomania: clinical characteristics and associated psychopathology. Psychol Med 21:93–108, 1991a

McElroy SL, Harrison G, Hudson JI, et al: Kleptomania: a report of 20 cases. Am J Psychiatry 148:652–657, 1991b

McElroy SL, Hudson JI, Pope HG Jr, et al: The DSM-III-R impulse control disorders not elsewhere classified: clinical characteristics and relationship to other psychiatric disorders. Am J Psychiatry 149:318–327, 1992

McElroy SL, Keck PE Jr, Pope HG Jr, et al: Compulsive buying: a report of 20 cases. J Clin Psychiatry 55:242–248, 1994

McElroy SL, Keck PE, Phillips KA: Kleptomania, compulsive buying, and binge-eating disorder. J Clin Psychiatry 56 (suppl 4): 14–26, 1995

McGrath P, Marshall PG: A comprehensive treatment program for a fire setting child. J Behav Ther Exp Psychiatry 10:69–72, 1979

McIntyre AW, Emsley RA: Shoplifting associated with normal-pressure hydrocephalus: report of a case. J Geriatr Psychiatry Neurol 3:229–230, 1990

Menninger KA: The Vital Balance. New York, Viking, 1963

Menninger KA, Mayman M: Episodic dyscontrol: a third order of stress adaptation. Bull Menninger Clin 20:153–165, 1956

Moak GS: Clinical perspectives on elderly first-offender shoplifters. Hospital and Community Psychiatry 39:648–651, 1988

Molnar G, Keitner L, Harwood BT: A comparison of partner and solo arsonists. J Forensic Sci 29:574–583, 1984

Monroe RR: Episodic Behavioral Disorders. Cambridge, MA, Harvard University Press, 1970

Monterosso J, Ainslie G: Beyond discounting: possible experimental models of impulse control. Psychopharmacology 146:339–347, 1999

Moskowitz JA: Lithium and lady luck: use of lithium carbonate in compulsive gambling. New York State Journal of Medicine 80:785–788, 1980

Narayan M, Nelson JC: Treatment of dementia with behavioral disturbance using divalproex or a combination of divalproex and a neuroleptic. J Clin Psychiatry 58:351–354, 1997

Neudecker A, Rufer M, Hand I, et al: Paroxetine versus multimodal behavioral therapy in the treatment of trichotillomania: a pilot study (NR579), in 2001 New Research Program and Abstracts, American Psychiatric Association 154th Annual Meeting, New Orleans, LA, May 5–10, 2001. Washington, DC, American Psychiatric Association, 2001

Ninan PT, Knight B, Kirk L, et al: A controlled trial of venlafaxine in trichotillomania: interim phase I results. Psychopharmacol Bull 34:221–224, 1998

Ninan PT, Rothbaum BO, Marsteller FA, et al: A placebo-controlled trial of cognitive-behavioral therapy and clomipramine in trichotillomania. J Clin Psychiatry 61:47–50, 2000

Oranje AP, Pureboom-Wynia JDR, De Raeymaechec CMJ: Trichotillomania in childhood. J Am Acad Dermatol 16:614–619, 1986

O'Sullivan RL, Keuthen NJ, Hayday CF, et al: The Massachusetts General Hospital (MGH) Hairpulling Scale, 2: reliability and validity. Psychother Psychosom 64:146–148, 1995

Rasanen P, Hakko H, Valsanen E: The mental state of arsonists as determined by forensic psychiatric examinations. Bull Am Acad Psychiatry Law 23:547–553, 1995

Rice ME, Harris GT: Firesetters admitted to a maximum psychiatric institution. Journal of Interpersonal Violence 6:461–475, 1991

Ristvedt SL, Christenson GA: The use of pharmacologic pain sensitization in the treatment of repetitive hair-pulling. Behav Res Ther 34:647–648, 1996

Ritchie EC, Huff T: Psychiatric aspects of arsonists. J Forensic Sci 44:733–740, 1999

Rix KJB: A psychiatric study of adult arsonists. Med Sci Law 34:21–34, 1994

Rothbaum BO, Ninan TA: Treatment of trichotillomania: behavior therapy versus clomipramine. Poster presented at the annual meeting of the Association for Advancement of Behavior Therapy, Boston, MA, November 1992

Roy A, Custer R, Lorenz V, et al: Depressed pathological gamblers. Acta Psychiatr Scand 77:163–165, 1988

Sarasalo E, Bergman B, Toth J: Personality traits and psychiatric and somatic morbidity among kleptomaniacs. Acta Psychiatr Scand 94:358–364, 1996

Shapiro BA, Warren J, Egol AB, et al: Practice parameters for intravenous analgesia and sedation for adult patients in the intensive care unit: an executive summary. Crit Care Med 23:1596–1600, 1995

Shaw SC, Fletcher AP: Aggression as an adverse drug reaction. Adverse Drug React Toxicol Rev 19:35–45, 2000

Sheard MH: Clinical pharmacology of aggressive behavior. Clin Neuropharmacol 11:483–492, 1988

Sheard MH, Marini JL, Bridges CI, et al: The effect of lithium on impulsive aggressive behavior in man. Am J Psychiatry 133:1409–1413, 1976

Singer BA: A case of kleptomania. Bull Am Acad Psychiatry Law 6:414–422, 1978

Slutske WS, Eisen S, True WR, et al: Common genetic vulnerability for pathological gambling and alcohol dependence in men. Arch Gen Psychiatry 57:666–673, 2000

Soothill KL, Pope PJ: Arson: a twenty-year cohort study. Med Sci Law 13:127–138, 1973

Soriano JL, O'Sullivan RL, Baer L, et al: Trichotillomania and self-esteem: a survey of 62 female hair pullers. J Clin Psychiatry 57:77–82, 1996

Soubrie P: Reconciling the role of central serotonin neurones in human and animal behavior. Behav Brain Sci 9:319–364, 1986

Stanley MA, Swann AC, Bowers TC, et al: A comparison of clinical features in trichotillomania and obsessive-compulsive disorder. Behav Res Ther 30:39–44, 1992

Stanley MA, Prather RC, Wagner AL, et al: Can the Yale-Brown Obsessive Compulsive Scale be used to assess trichotillomania? A preliminary report. Behav Res Ther 31:171–177, 1993

Stanley MA, Breckenridge JK, Swann AC: Fluvoxamine treatment of trichotillomania. J Clin Psychopharmacol 17:278–283, 1997

Steel Z, Blaszczynski A: Impulsivity, personality disorders and pathological gambling severity. Addiction 93:895–905, 1998

Stein DJ, Hollander E: Low-dose pimozide augmentation of serotonin reuptake blockers in the treatment of trichotillomania. J Clin Psychiatry 53:123–126, 1992

Stein DJ, Hollander E, Liebowitz MR: Neurobiology of impulsivity and the impulse control disorders. J Neuropsychiatry Clin Neurosci 5:9–17, 1993

Stein DJ, Simeon D, Frenkel M, et al. An open trial of valproate in borderline personality disorder. J Clin Psychiatry 56:506–510, 1995a

Stein DJ, Bouwer C, Hawkridge S, et al: Risperidone augmentation of serotonin reuptake inhibitors in obsessive-compulsive and related disorders. J Clin Psychiatry 58:119–122, 1997

Stewart LA: Profile of female firesetters: implications for treatment. Br J Psychiatry 163:248–256, 1993

Streichenwein SM, Thornby JI: A long-term, double-blind, placebo-controlled crossover trial of the efficacy of fluoxetine for trichotillomania. Am J Psychiatry 152:1192–1196, 1995

Stroud JD: Hair loss in children. Pediatr Clin North Am 30:641–657, 1983

Swedo SE, Leonard HL: Trichotillomania: an obsessive compulsive spectrum disorder? Psychiatr Clin North Am 15:777–790, 1992

Swedo SE, Leonard HL, Rapoport JL, et al: A double-blind comparison of clomipramine and desipramine in the treatment of trichotillomania (hair pulling). N Engl J Med 321:497–501, 1989

Swedo SE, Rapoport JL, Leonard HL, et al: Regional cerebral glucose metabolism of women with trichotillomania. Arch Gen Psychiatry 48:828–833, 1991

Swedo SE, Lenane MC, Leonard HL: Longterm treatment of (hair pulling) (letter). N Engl J Med 329:141–142, 1993

Sylvain C, Ladoceur R, Boisvert JM: Cognitive and behavioral treatment of pathological gambling: a controlled study. J Consult Clin Psychol 65:727–732, 1997

Symes BA, Nicki RM: A preliminary consideration of cue-exposure, response-prevention treatment for pathological gambling behavior: two case studies. Journal of Gambling Studies 13:145–157, 1997

Tardiff K: The current state of psychiatry in the treatment of violent patients. Arch Gen Psychiatry 49:493–499, 1992

Turnbull JM: Sexual relationships of patients with kleptomania. South Med J 80:995–997, 1987

Van Ameringen M, Mancini C, Oakman JM, et al: The potential role of haloperidol in the treatment of trichotillomania. J Affect Disord 56:219–226, 1999

Virkkunen M: On arson committed by schizophrenics. Acta Psychiatr Scand 50:152–160, 1974

Virkkunen M, DeLong J, Bartko J, et al: Relationship of psychobiological variables to recidivism in violent offender and impulsive fire setters. Arch Gen Psychiatry 46:600–603, 1989

Virkkunen M, Rawlings R, Takola R, et al: CSF biochemistries, glucose metabolism, and diurnal activity rhythms in alcoholic, violent offenders, fire setters, and healthy volunteers. Arch Gen Psychiatry 51:20–27, 1994

Virkkunen M, Eggert M, Rawlings R, et al: A prospective follow-up study of alcoholic violent offenders and fire setters. Arch Gen Psychiatry 53:523–529, 1996

Wiedemann G: Kleptomania: characteristics of 12 cases. European Psychiatry 13:67–77, 1998

Williams DT, Mehl R, Yudofsky S, et al: The effect of propranolol on uncontrolled rage outbursts in children and adolescents with organic brain dysfunction. J Am Acad Child Psychiatry 21:129–135, 1982

Winchel RM, Jones JS, Stanley B, et al: Clinical characteristics of trichotillomania and its response to fluoxetine. J Clin Psychiatry 53:304–308, 1992a

Winchel RM, Jones JS, Molcho A, et al: The Psychiatric Institute Trichotillomania Scale (PITS). Psychopharmacol Bull 28:463–476, 1992b

Wise MG, Hilty DM, Cerda GM: Delirium (Confusional States), in The American Psychiatric Publishing Textbook of Consultation-Liaison Psychiatry: Psychiatry in the Medically Ill, 2nd Edition. Edited by Wise MG, Rundell JR. Washington, DC, American Psychiatric Publishing, 2002, pp 257–272

Wolpe J: Psychotherapy by Reciprocal Inhibition. Stanford, CA, Stanford University Press, 1958

World Health Organization: International Classification of Diseases, 9th Revision, Clinical Modification. Ann Arbor, MI, Commission on Professional and Hospital Activities, 1978

Yates E: The influence of psycho-social factors on non-sensical shoplifting. International Journal of Offender Therapy and Comparative Criminology 30:203–211, 1986

Yudofsky SC, Williams D, Gorman J: Propranolol in the treatment of rage and violent behavior in patients with chronic brain syndromes. Am J Psychiatry 138:218–220, 1981

Yudofsky SC, Silver JM, Jackson W, et al: The Overt Aggression Scale for objective rating of verbal and physical aggression. Am J Psychiatry 143:35–39; 1986

Yudofsky SC, Kopecky HJ, Kunik M, et al: The Overt Agitation Severity Scale for the objective rating of agitation. J Neuropsychiatry Clin Neurosci 9:541–548, 1997

Personality Disorders

Katharine A. Phillips, M.D.

Shirley Yen, Ph.D.

John G. Gunderson, M.D.

All clinicians frequently encounter patients with personality disorders. These patients are commonly seen in a variety of treatment settings, both inpatient and outpatient. Studies indicate that 30%–50% of outpatients have a personality disorder (Koenigsberg et al. 1985) and that 15% of inpatients are hospitalized primarily for problems caused by a personality disorder; as many as half of the remaining inpatients have a comorbid personality disorder (Loranger 1990) that significantly affects their response to treatment. It has also been estimated that personality disorders are relatively common in the general population, the prevalence being between 10% and 13% (Lenzenweger et al. 1997; Weissman 1993).

Patients with personality disorders present with problems that are among the most complex and challenging that clinicians encounter. Some patients intensely desire relationships but fearfully avoid them because they anticipate rejection; others seek endless admiration and are engrossed with grandiose fantasies of limitless power, brilliance, or ideal love. Still others have a self-concept so disturbed that they feel they embody evil or do not exist. This complexity is amplified by the fact that these and other personality disorder characteristics are not simply a problem the person has but are in fact central to who the person is.

Personality disorders, according to DSM-IV (American Psychiatric Association 1994), are patterns of inflexible and maladaptive personality traits that cause subjective distress, significant impairment in social or occupational functioning, or both. These traits must also deviate markedly from the culturally expected and accepted range, or *norm*, and this deviation must be manifested in more than one of the following areas: cognition, affectivity, control over impulses and need gratification, and ways of relating to others. In addition, the deviation must have been stably present and enduring since adolescence or early adulthood, and it must be pervasive—that is, it must manifest itself across a broad range of situations, rather than in only one specific triggering situation or in response to a particular stimulus.

Although useful, this definition has ambiguities and limitations. It can be difficult, for example, to determine whether personality traits are inflexible or to differentiate deviance from the norm or sickness from health. Whether dependence on others, compulsive work habits, or passive resistance to demands is considered excessive or problematic depends to some extent on the personal, social, and cultural context in which each occurs. Furthermore, the stability of personality disorders has recently been called into question (Ferro et al. 1998).

Nonetheless, it is important that clinicians attempt to recognize personality disorders in their patients. First, personality disorders do, by definition, cause significant problems for those who have them. Persons with these disorders often suffer, and their relationships with others are problematic. They have difficulty responding flexibly and adaptively to the environment and to the changes and demands of life, and they lack resilience when under stress. Instead, their usual ways of responding tend to perpetuate and intensify their difficulties. However, these individuals are often oblivious to the fact that their personality causes them problems, and they may instead blame others for their difficulties or even deny that they have any problems at all.

Personality disorders also often cause problems for others and are costly to society. Individuals with personality disorders frequently have considerable difficulty in their family, academic, occupational, and other roles. They have elevated rates of separation, divorce, child custody proceedings, unemployment, homelessness (Caton et al. 1994), and perpetration of child abuse (Dinwiddie and Bucholz 1993). They also have increased rates of accidents (McDonald and Davey 1996); police contacts (Gandhi et al. 2001); emergency department visits; medical hospitalization (J.[H.] Reich et al. 1989); violence, including homicide (Miller et al. 1993; Raine 1993); self-injurious behavior

(Hillbrand et al. 1994); attempted suicide (Pirkis et al. 1999); and completed suicide (Brent et al. 1994; Hawton et al. 1993). A high percentage of criminals (70%–85% in some studies) (Jordan et al. 1996), 60%–70% of alcoholic individuals, and 70%–90% of persons who abuse drugs have a personality disorder.

Finally, personality disorders need to be identified because of their treatment implications. These disorders often need to be a focus of treatment or, at the very least, need to be taken into account when comorbid Axis I disorders are treated, because their presence often affects the prognosis and treatment response of the Axis I disorder. For example, patients with depressive disorders (Black et al. 1988; Nelson et al. 1994), bipolar disorder (Calabrese et al. 1993), panic disorder (J.H. Reich 1988), obsessive-compulsive disorder (Jenike et al. 1986), and substance abuse (Fals-Stewart 1992) often respond less well to pharmacotherapy when they have a comorbid personality disorder. The presence of a comorbid personality disorder is also associated with poor compliance with pharmacotherapy (Colom et al. 2000). Furthermore, personality disorders have been shown to predict the development and relapse of major depression (Alnæs and Torgersen 1997; Lewinsohn et al. 2000), and individuals with a personality disorder are less likely to remit from major depression (O'Leary and Costello 2001), bipolar disorder (Dunayevich et al. 2000), and generalized anxiety disorder (Yonkers et al. 2000).

As most clinicians are well aware, the characteristics of patients with personality disorders are likely to be manifested in the treatment relationship, regardless of whether the personality disorder is the focus of treatment. For example, some patients may be overly dependent on the clinician, others may not follow treatment recommendations, and still others may experience significant conflict about getting well. Although individuals with personality disorders tend to use psychiatric services extensively, they are more likely to be dissatisfied with the treatment they receive (Kelstrup et al. 1993; Kent et al. 1995).

General Considerations

Assessment Issues and Methods

The assessment of Axis II disorders is in some ways more complex than that of Axis I disorders. It can be difficult to assess multiple domains of experience and behavior (i.e., cognition, affect, intrapsychic experience, and interpersonal interactions) and to determine that traits are not only distressing, impairing, and of early onset, but also pervasive and enduring. Nonetheless, a personality disorder assessment is essential to the comprehensive evaluation and adequate treatment of all patients. What follows is a discussion of such an assessment and steps that can be taken to avoid commonly encountered problems.

Comprehensiveness of Evaluation

A skilled clinical interview is the mainstay of personality disorder diagnosis and requires the clinician to be familiar with DSM criteria, take a longitudinal view, and use multiple sources of information. A psychodynamic perspective may contribute depth to the assessment through its attention to defenses, attitudes, and development. However, because an open-ended approach may inadequately cover all Axis II disorders, the additional use of a self-report or semistructured (i.e., interviewer-administered) personality disorder assessment instrument can be useful. Such instruments systematically assess each personality disorder criterion

with the use of standard questions or probes. Although self-report instruments have the advantage of saving the interviewer time, they often yield false-positive diagnoses and allow contamination of Axis II traits by Axis I states (Widiger and Frances 1987). Semistructured interviews—which require the interviewer to use certain questions but allow further probing—facilitate accurate diagnosis in several ways: they allow the interviewer to attempt to differentiate Axis II traits from Axis I states, clarify contradictions or ambiguities in the patient's response, and determine that traits are pervasive rather than limited to a specific situation.

Nonetheless, even with the use of a structured interview, the interviewer must often use his or her own judgment. For example, is a given trait present in enough situations to be considered pervasive? How much distress or impairment is necessary to consider the criterion present? Is a given characteristic a personality trait or a symptom of an Axis I disorder (i.e., a state)? Another limitation is that agreement among existing instruments is fairly low, and the instruments do not indicate which disorder in any given patient is most severe or should be the focus of treatment.

Syntonicity of Traits

As was noted earlier, because personality disorders to some extent reflect who the person is—and not simply what he or she has—some patients are unaware of the traits that reflect their disorder or may not perceive them as problematic. This limited self-awareness can interfere with personality disorder assessment, especially if the questions asked have negative or unflattering implications. This problem can be minimized by the use of multiple sources of information (e.g., medical records and informants who know the patient well). Still, the fact that studies

have shown low concordance rates between patient-based and informant-based
interviews (Bernstein et al. 1997; Ferro
and Klein 1997) means that interviewers
will often need to rely on their personal
experience with the patient to reach a
conclusion.

State Versus Trait

Another potential problem in personality
disorder assessment is that the presence
of an Axis I disorder can complicate the
assessment of Axis II traits. For example,
a person with social withdrawal, low self-
esteem, and lack of motivation or energy
due to major depression might appear to
have avoidant or dependent personality
disorder, when in fact these features reflect the Axis I condition. Or a hypomanic
person with symptoms of grandiosity or
hypersexuality might appear narcissistic
or histrionic. In some cases, assessment of
Axis II disorders may need to wait until
the Axis I condition, such as florid psychosis or mania, has subsided. However,
the clinician can often differentiate personality traits from Axis I states during an
Axis I episode by asking the patient to describe his or her usual personality outside
Axis I episodes; the use of informants who
have observed the patient over time and
without an Axis I disorder can be helpful.
Prior systematic assessment of Axis I conditions is invaluable in terms of alerting
the clinician to which Axis II traits will
need particularly careful assessment. This
task can be very difficult, however, in
patients with Axis I conditions that are
chronic and of early onset.

Medical Illness Versus Trait

Similarly, the interviewer must ascertain
that what appear to be personality traits
are not symptoms of a medical illness. For
example, aggressive outbursts caused by a
seizure disorder should not be attributed

to borderline or antisocial personality
disorder; nor should the unusual perceptual experiences that can accompany temporal lobe epilepsy be attributed to schizotypal personality disorder. A medical
evaluation should be included in a thorough patient assessment.

Situation Versus Trait

The interviewer should also ascertain that
personality disorder features are pervasive—that is, not limited to only one situation or occurring in response to only one
specific trigger. Similarly, these features
should be enduring rather than transient.
Asking the patient for behavioral examples of traits can help determine that the
trait is indeed present in a wide variety of
situations and is expressed in many relationships.

Gender and Cultural Bias

Although most research suggests that
existing personality disorder criteria are
relatively free of gender bias, interviewers
can unknowingly allow such bias to affect
their assessments. It is important, for example, that histrionic, borderline, and dependent personality disorders be assessed
as carefully in men as in women and that
obsessive-compulsive, antisocial, and narcissistic personality disorders be assessed
as carefully in women as in men. Interviewers should also be careful to avoid
cultural bias when diagnosing personality
disorders, especially when evaluating such
traits as promiscuity, suspiciousness, or
recklessness, which may have different
norms in different cultures.

Diagnosing Personality Disorders
in Children and Adolescents

Because the personality of children and
adolescents is still developing, personality
disorders should be diagnosed with care in
this age group. It is in fact often preferable

to defer these diagnoses until late adolescence or early adulthood, at which time a personality disorder diagnosis may be appropriate if the features appear to be pervasive, stable, and likely to be enduring. The diagnosis, however, may prove to be wrong as any stage-specific difficulties of adolescence resolve and as the person further matures.

Treatment

Because personality disorders consist of deeply ingrained attitudes and behavior patterns that consolidate during development and have endured since early adulthood, they have always been believed to be very resistant to change. Moreover, as previously noted, treatment efforts are further confounded by the degree to which patients with a personality disorder do not recognize their maladaptive personality traits as undesirable or needing to be changed. Although these reasons have fostered a general wariness about the treatability of patients with personality disorders, there is increasing evidence from longitudinal studies that personality disorders are quite variable in their course and much more malleable than had been thought (Grilo et al. 1999).

Psychoanalysts pioneered the hope that persons with personality disorders could respond to treatment. The original conception of neurosis as a discrete set of symptoms related to a discrete developmental phase or to discrete conflicts was gradually replaced by the idea that more enduring defensive styles and identification processes were the building blocks of character traits. From this perspective, Wilhelm Reich (1949) and others developed the concepts of *character analysis* and *defense analysis*. These processes refer to an analyst's efforts to address the ways in which a person resists learning or the confrontations by which the analyst

draws attention to the maladaptive effects of the patient's character traits (i.e., his or her usual interpersonal and behavioral style). A parallel development in technique evolved from group therapy experience. Maxwell Jones (1953) identified the value of confrontations delivered within group settings in which peer pressure made it difficult for patients to ignore feedback or to leave the group. Here, too, a primary goal of treatment was to render more dystonic the ego-syntonic but maladaptive aspects of the patient's interpersonal and behavioral style. This general principle was subsequently adopted by other forms of sociotherapies, notably those within hospital milieus and family therapies.

Families or couples may present complications insofar as the designated patient's disordered interpersonal and behavioral patterns may serve functions for, or be complementary to, the disordered patterns of persons with whom the patient is closely associated. For example, a dependent person is apt to bond with an overly authoritarian partner, or an emotionally constricted obsessional person may find an emotionally expressive, hysterical person particularly compatible. Under these circumstances, treatment is primarily directed not at confronting the maladaptive aspects of one person's character traits but rather at identifying the way in which these aspects may be welcomed and reinforced in one setting but maladaptive and impairing in others.

Significant developments in the treatment of personality disorders involve the use of multiple modalities, the growth of an empirical base, and greater optimism about treatment effectiveness. The overall development of treatment strategies for personality disorders has involved a movement away from therapeutic nihilism to the present widespread but still inconsistent use of a full spectrum of treatment

TABLE 14–1. Evidence of treatment effectiveness for personality disorders

Personality disorder	Psychotherapies	Sociotherapies	Pharmacotherapies
Paranoid	–	–	±
Schizoid	+	+	–
Schizotypal	–	±	+
Antisocial	–	+	–
Borderline	+	+ +	+
Histrionic	+ +	–	–
Narcissistic	+ +	–	–
Avoidant	+ +	+	±
Dependent	+ +	+	–
Obsessive-compulsive	+ +	–	–

Note. – = no support; ± = uncertain support; + = modestly helpful; + + = significantly helpful.

modalities. A review of psychotherapy outcome studies, including psychodynamic/interpersonal, cognitive-behavioral, mixed, and supportive therapies, found that psychotherapy was associated with a significantly faster rate of recovery compared with the natural course of personality disorders (Perry et al. 1999).

An overview of knowledge about the potential usefulness of the three major types of psychiatric treatment—psychotherapies, sociotherapies, and pharmacotherapies—is provided in Table 14–1. It is expected that use of these therapies will increasingly be guided by more specific and empirically based information on which modalities, in what sequence, are most effective for treatment of each personality disorder.

One of the most significant developments in the field has been the use of cognitive-behavioral strategies. These strategies generally are more focused and structured than are psychodynamic therapies. They typically involve efforts to diminish traits such as impulsivity or to increase assertiveness by using relaxation techniques, role-playing exercises, and other behavioral strategies. Cognitive strategies involve first identifying specific internal mental schemes by which patients typically misunderstand certain situations or

misrepresent themselves, and then learning how to modify those internal schemes.

In the past decade, the use of pharmacotherapy for personality disorders has begun to be explored. To the prospect of using specific medications for specific disorders has been added that of identifying biological dimensions of personality psychopathology that may respond to different medication classes (Cloninger 1987; Coccaro and Kavoussi 1997; Siever and Davis 1991). For example, research has increasingly suggested that impulsivity and aggression may respond to serotonergic medications; mood instability and lability may respond to serotonergic medications, other antidepressants, and mood stabilizers; and psychosis-like experiences may respond to antipsychotics (Coccaro and Kavoussi 1997; Cornelius et al. 1993; Soloff et al. 1993).

Specific Personality Disorders

Paranoid Personality Disorder

Clinical Features

Persons with paranoid personality disorder have a pervasive, persistent, and inappropriate mistrust of others (Table 14–2). They are suspicious of others' motives and assume that others intend to harm, exploit, or trick them. Thus, they may question, without justification, the loyalty or trustworthiness of friends or sexual partners, and they are reluctant to confide in others for fear the information will be used against them. Persons with paranoid personality disorder appear guarded, tense, and hypervigilant, and they frequently scan their environment for clues of possible attack, deception, or betrayal. They often find "evidence" of such malevolence by misinterpreting benign events (such as a glance in their direction) as demeaning or threatening. In response to perceived or actual insults or betrayals, these individuals overreact, quickly becoming excessively angry and responding with counterattacking behavior. They are unable to forgive or forget such incidents and instead bear long-term grudges against their supposed betrayers; some persons with paranoid personality disorder are litigious. Whereas some individuals with this disorder appear quietly and tensely aloof and hostile, others are overtly angry and combative. Persons with this disorder are usually socially isolated and, because of their paranoia, often have difficulties with co-workers.

Differential Diagnosis

Unlike paranoid personality disorder, the Axis I disorders paranoid schizophrenia and delusional disorder, paranoid type, are both characterized by prominent and persistent paranoid delusions of psychotic proportions; paranoid schizophrenia is also accompanied by hallucinations and other core symptoms of schizophrenia. Although paranoid and schizotypal personality disorders both involve suspiciousness, paranoid personality disorder does not entail perceptual distortions and eccentric behavior.

TABLE 14–2. DSM-IV-TR diagnostic criteria for paranoid personality disorder

A. A pervasive distrust and suspiciousness of others such that their motives are interpreted as malevolent, beginning by early adulthood and present in a variety of contexts, as indicated by four (or more) of the following:

(1) suspects, without sufficient basis, that others are exploiting, harming, or deceiving him or her

(2) is preoccupied with unjustified doubts about the loyalty or trustworthiness of friends or associates

(3) is reluctant to confide in others because of unwarranted fear that the information will be used maliciously against him or her

(4) reads hidden demeaning or threatening meanings into benign remarks or events

(5) persistently bears grudges, i.e., is unforgiving of insults, injuries, or slights

(6) perceives attacks on his or her character or reputation that are not apparent to others and is quick to react angrily or to counterattack

(7) has recurrent suspicions, without justification, regarding fidelity of spouse or sexual partner

B. Does not occur exclusively during the course of schizophrenia, a mood disorder with psychotic features, or another psychotic disorder and is not due to the direct physiological effects of a general medical condition.

Note: If criteria are met prior to the onset of schizophrenia, add "premorbid," e.g., "paranoid personality disorder (premorbid)."

Treatment

Because they mistrust others, persons with paranoid personality disorder usually avoid psychiatric treatment. If they do seek treatment, the therapist immediately encounters the challenge of engaging them and keeping them in treatment.

This can best be accomplished by maintaining an unusually respectful, straightforward, and unintrusive style aimed at building trust. If a problem develops in the treatment relationship—for example, the patient accuses the therapist of some fault—it is best simply to offer a straightforward apology, if warranted, rather than to respond evasively or defensively. It is also best to avoid an overly warm style, because excessive warmth and expression of interest can exacerbate the patient's paranoid tendencies. A supportive psychotherapy that incorporates such an approach may be the best treatment for these patients.

Although group treatment or cognitive-behavioral treatment (Turkat and Maisto 1985) aimed at anxiety management and the development of social skills might be of benefit, these patients, because of their suspiciousness and fears of losing control and being criticized, tend to resist such approaches.

Antipsychotic medications are sometimes useful in the treatment of this disorder. Patients may view such treatment with mistrust; however, these medications are particularly indicated in the treatment of the overtly psychotic decompensations that these patients sometimes experience.

Schizoid Personality Disorder

Clinical Features

Schizoid personality disorder is characterized by a profound defect in the ability to relate to others in a meaningful way (Table 14–3). Persons with this disorder have little or no desire for relationships with others and, as a result, are extremely socially isolated. They prefer to engage in solitary, often intellectual, activities, such as computer games or puzzles, and they often create an elaborate fantasy world into which they retreat and which substitutes for relationships with others. As a result of their lack of interest in relationships, they have few or no close friends or confidants. They date infrequently and seldom marry, and they often work at jobs requiring little interpersonal interaction (e.g., in a laboratory). These individuals are also notable for their lack of affect. They usually appear cold, detached, aloof, and constricted, and they have particular discomfort when experiencing warm feelings. Few, if any, activities or experiences give them pleasure, which is reflected in their chronic anhedonia.

TABLE 14–3. DSM-IV-TR diagnostic criteria for schizoid personality disorder

---

A. A pervasive pattern of detachment from social relationships and a restricted range of expression of emotions in interpersonal settings, beginning by early adulthood and present in a variety of contexts, as indicated by four (or more) of the following:

    (1) neither desires nor enjoys close relationships, including being part of a family

    (2) almost always chooses solitary activities

    (3) has little, if any, interest in having sexual experiences with another person

    (4) takes pleasure in few, if any, activities

    (5) lacks close friends or confidants other than first-degree relatives

    (6) appears indifferent to the praise or criticism of others

    (7) shows emotional coldness, detachment, or flattened affectivity

B. Does not occur exclusively during the course of schizophrenia, a mood disorder with psychotic features, another psychotic disorder, or a pervasive developmental disorder and is not due to the direct physiological effects of a general medical condition.

Note: If criteria are met prior to the onset of schizophrenia, add "premorbid," e.g., "schizoid personality disorder (premorbid)."

Differential Diagnosis

Schizoid personality disorder shares the features of social isolation and restricted emotional expression with schizotypal personality disorder, but it lacks the latter disorder's characteristics of cognitive and perceptual distortion. Unlike individuals with avoidant personality disorder, who intensely desire relationships but avoid them because of exaggerated fears of rejection, persons with schizoid personality disorder have little or no interest in developing relationships with others.

Treatment

Persons with schizoid personality disorder, like those with schizotypal personality disorder, rarely seek treatment. They do not perceive the formation of any relationship—including a therapeutic relationship—as potentially valuable or beneficial. They may, however, occasionally seek treatment for an associated problem, such as depression, or they may be brought for treatment by others. Whereas some patients can tolerate only a supportive therapy or treatment aimed at the resolution of a crisis or associated Axis I disorder, others do well with insight-oriented psychotherapy aimed at effecting a basic shift in their comfort with intimacy and affects.

Development of a therapeutic alliance may be difficult and can be facilitated by an interested and caring attitude and an avoidance of early interpretation or confrontation. Some authors have suggested the use of so-called inanimate bridges, such as writing and artistic productions, to ease the patient into the therapy relationship. Incorporation of cognitive-behavioral approaches that encourage gradually increasing social involvement may be of value (Liebowitz et al. 1986). Although many patients may be unwilling to participate in a group, group therapy may also facilitate the development of social skills and relationships.

Schizotypal Personality Disorder

Clinical Features

Persons with schizotypal personality disorder experience cognitive or perceptual distortions, behave in an eccentric manner, and are socially inept and anxious (Table 14–4). Their cognitive and perceptual distortions include ideas of reference, bodily illusions, and unusual telepathic and clairvoyant experiences. These distortions, which are inconsistent with subcultural norms, occur frequently and are an important and pervasive component of the person's experience. They are in keeping with the odd and eccentric behavior characteristic of this disorder. These individuals may, for example, talk to themselves in public, gesture for no apparent reason, or dress in a peculiar or unkempt fashion. Their speech is often odd and idiosyncratic—unusually circumstantial, metaphorical, or vague, for instance—and their affect is constricted or inappropriate. Such an individual may, for example, laugh inappropriately when discussing his or her problems.

Persons with schizotypal personality disorder are socially uncomfortable and isolated, and they have few friends. This isolation is often due to their eccentric cognitions and behavior as well as their lack of desire for relationships, which stems in part from their suspiciousness of others. If they develop a relationship, they tend to remain distant or may even terminate it because of their persistent social anxiety and paranoia.

Differential Diagnosis

Schizotypal personality disorder shares the feature of suspiciousness with paranoid personality disorder and that of social isolation with schizoid personality

TABLE 14–4. DSM-IV-TR diagnostic criteria for schizotypal personality disorder

A. A pervasive pattern of social and interpersonal deficits marked by acute discomfort with, and reduced capacity for, close relationships as well as by cognitive or perceptual distortions and eccentricities of behavior, beginning by early adulthood and present in a variety of contexts, as indicated by five (or more) of the following:

  (1) ideas of reference (excluding delusions of reference)

  (2) odd beliefs or magical thinking that influences behavior and is inconsistent with subcultural norms (e.g., superstitiousness, belief in clairvoyance, telepathy, or "sixth sense"; in children and adolescents, bizarre fantasies or preoccupations)

  (3) unusual perceptual experiences, including bodily illusions

  (4) odd thinking and speech (e.g., vague, circumstantial, metaphorical, overelaborate, or stereotyped)

  (5) suspiciousness or paranoid ideation

  (6) inappropriate or constricted affect

  (7) behavior or appearance that is odd, eccentric, or peculiar

  (8) lack of close friends or confidants other than first-degree relatives

  (9) excessive social anxiety that does not diminish with familiarity and tends to be associated with paranoid fears rather than negative judgments about self

B. Does not occur exclusively during the course of schizophrenia, a mood disorder with psychotic features, another psychotic disorder, or a pervasive developmental disorder.

Note: If criteria are met prior to the onset of schizophrenia, add "premorbid," e.g., "schizotypal personality disorder (premorbid)."

disorder, but these latter two disorders lack the markedly peculiar behavior and significant cognitive and perceptual distortions typically present in schizotypal

personality disorder. Schizotypal personality disorder, although on a spectrum with Axis I schizophrenia, lacks enduring overt psychosis.

Treatment

Because they are socially anxious and somewhat paranoid, persons with schizotypal personality disorder usually avoid psychiatric treatment. They may, however, seek such treatment—or be brought for treatment by concerned family members—when they become depressed or overtly psychotic. As with patients with paranoid personality disorder, it is difficult to establish an alliance with schizotypal patients, and they are unlikely to tolerate exploratory techniques that emphasize interpretation or confrontation. A supportive relationship that counters cognitive distortions and ego-boundary problems may be useful (Stone 1985). This may involve an educational approach that fosters the development of social skills or encourages risk-taking behavior in social situations, or, if these efforts fail, encourages the development of activities with less social involvement. If the patient is willing to participate, cognitive-behavioral therapy and highly structured educational groups with a social skills focus may also be helpful.

   Several case series support the usefulness of low-dose antipsychotic medications in the treatment of schizotypal personality disorder (Goldberg et al. 1986; Serban and Siegel 1984). These medications may ameliorate the anxiety and psychosis-like features associated with this disorder, and they are particularly indicated in the treatment of the more overt psychotic decompensations that these patients can experience. In addition, results of an open-label trial suggested that fluoxetine may also diminish features of schizotypal personality disorder (Markovitz et al. 1991).

Antisocial Personality Disorder

Clinical Features

The central characteristic of antisocial personality disorder is a long-standing pattern of socially irresponsible behaviors that reflects a disregard for the rights of others (Table 14–5). Many persons with this disorder engage in repetitive unlawful acts. The more prevailing personality characteristics include a lack of interest in or concern for the feelings of others, deceitfulness, and, most notably, a lack of remorse over the harm they may cause others. These characteristics generally make these individuals fail in roles requiring fidelity (e.g., as a spouse or a parent), honesty (e.g., as an employee), or reliability in any social role. Some antisocial persons possess a glibness and charm that can be used to seduce, outwit, and exploit others. Although most antisocial persons are indifferent to their effects on others, a notable subgroup takes sadistic pleasure in being harmful. Antisocial personality disorder is associated with high rates of substance abuse (Dinwiddie et al. 1992).

Differential Diagnosis

The primary differential diagnostic issue involves narcissistic personality disorder. Indeed, these two disorders may be variants of the same basic type of psychopathology (Hare et al. 1991). However, the antisocial person, unlike the narcissistic person, is likely to be reckless and impulsive. In addition, narcissistic individuals' exploitiveness and disregard for others are attributable to their sense of uniqueness and superiority rather than to a desire for materialistic gains.

Treatment

It is clinically important to recognize antisocial personality disorder because an uncritical acceptance of these individuals' glib or shallow statements of good inten-

TABLE 14–5. DSM-IV-TR diagnostic criteria for antisocial personality disorder

A. There is a pervasive pattern of disregard for and violation of the rights of others occurring since age 15 years, as indicated by three (or more) of the following:
   (1) failure to conform to social norms with respect to lawful behaviors as indicated by repeatedly performing acts that are grounds for arrest
   (2) deceitfulness, as indicated by repeated lying, use of aliases, or conning others for personal profit or pleasure
   (3) impulsivity or failure to plan ahead
   (4) irritability and aggressiveness, as indicated by repeated physical fights or assaults
   (5) reckless disregard for safety of self or others
   (6) consistent irresponsibility, as indicated by repeated failure to sustain consistent work behavior or honor financial obligations
   (7) lack of remorse, as indicated by being indifferent to or rationalizing having hurt, mistreated, or stolen from another
B. The individual is at least age 18 years.
C. There is evidence of conduct disorder with onset before age 15 years.
D. The occurrence of antisocial behavior is not exclusively during the course of schizophrenia or a manic episode.

tions and collaboration can permit them to have a disruptive influence on treatment teams and other patients. However, there is little evidence to suggest that this disorder can be successfully treated by usual psychiatric interventions. Of interest, nonetheless, are reports suggesting that in confined settings, such as the military or prisons, depressive and introspective concerns may surface (Vaillant 1975). Under these circumstances, confrontation by peers may bring about changes in the antisocial person's social behaviors. It is also notable that some antisocial patients demonstrate an ability to form a therapeutic alliance with psychotherapists, which augurs well for these patients' future course (Woody et al. 1985). These findings contrast with the clinical tradition that emphasizes such persons' inability to learn from harmful consequences. Yet longitudinal follow-up studies have shown that the prevalence of this disorder diminishes with age as these individuals become more aware of the social and interpersonal maladaptiveness of their most noxious social behaviors.

Borderline Personality Disorder

Clinical Features

Borderline personality disorder is characterized by instability and dysfunction in affective, behavioral, and interpersonal domains. Central to the psychopathology of this disorder are a severely impaired capacity for attachment and predictably maladaptive behavior patterns related to separation (Gunderson 1996). When borderline patients feel cared for, held on to, and supported, depressive features (notably loneliness and emptiness) are most evident (Table 14–6). When there is the threat of losing such a sustaining relationship, the idealized image of a beneficent caregiver is replaced by a devalued image of a cruel persecutor. This shift is called *splitting*. An impending separation also evokes intense abandonment fears. To minimize these fears and to prevent the separation, rageful accusations of mistreatment and cruelty and angry self-destructive behaviors may occur. These behaviors often elicit a guilty or fearful protective response from others.

Another central feature of this disorder is extreme affective instability that often leads to impulsive (Herpertz et al. 1997) and self-destructive (Kemperman et al. 1997) behaviors. These episodes are usually brief and reactive and involve extreme alternations between mood states. The experience and expression of anger can be particularly difficult for the borderline patient. During periods of unusual stress, dissociative experiences, ideas of reference, or desperate impulsive acts (including substance abuse and promiscuity) commonly occur.

TABLE 14–6. DSM-IV-TR diagnostic criteria for borderline personality disorder

A pervasive pattern of instability of interpersonal relationships, self-image, and affects, and marked impulsivity beginning by early adulthood and present in a variety of contexts, as indicated by five (or more) of the following:

(1) frantic efforts to avoid real or imagined abandonment. **Note:** Do not include suicidal or self-mutilating behavior covered in Criterion 5.

(2) a pattern of unstable and intense interpersonal relationships characterized by alternating between extremes of idealization and devaluation

(3) identity disturbance: markedly and persistently unstable self-image or sense of self

(4) impulsivity in at least two areas that are potentially self-damaging (e.g., spending, sex, substance abuse, reckless driving, binge eating). **Note:** Do not include suicidal or self-mutilating behavior covered in Criterion 5.

(5) recurrent suicidal behavior, gestures, or threats, or self-mutilating behavior

(6) affective instability due to a marked reactivity of mood (e.g., intense episodic dysphoria, irritability, or anxiety usually lasting a few hours and only rarely more than a few days)

(7) chronic feelings of emptiness

(8) inappropriate, intense anger or difficulty controlling anger (e.g., frequent displays of temper, constant anger, recurrent physical fights)

(9) transient, stress-related paranoid ideation or severe dissociative symptoms

Differential Diagnosis

Borderline patients' intense feelings of being bad or evil are distinctly different from the idealized self-image of narcissistic persons. Although patients with borderline personality disorder, like persons with antisocial personality disorder, may be reckless and impulsive, their behaviors are primarily interpersonally oriented and aimed toward obtaining support rather than materialistic gains.

Treatment

Borderline patients are high utilizers of psychiatric outpatient, inpatient, and psychopharmacologic treatment (Bender et al. 2001). The extensive literature on the treatment of borderline personality disorder universally notes the extreme difficulties that clinicians encounter with these patients. These problems derive from the patients' appeal to their treaters' nurturing qualities and their rageful accusations in response to their treaters' perceived failures. Often therapists develop intense countertransference reactions that lead them to attempt to re-parent or reject borderline patients. As a consequence, regardless of the treatment approach used, personal maturity and considerable clinical experience are important assets.

As a result of the work of Kernberg (1968) and Masterson (1972), much of the treatment literature has focused on the value of intensive exploratory psychotherapies directed at modifying borderline patients' basic character structure. However, this literature has increasingly suggested that improvement may be related not to the acquisition of insight but to the corrective experience of developing a stable, trusting relationship with a therapist who fails to retaliate in response to these patients' angry and disruptive behaviors. Paralleling this development has been the suggestion that supportive psychotherapies or group therapies may bring about similar changes. Recent evidence has provided support for the effectiveness of an 18-month psychoanalytic treatment program in a partial hospital setting (Bateman and Fonagy 1999). In addition, a long-term, phased model of psychodynamic therapy that combined hospital-based and community-based strategies was reported to be more effective than hospital-based treatment alone (Chiesa and Fonagy 2000).

Treatment of borderline patients has now expanded to include pharmacological and cognitive-behavioral interventions (American Psychiatric Association 2001). Although no one medication has been found to have dramatic or predictable effects, studies indicate that many medications may diminish specific problems such as impulsivity, affective lability, or intermittent cognitive and perceptual disturbances (Table 14–7), as well as irritability and aggressive behavior (Coccaro and Kavoussi 1997; Cornelius et al. 1993; Cowdry and Gardner 1988; Salzman et al. 1995; Soloff 1989; Soloff et al. 1993). Linehan et al. (1991) demonstrated that behavioral treatment consisting of a once-weekly individual and once-weekly group regimen can effectively diminish the self-destructive behaviors and hospitalization of borderline patients. The success and cost benefits of this treatment, called *dialectical behavior therapy*, have led to its rapid adoption and modification in a variety of settings. In general, the profusion of treatment modalities and the introduction of empiricism point toward the increasing use of more focused treatment strategies.

Histrionic Personality Disorder

Clinical Features

Central to histrionic personality disorder is an overconcern with attention and appearance (Table 14–8). Persons with this disorder spend an excessive amount of

TABLE 14–7.　Medication efficacy in borderline personality disorder

Medication	Mood	Suicidality/ self-destructiveness	Impulsivity	Psychosis-like features
Monoamine oxidase inhibitors	+	+	+	?
Serotonin reuptake inhibitors	++	++	++	+
Tricyclic antidepressants	±	±	±	±
Antipsychotics	+	+	+	++
Mood stabilizers	+	+	+	+
Benzodiazepines	±	–	–	?

Note.　The information in this table should be considered tentative; some medications have received relatively little investigation, many medication trials have been small and open, and few of the medications listed have been directly compared with one another. ++ = clear improvement; + = modest improvement; ± = variable improvement or worsening; – = some worsening; ? = unknown. Most published studies of serotonin reuptake inhibitors have used fluoxetine.

time seeking attention and making themselves attractive. The desire to be found attractive may lead to inappropriately seductive or provocative dress and flirtatious behavior, and the desire for attention may lead to other flamboyant acts or self-dramatizing behavior. All of these features reflect these persons' underlying insecurity about their value as anything other than a fetching companion. Persons with histrionic personality disorder also display an effusive but labile and suspiciously shallow range of feelings. They are often overly impressionistic and given to hyperbolic descriptions of others (e.g., "She's wonderful" or "She's horrible"). More generally, these persons do not attend to detail or facts, and they are reluctant or unable to make reasoned critical analyses of problems or situations. Persons with this disorder often present with complaints of depression, somatic problems of unclear origin, and a history of disappointing romantic relationships.

Differential Diagnosis

This disorder can be confused with dependent, borderline, and narcissistic personality disorders. Histrionic individuals are often willing, even eager, to have others make decisions and organize their activities for them. However, unlike individuals with dependent personality disorder, histrionic persons are uninhibited and lively companions who willfully forgo appearing autonomous because they believe that others desire this. Unlike individuals with borderline personality disorder, they do not perceive themselves as bad, and they lack ongoing problems with rage or willful self-destructiveness. Individuals with narcissistic personality disorder also seek attention to sustain their self-esteem but differ in that their self-esteem is characterized by grandiosity, and the attention they crave must be admiring—for example, unlike the histrionic individual, they would not want to be described as "cute" or "silly."

Treatment

Individual psychodynamic psychotherapy, including psychoanalysis, remains the cornerstone of most treatment for persons with histrionic personality disorder. This treatment is directed at increasing

TABLE 14–8. DSM-IV-TR diagnostic criteria for histrionic personality disorder

A pervasive pattern of excessive emotionality and attention seeking, beginning by early adulthood and present in a variety of contexts, as indicated by five (or more) of the following:

(1) is uncomfortable in situations in which he or she is not the center of attention

(2) interaction with others is often characterized by inappropriate sexually seductive or provocative behavior

(3) displays rapidly shifting and shallow expression of emotions

(4) consistently uses physical appearance to draw attention to self

(5) has a style of speech that is excessively impressionistic and lacking in detail

(6) shows self-dramatization, theatricality, and exaggerated expression of emotion

(7) is suggestible, i.e., easily influenced by others or circumstances

(8) considers relationships to be more intimate than they actually are

patients' awareness of 1) how their self-esteem is maladaptively tied to their ability to attract attention at the expense of developing other skills, and 2) how their shallow relationships and emotional experience reflect unconscious fears of real commitments. Much of this increase in awareness occurs through analysis of the here-and-now doctor–patient relationship rather than through the reconstruction of childhood experiences. Therapists should be aware that the typical idealization and eroticization that such patients bring into treatment are the material for exploration, and thus therapists should be aware of countertransferential gratification.

Narcissistic Personality Disorder

Clinical Features

Because persons with narcissistic personality disorder have grandiose self-esteem,

they are vulnerable to intense reactions when their self-image is damaged (Table 14–9). They respond with strong feelings of hurt or anger to even small slights, rejections, defeats, or criticisms. As a result, persons with narcissistic personality disorder usually go to great lengths to avoid exposure to such experiences and, when that fails, react by becoming devaluative or rageful. Serious depression can ensue, which is the usual precipitant for their seeking clinical help. In relationships, narcissistic persons are often quite distant, try to sustain "an illusion of self-sufficiency" (Modell 1975), and may exploit others for self-serving ends. They are likely to feel that those with whom they associate need to be special and unique because they see themselves in these terms; thus, they usually wish to be associated only with persons, institutions, or possessions that will confirm their sense of superiority. The DSM-IV criteria are most accurate in identifying the arrogant, socially conspicuous forms of narcissistic personality disorder; however, there are other forms in which a conviction of personal superiority is hidden behind social withdrawal and a facade of self-sacrifice and even humility (Cooper and Ronningstam 1992).

Differential Diagnosis

Narcissistic personality disorder can be most readily confused with histrionic and antisocial personality disorders. Like persons with antisocial personality disorder, those with narcissistic personality disorder are capable of exploiting others but usually rationalize their behavior on the basis of the specialness of their goals or their personal virtue. In contrast, antisocial persons' goals are materialistic, and their rationalizations, if offered, are based on a view that others would do the same to them. The narcissistic person's excessive pride in achievements, relative constraint

TABLE 14–9.   DSM-IV-TR diagnostic criteria for narcissistic personality disorder

A pervasive pattern of grandiosity (in fantasy or behavior), need for admiration, and lack of empathy, beginning by early adulthood and present in a variety of contexts, as indicated by five (or more) of the following:

(1) has a grandiose sense of self-importance (e.g., exaggerates achievements and talents, expects to be recognized as superior without commensurate achievements)

(2) is preoccupied with fantasies of unlimited success, power, brilliance, beauty, or ideal love

(3) believes that he or she is "special" and unique and can only be understood by, or should associate with, other special or high-status people (or institutions)

(4) requires excessive admiration

(5) has a sense of entitlement, i.e., unreasonable expectations of especially favorable treatment or automatic compliance with his or her expectations

(6) is interpersonally exploitative, i.e., takes advantage of others to achieve his or her own ends

(7) lacks empathy: is unwilling to recognize or identify with the feelings and needs of others

(8) is often envious of others or believes that others are envious of him or her

(9) shows arrogant, haughty behaviors or attitudes

in expression of feelings, and disregard for other people's rights and sensitivities help distinguish him or her from persons with histrionic personality disorder. Perhaps the most difficult differential diagnostic problem is whether a person who meets criteria for narcissistic personality disorder has a stable personality disorder or an adjustment reaction. When the emergence of narcissistic traits has been defensively triggered by experiences of failure or rejection, these traits may diminish radically and self-esteem may be restored when new relationships or successes occur.

Treatment

Individual psychodynamic psychotherapy, including psychoanalysis, is the cornerstone of treatment for persons with narcissistic personality disorder. Following Kohut's lead, some therapists believe that the vulnerability to narcissistic injury indicates that intervention should be directed at conveying empathy for the patient's sensitivities and disappointments. This approach, in theory, allows a positive idealized transference to develop that will then be gradually disillusioned by the inevitable frustrations encountered in therapy—disillusionment that will clarify the excessive nature of the patient's reactions to frustrations and disappointments. An alternative view, explicated by Kernberg (1974), is that the vulnerability should be addressed earlier and more directly through interpretations and confrontations by which these persons will come to recognize their grandiosity and its maladaptive consequences. With either approach, the psychotherapeutic process usually requires a relatively intensive schedule over a period of years in which the narcissistic patient's hypersensitivity to slights is foremost in the therapist's mind and interventions.

Avoidant Personality Disorder

Clinical Features

Persons with avoidant personality disorder experience excessive and pervasive anxiety and discomfort in social situations and in intimate relationships (Table 14–10). Although strongly desiring relationships, they avoid them because they fear being ridiculed, criticized, rejected, or humiliated. These fears reflect their low self-esteem and hypersensitivity to negative evaluation by others. When they do enter into social situations or relationships, they feel inept and are self-conscious, shy, awk-

TABLE 14–10. DSM-IV-TR diagnostic criteria for avoidant personality disorder

A pervasive pattern of social inhibition, feelings of inadequacy, and hypersensitivity to negative evaluation, beginning by early adulthood and present in a variety of contexts, as indicated by four (or more) of the following:

(1) avoids occupational activities that involve significant interpersonal contact, because of fears of criticism, disapproval, or rejection
(2) is unwilling to get involved with people unless certain of being liked
(3) shows restraint within intimate relationships because of the fear of being shamed or ridiculed
(4) is preoccupied with being criticized or rejected in social situations
(5) is inhibited in new interpersonal situations because of feelings of inadequacy
(6) views self as socially inept, personally unappealing, or inferior to others
(7) is unusually reluctant to take personal risks or to engage in any new activities because they may prove embarrassing

ward, and preoccupied with being criticized or rejected. Their lives are constricted in that they tend to avoid not only relationships but also new activities because they fear that they will embarrass or humiliate themselves.

Differential Diagnosis

Schizoid personality disorder also involves social isolation, but the schizoid person does not desire relationships, whereas the avoidant person desires them but avoids them because of anxiety and fears of humiliation and rejection. Whereas avoidant personality disorder is characterized by avoidance of situations and relationships involving possible rejection or disappointment, Axis I social phobia usually consists of specific fears related to social performance (e.g., a fear of saying something in-

appropriate or of being unable to answer questions in social situations).

Treatment

Because of their excessive fear of rejection and criticism and their reluctance to form relationships, persons with avoidant personality disorder may be difficult to engage in treatment. Engagement in psychotherapy may be facilitated by the therapist's use of supportive techniques, sensitivity to the patient's hypersensitivity, and gentle interpretation of the defensive use of avoidance. Early in treatment, these patients may tolerate only supportive techniques; however, they may eventually respond well to many types of psychotherapy, including short-term, long-term, and psychoanalytic approaches. Clinicians treating these patients should be aware of the potential for countertransference reactions such as overprotectiveness, hesitancy to adequately challenge the patient, or excessive expectations for change.

Although few data exist, it seems likely that assertiveness and social skills training may increase patients' confidence and willingness to take risks in social situations. Cognitive techniques that gently challenge patients' pathological assumptions about their sense of ineptness may also be useful. Group experiences—perhaps, in particular, homogeneous supportive groups that emphasize the development of social skills—may prove useful for avoidant patients.

Some data suggest that avoidant personality disorder may improve with treatment with monoamine oxidase inhibitors or serotonin reuptake inhibitors (Deltito and Stam 1989; Versiani et al. 1992). Anxiolytics sometimes help patients better manage anxiety (especially severe anxiety) caused by facing previously avoided situations or trying new behaviors.

Dependent Personality Disorder

Clinical Features

Dependent personality disorder is characterized by an excessive need to be cared for by others, which leads to submissive and clinging behavior and excessive fears of separation from others (Table 14–11). Although these individuals are able to care for themselves, they so doubt their abilities and judgment, and they view others as so much stronger and more capable than they, that they can be quite disabled. These persons excessively rely on "powerful" others to initiate and perform tasks for them, make their decisions, assume responsibility for their actions, and guide them through life. Low self-esteem and doubt about their effectiveness lead them to avoid positions of responsibility. Because they feel unable to function without excessive guidance, they go to great lengths to maintain the dependent relationship. They may, for example, always agree with those on whom they depend, and they tend to be excessively clinging, submissive, passive, and self-sacrificing. If the dependent relationship ends, these individuals feel helpless and fearful because they feel incapable of caring for themselves, and they often indiscriminately find another person with whom to have a relationship so that they can be provided with direction and nurturance—an unfulfilling or even an abusive relationship may seem better than being on their own.

Differential Diagnosis

Although persons with borderline personality disorder also dread being alone and need ongoing support, dependent persons want others to assume a controlling function that would frighten the borderline patient. Moreover, persons with dependent personality disorder become appeasing rather than rageful or self-destructive

TABLE 14–11. DSM-IV-TR diagnostic criteria for dependent personality disorder

A pervasive and excessive need to be taken care of that leads to submissive and clinging behavior and fears of separation, beginning by early adulthood and present in a variety of contexts, as indicated by five (or more) of the following:

(1) has difficulty making everyday decisions without an excessive amount of advice and reassurance from others
(2) needs others to assume responsibility for most major areas of his or her life
(3) has difficulty expressing disagreement with others because of fear of loss of support or approval. **Note:** Do not include realistic fears of retribution.
(4) has difficulty initiating projects or doing things on his or her own (because of a lack of self-confidence in judgment or abilities rather than a lack of motivation or energy)
(5) goes to excessive lengths to obtain nurturance and support from others, to the point of volunteering to do things that are unpleasant
(6) feels uncomfortable or helpless when alone because of exaggerated fears of being unable to care for himself or herself
(7) urgently seeks another relationship as a source of care and support when a close relationship ends
(8) is unrealistically preoccupied with fears of being left to take care of himself or herself

when threatened with separation. Although both avoidant and dependent personality disorders are characterized by low self-esteem, rejection sensitivity, and an excessive need for reassurance, persons with dependent personality disorder seek out rather than avoid relationships, and they quickly and indiscriminately replace ended relationships instead of further withdrawing from others.

Treatment

Patients with dependent personality disorder often enter therapy with complaints of depression or anxiety that may be precipitated by the threatened or actual loss of a dependent relationship. They often respond well to various types of individual psychotherapy. Treatment may be particularly helpful if it explores the patients' fears of independence; uses the transference to explore their dependency; and is directed toward increasing patients' self-esteem, sense of effectiveness, assertiveness, and independent functioning. These patients often seek an excessively dependent relationship with the therapist, which can lead to countertransference problems that may actually reinforce their dependence. The therapist may, for example, overprotect or be overly directive with the patient, give inappropriate reassurance and support, or prolong the treatment unnecessarily. He or she may also have excessive expectations for change or withdraw from a patient who is perceived as too needy.

Group therapy and cognitive-behavioral therapy aimed at increasing independent functioning, including assertiveness and social skills training, may be useful for some patients. If the patient is in a relationship that is maintaining and reinforcing his or her excessive dependence, couples or family therapy may be helpful.

Obsessive-Compulsive Personality Disorder

Clinical Features

As Freud noted, and as DSM-IV criteria reflect, persons with obsessive-compulsive personality disorder are excessively orderly (Table 14–12). They are neat, punctual, overly organized, and overconscientious. Although these traits might be considered virtues, especially in cultures that subscribe to the Puritan work ethic, to qualify as obsessive-compulsive personality disorder the traits must be so extreme

that they cause significant distress or impairment in functioning. As Abraham (1923) noted, these individuals' perseverativeness is unproductive. For example, attention to detail is so excessive or time consuming that the point of the activity is lost, conscientiousness is so extreme that it causes rigidity and inflexibility, and perfectionism interferes with task completion. And although these individuals tend to work extremely hard, they do so at the expense of leisure activities and relationships. As Shapiro (1965) pointed out, the most characteristic thought of obsessive-compulsive persons is "I should"—a phrase that aptly reflects their severe superego and captures their overly high standards, drivenness, and excessive conscientiousness, perfectionism, rigidity, and devotion to work and duties.

These individuals also tend to be overly concerned with control—not only over the details of their own lives but also over their emotions and other people. They have difficulty expressing warm and tender feelings, often using stilted, distant phrasing that reveals little of their inner experience. And they may be obstinate and reluctant to delegate tasks or to work with others unless others submit exactly to their way of doing things, which reflects their need for interpersonal control as well as their fear of making mistakes. Their tendency to doubt and worry also manifests itself in their inability to discard worn-out or worthless objects that might be needed for future catastrophes, and, as Freud and Jones noted, persons with obsessive-compulsive personality are miserly toward themselves and others. A caricatured description of such persons is Rado's (1959) "living machines."

Differential Diagnosis

Obsessive-compulsive personality disorder differs from Axis I obsessive-compulsive disorder in that the latter disorder

TABLE 14–12. DSM-IV-TR diagnostic criteria for obsessive-compulsive personality disorder

A pervasive pattern of preoccupation with orderliness, perfectionism, and mental and interpersonal control, at the expense of flexibility, openness, and efficiency, beginning by early adulthood and present in a variety of contexts, as indicated by four (or more) of the following:

(1) is preoccupied with details, rules, lists, order, organization, or schedules to the extent that the major point of the activity is lost

(2) shows perfectionism that interferes with task completion (e.g., is unable to complete a project because his or her own overly strict standards are not met)

(3) is excessively devoted to work and productivity to the exclusion of leisure activities and friendships (not accounted for by obvious economic necessity)

(4) is overconscientious, scrupulous, and inflexible about matters of morality, ethics, or values (not accounted for by cultural or religious identification)

(5) is unable to discard worn-out or worthless objects even when they have no sentimental value

(6) is reluctant to delegate tasks or to work with others unless they submit to exactly his or her way of doing things

(7) adopts a miserly spending style toward both self and others; money is viewed as something to be hoarded for future catastrophes

(8) shows rigidity and stubbornness

consists of specific repetitive thoughts and ritualistic behaviors rather than personality traits. In addition, obsessive-compulsive disorder has traditionally been considered ego-dystonic, whereas obsessive-compulsive personality disorder has been considered ego-syntonic. These two disorders are sometimes, but not necessarily, comorbid.

Treatment

Persons with obsessive-compulsive personality disorder may seem difficult to treat because of their excessive intellectualization and difficulty expressing emotion. However, these patients often respond well to psychoanalytic psychotherapy or psychoanalysis. Therapists usually need to be relatively active in treatment. They should also avoid being drawn into interesting but affectless discussions that are unlikely to have therapeutic benefit. In other words, rather than intellectualizing with the patient, therapists should focus on the feelings these patients usually avoid. Other defenses common in this disorder, such as rationalization, isolation, undoing, and reaction formation, should also be identified and clarified. Power struggles that may occur in treatment offer opportunities to address the patient's excessive need for control.

Cognitive techniques may also be used to diminish the patient's excessive need for control and perfection. Although patients may resist group treatment because of their need for control, dynamically oriented groups that focus on feelings may provide insight and increase their comfort with exploring and expressing new affects.

References

Abraham K: Contributions to the theory of the anal character. Int J Psychoanal 4:400–418, 1923

Alnæs R, Torgersen S: Personality and personality disorders predict development and relapses of major depression. Acta Psychiatr Scand 95:336–342, 1997

American Psychiatric Association: Diagnostic and Statistical Manual of Mental Disorders, 4th Edition. Washington, DC, American Psychiatric Association, 1994

American Psychiatric Association: Practice guideline for the treatment of patients with borderline personality disorder. Am J Psychiatry 158(suppl):1–52, 2001

Bateman A, Fonagy P: Effectiveness of partial hospitalization in the treatment of borderline personality disorder: a randomized controlled trial. Am J Psychiatry 156:1563–1569, 1999

Bender DS, Dolan RT, Skodol AE, et al: Treatment utilization by patients with personality disorders. Am J Psychiatry 158:295–302, 2001

Bernstein DP, Kasapis C, Bergman A: Assessing Axis II disorders by informant interview. J Personal Disord 11:158–167, 1997

Black DW, Bell S, Hulbert J, et al: The importance of Axis II in patients with major depression: a controlled study. J Affect Disord 14:115–122, 1988

Brent DA, Johnson BA, Perper J, et al: Personality disorder, personality traits, impulsive violence, and completed suicide in adolescents. J Am Acad Child Adolesc Psychiatry 33:1080–1086, 1994

Calabrese JR, Woyshville MJ, Kimmel SE, et al: Predictors of valproate response in bipolar rapid cycling. J Clin Psychopharmacol 13:280–283, 1993

Caton CL, Shrout PE, Eagle PF, et al: Risk factors for homelessness among schizophrenic men: a case-control study. Am J Public Health 84:265–270, 1994

Chiesa M, Fonagy P: Cassel personality disorder study. Br J Psychiatry 176:485–491, 2000

Cloninger CR: A systematic method for clinical description and classification of personality variants. Arch Gen Psychiatry 44:573–588, 1987

Coccaro EF, Kavoussi RJ: Fluoxetine and impulsive aggressive behavior in personality-disordered subjects. Arch Gen Psychiatry 54:1081–1088, 1997

Colom F, Vieta E, Martínez-Arán A, et al: Clinical factors associated with treatment noncompliance in euthymic bipolar patients. J Clin Psychiatry 61:549–555, 2000

Cooper AM, Ronningstam E: Narcissistic personality disorder, in American Psychiatric Press Review of Psychiatry, Vol 11. Edited by Tasman A, Riba ME. Washington, DC, American Psychiatric Press, 1992, pp 80–97

Cornelius JR, Soloff PH, Perel JM, et al: Continuation pharmacotherapy of borderline personality disorder with haloperidol and phenelzine. Am J Psychiatry 150:1843–1848, 1993

Cowdry RW, Gardner DL: Pharmacotherapy of borderline personality disorder: alprazolam, carbamazepine, trifluoperazine, and tranylcypromine. Arch Gen Psychiatry 45:111–119, 1988

Deltito JA, Stam M: Psychopharmacological treatment of avoidant personality disorder. Compr Psychiatry 30:498–504, 1989

Dinwiddie SH, Bucholz KK: Psychiatric diagnoses of self-reported child abusers. Child Abuse Negl 17:465–476, 1993

Dinwiddie SH, Reich T, Cloninger CR: Psychiatric comorbidity and suicidality among intravenous drug users. J Clin Psychiatry 53:364–369, 1992

Dunayevich E, Sax KW, Keck PE Jr, et al: Twelve-month outcome in bipolar patients with and without personality disorders. J Clin Psychiatry 61:134–139, 2000

Fals-Stewart W: Personality characteristics of substance abusers: an MCMI cluster typology of recreational drug users treated in a therapeutic community and its relationship to length of stay and outcome. J Pers Assess 59:515–527, 1992

Ferro T, Klein DN: Family history assessment of personality disorders, I: concordance with direct interview and between pairs of informants. J Personal Disord 11:123–136, 1997

Ferro T, Klein D, Schwartz JE, et al: 30 month stability of personality disorder diagnosis in depressed outpatients. Am J Psychiatry 155:653–659, 1998

Gandhi N, Tyrer P, Evans K, et al: A randomized controlled trial of community oriented and hospital-oriented care for discharged psychiatric patients: influence of personality disorder on police contacts. J Personal Disord 15:94–102, 2001

Goldberg SC, Schulz C, Schulz PM, et al: Borderline and schizotypal personality disorders treated with low-dose thiothixene vs placebo. Arch Gen Psychiatry 43:680–686, 1986

Grilo CM, McGlashan TH, Oldham JM: Course and stability of personality disorders. J Pract Psychiatry Behav Health 1:61–75, 1999

Gunderson JG: The borderline patient's intolerance of aloneness: insecure attachment and therapist availability. Am J Psychiatry 153:752–758, 1996

Hare RD, Hart SD, Harpur TJ: Psychopathy and the DSM-IV criteria for antisocial personality disorder. J Abnorm Psychol 100:391–398, 1991

Hawton K, Fagg J, Platt S, et al: Factors associated with suicide after parasuicide in young people. BMJ 306:1641–1644, 1993

Herpertz S, Gretzer EM, Steinmeyer V, et al: Affective instability and impulsivity in personality disorder. J Affect Disord 44:31–37, 1997

Hillbrand M, Krystal JH, Sharpe KS, et al: Clinical predictors of self-mutilation in hospitalized forensic patients. J Nerv Ment Dis 182:9–13, 1994

Jenike MA, Baer L, Minichiello WE, et al: Coexistent obsessive-compulsive disorder and schizotypal personality disorder: a poor prognostic indicator (letter). Arch Gen Psychiatry 43:296, 1986

Jones M: The Therapeutic Community: A New Treatment in Psychiatry. New York, Basic Books, 1953

Jordan BK, Schlenger WE, Fairbank JA, et al: Prevalence of psychiatric disorders among incarcerated women. Arch Gen Psychiatry 53:513–519, 1996

Kelstrup A, Lund K, Lauritsen B, et al: Satisfaction with care reported by psychiatric inpatients. Relationship to diagnosis and medical treatment. Acta Psychiatr Scand 87:374–379, 1993

Kemperman I, Russ MJ, Shearin E: Self-injurious behavior and mood regulation in borderline patients. J Personal Disord 11:146–157, 1997

Kent S, Fogarty M, Yellowlees P: A review of studies of heavy users of psychiatric services. Psychiatr Serv 46:1247–1253, 1995

Kernberg OF: Treatment of patients with borderline personality organization. Int J Psychoanal 49:600–619, 1968

Kernberg OF: Further contributions to the treatment of narcissistic personalities. Int J Psychoanal 55:215–240, 1974

Koenigsberg HW, Kaplan RD, Gilmore MM, et al: The relationship between syndrome and personality disorder in DSM-III: experience with 2,462 patients. Am J Psychiatry 142:207–212, 1985

Lenzenweger MF, Loranger AW, Korfine L, et al: Detecting personality disorders in a nonclinical population. Arch Gen Psychiatry 54:345–351, 1997

Lewinsohn PM, Rhode P, Seeley JR, et al: Natural course of adolescent major depressive disorder in a community sample: predictors of recurrence in young adults. Am J Psychiatry 157:1584–1591, 2000

Liebowitz MR, Stone MH, Turkat ID: Treatment of personality disorders, in Psychiatry Update: American Psychiatric Association Annual Review, Vol 5. Edited by Frances AJ, Hales RE. Washington, DC, American Psychiatric Press, 1986, pp 356–393

Linehan MM, Armstrong HE, Suarez A, et al: Cognitive behavioral treatment of chronically parasuicidal borderline patients. Arch Gen Psychiatry 48:1060–1064, 1991

Loranger AW: The impact of DSM-III on diagnostic practice in a university hospital. Arch Gen Psychiatry 47:672–675, 1990

Markovitz PJ, Calabrese JR, Schulz SC, et al: Fluoxetine in the treatment of borderline and schizotypal personality disorders. Am J Psychiatry 148:1064–1067, 1991

Masterson JF: Treatment of the Borderline Adolescent: A Developmental Approach. New York, Wiley-Interscience, 1972

McDonald AS, Davey GCL: Psychiatric disorders and accidental injury. Clinical Psychology Review 16:105–127, 1996

Miller RJ, Zadolinnyj K, Hafner RJ: Profiles and predictors of assaultiveness for different psychiatric ward populations. Am J Psychiatry 150:1368–1373, 1993

Modell AH: A narcissistic defense against affects and the illusion of self-sufficiency. Int J Psychoanal 56:275–282, 1975

Nelson JC, Mazure CM, Jatlow PI: Characteristics of desipramine-refractory depression. J Clin Psychiatry 55:12–19, 1994

O'Leary D, Costello F: Personality and outcome in depression: an 18-month prospective follow-up study. J Affect Disord 63:67–78, 2001

Perry JC, Banon E, Ianni F: Effectiveness of psychotherapy for personality disorders. Am J Psychiatry 156:1312–1321, 1999

Pirkis J, Burgess P, Jolley D: Suicide attempts by psychiatric patients in acute inpatient, long-stay inpatient and community care. Soc Psychiatry Psychiatr Epidemiol 34: 634–644, 1999

Rado S: Obsessive behavior, in American Handbook of Psychiatry, Vol 1. Edited by Arieti S. New York, Basic Books, 1959, pp 324–344

Raine A: Features of borderline personality and violence. J Clin Psychology 49:277–281, 1993

Reich JH: DSM-III personality disorders and the outcome of treated panic disorder. Am J Psychiatry 145:1149–1152, 1988

Reich J[H], Boerstler H, Yates W, et al: Utilization of medical resources in persons with DSM-III personality disorders in a community sample. Int J Psychiatry Med 19:1–9, 1989

Reich W: On the technique of character analysis, in Character Analysis, 3rd Edition. New York, Simon & Schuster, 1949, pp 39–113

Salzman C, Wolfson AN, Schatzberg A, et al: Effect of fluoxetine on anger in symptomatic volunteers with borderline personality disorder. J Clin Psychopharmacol 15:23–29, 1995

Serban G, Siegel S: Response of borderline and schizotypal patients to small doses of thiothixene and haloperidol. Am J Psychiatry 141:1455–1458, 1984

Shapiro D: Neurotic Styles. New York, Basic Books, 1965

Siever LJ, Davis KL: A psychobiological perspective on the personality disorders. Am J Psychiatry 148:1647–1658, 1991

Soloff PH: Psychopharmacologic therapies in borderline personality disorder, in American Psychiatric Press Review of Psychiatry, Vol 8. Edited by Tasman A, Hales RE, Frances AJ. Washington, DC, American Psychiatric Press, 1989, pp 65–83

Soloff PH, Cornelius J, George A, et al: Efficacy of phenelzine and haloperidol in borderline personality disorder. Arch Gen Psychiatry 50:377–385, 1993

Stone M: Schizotypal personality: psychotherapeutic aspects. Schizophr Bull 11:576–589, 1985

Turkat I, Maisto S: Application of the experimental method to the formulation and modification of personality disorders, in Clinical Handbook of Psychological Disorders. Edited by Barlow D. New York, Guilford, 1985, pp 502–570

Vaillant GE: Sociopathy as a human process: a viewpoint. Arch Gen Psychiatry 32:178–183, 1975

Versiani M, Nardi AE, Mundim FD, et al: Pharmacotherapy of social phobia. A controlled study with moclobemide and phenelzine. Br J Psychiatry 161:353–360, 1992

Weissman MM: The epidemiology of personality disorders: a 1990 update. J Personal Disord 7:44–62, 1993

Widiger TA, Frances AJ: Interviews and inventories for the measurement of personality disorders. Clinical Psychology Review 7: 49–75, 1987

Woody GE, McLellan AT, Luborsky L, et al: Sociopathy and psychotherapy outcome. Arch Gen Psychiatry 42:1081–1086, 1985

Yonkers KA, Dyck IR, Warshaw M, et al: Factors predicting the clinical course of generalised anxiety disorder. Br J Psychiatry 176:544–549, 2000

CHAPTER 15

Disorders Usually First Diagnosed in Infancy, Childhood, or Adolescence

Charles W. Popper, M.D.

G. Davis Gammon, M.D.

Scott A. West, M.D.

Charles E. Bailey, M.D.

Childhood is recognized in psychiatry as a period of vulnerability and progressive development toward adult personality and character. The psychiatric disorders in children and adolescents are increasingly coming into focus as serious but treatable conditions and as precursors of adult psychopathology.

In this chapter, the discrete psychopathological entities that are usually first diagnosed in youth are discussed. These disorders often emerge in combinations, change in presentation during maturation, interact with one another over time, and can be obscured or amplified by intervening developmental events. As in DSM-IV-TR (American Psychiatric Association 2000), these childhood-onset disorders are described here as crystalline abstract entities, a presentation that does not respect the individuality of their appearance in each child, cradled in a particular family and society, and undergoing continual change.

The primary "work" of children is to change and grow, a task that reflects their push to interact and modify in multiple dimensions. Rigid crystallized descriptions of their disorders do not convey the liveliness and energy of children who are coping and growing in ways that are characteristic of these disorders and in ways quite independent of psychiatric states.

The main message of this chapter concerns the dynamic undercurrent: not the rigidity of diagnostic categories but the flux and change that these abstract entities produce in the lives of children—and of the adults they become.

Where were adult psychiatric patients during their childhoods? Part of the answer rests in the ability to observe and diagnose disorders in children. Not long ago, it was believed that mood disorders did not begin until mid- or late adolescence. Now it is known that all "adult" psychiatric disorders in DSM-IV-TR can begin during childhood. Any diagnosis can be used as a primary diagnostic label in a child. Even personality disorders, except for antisocial personality disorder, may be diagnosed in children if the characteristics of the personality disorder appear pervasive and unusually persistent. We also now know that all childhood-onset disorders can have major sequelae in adults or develop into adult disorders.

Medical conditions in children are crucial in evaluating their behavior; even mild or transient Axis III medical problems can cause flagrant behavioral symptoms, especially in young children (Cantwell and Baker 1988). The prevalence of psychiatric disorders is doubled in children with non–central nervous system (CNS) physical disabilities and diseases. On Axis IV, DSM-IV-TR provides a modified version of the Severity of Psychosocial Stressors Scale for children and adolescents. Parental absence or neglect, physical and sexual abuse, psychiatric disorders among caregivers, and even puberty exert age-specific effects on children. The Axis V Global Assessment of Functioning Scale incorporates features of the Children's Global Assessment Scale (Shaffer et al. 1983).

Developmental stage can influence the presentation, significance, and course of a psychiatric disorder. Coping functions and adaptive strengths change with development and are not related in a simple way to chronological age. Under the current DSM system, such developmental characteristics are not classified, and the clinician is left to personal judgment to assess the developmental stage of the individual and the developmental significance of presenting symptoms.

The DSM-IV-TR category "Disorders Usually First Diagnosed in Infancy, Childhood, or Adolescence" includes conditions that not only begin in childhood but also are typically *diagnosed* during childhood (Table 15–1). Some behavioral patterns

are normal at certain developmental stages but become pathological at later developmental stages (e.g., separation anxiety disorder, enuresis, encopresis, and oppositional defiant disorder). Most of the behaviors manifested in these disorders, however, are not "normal" at any age.

In this chapter, we do not discuss adjustment disorders in children (Newcorn and Strain 1992) or problems of parent–child relationships. Child development and child psychiatric treatment are discussed in Chapters 1 and 20, respectively. Important psychiatric disorders in youth, including mood and anxiety disorders, substance use disorders, eating disorders, and schizophrenia, also are described elsewhere in this volume. Although these conditions generally present with symptoms during childhood, they are frequently not diagnosed until the individual reaches maturity.

Disruptive Behavior Disorders

Attention-Deficit/ Hyperactivity Disorder

Children and adults with attention-deficit/hyperactivity disorder (ADHD) show the behavioral characteristics of impulsivity and motor hyperactivity and the cognitive characteristics of inattention. The DSM-IV-TR criteria (Table 15–2) no longer suggest that ADHD is a childhood disorder—a loose mix of scattered attention and annoying behaviors—or a problem that is confined to one setting. It is now understood that ADHD persists into adulthood in many individuals (Biederman 1998; Faraone et al. 2000a; T. Spencer et al. 1998a; Wender 1998), and this body of research characterizing the phenomenology, comorbidity, and treatment of adult populations is growing. Thus far, most

TABLE 15–1. DSM-IV-TR disorders usually first diagnosed in infancy, childhood, or adolescence

Mental retardation
  Mild mental retardation
  Moderate mental retardation
  Severe mental retardation
  Profound mental retardation
  Mental retardation, severity unspecified
Learning disorders
  Reading disorder
  Mathematics disorder
  Disorder of written expression
  Learning disorder not otherwise specified
Motor skills disorder
  Developmental coordination disorder
Pervasive developmental disorders
  Autistic disorder
  Rett's disorder
  Childhood disintegrative disorder
  Asperger's disorder
  Pervasive developmental disorder not
    otherwise specified
**Attention-deficit and disruptive behavior
  disorders**
  Attention-deficit/hyperactivity disorder
    Predominantly inattentive type
    Predominantly hyperactive-impulsive
      type
    Combined type
    Not otherwise specified
  Conduct disorder
  Oppositional defiant disorder
  Disruptive behavior disorder not
    otherwise specified
**Feeding and eating disorders of infancy or
  early childhood**
  Pica
  Rumination disorder of infancy
  Feeding disorder of infancy or early
    childhood
Tic disorders
  Tourette's disorder
  Chronic motor or vocal tic disorder
  Transient tic disorder
  Tic disorder not otherwise specified
Communication disorders
  Expressive language disorder
  Mixed receptive-expressive language
    disorder

TABLE 15–1. DSM-IV-TR disorders usually first diagnosed in infancy, childhood, or adolescence *(continued)*

  Phonological disorder
  Stuttering
  Communication disorder not otherwise
    specified
Elimination disorders
  Encopresis
  Enuresis
**Other disorders of infancy, childhood, or
  adolescence**
  Separation anxiety disorder
  Selective mutism
  Reactive attachment disorder of infancy or
    early childhood
  Stereotypic movement disorder
  Disorder of infancy, childhood, or
    adolescence not otherwise specified

findings concerning ADHD in adults have been consistent with previous findings on ADHD in children and adolescents (Biederman et al. 2000), where most of the available research remains concentrated at this time.

A current debate concerns whether ADHD should be conceptualized in dimensional terms, described by a set of numbers quantifying various symptoms and their severity, or in categorical terms, described as either present or absent—regardless of symptom severity. These two models support different concepts of the illness: ADHD as a diverse group of behavior management problems or as a disorder with a final common physiological pathway. Clinically, both models are useful. Indeed, the National Institute of Mental Health Consensus Statement (1998) concluded that although there are differing clinical models for ADHD, substantial evidence supports both the validity of the disorder and the adverse long-term effects that may result from lack of appropriate diagnosis and treatment.

TABLE 15–2.   DSM-IV-TR diagnostic criteria for attention-deficit/hyperactivity disorder

---

A. Either (1) or (2):
    (1) six (or more) of the following symptoms of **inattention** have persisted for at least 6 months
        to a degree that is maladaptive and inconsistent with developmental level:
        Inattention
        (a) often fails to give close attention to details or makes careless mistakes in schoolwork,
            work, or other activities
        (b) often has difficulty sustaining attention in tasks or play activities
        (c) often does not seem to listen when spoken to directly
        (d) often does not follow through on instructions and fails to finish schoolwork, chores,
            or duties in the workplace (not due to oppositional behavior or failure to understand
            instructions)
        (e) often has difficulty organizing tasks and activities
        (f) often avoids, dislikes, or is reluctant to engage in tasks that require sustained mental
            effort (such as schoolwork or homework)
        (g) often loses things necessary for tasks or activities (e.g., toys, school assignments,
            pencils, books, or tools)
        (h) is often easily distracted by extraneous stimuli
        (i) is often forgetful in daily activities
    (2) six (or more) of the following symptoms of **hyperactivity-impulsivity** have persisted for
        at least 6 months to a degree that is maladaptive and inconsistent with developmental level:
        Hyperactivity
        (a) often fidgets with hands or feet or squirms in seat
        (b) often leaves seat in classroom or in other situations in which remaining seated is
            expected
        (c) often runs about or climbs excessively in situations in which it is inappropriate
            (in adolescents or adults, may be limited to subjective feelings of restlessness)
        (d) often has difficulty playing or engaging in leisure activities quietly
        (e) is often "on the go" or often acts as if "driven by a motor"
        (f) often talks excessively
        Impulsivity
        (g) often blurts out answers before questions have been completed
        (h) often has difficulty awaiting turn
        (i) often interrupts or intrudes on others (e.g., butts into conversations or games)
B. Some hyperactive-impulsive or inattentive symptoms that caused impairment were present
    before age 7 years.
C. Some impairment from the symptoms is present in two or more settings (e.g., at school
    [or work] and at home).
D. There must be clear evidence of clinically significant impairment in social, academic, or
    occupational functioning.
E. The symptoms do not occur exclusively during the course of a pervasive developmental dis-
    order, schizophrenia, or other psychotic disorder and are not better accounted for by another
    mental disorder (e.g., mood disorder, anxiety disorder, dissociative disorder, or a personality
    disorder).
Code based on type:
    314.01   Attention-Deficit/Hyperactivity Disorder, Combined Type:
    if both Criteria A1 and A2 are met for the past 6 months
    314.00   Attention-Deficit/Hyperactivity Disorder, Predominantly Inattentive Type:
    if Criterion A1 is met but Criterion A2 is not met for the past 6 months
    314.01   Attention-Deficit/Hyperactivity Disorder, Predominantly Hyperactive-Impulsive
    Type: if Criterion A2 is met but Criterion A1 is not met for the past 6 months
Coding note: For individuals (especially adolescents and adults) who currently have symptoms
    that no longer meet full criteria, "in partial remission" should be specified.

Clinical Description

Symptoms of ADHD fall into three primary domains: motor hyperactivity, impulsivity, and inattention. These core symptoms may present in different ways at different ages, but they reflect the shared basic characteristics of the disorder (Table 15–3).

Measures of activity and attention are weakly correlated, and these symptom clusters appear to reflect independent dimensions of psychopathology. In factor analyses of behavioral ratings on Conners' Hyperactivity Scale and the Achenbach Child Behavioral Checklist (CBCL; Achenbach and Ruffle 2002), the "hyperactivity" factor emerges robustly as a distinct component of general childhood behavior, and "inattention" emerges as a separate factor, not as powerful but consistent in clinical and community samples of children. This separation between the cognitive and the behavioral factors is clinically useful. The DSM-IV-TR subtyping of ADHD into "predominantly inattentive," "predominantly hyperactive-impulsive," and "combined" types allows the diagnostic label of ADHD to designate three of the most pronounced symptom complexes. Each of these three DSM-IV-TR ADHD subtypes appears to have a distinct prognosis and response to treatment; therefore, a separate clinical assessment of inattention and hyperactivity-impulsivity is necessary when evaluating for ADHD.

The DSM-IV-TR diagnosis of ADHD not otherwise specified (NOS) subsumes conditions similar to ADHD that do not fulfill diagnostic criteria. Although ADHD NOS might be expected to be a diagnosis of convenience rather than a biologically distinct disorder, researchers employing quantitative electroencephalography and evoked response potentials have found electrophysiological characteristics that distinguish ADHD NOS from the three

main forms of ADHD (Kuperman et al. 1996). This finding suggests that an additional subtype of ADHD may indeed exist, currently hidden within the group of patients with ADHD NOS, and that further research in individuals with ADHD NOS may be warranted.

Although individuals with ADHD tend to be symptomatic in many if not all settings, the intensity of symptoms varies across settings. Symptoms tend to be more pronounced in settings with more environmental structure, such as classrooms and restaurants; during high levels of sensory stimulation; and during high emotional states. Children tend to experience more environmental demands at school—where they are expected to maintain concentration, focus, and inhibit their physical and mental impulses—than at home. Indeed, children with ADHD may appear quite different in different environments, with their symptoms often more apparent to observers in crowded waiting rooms or clinic hallways than to a physician in a quiet office.

Although DSM-IV-TR emphasizes the three core symptoms, pathological functioning is also seen in motivation, emotionality, anger control, and aggression. Motivational problems in ADHD can include variability, unpredictability, difficulty in sustaining interest and completing projects, and simple frustration and discouragement. Although these characteristics are considered in DSM-IV-TR to be associated features of ADHD, lack of motivation and difficulty in self-organization may produce more functional interference than do the core symptoms of ADHD. Emotional impulsivity is most obvious in anger and aggressive behavior, symptoms that can be regularly triggered in response to minor provocation. Exploratory behavior can seem aggressive, involving an energetic foraging into new places and things. On entering a room, a child with ADHD

TABLE 15–3. Different presentations of attention-deficit/hyperactivity disorder (ADHD) through the life cycle

Developmental stage	Characteristics of ADHD	Comments
Infancy	Frequent crying; difficult to soothe; sleep disturbances; feeding difficulties	May cry to an extent that interferes with nutritional intake; may be excessively drowsy and unresponsive or sleep poorly because of overreactivity and restlessness.
Preschool	Motor restlessness; insatiable curiosity; vigorous and sometimes destructive play; demanding of parental attention; low-level compliance (especially with boys); excessive temper tantrums; difficulty completing developmental tasks; decreased and/or restless sleep; delays in motor or language development; family difficulties	Often difficult to distinguish from normal behaviors in children at this age; the child seems as if "driven by a motor"; climbs on and gets into things constantly; often accidentally breaks toys and household objects; accidental injuries are also common; severity, frequency, and duration of tantrums far exceed those in children without ADHD.
School age	Easily distracted; engages in off-task activities; unable to sustain attention; impulsive; displays aggression; acts as a "class clown"; social deficits include having difficulty waiting for a turn, following rules, losing gracefully, curbing temper, showing consideration for others; frequently becomes overly excited or may act very silly	May call out in class inappropriately, fidget excessively, have difficulty staying in seat; assignments are frequently messy and disorganized with many mistakes. Symptoms affect academic performance and cause increasing difficulty in peer relationships and social interactions as the child grows older; failures in these areas may lead to poor self-esteem and depression.
Adolescence	Excessive motor activity (e.g., excessive running and climbing, not staying in seat) tends to decrease, although fidgetiness and inner restlessness may continue; problem behaviors include discipline problems, family conflict, anger and emotional lability, difficulty with authority, significant lags in academic performance; poor peer relationships; poor self-esteem; hopelessness; lethargy and lack of motivation, driving mishaps, speeding, accidents	Impulsive symptoms may lead adolescents to break rules and get into conflict with authority figures.

TABLE 15–3. Different presentations of attention-deficit/hyperactivity disorder (ADHD) through the life cycle *(continued)*

Developmental stage	Characteristics of ADHD	Comments
Adulthood	Difficulty with concentration and performing sedentary tasks; disorganization; forgetfulness; losing things; failure to plan; depending on others to maintain order; difficulty keeping track of several things at once; trouble both getting started on and finishing tasks; changing plans or jobs in midstream; misjudging time; restlessness; impulsivity; being "absent-minded"	May have employment difficulties, especially in desk jobs, which may lead to short durations of employment; higher incidence of antisocial acts and arrests than in the general population.

Source. Reprinted with permission from Conners CK, March JS, Frances A, et al. (eds.): "Treatment of Attention-Deficit/Hyperactivity Disorder: Expert Consensus Guidelines." *Journal of Attention Disorders* 4(suppl 1):7–128, 2001.

may immediately begin to touch and climb. These inclinations can lead to rough handling of objects, accidental breakage, intrusive entry into unsafe areas, physical injuries, and even accidental ingestions. Property damage may result without malicious intent.

However, it is important to remember that many children with ADHD do not have behavior problems, hyperactivity, or excessive aggression. The predominantly inattentive type of ADHD is very common and often is found in settings such as primary care offices and learning disorder clinics, where the threshold for evaluation does not require high levels of hyperactivity and/or aggression. In contrast to children with the predominantly hyperactive-impulsive type of ADHD, predominantly inattentive children show more manageable behavior, mild anxiety and shyness, more sluggishness and drowsiness, less impulsivity, less conduct disorder and problem behavior, and more mood and anxiety disorders (Gaub and Carlson 1997; Lahey et al. 1987).

Girls and women with ADHD have received more attention in recent years, as attempts have been made to closely examine populations other than preadolescent boys with ADHD. Historically, girls have been reported to have less impulsivity, hyperactivity, and comorbid conduct disorder than boys (Berry et al. 1985). However, factor analysis of behavioral data in adults with ADHD suggests that certain inattention and impulsivity items load on different factors in men than in women; that is, gender affects factor composition (M.A. Stein et al. 1995). Recent studies indicate that there are far more similarities than differences in core ADHD symptoms between boys and girls (Biederman et al. 1999a; Rucklidge and Tannock 2001). Moreover, these studies have found that girls are at higher risk for more psychological impairment, with

more fear, depression, mood swings, cognitive difficulties, and language problems than boys with ADHD. These recent data seem to dispel the myth that females suffer silently with minimal symptoms, because their outcome is often worse than that of males (Faraone et al. 2000b).

Although inattention and hyperactivity-impulsivity are currently the two defining dimensions of ADHD in DSM-IV-TR, the organizational deficits, motivational problems, and impaired time sense in ADHD deserve considerably more clinical attention and warrant further research because they might constitute additional dimensions of ADHD. Currently, the two-dimensional concept of ADHD has a high degree of clinical usefulness and scientific validity, but the construct of ADHD will likely become more differentiated and multidimensional as research continues.

Epidemiology

In the United States, approximately 6% of school-age children have ADHD (range = 3%–10%). ADHD is present in 30%–50% of children in child psychiatric outpatient clinics and inpatient treatment centers. The strong male predominance in ADHD (3–10 to 1) may be partly the result of diagnostic expectations rather than true predominance. Despite this potential bias, girls are generally reported to constitute up to 25% of children with ADHD and may constitute a higher proportion of the predominantly inattentive subtype.

The prevalence of childhood ADHD has been traditionally higher in the United States than in other countries, a difference that may be a result of diagnostic practices. In the past, about 2% of child psychiatric outpatients in Great Britain had a diagnosis of ADHD compared with 40% in the United States. Prevalence rates have become more uniform among countries as different internationally used diagnostic systems have come into greater concordance.

Etiology

No evidence indicates that there is only one attention deficit or that a single brain mechanism is responsible for all manifestations of ADHD. Similarly, there is no evidence of a single gene defect or a specific mechanism of genetic transmission in ADHD, and the hereditary component is likely to be polygenic. Different etiologies and different sites of pharmacological action may be relevant for different individuals or subpopulations with ADHD.

Genetics. Although family studies have suggested strong genetic and nongenetic contributions (Pauls 1991), the genetic factors appear to predominate (Faraone and Doyle 2001; Sherman et al. 1997). The prevalence of psychopathology is two to three times higher in the relatives of children with ADHD, even after controlling for socioeconomic class and family intactness. In adopted children with ADHD, biological parents have been found to have more psychopathology than adopting parents (Deutsch et al. 1982). Family members of children with ADHD show an increased prevalence of ADHD, conduct disorder and antisocial personality disorder, mood disorders, anxiety disorders, and substance abuse.

Although the extent of genetic influence appears to vary, several specific genes have been implicated in the development of ADHD (Sprich et al. 2000). Indeed, ADHD is most likely a polygenic disorder involving norepinephrine, dopamine, serotonin, γ-aminobutyric acid (GABA), and other neurotransmitters (Comings et al. 2000a).

General medical factors. Various medical factors can lead to the appearance of

ADHD or ADHD-like symptoms, including streptococcal infection, generalized resistance to thyroid hormone, hyperthyroidism, ordinary hunger, and even occasionally constipation. Certain psychiatric medications also may mimic ADHD by inducing anxiety, agitation, mood swings, behavioral activation, or disinhibition. These medications include psychostimulants, antidepressants, anticonvulsants, benzodiazepines, and substances such as caffeine and theophylline.

Pediatric autoimmune neuropsychiatric disorders associated with streptococcal infections (PANDAS), such as obsessive-compulsive disorder (OCD) and Tourette's disorder, also may present with ADHD symptoms. Indeed, about half of the preadolescent children diagnosed with PANDAS have symptoms of ADHD (Peterson et al. 2000).

Because nutrition is a critical factor in the development of the CNS, severe early malnutrition may be a common cause of ADHD worldwide. In children who experience severe malnutrition during the first year of life, 60% show inattention, impulsivity, and hyperactivity persisting at least into adolescence (Galler et al. 1983). In addition, pyloric stenosis is associated with the subsequent appearance of ADHD, even when corrected by age 2 months. At this time, the specific nutritional deficiencies that contribute to the etiology of ADHD are unknown.

Neuromedical factors. Neuromedical etiologies of ADHD include brain damage (often frontal cortex), neurological disorders, low birth weight, extreme perinatal anoxia, and exposure to neurotoxins. Intrauterine exposure to toxic substances, including alcohol, lead, cigarette smoke, and probably cocaine, can produce teratological effects on behavior. For example, fetal alcohol syndrome includes hyperactivity, impulsivity, and inattention as well as physical anomalies and diminished intelligence.

Children with ADHD have higher mean blood lead levels than do their siblings. A large-scale study in Ottawa, Ontario, showed a topological distribution of ADHD children living in public housing, perhaps reflecting the lead-containing paints in residential buildings.

Intrauterine exposure to cigarette smoke also may be associated with ADHD. In one study, 22% of the mothers of children with ADHD smoked during pregnancy, compared with 8% of the mothers of children without ADHD (Milberger et al. 1996).

Obstetrical complications during late pregnancy or delivery occasionally may result in ADHD. Generally, obstetrical difficulties and perinatal asphyxia are not highly correlated with the appearance of neurological disorders such as cerebral palsy (Nelson and Ellenberg 1986), and such events probably do not account for more than a small percentage of cases of ADHD. Furthermore, correlations between perinatal distress and ADHD may not reflect a causal link.

Overt neurological disorders, most commonly seizures and cerebral palsy, are present in approximately 5% of the children with ADHD, although they do not correlate with the severity of ADHD symptoms. Like children with other psychiatric disorders, children with ADHD may have multiple minor physical and neurological anomalies. Nonlocalizing neurological soft signs (such as clumsiness, left–right confusion, perceptual-motor dyscoordination, and dysgraphia) are common in children with ADHD. However, approximately 15% of the children without ADHD have up to five neurological soft signs, so the clinical relevance usually is presumed to be insignificant.

ADHD with onset after toddlerhood may indicate the presence of acquired neuropathological changes, such as traumatic brain injury, encephalitis, or CNS infection. Frontal lobe injury often results in ADHD symptoms, but brain lesions in a variety of other locations can lead to a clinical picture that resembles ADHD and responds to medication in a similar manner.

Right hemisphere syndrome. ADHD-like symptoms are present in 93% of the patients with right hemisphere syndrome (Voeller 1986). Typically evident from birth, right hemisphere syndrome is not a medical disorder, a result of injury or disease, or a learning disorder in the usual sense that involves a particular skill, such as reading or arithmetic. Instead, it consists of a series of right cortical deficits that can appear in healthy individuals who have difficulties with learning, memory, concentration, and organization (García-Sánchez et al. 1997). The entire right hemisphere appears to be involved, with no specific localization.

This syndrome, sometimes called nonverbal learning disorder, is readily identifiable in routine intelligence testing by a Verbal IQ score that is significantly higher than the Performance IQ score. Usually, a 15- to 20-point IQ difference can generate noticeable characteristics, and 20- to 50-point differences account for most severe cases. Extreme cases can involve differences of 100 points or more, with the level of intelligence of individuals with right hemisphere syndrome ranging from retarded to brilliant.

Misdiagnosis. Misidentification does not normally function as an etiological factor, but ADHD can be viewed as a special case because many psychiatric disorders may, on the surface, look similar to ADHD in their clinical presentation. Disorders that can look like ADHD include opposi-

TABLE 15–4. Psychiatric disorders often associated with attention-deficit/hyperactivity disorder

Conduct disorder
Oppositional defiant disorder
Anxiety disorders
Learning disorders
Motor skills disorder
Substance use disorders
Communication disorders
Bipolar disorder
Major depression
Posttraumatic stress disorder
Obsessive-compulsive disorder
Tourette's disorder
Schizophrenia
Mental retardation
Pervasive developmental disorders, including
  autistic disorder

Note. Various psychiatric states should be assessed clinically in individuals with attention-deficit/hyperactivity disorder, even though strong statistical associations have not been shown for each of these conditions.

the understanding of the etiology of the disorder. ADHD is unique, at least in psychiatry, in being a highly prevalent disorder that may frequently be misdiagnosed in a large proportion of cases. Although misdiagnosis can distort the understanding and treatment of any medical condition, ADHD is a special case because of the high frequency of diagnostic error. To minimize this possibility, structured assessments may be a critical tool to adequately tease apart complicated and at times overlapping symptom clusters. To accurately diagnose ADHD, all confounding and potentially comorbid diagnoses should be considered.

Conduct disorder and oppositional defiant disorder. Conduct disorder (not merely conduct problems or symptoms) is seen in 40%–70% of the children with ADHD, and about the same percentage of children with conduct disorder have ADHD (Kadesjo and Gillberg 2001; Soussignan and Tremblay 1996). Children whose conduct disorder is diagnosed before age 12 years nearly always meet criteria for ADHD, whereas about one-third of children with adolescent-onset conduct disorder meet ADHD criteria.

Anxiety disorders. About one-third of the children with ADHD have an anxiety disorder (MTA Cooperative Group 1999a), reflecting a two- to fourfold increase in prevalence compared with children in the general population (Bird et al. 1993; P. Cohen et al. 1993). Family genetic studies have suggested that the risk for anxiety disorders may be transmitted separately from the risk for ADHD (Perrin and Last 1996).

Mood disorders. Children with ADHD may have an increased prevalence of major depressive disorder, although these findings have been mixed. Nonetheless,

tional defiant disorder, conduct disorder, bipolar disorder, Tourette's disorder, posttraumatic stress disorder (PTSD), abuse or neglect, and even major depressive disorder (Table 15–4). For example, about 25% of the patients who traditionally might have been given diagnoses of ADHD are now given diagnoses of bipolar disorder.

Comorbidity

ADHD represents a true challenge in many individuals because of the valid and extensive comorbidity often present. Unfortunately, these comorbid conditions are often the only diagnosis made, causing particular concern when these diagnoses are the result of a primary diagnosis of ADHD, such as substance abuse and depression. Indeed, the high prevalence of comorbidity in ADHD poses a variety of problems for both diagnostic practice and whether minimal or robust, the connection is likely in part biological. Both ADHD and major depressive disorder are associated with decreased rapid eye movement (REM) latency, responsiveness to noradrenergic antidepressants, genetic interrelationships, anxiety disorders, and bipolar disorder.

More than half of the children with bipolar disorder also fulfill criteria for ADHD (West et al. 1995), and about 20%–25% of the children with ADHD also fulfill criteria for bipolar disorder (Biederman et al. 1996). Thus, certain children with ADHD may have precursor conditions of bipolar disorder or they may have true comorbid conditions that significantly affect the course of treatment (T. Spencer et al. 2001; West et al. 1995; Wozniak et al. 2001a).

Tic disorders. Tourette's disorder is overrepresented in patients with ADHD, and at least 25% of males with Tourette's disorder have ADHD. OCD in children also appears to be linked to ADHD, often in association with Tourette's disorder. More recently, children who have comorbid tic disorder with ADHD as well as those who have comorbid OCD with ADHD have been found to have PANDAS with antistreptococcal/antineuronal antibodies. About half of PANDAS cases also fulfill criteria for ADHD (Peterson et al. 2000).

Pervasive developmental disorders. Autism presents so commonly with ADHD that the DSM-III-R criteria (American Psychiatric Association 1987) for ADHD excluded its diagnosis in the presence of autism. That exclusion was removed in DSM-IV (American Psychiatric Association 1994), so patients with autistic disorder and ADHD can legitimately be treated with psychostimulants without the necessity of declaring autism to be a new indication for psychostimulants.

Psychotic agitation. Although psychotic agitation is relatively uncommon, accurate differential diagnosis of this condition is essential because psychostimulant or antidepressant treatment can exacerbate psychotic symptoms. Typically, patients with ADHD have absolutely no hallucinations, delusional thinking, or breakthroughs of primary process thinking. However, similar to patients with psychotic disorders, ADHD patients may have loose thought patterns, engage in self-endangering behavior, and show little awareness of their environment. The motor activity in ADHD appears continuous and endless, and the tempo of the impulsivity is roughly constant, in contrast to the irregular and less predictable body and affective tempo of psychotic children. Psychotic children may show anger and emotional overreactions that are primarily derived from cognitive distortions and can have a long duration (30 minutes to 5 hours). In contrast, emotional overreactions in patients with ADHD usually are based on misunderstandings and accidents, and tantrums in these patients usually resolve within 30 minutes. Generally, the long-term course of ADHD is gradual improvement (Biederman et al. 2000), in contrast to psychotic disorders, which typically worsen with time. Also of interest, however, is that some children of mothers with schizophrenia have motor and attention deficits and, according to follow-up studies, often grow up to become adults with schizophrenia; and their non-ADHD siblings have a low incidence of adult schizophrenia (Marcus et al. 1985).

Learning disorders. ADHD is associated with a high prevalence of all learning and communication disorders. Similarly, ADHD has a relatively high prevalence in samples of individuals with mental retardation. Language disorders and reading disorders (Purvis and Tannock 2000) may occur in patients with ADHD and are often not reflected in routine IQ testing and scores (Tirosh and Cohen 1998), suggesting a need for specific testing when clinically appropriate.

Psychosocial factors. Psychosocial factors such as situational anxiety, child abuse and neglect, and simple boredom can clinically manifest in symptoms that mimic ADHD. Examination of the course of illness distinguishes these conditions from ADHD.

Pathogenesis

Elucidating the pathophysiology of ADHD is a complex and ongoing task that is complicated by the remaining diagnostic and conceptual ambiguities. The large array of etiological factors, mechanisms, symptom overlap, comorbid disorders, developmental changes, and complications of illness—and especially their interactions—explain why it has been difficult to identify the core symptoms of ADHD as distinct from those of other disorders. The task of cleaning up the blur of diagnostic boundaries is an essential step in the formation of a definition of ADHD. Research on the etiology and pathophysiology is complicated by the incompleteness of this effort.

Although both biological and psychosocial factors are involved in shaping the appearance of ADHD in individuals, it appears that most cases of ADHD have a pronounced biological origin. A wide variety of biological findings in ADHD may contribute to the descriptive and etiological understanding of this disorder.

Neuropsychological studies. Many methodological and conceptual issues remain to be worked out, but the neuropsychological literature implicates disturbances in response inhibition and various executive functions in the pathogenesis of ADHD (see Tannock 1998 and Barkley 2000 for reviews; Barkley et al. 2001; Biederman 1998). The neuropsychological literature also has provided evidence for impairments in working memory (Barkley et al. 2001; Levy and Farrow 2001) and semantic processing (Tannock et al. 2000) in the pathogenesis of ADHD. These functional deficits contribute to a range of difficulties in structuring a narrative (Purvis and Tannock 1997), in accurately appraising the moment-to-moment consequences of actions and interactions with others (self-monitoring), and in coordinating complex intertwined activities (multitasking and multiprocessing).

Neurochemical and pharmacological studies. Neurochemical studies of ADHD were initially organized around the catecholamine hypothesis, beginning with norepinephrine as the crucial neurotransmitter (Wender 1971). This hypothesis has undergone numerous revisions over the years, but a strong emphasis remains on norepinephrine and dopamine (Biederman and Spencer 1999). Although much research in recent years has centered on dopamine, findings that ADHD can be treated with atomoxetine or clonidine (which lack direct dopamine effects) have refueled the norepinephrine theories. It has been suggested that norepinephrine neuronal projections are involved in alerting (i.e., signaling) the posterior attention system of the cortex to receive incoming stimuli and that the dopamine system might influence the cortical anterior attention system, which subserves executive functions that are linked to behavioral responses (Pliszka et al. 1996). These findings are consistent with a norepinephrine/attention and dopamine/activity model of ADHD—with "activity" encompassing hyperactivity, impulsivity, and behavioral self-control. Another chemical model suggests an association of norepinephrine with hyperactivity, dopamine with impulsivity, and serotonin with aggression (Castellanos et al. 1994a). Numerous such models are possible. Peripheral and possibly central epinephrine might be involved in the mechanism of psychostimulant action on attention and impulsivity, and roles of GABA (Pliszka et al. 1996), glutamate (Carlsson 2000), and acetylcholine are also being investigated.

Neuroanatomical studies. Quantitative magnetic resonance imaging (MRI) studies have identified several anatomical characteristics of ADHD, with consistent findings implicating abnormal structural changes in the frontal lobes, basal ganglia, and cerebellar vermis (Giedd et al. 2001). Total brain volume appears to be reduced by about 4%–5% in boys and girls with ADHD (Castellanos et al. 1994b, 2001); the lack of progressive change with age suggests an early and global disruption of brain growth, possibly implicating neurotrophic growth factors (Rapoport et al. 2001). The possibility of disrupted brain development in early gestation is consistent with findings of abnormal neuronal migration in some individuals with ADHD (Nopoulos et al. 2000). The anterior frontal cortex has been reported to be smaller on the right side (Castellanos et al. 1996), a finding corroborated with decreased blood flow in the frontal regions compared with healthy control subjects (Lou et al. 1998) and consistent with a defect in cortical-striatal-thalamic-cortical (CSTC) circuits in the right hemisphere. The caudate region shows abnormal structural asymmetry; this finding suggests that the caudate does not have its normal extent of developmental reduction in size and is consistent with a disruption of the normal developmental transfer of func-

tions from the basal ganglia to the frontal cortex (Castellanos et al. 1994b; Mataro et al. 1997; Pueyo et al. 2000). The putamen, which is involved in regulation of motoric behavior, also has been implicated in ADHD (Teicher et al. 2000). Another consistent finding is reduced cerebellar volume, particularly the posterior inferior lobe of the vermis, in both boys and girls with ADHD (Berquin et al. 1998; Castellanos et al. 2001). Cerebellar involvement in cognitive processes, possibly including executive functions as well as motor control and inhibition, suggests that a prefrontal-thalamic-cerebellar network may be involved in core symptoms of ADHD.

Neurophysiological studies. Although routine clinical electroencephalograms (EEGs) are interpreted as normal in most patients with ADHD, quantitative EEG data have shown that 93% of children with ADHD could be categorized as having either hyperarousal or hypoarousal relative to control subjects without ADHD (Chabot and Serfontein 1996). Studies of evoked potentials (event-related electrical waves in the brain) also have reported numerous findings in ADHD suggestive of abnormal arousal and attention. Some of these evoked potential characteristics have been found to change with age, correlate to specific ADHD symptoms or associated features (such as aggressive behavior), and be corrected by psychostimulants. An abnormality in the right frontal cortex associated with impaired attention and information processing (small P300 amplitude) may correlate with diminished effectiveness of psychostimulants in some patients.

These neurophysiological findings suggest that ADHD involves a disorder of arousal in addition to defects in attention, response inhibition, and executive functioning. The disorder of arousal may present as either hyperarousal or hypoarousal in different patients, and both may be linked to high or low autonomic reactivity. Both hyperarousal and hypoarousal appear associated with abnormalities in the function of frontal circuits. The data on arousal seem to imply that there are different forms of dysregulation of the frontal cortex in ADHD rather than a simple decrease in frontal activity, and such differences in arousal characteristics might be significant to ADHD subtyping.

Neuroimaging studies. An early positron emission tomography (PET) scan study of adults with ADHD found an overall reduction in global cerebral glucose metabolism of 8%, with the largest decreases observed in the premotor cortex and superior prefrontal cortex. More recent PET scan evidence of redistribution of blood flow, some following successful treatment with psychostimulants, further supports relative hypofrontality and compensatory redistribution of blood flow in patients with ADHD (Bush et al. 1999; Lou 1996; Lou et al. 1989; Matochik et al. 1994; Schweitzer et al. 2000). The newer generation of studies that examine structure–function correlations suggest significant roles of the right prefrontal and caudate areas in specific cognitive functions. For example, changes in performance on neuropsychological tasks that require response inhibition have been correlated with anatomical changes in the right frontostriatal neuronal circuits (Casey et al. 1997; Teicher et al. 2000).

Course and Prognosis

Although generalizations about the course and prognosis of ADHD are difficult, it is now recognized that most cases of ADHD are both congenital and lifelong. The symptoms of inattention, impulsivity, and hyperactivity are manifested in different ways as an individual develops, reflecting the developmental tasks and normal activities at different points in the life cycle (see Table 15–3). However, an adult with pronounced inattention, impulsivity, and hyperactivity does not necessarily have ADHD because the DSM-IV-TR diagnosis of ADHD in adults requires a history of ADHD during childhood. ADHD can be diagnosed by age 3 years, but it is usually difficult to recognize the disorder before age 5 years because a normal developmental stage of increased activity begins at about age 2 years. Identification is often delayed until elementary school, when demands for physical stillness and mental focus are greater, comparison with peers is easier, and more group stimulation is involved. Individuals with ADHD often experience their most challenging adjustments during the regimented school years. This is in part because they are not yet free to select areas of learning and schoolwork that are least affected by their cognitive, behavioral, and motivational symptoms. In addition to academic challenges and behavioral infractions, school-age children with ADHD may be significantly compromised in social skills and self-esteem.

The hyperactivity of ADHD often improves during childhood and early adolescence (Biederman 1998). In general, the symptoms of hyperactivity improve notably, impulsivity improves to a lesser degree, but the inattention does not seem to improve (Hart et al. 1995). Despite the improvement in some symptoms over time, social skills and general adaptive abilities appear to fall progressively further behind with age (Roizen et al. 1994). The prevalence of ADHD is estimated to decline by 50% about every 5 years until the mid-20s (J.C. Hill and Schoener 1996), regardless of the type and duration of treatment (Hart et al. 1995). Features of impulsivity persist into adolescence in

70% and into adulthood in 30%–50% of cases of childhood ADHD. These compelling data highlight the need for aggressive treatment in adolescents and adults who might have a reduction in symptoms but remain at high risk for poor functional outcomes.

Clearly, ADHD is not a benign or self-limited childhood disorder. By young adulthood, ADHD is associated with fewer completed years of schooling, more changes of residence, more cigarette smoking, more marijuana use, more alcohol use, more traffic violations, more speeding, more car accidents and crashes, more court appearances, and more felony convictions (T. Spencer et al. 1999; Wilens et al. 1998). In regard to psychiatric symptoms, young adults with ADHD have more mood disorders, suicide attempts, phobic anxiety, somatization symptoms, and psychosexual traumas.

Substance use disorders emerge in children with ADHD earlier and more often than in children without ADHD, and substance use continues into adulthood in about half of the patients with ADHD (Pomerleau et al. 1995). ADHD may be an independent risk factor for the development of substance abuse, including alcohol and nicotine (Biederman et al. 1997b; Sullivan and Rudnik-Levin 2001; Wilens et al. 1998). These findings contrast with other data that suggest that, in the absence of conduct disorder, ADHD does not appear to be associated with subsequent substance abuse (Disney et al. 1999; Lynskey and Fergusson 1995). The links between ADHD and substance abuse probably can be explained in some patients by psychiatric comorbidity, such as bipolar disorder or conduct disorder in children and antisocial personality or personality disorder in adults. Alternatively, characteristics such as risk-taking behavior, difficulty in anticipating or planning for consequences, or aggressive behavior may play a role. Despite

these conflicting data, it appears that treatment of ADHD may lead to significant reductions in substance abuse and dependence (Biederman et al. 1998; Greene et al. 1999; Wilens et al. 1998).

Although historically overemphasized, antisocial personality disorder in adulthood is one of the most common serious outcomes of ADHD. The high risk of antisocial outcome is likely to be concentrated in children with ADHD who have comorbid conduct disorder. Follow-up studies examining some of the populations with more severe ADHD and comorbid conduct disorder have reported that 25%–30% of these children eventually develop antisocial personality disorder. Although this is not likely generalizable to the entire ADHD population, when it occurs, it seems to be mediated by the interaction of hyperactivity-impulsivity symptoms with conduct disorder. Inattention does not appear to play a significant role in development of symptoms of criminality (August et al. 1983; Babinski et al. 1999).

Diagnostic Evaluation

Clinical evaluation includes assessing the specific symptoms of ADHD, considering similarly presenting disorders, and delineating concomitant psychiatric and neurological disorders. In addition to a routine and thorough psychiatric evaluation of the individual and a general family assessment, special emphasis is warranted in several areas. These include school reports of grades and behavior (including behavior on the bus and in the cafeteria) or work history, concomitant learning disorders and other common comorbid psychiatric disorders, social functioning and social skills, obstetrical history (maternal alcohol use, fetal overactivity, prenatal or perinatal injury), family residence (lead exposure in paints and car exhaust fumes), family psychiatric history (including ADHD in males), family medical history (thyroid disorder), medication use (barbiturates, benzodiazepines, psychostimulants, carbamazepine), history of child abuse or neglect, and potential risks of medication abuse by the patient or family members. Essential sources of information include the patient, parents, teachers, significant others, and treating physicians.

Physical examination and laboratory testing can identify physical anomalies and thyroid disorders. Neurological evaluation can uncover possible localizing symptoms, neuromaturational signs such as choreiform movements, overflow and mirror movements, tremor, gross and fine motor function, cerebral laterality, and baseline (premedication) frequency of tics or dystonias. Lead screening is appropriate when excessive lead exposure is suspected; the screening test is a plasma level of zinc protoporphyrin, which has replaced the free erythrocyte protoporphyrin because it has fewer false-positive results and is an indicator of long-term lead exposure. A plasma lead level is optional at initial screening because it reflects lead exposure over the previous 4 weeks only. A baseline sample of handwriting permits visual documentation of clinical change in the medical record. In the absence of suggestive symptoms, baseline (premedication) EEG, electrocardiogram, and thyroid evaluation are not essential and probably not cost-effective. Other laboratory tests, apart from those for the routine management of medications, are not necessary.

Educational testing and neuropsychological evaluation are useful to assess academic achievement, intelligence, cortical functioning, attention, impulsivity, and developmental skills, as well as symptoms of learning, motor skills, and communication disorders.

Comorbidity rates are sufficiently high that evaluations of ADHD should be initially based on the expectation that concurrent psychiatric disorders will be identified. ADHD is often diagnosed in association with conduct disorder, oppositional defiant disorder, bipolar disorder, depression, and learning disorders (Table 15–4). The differential diagnosis of ADHD is also challenging at times because of comorbid neurological disorders and the extensive phenomenological similarity to other psychiatric disorders and to normal behavior.

In addition to the comorbidity, ADHD is typically accompanied by certain "associated features," as described in DSM-IV-TR. For instance, when compared with adolescents with bipolar disorder, adolescents who have both bipolar disorder and ADHD are more likely to have mixed mania, irritability, higher scores on mania rating scales, and sometimes lower serum thyroxine concentrations. Such findings highlight the fact that clinically relevant features of ADHD are difficult to delineate but nonetheless can be helpful in clinical diagnosis.

Often in psychiatry, diagnostic confidence cannot be achieved, and a working diagnosis is used as a basis for treatment. With ADHD, this approach can lead to an empirical trial of psychostimulants. However, a positive treatment response to a psychostimulant does not necessarily imply a diagnosis of ADHD because patients with several other disorders also may show a therapeutic response to psychostimulants. On the other hand, a negative response to a psychostimulant does not rule out ADHD because patients with ADHD may respond only to certain psychostimulants or to another class of medications altogether. At times it may be helpful to keep the diagnostic process open ended and to expect that emerging clinical data will confirm or refute initial diagnostic impressions.

Currently, making a diagnosis of ADHD is much more complicated than in past decades. It is difficult to make a firm diagnosis of ADHD without assessing the presence or absence of many disorders (see Table 15–4). It is no longer easy to make this diagnosis in many patients in a single office visit, because the accumulation of adequate clinical data to address each of these possibilities requires careful evaluation and observation over time. In effect, ADHD is a diagnosis of exclusion. In the future, the continual refinement of specific and sensitive diagnostic criteria for ADHD across the life span will create a major advantage in diagnosing ADHD and differentiating it from other conditions.

Treatment

Various treatment methods are useful. Both multimodal and sequential approaches are generally needed. Certain interventions are specific to particular etiologies, but some treatments are helpful regardless of etiology. A major study of the multimodal treatment of ADHD (the MTA study) has solidified knowledge and provided important new insights into the roles and contributions of psychopharmacological and psychosocial treatments in the management of ADHD.

Psychostimulants remain the primary treatment for ADHD because they are more effective than alternative medications and modalities for improving inattention and other cognitive symptoms. The use of psychostimulants in ADHD is one of the oldest and most established psychopharmacological treatments. There have been more than 200 double-blind demonstrations of its efficacy and safety in children, with additional trials confirming its benefits in adult populations. The effect of psychostimulants in treating core symptoms of ADHD is as effective in girls as in boys. The effectiveness of these drugs has been shown to persist for at least 15 months (Gillberg et al. 1997; Sharp et al. 1999) and, in clinical use, appears to endure for many years.

A small percentage of patients may develop tolerance to psychostimulants after several months of treatment; the psychostimulants appear to become ineffective despite dose increases. If a therapeutic effect diminishes over time and is not due to intercurrent (including psychiatric) illness or stress, this problem generally can be clinically managed by alternating between two different psychostimulants every few weeks or months.

The "quieting" effects of psychostimulants on the impulsivity, hyperactivity, inattention, and emotional lability of ADHD are distinct from caffeine-induced focusing of attention, the antianxiety effect of benzodiazepines, or the tranquilization of antipsychotic agents. These agents act by different neurochemical and neurophysiological mechanisms, and they produce chemically different forms of "sedation." Children with ADHD can show a calming response to other medical psychostimulants (pseudoephedrine) and behavioral excitation to sedatives (benzodiazepines and barbiturates). Such "paradoxical" clinical effects may not be specific to hyperactive children. Under laboratory conditions, boys and men without ADHD show a qualitatively similar psychostimulant-induced reduction of motor behavior; however, the quantitative effect in hyperactive boys is significantly larger (Rapoport et al. 1980). The explanation of this apparent difference in the human laboratory, and of the clinical finding that not all people with ADHD respond "therapeutically" to psychostimulants, is uncertain. It appears that psychostimulant responsiveness is not specifically tied to diagnostic state but instead reflects more basic biological mechanisms.

In addition to reducing the core symptoms of inattention, impulsivity, and hyperactivity, psychostimulant treatment often appears to lead to enduring improvement in social skills and self-esteem. Improvements in academic performance, socialization, and school or work productivity are further enhanced by concurrent changes in external structure and support (Barkley and Cunningham 1978; Jensen et al. 2001b). Controlled follow-up studies examining physical growth also have found that most deficits are temporary and tend to normalize by late adolescence, even with continued treatment. This has been hypothesized to suggest that the growth deficits may be mediated by ADHD itself and not psychostimulants (T. Spencer et al. 1998c).

Some patients do not experience therapeutic effects from psychostimulants. Several factors can be considered in these cases. Some comorbid psychiatric disorders, including anxiety disorders or symptoms, bipolar disorder, and schizophrenia, are aggravated by psychostimulants. Most psychotic disorders or symptoms can be aggravated by psychostimulants. Any neurological condition or neurodevelopmental idiosyncrasy that occurs concomitantly with ADHD might lead to drug-induced neurotoxic symptoms, often at unexpectedly low doses of psychotropic medications. The presence of anxiety (and perhaps other internalizing symptoms) has been reported by numerous research groups to be associated with a weaker and less prevalent therapeutic effect of psychostimulants. Patients with internalizing disorders tend to be overly inhibited, whereas ADHD patients typically have deficits in inhibitory self-control (Oosterlaan and Sergeant 1996). It may be hypothesized that the fluctuating balance between these characteristics and the intermittent nature of anxiety contribute to the unevenness of psychostimulant effects in patients with ADHD and anxiety.

In some cases, the dosage of the psychostimulant may need to be reduced when ADHD with comorbid anxiety is treated in order to obtain stable therapeutic effects (Livingston et al. 1992).

Current concepts of the mechanism or mechanisms of psychostimulant action in ADHD are undergoing continual revision. The largely catecholaminergic, lesser serotonergic, possibly some cholinergic, and probably other pharmacological effects of the psychostimulants are consistent with many different (and conflicting) models of ADHD. Simple single neurotransmitter explanations are viewed as unlikely. Newer theories, incorporating nonpharmacological and neurophysiological findings, can become quite elaborate and interesting. For instance, the unexpected finding that methylphenidate slows right hemisphere processing (i.e., slower reaction time on neuropsychological tasks without a change in accuracy) seems to imply that the therapeutic effects of psychostimulants must be strong enough to outweigh their seemingly negative effects on right-sided functioning (Campbell et al. 1996).

In healthy individuals, the most serious risks of psychostimulants include tics and psychosis. Seizures are not induced by psychostimulants, and cardiac and cardiovascular effects are generally not clinically significant. Common side effects include delayed sleep onset, minor increase in blood pressure and heart rate, decreased appetite, reduced (or slowed) height and weight gain, tremor or adventitious movements, cognitive overfocusing, anxiety, dysphoria, irritability, nightmares, and social withdrawal. The risk of drug abuse (and drug dealing and stealing in schools) is a major liability.

Although psychostimulants are short-acting and may cause uneven (on–off) effects throughout the day, the commercial development of technologies for gradual medication release has created a broad range of longer-acting formulations with more sustained and even effects. These formulations may provide the convenience of once-daily administration (and enhanced compliance) for some patients, but many patients still require booster doses later in the day. Their sustained clinical effects can increase insomnia and other side effects, and the long-term safety of persistently elevated psychostimulant blood levels has not been adequately assessed.

Atomoxetine, a recently introduced selective norepinephrine reuptake inhibitor, has been found effective for both children and adults with ADHD (Michelson et al. 2001, 2003). Its selectivity enhances its favorable side-effect profile, and its long-lasting effects allow for once-daily administration. In contrast to the psychostimulants, atomoxetine is not an abusable drug when used alone but speculatively could be dangerous when used in combination with certain drugs of abuse.

In general, other nonpsychostimulant medications are not abusable but are notably less effective in treating ADHD, especially in treating symptoms of inattention. Tricyclic antidepressants (TCAs) are able to treat the core symptoms of ADHD but are typically less effective than psychostimulants for symptoms of inattention. Their efficacy has been shown in double-blind, placebo-controlled studies conducted by 11 separate research groups over the past 30 years. Low dosages of TCAs (e.g., nortriptyline 0.3–2.0 mg/kg/day) provide therapeutic effects that last 24 hours, allowing for convenient once-daily dosing.

Reports of sudden death during routine desipramine treatment in several children and adolescents (Popper and Elliott 1990; Riddle et al. 1991, 1995) have led to general concern about the use of TCAs in youths, particularly for treating non-

lethal disorders such as ADHD. The problem appears to be specific to desipramine; even imipramine has not been implicated, probably because its anticholinergic side effects are cardioprotective. Most of these cases of sudden death involved treatments for ADHD rather than mood disorders or enuresis, which is the most common pediatric use of TCAs. Some of the patients who died had significant preexisting cardiovascular risks, including one patient whose coronary artery anomaly could not have been identified before death unless invasive arteriography had been obtained. Desipramine treatment of ADHD is easy to avoid because so many other TCAs are readily available, and all appear to be equally effective in treating ADHD. TCAs may be reasonably considered if rebound effects of psychostimulants are disruptive, if tics emerge specifically during rebound, if once-a-day administration is needed for treatment adherence, if the child or family is potentially drug abusing, if a comorbid mood disorder is present, if sleep disturbance is prominent, and perhaps if a strong family psychiatric history of mood disorder exists.

Bupropion has been successfully used in adults with ADHD (Wender and Reimherr 1990), but findings in children are mixed (Casat et al. 1989; Clay et al. 1988; Conners et al. 1996). The anti-ADHD effects of bupropion appear to be smaller than those of standard psychostimulant drugs. In a controlled drug comparison study with methylphenidate, bupropion produced comparable but consistently weaker therapeutic effects (Barrickman et al. 1995). An unexpectedly high incidence of severe skin rash has been associated with bupropion treatment in children (Conners et al. 1996).

Monoamine oxidase inhibitor (MAOI) antidepressants usually are clinically effective, but they are not typically used for treating ADHD because of the dietary restrictions and potential risks. The newer MAOIs, such as L-deprenyl (selegiline) and moclobemide (available in Canada), are more isoenzyme specific than are the traditional MAOIs. Early findings suggested that moclobemide is effective in ADHD (Trott et al. 1992) and that L-deprenyl is not (Ernst et al. 1996; Feigin et al. 1996).

α_2-Agonists such as clonidine have become widely used to treat ADHD (Hunt et al. 1990), but the two randomized double-blind, placebo-controlled studies of clonidine in children with ADHD found only minor effects on ADHD (Jaselskis et al. 1992; Singer et al. 1995). A meta-analysis estimated that clonidine has some value (mean effect size = 0.58) for treating ADHD but less than that of psychostimulants (Connor et al. 1999). In general, clonidine appears to treat behavioral hyperactivity and impulsivity, as well as associated aggressive behavior and insomnia, but not the attentional symptoms (van der Meere et al. 1999). Its potentially serious adverse cardiovascular effects, including hypotension and bradycardia, are typically benign, but either one can result in syncope. Abrupt discontinuation (including running out of pills) can induce significant tachycardia and hypertension but also has been associated with severe ventricular tachyarrhythmias in adults (Jain and Misra 1991) and children (Coumel et al. 1978). Clinicians are advised to monitor blood pressure and heart rate before and during any treatment involving clonidine, alone or in combination with other drugs. Guanfacine is a similar agent with some pharmacological advantages (Hunt et al. 1995; Scahill et al. 2001), especially in terms of adverse effects.

Other medications for consideration include venlafaxine, β-adrenergic blockers, donepezil, and possibly modafinil or nicotine. Antipsychotic medications may be appropriate for treating ADHD in the context of significant comorbidity, including tic disorders, bipolar disorder, or other psychotic conditions.

In the nonpharmacological management of ADHD, various psychosocial interventions appear helpful in supporting the patient and family and in relieving some of the predictable problems associated with ADHD. Education of the patient and family members about ADHD, its treatment, and its management is necessary as well. Family members usually can be "coached" in behavioral management techniques that can be applied at home. For children, parents can be pivotal in exacerbating or diminishing symptoms; therefore, focused parent counseling is sensible in nearly all cases.

Education and support for parents and family members are crucial, and they can be provided through programmed group training sessions. National organizations for parents, such as ChADD, have many local chapters throughout the United States that can provide crucial support, education, and advocacy for families and patients.

Environmental management of sensory stimulation can reduce overstimulation from external sources, keep impulsivity and aggressivity in better control, and provide a sense of control and basis for self-esteem. Environmental measures can involve arranging the patient's home and job or school setting to reduce stimuli and distractions. For children at home, parents can be advised to establish quiet spaces, decorate with simple furniture and subdued colors, keep toys in the closet, permit only one friend to visit at a time, avoid supermarkets and parties, and encourage fine motor exercises (e.g., jigsaw puzzles). At work, adolescents and adults should be encouraged to make arrangements to use a quiet, small office space with no officemates; to have a minimum of visitors; to avoid chatting or visual contact with passersby; and to have few telephone interruptions. The work environment should be uncluttered and undistracting, containing few windows and no nearby refrigerator, radio or television, or sound-making machinery. These recommendations have not been evaluated in controlled studies, but they are commonly offered and appear clinically valuable.

Special education is generally required because children with ADHD are typically below achievement levels expected for school grade, even after accounting for IQ (Cantwell and Baker 1988). At school, beneficial accommodations include a small and self-contained classroom, small-group activities, thoughtful selection of seating location to minimize distractions, high teacher-to-student ratio, quiet ambience, routine and predictable structure, one-to-one tutoring, and use of a resource room. Arrangements for supervision or modifications at recess, in physical education class, on the bus, and in the cafeteria are sometimes helpful. Careful management of transitions to new schools and between programs requires administrative foresight and detail-oriented planning. It is essential to inform school officials about the child's strengths and problems, self-esteem, social skills, and useful environmental measures as well as to receive regular reports from school personnel about behavior and academic performance. An individualized educational plan (IEP) can be developed with the school to facilitate classroom arrangements, perhaps with concomitant interventions to accommodate specific learning disorders.

Contingent rewards, response-cost management, and time-outs can help build impulse control in children. Behavioral methods can be as effective as psychostimulants in modifying classroom behavior, but generalization beyond the treatment setting may be limited. Cogni-

tive-behavioral therapy is used for teaching problem-solving strategies, self-monitoring, verbal mediation (using internal speech) for self-praise and self-instruction, and seeing rather than glossing over errors.

Group treatments can be helpful for children and adolescents with ADHD who need training in social skills. Deficits in the development of social skills are commonly found in individuals with ADHD, including those without aggressive behavior, oppositional behavior, impulsivity, or hyperactivity. Other areas of adaptive functioning are also compromised, even in patients with predominantly inattentive ADHD. Children of normal intelligence (Full-Scale IQ of 101 ± 14) who have ADHD may have low-to-borderline scores on the Vineland Adaptive Behavior Scale (73 ± 14), and this discrepancy increases with age (Roizen et al. 1994). Social and adaptive dysfunctions only recently have been viewed as standard components of ADHD, and they may justify incorporation into the routine management of ADHD (M.A. Stein et al. 1995).

Reinforcement of smoking and drug abuse prevention attitudes is also very important in this population, along with the acquisition of alternative means of dealing with peer pressure, self-image, anxiety, and peers' opinions. Children with ADHD tend to be less future-oriented and less concerned about future health problems (and other delayed risks). Their novelty-seeking behavior also may interfere with subsequent smoking cessation efforts (Downey et al. 1997). Early intervention is particularly valuable for youths with ADHD, who generally start smoking earlier than their peers who do not have ADHD (Biederman et al. 1999b; Downey et al. 1997). Among youths with ADHD, appropriate treatment with psychiatric medications may result in up to an 85% reduction in subsequent substance abuse disorder (Biederman et al. 1999b). However, in view of the possible therapeutic effects of nicotine on ADHD symptoms (Levin et al. 1996), symptoms may worsen during smoking cessation, making it even more difficult for persons with ADHD to stop smoking. In a similar manner, preventive measures to stem alcohol and other substance use disorders are useful and often critical.

Nutritional therapy of ADHD has a murky history, involving a string of cures too good to be true and "new" treatments that have been used for years. Perhaps frustrated by behavioral methods and frightened by "mind drugs," parents are often interested in hearing physicians' views on nutritional and other unproven treatments of ADHD. Some of these parents seem willing to accept that their child has a "physical problem" but are not ready to acknowledge a "medical disorder." It is also striking that ADHD has attracted more medical and professional advocates of nutritional treatment than any other psychiatric and most other medical disorders. Numerous forms of elimination diets have been enthusiastically promulgated and enforced for years on the basis of anecdotes and repeated assertions, without the benefit of adequate testing or even attempts at controlled trials.

Although no dietary treatment of ADHD has been consistently shown to have clinical value, some studies cannot be readily dismissed. Several reasonable reports are consistent with a possible role of dietary factors in the etiology and treatment of ADHD. In a controlled trial that used dye washout periods and high-dose dye challenges, specific restriction of a set of food dyes (with no other restrictions) was found to be effective for treating a subgroup (5%–10%) of children with ADHD (Swanson and Kinsbourne 1980). In another controlled rechallenge study, a

diet that minimized the intake of certain "reactive" foods, preservatives, and artificial food dyes was found to produce a clinically and statistically significant improvement in children with ADHD (M. Boris and Mandel 1994); in this study, atopic children with ADHD appeared to be more likely to respond than other children with ADHD. In an EEG study examining children whose ADHD appeared to be aggravated by specific foods (as determined by previous deprivation and challenge), an increase was found in beta activity in the frontotemporal cortex during rechallenge with the sensitizing food (Uhlig et al. 1997). A controlled study of a low-antigen diet found no changes on attention or activity measures, but the children with ADHD reported significant subjective improvement (Schulte-Körne et al. 1996).

Other dietary treatments of ADHD have been examined but without convincing evidence of clinical value. The well-publicized Feingold diet, involving reduced dietary intake of salicylates and food dyes, has yielded contradictory findings in controlled trials. Data on salicylate elimination and challenge have indicated minimal effects (Perry et al. 1996). Sugar toxicity, sugar withdrawal, and reactive hypoglycemia have been reported to induce ADHD symptoms, but these claims do not appear to be valid unless perhaps there were preexisting nutritional deficiencies. It has been well documented that aspartame has no clinical effects on ADHD. Dietary treatments based on trace mineral content in hair analysis, particularly zinc deficiency and cadmium excess, have not been rigorously evaluated. Megavitamin treatments appear ineffective and can cause toxic effects.

Despite prevailing skepticism of dietary treatments of ADHD, some studies of dietary treatments of ADHD have produced enough suggestive evidence to warrant a measure of respect and to justify further disciplined research. Reasonably good evidence suggests that some foods or food dyes induce hyperactive behavior or other ADHD symptoms in a very small percentage of children (Arnold 2002). Some data seem to confirm the folklore that mood and sleep are influenced by a broad range of foods in children (Breakey 1997). Based on the involvement of iron in mechanisms affecting dopaminergic activity, a well-conducted open-label study suggested that boys with ADHD may respond to 30-day iron supplementation (Sever et al. 1997). Reduced blood levels of omega-3 and omega-6 fatty acids have been reported in children with ADHD (Arnold et al. 1994; Mitchell et al. 1987; Stevens et al. 1995, 1996), with these reductions possibly correlating to severity of symptoms. Double-blind, placebo-controlled studies in youths have suggested some effect of omega-6 γ-linolenic acid in treating ADHD (Arnold 2001), and recent data have suggested that relative zinc deficiency may explain why some patients with ADHD do not show a more robust response to psychostimulants (Arnold et al. 2000).

To monitor treatment effects in research and clinical practice, a variety of standardized scales have been developed. The best available instrument for adults is the Wender Utah Rating Scale, which is also useful in assessing ADHD symptoms in children (M.A. Stein et al. 1995). Other options are available for children as well. The Child Attention/Activity Profile (CAP) assesses both the inattention and the hyperactivity-impulsivity factors and is sensitive to psychostimulant effects (Edelbrock 1987). Early versions of the Conners' Parent Rating Scale and the Conners' Teacher Rating Scale (Rapoport et al. 1985) were widely used, but they functioned as nonspecific measures of "misbehavior" and conduct problems;

they were not as useful for monitoring specific ADHD symptoms or for the predominantly inattentive type of ADHD. However, Conners updates these scales to keep pace, and the current versions appear to function quite well (Conners 1997). The Home Situations Questionnaire can be used by parents or residential caregivers; it assesses behaviors in a variety of different settings and also can measure drug effects. All these instruments, although developed for drug research, can be applied to outcome assessment of ADHD for any treatment method. An additional method of assessment, which is one of the best but not as systematic or reproducible as the scales, is an arrangement for clinicians to receive reports on behavior and cognition from teachers as well as parents.

Certain performance tests, mostly variations on the Continuous Performance Test (CPT), have been used clinically to measure attentiveness and responsiveness to changing sensory cues. Although these tests, computerized or otherwise, have been used to monitor treatment and to adjust medication dosages, their usefulness is open to question. Attentional performance in a laboratory is not necessarily related to naturalistic behavior or cognitive functioning in different life spaces.

Multimodal treatment of ADHD is currently the standard of care for children, especially those with major psychiatric or neurological comorbidity, behavior disorders, aggression, disruptiveness, learning disorders, developmental disorders, or poor prognosis. However, appropriate pharmacological treatment remains the cornerstone of all effective treatment regimens. Indeed, numerous large- and small-scale studies have found that in the absence of appropriate pharmacotherapy, outcomes are often poor; but there is a lot to be gained by supporting medication treatment with appropriate cognitive, educational, psychosocial, and family interventions (Ialongo et al. 1993; Jensen et al. 2001b; Pelham et al. 1993; Vitiello et al. 2001).

Conduct Disorder

Conduct disorder is the most common diagnosis of child and adolescent patients in both clinic and hospital settings. This disorder entails repeated violations of personal rights or societal rules, including violent and nonviolent behaviors. The syndrome is not a single medical entity but consists of various forms of misbehavior—some more extreme than others but all with the core feature of basic disregard for people and property. The diagnostic criteria include offenses ranging from frequent lying, cheating, and truancy to vandalism, running away, car theft, arson, and rape (Table 15–5). The validity of a single categorical grouping has been questioned by proponents of more symptomatic or dimensional approaches to conduct problems. Conduct disorders can present with or derive from comorbid psychiatric disorder, such as mood disorders, psychosis, ADHD, substance abuse, organic impairment, mental retardation, psychodevelopmental (or personality) disorders, and learning disorders. However, in most cases, family, socioeconomic, and environmental factors appear to contribute heavily to the genesis of conduct disorder (Loeber et al. 2000).

Conduct disorder encompasses some of the most severe behavior disorders of childhood (Frick 1998). Only a fraction of the children with this disorder receive treatment. Many can be rehabilitated or habilitated, but some lead lives of delinquency or undergo long-term incarceration. Early onset has been found to be the strongest predictor of poor outcome in a variety of studies, forming the basis for the DSM-IV-TR subtyping of conduct disorder into early and late onset (Lahey et al. 1998c; Tolan 1987). Compared with adolescent-onset conduct disorder, childhood-onset conduct disorder is more predominantly seen in males and is more likely to be associated with physical aggression, ADHD, an early history of oppositional defiant disorder, and antisocial personality disorder in adulthood.

Clinical Description

Conduct disorder accounts for 50% of convicted juvenile delinquents and a higher proportion of incarcerated youths. These youths are often products of low socioeconomic status, unstable homes with family discord, maternal rejection, and absent or alcoholic fathers (DeKlyen et al. 1998; Farrington and Loeber 2000), but some youths with conduct disorder come from more favorable environments. As a group, youths with conduct disorder have measurably lower cognitive and moral development, more behavioral impulsivity, greater susceptibility to boredom and stimulus-seeking behavior, and in some cases lower nutritional status. Many of these patients tend to be overtly aggressive, even to the point of being homicidal, particularly toward parents but more generally toward authority figures (Fergusson et al. 1994; Vitiello and Stoff 1997). Outcome and course depend partially on involvement in a delinquency group, the nature of the delinquency group, the availability of alternative social supports, concurrent psychiatric disorders, and the age at onset.

A crucial feature of conduct disorder is the absence of impulsivity (Halperin et al. 1995). Impulsive anger in patients with conduct disorder typically derives from comorbid disorders, especially ADHD. Both impulsive and nonimpulsive anger can play a role in the conduct of illegal behavior. Dealing (selling) drugs requires

TABLE 15–5.   DSM-IV-TR diagnostic criteria for conduct disorder

A. A repetitive and persistent pattern of behavior in which the basic rights of others or major age-appropriate societal norms or rules are violated, as manifested by the presence of three (or more) of the following criteria in the past 12 months, with at least one criterion present in the past 6 months:

Aggression to people and animals
  (1) often bullies, threatens, or intimidates others
  (2) often initiates physical fights
  (3) has used a weapon that can cause serious physical harm to others (e.g., a bat, brick, broken bottle, knife, gun)
  (4) has been physically cruel to people
  (5) has been physically cruel to animals
  (6) has stolen while confronting a victim (e.g., mugging, purse snatching, extortion, armed robbery)
  (7) has forced someone into sexual activity

Destruction of property
  (8) has deliberately engaged in fire setting with the intention of causing serious damage
  (9) has deliberately destroyed others' property (other than by fire setting)

Deceitfulness or theft
  (10) has broken into someone else's house, building, or car
  (11) often lies to obtain goods or favors or to avoid obligations (i.e., "cons" others)
  (12) has stolen items of nontrivial value without confronting a victim (e.g., shoplifting, but without breaking and entering; forgery)

Serious violations of rules
  (13) often stays out at night despite parental prohibitions, beginning before age 13 years
  (14) has run away from home overnight at least twice while living in parental or parental surrogate home (or once without returning for a lengthy period)
  (15) is often truant from school, beginning before age 13 years

B. The disturbance in behavior causes clinically significant impairment in social, academic, or occupational functioning.

C. If the individual is age 18 years or older, criteria are not met for antisocial personality disorder.

Code based on age at onset:
  312.81   Conduct Disorder, Childhood-Onset Type: onset of at least one criterion characteristic of conduct disorder prior to age 10 years
  312.82   Conduct Disorder, Adolescent-Onset Type: absence of any criteria characteristic of conduct disorder prior to age 10 years
  312.89   Conduct Disorder, Unspecified Onset: age at onset is not known

Specify severity:
  Mild: few if any conduct problems in excess of those required to make the diagnosis **and** conduct problems cause only minor harm to others
  Moderate: number of conduct problems and effect on others intermediate between "mild" and "severe"
  Severe: many conduct problems in excess of those required to make the diagnosis **or** conduct problems cause considerable harm to others

much more thoughtful planning and effective action than does abusing drugs. The strong association between conduct disorder and impulsivity is most likely an artifact of the frequent comorbid presentation of ADHD and conduct disorder. In fact, many of the characteristics attributed to conduct disorder result from comorbid psychiatric disorders. The high rate of comorbidity has complicated delineation of the features specific to conduct disorder, of which impulsivity is just one example.

Across a diversity of presentations, children and adolescents with conduct disorder show alterations of mood (sullenness, anger) and cognition, including attention and learning disorders. Cognitive problems include a faulty sense of size and time, a distorted view of the consequences of previous events, difficulty in imagining the expectable outcome of future events, underestimation of risks, disrupted awareness of cause and effect (particularly in regard to their own behavior), reduced problem-solving ability, blocks in logical thinking, and impaired moral reasoning. Pathological defenses include minimizing, avoiding, lying, externalizing, unconscious manipulation, and denial. Interpersonal impairments may appear as suspiciousness or paranoia (with cognitive distortions sometimes triggering fights and resentments), a minimum of guilt and empathy, and difficulty in relating to professionals.

Although symptoms such as driving recklessly, carrying weapons, and showing impulsive and nonimpulsive violence may be observed, wanton dangerousness to the public is not typical of all youths with conduct disorder. However, dangerousness may be significant in the small subgroup of children whose aggressive or suicidal behavior is a direct response to hallucinations.

Embedded within the concept of conduct disorder is the stereotype of the young "hardened criminal" who is dangerous and sociopathic but has not yet been imprisoned. DSM-IV-TR makes no attempt to designate such youths. In attempts at a more precise description of these youths, researchers have considered various attributes hypothesized to be more specific to these individuals, including callousness, low emotional reactivity, and family history of antisocial personality disorder, illegal behavior, and career criminality (Barry et al. 2000).

Epidemiology

Although abundant epidemiological information about crime is available, the data about conduct disorder are very limited and contaminated by comorbidity. The prevalence estimates for conduct disorder range from 1% to 10%. Conduct disorder has been found to be more prevalent in youths residing in large cities, although adjustments for population size diminish this disparity (Wichstrøm et al. 1996). The prevalence of conduct disorders has been increasing in females in recent years, so that the traditional male predominance is decreasing over time (Zoccolillo et al. 1996). Conduct disorder is more prevalent in areas of low income, high crime, and social disorganization (Sampson et al. 1997). The epidemiology of conduct disorder will continue to vary, depending on diagnostic criteria used, population size and distribution, family and community structure, socioeconomic conditions, and information source.

Etiology

A wide variety of etiological factors have been described, reflecting the full range of explanatory models of behavioral causation and the importance of delinquency as a central societal concern. Early speculation centered on intrapsychic structures, such as "superego defects" (Aichhorn 1925/1955), and on parental influences on unconscious motivation (A.M. Johnson et al. 1941), such as "superego lacunae" and the "acting out" of parents' unverbalized antisocial wishes or impulses. These inferences were never subjected to large-scale or epidemiological studies in children or adults.

Sociological theories focus on the effects of social deprivation, substance abuse, local variations in behavioral norms, gang formation, status seeking, escape from social entrapment, early rejection by peers, and school failure. Researchers in the field of sociology use sophisticated mathematical modeling to determine the role of specific socialization experiences in the path that leads to delinquent behavior and drug use.

Parent, caregiver, and home microenvironment characteristics are believed to be particularly important in the presentation of conduct disorder. Proposed factors in the etiology of conduct disorder include fathers with antisocial personality disorder, absent or alcoholic fathers, large families, shifting caregivers, parental rejection, parental abandonment, parental role modeling of impulsive or injurious behaviors, inadequate limit setting, harsh discipline, inconsistent or unpredictable discipline, parental overstimulation or understimulation, parental manipulative behavior, separation from parents, institutional care, early onset of unsanctioned use of alcohol, proximity of a delinquent peer group, and chronic poverty. Empirical evidence for the validity of these factors (and their interactions) varies in strength. Each factor most likely contributes significantly in some cases.

Some counterintuitive findings are clinically instructive. Coming from a single-parent home does not appear to be a major risk factor. It is family discord rather than separation per se that appears to mediate the risk for conduct disorder (Rutter and Giller 1984). Although other factors associated with single-parent homes also appear to be mediating factors (Lahey et al. 1988a) it appears that keeping families together may, in some cases, have disas-trous developmental consequences.

Certain microenvironmental factors can also statistically protect a child. Intelligence and small family size repeatedly have been found to be protective factors against both the development and the persistence of conduct disorder. Adequate supervision at home, especially when parents are away, has been shown to reduce the risk of conduct disorder. After-school activities, involvement of neighbors and relatives, community centers, and extended school hours can provide this type of supervision.

Neurological factors appear significant in some individuals with conduct disorder, especially in more aggressive and violent children. Conduct disorder is associated with an increased prevalence of neurological symptoms, both hard and soft signs; neuropsychological deficits, especially inattention; and seizures. The degree of aggression correlates with a history of physical abuse, head and face injuries, neurological findings, and ADHD. Elevated bone lead levels are associated with aggression and conduct symptoms (Needleman et al. 1996). In extremely violent youths, severe learning and communication problems appear to be common. Psychomotor seizures occur in 20% of these individuals, compared with less than 1% in a general population of youths. Furthermore, psychotic symptoms appear in up to 60% of severely violent youths with conduct disorder (D.O. Lewis et al. 1988).

Course and Prognosis

The major outcome risk of conduct disorder in childhood is antisocial personality disorder in adulthood. In a 30-year follow-up study of 500 child guidance clinic patients (Robins 1966), antisocial behavior in childhood was found to predict maladjustment and a high prevalence (37%) of severe psychopathology in adulthood: antisocial behavior, alcohol abuse, psychiatric hospitalization, child neglect, nonsupport, financial dependency, and poor employment and military records. The children of these patients showed a high prevalence of truancy, running away, theft, and dropping out of high school. Of particular interest was the finding that the natural course of conduct disorder did not appear to be influenced by psychiatric treatment, lengthy incarceration, job or military experiences, or degree of religious involvement (Robins 1966). In contrast, marriage to a stable spouse, support from siblings and parents, and brief incarceration were found to be helpful in promoting stability.

Among youths with conduct disorder, childhood predictors of chronicity and unfavorable outcome in adulthood include early onsct, attentional problems, school failure, anxiety disorders (two or more in childhood), substance abuse, antisocial behavior, arson, socialization deficits, family discord, family history of antisocial personality disorder, and low socioeconomic status. Family risk factors appear to be more prognostically significant for the development of conduct disorder than for any other child psychiatric diagnosis (Fendrich et al. 1990).

Better socialization, positive social experiences, and adequate social skills—especially assertiveness and effective problem-solving—are useful in predicting a better long-term outcome (Jenkins 1973; Rutter and Giller 1984). The nature of involvement with peers is also a predictor of course and severity. Peer ratings of misbehavior and low popularity in first grade were found to predict delinquent behavior during adolescence (Tremblay et al. 1988). Furthermore, ratings of aggressivity made by a child's peers at age 8 years may predict certain features of the person's psychiatric, marital, and legal status at age 28–30 (Huesmann et al. 1984).

Complications of conduct disorder are numerous: school failure, school suspension, legal problems, injuries due to fighting or retaliation, accidents, sexually transmitted disease, teenage pregnancy, prostitution, being raped or murdered, criminal activity, imprisonment, fugitive status, abandonment of family, drug addiction, suicide, and homicide. Consequences of comorbid attention deficits and learning disorders can include low frustration tolerance, educational failure, loss of interest in school, underdevelopment of verbal skills, school dropout, and subsequent unemployment. Children with conduct disorder have a high rate of physical injuries, accidents, and illnesses, as well as emergency department visits and hospitalizations. At follow-up, the most common causes of mortality in conduct disorder were found to be suicide, motor vehicle accidents, and death from uncertain causes (Rydelius 1988).

Despite the extremely high incidence of major psychopathology, maladjustment, and incarceration, about half of the children with conduct disorder achieve a favorable adult adjustment (Loeber 1982; Rutter and Giller 1984). There is a tendency toward a reduction in antisocial symptoms after age 40 (Hare et al. 1988; Robins 1966). Although later onset, adequate supervision at home, and good socialization skills are predictors of better course and adult outcome, it is unknown to what degree the good outcomes are associated with the natural course of illness, life experiences, therapeutic intervention, comorbidity, or preexisting characteristics.

Diagnostic Evaluation

For youths with conduct disorder who have impaired verbal skills, use manipulative defenses, or become uncomfortable when talking with professionals, participation in interactive diagnostic interviews can be difficult. Specific verbal inquiries or repetitive questioning can elicit inconsistent or hostile responses. For these individuals, standard interviews can be ineffective or even counterproductive. Assessments based on highly verbal and structured interviews may overestimate the psychopathology and underestimate the interpersonal or intellectual strengths of these individuals.

Virtually any child psychiatric disorder can present with behavior problems or with comorbid conduct disorder. In assessing an individual with conduct disorder, it is essential to evaluate the full range of psychiatric diagnoses, neurological status, intelligence and neuropsychological features, educational skills and deficits, social adaptation and assertiveness, and family functioning.

The finding that up to 25% of children with conduct disorder also have bipolar disorder, but that there is no overrepresentation of conduct disorder with major depressive disorder, challenges the formerly common clinical belief that a diagnosis of conduct disorder is a signal that the child must be depressed. Instead, conduct disorder can be more appropriately interpreted as a signal that the child might have bipolar disorder. Conduct disorder can appear before or after the apparent onset of bipolar disorder, and the conduct disorder may persist or remit after the resolution of the bipolar symptoms (Kovacs et al. 1988; T. Spencer et al. 2001).

Substance abuse, although very common among patients with conduct disorder, is commonly underdiagnosed. It is not unusual for the substance abuse to remain undiagnosed until these patients present for treatment as adults (Schubiner et al. 2000; Whitmore et al. 1997).

In addition to comorbid bipolar disorder and substance abuse, it is clinically helpful to emphasize that learning and communication disorders are common

concomitants of conduct disorder and can contribute to a chronic course. Developmental deficits in social skills and other adaptive functions are often apparent, even in individuals who have predominantly inattentive ADHD. Mild mental retardation is often overlooked. Prepsychotic children and intermittently psychotic children may have or appear to have conduct disorder.

Treatment

Psychiatric treatment of conduct disorder depends more on individual variables than on diagnosis. Given the diversity of presentations and severities of conduct disorder, it is not surprising that treatment can move in several directions: legal sanctions, family interventions, social support, psychotherapeutic treatment of individual or family psychopathology, or pharmacological treatment (Kazdin 1987). The biopsychosocial treatment of conduct disorder can involve a large multidisciplinary team, conceivably including a psychiatrist, a psychologist, a pediatrician, a neurologist, an educational consultant, a speech and language specialist, an occupational and recreational supervisor, a social worker, a legal adviser, a parole officer, a school liaison person, and a case manager. The treatment site can be a home, school, hospital, residential school, or specialized delinquency program.

From the very start to the end of treatment, the quick establishment of a containment structure and an expectation of effective limit setting—to provide both safety and a holding environment for treatment—are essential. Limit setting at home may be compromised by parental conflict, parental absence, inconsistent discipline, vague or low behavioral expectations, or parental depression or other psychiatric illness. Creating or reinforcing limits can involve parent counseling, psychiatric treatment of parents, increased supervision at home, surveillance at school, or use of legal mechanisms. Guardianship, hearings before judges, counseling by parole officers, and brief incarceration may be essential for effective limit setting and for communicating the significance of behavioral violations. Treatment of conduct disorder typically requires the involved management of multiple systems (Kazdin 1997).

The possible primary and sustaining roles of comorbid mental disorders in most cases of conduct disorder require that mental health professionals evaluate and follow up psychiatric factors in essentially all cases. The minimum required would be a consultative role in a multimodal treatment program. A single treatment method can be decisive for some individuals with conduct disorder, but the vast majority of patients require multimodal treatment.

Pharmacological research on conduct disorder is quite limited, and most therapeutic effects have appeared to be more closely related to the comorbidity than to the conduct disorder itself. Indeed, the range of medications used in treatment reflects the range of comorbidity presenting with conduct disorder, and it appears to have little to do with specific treatment of conduct disorder per se. Pharmacotherapy can involve virtually any psychotropic drug, depending on the concomitant neuropsychiatric findings in the individual: psychostimulants for ADHD, lithium or anticonvulsants for bipolar disorders, antidepressants for depressive disorders, neuroleptics for psychotic features or impulsive behavior (Findling et al. 2000), and β-adrenergic blocking agents for severe aggression.

For treating comorbid ADHD and conduct disorder, a wide variety of medications could be useful, including psychostimulants, but the risks of comorbid substance abuse and drug dealing need to be considered. In a 4-year prospective study, 58% of the youths with comorbid conduct disorder and ADHD had their conduct symptoms remit with adequate treatment of their ADHD (Biederman et al. 2001b), a significant finding that emphasizes the importance of early and aggressive treatment of ADHD. Open trials of pemoline (Shah et al. 1994) also have indicated some therapeutic effects, but there is no evidence of the value of this drug in treating conduct disorder in the absence of ADHD. When using pemoline, the risks of drug-induced chemical hepatitis (potentially fulminant), substance abuse (although less than with short-acting psychostimulants), and drug dealing must be considered. Open-label clonidine also has been reported helpful in treating comorbid conduct disorder and ADHD (Schvehla et al. 1994).

A variety of psychotherapeutic treatments may be helpful, including cognitive-behavioral therapy for anger and impulse-control management (Faulstich et al. 1988) and individual psychotherapy for problem-solving skills (Kazdin et al. 1989; Kernberg and Chazan 1991). Group therapy, particularly in residential treatment or group-oriented facilities, often permits the "gang orientation" of these youths to be used in promoting positive change and improving socialization skills.

Youths with conduct disorder often have family members with externalizing behaviors and psychiatric disorders. Psychiatric treatment is often needed for the psychiatric disorders of the parents or siblings. A major focus of working with family members may involve maintaining effective limits and a focused orientation toward treatment (rather than punishment). Functional family therapy can be useful in some cases for reducing interpersonal manipulation (Patterson 1982) and for limiting projective identification between family members (Tolan et al. 1986).

School interventions can include individualized educational programming, vocational training, and remediation of language and learning disorders. Evidence indicates that the early treatment of learning disorders may help prevent the development of conduct disorder.

Oppositional Defiant Disorder

Children with oppositional defiant disorder show argumentative and disobedient behavior but, unlike children with conduct disorder, respect the personal "rights" of other people. Similar provocative and antiauthority behavior is common in children with conduct disorders and ADHD, but oppositional defiant disorder is a separate diagnosis in its own right. In addition, children may show oppositional or defiant behavior during major affective episodes (depression or hypomania) or more enduringly in chronic mood disorder. However, the term *oppositional defiant disorder* describes children whose provocative, antiauthority, or angry behavior occurs apart from psychosis or symptomatic periods of mood disorders (Table 15–6). Criteria for oppositional defiant disorder are often fulfilled in individuals with ADHD, conduct disorder, bipolar disorder, and other psychiatric diagnoses (Greene and Doyle 1999).

Clinical Description

Oppositional and defiant features can be normal for young children ages 18–36 months and for adolescents; the 6-month minimum duration criterion for oppositional defiant disorder is used to exclude ordinary developmental phenomena.

Anger-related symptoms are the presenting behavior problems, but management of anger appears to be a circumscribed problem. Unlike children with ADHD, the oppositional and angry behav-

---

TABLE 15–6.   DSM-IV-TR diagnostic criteria for oppositional defiant disorder

A. A pattern of negativistic, hostile, and defiant behavior lasting at least 6 months, during which four (or more) of the following are present:
    (1) often loses temper
    (2) often argues with adults
    (3) often actively defies or refuses to comply with adults' requests or rules
    (4) often deliberately annoys people
    (5) often blames others for his or her mistakes or misbehavior
    (6) is often touchy or easily annoyed by others
    (7) is often angry and resentful
    (8) is often spiteful or vindictive
    Note: Consider a criterion met only if the behavior occurs more frequently than is typically observed in individuals of comparable age and developmental level.
B. The disturbance in behavior causes clinically significant impairment in social, academic, or occupational functioning.
C. The behaviors do not occur exclusively during the course of a psychotic or mood disorder.
D. Criteria are not met for conduct disorder, and, if the individual is age 18 years or older, criteria are not met for antisocial personality disorder.

---

ior of these children does not lead to impulsivity throughout their behavior, affect, and cognition (Halperin et al. 1995). The anger is typically directed at parents and teachers, and a lesser degree of anger dyscontrol may be seen in peer relationships. Temper tantrums typically subside in minutes, at most in 30 minutes. Children with mood disorders can require considerably longer to reorganize after an angry outburst.

A crucial feature of oppositional struggling is the self-defeating stand that these children take in arguments. They may be willing to lose something they want (a privilege or toy) rather than lose a struggle. The oppositional struggle takes on a life of its own in the child's mind and becomes more important than the reality of the situation. This "holding onto" or "winning" the struggle may feel paramount to the child. "Rational" objections voiced to the child become counterproductive, and the child may experience these interventions as the adult continuing the argument.

Epidemiology

Approximately 6% of children have oppositional defiant disorder, with estimates ranging from 1% to 10%. Along with ADHD, it is the most prevalent psychiatric disorder in 5- to 9-year-old children (August et al. 1996). A male predominance of 2–3:1 was reported in a nonreferred epidemiological sample (Anderson et al. 1987). Oppositional defiant disorder is commonly seen in classrooms for emotionally disturbed and learning-disabled children.

Etiology

The etiology of oppositional defiant disorder is not well understood. The influences of comorbid diagnoses, especially comorbid mood disorders and ADHD, will be important to sort out in studies that attempt to establish etiology. Oppositional defiant disorder often appears to be a characteristic of a family rather than of a child (K.E. Fletcher et al. 1996). In the absence of direct studies of the etiology of oppositional defiant disorder, several psychosocial mechanisms have been hypothesized: 1) parental problems (too harsh or inadequate) in disciplining, structuring, and limit-setting; 2) identification by the child with an impulse-disordered or aggressive parent, who sets a role model for oppositional and defiant interactions with other people; 3) attachment deficits caused by parents' emotional or physical

unavailability (e.g., depression, separation, evening work hours); and 4) impairments in the development of affect regulation and social cognition.

Neurological, neurobiological, and temperamental factors also may contribute. Traumatic brain injury has been associated with oppositional and defiant symptoms that appear approximately 2 years after injury (Max et al. 1998). Elevated dehydroepiandrosterone sulfate levels in children were found to be highly specific to a diagnosis of oppositional defiant disorder, suggesting a potential role of adrenal androgen functioning (van Goozen et al. 2000). Reduced plasma levels of serotonin (5-hydroxyindoleacetic acid [5-HIAA]) and dopamine (homovanillic acid [HVA]) metabolites were found in boys with oppositional defiant disorder, with degree of reduction correlating to aggressive and delinquent behaviors (van Goozen et al. 1999).

Course and Prognosis

Oppositional defiant disorder can be diagnosed after age 3 years but usually appears in late childhood. Follow-up studies suggest that 40% of the children with oppositional defiant disorder retain the diagnosis for at least 4 years, and 93% retain psychiatric symptoms (Cantwell and Baker 1989). Some evidence suggests a developmental progression for some individuals with oppositional defiant disorder to conduct disorder in adolescence and antisocial personality disorder in adulthood (Langbehn et al. 1998). However, even though conduct disorder is often preceded by oppositional defiant disorder, oppositional defiant disorder does not generally develop into conduct disorder (Speltz et al. 1999). Parental use of physical discipline appears to be associated with a less favorable outcome at 2-year follow-up (Speltz et al. 1998).

Diagnostic Evaluation

Behavioral evidence of oppositional defiant disorder often can be obtained within 30 minutes by observing peer interactions (Matthys et al. 1995). Psychiatric evaluation of the child and family is needed to investigate family and psychosocial factors as well as to identify concurrent presentations with conduct disorder, ADHD, mood disorders, or psychotic disorders. It is also worthwhile to evaluate for a learning disorder, language disorder, or low intelligence; the persistence of these conditions can contribute to a child's oppositional behavior.

Treatment

Several studies in the psychology literature have reported that behavioral techniques can modify oppositional behavior. Different presentations of oppositional defiant disorder and different comorbidity may justify different behavioral approaches to treatment (Greene and Doyle 1999). Parent training has been particularly useful in ameliorating oppositional behavior in children (Danforth 1998). One large-scale study reported that psychoanalytic psychotherapy had greater effectiveness in treating oppositional defiant disorder (56%) than in treating conduct disorder (23%), especially if the patient and family did not drop out during the first year of treatment (Fonagy and Target 1994). No controlled studies support the typical practice of treating these children with individual or family psychotherapy.

Learning, Motor Skills, and Communication Disorders

Developmental problems and barriers to the acquisition or performance of specific skills are usually first diagnosed in childhood and can have major consequences for lifetime functioning. Three major domains of skills are addressed by DSM-IV-TR. The learning disorders involve a series of impairments in the learning of academic skills, particularly reading, mathematics, and expressive writing. Motor skills disorder entails difficulty with physical coordination. The communication disorders involve developmental problems with language and speech, specifically deficits of expressive language, receptive (plus expressive) language, stuttering, and articulation.

These disorders often occur in combination with other psychiatric comorbidity in individuals and families. In practice, these children commonly present with psychiatric or behavior problems, and the learning and communication disorders are uncovered secondarily.

Most of these disorders are defined by a particular skill or area of functioning that is impaired relative to general intelligence. DSM-IV-TR criteria specify that these diagnoses should be based on more than simple clinical observation; when possible, standardized test protocols are important for documenting the presence of a specific deficit. Depending on the disorder, formal measurements of both intelligence and specific skills may be required for diagnosis.

As a group, these disorders are present in 10%–15% of the school-age population. Most of these disorders have a male predominance of 3:1–4:1. Equal sex ratios are reported for reading disorder, mathematics disorder, and mixed receptive-expressive language disorder. All of these disorders run in families.

The etiology is unknown but is generally believed to be related to dysmaturation or early damage to the brain areas related to these specific processing functions. The strength of the direct evidence for genetic or biological abnormalities varies with each disorder, and nonbiological factors also are clearly involved in shaping outcome. There is no reason to assume that each disorder is due to a single pathological mechanism, and subtyping may become possible as the brain mechanisms involved become better understood. The clustering of these disorders in the same individuals suggests that these neuropsychological impairments reflect an early disruption in developmental processes, can involve wide-ranging but potentially related cerebral dysfunctions, and are likely to require multimodal educational remediation and subsequent educational accommodations.

These learning, motor skills, and communication disorders are commonly associated with high rates of comorbid psychiatric disorders and various psychological complications, including low self-esteem ("feeling stupid"), poor frustration tolerance, passivity, rigidity in new learning situations, truancy, and dropping out of school. Disruptive behavior disorder can be a complication of these disorders, but signs of developmental dysfunction may appear before school failure, in the preschool years. Although there has been considerable emphasis on the "emotional overlay" resulting from learning and communication disorders, there is an increasing awareness of the neuropsychiatric and sociofamilial antecedents of these disorders.

Over time, mild cases may "resolve" through persistent education and practice. Certain individuals may compensate by "overlearning," but others retain specific deficits in adulthood. Often, the associated behavioral symptoms and intrapsychic complications persist beyond the duration of the developmental deficits, and they may remain problematic during adult life (J. Cohen 1985).

Psychoeducational evaluation includes intelligence testing, a battery of specific achievement tests (of the full range of ac-

ademic skills, language, speech, and motor coordination), and observation of the child's behavior in the classroom. A general determination of the quality of teaching available at the school is needed before a diagnosis is made. It is also essential to evaluate for possible mental retardation, ADHD, mood disorder (causing low motivation), and other psychiatric and neurological disorders. Sensory perception tests are given to assess possible impairments of vision or hearing, which can aggravate or mimic features of these disorders.

Although children with these underdiagnosed and undertreated disorders have begun to receive remediation during childhood, the many types of psychoeducational and educational techniques in use nationwide have been too infrequently evaluated in comparative studies.

Psychopharmacological therapy is not helpful in treating learning, communication, or motor skills disorders. Aggressive management is required for psychological effects on self-esteem, patience, assertiveness, and flexibility. The evaluation and treatment of concurrent psychiatric disorders, as well as the management of secondary psychological complications, require more than a purely educational or neuropsychiatric perspective.

These neurodevelopmental disorders appear to be predominantly genetic or neuromaturational in origin; however, socioenvironmental factors are critical in the appearance of the complications of these disorders, so that psychosocial and interpersonal factors are central in treatment and prognosis.

Learning Disorders

The learning disorders involve deficits in the acquisition and performance of reading, writing (not handwriting but expressive writing), or arithmetic. These conditions are meant to designate individuals who have specific deficits in acquiring skills and neurointegrative processing, and so are qualitatively different from other slow learners.

Learning disorders are defined to exclude individuals whose slow learning is explainable by weak educational opportunities, low intelligence, motor or sensory (visual or auditory) handicaps, or neurological problems. In understanding the effect of these disorders, it is helpful to hold a broad psychiatric and neurological view of development in childhood and functioning in adulthood because the estimated 5%–10% of the population with learning disorders is at increased risk for other psychiatric disorders. People with learning disorders commonly have a comorbid communication or motor skills disorder, low self-esteem, motivational problems, and symptoms of anxiety.

The diagnosis of a learning disorder is often made initially during grade school. During the early school years, basic skills, attention, and motivation are building blocks for subsequent learning. Major impairments in these fundamental abilities require identification and remediation to avoid developmental derailment in multiple spheres of functioning. In later school years, organizational skills become increasingly significant: problems with note taking, time management, and book and paper arrangements may be signs of cortical deficits, even for individuals whose basic skills are well remedied. In high school and college, these students may have difficulty in learning foreign languages, writing efficiently, reading for fun, enjoying sports, pursuing intellectual studies, setting high personal goals, or striving to achieve their goals (J. Cohen 1985).

Reading Disorder

Learning to read can be compromised in many ways, but reading disorder is a spe-

---

TABLE 15–7. DSM-IV-TR diagnostic criteria for reading disorder

A. Reading achievement, as measured by individually administered standardized tests of reading accuracy or comprehension, is substantially below that expected given the person's chronological age, measured intelligence, and age-appropriate education.
B. The disturbance in Criterion A significantly interferes with academic achievement or activities of daily living that require reading skills.
C. If a sensory deficit is present, the reading difficulties are in excess of those usually associated with it.

Coding note: If a general medical (e.g., neurological) condition or sensory deficit is present, code the condition on Axis III.

---

cific neuropsychiatric form of reading disability. Commonly called developmental dyslexia, this learning disorder is characterized by a slow acquisition of reading skills resulting from demonstrable cognitive deficits, primarily in cortical function, in the presence of normal intelligence, educational opportunity, motivation, and emotional control. Slow reading speed, impaired comprehension, word omissions or distortions, and letter reversals result in functioning below the expected performance levels based on age and intelligence (Table 15–7).

Although the distinctiveness of this disorder was once questioned, reading disorder has been validated as a specific disorder. The historically influential Isle of Wight study (Rutter and Yule 1975) revealed a hump at the "slow" end of the curve for reading acquisition and no analog of "fast" learners at the high end of the curve; these findings were taken for many years to support reading disorder as an entity distinct from simple learning slowness or other causes of difficulty learning to read. In retrospect, these findings appear to have resulted from an artifact of the reading test used in the study (Van der Wissel and Zegers 1985). Subsequent data suggested that reading ability follows a normal distribution in the population, similar to blood pressure. Reading disability is determined by a cutoff score, just as is hypertension. Like many other medical conditions, reading disorder is now viewed as a lifelong condition with familial genetic transmission, heterogeneous etiology, and important environmental determinants of outcome.

Clinical description.   The "core" specific dysfunction in most dyslexic patients involves a defect in phonological processing. In phonological processing, words are decomposed (decoded) into their constituent units of sound (phonemes) and then mapped onto the appropriate groups of letters (graphemes). Impairment in the accuracy and speed of reading single words is the "gold standard" difficulty in reading disorder, and it arises specifically from the difficulty with phonological processing. Slow and inaccurate reading of phonetically "legal" nonsense words is the most accurate predictor of reading problems. Reading disorder seems to involve dysfunction of a largely "posterior" cortical system specialized for reading (Shaywitz et al. 1998). Contrary to earlier belief, support for specific visuospatial processing problems is currently rather limited.

The prominent features of reading disorder may present differently at different ages. Children with reading disorder frequently manifest early or preclinical signs of the disorder. Difficulties in learning the letters of the alphabet and the names of numbers, in learning to associate sounds with letters, and in rhyming words or being confused by words that sound alike are common. Additionally, mild language delays and mild expressive language difficul-

ties, such as difficulties with word finding, mispronunciation, and breaks in speech, may be early indicators of risk for reading disorder. They may be early indicators of more general language difficulties as well.

With increasing age, delays in reading acquisition, slow oral reading, and poor comprehension are appreciated. In the elementary school years, problems associating letters with sounds evolve into problems sounding out written words (particularly "legal" nonsense words) and translating spoken words into properly spelled (orthographically correct) words. Syllables may be elided or their letters reversed, as may letters of similar phonology or morphology, such as *b* and *d*. In oral reading or dictation, words may be left out, unfamiliar words creatively spelled, and familiar words substituted for unfamiliar words with similar general appearance. Difficulty with the reading of single words and especially difficulty in reading phonetically "legal" nonsense words are the strongest predictors of poor reading comprehension in elementary school.

Reading disorder is a lifelong disability. Of the children with reading disorder identified in the first grade, 74% have significantly impaired reading in the tenth grade. The spelling problems typically associated with reading disorder usually are lifelong and may be more severe and long lasting than the reading problem. Because reading disorder persists, strategies for accommodation will eventually supplant remediation because reading will be slower and laborious in most dyslexic patients.

Epidemiology.   Reading disorder is by far the most prevalent of the learning disorders, involving 80% of all individuals with learning disorders. Prevalence estimates for reading disorder vary widely; DSM-IV-TR cites a prevalence of 4% in the United States, but figures up to 17.5%

of the general population have been reported. Reading disorder was believed to show the 3:1–4:1 male predominance observed in most learning disorders, but more recent data suggest an equal prevalence in males and females (Shaywitz et al. 1990; Wadsworth et al. 1992). Reading disorder is familial, and current data suggest that from 23% to 65% of the affected children have an affected parent. Increased prevalence of reading disorder is associated with low socioeconomic class, large family size, and social disadvantage. Prevalence has been reported to vary with geographic region, but this may reflect different standards for classification or other differences in ascertainment. The prevalence of reading disorder may differ across countries, where demands for high-quality reading may vary and where reading may involve different linguistic structures or pictographic symbols.

Etiology.   Several lines of evidence lend support for the central role of the phonological processing deficits in reading disorder (Swank 1999). Measures of phonological processing are predictive of later reading success (Torgesen et al. 1994). Deficits in phonological awareness distinguish normal readers from dyslexic patients (Stanovitch and Siegel 1994). These deficits persist into adult life and continue to be associated with the degree of reading impairment (Bruck 1992). Interventions to improve phonological awareness have been found to promote reading acquisition (Foorman et al. 1997; Wise and Olson 1995).

Reading disorder appears to be related to dysfunction principally in the posterior superior temporal gyrus (Wernicke's area), the angular gyrus, the striate cortex, the inferior frontal gyrus (Broca's area), and the inferior lateral extrastriate cortex. These neurological structures appear to be involved in the rapid sequencing of spoken language into phonemes and in subsequent phonological and metaphonological processing.

MRI data show subtle variations in the morphology of the corpus callosum. The reduction in the anterior (genu) volume of the corpus callosum suggests potential difficulties with interhemispheric transfer (Hynd et al. 1995). These studies also found a significant correlation between corpus callosum volume and reading achievement. A recent functional MRI (fMRI) study suggested abnormalities of activation in the left prefrontal cortex and in the right cerebellum. Together, these findings suggest that structural changes in the anterior corpus callosum that interfere with interhemispheric transfer or coordination of information might play a role in reading disorder.

Despite the neurogenetic factors in the etiology of reading disorder, environmental factors exert a strong influence on its expression and clinical presentation. Although the main etiological factors appear to be neurological, symptom severity and duration may be affected by learning and experience. The phonological and orthographic demands of one's language, educational opportunity, and self-expectations may affect outcome. Reading disorder can be negatively influenced by maternal smoking, low birth weight, and prenatal and perinatal mishaps. In the positive direction, reading disorder can be beneficially influenced by educational opportunities; family support; and individual personality, drive, and ambition. In this sense, none of the neurological abnormalities can be assumed to be deterministic causes of reading disorder because educational and environmental factors interact to alter the expression of these neuronal lesions.

Course and prognosis.   For reading disorder and slow reading acquisition, adequate reading skills eventually may be acquired with sufficient time and effort. Educational interventions appear to accelerate this process, especially if family support and personal motivation are strong. The extent of residual symptoms in reading disorder and its associated features is quite variable.

Delayed acquisition of reading skills usually is identified in grade school. Typically, by third grade, the child with reading disorder is 1–2 years behind expectations and may fall farther behind unless remediation is received. Adolescents may become frustrated with learning, lose interest in school, and drop out of school; in addition, there may be an exacerbation (or clinical recognition) of conduct disorder or other concomitant psychiatric disorders. Although reading usually improves over time, spelling problems and delinquency may persist. In adulthood, the rate of unemployment and placement in unskilled jobs is elevated.

Some adults never attain substantial reading skills and may adapt by hiding the disability from their children, friends, and employers. They may not seek remedial education or may continue to resist remediation in adulthood, because of either embarrassment, pride, or the required effort. The associated feature of rejection of help may be both a cause and a complication of persistent reading problems. Mismanagement of this major problem in early learning can become a model for the child's subsequent approach to problem solving. Alternatively, proper management can teach the child how to persevere in the face of a seemingly hopeless personal problem.

Diagnostic evaluation. It can be useful to obtain neurological and psychiatric assessment (especially regarding disruptive behavior, ADHD, other learning and communication disorders, and social deprivation); hearing and vision tests; and IQ,

psychological, neuropsychological, and educational measurements (including reading speed, comprehension, and spelling). The new neuroimaging techniques are expected to contribute significantly to diagnostic assessment in the future.

The evaluation of students with reading disorder often includes an assessment that determines whether they will receive extra training or accommodations through a special education program at school. Among students whose reading achievement scores are substantially below their intelligence measures, most would be classified as qualifying for special education services because their reading achievement scores are below the cutoff scores. However, bright students with reading disorder might have substantial reading underachievement relative to their intelligence but not "qualify" for special education services because their reading achievement scores exceed the cutoff scores. To allow such students to receive intervention, the evaluation process that determines which students will receive special education requires thoughtfulness and flexibility.

Treatment. Early educational intervention may involve one of several remedial programs. Comparative studies of the different educational approaches to reading disorder are still limited, but growing evidence supports the use of phonologically based interventions. In an interesting approach to outcome measurement, an intensive 3-week program that emphasized phonological segmentation and comprehension was found to normalize lactate metabolism in the inferior frontal gyrus in dyslexic children at the end of treatment (Richards et al. 2000).

In addition to remediating the phonological and reading deficits, treatment should be directed at comorbid learning or communication disorders, disruptive behavior disorders (i.e., conduct disorder or ADHD), or mood or anxiety disorders. Self-esteem may need to be bolstered to help the child (or adult) tolerate the remedial efforts. Parental involvement is crucial in providing support for the educational program and for the child's persistent efforts in a criticism-free learning environment. Some parents may advocate alternative vitamin or dietary approaches, but no data support these options for treating learning disorders (Arnold 2002). Parents can be advised that it is beneficial for them to listen to their children read at home daily (Tizard et al. 1982).

The standard psychotropic medications are not useful in treating reading disorder. Somewhat unexpectedly, piracetam has been reported—in double-blind, placebo-controlled studies in which standardized reading tests were among the outcome measures—to improve reading in children with developmental reading disorder. Such studies have demonstrated that the improvements in children are modest but consistent and statistically significant, and the longer studies (5–9 months) showed more pronounced improvements in reading. Furthermore, five double-blind, placebo-controlled studies in adults with reading disorder confirmed the findings in children. Piracetam, a derivative of GABA, has been used outside the United States to treat cognitive changes in the elderly. It is not a psychostimulant and does not alter levels of alertness or arousal. With accumulating evidence that piracetam can modestly improve reading in children and adults with reading disorder, further investigation of nootropic agents (memory or learning enhancers) should be entertained.

Mathematics Disorder

The capacity for making simple mathematical calculations is critical in a con-

---

TABLE 15–8. DSM-IV-TR diagnostic criteria for mathematics disorder

A. Mathematical ability, as measured by individually administered standardized tests, is substantially below that expected given the person's chronological age, measured intelligence, and age-appropriate education.
B. The disturbance in Criterion A significantly interferes with academic achievement or activities of daily living that require mathematical ability.
C. If a sensory deficit is present, the difficulties in mathematical ability are in excess of those usually associated with it.

Coding note: If a general medical (e.g., neurological) condition or sensory deficit is present, code the condition on Axis III.

---

sumer economy and high-technology culture. Arithmetic, calculation (fractions, decimals, percentages), measurement (space, time, weight), and logical reasoning are basic skills.

Clinical description. Mathematics disorder can present with circumscribed deficits associated with fact retrieval or with more globalized deficits associated with problem conceptualization. Arithmetic facts may be deficient despite preserved mathematical conceptual knowledge (Hittmair-Delazer et al. 1995). Individuals with mathematics disorder (Table 15–8) have difficulty in learning to count, doing simple mathematical calculations, conceptualizing sets of objects, and thinking spatially (right/left, up/down, east/west). Deficits may be seen in copying shapes, mathematical memory, number and procedure sequencing, and the naming of mathematical concepts and operations. Also, reading and spelling problems may be seen in association with mathematics disorder.

Factors that produce slow academic development of mathematical abilities include neurological, genetic, psychological, and socioeconomic conditions as well as learning experiences. Typically, arithmetic ability correlates with IQ and classroom training. However, mathematics disorder is not defined to designate individuals who are merely slow learners or who have poor educational opportunities; instead, it labels individuals whose mathematical abilities are low for their IQ. In addition, individuals with mathematics disorder often have comorbid psychiatric disorders or symptoms, although descriptions of the psychiatric concomitants of this disorder are limited.

Epidemiology. Approximately 3%–6% of the population is affected by mathematics disorder, and the sex distribution appears to be equal (Gross-Tsur et al. 1996; C. Lewis et al. 1994; Shalev et al. 2000). As in other learning disabilities, psychiatric comorbidities are common, especially conduct disorder. Also, about 20% of the patients have dyslexia, and about 25% have ADHD; children comorbid for dyslexia were more profoundly impaired on math skills and other neuropsychological measures than were children with mathematics disorder alone or with mathematics disorder and comorbid ADHD (Shalev et al. 1997). Attentional problems may lead to arithmetic difficulties (Ehlers et al. 1997) in children who do not have mathematics disorder, but children with such difficulties need to be evaluated for this disorder. Lower socioeconomic classes show an overrepresentation of mathematics disorder as well as other learning disorders. Studies of genetic contributions are sparse. In a large study of patients with developmental dyscalculia, about half of the siblings (Shalev et al. 2001) and 42% of the first-degree relatives of the index child (Gross-Tsur et al. 1996) were reported to have learning disabilities; the risks of dyscalculia in the first-degree relatives of affected children exceeded the risks to first-degree relatives of control children by 5- to 10-fold.

Etiology. Etiological factors in this disorder are not well defined. Individuals with mathematics disorder appear to have a type of neurocortical abnormality that is linked to a deficit in processing speed in some areas of mathematics (Bull and Johnston 1997). Neuropsychological deficits in number manipulation, spatial relationships, and mathematical reasoning may be present. Both verbal (sequencing) and visuospatial deficits can contribute to mathematics disorder, suggesting that bilateral hemisphere dysfunction may be involved (Rourke 1993; Rourke and Strang 1983). Although gross neurological deficit in the language-dominant hemisphere is not typically demonstrable, evidence indicates that the left hemisphere may play a relatively more important role, at least in certain functional deficits (Shalev et al. 1995). For example, the left prefrontal region has been implicated in mathematics disorder (Tohgi et al. 1995). Subcortical mechanisms also have been proposed.

Course and prognosis. During the school years, the course of mathematics disorder usually entails a progressive increase in disability, because the learning of mathematical skills is based on the developmental completion of earlier steps. Some children perform well on rote arithmetic but fail later in trigonometry and geometry, which require more abstract and spatial thinking. Over time, most individuals with mathematics disorder show gradual improvement. As in other learning disorders, complications include low self-esteem, truancy, dropping out of school, symptoms of disruptive behavior disorders, and avoidance (or poor performance) of jobs that require mathematical skills.

Diagnostic evaluation. Evaluation for mathematics disorder includes psychiatric (i.e., disruptive behavior disorders, other learning disorders, and mental retardation), neurological, cognitive (i.e., intelligence, psychological, neuropsychological, and educational achievement testing), and social assessments. Standardized tests of arithmetic skills may need to be individually adjusted for the child's educational experience with an older (rote calculation) or newer (logical concept) mathematics curriculum.

Treatment. Treatment of mathematics disorder involves special education, with initial evaluation and subsequent monitoring of the possible need for psychiatric and neurological intervention. It is interesting that when mathematics disorder is accompanied by ADHD, salient auditory stimulation has been found to improve mathematical performance (Abikoff et al. 1996).

The mathematical skills of a fifth- or sixth-grader without mathematics disorder are quite sufficient for the practical requirements of most adults, although concomitant social and nonverbal deficits that accompany mathematics disorder may be more significant and enduring (Semrud-Clikeman and Hynd 1990). After the school years (and even during them), weakness in arithmetic skills is not socially stigmatic and may not be a direct source of personal distress. It is likely that this disorder is quietly present in many adults, who make accommodations in their lives and choice of work to manage a residue of dysfunctions that were more evident during school years.

Disorder of Written Expression

Disorder of written expression is not well characterized in the psychiatric literature, and its assessment and treatment are not

---

TABLE 15–9. DSM-IV-TR diagnostic criteria for disorder of written expression

A. Writing skills, as measured by individually administered standardized tests (or functional assessments of writing skills), are substantially below those expected given the person's chronological age, measured intelligence, and age-appropriate education.

B. The disturbance in Criterion A significantly interferes with academic achievement or activities of daily living that require the composition of written texts (e.g., writing grammatically correct sentences and organized paragraphs).

C. If a sensory deficit is present, the difficulties in writing skills are in excess of those usually associated with it.

Coding note: If a general medical (e.g., neurological) condition or sensory deficit is present, code the condition on Axis III.

---

well developed. Spelling, grammar, sentence and paragraph formation, organizational structure, and punctuation are the areas of difficulty (Table 15–9).

Clinical description. Symptoms include slow writing speed, low written yield, illegibility, letter reversals, word-finding and syntax errors, erasures, rewritings, spacing errors, and punctuation and spelling problems. A more generalized "developmental output failure" may be suggested by low productivity, refusal to complete work or submit assignments, and chronic underachievement (Levine et al. 1981). Ideational content and intellectual abstraction may be limited, although not necessarily. The "sense of audience," a social cognition of the interests and needs of the reader, may be impaired (Gregg and McAlexander 1989).

Epidemiology and etiology. The prevalence of disorder of written expression is not well delineated. There is a standard

3:1–4:1 male predominance. These deficits in written expression may result from underlying problems with graphomotor (hand and pencil control), fine motor, and visuomotor function; attention; memory; concept formation and organization (prioritizing and flow); and expressive language function. Other motor dysfunctions may be present. Like other learning disorders, disorder of written expression is presumed to result from neurocortical dysfunctions, which may be modified by environmental experiences.

Diagnostic evaluation. Formal methods for assessment and measurement of expressive writing have been developed (Brown et al. 2000), but adequate clinical screening can be obtained from samples of copied, dictated, and spontaneous writing. In evaluating disorder of written expression, it is worthwhile to screen for developmental coordination disorders and other motor abnormalities.

Treatment. Genuine remedial therapy is possible. Educational interventions traditionally have consisted of alternative writing formats and skill building. The wide availability of computers has promoted new methods in remediation. Pending more specific research, the psychiatric evaluation and intervention for the disorder of written expression resemble the approach to the other learning disorders.

Motor Skills Disorder

Developmental Coordination Disorder

Developmental coordination disorder, the only motor skills disorder recognized in DSM-IV-TR, involves deficits in the learning and performance of motor skills (Table 15–10). Integration of motor functions and memory of motor tasks also are im-

paired. Overall, about 5%–6% of children have significant impairments of gross or fine motor functions, which are apparent in running, throwing a ball, buttoning, holding a pencil, and moving with grace; the disorder also may manifest as generalized physical awkwardness. Although the learning of new motor skills may be slow or delayed, some already-learned motor skills may be performed very well, whereas other learned movements are performed poorly. Movements that require coordinated symmetrical or bilateral actions (such as jumping or swimming), good balance (ice skating), or continuous positional changes (running, tennis) may be particularly difficult. Most of these children have difficulties with handwriting (Miller et al. 2001a). Perceptual problems are common, especially visuospatial processing (Wilson and McKenzie 1998). None of the motor impairments in developmental coordination disorder can be explained by fixed or localizable neurological abnormalities or by mechanical interference. It was previously assumed that these children would "outgrow" their motor learning problems, but long-term data suggest that the impairments commonly persist into adulthood (Cantell and Kooistra 2002; Fox and Lent 1996).

Although this disorder is rarely the primary complaint leading to psychiatric evaluation, it is commonly found in association with many psychiatric disorders, especially learning disorders, speech and language disorders, and ADHD (E.L. Hill 1998; Kadesjo and Gillberg 2001; Trauner et al. 2000). Even so, the psychiatric literature on developmental coordination disorder remains sparse (Miyahara and Mobs 1995).

Three main areas of motor deficits have been defined: clumsiness, adventitious movements, and dyspraxia. *Clumsiness*, technically defined as a slowness or awkwardness in the movement of single

TABLE 15–10. DSM-IV-TR diagnostic criteria for developmental coordination disorder

A. Performance in daily activities that require motor coordination is substantially below that expected given the person's chronological age and measured intelligence. This may be manifested by marked delays in achieving motor milestones (e.g., walking, crawling, sitting), dropping things, "clumsiness," poor performance in sports, or poor handwriting.

B. The disturbance in Criterion A significantly interferes with academic achievement or activities of daily living.

C. The disturbance is not due to a general medical condition (e.g., cerebral palsy, hemiplegia, or muscular dystrophy) and does not meet criteria for a pervasive developmental disorder.

D. If mental retardation is present, the motor difficulties are in excess of those usually associated with it.

Coding note: If a general medical (e.g., neurological) condition or sensory deficit is present, code the condition on Axis III.

joints, involves disruption of the integration of agonist and antagonist muscle groups. Although it is defined in terms of dysfunction at the basic level of single-joint movements, clumsiness can reduce the capacity to perform more complex motor tasks, such as riding a bike or drawing. Clinically, clumsiness is easily observed in finger tapping or in picking up very small objects. Clumsiness may present alone or associated with ADHD, learning disorders, or mental retardation (especially trisomy 21/Down syndrome), and it sometimes is aggravated by anticonvulsants.

Adventitious movements are involuntary movements that occur during voluntary movements. Overflow movements (i.e., synkinesias) may include mirror movements (which occur in symmetrically active muscles) or motions seen in unrelated muscle groups (e.g., opening the mouth while reaching). Other adventitious movements include tics, tremor, and chorea. Clinically, adventitious movements can be observed while the child is performing specific tasks that emphasize voluntary control.

Dyspraxia, the impaired learning or performance of sequential voluntary movements (relative to age or verbal intelligence) that cannot be attributed to gross sensory deficits or mechanical limitations, does not improve when specific tasks are executed without time limits or hurry. The expression of developmental dyspraxia may involve a range of muscle movements, from localized (face, tongue, or hands) to global, and may depend partially on cerebral dominance (both in spatial vs. linguistic functions and in left- vs. right-sided tasks). This symptom is also seen in mental retardation, especially fragile X syndrome. Dyspraxia may be screened clinically by asking the child to imitate some unusual hand or finger positions and by pantomiming sequential tasks (e.g., taking a bottle out of a refrigerator, opening it, pouring the contents, and having a drink from the glass).

A common problem faced by parents of children with developmental coordination disorder is that physicians, especially in the absence of evidence of hard neurological findings, may indicate that children will simply outgrow the problems. Evidence indicates that some children with mild symptoms may show a generally improving course over time, but it appears that others show highly persistent symptoms. In general, longitudinal studies suggest the development and persistence of neurocognitive impairments, academic underachievement, reduced self-esteem, social withdrawal, and passivity, at least for individuals with more severe manifestations of developmental coordination disorder (Cantell and Kooistra 2002). Even children who learn basic motor skills appear to have difficulty later in learning new age-appropriate motor skills (Missiuna 2001).

These children often avoid voluntary physical activities and become less physically fit than their peers, potentially placing their long-term health at risk (Bouffard et al. 1996).

Formal treatment for developmental coordination disorder may seem questionable in clinical settings, especially for mild presentations, but the longitudinal data suggest that it is a risk factor for various forms of later psychopathology and possibly other health problems. More simply, "good hands" and athletic ability are crucial building blocks of self-esteem for children and adolescents and may be economically vital for some adults, so remediation is warranted to promote general development, even if special education funding is limited.

Communication Disorders

Speech problems (regarding sound production) are seen in about 15% of the general school-age population, and language problems (involving the communicative use of speech as well as other communicative modes) are seen in about 3%–7%. The frequent association of communication disorders, including disorders of speech or language, with the learning disorders highlights the general cerebral dysfunctions that characterize both groups of disorders. Some evidence suggests that language disorders may be developmental precursors of learning disorders rather than merely comorbid disorders of independent etiology (Snowling et al. 2000; Torgesen et al. 1994). Language disorders in young children may not become clinically evident until the appearance of learning disorders during the school years.

About 25%–50% of child psychiatric

patients have a communication disorder. About 50% of the children with communication disorders have concomitant psychiatric disorders, most notably ADHD, and in an additional 20%, learning disorders eventually appear (Beitchman et al. 1986; Cantwell and Baker 1987; Snowling et al. 2000; Tomblin et al. 2000). Children with developmental language disorders (and speech disorders) also tend to have motor deficits (E.L. Hill 1998; Trauner et al. 2000), and these deficits also may require treatment (Owen and McKinlay 1997). Language deficiencies observed in children with ADHD are typically higher-order executive deficiencies and not deficits in basic language processing (Purvis and Tannock 1997).

The usual development of language and speech skills occurs over many years, and there is a wide range of normal functioning. Speech and language may interact with other environmental factors in influencing development and adult skills. Sex differences in cortical maturation may relate to girls' developmental advantage in verbal skills (which lasts until adolescence), which is comparable to boys' advantage in spatial processing.

In speech and language disorders, deficits in articulation (diction or speech sound production), expression (oral language production and use), and reception (comprehension) may be evident by age 2–3 years. Early speech and language problems frequently improve during development, and these early delays are not strongly predictive of subsequent learning disorders. However, children with genuine early speech and language problems are at high risk for later learning disorders as well as persistent communication disorders. Most preschool children with communication disorders (70%) are placed in special education or repeat a grade within the first 10 years of schooling (Aram et al. 1984).

As in the learning disorders, recent

research in communication disorders is moving away from an emphasis on deficits in audioperceptual processing and toward a conceptualization based on language and symbolic functions. Sensory, perceptual, motor, and cognitive processes are closely connected in cerebral development. During the course of early development of the cerebral cortex, there is a progressive leftward lateralization of language functions, including speech (sound production), phonetic and syntactic analysis, and verbal (as well as nonverbal) sequence analysis. The right hemisphere appears to be more involved in sound recognition than the left. Lesion data and neurobiological theory have implicated the left perisylvian regions in the processing of phonemes and auditory information. These findings have been confirmed by MRI, single photon emission spectroscopy, and PET. The areas of the planum temporale and angular gyrus appear compromised in both children and adults with language impairments (Semrud-Clikeman 1997). Also, evidence is emerging of familial transmission of these specific and discrete deficits (Tallal et al. 2001).

Socioeconomic and cultural factors are associated with speech and language impairments (Tomblin et al. 1997a) and may contribute to their risk. Prematurity, CNS infections, and other pre- and perinatal risk factors may increase the severity of or account for speech and language impairments (Tomblin et al. 1997b).

Hearing loss plays a significant role in the etiology of the communication disorders (Bennett and Haggard 1999). Hearing is crucial in the development of speech and language, and impairments of hearing operate etiologically alongside genetic, neurological, environmental, and educational factors. Deafness is associated with clear reduction in communication skills, but milder hearing decrements also may be developmentally significant. A mild

hearing loss (25–40 decibels) resulting from chronic otitis media or perforation of the tympanic membrane may delay development of articulation, expressive and receptive language, and spelling. During the formative period for language development, fluctuating hearing capacity can diminish verbal intelligence and academic performance in a persistent way (Howie 1980).

Early middle-ear pathology may cause language or speech symptoms, particularly if the hearing impairment is chronic. Otitis media, a common infectious disease in children, may leave a residual hearing decrement in 20% of the American population. The degree of language and speech delay may correlate to the number of otitis episodes. Determinants of otitis media include socioeconomic class, allergies, and oropharyngeal (palate) or craniofacial malformations. Hearing loss also may result from genetic and metabolic disorders, chromosomal anomalies, low birth weight, perinatal anoxic damage, CNS infections, ototoxic medications (e.g., antibiotics, diuretics), and toxin exposures (e.g., alcohol, anticonvulsants). Sociofamilial as well as medical factors can contribute, via otitis media, to the appearance of communication disorders.

It has been speculated that the mechanisms involved in early influences on the development of the cerebral cortex may be useful in understanding the pathogenesis of learning disorders as well as communication disorders, and they may apply to a broader range of mental functions.

Speech and language skills are eventually acquired in virtually all children with communication disorders, but lower IQ and concomitant psychopathology appear to predict less favorable outcome. Complications include progressive academic impairments, psychological distress, low self-esteem, rigidity regarding learning, and dropping out of school.

Evaluation includes a medical, psychiatric, social, and developmental workup as well as language and speech assessment (Cantwell and Baker 1987). Because 20% of children have hearing deficits caused by otitis media, it is helpful to test for hearing acuity with methods such as audiometry or auditory evoked response (which does not require a young child's cooperation). Parents may give a history of few startle reactions, lack of sound imitation (at 6 months) or reactiveness (at 12 months), unintelligibility (at 2.5 years), loud speech, frequent misunderstandings ("Huh?"), speech avoidance, or communication-associated embarrassment or tension (e.g., blinking). Assessing family characteristics (e.g., family size, birth order, socioeconomic status, parental verbal skills, familial speech patterns, interpersonal stimulation), as well as observing free speech between parents and child, may be useful. The child's speech may be studied for language comprehension (linguistic structures), expression (structure and length of utterances), and logical reasoning. Auditory attention (e.g., keeping up with the flow of conversation, ability to hear in a crowd, lack of distractibility), discrimination (e.g., distinguishing similar sounds), and memory (e.g., the ability to repeat sequences of words or digits) can be assessed informally or formally. In neuropsychological tests, nonverbal measures of IQ (e.g., Leiter International Performance Scale, Columbia Scale of Mental Maturity) are used. Also, a neurological evaluation may be indicated for children with a communication disorder in whom a motor abnormality is suspected.

Treatment of communication disorders includes educational and behavioral interventions, as well as treatment of concomitant medical (e.g., hearing), neurological (e.g., seizures), and psychiatric problems. Aggressive treatment of otitis media is particularly indicated in these children, despite the uncertainty about the relation of this disease to language and speech development. It is particularly helpful to encourage social involvement, imitation, and imaginative play as a means of increasing verbal, communicative, and symbolic exercise. There is no evidence that use of nonverbal communication by child or parents inhibits the development of language skills, and it might even enhance such skills.

Expressive Language Disorder

In expressive language disorder, which involves a linguistic "encoding" problem, the symbolic production and communicative use of language are impaired. The individual cannot put the idea into words ("I can't get the words out") and also has problems in nonverbal expression. These individuals have similar difficulties with repeating, imitating, pointing to named objects, or acting on commands. Unlike autistic and pervasive developmental disorders, comprehension is typically normal in verbal and nonverbal communication. In verbal language, both semantic and syntactic errors occur so that word selection and sentence construction may be impaired; paraphrasing, narrating, and explaining are weak in intelligibility or coherence. The child with expressive language disorder may use developmentally earlier forms of language expression and may rely more on nonverbal communication for requests and comments. Short sentences and simple verbal structures may be used, even with nonverbal communications such as sign language (Paul et al. 1994). This feature implies a problem in symbolic development across language modalities, leading to a diverse group of delays in articulation, vocabulary, and grammar (Table 15–11).

Individuals with expressive language disorder generally learn language in a normal sequence but slowly. These children

TABLE 15–11. DSM-IV-TR diagnostic criteria for expressive language disorder

A. The scores obtained from standardized individually administered measures of expressive language development are substantially below those obtained from standardized measures of both nonverbal intellectual capacity and receptive language development. The disturbance may be manifest clinically by symptoms that include having a markedly limited vocabulary, making errors in tense, or having difficulty recalling words or producing sentences with developmentally appropriate length or complexity.

B. The difficulties with expressive language interfere with academic or occupational achievement or with social communication.

C. Criteria are not met for mixed receptive-expressive language disorder or a pervasive developmental disorder.

D. If mental retardation, a speech-motor or sensory deficit, or environmental deprivation is present, the language difficulties are in excess of those usually associated with these problems.

Coding note: If a speech-motor or sensory deficit or a neurological condition is present, code the condition on Axis III.

can adjust their speech to talk appropriately to young children (Fey et al. 1981), suggesting some facility and flexibility in the use of their language skills. There may be associated learning disorders, phonological disorder, inattentiveness, impulsivity, or aggressivity.

When frustrated, the child may have tantrums during the early years or may briefly refuse to speak when older. Problems in social interactions may lead to peer problems and overdependence on family members.

Approximately 1 in 1,000 children have a severe form of expressive language disorder, but mild forms may be 10 times more common. The standard 3:1–4:1

male predominance of some of the other developmental disorders is seen in this disorder.

DSM-IV-TR recognizes both congenital and acquired forms of expressive language disorder. Diverse etiologies involving neurological, genetic, environmental, and familial factors have been described. Teratogenic, perinatal, toxic, and metabolic influences are linked to certain cases. When hearing loss is present, the degree to which hearing is lost strongly correlates with the amount of language impairment (J.A.M. Martin 1980). Children with expressive language disorder are reported to have low cerebral blood flow to the left hemisphere (Raynaud et al. 1989).

Although expressive language disorder is often associated with seemingly secondary behavioral and attentional problems, a high incidence of various psychiatric problems is also observed in the relatives of those with the disorder, suggesting that concomitant psychiatric disorders may be present in children with difficulties in expressive language.

This condition usually causes parental concern by the time the child reaches age 2–3 years, when the child may appear to be bright but is not yet talking, has acquired only a small vocabulary, or is difficult to comprehend. The period from age 4 to age 7 years is crucial. By age 8, one of two developmental courses is usually established. The child may be progressing toward nearly normal speech, retaining only subtle defects and perhaps symptoms of other learning disorders. Alternatively, the child may remain disabled, show slow progress, and subsequently lose some previously achieved capacities. There appears to be a decrease in nonverbal IQ, possibly because of the failure of development of sequencing, categorization, and related higher cortical functions. The child may lose some of his or her earlier brightness and come to resemble a mentally retarded adolescent. In both courses, complications of expressive language disorder include shyness, withdrawal, and emotional lability.

Evaluation includes psychiatric (attentional and behavior problems), neurological, cognitive, and educational assessments. Intelligence is determined by a nonverbal measure of IQ. A test of hearing acuity is sensible, and workup for concomitant learning disorders is essential.

Few studies of language disorders in recent years have examined DSM-IV-TR expressive language disorder as a discrete entity. Instead, psychiatric research on language problems has focused on receptive or mixed receptive-expressive language disorder.

Mixed Receptive-Expressive Language Disorder

Mixed receptive-expressive language disorder is impaired development of language comprehension that entails impairments in both decoding (i.e., comprehension) and encoding (i.e., expression). Multiple cortical and subcortical deficits usually are observed, including sensory, integrative, recall, and sequencing functions (Table 15–12). Although receptive aphasia in adults leaves expression intact, a similar condition during development generally leaves a child impaired in the learning of a first verbal language, so that the learning of both receptive and expressive functions are disrupted. Depending on the nature of the deficits, nonverbal comprehension may be preserved or disrupted. Involving receptive and expressive language deficits, mixed receptive-expressive language disorder is considerably more severe and socially disruptive than simple expressive or receptive language disorders (Beitchman et al. 2001; D. Cohen et al. 1976; C.J. Johnson et al. 1999).

TABLE 15–12. DSM-IV-TR diagnostic criteria for mixed receptive-expressive language disorder

A. The scores obtained from a battery of standardized individually administered measures of both receptive and expressive language development are substantially below those obtained from standardized measures of nonverbal intellectual capacity. Symptoms include those for expressive language disorder as well as difficulty understanding words, sentences, or specific types of words, such as spatial terms.

B. The difficulties with receptive and expressive language significantly interfere with academic or occupational achievement or with social communication.

C. Criteria are not met for a pervasive developmental disorder.

D. If mental retardation, a speech-motor or sensory deficit, or environmental deprivation is present, the language difficulties are in excess of those usually associated with these problems.

Coding note: If a speech-motor or sensory deficit or a neurological condition is present, code the condition on Axis III.

Psychiatric comorbidity is often extensive, and mild presentations of mixed receptive-expressive language disorder are frequently overlooked or eclipsed by more evident social-emotional and learning difficulties, resulting in a lost opportunity for early intervention.

In mild cases, there may be slow "processing" of certain linguistic forms (e.g., unusual, uncommon, or abstract words; spatial or visual language) or slow comprehension of complicated sentences. There also may be difficulty in understanding humor and idioms and in "reading" situational cues. In severe cases, these difficulties may extend to simpler phrases or words, reflecting slow auditory processing. Muteness, echolalia, or neologisms may be observed. During the developmental period, the learning of expressive language skills becomes impaired by the slowness in receptive language processing.

The developmental type of mixed receptive-expressive language disorder may be distinguished from aphasia (which is not a developmental disorder but a loss of preexisting language functions), other acquired deficits (usually caused by neurological trauma or disease), or the absence of language (a rare condition usually associated with profound mental retardation). Although DSM-IV-TR considers the developmental and the acquired forms to be subtypes of mixed receptive-expressive language disorder, the developmental subtype corresponds more closely to the learning disorders.

Psychiatric comorbidity often includes learning and motor skills disorders, in addition to emotional and disruptive behavior disorders (Beitchman et al. 2001; C.J. Johnson et al. 1999). Mixed receptive and expressive language impairments at age 5 years are associated with aggressiveness and ADHD, and their presence predicts academic failure and antisocial outcome. A strong association with low socioeconomic status, unmarried parents, impaired hearing, and visuomotor deficits has been noted.

Mixed receptive-expressive language disorder may approach the severity of autistic disorder during adolescence because of social awkwardness, stereotypies, resistance to change, and low frustration tolerance (D. Cohen et al. 1976). However, these individuals typically have better social skills, environmental awareness, abstraction, and nonverbal communication than do those with autism.

About 3%–6% of school-age children have mixed receptive-expressive language disorder, but severe cases have a prevalence of 1 in 2,000. Unlike the male predominance of expressive language disorder and many of the learning disorders, an equal sex ratio is found in mixed receptive-expressive language disorder, although sex may influence the range and expression of concomitant social and behavioral difficulties.

The main etiology of mixed receptive-expressive language disorder appears to be neurobiological, usually genetic factors or cerebral damage. Neurological examination detects abnormalities in about two-thirds of cases. Electroencephalographic findings include a slight increase in nondiagnostic abnormalities, especially in the language-dominant hemisphere. Computed tomography (CT) scans may show abnormalities, but these are not uniform or diagnostic. Similarly, dichotic listening may be abnormal but without specific or lateralizing findings.

Evaluation includes assessment of nonverbal IQ, social skills, hearing acuity, articulation, receptive skills (understanding single words, word combinations, and sentences), nonverbal communication (vocalizations, gestures, and gazes), and expressive language skills. Expressive language skills can be measured in terms of the mean length of utterances, which is compared with developmental norms. Syntactic structures should be assessed and also compared with developmental norms. Standardized instruments are available to assess comprehension, with norms starting at age 18 months. Concomitant medical, neurological, and psychiatric (e.g., learning disorders, mood disorders, disruptive behavior disorders, autistic disorder and other pervasive developmental disorders, mental retardation, and selective mutism) diagnoses should be considered.

For treatment of expressive and receptive language problems, special education including speech and language therapy should be maintained until the symptoms improve. After a child is "mainstreamed," supplemental academic and language supports may be helpful. Psychiatric treatment for attention deficits, behavior problems, and other comorbidity, as well as speech therapy for phonological disorder, may be needed.

Phonological Disorder

Diction problems, especially for late-acquired sounds, may be seen in children who have normal vocabulary and grammar. This impairment in articulation and in learning sound production for speech includes substitutions ("wery" for "very"), omissions ("cayon" for "crayon"), additions ("blook" for "book"), sequencing ("aks" for "ask"), lisping (of sibilants), and distortions (Table 15–13). Speech may be slightly or largely unintelligible, or it may sound like "baby talk." The understandability of speech may be further compromised by problems that are not part of phonological disorder: accent, intonation (e.g., neurologically induced), stuttering, cluttering, physical conditions (orofacial disorders such as cleft palate), neurological disease, or psychotropic medication (especially neuroleptics).

Research suggests that children are born with innate *phonemic awareness* (Grigorenko et al. 2001; Petryshen et al. 2001) and *speech motor control*. Early in development, infant sounds are biologically determined and similar cross-culturally, but phonemic awareness permits a child in the first year of life to distinguish among, represent, recognize, and reproduce the constituent speech sounds (*phonemes*) of the language spoken in the environment. As an infant learns the sounds of the local language and environment, sound productions change and become culture-specific. Subsequent speech sound production depends on the development of speech motor control (tongue, lips, palate, larynx, jaw, breathing muscles), auditory perception (vowel and consonant phonemes, rhythm, intensity, intonation), and the ability to make sounds,

TABLE 15–13. DSM-IV-TR diagnostic criteria for phonological disorder

A. Failure to use developmentally expected speech sounds that are appropriate for age and dialect (e.g., errors in sound production, use, representation, or organization such as, but not limited to, substitutions of one sound for another [use of /t/ for target /k/ sound] or omissions of sounds such as final consonants).

B. The difficulties in speech sound production interfere with academic or occupational achievement or with social communication.

C. If mental retardation, a speech-motor or sensory deficit, or environmental deprivation is present, the speech difficulties are in excess of those usually associated with these problems.

Coding note: If a speech-motor or sensory deficit or a neurological condition is present, code the condition on Axis III.

contrasts, combinations, plural formations, and emphases.

With subsequent development, the child acquires increasing competence in rapidly "decoding" speech sounds in conversation and in accurately reproducing them. The child also acquires a *metaphonology*, a set of rules that governs the permissible combinations of phonemes and the subtleties of pronunciation. By age 8 years, a child has acquired all speech sounds and can reproduce and "blend" them in the allowed combinations. *Phonological receptivity*, which is maximal in the first year of life, deteriorates until preadolescence, when the acquisition of a second language becomes increasingly difficult.

Neuropsychological, neuroimaging, genetic, and other studies of the phonological processing deficit in dyslexia have burgeoned in recent years, whereas comparable research into the phonological deficits and motor control deficits in phonological disorder has been quite limited. Careful genetic studies have begun to identify gene loci that are involved in phonological processes and speech motor control, but their relevance to the clinical condition of DSM-IV-TR phonological disorder is unclear. These studies have identified potential sites that may pertain to phonological processes such as perceiving sounds (Grigorenko et al. 2000; Petryshen et al. 2000, 2001), but genetic studies have not yet focused on sound production or articulation. Other contributing factors in phonological disorder may include faulty speech models within the family and mild hearing impairment.

Age at diagnosis of phonological disorder is generally about 3 years, but the disorder may appear earlier or later depending on its severity. Approximately 6% of boys and 3% of girls have phonological disorder, but problems with articulation become less prevalent with age. Spontaneous recovery usually occurs by age 6–8, but individual or group speech therapy can help the speed and completeness of speech development (Almost and Rosenbaum 1998; Dodd and Bradford 2000; Gierut 1998). In addition to an evaluation of intelligence, a full language assessment should be done because many of these children have associated language disorders. "Communicative low self-esteem" is a potential complication.

Stuttering

Stuttering, the disruption of normal speech flow, is characterized by involuntary and irregular hesitations, prolongations, repetitions, or blocks on sounds, syllables, or words (Table 15–14). Unlike the case of cluttering or other dysfluencies in children, anxiety produces a noticeable aggravation of speech rhythm and rate in people who stutter. There may be a transient worsening during periods of perfor-

TABLE 15–14. DSM-IV-TR diagnostic criteria for stuttering

A. Disturbance in the normal fluency and time patterning of speech (inappropriate for the individual's age), characterized by frequent occurrences of one or more of the following:
   (1) sound and syllable repetitions
   (2) sound prolongations
   (3) interjections
   (4) broken words (e.g., pauses within a word)
   (5) audible or silent blocking (filled or unfilled pauses in speech)
   (6) circumlocutions (word substitutions to avoid problematic words)
   (7) words produced with an excess of physical tension
   (8) monosyllabic whole-word repetitions (e.g., "I-I-I-I see him")
B. The disturbance in fluency interferes with academic or occupational achievement or with social communication.
C. If a speech-motor or sensory deficit is present, the speech difficulties are in excess of those usually associated with these problems.
Coding note: If a speech-motor or sensory deficit or a neurological condition is present, code the condition on Axis III.

mance anxiety or "communicative stress" (e.g., during public speaking or a job interview). In laboratory studies, abnormalities of speech behavior and body movement are seen even during periods of apparently fluent speech.

Approximately 1%–2% of children have this speech disorder. Stuttering improves spontaneously in 50%–80% of cases, and about 0.8% of adolescents and adults continue to fulfill criteria for the disorder. A male predominance of approximately 2:1 is present in stuttering during childhood and increases to 3:1 or 4:1 in adulthood, reflecting the higher likelihood of remission of stuttering in females.

Etiological theories of stuttering are based on genetic, neurological, and behavioral concepts. There may be several etiological subgroups of stuttering. A strikingly higher concordance in monozygotic than dizygotic twins suggests a large genetic etiological factor (Felsenfeld et al. 2000). For 60% of the persons who stutter, the disorder runs in families, appearing in about 20%–40% of first-degree relatives (especially in males). Because the prevalence is lower in females but the familial prevalence is higher in the relatives of female stutterers, a sex threshold effect on penetrance (sex-specific difference in penetrance or in the genetic loading required for penetrance) is apparent.

Phonological disorder is overrepresented among people with stuttering, and poor phonological ability in young children contributes to the appearance of stuttering. Developmental improvement in phonological performance appears to contribute to its resolution (Paden and Yairi 1996). In contrast, although some patients also have expressive language disorder, expressive language seems to develop normally in most persons who stutter (Watkins et al. 1999).

Certain forms of acquired stuttering are clearly neurological in origin, such as stuttering that begins after a stroke (presumably caused by damage to fluency centers) or secondary to degenerative brain disease. These acquired forms may be transient, but they can persist, particularly if bilateral and multifocal brain disease is present. These neurologically based forms of stuttering have clinical characteristics that differ from the developmental form of stuttering: blocks and prolongations occur but are not primarily at initial syllables and substantive words, and associated grimacing and hand movements are unusual.

Stuttering often starts at age 2–4 years or, less commonly, at age 5–7 years. For toddlers, stuttering is usually a transient developmental symptom lasting less than 6 months, but about 25% of early-onset patients have persistent stuttering beyond age 12 years. For onset during latency, symptoms are usually stress related, and a benign course of 6 months' to 6 years' duration is typical.

At the onset, the child usually is unaware of the symptom. Symptoms usually appear gradually and then take on a waxing and waning course. The disorder may gradually improve during childhood and essentially resolve by mid-adolescence, or it may worsen and lead to a chronic course. Males tend to have more chronic forms of the disorder. Persons with persistent stuttering have greater phonological and articulation deficits (Paden et al. 1999).

Complications include fearful anticipation, eye blinking, tics, and avoidance of problematic words and situations. The child may experience negative emotional reactions of family and peers (embarrassment, guilt, anger), teasing, and social ostracism. Speech avoidance and poor self-image may affect language and social development and may lead to academic and occupational problems.

Evaluation of stuttering includes a workup for possible neurological causes (cortical, basal ganglial, cerebellar). A full developmental history and general evaluation of speech, language, and hearing are needed. Behavioral assessment includes delineating any restrictions in social interactions and activities. Referral for evaluation to a speech and language pathologist is indicated in all cases of stuttering. It is helpful to assess the dysfluency in monologue, conversation, play, and anxiety; to test the effects of slowed speech and focused attention on the dysfluency; and to observe parent–child interactions for communicative stress placed on the child (e.g., rapid questioning, interruptions, repeated corrections, frequent topic shifts).

Speech therapy involves some elements of behavior therapy, including modifying environmental and conversational factors that trigger stuttering, relaxation, rhythm control, feedback, and dealing with accessory body movements, as well as fostering self-esteem and social assertiveness. Specific therapies for stuttering include intensive smooth speech, intensive electromyography feedback, and home-based smooth speech; all have been reported to reduce stuttering frequency by 85%–90%, and these gains have persisted 6 years after treatment (Craig et al. 1996; Hancock et al. 1998). Other methods include imitation, role-playing, practice in speaking (while reading, choral reading, conversing), and talking in different settings (alone, in a group, in front of a classroom, on a telephone) and with different people (parents, relatives, friends, strangers).

Education and counseling of family members are advised. Psychotherapy is generally not indicated, but it might be considered if stuttering persists or begins in adolescence. Antianxiety drugs are generally of minimal value. Neuroleptics may be useful in some cases, but there are no controlled studies. Some studies have suggested the possible effectiveness of serotonin reuptake inhibitors for stuttering. A controlled trial found that clonidine did not improve stuttering (Althaus et al. 1995). Therefore, the role of pharmacotherapy seems limited at best, especially in view of the effectiveness of speech therapy.

Mental Retardation

Intelligence (e.g., as measured by IQ) might be considered an independent dimension that deserves its own separate DSM-IV-TR axis. However, the diagnosis of mental retardation encompasses more than low intelligence; it also requires deficits in adaptive functioning. The diagnostic concept of mental retardation as constituting low IQ plus adaptive deficits was developed by the American Association on Mental Retardation (1992) and essentially adopted by DSM-IV. It emphasizes that mental retardation is not an innate characteristic of an individual but the result of an interaction between personal intellectual capacities and the environment.

At least 90% of the individuals with low intelligence are identified by age 18 years, but the diagnosis of mental retardation requires onset during the developmental period. Furthermore, developmental understanding is basic to the treatment of mental retardation, although psychiatric treatment of mental retardation is typically provided by general and child psychiatrists.

The definition of mental retardation encompasses three features: 1) subaverage intelligence (e.g., IQ of 70 or below), 2) impaired adaptive functioning, and 3) childhood onset (Table 15–15). The system for subclassifying the severity of mental retardation in DSM-IV-TR is based on IQ scores, but the American Association on Mental Retardation (1992) instead subclassifies by the required "intensity and pattern of support systems" (intermittent, limited, extensive, and pervasive).

Mental retardation is diagnosed only if low intelligence is accompanied by impaired adaptive functioning. Low intelligence alone, or deficits in adaptive behavior alone, does not warrant a diagnosis of mental retardation.

Intelligence is routinely measured by standardized tests, such as the Wechsler Adult Intelligence Scale—Revised (WAIS-R), the Wechsler Intelligence Scale for Children—Third Edition (WISC-III) for 6- to 16-year-olds, the Stanford-Binet Intelligence Scale, 4th Edition, for 2- to 18-year-olds, or sections of the Bayley Scales

TABLE 15–15. DSM-IV-TR diagnostic criteria for mental retardation

A. Significantly subaverage intellectual functioning: an IQ of approximately 70 or below on an individually administered IQ test (for infants, a clinical judgment of significantly subaverage intellectual functioning).

B. Concurrent deficits or impairments in present adaptive functioning (i.e., the person's effectiveness in meeting the standards expected for his or her age by his or her cultural group) in at least two of the following areas: communication, self-care, home living, social/interpersonal skills, use of community resources, self-direction, functional academic skills, work, leisure, health, and safety.

C. The onset is before age 18 years.

Code based on degree of severity reflecting level of intellectual impairment:

    317   Mild Mental Retardation: IQ level 50–55 to approximately 70

    318.0   Moderate Mental Retardation: IQ level 35–40 to 50–55

    318.1   Severe Mental Retardation: IQ level 20–25 to 35–40

    318.2   Profound Mental Retardation: IQ level below 20 or 25

    319   Mental Retardation, Severity Unspecified: when there is strong presumption of Mental Retardation but the person's intelligence is untestable by standard tests

of Mental Development for children from age 2 months to 2.5 years. Specialized test protocols are being developed for infants. Major limitations of these standardized methods include cultural variations in question meaning and test performance, language and communicational differences among individuals, the unresponsiveness of standardized tests to "creative" responses, the dangers of using a rigid construct of intelligence that masks individual strengths, and overreliance on test findings in planning education. Even the concept of intel-

ligence may be questioned, in view of the wide varieties of cognition (verbal and nonverbal, conscious and unconscious, emotional and "other"). However, these standardized IQ tests are capable of providing a global assessment that is of clinical value, particularly when combined with an evaluation of adaptive behavior.

Adaptive capacities may be judged by many means, including standardized instruments for assessing social maturity and adaptive skills. For example, the Vineland Adaptive Behavior Scale is a multidimensional measure of adaptive behaviors in five "domains": communication, daily living skills, socialization, motor skills, and maladaptive behaviors (Balboni et al. 2001; Sparrow et al. 1984). Data are provided by a semistructured interview of a parent or caregiver. Age-dependent expected competency scores of adaptive skills are established for children up to age 18 years with different levels of mental retardation. Adaptive competence may be above or below the level of general intelligence.

The Vineland Adaptive Behavior Scale assesses typical performance (not optimal ability) of the "daily activities required for personal and social sufficiency" (Sparrow et al. 1984). For instance, in the socialization domain, coping skills, including manners, following rules, apologizing, keeping secrets, and controlling impulses, are assessed. Multidimensional scoring in different domains permits assessment of specific skills and deficits for an individual, facilitates the targeting of goals in different areas of adaptive functioning, helps in planning (for school, job, and residential placements), and allows measurement of changes in adaptive functioning over time. It is possible for scores in each domain to show more "scatter" than is shown by the intelligence subtests.

Because adaptive behavioral functioning may vary in different environments, a single measurement may be an oversimplification. In practice, it is rare that a single observer sees a patient in all settings or at all times of the day. This complicates the assessment of adaptive behavior in both standardized and global clinical methods. Clinicians typically use data from multiple sources to draw a composite picture of life functioning.

Because the diagnosis of mental retardation requires onset during childhood, an adult who experiences severe neurological damage is not classified as mentally retarded, even if both intelligence and adaptive skills are impaired. The adult-onset condition is diagnosed as dementia, which is an organic mental disorder (although certain dementias also can be designated as occurring in children). Disruption of the developmental process is required, by definition, for the diagnosis of mental retardation.

Mild forms of mental retardation, present in individuals with an IQ below 71 who do not meet adaptive functioning criteria for diagnosis, may receive a V code for borderline intellectual functioning.

Clinical Description

Developmental slowness may appear in mental retardation across all areas of functioning, but it is primarily evident in cognition and intellectual functioning. Certain clinical features depend on the degree of intellectual functioning in mental retardation (Table 15–16). Neurobiological, motor, sensory, and integrative features; parent–child attachment; self–other differentiation; and subsequent emotional development are commonly affected. Although other aspects of psychological development are often impaired secondarily, there can be a remarkable degree of preservation of psychological growth. There may be wide "scatter" among various subtests of intellectual and adaptive functions, reflecting significant strengths in particular areas.

Because there is a two- to fourfold increase in psychopathology among mentally retarded persons, many of these individuals have "dual diagnoses." Fully half or more of the persons with mental retardation have an additional psychiatric diagnosis (Gillberg et al. 1986; Gostason 1985; Stromme and Diseth 2000). Psychiatric comorbidity appears to increase with severity of mental retardation (Deb 1997; Molteni and Moretti 1999; Stromme and Diseth 2000). The frequency appears to be the same in both children and adults (Cherry et al. 1997), suggesting that the comorbid diagnoses are distinct clinical entities and do not represent age-related complications of mental retardation.

Any psychiatric diagnosis may occur in combination with mental retardation; DSM-IV-TR criteria do not exclude any psychiatric disorder. Interestingly, increased risk of suicide is not associated with mental retardation (Harris and Barraclough 1997) and might, for males, be below population average. Disorders that occur at relatively high rates with mental retardation include impulse-control disorders, anxiety disorders, mood disorders (Vanstraelen and Tyrer 1999), ADHD (Pearson et al. 2000), communication disorders, pervasive developmental disorders (including autistic disorder), stereotypic movement disorder (including self-injurious behavior [SIB]), pica, epilepsy (Airaksinen et al. 2000), and substance abuse (Burgard et al. 2000; B.H. King et al. 1994). Although most individuals with mental retardation do not drink alcohol, nearly half of the drinkers drink excessively (McGillicuddy and Blane 1999). PTSD and adjustment disorder may certainly be seen, and the full array of personality types and all personality disorders may appear. The same DSM-IV-TR criteria for defining these disorders may

TABLE 15–16. Clinical features of mental retardation

	Mild	Moderate	Severe	Profound
IQ	50–55 to approximately 70	35–40 to 50–55	20–25 to 35–40	<20 or 25
Age at death (years)	50s	50s	40s	About 20
Percentage of mentally retarded population	89	7	3	1
Socioeconomic class	Low	Less low	No skew	No skew
Academic level achieved by adulthood	Sixth grade	Second grade	Below first-grade level in general	Below first-grade level in general
Education	Educable	Trainable (self-care)	Untrainable	Untrainable
Residence	Community	Sheltered	Mostly living in highly structured and closely supervised settings	Mostly living in highly structured and closely supervised settings
Economic	Makes change; manages a job; budgets money with effort or assistance	Makes small change; usually able to manage change well	Can use coin machines; can take notes to shop owner	Dependent on others for money management

be applied without modification for the population with mental retardation. Unfortunately, some clinicians are less inclined to diagnose or evaluate psychiatric comorbidity in individuals with mental retardation. Mentally retarded people also receive less treatment for their concomitant psychiatric disorders, in part because of their low self-expectations (which may be derived from family and clinician attitudes), economic limitations, and difficulties in managing complex organizational systems.

Some clinical findings are primary cognitive and neurobiological features of mental retardation. Cognitively, there may be concreteness, egocentricity, distractibility, and short attention span. Sensory hyperreactivity may lead to "overflow" behaviors, stimulus avoidance, and the need to process stimuli at low levels of intensity.

Emotional features may include difficulty in expressing feelings and perceiving affect in self and others. Slow development of self–other differentiation may be clinically evident in affect management. Affective expression may be modified by physical disabilities, such as hypertonia or hypotonia. There may be cognitively based difficulty in "reading" facial expressions. With delays in speech and language development, limitations in communication may inhibit expression of negative affect, leading to instances of apparent affective hyperreactivity including impulsive anger, low frustration tolerance, and reactive agitation. In extreme cases, impulse dyscontrol may lead to violence and destructiveness. These behavioral manifestations may show only modest improvement over time, especially in patients with severe or profound mental retardation (Reid and Ballinger 1995). Interestingly, the usual signals of distress may not be evident in patients with severe or profound mental retardation, leading to

an underestimation of their discomfort and subjective stress in a variety of circumstances, including medical evaluation and procedures (Cavaliere et al. 1999).

The ordinary complexities of daily human interactions may test an individual's cognitive limits (Sigman 1985). Cognitive capacities may be taxed in the parallel processing of speech production; thought communication; listening; and the understanding of situational context, social cues, and emotional signals. Changes in daily situation may stretch cognitive capacities and coping abilities, sometimes leading to frustration. Resistance to novelty and environmental change may be viewed as an associated finding or a developmental consequence of mental retardation.

Medical comorbidity is approximately twice as frequent as in the general population (Ryan and Sunada 1997). Such medical problems (including associated neurological or metabolic disorders, physical disabilities, and sensory deficits) often are undertreated. When motor deficits are present, their specific characteristics should be identified and targeted for treatment. However, receiving adequate medical care may require organizational and social skills that exceed the grasp of some mentally retarded people.

Generalizations about mental retardation are increasingly coming into question as research permits the understanding and differentiation of specific mental retardation syndromes. Contrasting with the old notion that mental retardation is a nonspecific form of slow development, newer phenomenological data indicate that these syndromes share many commonalities but are not the same. For example, persons with trisomy 21 (Down syndrome) and fragile X syndrome tend to have quite different characteristics of language, cognition, social behavior, and adaptive skills (Bregman and Hodapp 1991; Lachiewicz et al. 1994) as well as different psychiatric comorbidity (Bregman 1991). Such findings suggest that individuals with mental retardation of different etiologies, not just of different severities, have distinct profiles of strengths and weaknesses that may be expected to influence their development.

Epidemiology

Prevalence figures in the United States range from 1% to 3%, depending mainly on the definition of adaptive functioning (Larson et al. 2001). Approximately 85%–90% of patients are mildly retarded (IQ = 55–70). There appears to be a male predominance at all levels of mental retardation of about 1.5:1, although ratios as high as 6:1 have been reported; there may be a female predominance in severe mental retardation (Katusic et al. 1996).

Diagnostic labeling is low before age 5 years, rises sharply during the early school years, peaks in the later school years (about age 15), and then declines during adulthood toward 1%. High prevalence rates during the school years usually are attributed to the adaptive and intellectual demands of school (especially social and abstract thinking) and the high degree of supervision in classrooms (increased recognition of the child's difficulties). The decline during adulthood usually is attributed to improving social and economic skills, less supervision at work, and possibly (in some cases) delayed intellectual development. Typically, more severe levels of mental retardation have an earlier age at diagnosis.

Socioeconomic class is a crucial variable. Severe and profound mental retardation are distributed uniformly across all socioeconomic classes, but mild mental retardation is more common in low socioeconomic classes (Stromme and Magnus 2000). In the lowest socioeconomic class, the prevalence of mental retardation in

the American school-age population is 10%–30%. This "multiply disadvantaged" poverty class consists of inhabitants of city slums and poor rural areas, migrant workers, and economically oppressed groups. This fact highlights the etiological role of genetic–environmental interactions in mental retardation, especially in cases for which there is no obvious cause (Croen et al. 2001; Thapar et al. 1994).

In underdeveloped countries, the quality of nutrition, hygiene, sanitation, prenatal care, and mass immunization influences the incidence of mental retardation, but prevalence is reduced by infant mortality. In technologically advanced countries, medical and social supports enhance survival and longevity, although the effect on quality of life is less clear.

Etiology

There are almost 1,000 recognized biological syndromes involving mental retardation, entailing disruptions in virtually any sector of brain biochemical or physiological functioning (Grossman 1983; Johnston et al. 2001). Disruption of neurogenesis, neuronal migration, cellular differentiation, intercellular communication, cytoskeleton organization, synaptic vesicle transport, and other cellular functions are typical arenas of pathological change. The most common anatomical features of mental retardation are dendritic abnormalities, which may range from generalized dysgenesis to highly syndrome-specific abnormalities or from multiform changes resulting from neuronal damage and reorganization to particular cytoarchitectural formations and changes over time (Kaufmann and Moser 2000).

Mild retardation is generally idiopathic and familial, but severe and profound retardation are typically genetic or related to brain damage. Specific syndromes of mental retardation, such as Down syndrome or fragile X syndrome, can be identified on the basis of consistent clinical features. Even in cases of nonspecific mental retardation, in which no consistent and distinctive features are present, specific causes might be identified; for example, eight gene sites have so far been linked with nonspecific X-linked mental retardation.

The most common form is idiopathic mental retardation, a "nonspecific" form that is associated with sociocultural or psychosocial disadvantage and typically is seen in the offspring of retarded parents ("familial"). The degree of retardation in this form is generally mild and sometimes moderate. Intellectual and adaptive deficits are presumed to be determined by a polygenic mechanism, although emphasis is currently placed on the role of intervening social factors. These individuals live in low socioeconomic circumstances, and their functioning is influenced by poverty, disease, deficiencies in health care, and impaired help seeking. Family size may exceed parental capacities for attention and positive stimulation of the children, inducing marked effects on several dimensions of development. Social disadvantage contributes heavily to the etiology of some forms of mild mental retardation. Nonetheless, the overrepresentation of various genetic, physical, and neurological abnormalities in individuals with mild mental retardation is a reminder that social forces are not the predominant etiological factors in mental retardation.

Moderate and severe forms of mental retardation are less likely to be idiopathic. Specific biomedical etiologies may be identified in 60%–70% of all cases of mental retardation and in a higher proportion of cases of severe or profound mental retardation. These moderate and severe cases usually are first diagnosed in infancy or early childhood, and 90% have prenatal causes. Major mechanisms include genetic

and neurodevelopmental damage. When biological causes are identifiable, there are more severe disabilities, physical limitations, and dependency.

In cases of idiopathic mental retardation, there is substantial evidence for a biological basis of brain abnormalities. Enlarged ventricles, similar to findings in schizophrenia, have been reported in 75% of the children with mental retardation of unknown cause (Prassopoulos et al. 1996). Infants with mental retardation show an abnormal thickening of the corpus callosum during development in the first year of life (Fujii et al. 1994).

Neurodevelopmental damage or dysmorphogenesis may be produced by a variety of mechanisms. Physical insults that are typically damaging to the brain are catastrophic in early development. Because the fetus has no demonstrable immunological response in early gestation, maternal infections (e.g., congenital AIDS or toxoplasmosis) may cause major damage. If rubella is contracted during the first month of pregnancy, there is a 50% rate of fetal abnormalities. Intrauterine exposure to toxins (e.g., lead), medications, and radiation may result in intrauterine growth retardation and other toxic effects on brain development (Herskowitz 1987). Similarly, intrauterine exposures to nicotine, alcohol, and cocaine are preventable causes of mental retardation (Drews et al. 1996). Intrauterine seizures can be a prenatal cause of brain damage and impaired brain development (Volpe 1987). Certain forms of maternal illness (toxemia or diabetes) also may be dangerous to the developing nervous system in utero.

At birth, obstetrical trauma and Rh isoimmunization may cause brain injury. Birth asphyxia is probably not a significant source of mental retardation; there has been a deemphasis on the role of perinatal hypoxia in the etiology of neuropsychiatric problems (Nelson 1991). Hypoxic changes typically result in maturational delays that are no longer diagnosed by age 7 years, except perhaps in severe and profound mental retardation. Prematurity (or low birth weight) is not typically causal, but it may be in extreme cases (e.g., <28 weeks' gestation or birth weight <1,500 g) (Vexler and Ferriero 2001). Taken together, low birth weight, low gestational age, and low Apgar scores contribute significantly to only about 4% of the children with mental retardation (Stromme 2000).

Several forms of neurodevelopmental damage may occur postnatally. Environmental factors are particularly crucial in underdeveloped countries, where distribution of medical care may be limited. Neurological infections and disease, including seizures, may contribute. Neurological trauma may result from falls, accidents, athletic injury, extreme fever, child abuse, and severe malnutrition.

Chromosomal factors can be identified in 10% of institutionalized individuals with mental retardation. Apart from polygenetic inheritance, the major chromosomal mechanisms include dominantly inherited single-gene defects, recessively inherited inborn errors of metabolism, recessive chromosomal aberrations, and early developmental (embryonic) gene alterations.

As mental retardation in general and the specific disorders are more intensively studied, there is an emerging picture of the extraordinary complexity of genetic and neurodevelopmental processes, as well as of sociodevelopmental processes, that contribute to the different presentations. Specific genetic mechanisms, molecular events, developmental courses, cognitive features, language abilities, and adaptive strengths and weaknesses are being identified for the various mental retardation syndromes. Two examples, trisomy 21 and fragile X syndrome (Hager-

man and Hagerman 2002), provide an interesting contrast to illustrate the distinctive qualities among different syndromes of mental retardation.

Course and Prognosis

Although biological factors of each mental retardation syndrome in each individual may determine certain aspects of development, the course and outcome of mental retardation generally depend largely on social, economic, health/medical, educational, and developmental circumstances. Whether the disorder is a mild familial form or the result of a severe inborn metabolic error, the course of mental retardation is influenced by interactions with environmental opportunities and barriers. Parental characteristics may entail advantages that are compensatory or disadvantages that are compounding. Such features of the microenvironment operate as intervening factors and may have a stronger influence on adult psychiatric outcome than the causative factors, except in extreme cases. The course and prognosis of mental retardation is much less predictable than originally believed.

Neurodevelopmental evaluation during the first year can predict intellectual outcome and neurological status in later childhood in nearly 90% of premature children (Largo et al. 1990). Premature infants with intracranial hemorrhage (demonstrated on ultrasound) are especially likely to have impaired cognitive and motor abilities later, especially if there are persistent signs of periventricular abnormalities (M.L. Williams et al. 1987).

Current data on the course of mental retardation reflect varying degrees of aggressivity in habilitative efforts. The prognosis in mental retardation may be expected to improve as therapeutic interventions become available to more members of the general public and as the mentally retarded individual's adaptive skills improve over the course of a lifetime.

The period between ages 18 and 26 has been identified as a particularly critical interval in development for people with mental retardation (Blacher 2001). During this time, most individuals experience a completion of their state-supported formal education and the transition toward personal independence. Vocational training and placement, setting up residential arrangements, and the establishment of a social matrix and self-expectations are prominent during this time. This time also coincides with a withdrawal of organized community supports.

At present, about two-thirds of mentally retarded individuals shed their diagnoses in adulthood, as adaptive skills increase (Grossman 1983). Typically, the global level of adaptive functioning is found to change over the course of months or years in response to changes in economic and social supports, living arrangements, work opportunities, and parental support.

For mental retardation at all levels of severity, and for cases of both idiopathic and known etiologies, the developmental course is slow but not "deviant." The normal sequence of cognitive developmental stages is observed. The speed of developmental change is slow, and there appears to be a "ceiling" on ultimate achievement. In addition, secondary emotional and social "complications" may influence the clinical presentation and outcome.

Excessively low or high expectations maintained by family, therapeutic team, or patient constitute significant obstacles to therapeutic improvement. The habitual resignation to low expectation of achievement has a chilling effect on self-esteem, hope, and outcome.

Common psychological complications include frequent experiencing of failure, low self-esteem, frustration in fulfillment of dependency needs and wishes for love, wavering parental support, regressive wishes for institutionalization, anticipation of failure (leading to avoidance of problem solving and challenges, reduced curiosity and exploration, and impaired mastery seeking and pride), defensive rigidity, and excessive caution (e.g., resistance to dealing with new people and places, including helping professionals). Additional psychosocial complications are impaired interactions and communications, inappropriate social assertiveness, and vulnerability to being exploited. Financial complications (poverty) entail further medical complications, including impaired care seeking (delayed treatment, excessive use of emergency facilities), rarity of preventive treatment (prenatal and well-baby care, periodic checkups), accidents and trauma, malnutrition, lead exposure, child abuse, prematurity, and teenage pregnancy. It is apparent that complications of mental retardation are numerous. A lack of aggressivity, integration, or continuity in the provision of care can hinder basic medical treatment. Institutionalization may promote passivity and excessive compliance. Societal ignorance and stigmatization may lead to avoidance by potential social companions and professionals.

Family complications may include parental disappointment, anger, guilt, overprotectiveness, infantilization, overinvolvement, or detachment. Siblings may experience annoyance at having to share in sibling care, loss of parents' attention, and parents' compensatory overexpectations as well as realistic fears concerning genetic risks for their own children. The effect on parents of having a child with mental retardation is, however, positive in many cases (Taanila et al. 1996).

Death is often sudden and unexpected among individuals with mental retardation, especially among patients with seizure disorders (Chaney and Eyman 2000; McKee and Bodfish 2000). Prenatal etiology of mental retardation and low IQ are also risk factors for early mortality (Chaney and Eyman 2000).

A major part of the care of mentally retarded individuals includes prevention and management of the numerous medical, psychological, and family complications. Another major component of care is the monitoring of overall speed of progress: a lack of developmental improvement raises the possibility of concomitant psychiatric diagnoses.

Diagnostic Evaluation

It cannot be overemphasized that all psychiatric diagnoses may co-occur with mental retardation and that all personality types may occur in mental retardation. Up to one-half of these patients may have ADHD. Mentally retarded individuals also may have unipolar and bipolar mood disorders, anxiety disorders, psychotic reactions, autistic disorder, and learning disorders (G. Masi et al. 2000a; Menolascino et al. 1986). Some psychiatric rating scales have been formally tested (Aman 1991), but some standard evaluation instruments might perform differently in this population (Borthwick-Duffy et al. 1997; Embregts et al. 2000). Many patients with mental retardation never receive psychiatric evaluation and endure their comorbid mental disorders without treatment (Stromme and Diseth 2000).

Sadness, depression, lack of enthusiasm, excessive anxiety, and "primary process" associations are not primary features of mental retardation; these symptoms should be evaluated as complications or as signs of concomitant disorders.

Medical evaluation should include physical examination (seeking physical stigmata) and laboratory tests, including thyroid function, lead testing, chromo-somal analysis, and molecular screening for amino and organic acids and mucopolysaccharides, among others. However, specialized studies are best ordered by a clinical geneticist or other specialist in mental retardation because the rates of positive findings are dramatically higher for these expensive tests if they have been ordered on the basis of specifically leading physical and clinical findings (Hunter 2000). X-ray studies of long bones and wrists should be obtained. Neurological evaluation should be performed to discover possible treatable causes of mental retardation, seizure disorders, and possibly deafness and blindness. Head and face size and symmetries, head shape (including hair patterns), eye and ear position, and asymmetries of motor and sensory function should be examined. A history of maternal miscarriage, toxic exposures, infections, and fetal size and activity should be elicited. Neuroimaging, such as MRI and perhaps EEG, may be appropriate for patients with neurological symptoms, abnormal cranial size (microcephaly or macrocephaly), or unusual cranial contour (Curry et al. 1997). Psychological testing, including neuropsychological evaluation, is commonly required. Adaptive skills of the individual should be measured (e.g., the Vineland Adaptive Behavior Scale) to target areas of remediation and strength.

Families of individuals with mental retardation experience considerable challenge. The burden of management can tax the efforts of any family (Cooper 1981), especially the parents (Figure 15–1). Because intensive intervention is required to minimize developmental complications, this burden can continue for many years. The growth-promoting characteristics of the family can be assessed (through interviews and home visit) by investigating the level of stimulation, emotional support, help seeking, decision making, future

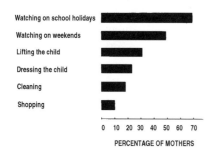

FIGURE 15–1. Caregiving burdens described by mothers of children with mental retardation.

The care of a child with mental retardation places practical responsibilities as well as emotional strains on the families.

Source. Adapted from Birch et al. 1970.

orientation, and financial planning for the mentally retarded individual.

Evaluation of these patients should be continued, sometimes over several years, to allow sequential assessments to fully characterize behavioral and physical features (Curry et al. 1997). It is not unusual for the etiological diagnosis to be changed during the course of such extended evaluations (Stromme 2000).

Treatment

Treatment of the multiple handicaps and complications commonly associated with mental retardation is typically multimodal, with a developmental orientation (Szymanski and King 1999). Long-term habilitative programs involve many specialists and agencies working collaboratively over time and across agency boundaries.

The vast majority of children and a sizable proportion of adults with mental retardation are able to live at home with their parents (Braddock et al. 2001). Out-of-home placements become more common as the child matures and continue to increase as the individual ages. Actual ac-

commodations and opportunities are often highly dependent on the local availability of resources and the choices made by responsible authorities in government or private agencies. The progressive trend away from the use of large centralized institutions has led to increased community-based placement in group homes. The group of residents is typically larger than the average family, requiring the homes to undergo special architectural and zoning accommodations. The transition from living with parents to living in a residential facility can be managed in a manner that promotes the satisfaction and well-being of all concerned, even when the aging of the patient's parents requires a late-life transition (Seltzer et al. 2001).

Psychiatric hospitalization may be required in certain cases, usually for the same reasons that justify inpatient management in the nonretarded population. Outreach programs may be an alternative to hospitalization for some patients with mental retardation and major psychiatric disorders (van Minnen et al. 1997).

Large state-operated psychiatric hospitals providing custodial care are still used in certain cases. Although many specialized chronic inpatient programs are well managed, some institutions have problems with neglect and physical abuse. In these settings, staff perpetrators tend to be new male employees with a history of perpetration, and the likelihood of such abuse being uncovered is increased by recent in-service training on abuse prevention (McCartney and Campbell 1998). Also, some custodial inpatient placements are clinically inappropriate, a problem that can be successfully challenged by class action lawsuit, resulting in improved patient adaptation (Dudley et al. 1997).

The specific psychiatric component includes the coordination of the primary diagnostic evaluation of medical and psychiatric conditions, parental guidance (behavioral management, educational and environmental planning, long-term monitoring, and advocacy), and the usual variety of psychiatric therapies for specific concomitant psychiatric disorders (Szymanski 1987; Szymanski and Tanguay 1980). Substance abuse treatment and prevention may be necessary, although research available to guide interventions is minimal (Christian and Poling 1997).

Behavior modification can be useful for treating symptoms of aggressivity, defiance, overactivity, asocial behavior, self-injury, stereotypies, and pica; in some cases, toilet training, dressing and grooming, and eating skills may be taught. Response-contingent procedures appear particularly effective (Didden et al. 1997). Educational and developmental training to enhance speech and language, motor, cognitive, occupational, social, recreational, sexual, and adaptive skills are commonly provided by specialized professionals (Felce and Emerson 2001). Cognitive training may be enhanced by methods that bring information from the periphery of attention ("out of focus") that is then faded into focus (Carlin et al. 2001). The individual may be trained to initiate task simplifications, request communicational clarifications, and perform environmental improvements. Parent counseling and education, as well as family support, are standard. Even within structured and protective residential programs, the average size of the social network of adults with mental retardation, excluding staff members, is two people (J. Robertson et al. 2001); thus, psychosocial skills training is useful, including concrete assistance in making and sustaining friendships. Cognitive-behavioral approaches to prevention of potential sexual and verbal abuse are appropriate (Khemka and Hickson 2000). Special attention is needed for managing the conflicts regarding standard of living

(economic) and behavioral expectations between home and treatment settings.

Although treatments based on abstract thinking may not be helpful, developmentally oriented psychotherapeutic interventions may be effective for crisis management or for achieving long-term psychosocial goals. For some adolescent or adult patients with mild mental retardation, verbal psychotherapy may be used to promote self–other differentiation, self-esteem, identity formation, interpersonal development, emotional and behavioral control, management of power, and expression of love and sexuality. Technical modifications include the use of briefer and clearer verbalizations, focus on current events and feelings, reinforcement of reality–fantasy differentiations, management of projections, teaching about the nature of emotional life, and free use of positive reinforcement. Brief frequent sessions may be more useful than standard formats. For children, play therapy may be used.

Pharmacotherapy may be helpful in the management of some symptoms associated with mental retardation as well as in the treatment of comorbid psychiatric disorders. Unfortunately, there is a paucity of controlled research in mental retardation, necessitating extrapolation from small open-label adult trials and studies conducted on other diagnostic groups (Aman et al. 2000). Behavioral manifestations may show only modest improvement over time, especially in patients with severe or profound mental retardation (Reid and Ballinger 1995). Treatment is primarily symptom-oriented or targets comorbid psychiatric conditions (Matson et al. 2000). Although controlled studies are still relatively few, atypical neuroleptics may be useful for treating aggressive and agitated behavior (Antonacci and de Groot 2000; Buitelaar 2000; Buitelaar et al. 2001; H. Williams et al. 2000). Less well-established treatments include use of β-adrenergic blockers or clonidine for agitation (Agarwal et al. 2001), psychostimulants for hyperactivity, TCAs for depressive disorders, serotonin reuptake inhibitors for mood and perseverative symptoms, anticonvulsants for seizures, mood stabilizers for bipolar disorders (Carta et al. 2001), and naltrexone for SIBs. Although published reports are few, electroconvulsive therapy may be used, and there does not appear to be an increased vulnerability to its adverse effects (Thuppal and Fink 1999).

Pervasive Developmental Disorders

The pervasive developmental disorders make up a neurobiologically diverse group of conditions characterized by deficits across many areas of functioning that lead to a remarkably pervasive but diffuse disruption of developmental processes. These multiply handicapped individuals typically have a developmental process that is not merely slow or limited but is "atypical" or "deviant." Anomalous strengths can emerge from this developmental process in some cases, but many of these individuals have mental retardation. Comorbidity may include any of the psychiatric disorders, and there may be an increased prevalence of OCD (often identified as "perseveration"), stereotypic movement disorder, tic disorders, ADHD, and mood disorders among individuals with a pervasive developmental disorder.

DSM-IV-TR recognizes several pervasive developmental disorders that differ in course of illness, symptoms, and severity. *Autistic disorder* involves an early onset of impairments in social interaction, communication deficits, and restricted activities and interests; there is some tendency toward partial improvement over time,

but unpredictable periods of rapid improvement appear between extended periods of minimal change. *Childhood disintegrative disorder* entails symptoms that are largely similar, but the symptoms follow at least 2 years of seemingly normal development; the child then loses early developmental gains and reaches a stable level of autistic-like functioning. *Rett's disorder*, an early-onset progressive disorder of females, is associated with mental retardation, generalized growth retardation, and multiple neurological symptoms (including stereotyped movements of the hands); this disorder appears similar to autistic disorder during early childhood, but it progressively takes on characteristics of a neurodegenerative or neurodevelopmental disorder. *Asperger's disorder* is largely similar to "high-functioning" autistic disorder in its relative preservation of language skills and intellect; despite some remaining skepticism about its validity as a distinct DSM-IV-TR disorder, several features of Asperger's disorder have been found that distinguish it from autism and other developmental disorders.

Early intervention and multiyear treatment of the pervasive developmental disorders emphasize communication and occupational functions. The treatment can be effective, although the benefits accrue slowly, and its value has not been well documented in controlled studies. General management requires a long-term, multimodal, developmentally oriented clinical program. Medical treatments are aimed at symptom relief and management of any comorbid neurological or psychiatric disorders.

Autistic Disorder

Autistic disorder, an early-onset pervasive developmental disorder, entails disabilities in virtually all psychological and behavioral sectors. In view of the severity of extreme cases of autistic disorder, it is remarkable that this condition was not documented until the late nineteenth century and not described until the mid-twentieth century. However, most individuals with autistic disorder do not have the massive, severe developmental impairments seen in the classically described cases.

Clinical Description

The DSM-IV-TR definition of autistic disorder puts particular emphasis on the impairments in social interaction and reciprocity, the difficulties with verbal and nonverbal communication (and related capacities such as symbolization), and the stereotyped pattern of behaviors and interests (Table 15–17).

Autistic disorder presents in a wide spectrum of severities. The classic form of "early infantile autism," described by Kanner (1943), was a severe infancy-onset disorder with profoundly disturbed social relationships (e.g., detachment, aloofness), communication disruption, motor abnormalities, affective atypicality, massive cognitive impairments, multiple behavioral oddities, distorted perception, and bizarre thoughts. These symptoms led to conceptualizations based on failed ego development or severe regression, and the bizarre thoughts and behaviors were viewed as suggestive of psychotic development. The notion of autistic disorder as a variant of schizophrenia or of any psychotic disorder is no longer considered heuristically useful.

Despite the extremely disrupted integration of brain functions, an almost chaotic form of disorganization, and cognitive and emotional confusion, autistic disorder is not associated with delusions, hallucinations, or loose associations. It is no longer viewed as a psychotic disorder, and emphasis is placed on the neurointegrative features of the disorganization and the idiosyncratic traits of the individual. In the relatively mild forms of autistic disorder, the social, communicative, and behavioral abnormalities are so subtle that they merge into the range of character pathology.

Children with autistic disorder may show limited social interactiveness, a seeming indifference to human warmth, little imitation or sharing, and rare smiling. Socially, these children appear passive and aloof, initially avoiding social contact, but they can come to enjoy and seek interpersonal experiences. Autistic children often have difficulty in comprehending verbal and nonverbal language and are often misinterpreted; typically, these issues need to be a focus of treatment. They often show persistent deficits in sensing or appreciating the feelings of other people and in understanding the process and nuances of social communication. Communicative speech and gesturing are limited and may be difficult to understand because of echolalia, pronoun reversals, and idiosyncratic meanings. Speech is typically late and unusual, and it sometimes fails to develop altogether. Phonological (i.e., sound production) and syntactic (i.e., grammar) functions may be relatively spared, with more significant impairments of semantics (i.e., sociocultural meanings) and pragmatics (i.e., rules of interpersonal exchange), as well as other aspects of communication. Imaginative and symbolic functions (e.g., use of toys in play) may be deeply affected. Rituals, stereotypies (e.g., rocking, whirling), self-stimulation, SIB, and unusual mannerisms are common. Autistic children often have an obsessive attachment to certain people or objects (resistance to change) and a lack of ordinary spontaneity. Affect may be "shallow," overly responsive to small changes, oblivious to large changes in the environment, and unpredictably labile and odd. Fear responses may be exaggerated or may be absent even when appropriate.

TABLE 15–17.   DSM-IV-TR diagnostic criteria for autistic disorder

---

A. A total of six (or more) items from (1), (2), and (3), with at least two from (1), and one each from (2) and (3):

   (1) qualitative impairment in social interaction, as manifested by at least two of the following:

       (a) marked impairment in the use of multiple nonverbal behaviors such as eye-to-eye gaze, facial expression, body postures, and gestures to regulate social interaction

       (b) failure to develop peer relationships appropriate to developmental level

       (c) a lack of spontaneous seeking to share enjoyment, interests, or achievements with other people (e.g., by a lack of showing, bringing, or pointing out objects of interest)

       (d) lack of social or emotional reciprocity

   (2) qualitative impairments in communication as manifested by at least one of the following:

       (a) delay in, or total lack of, the development of spoken language (not accompanied by an attempt to compensate through alternative modes of communication such as gesture or mime)

       (b) in individuals with adequate speech, marked impairment in the ability to initiate or sustain a conversation with others

       (c) stereotyped and repetitive use of language or idiosyncratic language

       (d) lack of varied, spontaneous make-believe play or social imitative play appropriate to developmental level

   (3) restricted repetitive and stereotyped patterns of behavior, interests, and activities, as manifested by at least one of the following:

       (a) encompassing preoccupation with one or more stereotyped and restricted patterns of interest that is abnormal either in intensity or focus

       (b) apparently inflexible adherence to specific, nonfunctional routines or rituals

       (c) stereotyped and repetitive motor mannerisms (e.g., hand or finger flapping or twisting, or complex whole-body movements)

       (d) persistent preoccupation with parts of objects

B. Delays or abnormal functioning in at least one of the following areas, with onset prior to age 3 years: (1) social interaction, (2) language as used in social communication, or (3) symbolic or imaginative play.

C. The disturbance is not better accounted for by Rett's disorder or childhood disintegrative disorder.

Impulsivity, agitation, and tantrum behavior is common, especially in the early years. Cognitive deficits include impairments in abstraction, sequencing, and integration. There may be distorted perception for smell, taste, or touch and underdevelopment of visual and auditory processing. Eating patterns may be restricted ("picky eating") or indiscriminate (pica).

Most individuals with autistic disorder show subnormal intelligence, but some show significant "increases" in measured IQ during the course of treatment or development. There are often dramatic inconsistencies, with extraordinary "scatter" of capabilities among different IQ subtests and over time. Unusual or special capacities ("savant" skills) may be present in particular areas, such as music, drawing, arithmetic, or calendar calculation.

Epidemiology

The available prevalence estimates for autistic disorder are based on criteria that emphasize the more severe forms of this disorder. When these criteria are used, prevalence is estimated at approximately 1 in 2,000. The less severe forms are more common, with estimates as high as 1 in 250. There is a male predominance of approximately 4:1–5:1, but females often have more severe symptoms. Contrary to early belief, increased prevalence is not associated with higher socioeconomic class or higher intelligence.

Etiology

Contrary to popular opinion, there is no significant evidence that psychosocial factors or parenting abnormalities cause autistic disorder or that exposure to mumps-measles-rubella vaccination increases the risk of autistic disorder.

Genetic and biological factors appear to play a significant role in autistic disorder (Folstein and Piven 1991), but what is inherited appears to be a spectrum of cognitive and social deficits rather than autism per se. The higher concordance in monozygotic than dizygotic twins (60%–91% vs. 0%) supports a genetic factor (Bailey et al. 1995). Family genetic studies establish higher rates of autism, social and communication deficits, and stereotyped behaviors (i.e., broader autism phenotype) in the relatives of autistic patients (Piven et al. 1997b). The reports of chromosome 15 abnormalities and the 2%–5% incidence of autism in individuals with fragile X syndrome initially led to optimism that genetic linkage studies might define genes for autistic disorder, but early attempts failed.

The probable overrepresentation of ADHD, obsessive-compulsive symptoms, and Tourette's disorder also may suggest that autistic disorder involves genetic factors that are related to the transmission of these disorders and, perhaps, the transmission of the syndrome entailing all three conditions (J.S. Stern and Robertson 1997). The first-degree (parents) and second-degree (aunts, uncles, and grandparents) relatives of individuals with autistic disorder have been reported to have sig-

nificantly higher rates of major depressive disorder and social phobia, in comparison with relatives of patients with Down syndrome (Piven and Palmer 1999). Shared genetic mechanisms may account for this overrepresentation.

Siblings of autistic children show a prevalence of autistic disorder of 2%–5% (more than 50 times the expected prevalence), and about 5%–25% of the siblings have delays in learning (usually language or speech disorder), mental retardation, or physical defects. Family studies have suggested autosomal recessive inheritance for certain cases of autistic disorder. Neuropathological studies have suggested that the neurodevelopmental changes begin early in gestation, probably during the second trimester (Bauman 1991). Decreased numbers of Purkinje cells and fetal cerebellar circuitry also have been reported.

Early neuroimaging studies have yielded findings that are inconsistent, nonspecific, nondiagnostic, or suggestive of general neuromaturational delays, adding little to the understanding of the pathogenesis of the pervasive developmental disorders. Failure to appreciate and properly correct for the effects of important covariates such as gender, age, performance IQ, and total brain volume in sample construction appears to have accounted for much of the inconsistency, but underlying etiological heterogeneity may play an important role as well. The most consistent neuroimaging findings implicate abnormalities in the temporal and parietal lobes of patients with autistic disorder.

A specific medical cause may be identified in some individuals. An elevated prevalence of early developmental problems, such as postnatal neurological infections, congenital rubella, and phenylketonuria, has been reported. About 2%–5% of autistic individuals appear to have fragile X syndrome. Seizure disorders are also common in autism, including both major motor seizures and complex partial seizures. Seizure onset typically is either during early childhood or during adolescence, and clinical seizures can be observed in up to 50% of autistic persons by age 20 years. Children with an early onset of seizures may show an increase in seizure symptoms during adolescence. Adolescence-onset seizures are observed more commonly in autistic disorder than in mental retardation.

Course and Prognosis

Autistic disorder is often apparent at birth or early infancy, and parents may seek a medical evaluation during the child's first year (often for deafness). Some symptoms are usually recognized, at least in retrospect, in more than 80% of children with autistic disorder by age 2 years. The DSM-IV-TR definition of autistic disorder requires an apparent onset before age 3 years.

The general course of autistic disorder is gradual improvement, but there is a high degree of irregularity and unpredictability in the speed of improvement. Periods of rapid developmental growth alternate with periods of slow, stable growth. The changes in maturational tempo occur abruptly or gradually. Developmental progress can be slow or rapid, and the periods of improvement may last for a couple of weeks or many months. Developmental change may be made in particular skills without improvement in other areas of functioning, or it may occur pervasively across many areas of functioning. Episodes of overt regression may occur during concurrent medical illness, situational stress, or puberty and even during periods of otherwise rapid developmental progress unexplained by environmental factors. Overall, predictors of good adaptive outcome include later onset, higher IQ, better language skills (especially vocabulary), and greater social and communicative skills.

The availability of educational and supportive services has a marked beneficial effect, just as in mental retardation. In the severe, classic forms, some adaptive skills can be learned. In the less severe forms, the acquired social skills and adaptations eventually may permit performance in an ordinary occupation. Even a relatively interactive and pleasant social life can be attained.

Over the years, the time course of change remains unpredictable. As adults, individuals with autistic disorder continue to show a gradual clearing of symptoms but retain clinical evidence of residual deficits (Rumsey et al. 1985a). Depending on the severity of the autistic disorder, perhaps 2%–15% achieve a nonretarded level of cognitive and adaptive functioning. Obsessive-compulsive features remain predominant in adulthood and may include stereotyped pacing, rocking, perseveration, and stuttering. Adults with autistic disorder remain socially aloof and often retain an oppositional streak. Expressive and receptive language often become normal, although speech may continue to have a singsong or monotonous sound. No delusions or hallucinations are evident. Autistic adults may achieve employment (generally in simple rote jobs) and the capacity for independent residence, but they rarely marry. The few outcome studies currently available describe the follow-up of severe and largely untreated cases; adult outcome may be better in less severe and more aggressively treated cases.

Diagnostic Evaluation

In addition to the standard psychiatric and behavioral evaluation, a workup of autistic disorder includes assessment of language skills, cognition, social skills, and adaptive functioning. Standardized scales and interviews have been developed to assess these areas of functioning (Tanguay 2000). Psychological and neuropsychological testing for mental retardation and mixed receptive-expressive language disorder are valuable, but it can be difficult to obtain reliable and consistent findings. Evaluation for communication disorders may be particularly formidable if the child's nonverbal skills are also impaired. An assessment of the home environment and emotional supportiveness of the family is essential.

Neurological examination includes consideration of possible inborn metabolic and degenerative diseases. Screening for phenylketonuria is probably cost-effective. MRI studies may be helpful in some cases as a part of the general neurological evaluation, but they cannot be used for diagnosis of autistic disorder at this time. It is typically worthwhile to obtain an EEG in view of the high prevalence of seizure disorders in this population, although the EEG patterns are often nonspecifically abnormal in the absence of seizures. Chromosomal analysis also should be considered to evaluate for relatively frequent genetic abnormalities, such as fragile X syndrome. In some cases, audiological examination for possible deafness and examinations for other sensory deficits may be considered.

Patients with autistic disorder also must be evaluated for psychiatric comorbidity, especially OCD, ADHD, tic disorders, mood disorders (particularly major depressive or dysthymic disorder), and psychotic disorders. Although ADHD may be functionally present and fulfill diagnostic criteria, it is not designated as a separate DSM-IV-TR disorder when it occurs in the context of a pervasive developmental disorder.

Differential diagnosis includes congenital deafness (although deaf children typically learn an alternate lip or sign language, lose their isolative behaviors, and develop sensitive expressive communication), congenital blindness (although blind children relate more socially), mental retardation (although children with mental retardation do not show the islands of special capacity that autistic children sometimes have), expressive and mixed receptive-expressive language disorder (although children with these disorders typically are more interactive and can communicate well in gestures), schizophreniform disorder, schizotypal personality disorder, and juvenile-onset schizophrenia (although children with schizophrenia typically have hallucinations, delusions, or thought disorder).

In many cases, particularly those involving less severe forms, it is difficult to make a definitive diagnosis of autistic disorder. The appearance of hallucinations, delusions, or clear thought disorder should lead to the consideration of a primary psychotic disorder rather than autism. However, children and adults with autistic disorder may have concomitant psychotic disorders, comorbid mood disorders, or anxiety disorders.

Treatment

Behavior therapy has been helpful in controlling unwanted symptoms, promoting social interactions, increasing self-reliance, and facilitating exploration (i.e., novelty-seeking behavior). Specialized assertiveness training may be helpful in enhancing adaptive skills. Special education, vocational training, the teaching of adaptive skills, and support in managing major life events are basic. Environmental management, especially predictable or programmed structure, has a particularly powerful effect.

Providing guidance to parents is critical, especially for those who are making the chronically afflicted child the emotional center of their lives. Although this attentiveness may have beneficial effects for the child, it is often driven by unjustified guilt, unrealistic pessimism, or narcissism. Parents can contribute to the child's learning of self-care and adaptive skills, arrange for special education and management with schools and other public agencies, and make long-term plans for the child's future. Because long-term treatment is essential, periodic medical reassessment is needed to monitor for the possible appearance of seizures or concomitant psychiatric disorders that may be masked by the autistic disorder.

A long-term program involving high levels of supervision and structure is generally required. Specialized day-care and group settings, incorporating elements of behavioral treatment in a naturalistic setting with a stable interpersonal network, are helpful in some cases (Landesman and Vietze 1987). At times, residential care is needed to provide a more enveloping structure of protection and supervision.

Most of the pharmacological studies of autistic disorder have been conducted in children, with little research concerning adults. No drug treatment of autistic disorder itself is available, but psychotropic medications can be used to target particular symptoms, symptom clusters, and comorbid disorders in individual patients. No psychotropic medications provide generally useful treatment for most cases of autistic disorder.

The symptoms most amenable to pharmacotherapy include perseverative behaviors (comparable to obsessive-compulsive symptoms), depressive disorders, aggressivity, impulsivity, destructiveness, bipolar disorders, anxiety, hyperactivity, hypoactivity, pica, and SIBs. Management of seizures is also approached medically. In general, the risk of overmedication requires continual attentiveness.

Although no single medication is generally indicated, different agents can pro-vide symptomatic benefit. Low doses of a nonsedating conventional neuroleptic (such as haloperidol) have been found helpful for promoting learning, controlling behavioral symptoms, reducing excessive activity levels, controlling aggressive and disruptive behavior, and enhancing the effects of behavior therapy and other interventions. However, the newer atypical antipsychotics, such as risperidone, appear to be more beneficial in some patients (McDougle et al. 1998), better tolerated, and less risky. Olanzapine is generally less satisfactory because of its tendency to aggravate obsessive-compulsive symptoms. Psychostimulants, anticonvulsants, and neuroleptics may be useful for symptoms of impulsivity. Psychostimulants are used for children who either are underactive or have concurrent ADHD. β-Blocking agents and perhaps clonidine might have some value in managing symptoms of impulsivity and aggression. Early reports on naltrexone, an opiate receptor–blocking agent, suggested that this drug could improve affective availability, promote social reciprocity, and reduce stereotyped motor behavior and SIBs; however, more recent data suggest that naltrexone has little or no clinically significant effects. Several preliminary reports have suggested that fluoxetine can be helpful in treating obsessional and depressive symptoms in patients with autistic disorder. Serotonin reuptake inhibitors also have been found to reduce anxiety symptoms in some children (Steingard et al. 1997). In a controlled study of adults with autism, fluvoxamine was significantly more beneficial than placebo (McDougle et al. 1997), and lithium has been found to be helpful as an adjunctive treatment, particularly when supplementing serotonin reuptake inhibitors. Other researchers have suggested possible benefits of H_1 (niaprazine) and H_2 (famotidine) blockers, corticotropin analogues, and inositol. Secretin has been reported to be helpful in this disorder, but controlled studies (Owley et al. 2001; W. Roberts et al. 2001) have not confirmed its utility. The efficacy of some popularly touted treatments for autistic disorder, including dimethylglycine (Bolman and Richmond 1999) and high-dose magnesium-pyridoxine (Findling et al. 1997), has also not been supported in controlled studies.

Childhood Disintegrative Disorder

Clinical Description

Childhood disintegrative disorder, as defined in DSM-IV-TR, differs from autistic disorder in time of onset, clinical course, and prevalence. In contrast to autistic disorder, childhood disintegrative disorder involves an early period of normal development until age 3–4 years. This phase is followed by a period of marked deterioration of adaptive, communicative, and social functioning (Table 15–18), usually occurring rapidly over the course of 6–9 months. Childhood disintegrative disorder may begin with behavioral symptoms, such as anxiety, anger, or outbursts, but the general loss of functions becomes pervasive and severe. The deterioration progresses to a syndrome that is symptomatically similar to autistic disorder, except that mental retardation (typically in the moderate-to-profound range) tends to be more frequent and pronounced (Volkmar and Rutter 1995), and significantly more children appear to develop seizures (Mouridsen et al. 1998). Over time, the deterioration remains stable, although some capacities may be regained to a limited degree. About 20% of individuals regain the ability to speak in sentences, but their communication skills remain impaired (A. E. Hill and Rosenbloom 1986). Most adults are completely dependent and re-

TABLE 15–18. DSM-IV-TR diagnostic criteria for childhood disintegrative disorder

A. Apparently normal development for at least the first 2 years after birth as manifested by the presence of age-appropriate verbal and nonverbal communication, social relationships, play, and adaptive behavior.

B. Clinically significant loss of previously acquired skills (before age 10 years) in at least two of the following areas:
 (1) expressive or receptive language
 (2) social skills or adaptive behavior
 (3) bowel or bladder control
 (4) play
 (5) motor skills

C. Abnormalities of functioning in at least two of the following areas:
 (1) qualitative impairment in social interaction (e.g., impairment in nonverbal behaviors, failure to develop peer relationships, lack of social or emotional reciprocity)
 (2) qualitative impairments in communication (e.g., delay or lack of spoken language, inability to initiate or sustain a conversation, stereotyped and repetitive use of language, lack of varied make-believe play)
 (3) restricted, repetitive, and stereotyped patterns of behavior, interests, and activities, including motor stereotypies and mannerisms

D. The disturbance is not better accounted for by another specific pervasive developmental disorder or by schizophrenia.

quire institutional care, and some have a shortened life span.

The syndromal validity of childhood disintegrative disorder has remained controversial (Mouridsen et al. 2000). Attempts to validate a distinction between autism and childhood disintegrative disorder have not been decisive. Comparisons of lifetime psychopathology in parents, neuroimaging studies, and genetic findings in childhood disintegrative disorder and childhood autistic disorder have uncovered mostly minor differences, except for a significantly higher rate of electroencephalographic abnormalities in childhood disintegrative disorder (Mouridsen et al. 1998, 1999a, 1999b, 2000).

Epidemiology

Childhood disintegrative disorder is rare, with prevalence estimates ranging from 1 to 4 in 100,000, which is about 1/100th the frequency of autistic disorder. There appears to be a male predominance of greater than 4:1.

Etiology

No specific neurobiological deficit or cause of childhood disintegrative disorder has been identified (Volkmar and Cohen 1989). Early associations of childhood disintegrative disorder with specific neurological and medical disorders have not been supported. Significant psychosocial or medical stressors have been reported in association with the onset or worsening of the disorder, but their etiological significance is unclear.

Diagnostic Evaluation and Treatment

The evaluation and treatment of childhood disintegrative disorder are essentially comparable to the approach to autistic disorder, although much more active support, behavioral treatment, neurological care, and medical monitoring are needed. Studies attempting to characterize this very rare disorder have been difficult to conduct, and research on the pathophysiology and treatment of this disorder has lagged behind research on the other specific pervasive developmental disorders. A change in the disease label is also needed because of the crudity of the term *disintegrative*, especially when used in speaking with parents about their child.

Rett's Disorder

Clinical Description

Rett's disorder is a progressive neurodevelopmental disorder and one of the most common causes of mental retardation in females.

Epidemiology

Its estimated prevalence ranges from 4 to 22 in 100,000 girls (Kozinetz et al. 1993; Skjeldal et al. 1997). Because Rett's disorder occurs almost exclusively in females, it had been proposed that Rett's disorder is caused by an X-linked dominant mutation with lethality in hemizygous males. This proposal has been confirmed with the discovery that Rett's disorder results from mutations in the X-linked methyl-CpG-binding protein 2 (*MECP2*) gene (Amir et al. 1999).

Etiology

Once considered a clearly neurodegenerative process, serial neurodevelopmental evaluations have provided support for an arrest of developmental functions at various stages, particularly during periods of rapid neuronal growth, pruning, and maturation (Naidu et al. 1995), and increasing support exists for Rett's disorder as a neurodevelopmental disorder that arises from a poorly understood failure in the epigenesis of neural systems (Johnston et al. 2001). Debate continues about the neurodevelopmental versus neurodegenerative nature of the disease process and course, but it is clear that the onset of Rett's disorder can be observed in very young girls and that progressive clinical decline is the hallmark.

The progressive clinical decline is not initially apparent. Typically, after 6–18 months of relatively normal development, the first social, language, neurological, and motor deficiencies become apparent. Initially, the clinical decline is gradual, but it becomes quite evident by age 4 years (Table 15–19). Head and body growth retardation, along with other developmental delays, can be seen during this phase. Then, starting during the early school years, there is a period of more rapid functional deterioration in which intellectual and communicative capacities diminish, and purposeful control of hand movements is replaced with apraxia, wringing, and washing motions. Following this rapid deterioration, these girls appear to have a pervasive developmental disorder, which usually is identified as autistic disorder or childhood disintegrative disorder (Moeschler et al. 1988). This rapid decline in functioning usually reaches an apparent plateau that may last for months or years. However, this plateau is eventually seen to be a gradual decline that is much slower than that of the previous stage. Gait and truncal ataxia, respiratory symptoms involving dysregulation of breathing functions, and scoliosis typically begin to emerge during this slow decline.

By age 3–5 years, girls with Rett's disorder are less likely to be viewed as having either autistic or childhood disintegrative disorder because of the progressive appearance of increasingly severe neurological symptoms. Mental retardation is generally apparent, and most patients have intelligence scores in the severely retarded range. Seizures, decreasing physical mobility, spasticity, muscle weakness, severe scoliosis, wasting, dystonia, and choreoathetosis may emerge. Typically, these girls are eventually confined to wheelchairs, often before adolescence. Feeding can become quite difficult because of compromised motor functioning (swallowing). Caregivers need to be aware of the high risk of aspiration, which may be compounded by the dysregulation of breathing. Seizures occur in 80% of these patients and add to the management

TABLE 15–19. DSM-IV-TR diagnostic criteria for Rett's disorder

A. All of the following:
  (1) apparently normal prenatal and perinatal development
  (2) apparently normal psychomotor development through the first 5 months after birth
  (3) normal head circumference at birth
B. Onset of all of the following after the period of normal development:
  (1) deceleration of head growth between ages 5 and 48 months
  (2) loss of previously acquired purposeful hand skills between ages 5 and 30 months with the subsequent development of stereotyped hand movements (e.g., hand-wringing or hand washing)
  (3) loss of social engagement early in the course (although often social interaction develops later)
  (4) appearance of poorly coordinated gait or trunk movements
  (5) severely impaired expressive and receptive language development with severe psychomotor retardation

problems. Some girls with Rett's disorder die suddenly of unexplained causes; some patients have a normal life span despite the severe symptoms and disabilities, but life expectancy is generally reduced.

The discovery of the gene for Rett's disorder is the result of a decade-long search. Extensive "exclusion" mapping studies of families with Rett's disorder mapped the locus of the putative gene(s) to Xq28. A systematic gene screening approach identified mutations in the *MECP2* gene as the cause of Rett's disorder (Amir et al. 1999). Subsequent studies confirmed the finding, and they have begun to better characterize the range of mutations and of their expression. In classic Rett's disorder, studies suggest that patterns of X chromosome inactivation may play a greater role in determining the clinical severity than the type of mutation; in variant presentations, however, the mutation may more strongly affect disease severity. Familial cases of Rett's disorder are rare and are due to X chromosomal inheritance from a carrier mother, who is often mildly affected. In sporadic cases of Rett's disorder, de novo mutations of the gene in the paternally derived X chromosome appear common (Trappe et al. 2001).

Diagnostic Evaluation

Data from neuroimaging studies are preliminary, but SPECT studies have suggested that bifrontal hypoperfusion correlates with severity of Rett's disorder. Diffuse atrophy (most notably in the prefrontal, posterior frontal, and anterior temporal regions) was noted in an MRI study. Abnormal EEG results are typically found after age 2 years; despite the high prevalence of seizures, the EEG findings are typically nonspecific. Taken together, the neurobiological abnormalities suggest an X-linked generalized atrophy with global dysfunction that correlates with severity of the symptoms.

Treatment

Treatment of Rett's disorder is supportive. Generally, these multiply handicapped patients require intensive care (Lindberg 1992). The role of psychopharmacotherapy is limited, but several reports have found carbamazepine to be more effective than other anticonvulsants for seizure control in girls with Rett's disorder. Lamotrigine might also be useful.

In contrast to childhood disintegrative disorder, Rett's disorder is an excellent example of rapid progress in recent research in the pervasive developmental disorders. Older findings will need to be reconsidered in light of the revolution that molecular genetics is catalyzing in this area.

Asperger's Disorder

Asperger's disorder is another pervasive developmental disorder that is similar to autistic disorder, except that language acquisition, cognitive development, learning skills, and even most adaptive behaviors are largely preserved (Table 15–20). The autistic features of impaired social interactions and stereotyped behaviors and interests are present but are generally more subtle (Klin et al. 2000). Rather than evidencing a relative lack of interest in other people or a general weakness in communication, conversational interactions may be merely impaired. These individuals may "interact" with others through seemingly endless monologues on a topic of extreme interest to themselves, without reading nonverbal and even verbal cues, continuing on without apparent awareness that the other person views the topic as eccentric or idiosyncratic. They may become quite knowledgeable, or at least collect large numbers of facts, about a topic. Even social communications might be learned as a set of rules and scripts. Such a child's "precocious" interest in particular topics can fascinate adults but may not engage peers or draw emotional sharing.

Because of its similarities to autism, the status of Asperger's disorder as a distinct form of pervasive developmental disorder is often questioned, and many specialists believe that it is a mild version of autistic disorder (i.e., high-functioning autism) rather than a separate and distinct disorder (Gillberg 1989; Rapin 1991; Szatmari 2000). Analysis of speech and communication patterns, cognitive batteries, and WISC findings (Ehlers et al. 1997) have supported the DSM-IV-TR interpretation that Asperger's and autistic disorders are distinct entities. However, the distinction is challenged by evidence suggesting that a spectrum of cognitive and social deficits (i.e., the "broad" autistic phenotype) may be inherited rather

---

TABLE 15–20. DSM-IV-TR diagnostic criteria for Asperger's disorder

A. Qualitative impairment in social interaction, as manifested by at least two of the following:
  (1) marked impairment in the use of multiple nonverbal behaviors such as eye-to-eye gaze, facial expression, body postures, and gestures to regulate social interaction
  (2) failure to develop peer relationships appropriate to developmental level
  (3) a lack of spontaneous seeking to share enjoyment, interests, or achievements with other people (e.g., by a lack of showing, bringing, or pointing out objects of interest to other people)
  (4) lack of social or emotional reciprocity
B. Restricted repetitive and stereotyped patterns of behavior, interests, and activities, as manifested by at least one of the following:
  (1) encompassing preoccupation with one or more stereotyped and restricted patterns of interest that is abnormal either in intensity or focus
  (2) apparently inflexible adherence to specific, nonfunctional routines or rituals
  (3) stereotyped and repetitive motor mannerisms (e.g., hand or finger flapping or twisting, or complex whole-body movements)
  (4) persistent preoccupation with parts of objects
C. The disturbance causes clinically significant impairment in social, occupational, or other important areas of functioning.
D. There is no clinically significant general delay in language (e.g., single words used by age 2 years, communicative phrases used by age 3 years).
E. There is no clinically significant delay in cognitive development or in the development of age-appropriate self-help skills, adaptive behavior (other than in social interaction), and curiosity about the environment in childhood.
F. Criteria are not met for another specific pervasive developmental disorder or schizophrenia.

---

than autism per se (Bailey et al. 1995). The view of Asperger's and autistic disorders as representing "parallel but potentially overlapping developmental trajectories" (Szatmari et al. 2000) is consistent with the concept of Asperger's disorder as a part of an autistic spectrum.

With the relative sparing of intelligence, language, and cognition, Asperger's disorder differs from autism in having a low prevalence of mental retardation. Also unlike in autism, verbal functioning is stronger than nonverbal functioning. Only 12% of the children with Asperger's disorder have IQ scores below 70. It is characteristic of these patients to misread nonverbal cues, have marked difficulties with peer interactions (especially in groups), focus repetitively in conversation on topics of interest only to themselves, appear not particularly empathic, and speak without normal inflection and tone variation; they may be relatively unexpressive affectively, and they tend to have few friends (Wing 1981). Even with these limitations, persons with Asperger's disorder are often quite sociable and talkative, and they may form affectionate bonds with family members (Frith 1991). Symptoms of right hemisphere syndrome are typical, and comorbid ADHD or developmental coordination disorder may be observed.

The course tends to be stable over time, often with some gradual gains (Szatmari et al. 1989, 2000). The verbal strengths may hide social deficits, especially from adults, who are often inclined to misinterpret behavioral abnormalities as laziness or stubbornness. Although social skills may improve with age, relative weakness in interpersonal interactions and lack of social spontaneity may become more limiting in later childhood and adolescence, leading to increasing isolation, anxiety, and depression. Nonetheless, long-term educational and occupational adjustment are markedly better than in autistic disorder, and financial and social independence are generally achieved.

Epidemiological data are limited, but the prevalence of the more severe presentations of Asperger's disorder is estimated at 5–15 in 100,000. The male predominance is 3:1–4:1.

The etiology of Asperger's disorder remains unknown. In some cases, it follows a familial pattern, consistent with genetic, psychosocial, or environmental transmission. A possible role of fetal exposure to alcohol has been raised (Aronson et al. 1997).

Neurobiological studies are extremely limited. About 30% of the patients with Asperger's disorder have nonspecific EEG abnormalities, and 15% show evidence of brain atrophy. In a recent SPECT study, abnormal right hemisphere metabolism was reported; although the significance of this finding is unclear, it lends some support to the concept of "right-hemisphere-only autistic disorder" (McKelvey et al. 1995; Szatmari et al. 1995).

Treatment includes social and motor skills training, remedial educational interventions when indicated, and vocational training (Attwood and Wing 1998). The relative sparing of language and intelligence allows individuals with Asperger's disorder to have a better outcome than do most persons with autistic disorder. For example, Temple Grandin is a productive member of society with good verbal skills who has Asperger's disorder (formerly diagnosed as autism). Her self-report (Grandin and Scariano 1986) shows that a high-functioning individual with a pervasive developmental disorder can vividly describe personal experiences and complex cognitions. Persons with Asperger's disorder, despite their relative handicaps in social functioning, can become quite expert and effective in their chosen activities, and perhaps they are even helped in these accomplishments by the highly focused nature of their interests.

Tic Disorders

Tics are sudden, rapid, nonrhythmic, stereotyped movements (motor tics) or vocalizations (vocal tics). Their form may be simple (motor: jerking movements, shrugging, eye blinking; vocal: grunting, sniffing, throat clearing) or complex (motor: grimacing, bending, banging; vocal: echolalia, odd inflections and accents). Tic movements are often preceded by a "premonitory urge"; these uncomfortable and irresistible somatosensory experiences, sometimes termed *sensory tics* (Kurlan et al. 1989), seem to motivate or compel about 30% of the movements and vocalizations.

Although tics are experienced as irresistible, they may be temporarily delayed or suppressed. The fact that tics may be consciously suppressed distinguishes them from choreiform movements (i.e., disruptions of normal synergistic movement by coordinated muscle groups, such as blinks or grimaces), athetosis (i.e., slow writhing), dystonias (i.e., abnormal muscle tone), other dyskinesias (i.e., disruptions of voluntary and involuntary motions), and other neurological movement disorders with which they may be confused. Instead, tics are brief and repetitive (but not rhythmic) motor or vocal responses. They are purposeless but may resemble purposeful acts. Although they involve recurrent movements of the same muscle groups, their location can change gradually over time.

Distinguishing tics from compulsive or impulsive symptoms can be challenging, particularly because OCD and ADHD often present comorbidly with Tourette's or chronic tic disorders. For example, patients with tics may be driven to recurrently touch surfaces, touch other people, touch their own genitals inappropriately, engage in SIBs such as head-banging or self-mutilating behaviors such as scratching a patch of skin to rawness (M.M. Robertson et al. 1989), or have aggressive or obscene verbal (coprolalic) or motoric (copropraxic) outbursts.

Individual tics or ticlike movements may be seen occasionally in children and adults without tic disorders, but such "twitches" (e.g., blinks, grimaces) and habits are not diagnosed as disorders unless they persist for at least 2 weeks.

DSM-IV-TR recognizes three discrete tic disorders: transient tic, chronic tic, and Tourette's disorders (Table 15–21). These conditions are closely related in descriptive, etiological, genetic, pathophysiological, and developmental characteristics.

Tic disorders are believed to arise from abnormal functioning of CSTC neural circuitry involved in motor control and sensorimotor integration. Genetic studies show that 50% of male (and 30% of female) first-degree relatives of patients with Tourette's disorder have transient tic disorder, chronic tic disorder, OCD (Hebebrand et al. 1997), and often ADHD. This overrepresentation suggests a genetic interrelationship among the three tic disorders, OCD, and perhaps ADHD. Environmental factors, including infections triggering autoimmune reactions against key portions of the brain, are also important in the developmental pathogenesis of these disorders. Because the symptoms of these disorders are subject to moment-to-moment influences from environmental and internal stimuli, tic disorders have been seen as prototypic illnesses for the study of interacting biopsychosocial influences (Chase et al. 1992; D. Cohen et al. 1988; Kurlan 1993).

Because the etiologies of the three tic disorders seem closely interrelated, it is appropriate that tic disorders are subtyped by clinical description and course rather than by etiology. Tourette's disorder is generally the most serious of these disorders and has been the best studied. Transient and chronic tic disorders are less well characterized.

Transient Tic Disorder

Transient tic disorder is diagnosed if daily tics persist for 4 weeks to 1 year, the threshold for the diagnosis of chronic tic disorder. Although a single symptomatic period may be observed in some patients, recurrent episodes may come and go for years.

Transient tics are usually motoric, but they are otherwise similar in appearance to chronic and Tourette's tics. Transient tic disorder may be relabeled later in its course if tics persist. These tics do not appear to be consistently associated with other symptoms, but situational or developmental anxiety may be prominent during episodes. Studies of comorbidity are sparse.

Up to 12% of children have tic symptoms, but the prevalence of transient tic disorder is undetermined.

Both genetic and psychosocial factors influence the appearance of transient tic disorder. Episodes are typically seen during periods of increased stress or excitement, which contribute to the transient presentation and the variability of symptom intensity. Even when tics present in apparent response to physical or emotional trauma, the individual generally has an underlying genetic vulnerability (Alegre et al. 1996).

The onset of single or recurrent epi-

TABLE 15–21.   DSM-IV-TR diagnostic criteria for tic disorders

---

Diagnostic criteria for transient tic disorder

A. Single or multiple motor and/or vocal tics (i.e., sudden, rapid, recurrent, nonrhythmic, stereo-typed motor movements or vocalizations)

B. The tics occur many times a day, nearly every day for at least 4 weeks, but for no longer than 12 consecutive months.

C. The onset is before age 18 years.

D. The disturbance is not due to the direct physiological effects of a substance (e.g., stimulants) or a general medical condition (e.g., Huntington's disease or postviral encephalitis).

E. Criteria have never been met for Tourette's disorder or chronic motor or vocal tic disorder.

Specify if: **Single Episode** or **Recurrent**

Diagnostic criteria for chronic motor or vocal tic disorder

A. Single or multiple motor or vocal tics (i.e., sudden, rapid, recurrent, nonrhythmic, stereotyped motor movements or vocalizations), but not both, have been present at some time during the illness.

B. The tics occur many times a day nearly every day or intermittently throughout a period of more than 1 year, and during this period there was never a tic-free period of more than 3 consecutive months.

C. The onset is before age 18 years.

D. The disturbance is not due to the direct physiological effects of a substance (e.g., stimulants) or a general medical condition (e.g., Huntington's disease or postviral encephalitis).

E. Criteria have never been met for Tourette's disorder.

Diagnostic criteria for Tourette's disorder

A. Both multiple motor and one or more vocal tics have been present at some time during the illness, although not necessarily concurrently. (A *tic* is a sudden, rapid, recurrent, nonrhythmic, stereotyped motor movement or vocalization.)

B. The tics occur many times a day (usually in bouts) nearly every day or intermittently throughout a period of more than 1 year, and during this period there was never a tic-free period of more than 3 consecutive months.

C. The onset is before age 18 years.

D. The disturbance is not due to the direct physiological effects of a substance (e.g., stimulants) or a general medical condition (e.g., Huntington's disease or postviral encephalitis).

---

sodes of transient tic disorder usually is during middle childhood (ages 5–10 years) or early adolescence. If episodes recur, the frequency and severity of symptoms typically diminish over the course of years. The tics usually do not interfere with functioning, although they may interact with anxiety and social stressors to produce interpersonal and self-esteem complications.

For mild presentations of transient tic disorder, medical workup is often omitted in actual practice. For more significant or persistent presentations, psychiatric, neu-rological, and medical evaluations should assess possible concomitant disorders such as mood and anxiety disorders (particularly OCD), ADHD, neurological co-morbidity (including other movement disorders), and general pediatric illnesses, including virus-induced tics (usually herpetic), autoimmune conditions, and post-traumatic tics from head trauma. Psychosocial sources of anxiety (that might aggravate tic severity), developmental details, and family genetic history should be ascertained.

Transient tic disorder typically does

not require treatment. It is usually helpful to advise the family to reduce attention to the symptom and criticism of the child. Behavioral techniques (e.g., relaxation), medications (e.g., minor tranquilizers), or brief psychotherapy may be helpful in certain cases for anxiety management and tic control. In the absence of significant comorbidity or psychosocial stressors, the patient and family may be provided with education and reassurance, and they may be encouraged to return for reevaluation if symptoms persist.

Chronic Motor or Vocal Tic Disorder

Chronic motor or vocal tic disorder is diagnosed if either a motor or a vocal tic persists for more than 1 year. Tourette's disorder is diagnosed if both motor and vocal tics are chronic.

Chronic tics usually are motoric and similar in form to those in other motor tic disorders. Chronic vocal tics are rare, are usually mild, and generally consist of grunts (e.g., diaphragmatic contractions) rather than true vocal or verbal tics. The persistence of chronic tics can be associated with anxiety or depressive disorders, both of which may aggravate tic disorders.

Prevalence data are not available for chronic tic disorders because the durational characteristics of tics have not been studied epidemiologically. Chronic tic disorder is probably less common than Tourette's disorder in clinical populations, but it is unclear whether this reflects general prevalence or referral bias (such as help seeking).

The intensity of chronic tics typically varies little over the course of weeks, although changes may be noted over the course of months or years. The onset is usually during early childhood (ages 5–10 years). In about two-thirds of individuals, the disorder ends during adolescence,

but some cases may persist in mild form for years or even decades. A subtype of chronic tic disorder also can appear in adulthood, typically after age 40.

Pediatric, neurological, and psychiatric evaluations, similar to the workup for transient tic disorder, are indicated. A child whose transient tics have persisted should be reevaluated after 6–12 months, so that comorbidity and psychosocial stressors can be reassessed and so that treatment can be considered.

Similar to transient tic disorder, both behavioral and pharmacological treatments are effective. Psychosocial interventions may be used to target anxiety or mood symptoms. Minor tranquilizers, or low doses of major tranquilizers, may be considered. Serotonin reuptake inhibitors may be appropriate to treat comorbid mood disorders or anxiety, especially comorbid OCD. Although systematic data are lacking, anecdotal information suggests that these medications are quite useful.

Tourette's Disorder

Tourette's disorder entails the presence of both vocal tics and multiple motor tics. Transient tic disorder is diagnosed during the first 12 months that both motor and verbal tics are observed, and the diagnosis is converted to Tourette's disorder beyond 1 year. The DSM-IV-TR definition of Tourette's disorder is considerably looser than the classic criteria and permits inclusion of a wider range of patients.

Although Tourette's disorder is often considered a lifelong disease, prevalence is 10-fold higher among children than adults, and longitudinal studies indicate that symptoms decline or fully resolve in 50% of affected individuals by age 18 years (Leckman et al. 1998), suggesting a more benign and less chronic outcome for many individuals.

Clinical Description

Both the motor and the vocal tics may be simple or complex. The behavioral component can be suppressed voluntarily, but then a premonitory sensory urge builds, usually with a subjective sense of tension. This sensation of craving before a tic is relieved temporarily when patients allow themselves to express their tics in action. Many patients experience their tics as a voluntary response to these premonitory urges, and they may feel more troubled by the continual pre-tic tension than by the tics themselves. They also may engage in self-reproach, faulting themselves for not controlling their "voluntary" behaviors.

Some patients find that they can control their tics during the day at school or work and then "let off the tension" later, when alone in their bedrooms. For these individuals, the use of the home as a haven for the release of symptoms can be an effective way to reduce the effect of their symptoms on their social and occupational life. However, some patients with severe Tourette's disorder feel that "saving" their tics in this manner is even more problematic because it interferes with the comfort of family members.

The symptoms of chronic tic and Tourette's disorders typically wax and wane over time. Anxiety and excitement typically lead to increased symptoms, relaxation and focused attention can reduce symptoms, and symptoms are typically minimal or absent during sleep. Severity varies widely. Mild cases may go undiagnosed (even in television personalities), whereas severe cases may be disabling and socially disfiguring. Increased symptom severity may be evident for several minutes during stressful situations, may last for months during periods of developmental anxiety and stress, or may last for years—particularly when associated with concomitant anxiety or mood disorders

(Coffey et al. 2000; Elstner et al. 2001), ADHD, or other comorbidity.

Vocal tics may be disguised, for example, in feigned coughing. Complex motor tics may appear to be purposeless, or they may be camouflaged by being blended into other purposeful movements.

Sometimes complex motor tics are self-destructive, such as scratching or cutting oneself, or violent, with temper tantrums and assaults.

Obsessive-compulsive features appear in about 20%–40% of patients, and full OCD presents in 7%–10%. Although the diagnostic criteria are clearly defined, the clinical boundaries between Tourette's disorder, ADHD, and OCD are blurred in the many patients who have combined features of these three disorders (Cath et al. 2001a, 2001b; Miguel et al. 2000).

Comorbid conduct, mood, and anxiety disorders are also common. Although disruptive behavior, mood, and anxiety disorders as well as cognitive dysfunctions may be accounted for by comorbidity with ADHD, the comorbid presentation of ADHD and Tourette's disorder appears to be a more severe condition than ADHD alone (J. Spencer et al. 2000).

Specific cognitive deficits that have been reported in Tourette's disorder consist of visual-motor integration problems, impaired fine motor skill, and executive dysfunction (Como 2001). The presence of comorbid conditions, notably ADHD and OCD, appears to significantly increase the likelihood that an individual with Tourette's disorder also will have learning problems or some demonstrable cognitive impairment, and they may, in fact, account for most such problems.

Neurological symptoms are typically observed in patients with Tourette's disorder, including soft signs in 50% of patients and choreiform movements in 30% of patients. Approximately 50% of patients show abnormal EEG findings, particularly immature patterns consisting of excess slow waves and posterior sharp waves. CT scans usually are normal.

Epidemiology

Up to 12% of children may have tic symptoms, which usually are transient. The general prevalence of tic disorders is currently estimated at 1%–2%, but it is probably higher in children and adolescents. Prevalence estimates for Tourette's disorder range from 1 in 350 to 1 in 2,000. A male predominance of 3:1–10:1 has been reported, but the actual ratio may be closer to 2:1. No socioeconomic skewing is apparent. Cross-cultural studies have suggested that Tourette's disorder presents similarly across cultures in its clinical features, comorbidity, family history, and treatment outcomes, consistent with a strong neurobiological etiology (Freeman et al. 2000; Staley et al. 1997).

Etiology

Genetic, biological, and psychosocial factors appear operative in Tourette's disorder and other tic disorders. Tics are noted in two-thirds of the relatives of patients with Tourette's disorder, and tic disorders are found in 5%–10% of their siblings. The higher concordance of Tourette's disorder in monozygotic (50%–56%) than dizygotic (10%) twins suggests a heritable component; when chronic tics are included in the ascertainment, the concordance between monozygotic twins is nearly 100%. Genetic studies show a link between Tourette's disorder, chronic tics, and OCD. There also may be a link between Tourette's disorder and ADHD, even in the absence of OCD (Sheppard et al. 1999).

Several segregation analyses of families of Tourette's patients have provided support for autosomal dominant transmission, with partial penetrance and gender threshold effects, of Tourette's disorder (Curtis et al. 1992; Pauls and Leckman 1986). Two studies have suggested more complex transmission (Walkup et al. 1996), perhaps even nonmendelian (Seuchter et al. 2000).

A gender threshold effect (Pauls and Leckman 1986), specifically involving a lower penetrance of Tourette's disorder in girls at a given level of genetic loading, could account for the higher prevalence in boys than in girls. A gender threshold effect also could explain findings that girls show a higher prevalence of Tourette's and chronic tic disorders in their families. When all presumed forms of the disorder were considered in the segregation analysis, the penetrance was estimated as essentially complete (100%) in males and 71% for females. Consistent with a gender threshold effect, males within affected families were more likely to have tic disorders, and females were more likely to have OCD (Pauls and Leckman 1986). In this model, about 10% of the individuals with Tourette's disorder were estimated to have a nonheritable form of the disorder, perhaps the result of an environmental exposure.

The search for candidate genes, while promising, has been inconclusive to date. Possible associations of Tourette's disorder with dopamine-related genes have been mixed (Rowe et al. 1998; Thompson et al. 1998). Examination of serotonin receptor genes suggests that this neurotransmitter system plays a minor role, if any (Brett et al. 1995).

PANDAS-associated Tourette's episodes are caused or triggered by group A β-hemolytic streptococcal infections, such as pharyngitis, upper respiratory infections, or subclinical streptococcal infections (Singer et al. 2000). Antibodies directed against group A β-hemolytic streptococcus also recognize and cross-react with neuronal antigens (epitopes) in the basal ganglia (Singer et al. 1998; Swedo 1994) and are believed to produce Sydenham's chorea, tic disorders, and OCD. They also might cause or contribute to some cases of anorexia nervosa (Sokol and Gray 1997). Consistent with this mechanism, MRI studies found enlargement of the basal ganglia in patients with streptococcal-related Tourette's disorder and OCD (Giedd et al. 2000).

A monoclonal antibody (D8/17) identifies a B lymphocyte antigen with expanded expression in nearly all patients with rheumatic fever as well as in most patients with childhood-onset Tourette's disorder or OCD (Hoekstra et al. 2001; T.K. Murphy et al. 1997). The antigen is believed to be a trait marker for susceptibility to this complication of group A β-hemolytic streptococcal infections, although it is also overexpressed in patients with autistic disorder. This finding provides further support for a role for group A β-hemolytic streptococcal infections in the pathogenesis of some cases of tic disorders and OCD.

Course and Prognosis

Tics usually appear first in middle childhood or early adolescence, although they may begin later in adult life or as early as 2 years. Tics typically wax and wane in intensity over time. They often worsen during times of psychosocial stress (including teasing and social ostracism), intrapsychic conflict, and positive or negative emotional excitement. Psychosocial stress may be particularly symptom inducing at the start of the school year, at times of parental separation and divorce, and during physical fatigue.

As many as 50% of affected individuals experience significant improvement or complete remission of their symptoms by age 18 years, consistent with a 10-fold higher prevalence of Tourette's disorder in children than in adults.

The clinical presentation of Tourette's disorder may change during the course of development (Leckman et al. 1998). The mean age at onset of tics (usually motor) is 5–7 years; earlier age at onset is associated with a stronger family history of tics (Freeman et al. 2000). Symptoms typically worsen with time but in a waxing and waning pattern. The progression in severity of the tics is sufficient to seriously jeopardize functioning in school in up to 22% of these children. Severity typically peaks at about age 10 years, and the onset of puberty is not usually associated with the onset or severity of tics.

Classic coprolalia, observed in 30%–60% of the patients with Tourette's disorder, usually first emerges in early adolescence. Copropraxia (complex obscene gestures) may appear later as coprolalia resolves.

Early in development, before the initial appearance of tics, 25%–50% of the children with Tourette's disorder show symptoms of impulsivity, hyperactivity, and inattention similar to ADHD. Obsessive-compulsive symptoms often follow the onset of simple tics by 5–10 years (Peterson et al. 2001a) and subsequently may elaborate extensively.

Comorbidity is an important determinant of outcome. Patients with only tic symptoms tend to have a relatively benign course, whereas patients with ADHD and/or OCD have courses complicated by aggressive and disruptive symptoms and social and academic failure (Budman et al. 2000; Coffey et al. 2000; T. Spencer et al. 1998b; Stephens and Sandor 1999). Concurrent mood and anxiety disorders often aggravate the course of tic disorders (Coffey et al. 2000).

In the autoimmune form of Tourette's disorder (PANDAS), tic symptoms usually begin with an acute and even dramatic onset at around age 7–8 years. Exacerbations may occur days to months after the onset of the streptococcal infection. The interval between first infection and initial appearance of tics may be weeks or months, but subsequently the interval between recurrent infections and symptom exacerbation typically decreases over time to a few days or weeks. Tic symptoms can be worsened by a "strep throat" or an "ordinary" upper respiratory infection. PANDAS can even be triggered by simple exposure to people with streptococcal infections, without any apparent clinical symptoms until the appearance or exacerbation of the neuropsychiatric syndrome.

Complications of severe Tourette's disorder may include impaired academic and social functioning and impaired self-esteem, interacting with the symptoms and complications that typically attend the comorbid disorders. Teasing, shame, self-consciousness, and social ostracism are common features in patients with predominantly internalizing comorbidities, whereas antisocial or criminal outcomes may be the manifestations with prominent externalizing comorbidity. Some patients may show a reluctance to involve themselves in socially demanding situations, particularly if their symptoms are severely socially disfiguring. Others may adopt an aggressive stance toward the world. Patients may avoid entering intimate relationships, marriage, and other interpersonally gratifying activities. The rate of unemployment is reportedly as high as 50% in adults with Tourette's disorder.

Diagnostic Evaluation

A complete psychiatric evaluation of the child and parents is indicated, including the assessment of possible ADHD, conduct disorder, OCD, learning disorders, pervasive developmental disorders, and mental retardation. A family genetic history should specifically include tic disorders, ADHD, OCD, and streptococcus-

related illnesses. Neurological examination is appropriate to rule out other movement disorders, including Wilson's disease. An EEG is helpful in ruling out myoclonic seizures and other neurological disorders. An assessment of baseline dyskinesias is necessary before neuroleptic drug treatments are started. School reports, including those addressing academic performance, general behavior, severity of tics, and social skills, are useful. The child's self-consciousness, management of teasing and social ostracism, and assertiveness may be assessed. The possibility of concurrent mood or anxiety disorder should be evaluated. Along with assessment of family psychopathology and stressors, direct evaluation of tic and related disorders in siblings and parents may be considered.

A careful history of potential post-streptococcal neuropsychiatric sequelae should be obtained. Antibodies to streptococcal enzymes streptolysin O and DNase B increase during infection, and elevated titers may persist for some months thereafter. Measurement of these titers can be obtained as evidence of a possible association between an infection and the appearance or exacerbation of tic symptoms. Throat or nasopharyngeal swabs may be cultured to confirm acute infection. However, the clinical utility of these studies in documenting or tracking PANDAS has not been established. Nonetheless, evaluation for antistreptococcal antibodies should be considered in children with tic disorders.

Treatment

Pharmacotherapy, behavior therapy, and sometimes psychotherapy and special education may be used, although longitudinal studies of complex interventions have yet to be conducted. Although medications may play a vital role in the management of Tourette's disorder, a child's adaptive capacities, comorbid diagnoses, coping mechanisms, interpersonal skills, and social support play a significant role in outcome. Also, in view of the studies suggesting a frequently benign resolution of Tourette's symptoms toward the end of adolescence, the presumption of extended or lifelong psychopharmacological treatment should be questioned or at least clinically tested in individual cases.

Neuroleptic drugs have been the cornerstone of pharmacotherapy. Although largely replaced by the newer atypical antipsychotic agents, studies of conventional neuroleptics have reported that approximately 60%–80% of Tourette's patients show clinically significant improvement. Low dosages of high-potency neuroleptics, such as haloperidol and pimozide, have been prescribed most commonly, but low-potency neuroleptics appear to be approximately as effective. The neuroleptic dosages are typically low in comparison to antipsychotic doses; dose elevations may be required gradually over time, but decreases in dosage also may be possible because of the waxing and waning of symptoms. Atypical antipsychotics, including olanzapine, risperidone, and ziprasidone, have been effective in controlled trials of Tourette's disorder (Bruggeman et al. 2001; Onofrj et al. 2000; Sallee et al. 2000). Despite the reduced incidence of adverse motor effects with the atypical antipsychotics, it is important to keep in mind that all neuroleptics carry a risk of inducing neuroleptic malignant syndrome (Latz and McCracken 1992; Steingard et al. 1992) and tardive tourettism (Bharucha and Sethi 1995).

Clonidine is an alternative treatment that has been reported to be helpful in about 50% of patients with Tourette's disorder, particularly for children with behavior disorders whose ADHD might be improved by clonidine. At low dosages,

clonidine stimulates α_2-adrenergic presynaptic receptors, leading acutely to decreased norepinephrine neurotransmission and, with chronic treatment, to increased dopamine use through an unknown indirect mechanism possibly involving serotonin. The clinical effect of clonidine might increase over the course of 2–3 months of treatment. Guanfacine, a similar α_2-adrenergic receptor agonist, has been found in controlled studies to be effective and safe in this population (Chappell et al. 1995; Scahill et al. 2001). The effects of long-term clonidine and guanfacine treatment are not well defined.

The use of stimulants and TCAs in treating Tourette's disorder remains controversial because of past findings that these agents may exacerbate or trigger tic disorders. Although some controlled findings suggest that these agents exacerbate tics in many children (Gadow et al. 1995; Riddle et al. 1995), many physicians have returned to using these agents with only occasional complaints of tic induction. With or without the use of stimulants and TCAs, continued vigilance regarding tic induction is advisable if over-the-counter sympathomimetic drugs are used by patients with Tourette's disorder. Similarly, special warnings are needed concerning the recreational use of cocaine and related drugs. At this time, it is acceptable practice to prescribe psychostimulants in treating chronic tic disorders with comorbid ADHD, and TCAs may be considered for patients with comorbid anxiety or depressive disorders.

Controlled trials support the use of various other agents in Tourette's disorder, including the selective MAOI selegiline (Feigin et al. 1996), the mixed dopamine agonist pergolide (Gilbert et al. 2000), the nicotinic receptor antagonist mecamylamine (Silver et al. 2001), the GABA receptor agonist baclofen (Singer et al. 2001), and the opioid agonist propoxyphene (Kurlan et al. 1991). Interestingly, botulinum toxin A, the neuromuscular blocking agent, was found in an open-label study to reduce motor tics and also to diminish the premonitory sensations (Kwak et al. 2000). Also, some evidence indicates that androgens and the opiate receptor antagonist naltrexone may worsen tics and associated obsessive-compulsive symptoms and therefore should be avoided.

If comorbid psychiatric disorders are present in patients with Tourette's disorder, treatment of the comorbidity may improve the symptoms of Tourette's disorder. This parallel improvement can be seen with most comorbid psychiatric disorders, including mood and anxiety disorders, ADHD, and other behavior disorders. Although there remains debate about the possible risk of tic induction or aggravation by use of psychostimulants, a growing body of literature supports their chronic use in treating ADHD with comorbid Tourette's disorder with little evidence of stimulant-induced tic exacerbation (Gadow et al. 1999).

Although psychotherapy is not a specific treatment of Tourette's disorder, it may be useful to help an individual deal with the stigma of illness and with self-esteem problems, promote interpersonal comfort and social skills, improve the opportunities for and the odds of successful marriage, and enhance functioning and satisfaction at work. In addition to enhancing adaptive skills, psychotherapy may reduce the anxiety that aggravates tic severity (O'Connor et al. 2001).

The family response to this disfiguring disorder is often significant, and its management is important for the welfare of both the family and the patient (D. Cohen et al. 1988). The Tourette Syndrome Association is a national organization that provides support and education to families and patients, funds and helps locate subjects for research, and advocates with public agencies.

Feeding and Eating Disorders of Infancy or Early Childhood

Anorexia nervosa and bulimia nervosa, usually first diagnosed in adolescence, are discussed in Chapter 17. Three additional eating disorders usually first diagnosed in childhood are pica, rumination disorder of infancy, and feeding disorder of infancy or early childhood.

Pica and rumination disorder are rarely treated as isolated entities by psychiatrists, but these disorders are significant medical conditions with definite psychiatric dimensions. Feeding disorder of infancy or early childhood corresponds to a subcategory of the pediatric diagnosis of nonorganic failure to thrive.

Pica

A pattern of eating nonfood materials can be seen in young children, individuals with severe or profound mental retardation, and pregnant women. Pica has been extensively documented in the pediatric literature but minimally documented in the psychiatric literature—despite its presumed biopsychosocial etiology and its potential for major behavioral, cognitive, neurological, and developmental complications.

Pica appears to be quite common in children, particularly young children, but is frequently underdiagnosed. When pica occurs in mentally retarded persons or in pregnant women, it can require a physician's vigilant inquiry to uncover. The psychiatric significance of pica is very different in these distinct populations.

Geophagia (the eating of clay or soil) is

TABLE 15–22. DSM-IV-TR diagnostic criteria for pica

A. Persistent eating of nonnutritive substances for a period of at least 1 month.
B. The eating of nonnutritive substances is inappropriate to the developmental level.
C. The eating behavior is not part of a culturally sanctioned practice.
D. If the eating behavior occurs exclusively during the course of another mental disorder (e.g., mental retardation, pervasive developmental disorder, schizophrenia), it is sufficiently severe to warrant independent clinical attention.

a similar phenomenon that is an ordinary and sanctioned activity in many cultures worldwide, especially in indigenous populations that live close to the soil. Even in some American locations, including the central Piedmont region of Georgia, chalk eating is a cultural norm (Grigsby et al. 1999). Such culturally determined forms of pica are not considered a mental disorder (Table 15–22). Whatever the basis for the pica, the risk of accidental poisoning is significant.

Clinical Description

Children and people with mental retardation may eat paper, paint, coins, string, rags, hair, feces, vomitus, leaves, bugs, worms, and cloth. Pica in children is typically observed in association with behavior and other medical problems, but such children are rarely brought for psychiatric treatment of the isolated problem of pica. Pica behavior can vary considerably across days, but some children have been documented to ingest 25–60 g of soil in a single day (Calabrese et al. 1997).

Pregnant women, apart from their common craving for fruit and sharp-tasting foods, have been reported at times to seek and eat starchy materials, refrigera-

tor frost, or substances containing minerals. Cultural geophagia commonly involves the eating of earth, clay, sand, and pebbles. Geophagia is also common in children and in pregnant women.

Epidemiology

Few epidemiological data are available on DSM-defined pica, but picalike behaviors are common. About 10%–20% of children in the United States exhibit picalike behavior at some point in their lives, and up to 50%–70% of children living in the inner cities have pica between ages 1 and 6 years. Boys and girls are equally involved. Epidemiological studies show that children with pica typically come from a low socioeconomic class, have pets at home, and show various behavioral abnormalities. Typically, they are not referred for treatment unless complications, such as lead poisoning, or concomitant disorders are identified. More than 50% of the children hospitalized for accidental ingestions have been found to have pica (Millican et al. 1968).

Mental retardation is associated with a high prevalence of pica. Approximately 20%–40% of institutionalized people with severe or profound mental retardation have pica. Gender prevalence is equal.

The prevalence of pica among pregnant women has been reported to vary geographically from 0% to 70%. In the lower socioeconomic classes of the United States, persistent nonnutritive eating is seen in about 60% of pregnant women. The specific eating of ice and freezer frost was reported by 8% of the pregnant women in the inner city of Washington, DC (Edwards et al. 1994). Most children with pica have mothers or siblings who also have pica.

Pica increases the risk of exposure to environmental toxins. Lead poisoning has been reported in as many as 92% of children living near a lead smelter in Brazil (Silvany-Neto et al. 1996). Households may become contaminated by toxins inadvertently brought home from job sites despite precautions to avoid occupational exposure and transportation of potentially toxic materials (Chiaradia et al. 1997). Even in affluent locations, pica is a major route of exposure to lead, pesticides, and organic toxins through the ingestion of house dust in carpets, mattresses, and sofas (J.W. Roberts and Dickey 1995).

Etiology

Childhood pica is sometimes interpreted as an ordinary part of exploratory learning or as a reflection of a young child's inability to differentiate food from inedible objects. The findings of increased childhood pica in households with pets and of the eating of pet food by children suggest that imitation can be an etiological factor. Most children with pica have parents with a history of pica; the disorder may be passed along by a variety of mechanisms, including cultural ones.

In individuals with severe or profound mental retardation, the primary mechanism is believed to be self-stimulation rather than impaired judgment. Children and adults with mental retardation and pica tend to engage in pica with a favorite object.

A nutritional etiology has been proposed for some adults, who are believed to have an instinctive craving for vitamins and minerals, especially iron and perhaps zinc or calcium. The eating is hypothesized to be an attempt to correct a nutritional deficiency. Evidence indicates that this mechanism operates in animals, but few data support this notion in humans. Eating of ice (or refrigerator frost) has been reported in pregnant women in association with iron deficiency, and prescription of iron supplements has been found to improve the anemia and reduce the ice

eating (Danford 1982). Pica can instead be a cause of malnutrition because the consumed objects or substances may interfere with the absorption of nutrients. Because anemia does not regularly induce pica in adults, it is more likely that pica causes nutritional imbalances in adults. The relevance of the nutritional deficiency theory of pica to children is undetermined.

Course and Prognosis

In children, pica usually starts at age 12–24 months and resolves by age 6 years. However, in mentally retarded persons, pica can endure and persist into adulthood. In pregnant women, geophagia usually resolves at the end of pregnancy, although it may recur in subsequent pregnancies.

Complications of pica are numerous and potentially severe. Constipation and gastrointestinal malabsorption are common. Fecal impaction may occur repetitively. Ingestion of foreign bodies or hair balls can lead to intestinal obstruction, potentially leading to intestinal perforation or biliary obstruction, which sometimes requires colostomy. Anemias can be produced by nutritional deficiencies and sometimes traumatic intestinal bleeding. Mineral toxicity, salt imbalances, parasitic infections, vomiting, poisoning, and dental injury may be seen. Ingestion of radioactively contaminated soil is also a public health concern (Simon 1998).

Ingestion of lead-containing paint, plaster, and earth can lead to toxic encephalopathy in severe cases, fatigue and weight loss (with constipation) in moderate cases, and learning impairments in mild cases. Approximately 80% of the children with severe lead poisoning have pica, and at least 30% of the children with pica show lead-related symptoms.

Lead intake by pregnant women can cause congenital plumbism. However, pica has developmental significance even without toxin ingestions: pregnant women who eat ice give birth to infants with smaller head circumferences than do women without pica (Edwards et al. 1994). Children with pica can have slow motor and mental development, growth retardation, seizures, and neurological deficits, as well as behavioral abnormalities both before and after the period of pica. A long-term follow-up study suggested that young children with pica are at increased risk for the subsequent development of bulimia nervosa, with an odds ratio of 6.7 (Marchi and Cohen 1990).

Diagnostic Evaluation

Evaluation of children with pica involves behavioral and psychiatric evaluation of the child and parents, psychosocial evaluation of the home (including caregiver availability and presence of pets), nutritional status, feeding history, lead exposure, and cultural values. The possibility of inadequate supervision of children or parental neglect needs assessment.

The diagnosis is often missed because children are typically brought for evaluation of other problems. Adults may not have directly observed the pica behavior in children or may volunteer such observations about their family only reluctantly.

Pica should be actively considered in children and adults (not only persons with mental retardation) with anemia, chronic constipation, fecal impaction, or accidental ingestions. Lead poisoning may be present in children with ADHD, unexplained fatigue or weight loss, learning impairments, mental retardation, or gingival "lead lines."

In view of the high risk of lead intoxication, it is reasonable to assess children with pica by obtaining both a zinc protoporphyrin and a plasma lead level. Debate remains about whether there is a developmentally "safe" minimal blood level of lead, and even the generally endorsed up-

per limits of acceptable plasma levels of lead (10 µg/dL) and zinc protoporphyrin (30 µg/dL) have been questioned. When identifying a child with pica, it is advisable to examine siblings and parents for pica as well.

Treatment

Behavior therapy has been used for children and mentally retarded individuals with pica. Rewarding appropriate eating, teaching the differentiation of edible foods, overcorrection (immediate enforcement of oral hygiene), and negative reinforcement (time-outs, physical restraint) have been successful, especially for mentally retarded people. Psychosocial interventions include promotion of maternal supervision and stimulation, improvement of play opportunities (new toys), and placement in day care.

Concomitant medical treatments may be required. Management of lead poisoning may be handled in the routine manner. It has been suggested that nutritional iron and zinc treatments produce short-term improvements in some individuals. Nutritional treatments have not been systematically assessed, although some preliminary evidence suggests that multivitamins might be able to reduce pica in some cases (Pace and Toyer 2000).

Psychosocial interventions also have not been evaluated, but improvements in personal and household hygiene appear to be beneficial. Removal of old or synthetic carpets and furniture, elimination of sources of dust and particulates, or even a family move away from a problematic home may be required in some cases.

Rumination Disorder of Infancy

Certain infants show a pleasurable relaxation as they regurgitate, rechew, drool, and reswallow their food, usually in the absence of caregivers and other sources of stimulation. Their continuing self-stimulation, apparent satisfaction, and languorous obliviousness highlight their full engrossment in rumination. Their obvious enjoyment and enthusiasm occur despite malnourishment and diminished weight gain and are in marked contrast to their parents' disgust at this activity.

This potentially fatal disorder of infants may reflect abnormal development of early self-stimulation and physiological regulation, and it is particularly apparent when infants are alone (Table 15–23). Rumination (merycism) may be a cause or result of disrupted parent–child attachments, and it can be associated with major developmental delays and mental retardation. It is recognized by gastroenterologists as a functional disorder of infancy (Rasquin-Weber et al. 1999).

The symptom of rumination is relatively common in adults with mental retardation; it has been reported in up to 10% of institutionalized adults with severe or profound mental retardation (Fredericks et al. 1998). In addition, patients with eating disorders are occasionally observed to ruminate (Eckern et al. 1999; Weakley et al. 1997). Rumination also may present in developmentally normal children (Reis 1994), adolescents (Khan et al. 2000), and adults (Parry-Jones 1994), seemingly as a transient response to situational stressors. The relation of these forms of rumination to the pathological condition of rumination disorder in infants is unclear.

Clinical Description

Rumination involves the continued eating of partially digested stomach contents that are regurgitated into the esophagus or mouth. It is different from vomiting, in which the stomach contents are expelled through the mouth.

Rumination may start with the infant's

TABLE 15–23. DSM-IV-TR diagnostic criteria for rumination disorder

A. Repeated regurgitation and rechewing of food for a period of at least 1 month following a period of normal functioning.

B. The behavior is not due to an associated gastrointestinal or other general medical condition (e.g., esophageal reflux).

C. The behavior does not occur exclusively during the course of anorexia nervosa or bulimia nervosa. If the symptoms occur exclusively during the course of mental retardation or a pervasive developmental disorder, they are sufficiently severe to warrant independent clinical attention.

placing fingers or clothes in the mouth to induce regurgitation, with rhythmic body or neck motions, or it may begin without any apparent initiating action. During rumination, the infant generally lies quietly, may look happy or "spacey," and may hold body and head in a characteristic arching position while sucking. No nausea, discomfort, or disgust is apparent. If observed, the infant usually stops and fixes visual attention on the intruder; when the infant is no longer aware of being observed, sucking and tongue movements restart in seconds. When he or she is not ruminating, the infant may appear apathetic and withdrawn, irritable and fussy, or seemingly normal.

Self-stimulatory behaviors are commonly seen in association with rumination disorder. Often, thumb sucking, cloth sucking, head banging, and body rocking are observed, lending support to the hypothesis that rumination can be an infantile form of self-stimulation.

Epidemiology

No prevalence figures are available, but rumination disorder is rare and decreasing in prevalence in the general population, perhaps because of improving infant and child care. The disorder has almost disappeared in some countries (Guedeney 1995). However, rumination disorder is not rare in infants with mental retardation. About 10% of institutionalized mentally retarded adults show similar medically unexplained symptoms. About 93% of the adults with rumination have severe or profound mental retardation. The few available studies consist of small samples and report contradictory findings on sex ratio. Both male predominance and equal sex prevalence have been reported.

Course and Prognosis

Regurgitation or vomiting (with reflux on barium fluoroscopy) is generally seen during the first 3 months of life, but rumination typically does not appear until age 3–12 months. It usually resolves by the end of the second year but may persist until the third or fourth year. In more persistent cases, the patient generally has mental retardation. Although people with mental retardation can also show a later onset of rumination disorder, the disorder typically emerges during childhood or adolescence.

Dehydration, electrolyte imbalance, slow weight gain, growth retardation, malnutrition, and tooth decay are seen in some individuals. Spontaneous remissions are common, but there is also a high risk of developmental delay and death. Reports in the literature from the 1950s indicate a 10%–25% mortality rate, with death from malnutrition. However, the risk of fatality depends on the availability of intervention, and the modern availability of parenteral hyperalimentation has probably led to a substantial reduction in deaths.

A major complication of rumination disorder of infancy is the parents' reaction to the symptoms. A parent's immediate response to observing rumination is typically acute anxiety and distress, which can lead to ongoing affective and cognitive responses that impair the formation of parental attachment to the child. The parents' frustration and disgust, particularly at the odor, may lead to further avoidance and understimulation of the child. This disruption of attachment can constitute a major complication in the child's development (Mayes et al. 1988).

The only available follow-up study of infants with rumination disorder indicated that about 50% have normal behavioral development and that 20% have severe developmental or medical pathology at age 5 years (Sauvage et al. 1985). Both mental retardation and pervasive developmental disorders are commonly associated with rumination disorder; they may be cause, effect, or concomitant disorders. Chronic malnutrition typically is not seen in rumination disorder. The course of rumination in adults with mental retardation has not been well described.

Diagnostic Evaluation

Evaluation includes behavioral and psychiatric evaluation of child and parents, with an emphasis on developmental history and psychosocial assessment, as well as eating history, nutritional status, and observation of parent–child interactions during feeding. Gastrointestinal disease needs to be considered, including gastroesophageal reflux, hiatal hernia, pyloric stenosis, other congenital anomalies, and infections. Gastrointestinal structural abnormalities (and other abnormalities) may be particularly common in individuals with cerebral palsy, physical anomalies, and developmental disorders.

The symptom of regurgitation in infants also can be due to anxiety; some children appear openly distressed during rumination. Usually, however, children with rumination disorder appear happy and enjoy the regurgitation, whereas children with gastrointestinal disorders vomit with discomfort and experience pain. Although this sounds like a simple distinction, the literature on rumination and reflux esophagitis is confounded by difficulties in this differential diagnosis. It is usually unclear whether reflux or rumination initiated the esophageal pathology. Clinically, it is advisable to carefully examine esophageal function in parallel with the psychiatric evaluation. In addition, diagnosticians should keep in mind that rumination occasionally presents in developmentally normal children and adults.

Treatment

There is no established treatment of rumination disorder of infancy, although various forms of behavior therapy, parental guidance, and medication (antispasmodics and tranquilizers) have been tried. Psychotherapy for the caregiver, dietary changes, and hand restraints have not been found to be particularly effective.

Behavioral techniques include cuddling and playing with the child before, during, and after mealtime to reduce social deprivation and behavioral withdrawal. Aversive conditioning (e.g., putting hot pepper sauce or lemon on the infant's tongue, electroshock) produces the most rapid symptom suppression, but it generally elicits strong caregiver resistance and usually cannot be applied immediately or consistently. Negative attention, such as shouting or slapping the child, can serve to reinforce the behavior, especially if other forms of reinforcement and attention are lacking or ineffective. A combination of a negative reinforcement (a scolding and putting the child down for 2 minutes) with a reward for nonrumination (parental attention and social interaction, such as being cleaned and played with) has been successfully used in outpatient treatment (Lavigne et al. 1981).

Temporary hospitalization is commonly used to provide a separation of the child from the primary caregiver, an alternative feeding environment for the child (to "decondition" the symptoms), and a period of relaxation for the parent (to permit anxiety reduction). Reassurance, education, and support of the parents help reduce their preexisting anxiety and avoidance, diminish their acute stress at times of the infant's rumination, and reestablish the parents' comfort in the feeding process. Psychiatric and psychosocial evaluation of the parents may be valuable. Ongoing clinical follow-up is useful to facilitate attachment between infant and mother, monitor the psychosocial environment at home, and provide support in the event of emerging mental retardation. There has been limited systematic assessment of the treatment interventions used in rumination disorder (Chatoor et al. 1984).

Feeding Disorder of Infancy or Early Childhood

In pediatrics, the diagnosis of failure to thrive indicates a retardation of body growth or milestone attainment as a result of inadequate nutritional intake. The "organic" forms of failure to thrive can result from chronic physical illness (congenital AIDS), neurological disease, sensory deficit, or virtually any serious pediatric disease. The "nonorganic" forms, constituting at least 80% of cases of failure to thrive, encompass 1) homeostatic disorders of infancy (sleep and feeding dysregulation), 2) pathological food refusal, 3) protein-calorie malnutrition, and 4) social and emotional factors interfering with adequate nutritional care (including reactive attachment disorder, which is discussed later in the chapter).

The DSM-IV-TR diagnosis of feeding disorder of infancy or early childhood does not include all forms of nonorganic failure to thrive but only the types of eating failure that occur in the context of adequate provision of food (Table 15–24). This disorder does not include cases of child neglect or cases of inadequate eating due to obviously defective parenting or feeding.

TABLE 15–24. DSM-IV-TR diagnostic criteria for feeding disorder of infancy or early childhood

---

A. Feeding disturbance as manifested by persistent failure to eat adequately with significant failure to gain weight or significant loss of weight over at least 1 month.

B. The disturbance is not due to an associated gastrointestinal or other general medical condition (e.g., esophageal reflux).

C. The disturbance is not better accounted for by another mental disorder (e.g., rumination disorder) or by lack of available food.

D. The onset is before age 6 years.

Clinical Description

Infants may gag when fed or refuse to open their mouths. Young children might decline to eat, or they may eat so slowly that their intake is drastically reduced. In infants, the retardation in weight gain is typically accompanied by motor, social, and linguistic delays as well as a problematic relationship with the feeder or caregiver (as a result if not a cause of the disorder). In early childhood, symptoms may include impaired interpersonal relationships and interactions, mood symptoms, behavior problems, developmental delays, unusual food preferences, excessively rigid or narrow food choices, and perhaps bizarre eating and foraging behaviors.

Epidemiology

About 25% of the infants in the general population are reported to have some type of feeding problem, but a prevalence of 80% is described in children with developmental delays (Manikam and Perman 2000). Approximately 1%–5% of pediatric hospital admissions are for nonorganic failure to thrive, and community-based estimates of the prevalence of nonorganic failure to thrive are approximately 1%–4%. Epidemiological data concerning the DSM-IV-TR diagnosis of feeding disorder of infancy or early childhood are not available.

Etiology

The relative loss of weight is due to malnutrition, but the malnutrition may have various causes (Woolston 1983). Both physical and psychosocial etiologies may be involved, although the definition of the disorder excludes cases that clearly result from overt medical problems or other psychiatric disorders.

Various mechanisms (and potential subtypes) include difficulties with physiological homeostasis, attachment to the caregiver, and autonomy from the caregiver, as well as posttraumatic responses (Chatoor et al. 1985).

Homeostatic control of sleep and feeding is an early developmental accomplishment that is generally easy to achieve. The lability of the autonomic nervous system, presumably seen in colicky infants, needs the calming and soothing responses of the caregiver to promote development of self-regulation. Even the physical requirements of eating may induce fatigue and interfere with feeding in some infants, especially those with medical conditions unrelated to feeding.

Attachment problems, reflected in impaired relatedness and reciprocal interactions with the caregiver, may operate to inhibit adequate feeding. The ordinary signals, including eye contact, smiling, vocal contact, visual stimulation, and physical touching, may not be provided (or responded to) by child or parent, undermining the reciprocal signaling that underlies effective feeding. Apathy might replace the enjoyment of feeding experienced by child and caregiver.

Autonomy struggles, reflecting the negotiation of separation from the feeder, may be manifest by the child's food refusal, "pickiness" about food choices, or undereating. Between ages 6 months and 3 years (the developmental period of separation and individuation), the child's agenda may effectively become "I will decide who puts food in my mouth." If the parent interprets the child's actions as rebellion or personal insult, a power struggle may become evident in feeding (before it becomes clear in other developmental arenas). Food refusal is often accompanied by other displays of autonomy and power, including temper tantrums and aggressivity (Chatoor 1989). The result is that the child's eating patterns become determined by the interpersonal and emotional struggle with the parent rather than nutritional needs or internal physiological hunger signals.

Additional socioemotional factors that might reduce nutritional intake and body growth include posttraumatic responses to medical procedures involving the mouth, child abuse, emotional deprivation, or family pathology. Maternal psychopathology appears to increase the risk of feeding problems, such as food refusal or pickiness, in infants.

Feeding disorder is distinct from general problems in feeding, but some findings on infants with feeding problems may be relevant. Although mood and anxiety disorders do not appear to be overrepresented in the mothers of children with feeding problems (Whelan and Cooper 2000), almost one-third of the children with a feeding disorder have mothers with current or past DSM-IV eating disorders (Whelan and Cooper 2000). Such moth-

ers appeared to have difficulty in tolerating normal child feeding behavior and appeared to react to it in a manner that reflected the mother's concerns about food and eating rather than the child's developmental needs (A. Stein et al. 1999). These mothers appear to show excessive concern about the weight, shape, and consistency of the food; concern about the shape and weight of the child; attitudes toward dieting and food restriction; uneasiness with child's use of food for nonnutritive purposes such as play; and discomfort with vomiting and mess.

Course and Prognosis

The untreated course of these disorders may depend on the specific subtype or mechanisms involved, but the expected outcome ranges from spontaneous remission to malnutrition, infection, susceptibility to chronic illness, and death. Both nutritional and psychosocial deprivation may result in long-term behavioral changes, hyperactivity, short stature, and lowered IQ. In some cases of prolonged food refusal, such as seen in the posttraumatic form, the lack of practice in chewing or eating may lead to oromotor delays. The relation of these feeding disorders to other psychiatric disorders in adulthood is undetermined, but some evidence indicates increased risk for later eating disorders (Jacobs and Isaacs 1986; Marchi and Cohen 1990).

Evaluation and Treatment

It is not clear from the DSM-IV-TR definition whether feeding disorder of infancy or early childhood includes cases in which food is available but the caregiver is simply an inept feeder. It is also unclear whether the reversal of the symptoms with appropriate care is characteristic.

In some cases, disturbed eating patterns based on power struggling may be approached by a behavioral-cognitive approach with the mother. However, in some cases, a more extensive psychotherapeutic approach is needed to address the mother's dependency and control issues (Chatoor 1989). Support for the mother of a temperamentally challenging infant might include modeling, direct coaching on how to read the infant's cues, teaching how to allow appropriate autonomy during meals, reducing the mother's distractions during feeding, fostering of self-feeding, tolerating mess, and using contingency management and praise.

In most cases of feeding disorder of infancy, however, the services of a multidisciplinary team, preferably in a hospital setting, are appropriate for evaluating and initiating treatment. Specialists in gastroenterology, nutrition, behavior, and development can be helpful. Many potential specialized procedures are available for evaluating feeding and swallowing disorders in children (Lefton-Greif and Loughlin 1996), but the medical workup of such children will depend on a variety of factors. Evaluation includes assessment of body growth as well as observations of the mother–child interactions in general and in feeding in particular.

Elimination Disorders

Encopresis

Encopresis includes fecal soiling of clothing, voiding in bed, and excretion onto the floor, occurring after age 4 years, when full bowel control is developmentally expected. Because "organic" causes of encopresis need to be excluded, medical examination for structural and other nonfunctional abnormalities must be obtained before the diagnosis is made (Table 15–25). Although the term *encopresis* is used loosely to denote both types of soiling, the medically ex-

plained cases are technically *fecal incontinence*, and the idiopathic ones are *encopresis* (Loening-Baucke 1996). Both biopsychiatric and psychodynamic theories have been proposed to explain the etiology of encopresis. However, if a specific neurobiological explanation were identified, the condition would no longer be idiopathic. *Idiopathic encopresis* would be a clearer term for this psychiatric disorder.

TABLE 15–25.   DSM-IV-TR diagnostic criteria for encopresis

A. Repeated passage of feces into inappropriate places (e.g., clothing or floor) whether involuntary or intentional.
B. At least one such event a month for at least 3 months.
C. Chronological age is at least 4 years (or equivalent developmental level).
D. The behavior is not due exclusively to the direct physiological effects of a substance (e.g., laxatives) or a general medical condition except through a mechanism involving constipation.

Code as follows:

787.6   **With Constipation and Overflow Incontinence**
307.7   **Without Constipation and Overflow Incontinence**

Behavior problems are found in one-third of the children with encopresis. Some of the psychological and behavioral difficulties appear to resolve when the encopresis improves. In such cases, encopresis appears to function as an etiological factor for the development of behavioral symptoms. In other cases, major psychiatric disorders appear comorbidly with encopresis and require concurrent treatment.

Most cases of encopresis result from chronic constipation that leads to overflow. The stool may be formed, semiformed, or liquid. At least some children have encopresis without constipation. Children who have encopresis with constipation have a longer colonic transit time (slower movement) than encopretic children without constipation (Benninga et al. 1994), suggesting that some additional mechanisms might be involved. Children with soiling showed a general increase in behavioral symptoms, as measured on the Child Behavior Checklist, which were comparable in magnitude for both the constipated and the nonconstipated children (Benninga et al. 1994).

Clinical Description

Encopresis is usually a result of chronic constipation and is generally accompanied by pain during defecation, smell, and embarrassment. Parents usually repeatedly ask the child to try to relieve the feces in the toilet. Encopresis during the daytime is much more common than nocturnal encopresis. Half of these patients have primary encopresis: these individuals have never established fecal continence. The other half have secondary encopresis: these children initially learned bowel control, were continent for at least 1 year, and then regressed, typically by age 8 years.

Primary encopresis may be viewed as reflecting slow development or an early developmental fixation. In fact, it is associated in boys with a high rate of developmental delays (and enuresis) compared with secondary encopresis. Secondary encopresis, in which control was learned and then lost, is associated more strongly with conduct disorder and psychosocial stressors than is primary encopresis (Foreman and Thambirajah 1996).

About 75%–90% of the children with encopresis have the DSM-IV-TR subtype designated as "with constipation and overflow incontinence." These "retentive" cases involve a low frequency of bowel movements, impaction, overflow of liquid around a partially hardened stool, and leakage of liquid into the clothing. The cause may be chronic constipation, inadequate bowel training (e.g., overly coercive), pain (e.g., from an anal fissure), or phobic avoidance of toilets. These retentive episodes usually extend for several days and are followed by painful defecation.

Encopresis without constipation and overflow incontinence can involve a variety of causes, including a lack of sphincter awareness or weak sphincter control. In cases of postbath soiling, physical stimulation may be causative. If soiling is deliberate and the child is typically impulsive or hostile, antisocial or major psychiatric disorders may be associated. Smearing may be accidental (the child who tries to hide the accident) or purposeful (defiant or vindictive).

Typically, children with encopresis experience shame and embarrassment, feel dirty, and have low self-esteem. They may endure accusations from their parents and siblings, fear discovery by their peers, and hide physically and emotionally.

Epidemiology

Encopresis is less common than enuresis. Prevalence is approximately 1.5% after age 5 years; the disorder diminishes with age and is rare in adolescents. There is a 4:1 male predominance. Slightly higher prevalence rates are associated with the lower socioeconomic classes and with mental retardation, particularly in moderate and severe cases. However, most cases of encopresis are not associated with low intelligence. Overall, neither social class nor intelligence appears to correlate with the presence of encopresis.

Etiology

Medical causes of fecal incontinence include hypothyroidism, hypercalcemia, anal fissure or malformation, rectal stenosis, lactase deficiency, overeating of fried and fatty foods, trauma or surgery, congenital aganglionic megacolon (although Hirschsprung's disease is usually associated with large feces rather than incontinence), meningomyelocele (tissue protrusion through a defect in the vertebral column), and other neuromedical disorders. Pathophysiological mechanisms include altered colon motility and contraction patterns, stretching and thinning of colon walls (megacolon), and decreased sensation or perception (usually appearing early in development). During infancy, fecal soiling may result from severe diaper rash: fecal withholding might help the infant avoid rectal pain. These medical causes of fecal soiling exclude the diagnosis of encopresis.

Abnormal secretion of gastrointestinal hormones or altered motility in the gastrointestinal tract could lead to constipation and overflow incontinence. Children with encopresis were reported to have normal secretion of gastrin and cholecystokinin; however, their levels of pancreatic polypeptide were found to reach their peak and remain abnormally high following meals, whereas postprandial motilin levels were diminished (H.P. Stern et al. 1995). These differences in hormone secretion and motility might explain the unusually chronic constipation associated with fecal overflow, although their association with encopresis also might be a result of the constipation.

Some encopretic children show neurodevelopmental symptoms, such as inattention, hyperactivity, impulsivity, low frustration tolerance, and dyscoordination. Neurodevelopmental theories of encopresis have been proposed, although most children with neurodevelopmental delays or disorders do not have encopresis, and most children with encopresis do not appear to have significant neurodevel-

opmental symptoms. Children with primary encopresis appear to have comorbid developmental delays and enuresis, whereas secondary enuresis is more likely to present with conduct disorder and psychosocial stressors (Foreman and Thambirajah 1996). This clustering supports a neurodevelopmental factor in the etiology of primary encopresis.

A familial occurrence of encopresis is well documented. About 15% of the children with encopresis have fathers who had encopresis during childhood. Unlike the findings in enuresis, psychosocial factors appear to be stronger than genetic factors in the familial transmission of encopresis.

Psychosocial stressors (suggestive of adverse circumstances) and conduct disorder (suggestive of family psychopathology) are associated with encopresis, specifically secondary enuresis (Foreman and Thambirajah 1996). Presumably, the loss of previously established sphincter control is secondary to intercurrent life events, such as disorder in the family and environment. In general, family psychopathology is overrepresented in encopresis and, in some cases, intrudes on the development of self-control and disrupts its consolidation.

Inadequate or punitive toilet training appears to be a cause of encopresis in some cases. Pathogenic toilet training approaches are those that usually are considered coercive, aggressive, perfectionistic, inconsistent, or neglectful. Some cases of encopresis reflect developmental complications. For example, encopresis can result from toilet-related fears that are not properly managed or from physical discomfort associated with inadequate physical support during toilet training (e.g., feet do not touch the ground). Stress-related factors appear causative in one-half of the cases of secondary encopresis; for example, frenetic rushing before school or during television commercials.

Course and Prognosis

Prevalence typically decreases over time throughout childhood, for both medically untreated and treated children. In children with chronic constipation and encopresis who also have concurrent psychiatric or medical disorders (unrelated to the encopresis), the disorder appearing comorbidly with encopresis can be the primary determinant of prognosis. For example, a more protracted course of encopresis is associated with the presence of conduct disorder, the use of soiling as a direct expression of anger, and parental disinterest in dealing with the problem.

Diagnostic Evaluation

Initial medical evaluation is required to evaluate possible structural abnormalities (e.g., anal fissure) and may involve barium enema. Psychiatric evaluation includes assessment of comorbid psychopathology, which is found in 35% of the children with encopresis. Typical comorbidity with encopresis includes conduct disorder, oppositional defiant disorder, psychotic disorders, mood disorders, and mental retardation.

Treatment

Many cases can be treated in a pediatric model by decompaction and behavioral treatment, but resistant cases may require psychiatric intervention. Pediatric management of cases may include bowel cleansing (laxatives, enemas), daily maintenance on mineral oil and high-fiber diets, counseling (education, reducing interpersonal struggles and negative affects, and rewards), and follow-up. Planned toilet sitting times can be helpful because bowel habits can be very susceptible to changes in daily routine in children (Youssef and Di Lorenzo 2001). Psychiatric comorbidity is higher among children who do not respond to these measures (Buttross 1999).

Although various behavioral treatments have been studied, relatively few have been well controlled (Brooks et al. 2000); none of these interventions are well established (McGrath et al. 2000). Cisapride, a serotonin type 4 (5-HT$_4$) receptor agonist used to treat gastroesophageal reflux, increases gastric motility and has been found helpful in a controlled trial for treating chronic constipation in children (Nurko et al. 2000); however, its tendency to induce QT prolongation makes this an undesirable treatment in routine cases.

In pediatric practice, approximately 50%–75% of the cases improve during the initial months of treatment (Levine 1982). Only 7% of the children with pediatrically treated encopresis and chronic constipation were encopretic at 7-year follow-up, and those patients had significant behavioral symptoms. In contrast, children whose chronic constipation (without encopresis) was pediatrically treated usually become asymptomatic. At 7-year follow-up, 70% of such children had a complete resolution of symptoms, and 25% had mild constipation occasionally; only 5% required occasional laxatives (Sutphen et al. 1995). Thus, a small but significant fraction of children with encopresis remain encopretic despite extended medical treatment (Rockney et al. 1996).

In resistant cases of encopresis, or if aggressive pediatric treatment becomes counterproductive, individual and family psychiatric interventions are indicated. The focus of treatment then shifts from the encopresis to a more general treatment of associated psychopathological disorders.

Enuresis (Not Due to a General Medical Condition)

Urinary incontinence in young children, and in older children after the completion of toilet training on an occasional basis, is a normal developmental phenomenon. Enuresis (not due to a general medical condition) is diagnosed when medically unexplained urinary incontinence is frequent, distressing, or interfering with activities (Table 15–26). Urinary bladder control is typically attained by age 3 or 4; therefore, DSM-IV-TR diagnosis requires a minimal age of 5 years. Before these presentations are designated as psychiatric disorders, a medical assessment of physical causes of enuresis (such as bladder infection or seizures) is required.

TABLE 15–26. DSM-IV-TR diagnostic criteria for enuresis

A. Repeated voiding of urine into bed or clothes (whether involuntary or intentional).
B. The behavior is clinically significant as manifested by either a frequency of twice a week for at least 3 consecutive months or the presence of clinically significant distress or impairment in social, academic (occupational), or other important areas of functioning.
C. Chronological age is at least 5 years (or equivalent developmental level).
D. The behavior is not due exclusively to the direct physiological effect of a substance (e.g., a diuretic) or a general medical condition (e.g., diabetes, spina bifida, a seizure disorder).

Specify type:
  Nocturnal Only
  Diurnal Only
  Nocturnal and Diurnal

Clinical Description

Bed-wetting is more common than daytime urinary incontinence. In the large majority of school-aged children, nocturnal enuresis is monosymptomatic (Varan et al. 1996), that is, not accompanied by daytime wetting or other urological conditions. Bed-wetting typically occurs 30 minutes to 3 hours after sleep onset, with the child either sleeping through the episode or being awakened by the moisture; however, for some children, enuresis may occur at any time during the night. Children with daytime (diurnal) enuresis usually have nocturnal enuresis too. About 30% of the children with nocturnal enuresis also have enuresis during the daytime (Kalo and Bella 1996).

Epidemiology

Enuresis is common, but prevalence figures vary widely, depending partially on quantitative aspects of the definitional criteria. Nocturnal enuresis may occur occasionally in 25% of boys, but more problematic enuresis persists beyond age 5 in 7%–10% of boys and 3% of girls. The male predominance persists but decreases with age. At age 10 years, 3%–5% of boys and 2%–3% of girls are still diagnosable. In adulthood, general prevalence is 1%. A correlation with socioeconomic status has been suggested but not established.

Etiology

The mechanisms involved in developing and maintaining bladder control are not well described, and multiple etiologies are believed to produce enuresis. Three major mechanisms include 1) low nocturnal release of vasopressin, which may lead to increased urine volume, associated with a possible circadian abnormality; 2) bladder abnormalities, such as small functional volume and/or detrusor hyperactivity; and 3) inability to achieve adequate arousal during sleep to experience bladder fullness sensations. These different mechanisms are not necessarily independent.

Some children with nocturnal enuresis do not have a normal nighttime release of vasopressin (antidiuretic hormone) and so may not have the usual reduction in the formation of urine at night (Rittig et al. 1989). The low overnight plasma levels of vasopressin (from 11:00 P.M. to 4:00 A.M.) are associated with increased urination volume and decreased osmolality (Aikawa et al. 1999).

Nocturnal polyuria has become recognized as a major factor in the etiology of many cases of "functional" enuresis. In fact, nocturnal bed-wetting sometimes can be induced in healthy children with ingestion of a water load at bedtime. In these cases, the wetting is elicited by a threshold volume that is specific to each individual and bears no correlation to bladder filling rate (Kirk et al. 1996).

Enuresis also can be caused by urological (urinary tract infection, especially in secondary enuresis in girls, or obstruction), anatomical (spinal disease, weak bladder or supporting musculature), physiological (abnormally low bladder pressure threshold or detrusor hyperactivity, leading to early emptying), metabolic (diabetes), and neurological (seizure disorder) mechanisms.

Disorders of sleep or diurnal rhythm may be etiological in some cases of functional enuresis. Although the nocturnal vasopressin changes can be interpreted in terms of a failure in diurnal regulation, some cases of enuresis are hypothesized to involve a failure of the reticular activating system to produce an adequate level of arousal during sleep to regulate bladder control (Neveus et al. 2000).

Approximately 50% of the children with functional enuresis have emotional or behavioral symptoms, but it is unclear whether this result represents cause, effect, or an associated finding (e.g., poor parental limit setting).

Functional enuresis also may be related to stress, trauma, or psychosocial crisis, such as the birth of a sibling, start of school, a move, hospitalization, a loss, parental absence, car accident, or developmental crisis. In contrast to other types of enuresis, stress-induced cases are equally prevalent in boys and girls. However, the roles of environmental stress, family support, and socioeconomic status have been questioned (Fergusson et al. 1986).

Some forms of functional enuresis may run in families, particularly in males. Approximately 65%–70% of the children with this disorder have a first-degree relative with functional enuresis. The chances of a child having enuresis are 77% if both parents have history of enuresis and 44% if one parent has such a history (Bakwin 1973).

Course and Prognosis

Enuresis remits spontaneously at a rate of approximately 15% per year (Forsythe and Butler 1989). Approximately 1% of boys (and fewer girls) still have this condition at age 18 years, generally with little associated psychopathology. The adolescent-onset form of enuresis, however, appears to have more associated psychopathology and a less favorable outcome. In adults, the onset of nocturnal enuresis, without daytime symptoms, often signifies serious urological pathology (Sakamoto and Blaivas 2001).

Diagnostic Evaluation

An initial medical assessment is required to rule out the various nonfunctional forms of enuresis. With extensive urological evaluation, about 20% of youths with nocturnal enuresis are found to have a urological abnormality. In certain cases, a sleep evaluation may be useful, but an EEG is not routinely required. Measurement of certain maturational indexes may be useful for identifying simple developmental variance.

Psychiatric evaluation of the child and parents includes assessment of associated psychopathology, recent psychosocial stressors, family concern about the symptom, and previous management of the symptoms. Inquiry about possible enuresis in the siblings is appropriate in view of their threefold increased risk. The proposed specific association of enuresis and depressive disorders has not been consistently supported in well-designed studies, but a stronger link has been found with ADHD.

Treatment

Most cases of functional enuresis are treated by pediatricians, who strongly prefer behavioral to pharmacological interventions for enuresis (Skoog et al. 1997). Behavioral methods for treating nocturnal enuresis include restriction of prebedtime fluid intake, planned mid-sleep awakenings for voiding in toilet, and rewards for successful nights.

Since the 1930s, nocturnal enuresis has been commonly treated by a simple device: a moisture-sensitive blanket that, during an enuretic episode, sounds a bell that arouses the patient from sleep. The "bell and pad" method has a high success rate (80%–90%), but it also has a high relapse rate (up to 15%–40%). A lower relapse rate usually can be achieved if the bell is set up to awaken the parents, who themselves then awaken the child. If relapse occurs, reinitiation of the bell system is often effective (Forsythe and Butler 1989). There is sometimes considerable resistance to the consistent use of the alarm system by either parent or child. One recent innovation has been the use of a noninvasive ultrasound device that detects bladder size and gives feedback when bladder volume reaches a critical size (Pretlow 1999). Other behavioral methods are in widespread use, but they have

not been as systematically tested.

Desmopressin, an analogue of the antidiuretic hormone vasopressin, has been successful in several double-blind trials in treating nocturnal enuresis (Glazener and Evans 2000a) and is now popularly prescribed by family practitioners and pediatricians. Its efficacy in 50%–80% of cases (Bonde et al. 1994; Caione et al. 1997; Wille 1986) is not as high as that of bell alarms, and the extent of improvement appears more limited. Only 60%–65% of patients with primary nocturnal enuresis have a marked reduction in wet nights (Skoog et al. 1997; Uygur et al. 1997).

TCAs can be helpful if a patient does not respond well to behavioral interventions, if daytime and nighttime enuresis are present, or if mood or anxiety disorder is associated. TCAs have been shown to be effective in many double-blind studies (Glazener and Evans 2000b), typically in low dosages (e.g., imipramine 25–125 mg or about 2 mg/kg nightly; EEG monitoring is absolutely mandatory; a daily dosage of 5 mg/kg is not to be exceeded). Some reports have suggested that the success rate is only 15% after discontinuation of antidepressants, but the success rate is probably higher if the dosage is tapered gradually. In view of the high rate of remission with placebo, it is sensible to attempt to lower the medication dosage every 4–6 months. In view of the high lethality of TCAs in overdose (particularly desipramine) and the reported sudden deaths during desipramine treatment (see "Treatment" subsection in the "Attention-Deficit/Hyperactivity Disorder" section earlier in this chapter), treatment of enuresis with desipramine should be avoided. Imipramine is much safer and is effective in treating enuresis. Carbamazepine is also efficacious in treating nocturnal enuresis (Al-Waili 2000). Also, access to pill bottles at home should be carefully controlled to minimize risks of overdose, which might result from the child's attempt to make treatment work faster, a suicide attempt, or accidental ingestion by younger siblings.

The mechanism for the effect of TCAs on enuresis is unknown, but it is not the anticholinergic properties (anticholinergic agents are not effective); it may be related to the antidepressant property (MAOIs are also effective). Consistent with a catecholamine/alertness hypothesis, pseudoephedrine was reported to provide statistically significant improvement in primary nocturnal enuresis (Varan et al. 1996). Selective serotonin reuptake inhibitors have not been examined for antienuretic properties. In patients with nocturnal polyuria (without enuresis), imipramine may produce reductions in urine osmolality as well as volume, suggesting that imipramine may have an antidiuretic effect that is independent of its antienuretic effect (Hunsballe et al. 1997).

For daytime enuresis, oxybutynin has been reported to produce significant improvement in 54% of cases (Caione et al. 1997). Oxybutynin treats enuresis mainly by acting as a smooth muscle relaxant through its effect of blocking cholinergic receptors on the detrusor muscle. By diminishing bladder muscle contraction, oxybutynin increases bladder capacity, allows delay of the need to urinate, and thereby reduces the urgency and frequency of involuntary voiding (and voluntary urination). Oxybutynin may be used in combination with desmopressin or even with TCAs (Kaneko et al. 2001) but may be less useful in patients with normal bladder function (Kosar et al. 1999).

Other interventions usually are not necessary in most cases of functional enuresis, although the presence of secondary enuresis might suggest possible benefits from counseling. Psychotherapy may be useful for the uncommon case in which the symptom of enuresis is interpersonally cathected (e.g., into an oppositional struggle or into expression of rage) or for patients with significant comorbid psychopathology.

Other Disorders of Infancy, Childhood, or Adolescence

Separation Anxiety Disorder

In addition to normal situational and developmental anxiety, children can show genuine anxiety disorders. These pathological states are common but are frequently dismissed by parents, pediatricians, and psychiatrists as mere "anxiety." Children are commonly imagined to be innately fearful, and adolescence is seen as naturally anxiety provoking. Anxiety is viewed as so ordinary in children that often due consideration is not given to the possibility of an anxiety disorder.

Separation anxiety, a normal developmental phenomenon at age 18–30 months, has been traditionally described in terms of attachment and separation theory (see Chapter 1). A nonpathological form of separation anxiety is sometimes observed in adults or children who have been geographically displaced and are feeling homesick; examples include students, soldiers, immigrants, refugees, and hospitalized patients (Van Tilburg et al. 1996).

In separation anxiety disorder, cognitive, affective, somatic, and behavioral symptoms appear in response to genuine or fantasied separation from attachment figures (Table 15–27). Separation anxiety disorder can present clinically in a variety of ways, including difficulty in falling asleep (prebedtime agitation) and school absenteeism (Bernstein and Borchardt 1991).

Separation anxiety disorder is the only anxiety disorder listed in DSM-IV-TR as a disorder usually first diagnosed in infancy,

---

TABLE 15–27.   DSM-IV-TR diagnostic criteria for separation anxiety disorder

---

A. Developmentally inappropriate and excessive anxiety concerning separation from home or from those to whom the individual is attached, as evidenced by three (or more) of the following:
  (1) recurrent excessive distress when separation from home or major attachment figures occurs or is anticipated
  (2) persistent and excessive worry about losing, or about possible harm befalling, major attachment figures
  (3) persistent and excessive worry that an untoward event will lead to separation from a major attachment figure (e.g., getting lost or being kidnapped)
  (4) persistent reluctance or refusal to go to school or elsewhere because of fear of separation
  (5) persistently and excessively fearful or reluctant to be alone or without major attachment figures at home or without significant adults in other settings
  (6) persistent reluctance or refusal to go to sleep without being near a major attachment figure or to sleep away from home
  (7) repeated nightmares involving the theme of separation
  (8) repeated complaints of physical symptoms (such as headaches, stomachaches, nausea, or vomiting) when separation from major attachment figures occurs or is anticipated
B. The duration of the disturbance is at least 4 weeks.
C. The onset is before age 18 years.
D. The disturbance causes clinically significant distress or impairment in social, academic (occupational), or other important areas of functioning.
E. The disturbance does not occur exclusively during the course of a pervasive developmental disorder, schizophrenia, or other psychotic disorder and, in adolescents and adults, is not better accounted for by panic disorder with agoraphobia.
Specify if:
  Early Onset: if onset occurs before age 6 years

---

childhood, or adolescence. Like other anxiety disorders in children, separation anxiety disorder can lead to social problems, academic underachievement, and interference with developing assertiveness skills and personal autonomy, often resulting in social awkwardness (or "immaturity") and sometimes a reluctance to date. Unlike many child psychiatric disorders, the anxiety disorders often cause more distress to the children than to the parents (although the parents may themselves be quite anxious because of their own anxiety disorders).

Clinical Description

The usual focus of the anxiety is fear of separation from a major attachment object, typically a parent or caregiver, but it can be a favorite toy or familiar place. Generally, even a young child can specify the attachment object that gives a sense of protection or safety (from anxiety). Common presentations include preoccupying or morbid fear of parents' death, clinging to parents, school avoidance, sleep refusal, resistance to being alone, nightmares, anticipatory worrying, cognitive disruption, or somatization. Although the anxiety is usually centered around separation from a parent, the fear can instead manifest as an anticipatory fear of being injured, kidnapped, or killed. Interference with autonomous functioning can extend to inability to sleep in one's own bed, visit friends, go on errands, or stay at camp.

Homesickness, a manifestation of separation anxiety, appears to be a distinct phenomenon from separation anxiety dis-

TABLE 15–28. Comparison of children with separation anxiety disorder and children with school-related phobic disorders

	Children with separation anxiety disorder	Children with phobic disorders
Age at referral (mean)	9 years	14 years
Sex ratio (M:F)	1:2	2:1
Low socioeconomic class (Hollingshead IV or V)	32%	68%
Concurrent DSM-III disorder	92%	63%
Concurrent anxiety disorder	50%	53%
Concurrent mood disorder	33%	32%
Maternal anxiety disorder	83%	57%
Maternal mood disorder	63%	14%

Note. These children were referred to an outpatient psychiatric clinic and were diagnosed with separation anxiety disorder or a phobic disorder (simple or social) regarding school. Although concomitant mood and anxiety disorders are common in both disorders, the children and mothers showed more psychopathology associated with separation anxiety disorder than with phobic disorders.
Source. Data from Last et al. 1987.

order. Homesickness may be freely described by young children ("I want my mommy") but can be difficult to admit for adolescents, especially boys. In contrast, the symptoms of separation anxiety disorder are often quite evident and freely admitted to parents by children.

More than 92% of the children with separation anxiety disorder have other DSM-IV-TR disorders, typically anxiety or mood disorders (Table 15–28). Many children with major depressive disorder also fulfill criteria for separation anxiety disorder.

The prominence of somatization with separation anxiety is similar to that of panic, phobic, generalized anxiety, and depressive disorders of adulthood. Children with separation anxiety disorder commonly experience stomachaches and palpitations, and they generally have more somatic complaints than do children with any other psychiatric disorder (Livingston et al. 1988). Separation anxiety disorder has many characteristics of phobic disorders, which often appear comorbidly. Separation anxiety disorder differs from other

anxiety disorders in its focus on separation and its early appearance (usually first diagnosed in childhood). It differs from phobic disorders in that the latter may be directed toward myriad potential sources of fear.

School absenteeism is reported in about 75% of the children with separation anxiety disorder, and separation anxiety disorder is reported in up to 50%–80% of school absentees (Klein and Last 1989); however, these conditions are quite distinct. The terms *school phobia, school avoidance,* and *school refusal* are misnomers: most school "phobics" are not in fact phobic, and the terms *avoidance* and *refusal* imply psychological mechanisms that may not apply. A more descriptively neutral and accurate label is *school absenteeism,* a term that has the advantage of highlighting a possible connection with job absenteeism. School absenteeism has a variety of etiologies (Table 15–29). Not all children with school absenteeism have separation anxiety, and not all children with separation anxiety disorder have school absenteeism (Last et al. 1987).

TABLE 15–29. Causes of school absenteeism

Separation anxiety disorder
Truancy (often associated with conduct
  disorder)
Psychiatric disorders usually first diagnosed
  in adulthood
  Mood disorders
    Major depressive disorder
    Bipolar disorder
  Other anxiety disorders
    Overanxious disorder
    Phobic disorder
    Panic disorder
    Obsessive-compulsive disorder
    Posttraumatic stress disorder
  Overt psychotic disorders (rare)
Sociocultural conformity
  Permission granted by family (e.g., overt or
    covert support to stay at home to take care
    of siblings, to earn money, or to avoid
    tests)
  Normative peer behavior in certain locales
    (spending time with peers rather than
    going to school)
Realistic fear of bodily harm in dangerous
  school settings
Drug-induced depression (e.g., propranolol,
  haloperidol)

Epidemiology

Separation anxiety disorder is common and tends to run in families. Epidemiological studies report a prevalence of 2%–5% among children (B. Masi et al. 2001) and a decrease with age. The sex ratio is equal or female predominant (2:1). Unlike the case in other anxiety disorders, 50%–75% of the families of children with separation anxiety disorder are of low socioeconomic status (Last et al. 1992; Velez et al. 1989).

School absenteeism is common, with 75% of adults admitting to this behavior during childhood. At some inner-city schools, absenteeism may be observed in more than 90% of students.

Etiology

The relation of separation anxiety disorder and school absenteeism to mood and other anxiety disorders has been an area of active research. There remains some debate about whether separation anxiety disorder in children exists entirely independently of associated major depressive disorder or other anxiety disorders. The comorbidity and familial and developmental relationships are extremely involved. Biological markers suggest that separation anxiety disorder is related to both depressive and panic disorders.

Another proposed etiological factor for separation anxiety disorder is PTSD. Separation anxiety disorder was the most common comorbid diagnosis in the 50% of sexually and/or physically abused boys who developed PTSD (Dykman et al. 1997). Also, children living with parental violence are at increased risk for separation anxiety disorder (Pelcovitz et al. 2000). It is unclear whether the appearance of separation anxiety disorder in this group is a result of traumatic abuse, PTSD, psychological grief, or concurrent depressive disorders or whether it is a marker for family chaos and abuse.

Course and Prognosis

Separation anxiety disorder may be diagnosed after the normative period of separation anxiety, but it is typically not observed before age 4 years. It is usually first recognized in early or mid childhood. Separation anxiety disorder is typically a chronic disorder, but exacerbations may occur at times of actual separations, deaths, illness, family moves, or natural disasters. Symptoms might be aggravated during episodes of comorbid psychiatric disorders. Symptoms also may worsen during or after medical illness, particularly chronic medical conditions with acute exacerbations. Multiple medical examinations are commonly sought by the child or parents.

School absentees often show academic underachievement and social avoidance, and they can be at risk for chronic unemployment in adulthood. Just as they have difficulty getting to school, they have difficulty getting to their jobs.

Long-term follow-up studies have suggested an increased risk for the development of other anxiety disorders, especially panic disorder with agoraphobia, and possibly depressive disorder (Klein and Last 1989). A follow-up study of children with separation anxiety disorder (who also had a communication disorder) found that 44% no longer had an anxiety disorder after 4 years; however, 11% still had separation anxiety disorder, and 33% had a different diagnosis, typically another anxiety disorder (Cantwell and Baker 1989). Also, separation anxiety disorder in childhood appears associated with early-onset panic disorder (Battaglia et al. 1995) but not in all studies (Hayward et al. 2000). Adults with panic disorder, especially those with agoraphobia, reported childhood symptoms of separation anxiety disorder even more often than did adults with generalized anxiety disorder or phobic disorder (Silove et al. 1995).

The majority (68%) of children of adults with agoraphobia were found to have diagnosable psychiatric disorders, especially anxiety disorders in general and separation anxiety disorder in particular (Capps et al. 1996). One-half of the children of parents with social phobia were found to have an anxiety disorder, and 19% of the total had separation anxiety disorder (Mancini et al. 1996).

A much simpler connection between childhood and adult anxiety disorders has more recently been examined. Perhaps because of the prominence of panic and other anxiety disorders in adults, the pres-ence of separation anxiety disorder in adults has been relatively underdiagnosed, and the developmental connection between childhood and adult separation anxiety disorder has not been emphasized. The symptoms appeared to persist from childhood, typically preceding the appearance of other anxiety disorders, and severity of childhood symptoms accounted for 33% of the variance in separation anxiety scores in adulthood (Manicavasagar et al. 2000).

Diagnostic Evaluation

The workup includes assessment of possible mood disorder or anxiety (simple or social phobia, panic) disorder. These disorders, as well as separation anxiety disorder, also should be evaluated in the parents.

Clinically, it is sometimes difficult to distinguish the presenting symptoms of separation anxiety disorder from ordinary acute anxiety. Both conditions can involve distractibility, distorted cognition, depersonalization, transient impairment in reality sense, motoric overactivity, and angry outbursts. However, the presence of separation anxiety disorder implies that separation-related psychodynamics are the primary trigger of the acute anxiety.

Treatment

The traditional treatment of separation anxiety disorder entails psychosocial interventions (individual psychotherapy combined with family therapy or parental guidance), often with antianxiety or antidepressant medication.

Antidepressants are commonly used for treating separation anxiety disorder. Fluoxetine has been reported in uncontrolled case series to be useful for treating separation anxiety disorder (Birmaher et al. 1994; Fairbanks et al. 1997; Manassis and Bradley 1994). In a controlled study, fluvoxamine was effective for children with anxiety disorders such as separation anxiety disorder (Research Unit on Pediatric Psychopharmacology Anxiety Study Group 2001). Although useful for treating social phobia, selective serotonin reuptake inhibitors have not been rigorously examined for treating separation anxiety per se or for treating school absenteeism. TCAs have been studied mainly in children with school absenteeism and separation anxiety disorder, and a substantial literature questions their usefulness for this indication (Klein et al. 1992). Newer antidepressants, such as bupropion or venlafaxine, have not been systematically examined.

Antidepressant treatments may be considered for children whose school absenteeism exceeds 2 weeks and is not explained by a medical problem, truancy, overt psychosis, sociocultural conformity, or realistic fear of physical danger. An open-label study of fluoxetine reported clinical improvement in all 10 children and adolescents with separation anxiety disorder and 8 of 10 youths with social phobia but only 1 of 7 with generalized anxiety disorder (Fairbanks et al. 1997). Antidepressants are probably effective in the many cases of school absenteeism in which the underlying etiology is separation anxiety disorder, mood disorder, phobic disorder, or panic disorder. However, the value of these treatments remains in question because the available studies are small; no large-scale investigations of antidepressants for treating either separation anxiety disorder or school absenteeism have been conducted.

Benzodiazepines (mainly alprazolam and clonazepam) and buspirone also have been used for children and parents with separation anxiety disorder, although with mixed success (Bernstein et al. 1990; Graae et al. 1994; Kranzler 1988; Simeon

et al. 1992). Clinically, these agents appear to be helpful for the "anticipatory" anxiety that can develop secondarily around "primary" anxiety symptoms, but adequate studies are needed.

If a parent has an anxiety or a mood disorder causing difficulty in separating from the child, the parent should receive direct psychiatric treatment as well as behavioral guidance for parenting. Antidepressant treatment of mood or anxiety disorders in a parent is commonly a part of the treatment of separation anxiety disorder in a child.

Cognitive-behavioral therapy and family management appear to be useful in controlled studies for treating separation anxiety disorder (P.M. Barrett 1998; P.M. Barrett et al. 1996; Kendall 1994; Kendall et al. 2001; Muris et al. 2001; Southam-Gerow et al. 2001) and school absenteeism (N.J. King et al. 1998). Goals of cognitive-behavioral treatment may include positive self-instruction and self-talk, cognitive restructuring, emotive imagery, graded exposure and desensitization, reduction in social anxiety, social problem solving, social skills training, and increasing levels of social participation. Parent involvement is also useful (Mendelowitz et al. 1999) to reinforce the child's successes, promote the child's social participation, and model appropriate behaviors. Forced school attendance appears to be highly effective for cases of school "refusal" (Blagg and Yule 1984), but it may be judged inappropriate in individual cases (e.g., panic disorder).

Psychodynamic aspects of individual and family psychotherapies have more regularly appearing characteristics for this disorder than for most childhood disorders. For children with separation anxiety disorder, the child's experience of psychotherapy is organized around the actual "separations within the therapy." It is advisable to pay special attention to planned and unplanned absences (vacations by the patient or therapist, school transitions, therapist or teacher pregnancy, parental unavailability, therapist illness, deaths) and to the termination of treatment. It is often useful to give the child a concrete object or souvenir, or a clearly verbalized image of the therapist's future activity, at the time of interruption or termination. Preventive verbal anticipation, preparation of the parents (who may also have separation anxiety) as well as the child, and active discussion of the practicalities surrounding expected separations are useful in the management of these cases.

A common pitfall in the treatment of separation anxiety disorder is an overemphasis by the parents and professionals on the presenting symptoms (e.g., poor school attendance) rather than on the child's broader problems and long-term development. A child's ability to attend school consistently or to manage anxiety quietly signifies behavioral improvement, but the child may be left with psychodevelopmental liabilities. It is essential to maintain a wide perspective on the psychopathology and the risk for adult impairment to prevent premature closure of therapeutic work.

Another pitfall in the treatment of this disorder in children and parents involves pathological compliance. Some parents and children have an overly "good" or "nice" presentation of self, and their perfectionistic manner of managing themselves can prevent them from exposing their deeper thoughts and feelings. "Pathological pleasantness" in a child or parents needs to be monitored during the course of treatment and not mistaken for substantial understanding, support, or change.

Limit setting in the treatment of separation anxiety disorder can be useful or disruptive. If the child has a panic disorder or major depressive episode, limit setting can be counterproductive and aggra-

vate the symptoms. Forcing a child with panic disorder to attend school can result in a temper tantrum or physical assault. However, "therapeutic coercion," sensitively applied, can be helpful in some cases of true separation anxiety disorder, particularly if the intervention is appropriately timed after drug treatment. For treating truancy (a far more common cause of school absenteeism), limit setting is certainly a useful and often necessary measure for establishing a routine daily structure in the child's life.

Selective Mutism

Children with selective mutism do not use speech in specific settings and show abnormalities of interpersonal behavior and social assertiveness. This uncommon disorder was initially described more than 100 years ago, but the medical literature on selective mutism consisted mainly of individual case reports until quite recently. The paucity of large-scale controlled studies impeded the accumulation of systematic and statistical descriptions, which are only now becoming available. This disorder, formerly viewed in almost exclusively psychodynamic terms, is now reconceptualized in view of findings of the prominent role of anxiety disorders and developmental delays.

Clinical Description

In selective mutism, children do not speak in one or several of the major environments in which they live. Even though they can talk without difficulty in certain places (usually at home), partial or total muteness appears selectively in unfamiliar places or particular social situations (Table 15–30). Typically, speech is normal at home when the child is alone with parents and siblings, and communication is constricted in the presence of teachers, peers, and strangers. When separated from a familiar or comfortable environment, these children might freely or hesitantly use gestural speech, nods, monosyllabic responses, written notes, or whispers, but they avoid full vocalization and verbal speech.

Although many children with selective mutism have normal language capabilities, developmental disorders or delays appear to be present in most of these children (Kristensen 2000). Approximately one-third of these children have a language disorder, and about one-half have a speech disorder or delayed speech development (Kolvin and Fundudis 1981). In addition, children with selective mutism have an increased prevalence of neurological disorders and mental retardation. The traditional assumption that children with selective mutism have normal speech, language, and biological development is not true in most cases.

TABLE 15–30. DSM-IV-TR diagnostic criteria for selective mutism

A. Consistent failure to speak in specific social situations (in which there is an expectation for speaking, e.g., at school) despite speaking in other situations.

B. The disturbance interferes with educational or occupational achievement or with social communication.

C. The duration of the disturbance is at least 1 month (not limited to the first month of school).

D. The failure to speak is not due to a lack of knowledge of, or comfort with, the spoken language required in the social situation.

E. The disturbance is not better accounted for by a communication disorder (e.g., stuttering) and does not occur exclusively during the course of a pervasive developmental disorder, schizophrenia, or other psychotic disorder.

Anxiety disorders are highly prevalent among these children (Kristensen 2000). Many children with selective mutism have school absenteeism, problems with separation, anxiety, and obsessive-compulsive features. Most children had behavioral abnormalities that were observed before age 6 years.

Usually, widespread impairments of social behavior and, sometimes, behavioral control are seen. Many of these children show early and persistent shyness, submissiveness, excessive dependency, timidity in activities involving personal assertiveness, clinging to parents, sulky behavior with strangers, temper tantrums, and regressive behaviors. At times, these children may show streaks of oppositionality, demanding and controlling behavior, passive-aggressiveness, and defiance.

Epidemiology

An estimated prevalence of 180 per 100,000 children has recently been reported (Kopp and Gillberg 1997), indicating a higher prevalence than generally was reported in the past (when more stringent definitional criteria were used). Teachers describe up to 2% prevalence of mute behavior in class (Kumpulainen et al. 1998). There is a slight female predominance, with a sex ratio of 1:1–1:2. An increased prevalence of selective mutism in children from immigrant families is also reported.

Etiology

Although traditional views of the etiology of selective mutism have been predominantly psychodynamic in nature, more recent findings suggest a variety of biological factors. The association of selective mutism with a history of early-onset shyness or a family history of shyness is consistent with a psychodynamic model, but it is also consistent with a constitutional or temperamental contribution to childhood shyness, anxiety disorders, or mood disorders.

In addition to the well-established association of selective mutism with anxiety disorders, comorbidity studies have indicated that most children with selective mutism also have a developmental disorder or delay (Kristensen 2000). The association of selective mutism with communication disorders, mental retardation, pervasive developmental disorder, and neurological disorder suggests a neuro-developmental etiological factor. These conditions can potentially aggravate the speech of a child with selective mutism. Interestingly, more than 30% of the children with selective mutism also have a comorbid elimination disorder (Kristensen 2000). The co-occurrence of an anxiety disorder and a developmental disorder or delay was reported in 46% of the children with selective mutism and 1% of the control subjects (Kristensen 2000).

A posttraumatic etiology is supported by the data suggesting a high prevalence of physical and sexual abuse, parental violence, and early mouth trauma. An etiology related to separation anxiety is consistent with some overt behavioral symptoms, as well as strong maternal ties, family history of mood disorder, and history of loss (e.g., through geographic move or sociopolitical change). In family studies, relatives of children with selective mutism are found to be taciturn and also to have an elevated prevalence of speech and language disorders (Steinhausen and Adamek 1997).

Course and Prognosis

Selective mutism typically starts at ages 3–5, when developmentally normal children may still show brief periods of mutism on meeting strangers or in new settings. Although the gradual emergence of early "shyness" may be identified retro-

spectively (Kolvin and Fundudis 1981), selective mutism is typically diagnosed at ages 5–8, when symptoms become obvious at school. If school attendance is adequate and social behavior is compliant, recognition and referral for treatment may be delayed or avoided.

Symptoms may last for several weeks, months, or years. Some children improve without therapy. About 50% of children are no longer selectively mute by age 10, but the prognosis appears less encouraging if speech behaviors do not improve by then (Kolvin and Fundudis 1981).

The long-term outcome is not known. The abnormal social behavior, interpersonal manipulations, shyness, and aggressivity appear to persist beyond the period of symptomatic muteness. Further information about the natural course of illness may be derived from studies on comorbidity. Selective mutism may be related to mood, separation anxiety, and phobic disorders. The finding that 97% of the children with selective mutism fulfill criteria for social phobia has led to the proposal that selective mutism may be a symptom or form of social phobia (Black and Uhde 1992).

Diagnostic Evaluation

A full psychiatric evaluation of the child and parents is warranted, with special attention to mood and anxiety disorders (Anstendig 1999). Neurological assessment is helpful to consider possible brain damage, mental retardation, pervasive developmental disorder, expressive language disorder, receptive aphasia, and deafness. Speech and language evaluation is needed, including examination of familial patterns of communication, silence, and anger. The child and family should be assessed for physical and sexual abuse, antisocial behavior, shyness, psychosocial deprivation, and mental retardation. At times, a home visit is helpful to evaluate the communication environment; in some cases, it may be essential to evaluate the child's speech because home may be the only place where the child is willing to talk (Cleator and Hand 2001). Differential diagnosis includes anxiety disorders such as social phobia, disuse of speech in schizophrenia (alogia) or schizotypal personality, deafness, aphasia, and hysteria.

Treatment

Selective mutism was notoriously difficult to treat until serotonin reuptake inhibitors were shown to produce substantial improvement in both mutism and global functioning of these children, as rated by parents (Black and Uhde 1994; J.S. Carlson et al. 1999). This finding was particularly striking in view of the inability of TCAs to treat this condition. However, most fluoxetine-treated children were still quite symptomatic after 12 weeks of treatment (Black and Uhde 1994), and the therapeutic effect appeared to decrease with increasing age (Dummit et al. 1996); therefore, the use of other methods is necessary. Anxiolytics or atypical neuroleptics might be helpful as adjuvants, and MAOIs might be considered in treatment-resistant cases (Golwyn and Sevlie 1999).

After pharmacotherapy, behavior therapy appears to have the next best outcome (Krohn et al. 1992; Labbe and Williamson 1984). Contingency management, positive reinforcement, desensitization, and assertiveness training generally have been used. At present, behavior therapy probably should be used in combination with a selective serotonin reuptake inhibitor. Speech and language therapy are often indicated for children with selective mutism, especially in view of their communication disorders and neurodevelopmental problems.

Parent counseling can be effective. Parents and teachers often make accom-

modations to the child's muteness; however, it is generally useful to maintain a clear expectation that the child talk and communicate, at least for a structured period each day at home, at each school period, and at each treatment session. It is important for the parents to be explicit with the child about the expectation of talking at school and in therapy. Most parents and teachers need to be supported and repeatedly reminded to refrain from reinforcing the child's passivity or contributing to the secondary gain.

Reactive Attachment Disorder of Infancy or Early Childhood

Following exposure to severe and prolonged neglect or physical or emotional abuse, infants and young children may show a variety of disturbances in interpersonal relatedness, social behavior, emotional reactivity and excitabilty, and cognition. Such disturbances are inferred to arise from disordered development of early interpersonal attachment (Table 15–31). Reactive attachment disorder encompasses both increased and decreased social interactiveness after trauma in infancy or early childhood.

The grossly pathological care that may lead to this posttraumatic syndrome includes physical or sexual abuse, neglect, the absence of stable attachment figures (such as in some institutional or foster care settings), the failure of an emotionally disturbed caregiver to read or respond to a child's emotional or physical needs, or the failure of caregivers to become attached to the child (Tibbits-Kleber and Howell 1985). According to DSM-IV-TR, any failure of normal development may be labeled as reactive attachment disorder if preceded by gross failures in child care.

The hallmark of reactive attachment disorder is the appearance of profoundly disturbed interpersonal relationships fol-

---

TABLE 15–31.   DSM-IV-TR diagnostic criteria for reactive attachment disorder of infancy or early childhood

---

A. Markedly disturbed and developmentally inappropriate social relatedness in most contexts, beginning before age 5 years, as evidenced by either (1) or (2):

   (1) persistent failure to initiate or respond in a developmentally appropriate fashion to most social interactions, as manifest by excessively inhibited, hypervigilant, or highly ambivalent and contradictory responses (e.g., the child may respond to caregivers with a mixture of approach, avoidance, and resistance to comforting, or may exhibit frozen watchfulness)

   (2) diffuse attachments as manifest by indiscriminate sociability with marked inability to exhibit appropriate selective attachments (e.g., excessive familiarity with relative strangers or lack of selectivity in choice of attachment figures)

B. The disturbance in Criterion A is not accounted for solely by developmental delay (as in mental retardation) and does not meet criteria for a pervasive developmental disorder.

C. Pathogenic care as evidenced by at least one of the following:

   (1) persistent disregard of the child's basic emotional needs for comfort, stimulation, and affection

   (2) persistent disregard of the child's basic physical needs

   (3) repeated changes of primary caregiver that prevent formation of stable attachments (e.g., frequent changes in foster care)

D. There is a presumption that the care in Criterion C is responsible for the disturbed behavior in Criterion A (e.g., the disturbances in Criterion A began following the pathogenic care in Criterion C).

Specify type:

   Inhibited Type: if Criterion A1 predominates in the clinical presentation

   Disinhibited Type: if Criterion A2 predominates in the clinical presentation

---

lowing grossly inadequate early care in childhood (with or without evidence of their linkage). The pediatric label of nonorganic failure to thrive is a broader diagnostic category that encompasses 1) cases of reactive attachment disorder that involve physical growth retardation, 2) the DSM-IV-TR category of feeding and eating disorders of infancy or early childhood, and 3) some cases of retarded physical growth without prominent social abnormalities.

Clinical Description

In attachment disorders, a variety of behavioral, cognitive, and affective presentations may be seen at different ages. In children, odd social responsiveness, weak interpersonal attachment, apathy or inappropriate excitability, and mood abnormalities are common. In early infancy, diagnosis is based on the failure to achieve developmentally expected milestones: lack of eye tracking or responsive smiling by age 2 months and failure to play simple games or to reach out to be picked up by 5 months.

Children with reactive attachment disorder may present with inhibited or disinhibited subtypes, which are recognized by DSM-IV-TR. *Inhibited* infants with reactive attachment disorder may appear lethargic or show little activity. Their body movements are weak. Sleep is excessive and disrupted, and weight gain is slow. They may seem spacey and unengaged or, alternatively, hypervigilant and avoidant. The infants have little interactive interest in the environment and often resist being held. As young children, individuals with reactive attachment disorder may appear withdrawn, passive, or disinterested in people, or they may respond to interpersonal stimuli in odd or inconsistent ways. Children who have the inhibited subtype of reactive attachment disorder seem to have closed down on incoming stimulation, interpersonal and otherwise, as if their general responsiveness were diminished and their reactivity were inhibited.

Children with the *disinhibited* form of reactive attachment disorder may exhibit overly rapid familiarity. They may show inappropriate touching or clinging, excessive interest, and a sort of unmodulated "enthusiasm" with people, even in a first-time meeting. They readily switch their intense "attachment" from one person to another, behaving as though people are interchangeable parts ("indiscriminate sociability") and repetitively reenacting a few rigid "scripts" in their interactions ("I love you. Take me home"). The behavior of these children appears to convey the message "I wish you would take care of me forever." Their immediate emotional involvement may seem initially gratifying to a stranger, but it is also experienced as weird or unusual.

Epidemiology

Adequate epidemiological data are unavailable. The prevalence of reactive attachment disorder is estimated at about 1% (Zeanah and Embe 1995), largely on the basis of approximately 1%–5% of pediatric hospital admissions that are due to nonorganic failure to thrive. There is a much higher prevalence in certain groups of children—for example, orphans raised in overcrowded institutions in countries ravaged by social chaos or war.

Etiology

The etiology of reactive attachment disorder is written into its DSM-IV-TR definition. Previous abuse, neglect, or grossly impaired caregiving is definitionally required, and the disease label suggests that a disruption of caregiver–child bonding is the crucial mechanism. Although it emphasizes the interpersonal or social effects on the child, the definition implies that the parenting is the cause of the child's problem.

Children who are adopted from institutional care are at increased risk for reactive attachment disorder. Although the large majority of children adopted from such facilities do not have behavior problems, it appears that both earlier age and longer duration of deprivation can increase the risk of subsequent insecure attachment, socialization disturbances, impulsive and disruptive behaviors, and autistic-like changes (L. Fisher et al. 1997; Rutter et al. 1999).

The foster care system is another source of children with reactive attachment disorder. Entry into the foster care system begins with a disruption of the primary attachment relationships, and the system itself often contributes to the problem by supplying a sequence of multiple caregivers with multiple relationship disruptions. Thus, the system designed to manage the problem is, at times, another factor contributing to the maintenance of this psychopathology.

Course and Prognosis

If this disorder is untreated, the course may vary from spontaneous remission to malnutrition, infection, or death. Both nutritional and psychosocial deprivation may result in long-term behavioral changes, hyperactivity, short stature, and lowered IQ. If emotional deprivation continues but enforced feeding is provided, children may show improved weight gain. However, even when body growth is preserved, ongoing emotional deprivation can cause depressive-type changes and developmental delays in infants.

For those children with the disinhibited type of reactive attachment disorder, the feature of indiscriminate sociability may persist in these children, even after subsequent environmental improvement and return to developmental trajectories have been achieved. Adopting parents are not generally concerned about this behavior, suggesting that it is accepted as a personality trait rather than viewed as maladaptive psychopathology.

Diagnostic Evaluation

A diagnosis of reactive attachment disorder should be considered whenever a child shows socially unusual behavior, including disruptive behavior (such as conduct disorder or oppositional defiant disorder). Early history and sociability factors might, in some cases, be submerged under a complex history of behavior problems.

In infants and younger children, professional observation of mother–child interactions in the medical setting and at home might be required. A home visit is central to evaluation and diagnosis. Psychiatric evaluation of the parents is essential. When possible, siblings should be assessed regarding their psychosocial experiences, social functioning, and possible psychiatric disorders. Medical assessment of the child is required to rule out chronic physical illness (organic failure to thrive), homeostatic sleep and feeding disorders, food refusal, malnutrition, neurological disease, and sensory deficit.

The diagnosis is essentially confirmed by the child's symptomatic improvement following the provision of adequate care. The evaluation of the child's response can be most readily conducted in a hospital, which permits direct evaluation of the child and the parent–child interactions. Hospitalization also allows a multidisciplinary team to make the observations necessary for diagnosis. An alternative to hospitalization is a planned parent–child separation, which involves removal of the child to a different environment in which the caregiver can provide care and make observations.

Although home visits can contribute to the evaluation of any psychiatric patient (including adults), reactive attachment disorder is the only psychiatric disorder for which a home visit is virtually required. In practice, however, parents may be reluctant to allow even one home visit. Parents may be defensive, angry, and ashamed concerning the professional's interest in home visits.

Treatment

Basic medical care, provision of adequate caregiving, parental education, and parental psychiatric treatment are generally needed to treat reactive attachment disorder of infancy or early childhood. Medical hospitalization, which is useful in evaluation, is generally justified for performing this massive intervention.

The use of hospitalization is much preferable to parent–child separation for infants or very young children, but it can be useful for children at any age. Both removal from the home environment and hospitalization permit the establishment of normal feeding and physiological patterns as well as the opportunity for evaluating and expanding the parents' caregiving capacities.

Given the complexity of medical and psychiatric problems, the need for proficiency in baby care and nurturance, the required sensitivity in managing the parents, and the frequent need for social services and legal procedures, it is a major advantage for treatment to be delivered by a specialized team working in a hospital. This multidisciplinary team typically provides care on a pediatric inpatient unit and in an outpatient clinic, with a determined emphasis on coordination and continuity.

Hospitalization or treatment intervention typically leads to a major improvement in the clinical status of the child. This improvement in response to treatment is considered confirmation of the diagnosis of reactive attachment disorder. Clinical nonresponsiveness implies the presence of a different disorder, an additional disorder, or persistent physical damage resulting from extreme medical complications that occurred before treatment was begun.

Stereotypic Movement Disorder

Certain repetitive and purposeless motor behaviors may be seen in young children, sensory-deprived (deaf or blind) people, or individuals with mental retardation, pervasive developmental disorders, and some psychotic disorders (e.g., schizophrenia, mood disorders with psychomotor changes). Many stereotypies appear to have a self-stimulatory component, but the diagnosis of stereotypic movement disorder is made only if these repetitive behaviors cause functional interference or physical injury (Table 15–32). SIB is a common and clinically important form of stereotypic behavior.

Clinical Description

Examples of stereotypies include head banging, body rocking, hand flapping, whirling, stereotyped laughter, thumb sucking, hair fingering, facial touching, eye poking, object biting, self-biting, self-scratching, self-hitting, teeth grinding, and breath holding. Although one behavioral stereotypy may predominate, it is typical for several stereotypies to co-occur. Different stereotypies may become prominent at different times. The rhythm of the repetitive behavior may be slow and gentle, fast and energetic, or even violently energized. Sometimes waves of increasing and decreasing energy may be seen over the course of several minutes.

TABLE 15–32. DSM-IV-TR diagnostic criteria for stereotypic movement disorder

A. Repetitive, seemingly driven, and nonfunctional motor behavior (e.g., hand shaking or waving, body rocking, head banging, mouthing of objects, self-biting, hitting own body).
B. The behavior markedly interferes with normal activities or results in self-inflicted bodily injury that requires medical treatment (or would result in an injury if preventive measures were not used).
C. If mental retardation is present, the stereotypic or self-injurious behavior is of sufficient severity to become a focus of treatment.
D. The behavior is not better accounted for by a compulsion (as in obsessive-compulsive disorder), a tic (as in tic disorder), a stereotypy that is part of a pervasive developmental disorder, or hair pulling (as in trichotillomania).
E. The behavior is not due to the direct physiological effects of a substance or a general medical condition.
F. The behavior persists for 4 weeks or longer.
Specify if:
  With Self-Injurious Behavior: if the behavior results in bodily damage that requires specific treatment (or that would result in bodily damage if protective measures were not used)

Frequency may increase during periods of tension, frustration, boredom, and isolation, as well as just before bedtime.

Two of the most common presentations are head banging and body rocking. Head banging may last for hours, particularly at bedtime or on morning awakening. The head banging can be soft and quiet, occurring during periods of isolation or boredom, and appear to have a self-stimulatory and pleasurable quality. Alternatively, head banging may occur during a clearly unpleasurable state. During a temper tantrum, a child may thrash on the floor, with limbs flailing and head banging vigorously against the floor or wall.

Body rocking may be slow swaying, with quiet murmuring or singing, or it may be violent enough to move a child's bed across the room. Whether pleasurable or unpleasurable, there is typically a self-absorbed quality of mentation.

Epidemiology

Approximately 15%–20% of a normal pediatric population may have a history of transient stereotypies, but no data are available regarding the prevalence of stereotypic movement disorder with physical injury or functional interference in the general population. Stereotypic behaviors appear to show equal sex prevalence. There are no data regarding socioeconomic influences. The prevalence is higher in individuals with mental retardation. Among institutionalized people with severe and profound mental retardation, about 60% have stereotypic movement disorder, and 15% engage in SIBs (Schroeder et al. 1979).

Etiology

Stereotypic movement disorder has no clear etiology, but several theories have been advanced, and multiple contributing or interacting factors are probably involved.

Organic influences are supported by the increased incidence of stereotypic movement disorder in individuals with abnormal brain structure or function, such as mental retardation, auditory or visual sensory deficit (blindness, deafness), brain disease (seizures, postinfection, metabolic abnormality), psychotic disorder, and drug-induced psychosis (amphetamines). A presumed final common pathway might involve disruption of the balance among elements of basal ganglia

motor circuitry (Canales and Graybiel 2000). Neurochemical mechanisms involving serotonin (regarding impulse control) and opioids (controlling pain) have been proposed (Villalba and Harrington 2000), and purinergic systems (regulating aggression) also have been suggested (Lara et al. 2000).

An etiological role of self-stimulation (or autoerotic stimulation) is suggested by the characteristic self-absorbed and apparently pleasurable appearance and by the occurrence of this behavior during periods of boredom or physical isolation. Self-stimulation through repetitive physical activity may be satisfying if normal forms of stimulation are unavailable or ineffective.

Although stereotypic movement disorder is overrepresented among individuals with a history of neglect, understimulation, and mental retardation, these behaviors can be seen in patients with normal intelligence and normal caregiving experiences. Body rocking, for example, has been observed in 3%–25% of college students, although the movements appear to be more associated with situational factors and smaller in physical amplitude than similar stereotypies seen in people with mental retardation (Berkson et al. 1999). Thumb sucking and body rocking in persons of normal intelligence appear to be associated with a lifetime diagnosis of mood or anxiety disorders (Castellanos et al. 1997) and with obsessive-compulsive, perfectionistic, or impulsive-aggressive traits (Niehaus et al. 2000; Wilhelm et al. 1999).

Course and Prognosis

Certain stereotypies, such as head banging and body rocking, begin as early as 6–12 months. These behaviors typically resolve in 80% of children without mental disorders by age 4 years, although more subtle habits may persist, such as finger tapping or teeth grinding (DeLissovoy 1962). In people with mental retardation or pervasive developmental disorders, such early-onset stereotypies may persist for years. Later-onset stereotypies may be descriptively similar, but they appear episodically and only during periods of anxiety or stress.

Diagnostic Evaluation

When the disorder begins during infancy or in very early childhood, evaluation for concurrent mental retardation and other developmental disabilities is appropriate. For disorders with later onset, it is necessary to evaluate for agitation or anxiety associated with psychosis or mood disorders as well as for mental retardation and pervasive developmental disorders. In some cases, the use of psychostimulant medications and other dopamine agonists may aggravate or produce stereotypic behaviors; therefore, evaluation of current medication use is appropriate.

Stereotypic movement disorder is not diagnosed if the symptoms can be explained by concomitant tic disorder or OCD. Stereotypies may be distinguished from tics or compulsions when they have a self-stimulatory or pleasurable component. Although tics or compulsions may carry a tension-discharging function, they are not experienced as pleasurable.

Treatment

The symptoms of stereotypic movement disorder are often treatment resistant. Behavioral techniques, especially overcorrection, have been found most effective. Interventions involving anxiety reduction, sensory stimulation, and the offering of alternatives to self-stimulation are also helpful.

Although behavioral methods usually rely on reward systems when possible, positive reinforcement in treating stereotypic movement disorder is generally not effective when used alone. Overcorrec-

tion has the best empirical support, but it is a coercive treatment that may invoke anger, oppositionalism, and symptom substitution.

Blocking pleasurable feedback from self-stimulation can be useful. The particular technique depends on the sensory mode of predominant self-stimulation. For self-stimulation based on sound, white noise or tape-recorded music may be considered. For rocking, a vibrator taped to the hand may distract from other kinesthetic self-stimulation. For finger waving, beads on a string may provide alternative proprioceptive stimulation. For visual stimulation, ambient lighting may be altered or a bubble-blower may be provided. Such distraction from self-stimulation and use of stimuli substitution can be helpful in some individuals (Baroff 1986).

Pharmacological treatment has been extensively explored, but no single approach has emerged as consistently helpful. Case reports suggest that serotonin reuptake inhibitors, atypical antipsychotics, and the opiate blocker naltrexone have some value in certain patients with mental retardation (C. Turner et al. 1999).

When stereotypies originate from a psychotic disorder, increased attention may be unhelpful or counterproductive. Treatment with antipsychotic or other sedative medications may be needed.

Some clinicians use simple and practical management techniques, such as directing a child to bang his or her head on a soft surface, combined with interventions for stress reduction. Controlled studies of most treatments of stereotypic movement disorder are lacking.

Complexity and the Capacity for Change

Rarely can a child psychiatric disorder be viewed as a single or simple disturbance.

Although each DSM-IV-TR disorder has been discussed here in isolation, multiple concurrent diagnoses are typical in children and adolescents. Moreover, early-onset psychiatric disorders typically induce developmental complications that manifest across multiple domains of functioning, producing cumulative and enduring impairments in adaptation. These disorders and their multiply interacting complications tend to organize and snowball into final common pathways of child psychopathology, including academic impairment (declining school grades, progressive learning delays, school failure, dropout), compromised peer and family relationships (aggressive behavior, isolation, ostracism, retaliation), damaged self-concept (disturbed self-esteem, disordered social assertiveness, identity diffusion), demoralization, societal marginalization or criminal outcome, and chronic dissatisfaction and underachievement.

Even more than in adult psychiatry, the developmental complications of child psychiatric illness make it difficult to place a precise definitional boundary around the core features of a psychiatric disorder in a child. The delineation of a child psychiatric disorder—whose core features can be distinguished from its developmental complications and comorbidity—is a task that is best approached in successive approximations. DSM-IV-TR provides a snapshot in the progressive elaboration and scientific clarification of psychopathology in youth.

Instilling Hope

Even in children with genetically severe psychiatric disorders or extreme psychosocial circumstances, a supportive set of environmental modifiers (including pharmacotherapy and psychosocial treatment) may be the dominant influence on long-term outcome. Children and parents find it difficult to believe that many pathogenic forces and problematic symptoms in a child can be "washed over" by later developmental experiences and opportunities.

During a crisis or its aftermath, it is often difficult for the clinician to accurately estimate the inner personal strengths of a child and the supportive capacities of a family or to reasonably gauge a child's prognosis. Failure by the clinician to gain this perspective can undermine a child's sense of confidence in the future.

Timely treatment can dramatically improve prognosis, although this may depend critically on the family's and the child's ability to seek and use treatment. A child with a psychiatric disorder—even severe—who is brought into treatment promptly and responds well to therapy may experience minimal interference with functioning and perhaps little detriment in long-term personal development, family life, education, work achievement, initiative, or lifetime satisfaction. On the other hand, a child who does not or cannot make use of treatment is more likely to have a life of chronic dissatisfaction, underachievement, and lower income, even if the psychiatric disorder is relatively mild. The ability to seek treatment can, in many cases, play a more decisive role in determining the prognosis than either the diagnosis or the severity of illness.

Understanding the disorder is a key element for succeeding in treatment and no less for children than for adults. For a child to be effectively involved in treatment, he or she must understand his or her illness in terms that are age- and intellect-appropriate. During the course of treatment, the child enters progressively higher levels of cognitive functioning and self-awareness. Over the years, the child will be required to repeatedly revise and reformulate his or her understanding of the disorder, of the treatment, and of himself or herself.

For better and for worse, the psychiatric disorders of children and adolescents are traditionally described from the point of view of the medical model of disease. In psychiatry, we have come to define "disorders" on the basis of functional interference, pathological causes, and long-term developmental consequences.

If we are embedded in a medical model of the psychiatric disorders usually first diagnosed in youth, young patients will see that we do not perceive an important side of their beings and the promise of their realistic hopes. They will come to feel, correctly, that we do not understand them. If, instead, we view these individuals as having medical conditions that are part of "the human condition" that they can struggle against and use their abilities to overcome, we will be able to understand these children—and the adults they become—in a more accurate, balanced, and complete way.

References

Abikoff H, Courtney ME, Szeibel PJ, et al: The effects of auditory stimulation on the arithmetic performance of children with ADHD and nondisabled children. J Learn Disabil 29:238–246, 1996

Achenbach TM, Ruffle T: Medical Practitioners' Guide for the Child Behavior Checklist and Related Forms. Burlington, VT, University of Vermont College of Medicine, Department of Psychiatry, 2002

Agarwal V, Sitholey P, Kumar S, et al: Double-blind, placebo-controlled trial of clonidine in hyperactive children with mental retardation. Ment Retard 39:259–267, 2001

Aichhorn A: Wayward Youth (1925). New York, Meridian Books, 1955

Aikawa T, Kasahara T, Uchiyama M: Circadian variation of plasma arginine vasopressin concentration, or arginine vasopressin in enuresis. Scand J Urol Nephrol Suppl 202:47–49, 1999

Airaksinen EM, Matilainen R, Mononen T, et al: A population-based study on epilepsy in mentally retarded children. Epilepsia 41:1214–1220, 2000

Al-Waili NS: Carbamazepine to treat primary nocturnal enuresis: double-blind study. Eur J Med Res 5:40–44, 2000

Alegre S, Chacon J, Redondo L, et al: Post-traumatic tics. Rev Neurol 24:1280–1282, 1996

Almost D, Rosenbaum P: Effectiveness of speech intervention for phonological disorders: a randomized controlled trial. Dev Med Child Neurol 40:319–325, 1998

Althaus M, Vink HJ, Minderaa RB, et al: Lack of effect of clonidine on stuttering in children. Am J Psychiatry 152:1087–1089, 1995

Aman MG, Kern RA: The efficacy of folic acid in fragile X syndrome and other developmental disabilities. J Child Adolesc Psychopharmacol 1:285–295, 1991

Aman MG, Collier-Crespin A, Lindsay RL: Pharmacotherapy of disorders in mental retardation. Eur Child Adolesc Psychiatry 9 (suppl 1):98–107, 2000

American Association on Mental Retardation: Mental Retardation: Definition, Classification, and Systems of Supports, 9th Edition. Washington, DC, American Association on Mental Retardation, 1992

American Psychiatric Association: Diagnostic and Statistical Manual of Mental Disorders, 3rd Edition, Revised. Washington, DC, American Psychiatric Association, 1987

American Psychiatric Association: Diagnostic and Statistical Manual of Mental Disorders, 4th Edition. Washington, DC, American Psychiatric Association, 1994

American Psychiatric Association: Diagnostic and Statistical Manual of Mental Disorders, 4th Edition, Text Revision. Washington, DC, American Psychiatric Association, 2000

Amir RE, Van den Veyver IB, Wan M, et al: Rett syndrome is caused by mutations in X-linked MECP2, encoding methyl-CpG-binding protein 2. Nat Genet 23:127–128, 1999

Anderson JC, Williams S, McGee R, et al: DSM-III disorders in preadolescent children: prevalence in a large sample from the general population. Arch Gen Psychiatry 44:69–76, 1987

Anstendig KD: Is selective mutism an anxiety disorder? Rethinking its DSM-IV classification. J Anxiety Disord 13:417–434, 1999

Antonacci DJ, de Groot CM: Clozapine treatment in a population of adults with mental retardation. J Clin Psychiatry 61:22–25, 2000

Aram DM, Ekelman BL, Nation JE: Preschoolers with language disorder: 10 years later. Journal of Speech and Hearing Research 27:232–244, 1984

Arnold LE: Alternative treatments for adults with attention-deficit hyperactivity disorder (ADHD), in Adult Attention Deficit Disorders: Brain Mechanisms and Life Outcomes. Edited by Wasserstein J, Wolfe LE, Lefever FF. New York, New York Academy of Sciences, 2001, pp 310–341

Arnold LE: Treatment alternatives for attention-deficit/hyperactivity disorder, in Attention Deficit Hyperactivity Disorder: State of the Science; Best Practices. Edited by Jensen PS, Cooper J. Kingston, NJ, Civic Research Institute, 2002

Arnold LE, Kleykamp D, Votolato N, et al: Potential link between dietary intake of fatty acids and behavior: pilot exploration of serum lipids in attention-deficit hyperactivity disorder. J Child Adolesc Psychopharmacol 4:171–182, 1994

Arnold LE, Pinkham SM, Votolato N: Does zinc moderate essential fatty acid and amphetamine treatment of attention-deficit/hyperactivity disorder? J Child Adolesc Psychopharmacol 10:111–117, 2000

Aronson M, Hagberg B, Gillberg C: Attention deficits and autistic spectrum problems in children exposed to alcohol during gestation: a follow-up study. Dev Med Child Neurol 39:583–587, 1997

Attwood T, Wing L: Asperger's Syndrome: A Guide for Parents and Professionals. London, England, Jessica Kingsley Publishers, 1998

August GJ, Stewart MA, Holmes CS: A four-year follow-up of boys with and without conduct disorder. Br J Psychiatry 143:192–198, 1983

August GJ, Realmuto GM, MacDonald AW, et al: Prevalence of ADHD and comorbid disorders among elementary school children screened for disruptive behavior. J Abnorm Child Psychol 24:571–595, 1996

Babinski LM, Hartsough CS, Lambert NM: Childhood conduct problems, hyperactivity-impulsivity, and inattention as predictors of adult criminal activity. J Child Psychol Psychiatry 40:347–355, 1999

Bailey A, Le Couteur A, Gottesman I, et al: Autism as a strongly genetic disorder: evidence from a British twin study. Psychol Med 25:63–77, 1995

Bakwin H: The genetics of enuresis, in Bladder Control and Enuresis. Edited by Kolvin RC, MacKeith RC, Meadow SR. London, England, W Heinemann Medical Books, 1973, pp 73–78

Balboni G, Pedrabissi L, Molteni M, et al: Discriminant validity of the Vineland Scales: score profiles of individuals with mental retardation and a specific disorder. Am J Ment Retard 106:162–172, 2001

Barkley RA: Genetics of childhood disorders, XVII: ADHD, part 1: the executive functions and ADHD. J Am Acad Child Adolesc Psychiatry 39:1064–1068, 2000

Barkley RA, Cunningham CE: Do stimulant drugs improve the academic performance of hyperkinetic children? A review of outcome studies. Clin Pediatr 17:85–92, 1978

Barkley RA, Edwards G, Laneri M, et al: Executive functioning, temporal discounting, and sense of time in adolescents with attention deficit hyperactivity disorder (ADHD) and oppositional defiant disorder (ODD). J Abnorm Child Psychol 29:541–556, 2001

Baroff GS: Mental Retardation: Nature, Cause and Management. New York, Hemisphere, 1986

Barrett PM: Evaluation of cognitive-behavioral group treatments for childhood anxiety disorders. J Clin Child Psychol 27:459–468, 1998

Barrett PM, Dadds MR, Rapee RM: Family treatment of childhood anxiety: a controlled trial. J Consult Clin Psychol 64:333–342, 1996

Barrickman LL, Perry PJ, Allen AJ, et al: Bupropion versus methylphenidate in the treatment of attention-deficit hyperactivity disorder. J Am Acad Child Adolesc Psychiatry 34:649–657, 1995

Barry CT, Frick PJ, DeShazo TM, et al: The importance of callous-unemotional traits for extending the concept of psychopathy to children. J Abnorm Psychol 109:335–340, 2000

Battaglia M, Bertella S, Politi E, et al: Age at onset of panic disorder: influence of familial liability to the disease and of childhood separation anxiety disorder. Am J Psychiatry 152:1362–1364, 1995

Bauman ML: Microscopic neuroanatomical abnormalities in autism. Pediatrics 87 (suppl):791–796, 1991

Beitchman JH, Nair R, Clegg M, et al: Prevalence of psychiatric disorders in children with speech and language disorders. Journal of the American Academy of Child Psychiatry 25:528–535, 1986

Beitchman JH, Wilson B, Johnson CJ, et al: Fourteen-year follow-up of speech/language-impaired and control children: psychiatric outcome. J Am Acad Child Adolesc Psychiatry 40:75–82, 2001

Bennett KE, Haggard MP: Behaviour and cognitive outcomes from middle ear disease. Arch Dis Child 80:28–35, 1999

Benninga MA, Buller HA, Heymans HS, et al: Is encopresis always the result of constipation? Arch Dis Child 71:186–193, 1994

Berkson G, Rafaeli-Mor N, Tarnovsky S: Body-rocking and other habits of college students and persons with mental retardation. Am J Ment Retard 104:107–116, 1999

Bernstein GA, Borchardt CM: Anxiety disorders of childhood and adolescence: a critical review. J Am Acad Child Adolesc Psychiatry 30:519–532, 1991

Bernstein GA, Garfinkel BD, Borchardt CM: Comparative studies of pharmacotherapy for school refusal. J Am Acad Child Adolesc Psychiatry 29:773–781, 1990

Berquin PC, Giedd JN, Jacobsen LK, et al: Cerebellum in attention-deficit hyperactivity disorder: a morphometric MRI study. Neurology 50:1087–1093, 1998

Berry CA, Shaywitz SE, Shaywitz BA: Girls with attention deficit disorder: a silent minority? A report on behavioral and cognitive characteristics. Pediatrics 76:801–809, 1985

Bharucha KJ, Sethi KD: Tardive tourettism after exposure to neuroleptic therapy. Mov Disord 10:791–793, 1995

Biederman J: Attention-deficit/hyperactivity disorder: a life-span perspective. J Clin Psychiatry 59 (suppl 7):4–16, 1998

Biederman J, Spencer T: Attention-deficit/hyperactivity disorder (ADHD) as a noradrenergic disorder. Biol Psychiatry 46:1234–1242, 1999

Biederman J, Faraone S, Mick E, et al: Attention-deficit hyperactivity disorder and juvenile mania: an overlooked comorbidity? J Am Acad Child Adolesc Psychiatry 35:997–1008, 1996

Biederman J, Wilens T, Mick E, et al: Is ADHD a risk factor for psychoactive substance use disorders? Findings from a four-year prospective follow-up study. J Am Acad Child Adolesc Psychiatry 36:21–29, 1997b

Biederman J, Wilens TE, Mick E, et al: Does attention-deficit hyperactivity disorder impact the developmental course of drug and alcohol abuse and dependence? Biol Psychiatry 44:269–273, 1998

Biederman J, Faraone SV, Mick E, et al: Clinical correlates of ADHD in females: findings from a large group of girls ascertained from pediatric and psychiatric referral sources. J Am Acad Child Adolesc Psychiatry 38:966–975, 1999a

Biederman J, Wilens T, Mick E, et al: Pharmacotherapy of attention-deficit/hyperactivity disorder reduces risk for substance use disorder (abstract). Pediatrics 104:e20, 1999b

Biederman J, Mick E, Faraone SV: Age-dependent decline of symptoms of attention deficit hyperactivity disorder: impact of remission definition and symptom type. Am J Psychiatry 157:816–818, 2000

Biederman J, Mick E, Faraone SV, et al: Patterns of remission and symptom decline in conduct disorder: a four-year prospective study of an ADHD sample. J Am Acad Child Adolesc Psychiatry 40:290–298, 2001b

Birch HG, Richardson SA, Baird D, et al: Mental Subnormality in the Community: A Clinical and Epidemiological Study. Baltimore, MD, Williams & Wilkins, 1970

Bird HR, Gould MS, Staghezza BM: Patterns of diagnostic comorbidity in a community sample of children aged 9 through 16 years. J Am Acad Child Adolesc Psychiatry 32:361–368, 1993

Birmaher B, Waterman GS, Ryan N, et al: Fluoxetine for childhood anxiety disorders. J Am Acad Child Adolesc Psychiatry 33:993–999, 1994

Blacher J: Transition to adulthood: mental retardation, families, and culture. Am J Ment Retard 106:173–188, 2001

Black B, Uhde TW: Elective mutism as a variant of social phobia. J Am Acad Child Adolesc Psychiatry 31:1090–1094, 1992

Black B, Uhde TW: Treatment of elective mutism with fluoxetine: a double-blind, placebo-controlled study. J Am Acad Child Adolesc Psychiatry 33:1000–1006, 1994

Blagg N, Yule W: The behavioral treatment of school refusal: a comparative study. Behav Res Ther 22:119–127, 1984

Bolman WM, Richmond JA: A double-blind, placebo-controlled, crossover pilot trial of low dose dimethylglycine in patients with autistic disorder. J Autism Dev Disord 29:191–194, 1999

Bonde HV, Andersen JP, Rosenkilde P: Nocturnal enuresis: change of nocturnal voiding pattern during alarm treatment. Scand J Urol Nephrol 28:349–352, 1994

Boris M, Mandel FS: Foods and additives are common causes of the attention deficit hyperactive disorder in children. Ann Allergy 72:462–468, 1994

Borthwick-Duffy SA, Lane KL, Widaman KF: Measuring problem behaviors in children with mental retardation: dimensions and predictors. Res Dev Disabil 18:415–433, 1997

Bouffard M, Watkinson EJ, Thompson LP, et al: A test of the activity deficit hypothesis with children with movement difficulties. Adapted Physical Activity Quarterly 13:61–73, 1996

Braddock D, Emerson E, Felce D, et al: Living circumstances of children and adults with mental retardation or developmental disabilities in the United States, Canada, England and Wales, and Australia. Mental Retardation and Developmental Disabilities Research Reviews 7:115–121, 2001

Breakey J: The role of diet and behaviour in childhood. J Paediatr Child Health 33:190–194, 1997

Bregman JD: Current developments in the understanding of mental retardation, part 2: psychopathology. J Am Acad Child Adolesc Psychiatry 30:861–872, 1991

Bregman JD, Hodapp RM: Current developments in the understanding of mental retardation, part 1: biological and phenomenological perspectives. J Am Acad Child Adolesc Psychiatry 30:707–719, 1991

Brett PM, Curtis D, Robertson MM, et al: Exclusion of the 5-HT1A serotonin neuroreceptor and tryptophan oxygenase genes in a large British kindred multiply affected with Tourette's syndrome, chronic motor tics, and obsessive-compulsive behavior. Am J Psychiatry 152:437–440, 1995

Brooks RC, Copen RM, Cox DJ, et al: Review of the treatment literature for encopresis, functional constipation, and stool-toileting refusal. Ann Behav Med 22:260–267, 2000

Brown MB, Giandenoto MJ, Bolen LM: Diagnosing written language disabilities using the Woodcock-Johnson Tests of Educational Achievement—Revised and the Wechsler Individual Achievement Test. Psychol Rep 87:197–204, 2000

Bruck M: Persistence of dyslexics' phonologic awareness deficits. Dev Psychol 28:874–886, 1992

Bruggeman R, van der Linden C, Buitelaar JK, et al: Risperidone versus pimozide, I: Tourette's disorder: a comparative double-blind parallel-group study. J Clin Psychiatry 62:50–56, 2001

Budman CL, Bruun RD, Park KS, et al: Explosive outbursts in children with Tourette's disorder. J Am Acad Child Adolesc Psychiatry 39:1270–1276, 2000

Buitelaar JK: Open-label treatment with risperidone of 26 psychiatrically hospitalized children and adolescents with mixed diagnoses and aggressive behavior. J Child Adolesc Psychopharmacol 10:19–26, 2000

Buitelaar JK, van der Gaag RJ, Cohen-Kettenis P, et al: A randomized controlled trial of risperidone in the treatment of aggression in hospitalized adolescents with subaverage cognitive abilities. J Clin Psychiatry 62:239–248, 2001

Bull R, Johnston RS: Children's arithmetical difficulties: contributions from processing speed, item identification, and short-term memory. J Exp Child Psychol 65:1–24, 1997

Burgard JF, Donohue B, Azrin NH, et al: Prevalence and treatment of substance abuse in the mentally retarded population: an empirical review. J Psychoactive Drugs 32:293–298, 2000

Bush G, Frazier JA, Rauch SL, et al: Anterior cingulate cortex dysfunction in attention-deficit/hyperactivity disorder revealed by fMRI and the Counting Stroop. Biol Psychiatry 45:1542–1552, 1999

Buttross S: Encopresis in the child with a behavioral disorder: when the initial treatment does not work. Pediatr Ann 28:317–321, 1999

Caione P, Arena F, Biraghi M, et al: Nocturnal enuresis and daytime wetting: a multicentric trial with oxybutynin and desmopressin. Eur Urol 31:459–463, 1997

Calabrese EJ, Stanek EJ, James RC, et al: Soil ingestion: a concern for acute toxicity in children. Environ Health Perspect 105:1354–1358, 1997

Campbell L, Malone MA, Kershner JR, et al: Methylphenidate slows right hemisphere processing in children with attention-deficit/hyperactivity disorder. J Child Adolesc Psychopharmacol 6:229–239, 1996

Canales JJ, Graybiel AM: A measure of striatal function predicts motor stereotypy. Nat Neurosci 3:377–383, 2000

Cantell M, Kooistra L: Long-term outcomes of developmental coordination disorder, in Developmental Coordination Disorder. Edited by Cermak SA, Larkin D. Albany, NY, Singular Publishing Group, 2002

Cantwell DP, Baker L: Developmental Speech and Language Disorders. New York, Guilford, 1987

Cantwell DP, Baker L: Issues in classification of child and adolescent psychopathology. J Am Acad Child Adolesc Psychiatry 27:521–533, 1988

Cantwell DP, Baker L: Stability and natural history of DSM-III childhood diagnoses. J Am Acad Child Adolesc Psychiatry 28:691–700, 1989

Capps L, Sigman M, Sena R, et al: Fear, anxiety and perceived control in children of agoraphobic parents. J Child Psychol Psychiatry 37:445–452, 1996

Carlin MT, Soraci SA, Dennis NA, et al: Enhancing free-recall rates of individuals with mental retardation. Am J Ment Retard 106:314–326, 2001

Carlson JS, Kratochwill TR, Johnston HF: Sertraline treatment of 5 children diagnosed with selective mutism: a single-case research trial. J Child Adolesc Psychopharmacol 9:293–306, 1999

Carlsson ML: On the role of cortical glutamate in obsessive-compulsive disorder and attention-deficit hyperactivity disorder, two phenomenologically antithetical conditions. Acta Psychiatr Scand 102:401–413, 2000

Carta MG, Hardoy MC, Dessi I, et al: Adjunctive gabapentin in patients with intellectual disability and bipolar spectrum disorders. J Intellect Disabil Res 45:139–145, 2001

Casat CD, Pleasants DZ, Schroeder DH, et al: Bupropion in children with attention deficit disorder. Psychopharmacol Bull 25:187–201, 1989

Casey BJ, Castellanos FX, Giedd JN, et al: Implication of right frontostriatal circuitry in response inhibition and attention-deficit/hyperactivity disorder. J Am Acad Child Adolesc Psychiatry 36:374–383, 1997

Castellanos FX, Elia J, Kruesi MJ, et al: Cerebrospinal fluid monoamine metabolites in boys with attention-deficit hyperactivity disorder. Psychiatry Res 52:305–316, 1994a

Castellanos FX, Giedd JN, Eckburg P, et al: Quantitative morphology of the caudate nucleus in attention deficit hyperactivity disorder. Am J Psychiatry 151:1791–1796, 1994b

Castellanos FX, Giedd JN, Marsh WL, et al: Quantitative brain magnetic resonance imaging in attention-deficit hyperactivity disorder. Arch Gen Psychiatry 53:607–616, 1996

Castellanos FX, Ritchie GF, Marsh WL, et al: DSM-IV stereotypic movement disorder: persistence of stereotypies of infancy in intellectually normal adolescents and adults. J Clin Psychiatry 58:177–178, 1997

Castellanos FX, Giedd JN, Berquin PC, et al: Quantitative brain magnetic resonance imaging in girls with attention-deficit/hyperactivity disorder. Arch Gen Psychiatry 58:289–295, 2001

Cath DC, Spinhoven P, van Woerkom TC, et al: Gilles de la Tourette's syndrome with and without obsessive-compulsive disorder compared with obsessive-compulsive disorder without tics: which symptoms discriminate? J Nerv Ment Dis 189:219–228, 2001a

Cath DC, Spinhoven P, Hoogduin CA, et al: Repetitive behaviors in Tourette's syndrome and OCD with and without tics: what are the differences? Psychiatry Res 101:171–185, 2001b

Cavaliere F, Cormaci S, Cormaci M, et al: Clinical and hormonal response to general anaesthesia in patients affected by different degrees of mental retardation. Minerva Anestesiol 65:499–505, 1999

Chabot RJ, Serfontein G: Quantitative electroencephalographic profiles of children with attention deficit disorder. Biol Psychiatry 40:951–963, 1996

Chaney RH, Eyman RK: Patterns in mortality over 60 years among persons with mental retardation in a residential facility. Ment Retard 38:289–293, 2000

Chappell PB, Riddle MA, Scahill L, et al: Guanfacine treatment of comorbid attention deficit hyperactivity disorder and Tourette's syndrome: preliminary clinical experience. J Am Acad Child Adolesc Psychiatry 34:1140–1146, 1995

Chase TN, Friedhoff AJ, Cohen DJ (eds): Tourette Syndrome: Genetics, Neurobiology, and Treatment (Advances in Neurology Series, Vol 58). New York, Raven, 1992

Chatoor I: Infantile anorexia nervosa: a developmental disorder or separation and individuation. J Am Acad Psychoanal 17:43–64, 1989

Chatoor I, Dickson L, Einhorn A: Rumination: etiology and treatment. Pediatr Ann 13:924–929, 1984

Chatoor I, Dickson L, Schaefer S, et al: A developmental classification of feeding disorders associated with failure to thrive: diagnosis and treatment, in New Directions in Failure to Thrive: Research and Clinical Practice. Edited by Drotar D. New York, Plenum, 1985

Cherry KE, Matson JL, Paclawskyj TR: Psychopathology in older adults with severe and profound mental retardation. Am J Ment Retard 101:445–458, 1997

Chiaradia M, Gulson BL, MacDonald K: Contamination of houses by workers occupationally exposed in a lead-zinc-copper mine and impact on blood lead concentrations in the families. Occup Environ Med 54:117–124, 1997

Christian L, Poling A: Drug abuse in persons with mental retardation: a review. Am J Ment Retard 102:126–136, 1997

Clay TH, Gualtieri CT, Evans RW, et al: Clinical and neuropsychological effects of the novel antidepressant bupropion. Psychopharmacol Bull 24:143–148, 1988

Cleator H, Hand L: Selective mutism: how a successful speech and language assessment really is possible. Int J Lang Commun Disord 36(suppl):126–131, 2001

Coffey BJ, Biederman J, Smoller JW, et al: Anxiety disorders and tic severity in juveniles with Tourette's disorder. J Am Acad Child Adolesc Psychiatry 39:562–568, 2000

Cohen D, Caparulo B, Shaywitz B: Primary childhood aphasia and childhood autism: clinical, biological, and conceptual observations. Journal of the American Academy of Child Psychiatry 4:604–645, 1976

Cohen D, Bruun R, Leckman J: Tourette's Syndrome and Tic Disorders: Clinical Understanding and Treatment. New York, Wiley, 1988

Cohen J: Learning disabilities and adolescence: developmental considerations, in Adolescent Psychiatry, Vol 12. Edited by Feinstein SC, Sugar M, Esman AH, et al. Chicago, IL, University of Chicago Press, 1985

Cohen P, Cohen J, Kasen S, et al: An epidemiological study of disorders in late childhood and adolescence, I: age- and gender-specific prevalence. J Child Psychol Psychiatry 34:851–867, 1993

Comings DE, Gade-Andavolu R, Gonzalez N, et al: Comparison of the role of dopamine, serotonin, and noradrenaline genes in ADHD, ODD and conduct disorder: multivariate regression analysis of 20 genes. Clin Genet 57:178–196, 2000a

Como PG: Prospective, longitudinal study of tic, obsessive-compulsive, and attention-deficit/hyperactivity disorders in an epidemiological sample. Adv Neurol 85:103–111, 2001

Conners CK: Conners' Rating Scales—Revised (CRS-R). North Tonawanda, NY, MHS Inc, 1997

Conners CK, Casat CD, Gualtieri CT, et al: Bupropion hydrochloride in attention deficit disorder with hyperactivity. J Am Acad Child Adolesc Psychiatry 35:1314–1321, 1996

Connor DF, Fletcher KE, Swanson JM: A meta-analysis of clonidine for symptoms of attention-deficit hyperactivity disorder. J Am Acad Child Adolesc Psychiatry 38:1551–1559, 1999

Cooper B (ed): Assessing the Handicaps and Needs of Mentally Retarded Children. New York, Academic Press, 1981

Coumel P, Fidelle J, Lucet V, et al: Catecholamine induced severe ventricular arrhythmia with Adam-Stokes syndrome in children: a report of 4 cases. British Heart Journal 409(suppl):28–37, 1978

Craig A, Hancock K, Chang E, et al: A controlled trial for stuttering in persons aged 9 to 14 years. J Speech Hear Res 39:808–826, 1996

Croen LA, Grether JK, Selvin S: The epidemiology of mental retardation of unknown cause. Pediatrics 107:E86, 2001

Curry CJ, Stevenson RE, Aughton D, et al: Evaluation of mental retardation: recommendations of a consensus conference: American College of Medical Genetics. Am J Med Genet 72:468–477, 1997

Curtis D, Robertson MM, Gurling HM: Autosomal dominant gene transmission in a large kindred with Gilles de la Tourette syndrome. Br J Psychiatry 160:845–849, 1992

Danford DE: Pica and nutrition. Annu Rev Nutr 2:303–322, 1982

Danforth JS: The outcome of parent training using the behavior management flow chart with mothers and their children with oppositional defiant disorder and attention-deficit hyperactivity disorder. Behav Modif 22:443–473, 1998

Deb S: Mental disorder in adults with mental retardation and epilepsy. Compr Psychiatry 38:179–184, 1997

DeKlyen M, Speltz ML, Greenberg MT: Fathering and early onset conduct problems: positive and negative parenting, father-son attachment, and the marital context. Clinical Child and Family Psychology Review Mar 1:3–21, 1998

DeLissovoy V: Head banging in early childhood. Child Dev 33:43–56, 1962

Deutsch CK, Swanson JM, Bruell JH, et al: Overrepresentation of adoptees in children with the attention deficit disorder. Behav Genet 12:231–238, 1982

Didden R, Duker PC, Korzilius H: Meta-analytic study on treatment effectiveness for problem behaviors with individuals who have mental retardation. Am J Ment Retard 101:387–399, 1997

Disney ER, Elkins IJ, McGue M, et al: Effects of ADHD, conduct disorder, and gender on substance use and abuse in adolescence. Am J Psychiatry 156:1515–1521, 1999

Dodd B, Bradford A: A comparison of three therapy methods for children with different types of developmental phonological disorder. Int J Lang Commun Disord 35:189–209, 2000

Downey KK, Stelson FW, Pomerleau OF, et al: Adult attention deficit hyperactivity disorder: psychological test profiles in a clinical population. J Nerv Ment Dis 185:32–38, 1997

Drews CD, Murphy CC, Yeargin-Allsopp M, et al: The relationship between idiopathic mental retardation and maternal smoking during pregnancy. Pediatrics 97:547–553, 1996

Dudley JR, Calhoun ML, Ahlgrim-Delzell L, et al: A consumer satisfaction survey of people with mental retardation and mental illness. Psychiatr Serv 48:1075–1077, 1997

Dummit ES, Klein RG, Tancer NK, et al: Fluoxetine treatment of children with selective mutism: an open trial. J Am Acad Child Adolesc Psychiatry 35:615–621, 1996

Dykman RA, McPherson B, Ackerman PT, et al: Internalizing and externalizing characteristics of sexually and/or physically abused children. Integr Physiol Behav Sci 32:62–74, 1997

Eckern M, Stevens W, Mitchell J: The relationship between rumination and eating disorders. Int J Eat Disord 26:414–419, 1999

Edelbrock C: Behavioral checklists and rating scales, in Basic Handbook of Child Psychiatry, Vol 5. Edited by Noshpitz JD, Call JD, Cohen RL, et al. New York, Basic Books, 1987

Edwards CH, Johnson AA, Knight EM, et al: Pica in an urban environment. J Nutr 124 (suppl 6):954S–962S, 1994

Ehlers S, Nyden A, Gillberg C, et al: Asperger syndrome, autism and attentional disorders: a comparative study of the cognitive profiles of 120 children. J Child Psychol Psychiatry 38:207–217, 1997

Elstner K, Selai CE, Trimble MR, et al: Quality of life (QOL) of patients with Gilles de la Tourette's syndrome. Acta Psychiatr Scand 103:52–59, 2001

Embregts PJ: Reliability of the Child Behavior Checklist for the assessment of behavioral problems of children and youth with mild mental retardation. Res Dev Disabil 21:31–41, 2000

Ernst M, Liebenauer LL, Jons PH, et al: Selegiline in adults with attention deficit hyperactivity disorder: clinical efficacy and safety. Psychopharmacol Bull 32:327–334, 1996

Fairbanks JM, Pine DS, Tancer NK, et al: Open fluoxetine treatment of mixed anxiety disorders in children and adolescents. J Child Adolesc Psychopharmacol 7:17–29, 1997

Faraone SV, Doyle AE: The nature and heritability of attention-deficit/hyperactivity disorder. Child Adolesc Psychiatr Clin North Am 10:299–316, 2001

Faraone SV, Biederman J, Spencer T, et al: Attention-deficit/hyperactivity disorder in adults: an overview. Biol Psychiatry 48:9–20, 2000a

Faraone SV, Biederman J, Mick E, et al: Family study of girls with attention deficit hyperactivity disorder. Am J Psychiatry 157:1077–1083, 2000b

Farrington DP, Loeber R: Epidemiology of juvenile violence. Child Adolesc Psychiatr Clin N Am 9:733–748, 2000

Faulstich ME, Moore JR, Roberts RW, et al: A behavioral perspective on conduct disorders. Psychiatry 51:116–130, 1988

Feigin A, Kurlan R, McDermott MP, et al: A controlled trial of deprenyl in children with Tourette's syndrome and attention deficit hyperactivity disorder. Neurology 46:965–968, 1996

Felce D, Emerson E: Living with support in a home in the community: predictors of behavioral development and household and community activity. Mental Retardation and Developmental Disabilities Research Reviews 7:75–83, 2001

Felsenfeld S, Kirk KM, Zhu G, et al: A study of the genetic and environmental etiology of stuttering in a selected twin sample. Behav Genet 30:359–366, 2000

Fendrich M, Warner V, Weissman MM: Family risk factors, parental depression, and psychopathology in offspring. Dev Psychol 26:40–50, 1990

Fergusson DM, Horwood LJ, Shannon FT: Factors related to the age of attainment of nocturnal bladder control. Pediatrics 78: 884–890, 1986

Fergusson DM, Horwood LJ, Lynskey MT: Structure of DSM-III-R criteria for disruptive childhood behaviors: confirmatory factor models. J Am Acad Child Adolesc Psychiatry 33:1145–1157, 1994

Fey M, Leonard L, Wilcox K: Speech style modification in language-impaired children. Journal of Speech and Hearing Disorders 46:91–96, 1981

Findling RL, Maxwell K, Scotese-Wojtila L, et al: High-dose pyridoxine and magnesium administration in children with autistic disorder: an absence of salutary effects in a double-blind, placebo-controlled study. J Autism Dev Disord 27:467–478, 1997

Findling RL, McNamara NK, Branicky LA, et al: A double-blind pilot study of risperidone in the treatment of conduct disorder. J Am Acad Child Adolesc Psychiatry 39:509–516, 2000

Fisher L, Ames EW, Chisholm K, et al: Problems reported by parents of Romanian orphans adopted to British Columbia. International Journal of Behavioral Development 20:67–82, 1997

Fletcher KE, Fischer M, Barkley RA, et al: A sequential analysis of the mother-adolescent interactions of ADHD, ADHD + ODD, and normal teenagers during neutral and conflict discussions. J Abnorm Child Psychol 24:271–297, 1996

Folstein SE, Piven J: Etiology of autism: genetic influences. Pediatrics 87(suppl):767–773, 1991

Fonagy P, Target M: The efficacy of psychoanalysis for children with disruptive disorders. J Am Acad Child Adolesc Psychiatry 33:45–55, 1994

Foorman BR, Francis DJ, Beeler T, et al: Early interventions for children with problems: study designs and preliminary findings. Learning Disabilities 8:63–71, 1997

Foreman DM, Thambirajah MS: Conduct disorder, enuresis and specific developmental delays in two types of encopresis: a case-note study of 63 boys. Eur Child Adolesc Psychiatry 5:33–37, 1996

Forsythe WI, Butler RJ: Fifty years of enuretic alarms. Arch Dis Child 64:879–885, 1989

Fox AM, Lent B: Clumsy children: primer on developmental coordination disorder. Can Fam Physician 42:1965–1971, 1996

Fredericks DW, Carr JE, Williams WL: Overview of the treatment of rumination disorder for adults in a residential setting. J Behav Ther Exp Psychiatry 29:31–40, 1998

Freeman RD, Fast DK, Burd L, et al: An international perspective on Tourette syndrome: selected findings from 3,500 individuals in 22 countries. Dev Med Child Neurol 42:436–447, 2000

Frick PJ: Conduct Disorders and Severe Antisocial Behavior. New York, Plenum, 1998

Frith U (ed): Autism and Asperger Syndrome. Cambridge, England, University of Cambridge, 1991

Fujii Y, Konishi Y, Kuriyama M, et al: Corpus callosum in developmentally retarded infants. Pediatr Neurol 11:219–223, 1994

Gadow KD, Sverd J, Sprafkin J, et al: Efficacy of methylphenidate for attention deficit hyperactivity disorder in children with tic disorder. Arch Gen Psychiatry 52:444–455, 1995

Gadow KD, Sverd J, Sprafkin J, et al: Long-term methylphenidate therapy in children with comorbid attention-deficit hyperactivity disorder and chronic multiple tic disorder. Arch Gen Psychiatry 56:330–336, 1999

Galler JR, Ramsey F, Solimano G, et al: The influence of early malnutrition on subsequent behavioral development, II: classroom behavior. Journal of the American Academy of Child Psychiatry 22:16–22, 1983

García-Sánchez C, Estévez-González A, Suárez-Romero E, et al: Right hemisphere dysfunction in subjects with attention-deficit disorder with and without hyperactivity. J Child Neurol 12:107–115, 1997

Gaub M, Carlson CL: Behavioral characteristics of DSM-IV ADHD subtypes in a school-based population. J Abnorm Child Psychol 25:103–111, 1997

Giedd JN, Rapoport JL, Garvey MA, et al: MRI assessment of children with obsessive-compulsive disorder or tics associated with streptococcal infection. Am J Psychiatry 157:281–283, 2000

Giedd JN, Blumenthal J, Molloy E: Brain imaging of attention deficit/hyperactivity disorder. Ann N Y Acad Sci 931:33–49, 2001

Gierut JA: Treatment efficacy: functional phonological disorders in children. J Speech Lang Hear Res 41:S85–100, 1998

Gilbert DL, Sethuraman G, Sine L, et al: Tourette's syndrome improvement with pergolide in a randomized, double-blind, crossover trial. Neurology 54:1310–1315, 2000

Gillberg C: Asperger syndrome in 23 Swedish children. Dev Med Child Neurol 31:520–531, 1989

Gillberg C, Persson E, Grufman M, et al: Psychiatric disorders in mildly and severely mentally retarded urban children and adolescents: epidemiological aspects. Br J Psychiatry 149:68–74, 1986

Gillberg C, Melander H, von Knorring AL, et al: Long-term stimulant treatment of children with attention-deficit hyperactivity disorder symptoms: a randomized, double-blind, placebo-controlled trial. Arch Gen Psychiatry 54:857–864, 1997

Glazener CM, Evans JH: Desmopressin for nocturnal enuresis in children. Cochrane Database Syst Rev 2:CD002112, 2000a

Glazener CM, Evans JH: Tricyclic and related drugs for nocturnal enuresis in children. Cochrane Database Syst Rev 3:CD002117, 2000b

Golwyn DH, Sevlie CP: Phenelzine treatment of selective mutism in four prepubertal children. J Child Adolesc Psychopharmacol 9:109–113, 1999

Gostason R: Psychiatric illness among the mentally retarded: a Swedish population study. Acta Psychiatr Scand 318 (suppl):1–117, 1985

Graae F, Milner J, Rizzotto L, et al: Clonazepam in childhood anxiety disorders. J Am Acad Child Adolesc Psychiatry 33:372–376, 1994

Grandin T, Scariano MM: Emergence Labeled Autistic. Novato, CA, Arena Press, 1986

Greene RW, Doyle AE: Toward a transactional conceptualization of oppositional defiant disorder: implications for assessment and treatment. Clinical Child and Family Psychology Review 2:129–148, 1999

Greene RW, Biederman J, Faraone SV, et al: Further validation of social impairment as a predictor of substance use disorders: findings from a sample of siblings of boys with and without ADHD. J Clin Child Psychol 28:349–354, 1999

Gregg N, McAlexander PA: The relation between sense of audience and specific learning disabilities: an exploration. Annals of Dyslexia 39:206–226, 1989

Grigorenko EL, Sternberg RJ, Ehrman ME: A theory-based approach to the measurement of foreign language learning ability: the canal-F theory and test. Modern Language Journal 84:390–405, 2000

Grigorenko EL, Wood FB, Meyer MS, et al: Linkage studies suggest a possible locus for developmental dyslexia on chromosome 1p. Am J Med Genet 105:120–129, 2001

Grigsby RK, Thyer BA, Waller RJ, et al: Chalk eating in middle Georgia: a culture-bound syndrome of pica? South Med J 92:190–192, 1999

Gross-Tsur V, Manor O, Shalev RS: Developmental dyscalculia: prevalence and demographic features. Dev Med Child Neurol 38:25–33, 1996

Grossman HJ (ed): Classification in Mental Retardation. Washington, DC, American Association on Mental Deficiency, 1983

Guedeney A: An update on merycism and early depression: a critical review of the literature and a psychopathological hypothesis [in French]. Psychiatr Enfant (Paris) 38:345–363, 1995

Hagerman RJ, Hagerman PJ: Fragile X Syndrome: Diagnosis, Treatment, and Research, 3rd Edition. Baltimore, MD, Johns Hopkins University Press, 2002

Halperin JM, Newcorn JH, Matier K, et al: Impulsivity and the initiation of fights in children with disruptive behavior disorders. J Child Psychol Psychiatry 36:1199–1211, 1995

Hancock K, Craig A, McCready C, et al: Two- to six-year controlled-trial stuttering outcomes for children and adolescents. J Speech Lang Hear Res 41:1242–1252, 1998

Hare RD, McPherson LM, Forth AE: Male psychopaths and their criminal careers. J Consult Clin Psychol 56:710–714, 1988

Harris EC, Barraclough B: Suicide as an outcome for mental disorders: a meta-analysis. Br J Psychiatry 170:205–228, 1997

Hart EL, Lahey BB, Loeber R, et al: Developmental change in attention-deficit hyperactivity disorder in boys: a four-year longitudinal study. J Abnorm Child Psychol 23: 729–749, 1995

Hayward C, Killen JD, Kraemer HC, et al: Predictors of panic attacks in adolescents. J Am Acad Child Adolesc Psychiatry 39: 207–214, 2000

Hebebrand J, Klug B, Fimmers R, et al: Rates for tic disorders and obsessive compulsive symptomatology in families of children and adolescents with Gilles de la Tourette syndrome. J Psychiatr Res 31:519–530, 1997

Herskowitz J: Developmental neurotoxicology, in Psychiatric Pharmacosciences of Children and Adolescents. Edited by Popper C. Washington, DC, American Psychiatric Press, 1987, pp 81–124

Hill AE, Rosenbloom L: Disintegrative psychosis of childhood: teenage follow-up. Dev Med Child Neurol 28:34–40, 1986

Hill EL: A dyspraxic deficit in specific language impairment and developmental coordination disorder? Evidence from hand and arm movements. Dev Med Child Neurol 40:388–395, 1998

Hill JC, Schoener EP: Age-dependent decline of attention deficit hyperactivity disorder. Am J Psychiatry 153:1143–1146, 1996

Hittmair-Delazer M, Sailer U, Benke T: Impaired arithmetic facts but intact conceptual knowledge: a single case study of dyscalculia. Cortex 31:139–147, 1995

Hoekstra PJ, Bijzet J, Limburg PC, et al: Elevated D8/17 expression on B lymphocytes, a marker of rheumatic fever, measured with flow cytometry in tic disorder patients. Am J Psychiatry 158:605–610, 2001

Howie VM: Developmental sequelae of chronic otitis media: a review. J Dev Behav Pediatr 1:34–38, 1980

Huesmann LR, Eron LD, Lefkowitz MM, et al: The stability of aggression over time and generations. Dev Psychol 20:1120–1134, 1984

Hunsballe JM, Rittig S, Pedersen EB, et al: Single dose imipramine reduces nocturnal urine output in patients with nocturnal enuresis and nocturnal polyuria. J Urol 158:830–836, 1997

Hunt RD, Capper L, O'Connell P: Clonidine in child and adolescent psychiatry. J Child Adolesc Psychopharmacol 1:87–102, 1990

Hunt RD, Arnsten AF, Asbell MD: An open trial of guanfacine in the treatment of attention-deficit hyperactivity disorder. J Am Acad Child Adolesc Psychiatry 34: 50–54, 1995

Hunter AG: Outcome of the routine assessment of patients with mental retardation in a genetics clinic. Am J Med Genet 90: 60–68, 2000

Hynd GW, Hall J, Novey ES: Dyslexia and corpus callosum morphology. Arch Neurol 52:32–38, 1995

Ialongo NS, Horn WF, Pascoe JM, et al: The effects of multimodal intervention with ADHD children: a 9-month follow-up. J Am Acad Child Adolesc Psychiatry 32: 182–189, 1993

Jacobs BW, Isaacs S: Pre-pubertal anorexia nervosa. J Child Psychol Psychiatry 27:237–250, 1986

Jain P, Misra A: Nonsustained ventricular tachycardia following clonidine withdrawal (letter). Postgrad Med J 33:403–404, 1991

Jaselskis CA, Cook EH, Fletcher K, et al: Clonidine treatment of hyperactive and impulsive children with autistic disorder. J Clin Psychopharmacol 12:322–327, 1992

Jenkins RL: Behavior Disorders of Childhood and Adolescence. Springfield, IL, Charles C Thomas, 1973

Jensen PS, Hinshaw SP, Swanson JM, et al: Findings from the NIMH Multimodal Treatment Study of ADHD (MTA): implications and applications for primary care providers. J Dev Behav Pediatr 22: 60–73, 2001b

Johnson AM, Falstein EI, Szurek SA, et al: School phobia. Am J Orthopsychiatry 11: 702–711, 1941

Johnson CJ, Beitchman JH, Young A, et al: Fourteen-year follow-up of children with and without speech/language impairments: speech/language stability and outcomes. J Speech Lang Hear Res 42:744–760, 1999

Johnston MV, Nishimura A, Harum K, et al: Sculpting the developing brain. Adv Pediatr 48:1–38, 2001

Kadesjo B, Gillberg C: The comorbidity of ADHD in the general population of Swedish school-age children. J Child Psychol Psychiatry 42:487–492, 2001

Kalo BB, Bella H: Enuresis: prevalence and associated factors among primary school children in Saudi Arabia. Acta Paediatr 85:1217–1222, 1996

Kaneko K, Fujinaga S, Ohtomo Y, et al: Combined pharmacotherapy for nocturnal enuresis. Pediatr Nephrol 16:662–664, 2001

Kanner L: Autistic disturbances of affective contact. Nervous Child 2:217–250, 1943

Katusic SJ, Colligan RC, Beard CM, et al: Mental retardation in a birth cohort, 1976–1980, Rochester, Minnesota. Am J Ment Retard 100:335–344, 1996

Kaufmann WE, Moser HW: Dendritic anomalies in disorders associated with mental retardation. Cereb Cortex 10:981–991, 2000

Kazdin AE: Conduct Disorders in Childhood and Adolescence. Newbury Park, CA, Sage, 1987

Kazdin AE: Practitioner review: psychosocial treatments for conduct disorder in children. J Child Psychol Psychiatry 38:161–178, 1997

Kazdin AE, Bass D, Siegel T, et al: Cognitive-behavioral therapy and relationship therapy in the treatment of children referred for antisocial behavior. J Consult Clin Psychol 57:522–535, 1989

Kendall PC: Treating anxiety disorders in children: results of a randomized clinical trial. J Consult Clin Psychol 62:100–110, 1994

Kendall PC, Brady EU, Verduin TL: Comorbidity in childhood anxiety disorders and treatment outcome. J Am Acad Child Adolesc Psychiatry 40:787–794, 2001

Kernberg PF, Chazan SE: Children With Conduct Disorders: A Psychotherapy Manual. New York, Basic Books, 1991

Khan S, Hyman PE, Cocjin J, et al: Rumination syndrome in adolescents. J Pediatr 136: 528–531, 2000

Khemka I, Hickson L: Decision-making by adults with mental retardation in simulated situations of abuse. Ment Retard 38: 15–26, 2000

King BH, DeAntonio C, McCracken JT, et al: Psychiatric consultation in severe and profound mental retardation. Am J Psychiatry 151:1802–1808, 1994

King NJ, Tonge BJ, Heyne D, et al: Cognitive-behavioral treatment of school-refusing children: a controlled evaluation. J Am Acad Child Adolesc Psychiatry 37:395–403, 1998

Kirk J, Rasmussen PV, Rittig S, et al: Provoked enuresis-like episodes in healthy children 7 to 12 years old. J Urol 156:210–213, 1996

Klein RG, Last CG: Anxiety Disorders in Children. Newbury Park, CA, Sage, 1989

Klein RG, Koplewicz HS, Kanner A: Imipramine treatment of children with separation anxiety disorder. J Am Acad Child Adolesc Psychiatry 31:21–28, 1992

Klin A, Volkmar FR, Sparrow SS (eds): Asperger Syndrome. New York, Guilford, 2000

Kolvin I, Fundudis T: Elective mute children: psychological development and background factors. J Child Psychol Psychiatry 22:219–232, 1981

Kopp S, Gillberg C: Selective mutism: a population-based study: a research note. J Child Psychol Psychiatry 38:257–262, 1997

Kosar A, Arikan N, Dincel C: Effectiveness of oxybutynin hydrochloride in the treatment of enuresis nocturna: a clinical and urodynamic study. Scand J Urol Nephrol 33:115–118, 1999

Kovacs M, Paulauskas S, Gatsonis C, et al: Depressive disorders in childhood, III: a longitudinal study of comorbidity with and risk for conduct disorders. J Affect Disord 15:205–217, 1988

Kozinetz CA, Skender ML, MacNaughton N, et al: Epidemiology of Rett syndrome: a population-based registry. Pediatrics 91: 445–450, 1993

Kranzler HR: Use of buspirone in an adolescent with overanxious disorder. J Am Acad Child Adolesc Psychiatry 27:789–790, 1988

Kristensen H: Selective mutism and comorbidity with developmental disorder/delay, anxiety disorder, and elimination disorder. J Am Acad Child Adolesc Psychiatry 39: 249–256, 2000

Krohn DD, Weckstein SM, Wright HL: A study of the effectiveness of a specific treatment for elective mutism. J Am Acad Child Adolesc Psychiatry 31:711–718, 1992

Kumpulainen K, Rasanen E, Raaska H, et al: Selective mutism among second-graders in elementary school. Eur Child Adolesc Psychiatry 7:24–29, 1998

Kuperman S, Johnson B, Arndt S, et al: Quantitative EEG differences in a nonclinical sample of children with ADHD and undifferentiated ADD. J Am Acad Child Adolesc Psychiatry 35:1009–1017, 1996

Kurlan R (ed): Handbook of Tourette's Syndrome and Related Tic and Behavioral Disorders. New York, Marcel Dekker, 1993

Kurlan R, Lichter D, Hewitt D: Sensory tics in Tourette's syndrome. Neurology 39:731–734, 1989

Kurlan R, Majumdar L, Deeley C, et al: A controlled trial of propoxyphene and naltrexone in patients with Tourette's syndrome. Ann Neurol 30:19–23, 1991

Kwak CH, Hanna PA, Jankovic J: Botulinum toxin in the treatment of tics. Arch Neurol 57:1190–1193, 2000

Labbe EE, Williamson DA: Behavioral treatment of elective mutism: a review of the literature. Clin Psychol Rev 4:273–294, 1984

Lachiewicz AM, Spiridigliozzi GA, Gullion CM, et al: Aberrant behaviors of young boys with fragile X syndrome. Am J Ment Retard 98:567–579, 1994

Lahey BB, Schaughency EA, Hynd GW, et al: Attention deficit disorder with and without hyperactivity: comparison of behavioral characteristics of clinic-referred children. J Am Acad Child Adolesc Psychiatry 26:718–723, 1987

Lahey BB, Hartdagen S, Frick PJ, et al: Conduct disorder: parsing the confounded relation to parental divorce and antisocial personality. J Abnorm Psychol 97:334–337, 1988a

Lahey BB, Loeber R, Quay HC, et al: Validity of DSM-IV subtypes of conduct disorder based on age of onset. J Am Acad Child Adolesc Psychiatry 37:435–442, 1998c

Landesman S, Vietze P: Living Environments and Mental Retardation. Washington, DC, American Association on Mental Deficiency, 1987

Langbehn DR, Cadoret RJ, Yates WR, et al: Distinct contributions of conduct and appositional defiant symptoms to adult antisocial behavior: evidence from an adoption study. Arch Gen Psychiatry 55:821–829, 1998

Lara DR, Belmonte-de-Abreu P, Souza DO: Allopurinol for refractory aggression and self-inflicted behaviour. J Psychopharmacol 14:81–83, 2000

Largo RH, Graf S, Kundu S, et al: Predicting developmental outcome at school age from infant tests of normal, at-risk, and retarded infants. Dev Med Child Neurol 32:30–45, 1990

Larson SA, Lakin KC, Anderson L, et al: Prevalence of mental retardation and developmental disabilities: estimates from the 1994/1995 National Health Interview Survey Disability Supplements. Am J Ment Retard 106:231–252, 2001

Last CG, Francis G, Hersen M, et al: Separation anxiety and school phobia: a comparison using DSM-III criteria. Am J Psychiatry 144:653–657, 1987

Last CG, Perrin S, Hersen M, et al: DSM-III-R anxiety disorders in children: sociodemographic and clinical characteristics. J Am Acad Child Adolesc Psychiatry 31: 1070–1076, 1992

Latz SR, McCracken JT: Neuroleptic malignant syndrome in children and adolescents: two case reports and a warning. J Child Adolesc Psychopharmacol 2:123–129, 1992

Lavigne JV, Burns WJ, Cotter PD: Rumination in infancy: recent behavioral approaches. Int J Eat Disord 1:70–82, 1981

Leckman JF, Zhang H, Vitale A, et al: Course of tic severity in Tourette syndrome: the first two decades. Pediatrics 102:14–19, 1998

Lefton-Greif MA, Loughlin GM: Specialized studies in pediatric dysphagia. Semin Speech Lang 17:311–329, 1996

Levin ED, Conners CK, Sparrow E, et al: Nicotine effects on adults with attention-deficit/hyperactivity disorder. Psychopharmacology (Berl) 123:55–63, 1996

Levine MD: Encopresis: its potentiation, evaluation, and alleviation. Pediatr Clin North Am 29:315–330, 1982

Levine MD, Oberklaid F, Meltzer LJ: Developmental output failure: a study of low productivity in school-aged children. Pediatrics 67:18–25, 1981

Levy F, Farrow M: Working memory in ADHD: prefrontal/parietal connections. Current Drug Targets 2:347–352, 2001

Lewis C, Hitch GJ, Walker P: The prevalence of specific arithmetic difficulties and specific reading difficulties in 9 to 10 year old and girls. J Child Psychol Psychiatry 35: 283–292, 1994

Lewis DO, Pincus JH, Bard B, et al: Neuropsychiatric, psychoeducational and family characteristics of 14 juveniles condemned to death in the United States. Am J Psychiatry 145:584–589, 1988

Lindberg B: Understanding Rett Syndrome: A Practical Guide for Parents, Teachers, and Therapists. Göttingen, Germany, Hogrefe & Huber, 1992

Livingston R, Taylor JL, Crawford SL: A study of somatic complaints and psychiatric diagnosis in children. J Am Acad Child Adolesc Psychiatry 27:185–187, 1988

Livingston RL, Dykman RA, Ackerman PT: Psychiatric comorbidity and response to two doses of methylphenidate in children with attention deficit disorder. J Child Adolesc Psychopharmacol 2:115–122, 1992

Loeber R: The stability of antisocial and delinquent childhood behavior. Child Dev 53: 1431–1446, 1982

Loeber R, Green SM, Lahey BB, et al: Findings on disruptive behavior disorders from the first decade of the developmental trends study. Clinical Child and Family Psychology Review Vol 3, 2000

Loening-Baucke V: Encopresis and soiling. Pediatr Clin North Am 43:279–298, 1996

Lou HC: Etiology and pathogenesis of attention-deficit hyperactivity disorder (ADHD): significance of prematurity and perinatal hypoxic-haemodynamic encephalopathy. Acta Paediatr 85:1266–1271, 1996

Lou HC, Henriksen L, Bruhn P, et al: Striatal dysfunction in attention deficit and hyperkinetic disorder. Arch Neurol 46:48–52, 1989

Lou HC, Andresen J, Steinberg B, et al: The striatum in a putative cerebral network activated by verbal awareness in normals and in ADHD children. Eur J Neurol 5: 67–74, 1998

Lynskey MT, Fergusson DM: Childhood conduct problems, attention deficit behaviors, and adolescent alcohol, tobacco, and illicit drug use. J Abnorm Child Psychol 23:281–302, 1995

Manassis K, Bradley S: Fluoxetine in anxiety disorders. J Am Acad Child Adolesc Psychiatry 33:761–762, 1994

Mancini C, van Ameringen M, Szatmari P, et al: A high-risk pilot study of the children of adults with social phobia. J Am Acad Child Adolesc Psychiatry 35:1511–1517, 1996

Manicavasagar V, Silove D, Curtis J, et al: Continuities of separation anxiety from early life into adulthood. J Anxiety Disord 14: 1–18, 2000

Manikam R, Perman JA: Pediatric feeding disorders. J Clin Gastroenterol 30:34–46, 2000

Marchi M, Cohen P: Early childhood eating behaviors and adolescent eating disorders. J Am Acad Child Adolesc Psychiatry 29: 112–117, 1990

Marcus J, Hans SL, Mednick SA, et al: Neurological dysfunctioning in offspring of schizophrenics in Israel and Denmark. Arch Gen Psychiatry 42:753–761, 1985

Martin JAM: Syndrome delineation in communication disorders, in Language and Language Disorders in Children. Edited by Hersov LA, Berger M. Oxford, England, Pergamon, 1980

Masi B, Mucci M, Millepiedi S: Separation anxiety disorder in children and adolescents: epidemiology, diagnosis, and management. CNS Drugs 15:93–104, 2001

Masi G, Favilla L, Mucci M: Generalized anxiety disorder in adolescents and young adults with mild mental retardation. Psychiatry 63:54–64, 2000a

Mataro M, Garcia-Sanchez C, Junque C, et al: Magnetic resonance imaging measurement of the caudate nucleus in adolescents with attention-deficit hyperactivity disorder and its relationship with neuropsychological and behavioral measures. Arch Neurol 54:963–968, 1997

Matochik JA, Liebenauer LL, King AC, et al: Cerebral glucose metabolism in adults with attention deficit hyperactivity disorder after chronic stimulant treatment. Am J Psychiatry 151:658–664, 1994

Matson JL, Bamburg JW, Mayville EA, et al: Psychopharmacology and mental retardation: a 10 year review (1990–1999). Res Dev Disabil 21:263–296, 2000

Matthys W, Van Loo P, Pachen V, et al: Behavior of conduct disordered children in interaction with each other and with normal peers. Child Psychiatry Hum Dev 25: 183–195, 1995

Max JE, Castillo CS, Bokura H, et al: Oppositional defiant disorder symptomatology after traumatic brain injury: a prospective study. J Nerv Ment Dis 186:325–332, 1998

Mayes SD, Humphrey FJ 2d, Handford HA, et al: Rumination disorder: differential diagnosis. J Am Acad Child Adolesc Psychiatry 27:300–302, 1988

McCartney JR, Campbell VA: Confirmed abuse cases in public residential facilities for persons with mental retardation: a multi-state study. Ment Retard 36:465–473, 1998

McDougle CJ, Holmes JP, Bronson MR, et al: Risperidone treatment of children and adolescents with pervasive developmental disorders: a prospective open-label study. J Am Acad Child Adolesc Psychiatry 36: 685–693, 1997

McDougle CJ, Holmes JP, Carlson DC, et al: A double-blind, placebo-controlled study of risperidone in adults with autistic disorder and other pervasive developmental disorders. Arch Gen Psychiatry 55:633–641, 1998

McGillicuddy NB, Blane HT: Substance use in individuals with mental retardation. Addict Behav 24:869–878, 1999

McGrath ML, Mellon MW, Murphy L: Empirically supported treatments in pediatric psychology: constipation and encopresis. J Pediatr Psychol 25:225–254, 2000

McKee JR, Bodfish JW: Sudden unexpected death in epilepsy in adults with mental retardation. Am J Ment Retard 105:229–235, 2000

McKelvey JR, Lambert R, Mottron L, et al: Right-hemisphere dysfunction in Asperger's syndrome. J Child Neurol 10:310–314, 1995

Mendelowitz SL, Manassis K, Bradley S, et al: Cognitive-behavioral group treatments in childhood anxiety disorder: the role of parental involvement. J Am Acad Child Adolesc Psychiatry 38:1223–1229, 1999

Menolascino FJ, Levitas A, Greiner C: The nature and types of mental illness in the mentally retarded. Psychopharmacol Bull 22:1060–1071, 1986

Michelson D, Faries D, Wernicke J, et al: Atomoxetine in the treatment of children and adolescents with attention-deficit/hyperactivity disorder: a randomized, placebo-controlled, dose-response study (abstract). Pediatrics 108:E83, 2001

Michelson D, Adler L, Spencer T, et al: Atomoxetine in adults with ADHD: two randomized, placebo-controlled studies. Biol Psychiatry 53:112–120, 2003

Miguel EC, do Rosario-Campos MC, Prado HS, et al: Sensory phenomena in obsessive-compulsive disorder and Tourette's disorder. J Clin Psychiatry 61:150–156, 2000

Milberger S, Biederman J, Faraone SV, et al: Is maternal smoking during pregnancy a risk factor for attention deficit hyperactivity disorder in children? Am J Psychiatry 153: 1138–1142, 1996

Miller LT, Missiuna CA, Macnab JJ, et al: Clinical description of children with developmental coordination disorder. Canadian Journal of Occupational Therapy 68:5–15, 2001a

Millican FK, Layman EM, Lourie RS, et al: Study of an oral fixation: pica. Journal of the American Academy of Child Psychiatry 7:79–107, 1968

Missiuna C (ed): Children With Developmental Coordination Disorder: Strategies for Success. New York, Haworth, 2001

Mitchell EA, Aman MG, Turbott SH, et al: Clinical characteristics and serum essential fatty acid levels in hyperactive children. Clin Pediatr 26:406–411, 1987

Miyahara M, Mobs I: Developmental dyspraxia and developmental coordination disorder. Neuropsychol Rev 5:245–268, 1995

Moeschler JB, Charman CD, Berg SZ, et al.: Rett syndrome: natural history and management. Pediatrics 82:1–10, 1988

Molteni M, Moretti G: Minor psychiatric disorders as possible complication of mental retardation. Psychopathology 32:107–112, 1999

Mouridsen SE, Rich B, Isager T: Validity of childhood disintegrative psychosis: general findings of a long-term follow-up study. Br J Psychiatry 172:263–267, 1998

Mouridsen SE, Rich B, Isager T: Epilepsy in disintegrative psychosis and infantile autism: a long-term validation study. Dev Med Child Neurol 41:110–114, 1999a

Mouridsen SE, Rich B, Isager T: The natural history of somatic morbidity in disintegrative psychosis and infantile autism: a validation study. Brain Dev 21:447–452, 1999b

Mouridsen SE, Rich B, Isager T: A comparative study of genetic and neurobiological findings in disintegrative psychosis and infantile autism. Psychiatry Clin Neurosci 54: 441–446, 2000

MTA Cooperative Group: A 14-month randomized clinical trial of treatment strategies for attention-deficit/hyperactivity disorder. The MTA Cooperative Group: Multimodal Treatment Study of Children With ADHD. Arch Gen Psychiatry 56: 1073–1086, 1999a

Muris P, Mayer B, Bartelds E, et al: The revised version of the Screen for Child Anxiety Related Emotional Disorders (SCARED-R): treatment sensitivity in an early intervention trial for childhood anxiety disorders. Br J Clin Psychol 40:323–336, 2001

Murphy TK, Goodman WK, Fudge MW, et al: B lymphocyte antigen D8/17: a peripheral marker for childhood-onset obsessive-compulsive disorder and Tourette's syndrome? Am J Psychiatry 154:402–407, 1997

Naidu S, Hyman S, Harris EL, et al: Rett syndrome studies of natural history and search for a genetic marker. Neuropediatrics 26:63–66, 1995

National Institute of Mental Health (NIMH) Consensus Statement: Diagnosis and treatment of attention deficit hyperactivity disorder (ADHD). NIH Consens Statement 16:1–37, 1998

Needleman HL, Riess JA, Tobin MJ, et al: Bone lead levels and delinquent behavior. JAMA 275:363–369, 1996

Nelson KB: Prenatal and perinatal factors in the etiology of autism. Pediatrics 87 (suppl):761–766, 1991

Nelson KB, Ellenberg JH: Antecedents of cerebral palsy: multivariate analysis of risk. N Engl J Med 315:81–86, 1986

Neveus T, Lackgren G, Tuvemo T, et al: Enuresis: background and treatment. Scand J Urol Nephrol Suppl 206:1–44, 2000

Newcorn JH, Strain J: Adjustment disorder in children and adolescents. J Am Acad Child Adolesc Psychiatry 31:318–327, 1992

Niehaus DJ, Emsley RA, Brink P, et al: Stereotypies: prevalence and association with compulsive and impulsive symptoms in college students. Psychopathology 33:31–35, 2000

Nopoulos P, Berg S, Castellenos FX, et al: Developmental brain anomalies in children with attention-deficit hyperactivity disorder. J Child Neurol 15:102–108, 2000

Nurko S, Garcia-Aranda JA, Worona LB, et al: Cisapride for the treatment of constipation in children: a double-blind study. J Pediatr 136:35–40, 2000

O'Connor KP, Brault M, Robillard S, et al: Evaluation of a cognitive-behavioural program for the management of chronic tic and habit disorders. Behav Res Ther 39:667–681, 2001

Onofrj M, Paci C, D'Andreamatteo G, et al: Olanzapine in severe Gilles de la Tourette syndrome: a 52-week double-blind crossover study vs. low-dose pimozide. J Neurol 247:443–446, 2000

Oosterlaan J, Sergeant JA: Inhibition in ADHD, aggressive, and anxious children: a biologically based model of child psychopathology. J Abnorm Child Psychol 24:19–36, 1996

Owen SE, McKinlay IA: Motor difficulties in children with developmental disorders of speech and language. Child Care Health Dev 23:315–325, 1997

Owley T, McMahon W, Cook EH, et al: Multisite, double-blind, placebo-controlled trial of porcine secretin in autism. J Am Acad Child Adolesc Psychiatry 40:1293–1299, 2001

Pace GM, Toyer EA: The effects of a vitamin supplement on the pica of a child with severe mental retardation. J Appl Behav Anal 33:619–622, 2000

Paden EP, Yairi E: Phonological characteristics of children whose stuttering persisted or recovered. J Speech Hear Res 39:981–990, 1996

Paden EP, Yairi E, Ambrose NG: Early childhood stuttering, II: initial status of phonological abilities. J Speech Lang Hear Res 42:1113–1124, 1999

Parry-Jones B: Merycism or rumination disorder: a historical investigation and current assessment. Br J Psychiatry 165:303–314, 1994

Patterson GR: Coercive Family Processes. Eugene, OR, Castalia, 1982

Paul R, Cohen D, Caparulo B: A longitudinal study of patients with severe, specific developmental language disorders. Journal of the American Academy of Child Psychiatry 22:525–534, 1994

Pauls DL: Genetic factors in the expression of attention-deficit hyperactivity disorder. J Child Adolesc Psychopharmacol 1:353–360, 1991

Pauls DL, Leckman JF: The inheritance of Gilles de la Tourette's syndrome and associated behaviors. N Engl J Med 315:993–997, 1986

Pearson DA, Lachar D, Loveland KA, et al: Patterns of behavioral adjustment and maladjustment in mental retardation: comparison of children with and without ADHD. Am J Ment Retard 105:236–251, 2000

Pelcovitz D, Kaplan SJ, DeRosa RR, et al: Psychiatric disorders in adolescents exposed to domestic violence and physical abuse. Am J Orthopsychiatry 70:360–369, 2000

Pelham WE, Carlson C, Sams SE, et al: Separate and combined effects of methylphenidate and behavior modification of boys with attention deficit hyperactivity disorder in the classroom. J Consult Clin Psychol 61:506–515, 1993

Perrin S, Last CG: Relationship between ADHD and anxiety in boys: results from a family study. J Am Acad Child Adolesc Psychiatry 35:988–996, 1996

Perry CA, Dwyer J, Gelfand JA, et al: Health effects of salicylates in foods and drugs. Nutr Rev 54:225–240, 1996

Peterson BS, Leckman JF, Tucker D, et al: Preliminary findings of antistreptococcal antibody titers and basal ganglia volumes in tic, obsessive-compulsive, and attention deficit/hyperactivity disorders. Arch Gen Psychiatry 57:364–372, 2000

Peterson BS, Pine DS, Cohen P, et al: Prospective, longitudinal study of tic, obsessive-compulsive, and attention-deficit/hyperactivity disorders in an epidemiological sample. J Am Acad Child Adolesc Psychiatry 40:685–695, 2001a

Petryshen TL, Kaplan BJ, Liu MF, et al: Absence of significant linkage between phonological coding dyslexia and chromosome 6p23–21.3, as determined by use of quantitative-trait methods: confirmation of qualitative analyses. Am J Hum Genet 66:708–714, 2000

Petryshen TL, Kaplan BJ, Fu Liu M, et al: Evidence for a susceptibility locus on chromosome 6q influencing phonological coding dyslexia. Am J Med Genet 105:507–517, 2001

Piven J, Palmer P: Psychiatric disorder and the broad autism phenotype: evidence from a family study of multiple-incidence autism families. Am J Psychiatry 156:557–563, 1999

Piven J, Palmer P, Jacobi D, et al: Broader autism phenotype: evidence from a family history study of multiple-incidence autism families. Am J Psychiatry 154:185–190, 1997b

Pliszka SR, McCracken JT, Maas JW: Catecholamines in attention-deficit hyperactivity disorder: current perspectives. J Am Acad Child Adolesc Psychiatry 35:264–272, 1996

Pomerleau OF, Downey KK, Stelson FW, et al: Cigarette smoking in adult patients diagnosed with attention deficit hyperactivity disorder. J Subst Abuse 7:373–378, 1995

Popper CW, Elliott GR: Sudden death and tricyclic antidepressants: clinical considerations for children. J Child Adolesc Psychopharmacol 1:125–132, 1990

Prassopoulos P, Cavouras D, Ioannidou M, et al: Study of subarachnoid spaces in children with idiopathic mental retardation. J Child Neurol 11:197–200, 1996

Pretlow RA: Treatment of nocturnal enuresis with an ultrasound bladder volume controlled alarm device. J Urol 162:1224–1228, 1999

Pueyo R, Maneru C, Vendrell P, et al: Attention deficit hyperactivity disorder: cerebral asymmetry observed on magnetic resonance. Rev Neurol 30:920–925, 2000

Purvis KL, Tannock R: Language abilities in children with attention deficit hyperactivity disorder, reading abilities, and normal controls. J Abnorm Child Psychol 25:133–144, 1997

Purvis KL, Tannock R: Phonological processing, not inhibitory control, differentiates ADHD and reading disability. J Am Acad Child Adolesc Psychiatry 39:485–494, 2000

Rapin I: Autistic children: diagnosis and clinical features. Pediatrics 87 (suppl):751–760, 1991

Rapoport JL, Buchsbaum MS, Weingartner H, et al: Dextroamphetamine: its cognitive and behavioral effects in normal and hyperactive boys and normal men. Arch Gen Psychiatry 37:933–943, 1980

Rapoport JL, Conners CK, Reatig N: Rating scales and assessment instruments for use in pediatric psychopharmacology research. Psychopharmacol Bull 21:713–1125, 1985

Rapoport JL, Castellanos FX, Gogate N, et al: Imaging normal and abnormal brain development: new perspectives for child psychiatry. Aust N Z J Psychiatry 35:272–281, 2001

Rasquin-Weber A, Hyman PE, Cucchiara S, et al: Childhood functional gastrointestinal disorders. Gut 45:II60–II68, 1999

Raynaud C, Billard C, Tzongrig H, et al: Study of rCBF developmental dysphasia children at rest and during verbal stimulation. J Cereb Blood Flow Metab 1 (suppl):S323, 1989

Reid AH, Ballinger BR: Behaviour symptoms among severely and profoundly mentally retarded patients: a 16–18 year follow-up study. Br J Psychiatry 167:452–455, 1995

Reis S: Rumination in two developmentally normal children: case report and review of the literature. J Fam Pract 38:521–523, 1994

Research Unit on Pediatric Psychopharmacology Anxiety Study Group: Fluvoxamine for the treatment of anxiety disorders in children and adolescents. N Engl J Med 344: 1279–1285, 2001

Richards TL, Corina D, Serafini S, et al: The effects of phonologically driven treatment for dyslexia on lactate levels as measured by proton MSRI. Am J Neuroradiol 25: 40–47, 2000

Riddle MA, Nelson JC, Kleinman CS, et al: Sudden death in children receiving Norpramin: a review of three reported cases and commentary. J Am Acad Child Adolesc Psychiatry 30:104–108, 1991

Riddle MA, Lynch KA, Scahill L, et al: Methylphenidate discontinuation and reinitiation during long-term treatment of children with Tourette's disorder and attention-deficit/hyperactivity disorder: a pilot study. J Child Adolesc Psychopharmacol 5:205–214, 1995

Rittig S, Knudsen UB, Norgaard JP, et al: Abnormal diurnal rhythm of plasma vasopressin and urinary output in patients with enuresis. Am J Physiol 256:F664–F671, 1989

Roberts JW, Dickey P: Exposure of children to pollutants in house dust and indoor air. Rev Environ Contam Toxicol 143:59–78, 1995

Roberts W, Weaver L, Brian J, et al: Repeated doses of porcine secretin in the treatment of autism: a randomized, placebo-controlled trial. Pediatrics 107:E71, 2001

Robertson J, Emerson E, Gregory N, et al: Social networks of people with mental retardation in residential settings. Ment Retard 39:201–214, 2001

Robertson MM, Trimble MR, Lees AJ: Self-injurious behaviour and the Gilles de la Tourette syndrome: a clinical study and review of the literature. Psychol Med 19: 611–625, 1989

Robins LN: Deviant Children Grown Up. Baltimore, MD, Williams & Wilkins, 1966

Rockney RM, McQuade WH, Days AL, et al: Encopresis treatment outcome: long-term follow-up of 45 cases. J Dev Behav Pediatr 17:380–385, 1996

Roizen NJ, Blondis TA, Irwin M, et al: Adaptive functioning in children with attention-deficit hyperactivity disorder. Arch Pediatr Adolesc Med 148:1137–1142, 1994

Rourke BP: Arithmetic disabilities, specific and otherwise: a neuropsychological perspective. J Learn Disabil 26:214–226, 1993

Rourke BP, Strang JD: Subtypes of reading and arithmetic disabilities: a neuropsychological analysis, in Developmental Neuropsychiatry. Edited by Rutter M. New York, Guilford, 1983

Rowe DC, Stever C, Gard JM, et al: The relation of the dopamine transporter gene (DAT1) to symptoms of internalizing disorders in children. Behav Genet 28:215–225, 1998

Rucklidge JJ, Tannock R: Psychiatric, psychosocial, and cognitive functioning of female adolescents with ADHD. J Am Acad Child Adolesc Psychiatry 40:530–540, 2001

Rumsey JM, Rapoport JL, Sceery WR: Autistic children as adults: psychiatric, social, and behavioral outcomes. Journal of the American Academy of Child Psychiatry 24:465–473, 1985a

Rutter M, Giller H: Juvenile Delinquency: Trends and Perspectives. New York, Guilford, 1984

Rutter M, Yule W: The concept of specific reading retardation. J Child Psychol Psychiatry 16:181–197, 1975

Rutter M, Anderson-Wood L, Beckett C, et al: Quasi-autistic patterns following severe early global privation. J Child Psychol Psychiatry 40:537–550, 1999

Ryan R, Sunada K: Medical evaluation of persons with mental retardation referred for psychiatric assessment. Gen Hosp Psychiatry 19:274–280, 1997

Rydelius A: The development of antisocial behavior and sudden violent death. Acta Psychiatr Scand 77:398–403, 1988

Sakamoto K, Blaivas JG: Adult onset nocturnal enuresis. J Urol 165:1914–1917, 2001

Sallee FR, Kurlan R, Goetz CG, et al: Ziprasidone treatment of children and adolescents with Tourette's syndrome: a pilot study. J Am Acad Child Adolesc Psychiatry 39:292–299, 2000

Sampson RJ, Raudenbusch SW, Earls F: Neighborhoods and violent crime: a multilevel study of collective efficacy. Science 277:918–924, 1997

Sauvage D, Leddet I, Hameury L, et al: Infantile rumination: diagnosis and follow-up of twenty cases. Journal of the American Academy of Child Psychiatry 24:197–203, 1985

Scahill L, Chappell PB, Kim YS, et al: A placebo-controlled study of guanfacine in the treatment of children with tic disorders and attention deficit hyperactivity disorder. Am J Psychiatry 158:1067–1074, 2001

Schroeder S, Schroeder C, Smith B, et al: Prevalence of self-injurious behaviors in a large state facility for the retarded: a three-year follow-up study. Journal of Autism and Childhood Schizophrenia 8:261–269, 1979

Schubiner H, Tzelepis A, Milberger S, et al: Prevalence of attention-deficit/hyperactivity disorder and conduct disorder among substance abusers. J Clin Psychiatry 61:244–251, 2000

Schulte-Körne G, Deimel W, Gutenbrunner C, et al: Effect of an oligo-antigen diet on the behavior of hyperkinetic children [in German]. Zeitschrift fur Kinder und Jugendpsychiatrie 24:176–183, 1996

Schvehla TJ, Mandoki MW, Sumner GS: Clonidine therapy for comorbid attention deficit hyperactivity disorder and conduct disorder: preliminary findings in a children's inpatient unit. South Med J 87:692–695, 1994

Schweitzer JB, Faber TL, Grafton ST, et al: Alterations in the functional anatomy of working memory in adult attention deficit hyperactivity disorder. Am J Psychiatry 157:278–280, 2000

Seltzer MM, Krauss MW, Hong J, et al: Continuity or discontinuity of family involvement following residential transitions of adults who have mental retardation. Ment Retard 39:181–194, 2001

Semrud-Clikeman M: Evidence from imaging on the relationship between brain structure and developmental language disorders. Semin Pediatr Neurol 4:117–124, 1997

Semrud-Clikeman M, Hynd GW: Right hemispheric dysfunction in nonverbal learning disabilities: social, academic, and adaptive functioning in adults and children. Psychol Bull 107:196–209, 1990

Seuchter SA, Hebebrand J, Klug B, et al: Complex segregation analysis of families ascertained through Gilles de la Tourette syndrome. Genet Epidemiol 18:33–47, 2000

Sever Y, Ashkenazi A, Tyano S, et al: Iron treatment in children with attention deficit hyperactivity disorder: a preliminary report. Neuropsychobiology 35:178–180, 1997

Shaffer D, Gould MS, Brasic J, et al: A Children's Global Assessment Scale (CGAS). Arch Gen Psychiatry 40:1228–1231, 1983

Shah MR, Seese LM, Abikoff H, et al: Pemoline for children and adolescents with conduct disorder: a pilot investigation. J Child Adolesc Psychopharmacol 4:255–261, 1994

Shalev RS, Manor O, Amir N, et al: Developmental dyscalculia and brain laterality. Cortex 31:357–365, 1995

Shalev RS, Manor O, Gross-Tsur V: Neuropsychological aspects of developmental dyscalculia. Math Cognition 33:105–120, 1997

Shalev RS, Auerbach J, Manor O, et al: Developmental dyscalculia: prevalence and prognosis. Eur Child Adolesc Psychiatry 9 (suppl 2):58–64, 2000

Shalev RS, Manor O, Kerem B, et al: Developmental dyscalculia is a familial learning disability. J Learn Disabil 34:59–65, 2001

Sharp WS, Walter JM, Marsh WL, et al: ADHD in girls: clinical comparability of a research sample. J Am Acad Child Adolesc Psychiatry 38:40–47, 1999

Shaywitz SE, Shaywitz BA, Fletcher JM, et al: Prevalence of reading disability in boys and girls: results of the Connecticut Longitudinal Study. JAMA 264:998–1002, 1990

Shaywitz SE, Shaywitz BA, Pugh KR, et al: Functional disruption in the organization of the brain for reading in dyslexia. Proc Natl Acad Sci U S A 95:2636–2641, 1998

Sheppard DM, Bradshaw JL, Purcell R, et al: Tourette's and comorbid syndromes: obsessive compulsive and attention deficit hyperactivity disorder: a common etiology? Clin Psychol Rev 19:531–552, 1999

Sherman DK, Iacono WG, McGue MK: Attention-deficit hyperactivity disorder dimensions: a twin study of inattention and impulsivity-hyperactivity. J Am Acad Child Adolesc Psychiatry 36:745–753, 1997

Sigman M (ed): Children With Emotional Disorders and Developmental Disabilities: Assessment and Treatment. Orlando, FL, Grune & Stratton, 1985

Silove D, Harris M, Morgan A, et al: Is early separation anxiety a specific precursor of panic disorder-agoraphobia? A community study. Psychol Med 25:405–411, 1995

Silvany-Neto AM, Carvalho FM, Tavares TM, et al: Lead poisoning among children of Santo Amaro, Bahia, Brazil in 1980, 1985, and 1992. Bulletin of the Pan American Health Organization 30:51–62, 1996

Silver AA, Shytle RD, Sheehan KH, et al: Multicenter, double-blind, placebo-controlled study of mecamylamine monotherapy for Tourette's disorder. J Am Acad Child Adolesc Psychiatry 40:1103–1110, 2001

Simeon JG, Ferguson HB, Knott V, et al: Clinical, cognitive, and neurophysiological effects of alprazolam in children and adolescents with overanxious and avoidant disorder. J Am Acad Child Adolesc Psychiatry 31:29–33, 1992

Simon SL: Soil ingestion by humans: a review of history, data, and etiology with application to risk assessment of radioactively contaminated soil. Health Phys 74:647–672, 1998

Singer HS, Brown J, Quaskey S, et al: The treatment of attention-deficit hyperactivity disorder in Tourette's syndrome: a double-blind placebo-controlled study with clonidine and desipramine. Pediatrics 95:74–81, 1995

Singer HS, Giuliano JD, Hansen BH, et al: Antibodies against human putamen in children with Tourette syndrome. Neurology 50:1618–1624, 1998

Singer HS, Giuliano JD, Zimmerman AM, et al: Infection: a stimulus for tic disorders. Pediatr Neurol 22:380–383, 2000

Singer HS, Wendlandt J, Krieger M, et al: Baclofen treatment in Tourette syndrome: a double-blind, placebo-controlled, crossover trial. Neurology 56:599–604, 2001

Skjeldal OH, von Tetzchner S, Aspelund F, et al: Rett syndrome: geographic variation in prevalence in Norway. Brain Dev 19:258–261, 1997

Skoog SJ, Stokes A, Turner KL: Oral desmopressin: a randomized double-blind placebo controlled study of effectiveness in children with primary nocturnal enuresis. J Urol 158:1035–1040, 1997

Snowling M, Bishop DV, Stothard SE: Is preschool language impairment a risk factor for dyslexia in adolescence? J Child Psychol Psychiatry 41:587–600, 2000

Sokol MS, Gray NS: An infection-triggered, autoimmune subtype of anorexia nervosa. J Am Acad Child Adolesc Psychiatry 36:1128–1133, 1997

Soussignan R, Tremblay R: Other disorders of conduct, in Hyperactivity Disorders of Childhood. Edited by Sandberg S. Cambridge, England, Cambridge University Press, 1996

Southam-Gerow MA, Kendall PC, Weersing VR: Examining outcome variability: correlates of treatment response in a child and adolescent anxiety clinic. J Clin Child Psychol 30:422–436, 2001

Sparrow SS, Balla DA, Cicchetti DV: Vineland Adaptive Behavior Scales. Circle Pines, MN, American Guidance Service, 1984

Speltz ML, Coy K, DeKlyen M, et al: Early onset oppositional defiant disorder: what factors predict its course? Seminars in Clinical Neuropsychiatry 3:302–319, 1998

Speltz ML, McClellan J, DeKlyen M, et al: Preschool boys with oppositional defiant disorder: clinical presentation and diagnostic change. J Am Acad Child Adolesc Psychiatry 38:838–845, 1999

Spencer J, O'Brien J, Riggs K, et al: Motion processing in autism: evidence for a dorsal stream deficiency. Neuroreport 11:2765–2767, 2000

Spencer T, Biederman J, Wilens TE, et al: Adults with attention-deficit/hyperactivity disorder: a controversial diagnosis. J Clin Psychiatry 59 (suppl 7):59–68, 1998a

Spencer T, Biederman J, Harding M, et al: Disentangling the overlap between Tourette's disorder and ADHD. J Child Psychol Psychiatry 39:1037–1044, 1998b

Spencer T, Biederman J, Wilens T: Growth deficits in children with attention deficit hyperactivity disorder. Pediatrics 102:501–506, 1998c

Spencer T, Biederman J, Wilens T: Attention-deficit hyperactivity disorder and comorbidity. Pediatr Clin North Am 46:915–927, 1999

Spencer T, Biederman J, Wozniak J, et al: Parsing pediatric bipolar disorder from its associated comorbidity with the disruptive behavior disorders. Biol Psychiatry 49:1062–1070, 2001

Sprich S, Biederman J, Crawford MH: Adoptive and biological families of children and adolescents with ADHD. J Am Acad Child Adolesc Psychiatry 39:1432–1437, 2000

Staley D, Wand R, Shady G: Tourette disorder: a cross-cultural review. Compr Psychiatry 38:6–19, 1997

Stanovich KE, Siegel LS: Phenotypic performance profile of children with reading disabilities: a regression-based test of the phonological-core-variable-difference model. Journal of Educational Psychology 86:24–53, 1994

Stein A, Woolley H, McPherson K: Conflict between mothers with eating disorders and their infants during mealtimes. Br J Psychiatry 175:455–461, 1999

Stein MA, Sandoval R, Szumowski E, et al: Psychometric characteristics of the Wender Utah Rating Scale (WURS): reliability and factor structure for men and women. Psychopharmacol Bull 31:425–433, 1995

Steingard R, Khan A, Gonzalez A, et al: Neuroleptic malignant syndrome: review of experience with children and adolescents. J Child Adolesc Psychopharmacol 2:183–198, 1992

Steingard RJ, Zimnitzky B, DeMaso DR, et al: Sertraline treatment of transition-associated anxiety and agitation in children with autistic disorder. J Child Adolesc Psychopharmacol 7:9–15, 1997

Steinhausen HC, Adamek R: The family history of children with elective mutism: a research report. Eur Child Adolesc Psychiatry 6:107–111, 1997

Stephens RJ, Sandor P: Aggressive behaviour in children with Tourette syndrome and comorbid attention-deficit hyperactivity disorder and obsessive-compulsive disorder. Can J Psychiatry 44:1036–1042, 1999

Stern HP, Stroh SE, Fiedorek SC, et al: Increased plasma levels of pancreatic polypeptide and decreased plasma levels of motilin in encopretic children. Pediatrics 96:111–117, 1995

Stern JS, Robertson MM: Tics associated with autistic and pervasive developmental disorders. Neurol Clin 15:345–355, 1997

Stevens LJ, Zentall SS, Deck JL, et al: Essential fatty acid metabolism in boys with attention-deficit hyperactivity disorder. Am J Clin Nutr 62:761–768, 1995

Stevens LJ, Zentall SS, Abate ML, et al: Omega-3 fatty acids in boys with behavior, learning, and health problems. Physiol Behav 59:915–920, 1996

Stromme P: Aetiology in severe and mild mental retardation: a population-based study of Norwegian children. Dev Med Child Neurol 42:76–86, 2000

Stromme P, Diseth TH: Prevalence of psychiatric diagnoses in children with mental retardation: data from a population-based study. Dev Med Child Neurol 42:266–270, 2000

Stromme P, Magnus P: Correlations between socioeconomic status, IQ and aetiology in mental retardation: a population-based study of Norwegian children. Soc Psychiatry Psychiatr Epidemiol 35:12–18, 2000

Sullivan MA, Rudnik-Levin F: Attention deficit/hyperactivity disorder and substance abuse: diagnostic and therapeutic considerations. Ann N Y Acad Sci 931:251–270, 2001

Sutphen JL, Borowitz SM, Hutchison RL, et al: Long-term follow-up of medically treated childhood constipation. Clin Pediatr (Phila) 34:576–580, 1995

Swank LK: Specific developmental disorders: the language-learning continuum. Child Adolesc Psychiatr Clin North Am 8:89–112, 1999

Swanson JM, Kinsbourne M: Food dyes impair performance of hyperactive children on a laboratory learning test. Science 207: 1485–1487, 1980

Swedo SE: Sydenham's chorea: a model for childhood autoimmune neuropsychiatric disorders. JAMA 272:1788–1791, 1994

Szatmari P: The classification of autism, Asperger's syndrome, and pervasive developmental disorder. Can J Psychiatry 45: 731–738, 2000

Szatmari P, Bremner R, Nagy J: Asperger's syndrome: a review of clinical features. Can J Psychiatry 34:554–560, 1989

Szatmari P, Archer L, Fisman S, et al: Asperger's syndrome and autism: differences in behavior, cognition, and adaptive functioning. J Am Acad Child Adolesc Psychiatry 34:1662–1671, 1995

Szatmari P, Bryson SE, Streiner DL, et al: Two-year outcome of preschool children with autism or Asperger's syndrome. Am J Psychiatry 157:1980–1987, 2000

Szymanski LS: Prevention of psychosocial dysfunction in persons with mental retardation. Ment Retard 25:215–218, 1987

Szymanski L, King BH: Summary of the Practice Parameters for the Assessment and Treatment of Children, Adolescents, and Adults With Mental Retardation and Comorbid Mental Disorders. American Academy of Child and Adolescent Psychiatry. J Am Acad Child Adolesc Psychiatry 38:1606–1610, 1999

Szymanski LS, Tanguay LS (eds): Emotional Disorders of Mentally Retarded Persons. Baltimore, MD, University Park Press, 1980

Taanila A, Kokkonen J, Järvelin MR: The long-term effects of children's early onset disability on marital relationships. Dev Med Child Neurol 38:567–577, 1996

Tallal P, Hirsch LS, Realpe-Bonilla T, et al: Familial aggregation in specific language impairment. J Speech Lang Hear Res 44: 1172–1182, 2001

Tanguay PE: Pervasive developmental disorders: a 10-year review. J Am Acad Child Adolesc Psychiatry 39:1079–1095, 2000

Tannock R: Attention deficit hyperactivity disorder: advances in cognitive, neurobiological, and genetic research. J Child Psychol Psychiatry 39:65–99, 1998

Tannock R, Martinussen R, Frijters J: Naming speed performance and stimulant effects indicate effortful, semantic processing deficits in attention-deficit/hyperactivity disorder. J Abnorm Child Psychol 28:237–252, 2000

Teicher MH, Anderson CM, Polcari A, et al: Functional deficits in basal ganglia of children with attention-deficit/hyperactivity disorder shown with functional magnetic resonance imaging relaxometry. Nat Med 6:470–473, 2000

Thapar A, Gottesman II, Owen MJ, et al: The genetics of mental retardation. Br J Psychiatry 164:747–758, 1994

Thompson M, Comings DE, Feder L, et al: Mutation screening of the dopamine D1 receptor gene in Tourette's syndrome and alcohol dependent patients. Am J Med Genet 81:241–244, 1998

Thuppal M, Fink M: Electroconvulsive therapy and mental retardation. J ECT 15:140–149, 1999

Tibbits-Kleber AL, Howell RJ: Reactive attachment disorder of infancy (RAD). J Clin Child Psychol 14:304–310, 1985

Tirosh E, Cohen A: Language deficit with attention-deficit disorder: a prevalent comorbidity. J Child Neurol 13:493–497, 1998

Tizard J, Schofield WN, Hewison J: Collaboration between teachers and parents in assisting children's reading. Br J Educ Psychol 52:1–15, 1982

Tohgi H, Saitoh K, Takahashi S, et al: Graphia and acalculia after a left prefrontal (F1, F2) infarction. J Neurol Neurosurg Psychiatry 58:629–632, 1995

Tolan PH: Implications of age of onset for delinquency risk. J Abnorm Child Psychol 15:47–63, 1987

Tolan PH, Cromwell RE, Brasswell M: Family therapy with delinquents: a critical review of the literature. Fam Process 25:619–650, 1986

Tomblin JB, Smith E, Zhang X: Epidemiology of specific language impairment: prenatal and perinatal risk factors. J Commun Disord 30:325–343, 1997a

Tomblin JB, Records NL, Buckwalter P, et al: Prevalence of specific language impairment in kindergarten children. J Speech Lang Hear Res 40:1245–1260, 1997b

Tomblin JB, Zhang X, Buckwalter P, et al: The association of reading disability, behavioral disorders, and language impairment among second-grade children. J Child Psychol Psychiatry 41:473–482, 2000

Torgesen JK, Wagner RK, Rashotte CA: Longitudinal studies of phonologic processing and reading. J Learn Disabil 27:276–286, 1994

Trappe R, Laccone F, Cobilanschi J, et al: MECP2 mutations in sporadic cases of Rett syndrome are almost exclusively of paternal origin. Am J Hum Genet 68:1093–1101, 2001

Trauner D, Wulfeck B, Tallal P, et al: Neurological and MRI profiles of children with developmental language impairment. Dev Med Child Neurol 42:470–475, 2000

Tremblay RE, LeBlanc M, Schwartzman AE: The pediatric power of first-grade peer and teacher ratings of behavior: sex differences in antisocial behavior and personality at adolescence. J Abnorm Child Psychol 16:571–583, 1988

Trott GE, Friese HJ, Menzel M, et al: Use of moclobemide in children with attention deficit hyperactivity disorder. Psychopharmacology 106:S134–S136, 1992

Turner C, Panksepp J, Bekkedal M, et al: Paradoxical effects of serotonin and opioids in pemoline-induced self-injurious behavior. Pharmacol Biochem Behav 63:361–366, 1999

Uhlig T, Merkenschlager A, Brandmaier R, et al: Topographic mapping of brain electrical activity in children with food-induced attention deficit hyperkinetic disorder. Eur J Pediatr 156:557–561, 1997

Uygur MC, Ozgü IH, Ozen H, et al: Long-term treatment of nocturnal enuresis with desmopressin intranasal spray. Clin Pediatr (Phila) 36:455–459, 1997

van der Meere J, Gunning B, Stemerdink N: The effect of methylphenidate and clonidine on response inhibition and state regulation in children with ADHD. J Child Psychol Psychiatry 40:291–298, 1999

Van der Wissel A, Zegers FE: Reading retardation revisited. Br J Dev Psychol 3:3–19, 1985

van Goozen SH, Matthys W, Cohen-Kettenis PT, et al: Plasma monoamine metabolites and aggression: two studies of normal and oppositional defiant disorder children. Eur Neuropsychopharmacol 9:141–147, 1999

van Goozen SH, van den Ban E, Matthys W, et al: Increased adrenal androgen functioning in children with oppositional defiant disorder: a comparison with psychiatric and normal controls. J Am Acad Child Adolesc Psychiatry 39:1446–1451, 2000

van Minnen A, Hoogduin CA, Broekman TG: Hospital vs. outreach treatment of patients with mental retardation and psychiatric disorders: a controlled study. Acta Psychiatr Scand 95:515–522, 1997

Van Tilburg MA, Vingerhoets AJ, Van Heck GL: Homesickness: a review of the literature. Psychol Med 26:899–912, 1996

Vanstraelen M, Tyrer SP: Rapid cycling bipolar affective disorder in people with intellectual disability: a systematic review. J Intellect Disabil Res 43:349–359, 1999

Varan B, Saatçi U, Ozen S, et al: Efficacy of oxybutynin, pseudoephedrine and indomethacin in the treatment of primary nocturnal enuresis. Turk J Pediatr 38:155–159, 1996

Velez CN, Johnson J, Cohen P: A longitudinal analysis of selected risk factors for childhood psychopathology. J Am Acad Child Adolesc Psychiatry 28:861–864, 1989

Vexler ZS, Ferriero DM: Molecular and biochemical mechanisms of perinatal brain injury. Seminars in Neonatology 6:99–108, 2001

Villalba R, Harrington CJ: Repetitive self-injurious behavior: a neuropsychiatric perspective and review of pharmacologic treatments. Semin Clin Neuropsychiatry 5:215–226, 2000

Vitiello B, Stoff DM: Subtypes of aggression and their relevance to child psychiatry. J Am Acad Child Adolesc Psychiatry 36:307–315, 1997

Vitiello B, Severe JB, Greenhill LL, et al: Methylphenidate dosage for children with ADHD over time under controlled conditions: lessons from the MTA. J Am Acad Child Adolesc Psychiatry 40:188–196, 2001

Voeller K: Right-hemisphere deficit syndrome in children. Am J Psychiatry 143:1004–1009, 1986

Volkmar FR, Cohen DJ: Disintegrative disorder or "late onset" autism (abstract). J Child Psychol Psychiatry 30:717, 1989

Volkmar FR, Rutter M: Childhood disintegrative disorder: results of the DSM-IV field trial. J Am Acad Child Adolesc Psychiatry 34:1092–1095, 1995

Volpe JJ: Neurology of the Newborn. Philadelphia, PA, WB Saunders, 1987

Wadsworth SJ, DeFries JC, Stevenson J, et al: Gender ratios among reading-disabled children and their siblings as a function of parent impairment. J Child Psychol Psychiatry 33:1229–1239, 1992

Walkup JT, LaBuda MC, Singer HS, et al: Family study and segregation analysis of Tourette syndrome: evidence for a mixed model of inheritance. Am J Hum Genet 59:684–693, 1996

Watkins RV, Yairi E, Ambrose NG: Early childhood stuttering, III: initial status of expressive language abilities. J Speech Lang Hear Res 42:1125–1135, 1999

Weakley MM, Petti TA, Karwisch G: Case study: chewing gum treatment of rumination in an adolescent with an eating disorder. J Am Acad Child Adolesc Psychiatry 36:1124–1127, 1997

Wender PH: Minimal Brain Dysfunction in Children. New York, Wiley, 1971

Wender PH: Attention-deficit hyperactivity disorder in adults. Psychiatr Clin North Am 21:761–774, 1998

Wender PH, Reimherr FW: Bupropion treatment of attention-deficit hyperactivity disorder in adults. Am J Psychiatry 147:1018–1020, 1990

West SA, Strakowski SM, Sax KW, et al: The comorbidity of attention-deficit hyperactivity disorder in adolescent mania: potential diagnostic and treatment implications. Psychopharmacol Bull 31:347–351, 1995

Whelan E, Cooper PJ: The association between childhood feeding problems and maternal eating disorder: a community study. Psychol Med 30:69–77, 2000

Whitmore EA, Mikulich SK, Thompson LL, et al: Influences on adolescent substance dependence: conduct disorder, depression, attention deficit hyperactivity disorder, and gender. Drug Alcohol Depend 47:87–97, 1997

Wichstrøm L, Skogen K, Oia T: Increased rate of conduct problems in urban areas: what is the mechanism? J Am Acad Child Adolesc Psychiatry 35:471–479, 1996

Wilens T, Spencer T, Frazier J, et al: Psychopharmacology in children and adolescents, in Handbook of Child Psychopathology. Edited by Ollendick T, Hersen M. New York, Plenum, 1998, pp 603–636

Wilhelm K, Parker G, Dewhurst-Savellis J, et al: Psychological predictors of single and recurrent major depressive episodes. J Affect Disord 54:139–147, 1999

Wille S: Comparison of desmopressin and enuresis alarm for nocturnal enuresis. Arch Dis Child 61:30–33, 1986

Williams H, Clarke R, Bouras N, et al: Use of the atypical antipsychotics olanzapine and risperidone in adults with intellectual disability. J Intellect Disabil Res 44:164–169, 2000

Williams ML, Lewandowski LJ, Coplan J, et al: Neurodevelopmental outcome of preschool children both preterm with and without intracranial hemorrhage. Dev Med Child Neurol 29:243–249, 1987

Wilson PH, McKenzie BE: Information processing deficits associated with developmental coordination disorder: a meta-analysis of research findings. J Child Psychol Psychiatry 39:829–840, 1998

Wing L: Asperger's syndrome: a clinical account. Psychol Med 11:115–130, 1981

Wise BW, Olson RK: Computer-based phonologic awareness and reading instruction. Annals of Dyslexia 45:99–122, 1995

Woolston JL: Eating disorders in infancy and early childhood. Journal of the American Academy of Child Psychiatry 22:114–121, 1983

Wozniak J, Biederman J, Richards JA: Diagnostic and therapeutic dilemmas in the management of pediatric bipolar disorder. J Clin Psychiatry 14:10–15, 2001a

Youssef NN, Di Lorenzo C: Childhood constipation: evaluation and treatment. J Clin Gastroenterol 33:199–205, 2001

Zeanah CH, Embe RN: Attachment disorders in infancy and childhood, in Child and Adolescent Psychiatry, 3rd Edition. Edited by Rutter M, Hersov L, Taylor E. London, England, Blackwell, 1995

Zoccolillo M, Tremblay R, Vitaro F: DSM-III-R and DSM-III criteria for conduct disorder in preadolescent girls: specific but insensitive. J Am Acad Child Adolesc Psychiatry 35:461–470, 1996

Sleep Disorders

Thomas C. Neylan, M.D.

Charles F. Reynolds III, M.D.

David J. Kupfer, M.D.

The 2001 Sleep in America Poll showed that 69% of adult Americans experience frequent sleep problems. Approximately two-thirds of adults average less than 8 hours of sleep per night, and a full one-third habitually sleep less than 7 hours (National Sleep Foundation 2001). Furthermore, this survey showed that Americans are working more and spending less time sleeping or in recreation than 5 years before. Despite increased attention to the health consequences of disturbed sleep and the phenomenal growth of organized sleep medicine, sleep disturbances remain pandemic and mostly undertreated. In this chapter we provide a broad overview of sleep disorders and summarize current treatment guidelines for each disorder.

Normal Human Sleep

The brain has three major states of activity and function: wakefulness, rapid eye movement (REM) sleep, and non-REM sleep. REM sleep, identified in 1953 by Aserinsky and Kleitman, is a dramatic physiological state in that the brain becomes electrically and metabolically activated with frequencies approaching those of wakefulness. Perhaps as a defense to preserve sleep, there is a generalized muscle atonia that is detected polysomnographically by the disappearance of electromyographic activity. REMs occur in phasic bursts and are accompanied by fluctuations in respiratory and cardiac rate. Finally, dreaming in REM sleep is frequently vivid and affectively charged and is associated with activation of the amygdala (L.D. Sanford et al. 2001), which is thought to regulate emotionally influenced memory (Macquet et al. 1996).

Healthy sleep in humans consists of recurring 70- to 120-minute cycles of non-REM and REM sleep characterized polysomnographically by the electroencephalogram (EEG), the electrooculogram (EOG), and the electromyogram (EMG) (Rechtschaffen and Kales 1968).

Supported in part by the General Clinical Research Center (UCSF: 5M01RR-00079) and National Institutes of Mental Health grants MH57157 (TCN); M01RR00056, P30MH05247, ROIMH37869, MH43832 (CFR); P30MH30915, ROIMH59769 (DJK).

The conventional EEG lead used for sleep staging is either C3 or C4 (Jasper 1958). Eye movements are detected by the EOG because of the presence of an electrical dipole between the cornea and the retina. Typically, sleep progresses from wakefulness through the four stages of non-REM sleep until the onset of the first REM period. In the healthy adult, the deepest stages of sleep, non-REM Stages III and IV (collectively referred to as *slow-wave sleep)*, occur in the first two non-REM periods. In contrast, the REM periods in the first half of the sleep period are brief and lengthen in successive cycles.

During wakefulness, the EEG is characterized by low-voltage fast activity consisting of a mix of alpha (8–13 Hz) and beta (>13 Hz) frequencies. *Stage I* of non-REM sleep is a transitional stage between wakefulness and sleep during which the predominant alpha rhythm disappears, giving way to the slower theta (4–7 Hz) frequencies. Tonic electromyographic activity decreases, and the eyes move in a slow, rolling pattern. *Stage II* is characterized by a background theta rhythm and the episodic appearance of sleep spindles (i.e., brief bursts of 12- to 14-Hz activity) and K complexes (i.e., a high-amplitude, slow-frequency electronegative wave followed by an electropositive wave). Muscle tone remains diminished, and eye movements are rare. *Stages III* and *IV* are defined as epochs of sleep consisting of greater than 20% and 50%, respectively, of high-amplitude activity in the delta band (0.5–3.0 Hz). Muscle tone is nearly nonexistent, and eye movements are absent.

Sleep and Circadian Rhythms

The timing of our daily sleep–wake cycle is mainly under the control of the supra-chiasmatic nucleus (SCN) in the hypothalamus, which establishes a daily, or circadian, rhythm. Destruction of the SCN eliminates circadian rhythmicity (Moore and Eichler 1972; Rusak and Zucker 1979), although sleep cycles persist. Hence, sleep is also regulated by a homeostatic drive that causes us to feel sleepy after sustained wakefulness. The circadian oscillator promotes sleepiness both in the afternoon and at night in those with a typical sleep–wake schedule. Thus, the interaction of circadian and homeostatic regulation explains the observation that a person may feel subjectively more alert at 7:00 P.M. than at 4:00 P.M. despite having had a longer period of sustained wakefulness. The circadian oscillator reacts and entrains to environmental cues (e.g., the light–dark cycle) that are called *zeitgebers* (literally, "time-givers"). The discovery of several genes responsible for familial forms of circadian rhythm disorders, including the "Clock" gene, has provided new insight into the mechanism of genetic regulation of circadian rhythms (Toh et al. 2001). These circadian pacemaker genes may control the oscillations of various systems, such as neuroendocrine activity and thermoregulation. Exposure to bright light may affect the regulation of these genes, thus allowing a shift in the circadian timing of multiple systems.

Ontogeny of Sleep Stages

During the first 3 years of life, the sleep–wake rhythm develops from an ultradian to a circadian pattern, with the principal sleep phase occurring at night. Sleep in prepubertal children is characterized by large percentages of REM and high-amplitude slow-wave sleep. During adolescence, a precipitous decrease in slow-wave sleep (Feinberg 1974) occurs during a period of rapid neuronal senescence and synaptic pruning (Feinberg 1982; Huttenlocher 1979). In the third through sixth decades, there is a gradual and slight decline in sleep efficiency and total sleep time. With advancing age, sleep becomes more fragmented and lighter in depth. There are more transient arousals, as well as sleep stage shifts, and there is also a gradual disappearance of slow-wave sleep (Gillin and Ancoli-Israel 1992). In addition, the diurnal sleep–wake pattern decays as sleep is redistributed into the light phase in the form of frequent naps (Buysse et al. 1992).

Sleep Pharmacology

Prior to the 1960s, when benzodiazepines were introduced, barbiturates were the most commonly prescribed sedative-hypnotic medications. Because of their superior tolerability and safety, benzodiazepines quickly supplanted the barbiturates. Currently, benzodiazepines and atypical sedative-hypnotics are used to induce sleep onset and to improve overall sleep continuity (Table 16–1). Within the class of benzodiazepines, the duration of action and the presence of active metabolites are the main variables to consider when using these agents. Long-acting benzodiazepines such as flurazepam, which have active metabolites with half-lives in excess of 200 hours, often cause problems with daytime alertness and are associated with more errors while driving an automobile as compared with short-acting agents. Short-half-life benzodiazepines such as triazolam are useful for sleep-onset insomnia but will not benefit those with sleep maintenance difficulties in the latter half of the night. Furthermore, short-half-life agents produce more pronounced and rapid rebound anxiety and insomnia. However, slow tapering of these agents can prevent the discontinuation syndrome. In general, it is thought that sedative-hypnotic therapy should be limited to agents with short and intermediate half-lives. The adverse effects of using long-duration sedative-hypnotics for periods of insomnia include impaired memory and psychomotor performance and an increased risk of motor vehicle accidents (Menzin et al. 2001). For example, the use of benzodiazepines and other sedatives increases the risk of hip fracture in elderly patients.

Zolpidem is a short-half-life nonbenzodiazepine drug that binds selectively to the type 1 benzodiazepine receptor (Langer et al. 1987). It has no effect on nocturnal respiratory function in patients with obstructive lung disease (Girault et al. 1996). In therapeutic doses, it has minimal effects on sleep architecture and does not cause rebound insomnia after discontinuation (Kryger et al. 1991; Merlotti et al. 1989). Like triazolam, zolpidem causes short-term impairment of memory that is reversible with flumazenil (Wesensten et al. 1995). Zaleplon has a mechanism of action similar to that of zolpidem. The primary difference is its very short duration of action, which makes it potentially useful for the management of sleep-onset insomnia and early-morning awakening (Weitzel et al. 2000).

A number of medications used in the treatment of insomnia are not approved by the U.S. Food and Drug Administration (FDA) for the treatment of insomnia (Table 16–2). Antihistamines are often used despite having poorer efficacy relative to the benzodiazepines and more adverse daytime effects. Trazodone is a sedating antidepressant that is frequently used as a sedative. It has been found to improve sleep continuity and subjective sleep quality. Although trazodone is frequently recommended because of its putative absence of tolerance effects, data on its long-term efficacy have not been obtained. Trazodone's major side effects in-

TABLE 16–1. Hypnotic agents

Generic	Trade	Onset	Half-life (h)[a]	Active metabolites	Dose (mg)
Benzodiazepines					
Flurazepam	Dalmane	Rapid	40–250	Yes	15, 30
Quazepam	Doral	Rapid	40–250	Yes	7.5, 15
Estazolam	ProSom	Rapid	10–24	Yes	0.5, 1, 2
Temazepam	Restoril	Intermediate	8–22	No	7.5, 15
Triazolam	Halcion	Rapid	<6	No	0.125, 0.25, 0.50
Imidazopyridine					
Zolpidem	Ambien	Rapid	2.5	No	5, 10
Pyrazolopyrimidine					
Zaleplon	Sonata	Rapid	1	No	5, 10, 20

[a]Parent compound and active metabolites.

TABLE 16–2. Unapproved agents used in the treatment of insomnia

Agent	Advantages	Disadvantages
Antidepressants		
Amitriptyline	No tolerance	Anticholinergic delirium, increased risk of falls, daytime sedation
Doxepin	No tolerance	Increased risk of falls, daytime sedation
Trazodone	No tolerance, no anticholinergic effects	Increased risk of falls, daytime sedation
Antipsychotics		
Haloperidol	No tolerance, few anticholinergic effects	Extrapyramidal effects, increased risk of falls, not very sedating
Thioridazine	No tolerance	Extrapyramidal effects, increased risk of falls, anticholinergic delirium
Barbiturates	No pertinent advantages over benzodiazepines	High risk of addiction, dangerous withdrawal syndrome, overdose potential, daytime sedation
Miscellaneous		
Chloral hydrate	Less addictive than benzodiazepines	Overdose potential, tolerance to hypnotic effects over time, nausea
Diphenhydramine	No tolerance	Anticholinergic delirium, increased risk of falls, daytime sedation, memory impairment

clude priapism, hypotension, and morning hangover. Melatonin has been used to treat insomnia despite warnings from multiple experts in sleep medicine. The safety of over-the-counter melatonin is unknown, given the lack of regulatory oversight by the FDA.

Clinical Manifestations and Evaluation of Sleep Disorders

In community and clinical studies, insomnia has been associated with poor job performance, fatigue, accidents, impaired physical well-being, and increased use of alcohol (Ford and Kamerow 1989; Gallup Organization 1995; Kales et al. 1984; Mellinger et al. 1985; National Commission on Sleep Disorders Research 1993).

Conservative estimates of the total annual cost of insomnia in the United States range from $92.5 to $107.5 billion (Stoller 1994). The chief complaint usually is related to disrupted or too little sleep, excessive sleepiness, or adverse events associated with the sleep period.

A thorough medical and psychiatric history is essential for diagnosing conditions that have an impact on sleep–wake function. The entire 24-hour period should be explored with respect to sleep–wake habits. Patients with insomnia should be questioned about their views on what constitutes healthy sleep. Very often patients who by virtue of their constitution are short sleepers are subjectively distressed by their inability to sleep for the popular standard of 8 hours. The severity of insomnia can be understood only in terms of its impact on daytime function such as mood, fatigue, muscle aches, attention, and concentration. Asking patients about the total number of hours of sleep typically obtained has limited value, given the overlap between good and poor sleepers. Self-rating instruments such as the Pittsburgh Sleep Quality Index (Buysse et al. 1989) are useful for measuring subjective sleep quality. A 2-week sleep–wake log is invaluable for obtaining a history of irregular sleep–wake patterns; napping; use of stimulants, hypnotics, or alcohol; diet; activity during the day; number of arousals; and perceived length of sleep time and its relationship to daytime mood and alertness.

Approximately 4%–5% of the general population complains of excessive sleepiness. Sleepiness relates to the propensity to sleep, such as after sleep deprivation. Clinically, it is more alarming than insomnia because of the higher degree of psychosocial impairment as well as the high rate of automobile and occupational accidents (Guilleminault and Carskadon 1977; Mitler et al. 1988; Roth et al. 1994). Patients should be asked about symptoms of morning headaches, cataplexy, hypnagogic or hypnopompic hallucinations, sleep paralysis, automatic behavior, or sleep drunkenness. In addition, they should be questioned carefully about falling asleep while driving or while performing any other potentially dangerous activity. Additional history should be obtained from bed partners for events that are usually not perceived by the patients, such as snoring, respiratory pauses longer than 10 seconds, unusual body movements, or somnambulism.

Patients who complain of disturbances associated with the sleep period should be questioned about nocturnal incontinence or polyuria, orthopnea, paroxysmal nocturnal dyspnea, headaches that interrupt sleep, jaw clenching or bruxism, sleeptalking, somnambulism, and, in the case of

TABLE 16–3. Practice guidelines for the use of polysomnography in the evaluation of insomnia

Polysomnography is not routinely indicated for transient or chronic insomnia.

Polysomnography is indicated when sleep apnea or myoclonus is suspected, particularly in older patients.

Polysomnography should be considered if the diagnosis is uncertain *and* behavior or drug therapy is ineffective.

Polysomnography is indicated for patients with confusional or violent arousals, particularly if the clinical diagnosis is uncertain.

Polysomnography should be considered for circadian rhythm disorders if the clinical diagnosis is uncertain.

Source.   Data from Chesson et al. 2000.

males, painful nocturnal erections (Aldrich 1994).

Polysomnography remains the principal diagnostic tool in the field of sleep medicine. A thorough polysomnographic study provides data on sleep continuity, sleep architecture, REM physiology, sleep-related respiratory impairment, oxygen desaturation, cardiac arrhythmias, and periodic movements. Additional measures may include nocturnal penile tumescence, temperature, and infrared video monitoring. The routine use of polysomnography in the evaluation of hypersomnolent patients is well justified given the high incidence of sleep apnea and narcolepsy in this group. Polysomnography should be used in any patient with a parasomnia in which there is clinical suspicion of sleep apnea or nocturnal seizure disorder. Practice guidelines for the use of polysomnography in the evaluation of chronic insomnia have been developed by the American Academy of Sleep Medicine (Chesson et al. 2000; Table 16–3).

The Multiple Sleep Latency Test (MSLT; Carskadon et al. 1986) is the most objective and valid measure of excessive sleepiness. Other measures such as the Stanford Sleepiness Scale (Hoddes et al. 1973) and the Maintenance of Wakefulness Test (Mitler et al. 1982) are less reliable, although they are easy and inexpensive to use. The Epworth Sleepiness Scale measures daytime sleepiness in eight common real-life situations (Johns 1991). In the MSLT, the patient is given the opportunity to fall asleep in a darkened room for five 20-minute periods in 2-hour intervals across the patient's usual period of wakefulness. The average latency to sleep onset, measured polysomnographically, is a direct measure of the propensity to fall asleep. Multiple studies have shown that an average sleep latency of less than 5 minutes indicates a pathological degree of sleepiness associated with a high rate of intrusive sleep episodes during the wake period and decrements in work performance (Carskadon et al. 1981; Dement et al. 1978; Nicholson and Stone 1986). The detection of sleep-onset REM periods in the MSLT has become a cornerstone in the diagnosis of narcolepsy (Mitler 1982).

Classification of Sleep Disorders

DSM-IV-TR (American Psychiatric Association 2000) divides sleep disorders into four major categories: primary sleep disorders, sleep disorders related to another mental disorder, sleep disorder due to a general medical condition, and substance-induced sleep disorder.

Primary Sleep Disorders

Dyssomnias

Primary Insomnia

Primary insomnia is the term used to describe difficulty initiating or maintaining

sleep, or nonrestorative sleep, lasting at least a month in duration. By definition, primary insomnia results in significant daytime impairment and is not secondary to another sleep disorder. Sleep fragmentation can usually be validated by polysomnography, which shows prolonged sleep latencies, decreased sleep efficiency, and a predominance of the lighter stages of non-REM sleep (Hauri and Fisher 1986; Hauri and Olmstead 1980). An overview of the evaluation of chronic insomnia is provided in Table 16–4.

TABLE 16–4. Evaluation of chronic insomnia

Step 1	Evaluate for a general medical condition that may adversely affect sleep.
Step 2	Evaluate whether medications or substance use is disrupting sleep.
Step 3	Evaluate whether another mental disorder such as depression, schizophrenia, or anxiety disorder is causing sleep disruption.
Step 4	Consider a breathing-related sleep disorder, particularly if the patient snores or is obese.
Step 5	Consider a sleep–wake schedule disorder if the patient has an irregular schedule or is involved in shift work.
Step 6	Consider a parasomnia diagnosis if the patient complains of behavioral or mental events that occur during sleep.
Step 7	If insomnia has persisted for more than a month and is not related to the above disorders, then the diagnosis is primary insomnia.
Step 8	If insomnia is not described by the above criteria, then the diagnosis of dyssomnia not otherwise specified is used.

Source. Data from Reynolds et al. 1995.

There are several effective treatment approaches to chronic insomnia that do not involve the use of hypnotics (Chesson et al. 1999a). Education about normal sleep and counseling around habits for promoting good sleep hygiene are a good but insufficient intervention when used alone (Hauri 1989; Morin et al. 1994). Various relaxation therapies such as hypnosis, meditation, deep breathing, and progressive muscle relaxation can be helpful. These techniques, in contrast to the use of hypnotics, are not immediately beneficial but require several weeks of practice to improve sleep (McClusky et al. 1991). Success is dependent on a high degree of motivation in patients, who must devote considerable time to practicing these techniques. Those who succeed in learning these techniques have a greater satisfaction with maintenance treatment than do patients chronically using hypnotics (Bootzin and Perlis 1992; Morin et al. 1992, 1999). Furthermore, responders to behavioral interventions have sustained benefits after 6 months (G.D. Jacobs et al. 1996).

Sleep restriction therapy is aimed at reducing the amount of wake time spent in bed (Spielman et al. 1987). Patients are asked to record in a sleep diary the amount of time they estimate they are asleep. They are then instructed to restrict their time in bed to a degree commensurate to their estimate of their total sleep time. Patients often have their usual difficulties with sleep fragmentation during the first few nights and become sleep deprived. Sleep deprivation helps consolidate sleep on subsequent nights, thereby improving sleep efficiency. Increases in length of time in bed can subsequently be titrated to the presence of daytime fatigue.

Hypnotics should be considered only after a thorough diagnostic assessment of secondary causes of insomnia, after sleep hygiene has been improved, and after behavioral treatments have been attempted. If these approaches are unsuccessful, then hypnotics can be used, starting with very low doses and limiting use to short periods. Long-term efficacy studies of behavioral and pharmacological interventions in insomnia are clearly needed.

Primary Hypersomnia

The diagnosis of primary hypersomnia is characterized by prolonged nocturnal sleep and severe daytime sleepiness that can be objectively documented by a short mean sleep latency on the MSLT. Primary hypersomnia is a diagnosis of exclusion, made when other disorders causing excessive sleepiness have been ruled out. A recurrent form of primary hypersomnia is characterized by intermittent attacks of hypersomnolence and hyperphagia, often associated with indiscrete hypersexuality, poor social judgment, mood disturbance, and hallucinations. Between episodes there can be a complete remission of symptoms. This pattern of primary hypersomnia occurs most frequently in males in their late adolescence and early 20s, after which time there is a gradual decline in the frequency and duration of the episodes. The pathophysiology of primary hypersomnia is postulated to involve an underlying disturbance of limbic and hypothalamic function. Several abnormal laboratory findings have been documented, including slowing of background rhythm on the EEG, altered secretory pattern of growth hormone and thyroid-stimulating hormone, and elevated cerebrospinal-fluid serotonin and dopamine metabolites. Treatment usually involves the use of psychostimulants to reduce daytime hypersomnolence.

Narcolepsy

Narcolepsy is a common cause of daytime hypersomnolence in which REM sleep repeatedly and suddenly intrudes into wakefulness. It represents an impairment in the ability to maintain a stable neural state; REM is no longer segregated in its usual ultradian rhythm during sleep. The clinical phenomenology of narcolepsy is best understood through a consideration of normal REM physiology (e.g., activated EEG, generalized atonia, dream cognition). Both cataplexy and sleep paralysis involve muscle atonia occurring at a time when the patient is cognizant of the environment and subjectively feels awake. Hypnagogic hallucinations are not well understood but are thought to be related to the dreamlike perceptual phenomenon of REM sleep. Nocturnal sleep is characterized by short REM latency and frequent arousals and shifts from non-REM sleep to REM sleep to wakefulness (Rechtschaffen et al. 1963).

Recent advances in molecular biology have clarified the pathophysiology of narcolepsy. Canine narcolepsy is caused by a mutation in the hypocretin gene (Lin et al. 1999). Preprohypocretin knockout mice have symptoms suggestive of narcolepsy. Finally, human narcolepsy has been found to be associated with generalized deficiency of hypocretin (Nishino et al. 2000; Peyron et al. 2000; Thannickal et al. 2000). It is possible that decreased tone of monoaminergic cells and increased cholinergic sensitivity, characteristic of narcolepsy (Nishino and Mignot 1997), are caused by the absence of excitatory inputs from hypocretin cells in the hypothalamus (Hungs and Mignot 2001). Low hypocretin levels in cerebrospinal fluid, which have been reported in studies of narcolepsy, may be an additional diagnostic tool in the evaluation of hypersomnolence (Nishino et al. 2000).

The treatment of narcolepsy primarily involves the use of dopaminomimetic stimulants such as dextroamphetamine, methamphetamine, methylphenidate, or pemoline. These agents can release presynaptic pools of monoamines, block their reuptake, or inhibit monoamine oxidase metabolism of norepinephrine and dopamine. Discontinuation of agents that release dopamine appears to result in rebound insomnia. Additional agents used to treat narcolepsy include γ-hydroxybutyrate and modafinil. Modafinil, an atypical psychostimulant that affects postsynaptic α_1-adrenergic receptors, promotes wakefulness and is rarely associated with substance dependence (Besset et al. 1996). Modafinil is less effective than amphetamine in controlling cataplexy (Shelton et al. 1995). REM-suppressing agents such as tricyclic antidepressants and γ-hydroxybutyrate have been found to control cataplexy. An important nonpharmacological approach is the use of scheduled naps throughout the wake period (Helmus et al. 1997).

Sleep Apnea

Sleep-disordered breathing is an age-related disorder affecting approximately 24% of community-dwelling individuals over age 65 years (Ancoli-Israel et al. 1991) and 42% of elderly persons living in nursing homes (Ancoli-Israel 1989). The estimated prevalence of apnea in a random sample of employed middle-aged subjects is 9% for women and 24% for men (Young et al. 1993). Although occasionally causing insomnia, sleep apnea is typically an occult disorder that causes daytime somnolence, impaired concentration and intellectual functioning, and morning headaches. It is associated with obesity, loud snoring, systemic and pulmonary hypertension, cardiac arrhythmias, nocturnal cardiac ischemia, myocardial infarction, and excessive mortality (Schafer et al. 1997; Strollo and Rogers 1996; Yamashiro and Kryger 1994). It can be caused by an impairment in central respiratory drive (central apnea), intermittent upper airway obstruction (obstructive apnea), or a combination of the two (mixed apnea). Patients with this disorder experience frequent respiratory pauses during sleep that are associated with oxygen desaturation. The apneic events are terminated by loud gasping, thrashing movements, and arousal on EEG. Patients, who usually have no awareness of these events, are often brought to clinical attention by alarmed bed partners (Guilleminault 1982).

Sleep apnea is quantified polysomnographically by measuring air flow with nasal cannulas; respiratory effort with thoracic and abdominal strain gauges, diaphragmatic or intercostal EMG, or an esophageal pressure gauge; oxygen saturation with an oximeter; and sleep architecture with a standard sleep montage (i.e., EEG, EOG, EMG). Patients with severe sleep apnea typically have evidence of pathological sleepiness as measured by latencies to sleep onset of less than 5 minutes on the MSLT. Ball et al. (1997) found that an effort by sleep specialists to increase awareness of obstructive sleep apnea among primary care physicians was successful in dramatically increasing case recognition and treatment of the disorder.

The clinical impact of sleep apnea is related to two phenomena: hypoxia and sleep fragmentation. Cerebral hypoxia can lead to intellectual deterioration, impaired attention and memory, and personality changes. Successful treatment improves neurocognitive performance on most, but not all, measures, which suggests that permanent anoxic injury occurs in some patients (Bedard et al. 1993).

There are a variety of behavioral, medical, pharmacological, and surgical treatments for sleep apnea. Behavioral approaches include weight loss, abstinence from sedative-hypnotics, and sleep-position training (which helps the patient avoid the supine position during sleep). Mechanical approaches include use of tongue-retaining devices, orthodontic appliances that advance the mandible (Loube and Strauss 1997; Nakazawa et al. 1992), and nasal continuous positive airway pressure (CPAP). Surgical techniques aim to increase the lumen size of the oropharynx and include uvulopalatopharyngoplasty (UPPP), maxillomandibular and hyoid advancement, and chronic tracheostomy (Powell et al. 1994).

To date, nasal CPAP remains the initial treatment of choice for moderate to severe sleep apnea. CPAP acts as a pneumatic splint that maintains the patency of the oropharynx during respiration (Sullivan and Grunstein 1994). The air pressure required to maintain airway patency should be directly titrated in the sleep laboratory. Reports of long-term compliance are variable, ranging from 25% to 70% (Guilleminault et al. 1992). Nightly compliance is required for optimal benefit.

Circadian Rhythm Sleep Disorder

The sleep–wake cycle, under the circadian control of endogenous regulators or oscillators, can be disrupted by a misalignment between biological rhythms and external demands on waking behavior. Circadian rhythm sleep disorders present with either insomnia or hypersomnolence, depending on the juxtaposition of performance demands and the underlying circadian cycle.

Shift workers have higher rates of on-the-job sleepiness, as well as higher rates of drug use and divorce (Regestein and Monk 1991). The *jet lag type* is one of the most common of the circadian rhythm sleep disorders. Travelers flying across multiple time zones must re-entrain their circadian sleep–wake rhythms with respect to both social schedule and the acquired light–dark cycle. Patients with *delayed sleep phase type disorder* are described as night owls, with an innate preference for beginning sleeping in the late hours of night and sleeping until the late morning or early afternoon. They experience sleep-onset insomnia and morning hypersomnolence when forced to comply with a conventional sleep–wake schedule. There are reports of patients with a phase advance in their sleep–wake schedule who experience hypersomnolence in the early evening hours, as well as midnight arousal. Typically these are older patients, because with age there is a tendency for the sleep–wake cycle to advance relative to clock time. The general treatment approach is to promote good sleep hygiene, with the goal of properly aligning patients' circadian systems with their sleep–wake schedules. Treatment may also involve manipulation or augmentation of external *zeitgebers*, such as with the use of bright-light therapy.

Phototherapy. Bright light has been found to be effective in treating delayed sleep phase type disorder (Rosenthal et al. 1990) and jet lag (Daan and Lewy 1984). Furthermore, it has been found to improve alertness and cognitive performance in night shift workers (Campbell et al. 1995a). In one method of therapy, patients are instructed to sit 3 feet away from a bright-light source of at least 2,500-lux intensity. Typically, patients require between 30 minutes and 2 hours of exposure, depending on therapeutic response. Side effects include eyestrain, headache, and mild psychomotor agitation. At present, there is no evidence that long-term use of bright-light therapy results in any ocular damage (Gallin et al. 1995). The timing of exposure depends on the direction in which patients wish to shift their sleep–wake schedule. Morning or evening exposure will phase-advance or phase-delay the sleep–wake schedule, respectively.

Dyssomnia Not Otherwise Specified

The category of dyssomnia not otherwise specified (NOS) includes the phenomenon of *nocturnal myoclonus*, which is characterized by periodic leg movements of sufficient severity to cause sleep continuity disturbance, leading to complaints of either insomnia or daytime sleepiness. Nocturnal myoclonus consists of repetitive, brief leg jerks that occur in regular 20- to 40-second intervals. These movements are frequently associated with transient arousals that lead to sleep fragmentation and a predominance of the lighter stages of non-REM sleep (Karadeniz et al. 2000).

Restless legs syndrome is a syndrome that causes sleep-onset insomnia. It is typically characterized by deep paresthesias in the calf muscles, prompting the urge to keep the legs in motion.

The most common treatments involve the use of benzodiazepines or dopaminomimetics such as L-dopa or bromocriptine (Montplaisir et al. 1992; Trenkwalder et al. 1995).

Parasomnias
Sleepwalking and Night Terrors

Sleepwalking and *night terrors* are found normally in young children and are associated with psychopathology only if persisting into adulthood. Typically, they involve a partial arousal from sleep during the first third of the night, a period characterized by a predominance of slow-wave sleep (Gaudreau et al. 2000). In sleepwalking, subjects become partially aroused and ambulatory; they are typically difficult to awaken and have amnesia for the events. Night terrors involve an emergence of intense fear associated with autonomic arousal in which patients are inconsolable, difficult to awaken fully, and unable to assign specific cognitions associated with the anxiety. Treatment is directed toward reducing stress, anxiety, and sleep deprivation, all of which are known to exacerbate these disorders. In extreme cases, low-dose benzodiazepines are indicated and effective.

Nightmare Disorder

Nightmare disorder, formerly known as *dream anxiety disorder,* occurs in 10%–50% of children. The incidence of the disorder peaks between the ages of 3 and 6 (Leung and Robson 1993) and declines with age (Hartmann 1984).

REM Sleep Behavior Disorder

REM sleep behavior disorder, which is listed as a parasomnia NOS in DSM-IV, occurs when there is incomplete or absent muscle atonia during REM sleep. The disorder is characterized by prominent motor activity during dreaming. Several dramatic cases have involved patients who suddenly assaulted their bed partners in response to frightening dreams. Benzodiazepines, particularly clonazepam, and carbamazepine have been found to be useful in reducing these events (Bamford 1993; Mahowald and Schenck 1994).

Sleep Disorders Related to Another Mental Disorder

Mood Disorders

Sleep disturbance is verifiable in 90% of patients with major depression and is characterized by sleep fragmentation, decreased quantity and altered distribution of delta sleep, reduced duration of the first non-REM period (i.e., REM latency), redistribution of REM sleep into the first half of the night, and increased number of REMs per minute of REM sleep (Kupfer and Foster 1972; Kupfer and Reynolds 1992; Reynolds and Kupfer 1987). Multiple studies have shown that disturbed sleep antedates the development of major depression (Breslau et al. 1996; Chang et al. 1997; Ford and Kamerow 1989; Roberts et al. 2000).

Antidepressant medications vary in their effects on sleep continuity and architecture. Tricyclic antidepressants have different effects on sleep latency and stage I and stage II sleep, but all increase slow-wave sleep, suppress REM sleep, and prolong REM latency. Selective serotonin reuptake inhibitors decrease sleep continuity, increase REM latency, and usually decrease REM time (Hendrickse et al. 1994; Nicholson and Pascoe 1988; Saletu et al. 1991). Trazodone increases slow-wave sleep, increases REM latency, decreases REM time, and improves sleep continuity (Muratorio et al. 1974; Scharf and Sachais 1990). Nefazodone improves sleep continuity but, in contrast to most other antidepressants, modestly increases REM sleep (Armitage et al. 1994; Rickels et al. 1994; Sharpley et al. 1992; Ware et al. 1994). Bupropion decreases sleep continuity and slow-wave sleep and, like nefazodone, increases REM sleep (Nofzinger et al. 1995).

Schizophrenia

Patients with schizophrenia have been found to have prolonged sleep latencies, sleep fragmentation with multiple arousals, decreased slow-wave sleep, variability in REM latency, and decreased REM rebound after REM sleep deprivation (Benson and Zarcone 1993; Ganguli et al. 1987; Keshavan et al. 1990b; Martin et al. 2001; Zarcone et al. 1987).

Diminished slow-wave sleep is one of the most replicated and stable findings in schizophrenia (Feinberg and Hiatt 1978; Keshavan et al. 1996, 1998; Maixner et al. 1998), although it has not been observed in all studies (Lauer et al. 1997). It has been found to be associated with poor performance on neuropsychological tests of attention (Orzack et al. 1977) and with negative symptoms (Ganguli et al. 1987; Keshavan et al. 1995b).

Anxiety Disorders

Sleep in patients with generalized anxiety disorder is similar to that in patients with primary insomnia in that there are prolonged sleep latencies and increased sleep fragmentation. Subjective sleep quality is significantly impaired in subjects with social phobia (Stein et al. 1993). Sleep in patients with anxiety disorders differs from that seen in patients with major depression: patients with anxiety disorders exhibit normal REM latencies and decreased REM percentage (Reynolds et al. 1983b). It has been suggested that patients with symptoms of both depression and anxiety may be segregated with respect to sleep variables on the basis of the presence or absence of a family history of depression (Sitaram et al. 1984). Furthermore, sleep deprivation does not result in symptomatic improvement in patients with anxiety disorders (Labbate et al. 1998), in contrast to the case in depressive patients.

Multiple studies have demonstrated that patients with PTSD have significant sleep continuity disturbance and increased REM phasic activity such as eye movements (Mellman et al. 1995a, 1995b; Ross et al. 1994; Woodward et al. 1996); these symptoms are directly correlated with PTSD symptom severity. Several studies suggest that nightmares may be uniquely related to exposure to traumatic stress. Neylan et al. (1998) conducted a secondary data analysis of the questionnaire items that address complaints about sleep from the National Vietnam Veterans Readjustment Study (Kulka et al. 1990), a major population-based study that sampled to represent the entire group of 3.1 million men and women who served in the Vietnam War. The results show that complaints of frequent nightmares are relatively rare and are found exclusively in subjects with PTSD (Neylan et al. 1998). These results support the hypothesis published by Ross et al. (1989), who stated that nightmares and disturbances of REM sleep are a hallmark of PTSD.

Dementia

Patients with dementia of the Alzheimer's type have more sleep fragmentation (Grace et al. 2000), less delta and REM sleep (Vitiello and Prinz 1988), and little to no spindle and K-complex activity (Reynolds et al. 1985a; Smirne et al. 1977) in comparison with age-matched control subjects. Patients with dementia have more sleep-related phenomena, such as sundowning and nocturnal wanderings, that provoke attempts to consolidate nocturnal sleep with hypnotics as well as prompt families to institutionalize their elderly relatives (J.R.A. Sanford 1975).

Studies examining the relationship between sleep, aging, and dementia suggest an important relationship between normal sleep–wake function and cognition. The severity of dementia has been found to correlate with severity of sleep disturbances (Bliwise et al. 1995). Feinberg et al. (1967) suggested that the sleep EEG is an indicator of the functional integrity of the cerebral cortex. An important unanswered question is whether sleep loss in aging is related to cognitive impairment or whether the two emerge secondary to some underlying, independent biological process.

Sleep Disorder Due to a General Medical Condition

Sleep can be adversely affected by multiple medical disorders, particularly those that compromise cardiopulmonary function or cause chronic pain. Endocrine disorders such as diabetes and hyperthyroidism can cause significant sleep continuity disturbance. Hot flashes associated with normal menopause can occur in sleep and cause arousals. Patients may complain of insomnia, hypersomnia, parasomnia, or a combination of symptoms.

Sleep and Seizures

Non-REM sleep has a well-known activating effect on seizure activity. EEG synchronization may explain the higher prevalence of seizures and interictal discharges seen in non-REM sleep (Shouse 1994). Although complaints of insomnia are unusual, sleep can be sufficiently fragmented to cause daytime fatigue and hypersomnolence (Bazil et al. 2000).

Sleep and Parkinson's Disease

Sleep disturbance is reported in approximately 50% of patients with Parkinson's disease (Shulman et al. 2001). Sleep in Parkinson's disease is characterized by an increased number of awakenings, a decreased amount of delta and REM sleep, and a scarcity of sleep spindles. The resting tremor usually subsides with the onset of stage I sleep, but, depending on the severity of the disorder, it can persist into stage II or reemerge during sleep stage changes (April 1966). Dopaminomimetic drugs such as L-dopa have dose-dependent effects on sleep and promote daytime somnolence (Schäfer and Greulich 2000).

Substance-Induced Sleep Disorder

Substance-induced sleep disorder is related to both direct and indirect toxic ef-

fects on sleep. Both alcohol- and hypnotic-induced sleep disorders involve the development of tolerance to the sleep-inducing effects of the agent, as well as increased arousals during withdrawal periods. Many studies have shown that acute alcohol administration causes REM sleep suppression in the first half of the night followed by a rebound increase of REM sleep and arousals in the second half. Acute alcohol use in high doses suppresses REM sleep for the entire night (Knowles et al. 1968). During acute withdrawal, there is marked sleep continuity disturbance and prominent REM sleep rebound (Johnson et al. 1970). Abstinent alcoholic subjects have been shown to have decreased slow-wave sleep and increased sleep stage changes for many months after alcohol withdrawal (Adamson and Burdick 1973).

Stimulants cause sleep-onset insomnia during usage and rebound hypersomnia during withdrawal. Food allergy– and toxin-induced sleep disorders presumably involve indirect toxic effects on the physiological substrate regulating sleep. In all of these disorders, careful removal of the offending agent either eliminates the problem or exposes an additional sleep disorder.

Conclusions

Careful assessment and treatment of sleep disorders can dramatically improve the quality of psychiatric care. Disordered sleep has protean effects on mood, attention, memory, and general sense of vigor. Furthermore, disturbance in sleep has clear prognostic value and must be addressed to optimize clinical care. The search for the core function of sleep remains an exciting area for scientific research, with clear implications for our understanding of basic brain homeostatic mechanisms.

References

Adamson J, Burdick JA: Sleep of dry alcoholics. Arch Gen Psychiatry 28:146–149, 1973

Aldrich MS: Cardinal manifestations of sleep disorders, in Principles and Practice of Sleep Medicine, 2nd Edition. Edited by Kryger MH, Roth T, Dement WC. Philadelphia, PA, WB Saunders, 1994, pp 413–425

American Psychiatric Association: Diagnostic and Statistical Manual of Mental Disorders, 4th Edition, Text Revision. Washington, DC, American Psychiatric Association, 2000

Ancoli-Israel S: Epidemiology of sleep disorders. Clin Geriatr Med 5:347–362, 1989

Ancoli-Israel S, Kripke DF, Klauber MR, et al: Sleep disordered breathing in community dwelling elderly. Sleep 14:486–495, 1991

April RS: Observations on parkinsonian tremor in all-night sleep. Neurology (New York) 16:720–724, 1966

Armitage R, Rush AJ, Trivedi M, et al: The effects of nefazodone on sleep architecture in depression. Neuropsychopharmacology 10:123–127, 1994

Aserinsky E, Kleitman N: Regularly occurring periods of eye motility and concomitant phenomena during sleep. Science 118:273–274, 1953

Ball EM, Simon RD Jr, Tall AA, et al: Diagnosis and treatment of sleep apnea within the community: the Walla Walla Project. Arch Intern Med 157:419–424, 1997

Bamford CR: Carbamazepine in REM sleep behavior disorder. Sleep 16:33–34, 1993

Bazil CW, Castro LH, Walczak TS: Reduction of rapid eye movement sleep by diurnal and nocturnal seizures in temporal lobe epilepsy. Arch Neurol 57:363–368, 2000

Bedard MA, Montplaisir J, Malo J, et al: Persistent neuropsychological deficits and vigilance impairment in sleep apnea syndrome after treatment with continuous positive airway pressure (CPAP). J Clin Exp Neuropsychol 15:330–341, 1993

Benson KL, Zarcone VP Jr: Rapid eye movement sleep eye movements in schizophrenia and depression. Arch Gen Psychiatry 50:474–482, 1993

Besset A, Chetrit M, Carlander B, et al: Use of modafinil in the treatment of narcolepsy: a long term follow-up study. Neurophysiol Clin 26:60–66, 1996

Bixler EO, Kales A, Soldatos CR, et al: Prevalence of sleep disorders in the Los Angeles metropolitan area. Am J Psychiatry 136:1257–1262, 1979

Bliwise DL, Hughes M, McMahon PM, et al: Observed sleep/wakefulness and severity of dementia in an Alzheimer's disease special care unit. J Gerontol A Biol Sci Med Sci 50:M303–M306, 1995

Bootzin RR, Perlis ML: Nonpharmacologic treatments of insomnia. J Clin Psychiatry 53 (suppl):37–41, 1992

Breslau N, Roth T, Rosenthal L, et al: Sleep disturbance and psychiatric disorders: a longitudinal epidemiological study of young adults. Biol Psychiatry 39:411–418, 1996

Buysse DJ, Reynolds CF, Monk TH, et al: The Pittsburgh Sleep Quality Index: a new instrument for psychiatric practice and research. Psychiatry Res 28:193–213, 1989

Buysse DJ, Browman KE, Monk TH, et al: Napping and 24-hour sleep/wake patterns in healthy elderly and young adults. J Am Geriatr Soc 40:779–786, 1992

Campbell SS, Dijk DJ, Boulos Z, et al: Light treatment for sleep disorders: consensus report, III: alerting and activating effects. J Biol Rhythms 10:129–132, 1995a

Carskadon MA, Harvey K, Dement WC: Sleep loss in young adolescents. Sleep 4:299–312, 1981

Carskadon MA, Dement WC, Mitler MM, et al: Guidelines for the Multiple Sleep Latency Test (MSLT): a standard measure of sleepiness. Sleep 9:519–524, 1986

Chang PP, Ford DE, Mead LA, et al: Insomnia in young men and subsequent depression: the Johns Hopkins Precursors Study. Am J Epidemiol 146:105–114, 1997

Chesson AL, Anderson WM, Littner M, et al: Practice parameters for the nonpharmacologic treatment of chronic insomnia: an American Academy of Sleep Medicine report. Standards of Practice Committee of the American Academy of Sleep Medicine. Sleep 22:1128–1133, 1999a

Chesson A, Hartse K, Anderson WM, et al: Practice parameters for the evaluation of chronic insomnia. An American Academy of Sleep Medicine report. Standards of Practice Committee of the American Academy of Sleep Medicine. Sleep 23: 237–241, 2000

Daan S, Lewy AJ: Scheduled exposure to daylight: a potential strategy to reduce "jet lag" following transmeridian flight. Psychopharmacol Bull 20:566–568, 1984

Dement WC, Carskadon MA, Richardson GS: Excessive daytime sleepiness in the sleep apnea syndrome, in Sleep Apnea Syndromes. Edited by Guilleminault C, Dement WC. New York, Alan R Liss, 1978, pp 23–46

Feinberg I: Changes in sleep cycle patterns with age. J Psychiatr Res 10:283–306, 1974

Feinberg I: Schizophrenia: caused by a fault in programmed synaptic elimination during adolescence? J Psychiatr Res 17:319–334, 1982

Feinberg I, Hiatt JF: Sleep patterns in schizophrenia: a selective review, in Sleep Disorders: Diagnosis and Treatment. Edited by Williams RC, Karacan I. New York, Wiley, 1978, pp 205–231

Feinberg I, Koresko RL, Heller N: EEG sleep patterns as a function of normal and pathological aging in man. J Psychiatr Res 5:107–144, 1967

Ford DE, Kamerow DB: Epidemiologic study of sleep disturbances and psychiatric disorders: an opportunity for prevention? JAMA 262:1479–1484, 1989

Gallin PF, Terman M, Reme CE, et al: Ophthalmologic examination of patients with seasonal affective disorder, before and after bright light therapy. Am J Ophthalmol 119:202–210, 1995

Gallup Organization: Sleep in America. Princeton, NJ, Gallup, 1995

Ganguli R, Reynolds CF, Kupfer DJ: Electroencephalographic sleep in young, never-medicated schizophrenics: a comparison with delusional and nondelusional depressives and with healthy controls. Arch Gen Psychiatry 44:36–44, 1987

Gaudreau H, Joncas S, Zadra A, et al: Dynamics of slow-wave activity during the NREM sleep of sleepwalkers and control subjects. Sleep 23:755–760, 2000

Gillin JC, Ancoli-Israel S: The impact of age on sleep and sleep disorders, in Clinical Geriatric Psychopharmacology, 2nd Edition. Edited by Salzman C. Baltimore, MD, Williams & Wilkins, 1992, pp 213–234

Girault C, Muir JF, Mihaltan F, et al: Effects of repeated administration of zolpidem on sleep, diurnal and nocturnal respiratory function, vigilance, and physical performance in patients with COPD. Chest 110:1203–1211, 1996

Grace JB, Walker MP, McKeith IG: A comparison of sleep profiles in patients with dementia with Lewy bodies and Alzheimer's disease. Int J Geriatr Psychiatry 15:1028–1033, 2000

Guilleminault C: Sleep and breathing, in Sleep and Waking Disorders: Indications and Techniques. Edited by Guilleminault C. Menlo Park, CA, Addison-Wesley, 1982, pp 155–182

Guilleminault C, Carskadon M: Relationship between sleep disorders and daytime complaints, in Sleep 1976. Edited by Koeller WP, Oevin PW. Basel, Switzerland, S Karger, 1977, pp 95–100

Guilleminault C, Stoohs R, Quera-Salva MA: Sleep-related obstructive and nonobstructive apneas and neurologic disorders. Neurology 42 (suppl 6):53–60, 1992

Hartmann E: The Nightmare: The Psychology and Biology of Terrifying Dreams. New York, Basic Books, 1984

Hauri P: Primary insomnia, in Treatment of Psychiatric Disorders, Vol 3. Washington, DC, American Psychiatric Association, 1989, pp 2424–2433

Hauri P, Fisher J: Persistent psychophysiologic (learned) insomnia. Sleep 9:38–53, 1986

Hauri P, Olmstead P: Childhood-onset insomnia. Sleep 3:59–65, 1980

Helmus T, Rosenthal L, Bishop C, et al: The alerting effects of short and long naps in narcoleptic, sleep deprived, and alert individuals. Sleep 20:251–257, 1997

Hendrickse WA, Roffwarg HP, Grannemann BD, et al: The effects of fluoxetine on the polysomnogram of depressed outpatients: a pilot study. Neuropsychopharmacology 10:85–91, 1994

Hoddes E, Zarcone VP, Smythe H, et al: Quantification of sleepiness: a new approach. Psychophysiology 10:431–436, 1973

Hungs M, Mignot E: Hypocretin/orexin, sleep and narcolepsy. Bioessays 23:397–408, 2001

Huttenlocher PR: Synaptic density in human frontal cortex: developmental changes and effects of aging. Brain Res 163:195–205, 1979

Jacobs GD, Benson H, Friedman R: Perceived benefits in a behavioral-medicine insomnia program: a clinical report. Am J Med 100:212–216, 1996

Jasper NH: The ten-twenty electrode system of the International Federation. Electroencephalogr Clin Neurophysiol 10:371–375, 1958

Johns MW: A new method for measuring daytime sleepiness: the Epworth sleepiness scale. Sleep 14:540–555, 1991

Johnson LC, Burdick JA, Smith J: Sleep during alcohol intake and withdrawal in the chronic alcoholic. Arch Gen Psychiatry 22:406–418, 1970

Kales JD, Kales A, Bixler EO, et al: Biopsychobehavioral correlates of insomnia, V: clinical characteristics and behavioral correlates. Am J Psychiatry 141:1371–1376, 1984

Karadeniz D, Ondze B, Besset A, et al: EEG arousals and awakenings in relation with periodic leg movements during sleep. J Sleep Res 9:273–277, 2000

Keshavan MS, Reynolds CF, Kupfer KJ: Electroencephalographic sleep in schizophrenia: a critical review. Compr Psychiatry 31:34–47, 1990b

Keshavan MS, Miewald J, Haas G, et al: Slow-wave sleep and symptomatology in schizophrenia and related psychotic disorders. J Psychiatr Res 29:303–314, 1995b

Keshavan MS, Reynolds CF III, Miewald JM, et al: A longitudinal study of EEG sleep in schizophrenia. Psychiatry Res 59:203–211, 1996

Keshavan MS, Reynolds CF III, Miewald MJ, et al: Delta sleep deficits in schizophrenia: evidence from automated analyses of sleep data. Arch Gen Psychiatry 55:443–448, 1998

Knowles JB, Laverty SG, Kuechler HA: The effects of alcohol on REM sleep. Quarterly Journal of Studies on Alcohol 29:342–349, 1968

Kryger MH, Steljes D, Pouliot Z, et al: Subjective versus objective evaluation of hypnotic efficacy: experience with zolpidem. Sleep 14:399–407, 1991

Kulka RA, Schlenger WE, Fairbank JA, et al: The National Vietnam Veterans Readjustment Study: Tables and Findings and Technical Appendices. New York, Brunner/Mazel, 1990

Kupfer DJ, Foster FG: Interval between onset of sleep and rapid-eye-movement sleep as an indicator of depression. Lancet 2:684–686, 1972

Kupfer DJ, Reynolds CF: Sleep and affective disorders, in Handbook of Affective Disorders, 2nd Edition. Edited by Paykel ES. New York, Guilford, 1992, pp 311–323

Labbate LA, Johnson MR, Lydiard RB, et al: Sleep deprivation in social phobia and generalized anxiety disorder. Biol Psychiatry 43:840–842, 1998

Langer SZ, Arbilla S, Scatton B, et al: Receptors involved in the mechanism of action of zolpidem, in Imidazopyridines in Sleep Disorders: A Novel Experimental and Therapeutic Approach. Edited by Sauvanet JP, Langer SZ, Morselli PL. New York, Raven, 1987, pp 55–72

Lauer CJ, Schreiber W, Pollmacher T, et al: Sleep in schizophrenia: a polysomnographic study on drug-naive patients. Neuropsychopharmacology 16:51–60, 1997

Leung AK, Robson WL: Nightmares. J Natl Med Assoc 85:233–235, 1993

Lin L, Faraco J, Li R, et al: The sleep disorder canine narcolepsy is caused by a mutation in the hypocretin (orexin) receptor 2 gene. Cell 98:365–376, 1999

Loube MD, Strauss AM: Survey of oral appliance practice among dentists treating obstructive sleep apnea patients. Chest 111:382–386, 1997

Macquet P, Peters J, Aerts J, et al: Functional neuroanatomy of human rapid-eye-movement sleep and dreaming. Nature 383:163–166, 1996

Mahowald MW, Schenck CH: REM sleep behavior disorder, in Principles and Practice of Sleep Medicine, 2nd Edition. Edited by Kryger MH, Roth T, Dement WC. Philadelphia, PA, WB Saunders, 1994, pp 574–588

Maixner S, Tandon R, Eiser A, et al: Effects of antipsychotic treatment on polysomnographic measures in schizophrenia: a replication and extension. Am J Psychiatry 155:1600–1602, 1998

Martin J, Jeste DV, Caliguiri MP, et al: Actigraphic estimates of circadian rhythms and sleep/wake in older schizophrenia patients. Schizophr Res 47:77–86, 2001

McClusky HY, Milby JB, Switzer PK, et al: Efficacy of behavioral versus triazolam treatment in persistent sleep-onset insomnia. Am J Psychiatry 148:121–126, 1991

Mellinger GD, Balter MB, Uhlenhuth EH: Insomnia and its treatment: prevalence and correlates. Arch Gen Psychiatry 42:225–232, 1985

Mellman TA, David D, Kulick-Bell R, et al: Sleep disturbance and its relationship to psychiatric morbidity after Hurricane Andrew. Am J Psychiatry 152:1659–1663, 1995a

Mellman TA, Kulick-Bell R, Ashlock LE, et al: Sleep events among veterans with combat-related posttraumatic stress disorder. Am J Psychiatry 152:110–115, 1995b

Menzin J, Lang KM, Levy P, et al: A general model of the effects of sleep medications on the risk and cost of motor vehicle accidents and its application to France. Pharmacoeconomics 19:69–78, 2001

Merlotti L, Roehrs T, Koshorek G, et al: The dose effects of zolpidem on the sleep of healthy normals. J Clin Psychopharmacol 9:9–14, 1989

Mitler MM: The Multiple Sleep Latency Test as an evaluation for excessive somnolence, in Disorders of Sleeping and Waking: Indications and Techniques. Edited by Guilleminault C. Menlo Park, CA, Addison-Wesley, 1982, pp 145–153

Mitler MM, Gujavarty KS, Browman CP: Maintenance of wakefulness test: a polysomnographic technique for evaluating treatment efficacy in patients with excessive somnolence. Electroencephalogr Clin Neurophysiol 53:658–661, 1982

Mitler MM, Carskadon MA, Czeisler CA, et al: Catastrophes, sleep, and public policy: consensus report. Sleep 11:100–109, 1988

Montplaisir J, Lapierre O, Warnes H, et al: The treatment of the restless legs syndrome with or without periodic leg movements in sleep. Sleep 15:391–395, 1992

Moore RY, Eichler VB: Loss of a circadian adrenal corticosterone rhythm following suprachiasmatic lesions in the rat. Brain Res 42:210–216, 1972

Morin CM, Gaulier B, Barry T, et al: Patients' acceptance of psychological and pharmacological therapies for insomnia. Sleep 15:302–305, 1992

Morin CM, Culbert JP, Schwartz SM: Nonpharmacological interventions for insomnia: a meta-analysis of treatment efficacy. Am J Psychiatry 151:1172–1180, 1994

Morin CM, Colecchi C, Stone J, et al: Behavioral and pharmacological therapies for late-life insomnia: a randomized controlled trial. JAMA 281:991–999, 1999

Muratorio A, Maggini C, Coccagna G, et al: Polygraphic study of the all-night sleep pattern in neurotic and depressed patients treated with trazodone. Mod Probl Pharmacopsychiatry 9:182–189, 1974

Nakazawa Y, Sakamoto T, Yasutake R, et al: Treatment of sleep apnea with prosthetic mandibular advancement (PMA). Sleep 15:499–504, 1992

National Commission on Sleep Disorders Research: Wake Up, America: A National Sleep Alert. Submitted to the United States Congress, January 1993

National Sleep Foundation: 2001 Sleep in America Poll. Washington, DC, National Sleep Foundation, 2001

Neylan TC, Marmar CR, Metzler TJ, et al: Sleep disturbances in the Vietnam generation: an analysis of sleep measures from the National Vietnam Veteran Readjustment Study. Am J Psychiatry 155:929–933, 1998

Nicholson AN, Pascoe PA: Studies on the modulation of the sleep-wakefulness continuum in man by fluoxetine, a 5-HT uptake inhibitor. Neuropharmacology 27:597–602, 1988

Nicholson AN, Stone BM: Impaired performance and the tendency to sleep. Eur J Clin Pharmacol 30:27–32, 1986

Nishino S, Mignot E: Pharmacological aspects of human and canine narcolepsy. Progress in Neurobiology 52:27–78, 1997

Nishino S, Ripley B, Overeem S, et al: Hypocretin (orexin) deficiency in human narcolepsy. Lancet 355:39–40, 2000

Nofzinger EA, Reynolds CF III, Thase ME, et al: REM sleep enhancement by bupropion in depressed men. Am J Psychiatry 152:274–276, 1995

Orzack MH, Hartmann EL, Kornetsky C: The relationship between attention and slow-wave sleep in chronic schizophrenia. Psychopharmacol Bull 13:59–61, 1977

Peyron C, Faraco J, Rogers W, et al: A mutation in a case of early onset narcolepsy and a generalized absence of hypocretin peptides in human narcoleptic brains. Nat Med 6:991–997, 2000

Powell NB, Guilleminault C, Riley RW: Surgical therapy for obstructive sleep apnea, in Principles and Practice of Sleep Medicine, 2nd Edition. Edited by Kryger MH, Roth T, Dement WC. Philadelphia, PA, WB Saunders, 1994, pp 706–771

Rechtschaffen A, Kales A: A Manual of Standardized Terminology, Techniques, and Scoring System for Sleep Stages of Human Subjects. Bethesda, MD, U.S. Department of Health, Education and Welfare, Public Health Service, 1968, pp 1–60

Rechtschaffen A, Wolpert EA, Dement WC, et al: Nocturnal sleep of narcoleptics. Electroencephalogr Clin Neurophysiol 15:599–609, 1963

Regestein QR, Monk TH: Is the poor sleep of shift workers a disorder? Am J Psychiatry 148:1487–1493, 1991

Reynolds CF III, Kupfer DJ: Sleep research in affective illness: state of the art circa 1987. Sleep 10:199–215, 1987

Reynolds CF III, Christiansen CL, Taska LS, et al: Sleep in narcolepsy and depression: does it all look alike? J Nerv Ment Dis 171:290–295, 1983b

Reynolds CF III, Kupfer DJ, Taska LS, et al: EEG sleep in elderly depressed, demented, and healthy subjects. Biol Psychiatry 20:431–442, 1985a

Reynolds CF III, Buysse DJ, Kupfer DJ: Disordered sleep: developmental and biopsychosocial perspectives on the diagnosis and treatment of persistent insomnia, in Psychopharmacology: The Fourth Generation of Progress. Edited by Bloom FE, Kupfer DJ. New York, Raven, 1995, pp 1617–1629

Rickels K, Schweizer E, Clary C, et al: Nefazodone and imipramine in major depression: a placebo-controlled trial. Br J Psychiatry 164:802–805, 1994

Roberts RE, Shema SJ, Kaplan GA, et al: Sleep complaints and depression in an aging cohort: a prospective perspective. Am J Psychiatry 157:81–88, 2000

Rosenthal NE, Joseph-Vanderpool JR, Levendosky AA, et al: Phase-shifting effects of bright morning light as treatment for delayed sleep phase syndrome. Sleep 13:354–361, 1990

Ross RJ, Ball WA, Sullivan KA, et al: Sleep disturbance as the hallmark of posttraumatic stress disorder. Am J Psychiatry 146:697–707, 1989

Ross RJ, Ball WA, Dinges DF, et al: Rapid eye movement sleep disturbance in posttraumatic stress disorder. Biol Psychiatry 35: 195–202, 1994

Roth T, Roehrs T, Carskadon M, et al: Daytime sleepiness and alertness, in Principles and Practice of Sleep Medicine, 2nd Edition. Edited by Kryger MH, Roth T, Dement WC. Philadelphia, PA, WB Saunders, 1994, pp 40–49

Rusak B, Zucker I: Neural regulation of circadian rhythms. Physiol Rev 59:449–526, 1979

Saletu B, Frey R, Krupka M, et al: Sleep laboratory studies on the single-dose effects of serotonin reuptake inhibitors paroxetine and fluoxetine on human sleep and awakening qualities. Sleep 14:439–447, 1991

Sanford JRA: Tolerance of debility in elderly dependants by supporters at home: its significance for hospital practice. BMJ 3: 471–473, 1975

Sanford LD, Silvestri AJ, Ross RJ, et al: Influence of fear conditioning on elicited ponto-geniculo-occipital waves and rapid eye movement sleep. Archives Italiennes de Biologie 139:169–183, 2001

Schäfer D, Greulich W: Effects of parkinsonian medication on sleep. Journal of Neurology 247(suppl 4):IV/24–IV/7, 2000

Schafer H, Koehler U, Ploch T, et al: Sleep-related myocardial ischemia and sleep structure in patients with obstructive sleep apnea and coronary heart disease. Chest 111:387–393, 1997

Scharf MB, Sachais BA: Sleep laboratory evaluation of the effects and efficacy of trazodone in depressed insomniac patients. J Clin Psychiatry 51:13–17, 1990

Sharpley AL, Walsh AES, Cowen PJ: Nefazodone—a novel antidepressant—may increase REM sleep. Biol Psychiatry 31: 1070–1073, 1992

Shelton J, Nishino S, Vaught J, et al: Comparative effects of modafinil and amphetamine on daytime sleepiness and cataplexy of narcoleptic dogs. Sleep 18:817–826, 1995

Shouse MN: Epileptic seizure manifestations during sleep, in Principles and Practice of Sleep Medicine, 2nd Edition. Edited by Kryger MH, Roth T, Dement WC. Philadelphia, PA, WB Saunders, 1994, pp 801–814

Shulman LM, Taback RL, Bean J, et al: Comorbidity of the nonmotor symptoms of Parkinson's disease. Mov Disord 16:507–510, 2001

Sitaram N, Gillin JC, Bunney WE Jr: Cholinergic and catecholaminergic receptor sensitivity in affective illness: strategy and theory, in Neurobiology of Mood Disorders. Edited by Post RM, Ballenger JC. Baltimore, MD, Williams & Wilkins, 1984, pp 629–651

Smirne S, Come G, Franceschi M, et al: Sleep in presenile dementia, in Communications in EEG. International Federation of Societies for Electroencephalography and Clinical Neurophysiology, 9th Congress, 1977, pp 521–522

Spielman A, Saskin P, Thorpy M: Treatment of chronic insomnia by restriction of time in bed. Sleep 10:45–56, 1987

Stein MB, Kroft CD, Walker JR: Sleep impairment in patients with social phobia. Psychiatry Res 49:251–256, 1993

Stoller MK: Economic effects of insomnia. Clin Ther 16:873–897, 1994

Strollo PJ Jr, Rogers RM: Obstructive sleep apnea. N Engl J Med 334:99–104, 1996

Sullivan CE, Grunstein RR: Continuous positive airway pressure in sleep-disordered breathing, in Principles and Practice of Sleep Medicine, 2nd Edition. Edited by Kryger MH, Roth T, Dement WC. Philadelphia, PA, WB Saunders, 1994, pp 694–705

Thannickal TC, Moore RY, Nienhuis R, et al: Reduced number of hypocretin neurons in human narcolepsy. Neuron 27:469–474, 2000

Toh KL, Jones CR, He Y, et al: An hPer2 phosphorylation site mutation in familial advanced sleep phase syndrome. Science 291:1040–1043, 2001

Trenkwalder C, Stiasny K, Pollmacher T, et al: L-dopa therapy of uremic and idiopathic restless legs syndrome: a double-blind, crossover trial. Sleep 18:681–688, 1995

Vitiello MV, Prinz PN: Aging and sleep disorders, in Sleep Disorders: Diagnosis and Treatment, 2nd Edition. Edited by Williams RL, Karacan I, Moore CA. New York, Wiley, 1988, pp 293–312

Ware JC, Rose FV, McBrayer RH: The acute effects of nefazodone, trazodone and buspirone on sleep and sleep-related penile tumescence in normal subjects. Sleep 17:544–550, 1994

Weitzel KW, Wickman JM, Augustin SG, et al: Zaleplon: a pyrazolopyrimidine sedative-hypnotic agent for the treatment of insomnia. Clin Ther 22:1254–1267, 2000

Wesensten NJ, Balkin TJ, Davis HQ, et al: Reversal of triazolam- and zolpidem-induced memory impairment by flumazenil. Psychopharmacology 121:242–249, 1995

Woodward SH, Friedman MJ, Bliwise DL: Sleep and depression in combat-related PTSD inpatients. Biol Psychiatry 39:182–192, 1996

Yamashiro Y, Kryger MH: Why should sleep apnea be diagnosed and treated? Clinical Pulmonary Medicine 1:250–259, 1994

Young T, Palta M, Dempsey J, et al: The occurrence of sleep-disordered breathing among middle-aged adults. N Engl J Med 328:1230–1235, 1993

Zarcone VP Jr, Benson KL, Berger PA: Abnormal rapid eye movement latencies in schizophrenia. Arch Gen Psychiatry 44:45–48, 1987

CHAPTER 17

Eating Disorders

Anorexia Nervosa, Bulimia Nervosa, and Obesity

Katherine A. Halmi, M.D.

The eating disorders *anorexia nervosa* and *bulimia nervosa* and the condition of *obesity* have been known since earliest times in Western civilization. Well-documented case reports of anorexia nervosa are found in literature describing early Christian saints. Although binge eating and purging behavior are certainly described in Roman civilization, the disorder bulimia nervosa as we define it today has not been so well documented.

Physiology and Behavioral Pharmacology of Eating

A Systems Conceptualization

Eating behavior is now known to reflect an interaction between an organism's physiological state and environmental conditions. Salient physiological variables include the balance of various neuropeptides and neurotransmitters, metabolic state, metabolic rate, condition of the gastrointestinal tract, amount of storage tissue, and sensory receptors for taste and smell. Environmental conditions include features of the food such as taste, texture,

novelty, accessibility, and nutritional composition, as well as other external conditions such as ambient temperature, presence of other people, and stress.

To understand eating behavior, it is also important to recognize the role of conditioned (learned) components in the initiation and termination of nutrient ingestion. Because of methodological complexities, this area has received little study. Booth (1985) provided the best discussion of conditioned appetites and satieties because he focused attention on the interaction between psychological and physiological phenomena.

Neurotransmitters

Biogenic Amines

Underweight anorexia nervosa patients and persons without eating disorders in times of dieting have reduced central and peripheral norepinephrine activity (Pirke 1996). This is confirmed by hypothermia, bradycardia, and hypotension.

Some evidence indicates that serotonin neuronal activity is involved in behavioral inhibition (Soubrie 1986), obsessive-

759

compulsive disorder (OCD) (Barr et al. 1992), anxiety and fear (Charney et al. 1990), and depression (Grahame-Smith 1992); serotonin neuronal activity also has well-established involvement with satiety for food intake. Anorexia nervosa has comorbid or coexisting disturbances of behavioral inhibition, obsessive-compulsive problems, excessive anxiety and fear, and depression. Bulimia nervosa is frequently characterized by behavioral disinhibition and depression.

Dopamine seems to play a more complicated role in eating behavior. Low doses of dopamine and dopamine agonist stimulate feeding, whereas higher doses inhibit feeding. Glucose administration suppresses firing in substantia nigra dopamine neurons. There is evidence of increased hypothalamic dopamine turnover during feeding. This finding suggests that central dopamine mechanisms mediate the rewarding effects of food as they mediate the rewarding effects of intracranial self-stimulation and the self-stimulation of psychoactive drugs.

Peptides and Opioids

Corticotropin-releasing factor (CRF) acts within the PVN to inhibit feeding. Norepinephrine seems to inhibit the CRF inhibitory feeding effect. The pancreatic polypeptide neuropeptide Y increases both food and water intake when injected into the PVN. Another pancreatic polypeptide, peptide YY, is a more potent stimulator of feeding than neuropeptide Y (Morley and Levine 1985).

Opioid antagonism decreases feeding in many species but has no effect in reducing food intake in other species. Under some physiological conditions, such as starving or insulin-induced hypoglycemia, naloxone fails to inhibit feeding. Stress-induced eating is probably driven by activation of the opioid system. Dynorphin, an endogenous κ opioid receptor ligand,

enhances feeding. Again, the major site of action for dynorphin appears to be the PVN (Morley and Levine 1985).

Vasopressin and oxytocin are neuropeptides distributed in the brain and function as long-acting neuromodulators with complex behavioral effects that are often reciprocal. Oxytocin antagonizes vasopressin's consolidation of learning acquired during aversive conditioning (Bohus et al. 1978). The dysregulation of secretion of these hormones in anorexia nervosa (Demitrek et al. 1992) may enhance the retention of cognitive distortions of the aversive consequences of eating.

Peripheral Satiety Network

Several peptides are released by ingested food from the gastrointestinal tract. Some of these peptides, such as CCK, bombesin, and glucagon, when administered parenterally to humans, have produced satiety. However, their usefulness as therapeutic agents at present is limited because of their restricted absorption from the gut and because the high doses required induce adverse effects such as nausea.

Leptin is a protein hormone secreted by adipose tissue cells and believed to act as an afferent signal and regulator of body fat stores (Zhang et al. 1994). Leptin activates receptors and is coded by the *DB* gene in the hypothalamus and OB receptors in the choroid plexus (Tartaglia et al. 1995). Defects in the leptin coding sequence in rodents result in leptin deficiency and defects in leptin receptors, which are associated with obesity (Chen et al. 1996). Leptin is positively correlated with fat mass in humans in all weight ranges (Considine et al. 1996). Underweight patients with anorexia nervosa have significantly reduced plasma and cerebrospinal fluid (CSF) leptin concentrations compared with normal-weight control subjects (Mantzoros et al. 1997). These levels reach normal values with weight restoration. Because acute fasting-induced weight loss provokes a decline in leptin concentration that is disproportionate to the amount of fat loss (Boden et al. 1996), it has been hypothesized that leptin is a protecting regulator against starvation. Reduced leptin concentrations induce a variety of neuroendocrine responses, including decreased thyroid thermogenesis, increased secretion of stress steroid, and decreased procreation (Ahima et al. 1996).

Anorexia Nervosa

Definition

Anorexia nervosa is a disorder characterized by preoccupation with body weight and food, behavior directed toward losing weight, peculiar patterns of handling food, weight loss, intense fear of gaining weight, disturbance of body image, and amenorrhea. DSM-IV-TR (American Psychiatric Association 2000a) criteria for anorexia nervosa are shown in Table 17–1.

Clinical Features

Individuals with anorexia nervosa typically express an intense fear of gaining weight, tend to be preoccupied with thoughts of food, and worry irrationally about fatness. Denial of their own clearly observable symptoms is characteristic of anorexic patients. They frequently look in mirrors to make sure they are thin, and they incessantly express concern about looking fat and feeling flabby. Collecting recipes and preparing elaborate meals for their families are other behaviors that reflect their preoccupation with food. Peculiar handling of food is frequent in individuals with anorexia. They will hide carbohydrate-rich foods and hoard large quantities of candies, carrying them in their pockets and purses. Often they will try to

TABLE 17–1. DSM-IV-TR diagnostic criteria for anorexia nervosa

A. Refusal to maintain body weight at or above a minimally normal weight for age and height (e.g., weight loss leading to maintenance of body weight less than 85% of that expected; or failure to make expected weight gain during period of growth, leading to body weight less than 85% of that expected).

B. Intense fear of gaining weight or becoming fat, even though underweight.

C. Disturbance in the way in which one's body weight or shape is experienced, undue influence of body weight or shape on self-evaluation, or denial of the seriousness of the current low body weight.

D. In postmenarcheal females, amenorrhea, i.e., the absence of at least three consecutive menstrual cycles. (A woman is considered to have amenorrhea if her periods occur only following hormone, e.g., estrogen, administration.)

Specify type:

Restricting Type: during the current episode of anorexia nervosa, the person has not regularly engaged in binge-eating or purging behavior (i.e., self-induced vomiting or the misuse of laxatives, diuretics, or enemas)

Binge-Eating/Purging Type: during the current episode of anorexia nervosa, the person has regularly engaged in binge-eating or purging behavior (i.e., self-induced vomiting or the misuse of laxatives, diuretics, or enemas)

dispose of their food surreptitiously to avoid eating. Anorexic persons will spend a great deal of time cutting food into small pieces and rearranging the food on their plates.

Anorexic patients' fear that they are gaining weight exists even in the face of increasing cachexia, and they characteristically show disinterest in and even resistance to treatment. Persons with this disorder lose weight by drastically reducing their total food intake and disproportionately decreasing the intake of high-carbohydrate and fatty foods. Some individuals with anorexia will develop rigorous exercise programs, and others simply will be as active as possible at all times. Self-induced vomiting and laxative and diuretic abuse are other purging behaviors by which anorexic persons attempt to lose weight. Weight loss and a refusal to maintain body weight over a minimal normal weight for age and height are the most characteristic features of this disorder. Anorexic individuals have a disturbance in the way in which they experience their body weight and shape. They often fail to recognize that their degree of emaciation is dangerous. Their cognition is so distorted that they judge their self-worth predominantly by body shape and weight.

Obsessive-compulsive behavior often develops after the onset of anorexia nervosa. An obsession with cleanliness, an increase in housecleaning activities, and a more compulsive approach to studying are not uncommonly observed in these patients.

Amenorrhea can appear before noticeable weight loss has occurred. Poor sexual adjustment is frequently present in patients with anorexia. Many adolescent patients with anorexia have delayed psychosocial sexual development, and adults often have a markedly decreased interest in sex with the onset of anorexia nervosa.

Patients with anorexia nervosa can be divided into two groups: those who binge eat and purge and those who merely restrict food intake to lose weight. There is a relatively frequent association with impulsive behavior such as suicide attempts, self-mutilation, stealing, and substance abuse (including alcohol abuse) among bulimic anorexic individuals, who are also less likely to be regressed in their sexual activity and may in fact be promiscuous.

Bulimic anorexic patients are more likely to have discrete personality disorder diagnoses (Halmi 1987).

Medical Complications

Most of the physiological and metabolic changes in anorexia nervosa are secondary to the starvation state or purging behavior and are reversed with nutritional rehabilitation. We often find abnormalities in hematopoiesis, such as leukopenia and relative lymphocytosis, in acutely emaciated anorexic patients. Individuals with anorexia nervosa who engage in self-induced vomiting or who abuse laxatives and diuretics are liable to develop hypokalemic alkalosis. These patients often have elevated serum bicarbonate levels, hypochloremia, and hypokalemia. Patients with electrolyte disturbances have physical symptoms of weakness and lethargy and, at times, have cardiac arrhythmias. The latter condition may threaten sudden cardiac arrest, a frequent cause of death in patients who purge. Other complications of bingeing and purging are discussed in the section on bulimia nervosa.

Elevation of serum enzymes reflects fatty degeneration of the liver and is observed both in the emaciated anorexic phase and during refeeding. Elevated serum cholesterol levels tend to occur more frequently in younger patients. Carotenemia is often observed in malnourished anorexic patients. All of these physiological changes reverse themselves with nutritional rehabilitation (Halmi and Falk 1981). Amenorrhea, which is a major diagnostic criterion for anorexia nervosa, is not related simply to weight loss and is discussed in the section "Etiology and Pathogenesis" later in this chapter.

Epidemiology, Course, and Prognosis

The incidence of anorexia nervosa has increased in the past 30 years both in the

United States and in Western Europe. In Monroe County, New York, the average annual incidence rate of 0.35 per 100,000 population in the 1960s increased to 0.64 per 100,000 in the 1970s (Jones et al. 1980). An incidence study in northeastern Scotland in the 1980s found four cases of anorexia nervosa per 100,000 population per annum (Szmukler 1985). A more recent incidence study conducted in northeastern Scotland (Eagles et al. 1995), reported that between 1965 and 1991, the incidence of anorexia nervosa increased nearly sixfold (from 3 per 100,000 to 17 per 100,000 cases). These studies probably underestimate the true incidence of the disorder, because not all cases come to the attention of health care providers. Only 4%–6% of the anorexic population is male (Halmi 1974).

In a community epidemiological survey in Canada, Woodside et al. (2001) found that men with eating disorders were very similar to women with the same diagnoses. The pattern of familial aggregation of eating disorders in males with anorexia nervosa was found to be highly similar to the pattern observed in recent family studies of affected females (Strober et al. 2001).

The course of anorexia nervosa varies from a single episode with weight and psychological recovery to nutritional rehabilitation with relapses to an unremitting course resulting in death. Two of the most methodologically satisfying long-term follow-up studies have shown a mortality rate of 6.6% at 10 years after a well-defined treatment program (Halmi et al. 1991) and a mortality rate of 18% at 30-year follow-up (Theander 1985).

A prospective 5-year study of 95 patients with anorexia nervosa in Australia found that 3 had died, 56 patients had no eating disorder diagnosis, and the remainder had a continuation of their illness with psychosocial difficulties (Ben-Tovin et al.

2001). All of these outcome studies indicate that anorexia nervosa is a serious, chronic disorder.

Etiology and Pathogenesis

A specific etiology and pathogenesis leading to the development of anorexia nervosa are unknown. Anorexia nervosa begins after a period of severe food deprivation, which may be due to any of the following:

- Willful dieting for the purpose of being more attractive
- Willful dieting for the purpose of being more professionally competent (e.g., ballet dancers, gymnasts, jockeys)
- Food restriction secondary to severe stress
- Food restriction secondary to severe illness and/or surgery
- Involuntary starvation

Previous periods of severe food restriction are often reported, and a history of earlier dieting is not unusual. The question is, what is unique about the individual who goes on to develop anorexia nervosa?

The psychological theories concerning the causes of anorexia have centered mostly on phobic mechanisms and psychodynamic formulations. Crisp (1976) postulated that anorexia nervosa constitutes a phobic avoidance response to food resulting from the sexual and social tension generated by the physical changes associated with puberty.

A cognitive and perceptual developmental defect was postulated by Bruch (1962) as the cause of anorexia nervosa. She described the disturbances of body image (denial of emaciation), disturbances in perception (lack of recognition or denial of fatigue, weakness, hunger), and a sense of ineffectiveness as being caused by untoward learning experiences.

Russell (1969) suggested that the

amenorrhea may be caused by a primary disturbance of hypothalamic function and that the full expression of this disturbance is induced by psychological stress. He thought that the malnutrition of anorexia nervosa perpetuates the amenorrhea but is not primarily responsible for the endocrine disorder. This hypothesis is supported by the fact that the return of normal menstrual cycles lags behind the return to a normal body weight; the resumption of menses in anorexia nervosa is associated with marked psychological improvement (Falk and Halmi 1982).

Although assessment of neurotransmitter function in the brain in humans has serious methodological problems, preliminary indirect studies indicate that a dysregulation of all three of these neurotransmitters probably occurs. Kaye et al. (1984b) showed a decreased serotonin turnover in bulimic anorexic patients compared with restricting anorexic patients. In addition, Kaye et al. (1984a) showed low CSF norepinephrine levels in long-term anorexic patients who have attained a weight within at least 15% of their normal weight range. Owen et al. (1983) showed that individuals with anorexia have a blunted growth hormone response to L-dopa, indicating a defect at the postsynaptic dopamine receptor sites. More recently, Brambilla et al. (2001) reported a blunted growth hormone response to the postsynaptic D_2 receptor stimulation with apomorphine in underweight anorexic patients. They suggested that the postsynaptic D_2 receptors are downregulated in anorexia nervosa because of a peripheral negative feedback linked to a hyperfunctioning somatotropic axis or to a hypothalamic presynaptic dopamine hypersecretion and/or reduced dopamine reuptake. In this study, growth hormone responses did not correlate with body mass index (BMI) but did correlate negatively with scores on the Eating Disorder Inventory Scale. Thus, dopamine alteration in anorexia nervosa may be linked to psychopathological parameters.

There is increasing evidence for genetic influences in the development of anorexia nervosa. Strober et al. (1985) found increased rates of anorexia nervosa, bulimia nervosa, and subclinical anorexia nervosa in first- and second-degree relatives of anorexic probands compared with the relatives of nonanorexic psychiatrically ill control probands. They proposed that the pattern of familial clustering of these disorders represents variable expressions of a common underlying psychopathology.

Another study providing evidence that both anorexia nervosa and bulimia nervosa are familial and that clustering of the disorder in families may arise partly from genetic transmission of risk was done by Lilenfeld et al. (1998). In a large epidemiological sample of twins obtained from the Virginia Twin Registry, a strong association between anorexia nervosa and bulimia nervosa was found; the co-twin of a twin affected with anorexia nervosa was 2.6 times more likely to have a lifetime diagnosis of bulimia nervosa compared with co-twins of unaffected twins. This evidence suggested some sharing of familial risk and liability factors between anorexia nervosa and bulimia nervosa (Kendler et al. 1991; Walters and Kendler 1995).

More recent family and twin studies examining comorbidity between eating disorders and other psychiatric diagnoses were reviewed in detail by Lilenfeld et al. (1997). Studies of major affective illness in anorexia nervosa probands reported familial risk estimates in the range of 7%–25%, with relative estimates in the range of 2.1–3.4. Family studies show relatively low rates of substance abuse among relatives of restricting anorexia nervosa probands and independent familial transmission of OCD and anorexia nervosa (Lilenfeld et al. 1998). In another study, the morbidity risk for obsessive-compulsive spectrum disorders was significantly higher among 436 relatives of eating disorder probands than among 358 relatives of comparison subjects (9.69% vs. 0%). The eating disorder probands and comparison subjects did not differ in familial risk for eating disorders (Bellodi et al. 2001).

In a study comparing the mothers of 57 anorexic patients with those of age- and sex-matched control subjects, Halmi et al. (1991) found a significantly greater prevalence of OCD in the mothers of the anorexic patients. Serotonin dysregulation may be a link between the OCD of the mothers and the anorexia nervosa in their daughters.

Treatment

A multifaceted treatment endeavor with medical management and behavioral, individual, cognitive, and family therapy is necessary to treat anorexia nervosa. The first step in treatment is to obtain the anorexic patient's cooperation in a treatment program. Most patients with anorexia nervosa are disinterested and even resistant to treatment and are brought to the therapist's office unwillingly by relatives or friends. For these patients, it is important to emphasize the benefits of treatment and to reassure them that treatment can bring about a relief of insomnia and depressive symptoms, a decrease in the obsessive thoughts about food and body weight that interfere with the ability to concentrate on other matters, an increase in physical well-being and energy, and an improvement in peer relationships.

The immediate aim of treatment should be to restore the patient's nutritional state to normal. Mere emaciation or the state of being mildly underweight (15%–25%) can cause irritability, depression, preoccupation with food, and sleep disturbance. It is exceedingly difficult to

achieve behavioral change with psychotherapy in a patient who is experiencing the psychological effects of emaciation. Outpatient therapy as an initial approach has the best chance for success in patients with anorexia who 1) have had the illness for less than 6 months, 2) are not bingeing and vomiting, and 3) have parents who are likely to cooperate and effectively participate in family therapy.

The more severely ill patient with anorexia may present an extremely difficult medical-management challenge and should be hospitalized and undergo daily monitoring of weight, food and calorie intake, and urine output. In the patient who is vomiting, frequent assessment of serum electrolytes is necessary. Behavior therapy is most effective in the medical management and nutritional rehabilitation of the patient with anorexia, although there are times when other target behaviors can be changed with this approach. Behavior therapy can be used in both outpatient and inpatient settings.

The operant conditioning paradigm has been the most effective form of behavior therapy for the treatment of anorexia nervosa. This can be used both in the context of a structured ward setting and in an individualized treatment program set up after a behavioral analysis of the patient has been completed. Positive reinforcements are used and consist of increased physical activity, visiting privileges, and social activities contingent on weight gain. An individual behavioral analysis may show other positive reinforcements to be more clinically relevant in the particular cases. The timing of reinforcement is important in behavior therapy. An adolescent patient needs at least a daily reinforcement for weight increase, which should be approximately 0.5 lb or 0.1 kg per day. Making positive reinforcements contingent only on weight gain is helpful in reducing the staff–patient arguments and stressful interactions concerning how and what the patient is eating because weight is an objective measure. In addition to being used to induce weight gain, behavior therapy can be used to stop vomiting. A response-prevention technique is used when bingeing and purging patients are required to stay in an observed dayroom area for 2–3 hours after every meal. Very few patients vomit in front of other people, and thus the emesis response is prevented and, eventually, stopped completely.

Cognitive therapy techniques for treating anorexia nervosa were developed by Garner and Bemis (1982). The assessment of cognition is a first step in cognitive therapy. Patients are asked to write down their thoughts on an assessment form so that cognitions can be examined for systematic distortions in the processing and interpretation of events. Cognitive techniques include operationalizing beliefs, decentering, using the "what if" technique, evaluating autonomic thoughts, testing prospective hypotheses, reinterpreting body image misperception, examining underlying assumptions, and modifying basic assumptions.

Cognitive-behavioral treatment for prevention of relapse of anorexia nervosa was further developed by Kleifield et al. (1996), who created an easy-to-use treatment manual. The cognitive-behavioral treatment is based on two core assumptions about the disorder. The first assumption is that anorexia nervosa has a significant positive functioning in the patient's life and develops as a way of coping with adverse experiences often associated with developmental transitions and distressing life events. The anorexic patient's deficient coping abilities produce anxiety and fear, and the patient is distracted from these anxieties by an overwhelming preoccupation with food and weight. The anorexic condition is also a reinforcing one,

in that the patient experiences a surge of confidence and a sense of competence and control after being successful in dieting. The second assumption is that food restriction and ritualistic food avoidance behaviors become independent of the events or issues provoking them. The anorexic patient's extreme anxiety about gaining weight and becoming fat is alleviated by not eating. The relief of anxiety about gaining weight—the anxiety being alleviated through avoidance of food—is another strong reinforcement and thus a key factor in the persistence with which these patients pursue food restriction.

On the basis of the aforementioned assumptions, two separate pathways are taken in treatment. First, the dietary restriction is regarded as a food phobia, and change in eating behavior is a primary objective. Behavioral methods such as monitoring food intake and the details surrounding food intake, along with techniques such as increasing exposure, are used to increase the patient's food intake gradually. Cognitive-behavioral methods are used to reduce the anxiety associated with behavioral change. Cognitive techniques such as cognitive restructuring and problem solving help the patient deal with distorted and overvalued beliefs about food and thinness and cope with life's stresses.

A family analysis should be done on all patients with anorexia who are living with their families. On the basis of this analysis, a clinical judgment should be made regarding what type of family therapy or counseling is clinically advisable. In some cases, family therapy will not be possible. However, in those cases, issues of family relationships must be dealt with in individual therapy and, in some cases, in brief counseling sessions with immediate family members. A controlled family therapy study by Russell et al. (1987) showed that patients with anorexia younger than 18 benefited from family therapy and patients older than 18 did worse in family therapy compared with the control therapy. There are no controlled studies of the combination of individual and family therapy. In actual practice, many clinicians provide individual therapy and some sort of family counseling in managing anorexia nervosa.

A multifaceted treatment approach is necessary for effective care of patients with anorexia nervosa. As medical rehabilitation proceeds, an associated improvement in psychological state occurs. Behavioral contingencies are useful for inducing weight gain and changing the medical condition of the patient. Cyproheptadine may be helpful in facilitating weight gain and decreasing depressive symptomatology in the restricting anorexic patient. If an anorexic patient has a predominance of depressive symptoms and is within 80% of a normal weight range, fluoxetine should be useful for treating the depression.

Severely obsessive-compulsive, anxious, and agitated anorexic patients are likely to require chlorpromazine or an atypical antipsychotic medication such as risperidone or olanzapine. All patients need cognitive individual psychotherapy. The more severely ill patients need hospitalization initially, followed by a well-planned continued outpatient treatment program (Garner and Garfinkel 1985). Prevention of relapse is a major part of the treatment of anorexia nervosa. Multicenter controlled treatment studies are being conducted to test the efficacy of a specific cognitive-behavioral therapy (CBT) and serotonin reuptake inhibitors in the prevention of relapse in this disorder.

Bulimia

Definition

Bulimia is a term that means "binge eating." This behavior has become a common practice among female students in universities and, more recently, in high schools. Not all persons who engage in binge eating require a psychiatric diagnosis. Bulimia can occur in anorexia nervosa; when this happens, the patient, under the DSM-IV-TR system, should have a diagnosis of *anorexia nervosa, binge-eating/purging type.* Bulimia also can occur in a normal-weight condition associated with psychological symptomatology. In that case, a diagnosis of *bulimia nervosa* applies (Table 17–2). Normal-weight bingeing and purging patients can fall into two categories: 1) normal-weight bulimic patients who have never had a history of anorexia nervosa and 2) those who have had a history of anorexia nervosa. Unfortunately, the DSM-IV-TR classification system does not separate these two subgroups of bulimic patients. The term *bulimia nervosa* implies a psychiatric impairment and therefore is a better label than simply *bulimia.*

Bulimia nervosa is a disorder in which the behavior of bulimia or binge eating is the predominant behavior. Binge eating is defined as an episodic, uncontrolled, rapid ingestion of large quantities of food over a short period. Abdominal pain or discomfort, self-induced vomiting, sleep, or social interruption terminates the bulimic episode. Feelings of guilt, depression, or self-disgust follow. Bulimic patients often use cathartics for weight control and have an eating pattern of alternate binges and fasts. Bulimic patients have a fear of not being able to stop eating voluntarily. The food consumed during a binge usually has a highly dense calorie content and a texture that facilitates rapid eating. Frequent weight fluctuations occur but without the severity of weight loss present in anorexia nervosa.

Bulimia is also encountered in DSM-IV-TR *binge-eating disorder* (BED), which did not exist in DSM-III-R (American Psychiatric Association 1987). This disor-

TABLE 17–2. DSM-IV-TR diagnostic criteria for bulimia nervosa

A. Recurrent episodes of binge eating. An episode of binge eating is characterized by both of the following:
   (1) eating, in a discrete period of time (e.g., within any 2-hour period), an amount of food that is definitely larger than most people would eat during a similar period of time and under similar circumstances
   (2) a sense of lack of control over eating during the episode (e.g., a feeling that one cannot stop eating or control what or how much one is eating)
B. Recurrent inappropriate compensatory behavior in order to prevent weight gain, such as self-induced vomiting; misuse of laxatives, diuretics, enemas, or other medications; fasting; or excessive exercise.
C. The binge eating and inappropriate compensatory behaviors both occur, on average, at least twice a week for 3 months.
D. Self-evaluation is unduly influenced by body shape and weight.
E. The disturbance does not occur exclusively during episodes of anorexia nervosa.
Specify type:
   Purging Type: during the current episode of bulimia nervosa, the person has regularly engaged in self-induced vomiting or the misuse of laxatives, diuretics, or enemas
   Nonpurging Type: during the current episode of bulimia nervosa, the person has used other inappropriate compensatory behaviors, such as fasting or excessive exercise, but has not regularly engaged in self-induced vomiting or the misuse of laxatives, diuretics, or enemas

TABLE 17–3. DSM-IV-TR diagnostic criteria for eating disorder not otherwise specified

The eating disorder not otherwise specified category is for disorders of eating that do not meet the criteria for any specific eating disorder. Examples include
1. For females, all of the criteria for anorexia nervosa are met except that the individual has regular menses.
2. All of the criteria for anorexia nervosa are met except that, despite significant weight loss, the individual's current weight is in the normal range.
3. All of the criteria for bulimia nervosa are met except that the binge eating and inappropriate compensatory mechanisms occur at a frequency of less than twice a week or for a duration of less than 3 months.
4. The regular use of inappropriate compensatory behavior by an individual of normal body weight after eating small amounts of food (e.g., self-induced vomiting after the consumption of two cookies).
5. Repeatedly chewing and spitting out, but not swallowing, large amounts of food.
6. Binge-eating disorder: recurrent episodes of binge eating in the absence of the regular use of inappropriate compensatory behaviors characteristic of bulimia nervosa.

der is listed as an example under the category "eating disorder not otherwise specified" (Tables 17–3 and 17–4). Insufficient data are currently available to make BED a distinct Axis I diagnosis. Preliminary field studies show that most persons who meet criteria for BED are obese. In the next 5 years, epidemiological studies will determine whether BED is a distinct disorder or merely the nonpurging type of bulimia.

Clinical Features

Bulimia nervosa usually begins after a period of dieting of a few weeks to a year or longer. The dieting may or may not have been successful in achieving weight loss. Most binge-eating episodes are followed by self-induced vomiting. Episodes are

---

TABLE 17–4. DSM-IV-TR research
criteria for binge-eating disorder

A. Recurrent episodes of binge eating. An
episode of binge eating is characterized by
both of the following:
  (1) eating, in a discrete period of time
      (e.g., within any 2-hour period), an
      amount of food that is definitely
      larger than most people would eat in
      a similar period of time under similar
      circumstances
  (2) a sense of lack of control over eating
      during the episode (e.g., a feeling that
      one cannot stop eating or control what
      or how much one is eating)
B. The binge-eating episodes are associated
   with three (or more) of the following:
  (1) eating much more rapidly than nor-
      mal
  (2) eating until feeling uncomfortably full
  (3) eating large amounts of food when not
      feeling physically hungry
  (4) eating alone because of being embar-
      rassed by how much one is eating
  (5) feeling disgusted with oneself,
      depressed, or very guilty after
      overeating
C. Marked distress regarding binge eating is
   present.
D. The binge eating occurs, on average, at
   least 2 days a week for 6 months.
   Note: The method of determining frequency differs from that used for bulimia
   nervosa; future research should address
   whether the preferred method of setting
   a frequency threshold is counting the
   number of days on which binges occur or
   counting the number of episodes of binge
   eating.
E. The binge eating is not associated with the
   regular use of inappropriate compensatory behaviors (e.g., purging, fasting,
   excessive exercise) and does not occur
   exclusively during the course of anorexia
   nervosa or bulimia nervosa.

---

less frequently followed by use of laxatives. A minority of bulimic patients use

diuretics for weight control. The average
length of a bingeing episode is about
1 hour. Most patients learn to vomit by
sticking their fingers down their throat,
and after a short time they learn to vomit
on a reflex basis. Some patients have abra-
sions and scars on the backs of their hands
(called *Russell's sign*) from their persistent efforts to induce vomiting. Most bulimic patients do not eat regular meals and
have difficulty feeling satiety at the end of
a normal meal. Bulimic patients usually
prefer to eat alone and at their homes. Approximately one-third to one-fifth of bulimic patients will choose a weight within a
normal weight range as their ideal body
weight. About one-fourth to one-third of
the patients with bulimia nervosa have
had a history of anorexia nervosa.

Most bulimic patients have depressive
signs and symptoms. They have problems
with interpersonal relationships, self-
concept, and impulsive behaviors and
show high levels of anxiety and compulsivity. Chemical dependency is not unusual in this disorder, alcohol abuse being
the most common. Bulimic individuals
will abuse amphetamines to reduce their
appetite and to lose weight. Impulsive
stealing usually occurs after the onset of
binge eating; however, about one-fourth
of patients actually begin stealing before
the onset of bulimia. Food, clothing, and
jewelry are the items most commonly
stolen.

Medical Complications

Individuals with bulimia nervosa who engage in self-induced vomiting and abuse
purgatives or diuretics are susceptible to
hypokalemic alkalosis. These patients
have electrolyte abnormalities, including
elevated serum bicarbonate levels, hypochloremia, hypokalemia, and, in a few
cases, low serum bicarbonate levels, indicating a metabolic acidosis. The latter is

particularly likely among bulimic individuals who abuse laxatives. It is important to remember that fasting can promote dehydration, which results in volume depletion. This, in turn, can promote generation of aldosterone, which stimulates further potassium excretion from the kidneys. Thus, there can be an indirect renal loss of potassium as well as a direct loss through self-induced vomiting. Patients with electrolyte disturbances have physical symptoms of weakness and lethargy and at times have cardiac arrhythmias. The latter, of course, can lead to a sudden cardiac arrest. Patients with bulimia nervosa can have severe attrition and erosion of the teeth, causing an irritating sensitivity, pathological pulp exposures, loss of integrity of the dental arches, diminished masticatory ability, and an unaesthetic appearance.

Parotid gland enlargement associated with elevated serum amylase levels is commonly observed in patients who binge and vomit. In fact, the serum amylase level is an excellent way to follow reduction of vomiting in patients with eating disorders who deny purging episodes. Acute dilatation of the stomach is a rare emergency condition for patients who binge. Esophageal tears also can occur through the process of self-induced vomiting. A complication of shock can result subsequent to the esophageal tear and should be treated by experienced medical and surgical personnel. Severe abdominal pain in the patient with bulimia nervosa should alert the physician to a diagnosis of gastric dilatation and the need for nasogastric suction, X rays, and surgical consultation.

Cardiac failure caused by cardiomyopathy from ipecac intoxication is a medical emergency that is being reported more frequently and that usually results in death. Symptoms of precordial pain, dyspnea, and generalized muscle weakness associated with hypotension, tachycardia, and abnormalities on the electrocardiogram should alert one to possible ipecac intoxication. Other laboratory findings may include elevated liver enzymes and an increased erythrocyte sedimentation rate. Obviously, at this point the patient should be under a cardiologist's care. An echocardiogram will show a cardiomyopathy contraction pattern associated with congestive heart failure.

Other mechanisms for cardiac arrhythmias and sudden death in bulimic patients probably exist. The arrhythmias noted here are associated with electrolyte disturbances and ipecac intoxication. More recent studies have shown arrhythmias associated with bingeing behavior even when serum electrolytes are within normal limits.

Epidemiology, Course, and Prognosis

No satisfactory incidence studies on bulimia nervosa have been reported. This is not surprising, given the fact that this disorder emerged only in 1980 as the distinct diagnostic entity presented in DSM-III (American Psychiatric Association 1980). In DSM-III, bulimia nervosa was referred to as "bulimia," and the criteria did not allow one to distinguish between occasional binge eating episodes and the truly incapacitating disorder of bulimia nervosa. The bulimia nervosa diagnostic criteria have been revised every few years, and this may account for the disparity in reported prevalence rates for this disorder. Studies that used strict criteria found prevalence rates between 1 and 3.8 per 100 females (Hart and Ollendick 1985; Schotte and Stunkard 1987). In a study combining surveys and interviews of women in the first year of college, Kurth et al. (1995) found the prevalence of bulimia nervosa to be 2%. In a Canadian community sample, in a study in which a structured interview was used, prevalence rates of this disorder were 1% (Garfinkel et al. 1995). Hoek (1991) found a 1-year prevalence rate of bulimia nervosa of 0.17% among adolescent girls and young women ages 15–29 years in a primary care health delivery system. The prevalence of males in the bulimia nervosa population varies between 10% and 15%. In most studies, the average age at onset of bulimia nervosa is 18 years (range = 12–35 years). These studies have shown a much higher representation of the social classes IV and V in patients with bulimia nervosa compared with patients with anorexia nervosa.

There are virtually no long-term follow-up studies on patients with bulimia nervosa. Thus, little information is available on the natural course of this disorder and on outcome predictors.

Etiology and Pathogenesis

Fairburn and Cooper (1984) found that a rigid diet was the most commonly reported precipitant of binge-eating behavior and that a gross bingeing bout was the most common precipitant for vomiting behavior. This finding may shed some light on the physiological mechanisms involved in binge eating and purging. For example, the period of strict dieting may influence peptide and neurotransmitter secretion, which may in turn affect appetite and satiety mechanisms. Studies of satiety responses in individuals with eating disorders have shown that the perceptions of hunger and of satiety are disturbed in patients who binge and purge (Halmi and Sunday 1991). Another study showed distinct differences in taste preferences for sweetness and "fattiness" in restricting anorexic patients, bulimic anorexic patients, normal-weight bulimic patients, and control subjects (Sunday

and Halmi 1990). Further identification of disturbances in the psychological processes of hunger, satiety, and taste could provide important clues concerning impaired central mechanisms. Evidence for dysregulation of serotonergic neurotransmission in bulimia nervosa consists of blunted prolactin response to the serotonin receptor agonist m-chlorophenylpiperazine (m-CPP), 5-hydroxytryptophan, and *dl*-fenfluramine and enhanced migrainelike headache response to m-CPP challenge. Low levels of CSF 5-hydroxyindoleacetic acid are associated with impulsive and aggressive behaviors and are also present in bulimia nervosa patients (Jimerson et al. 1997; Levitan et al. 1997). In a large interview study by Braun et al. (1994), 31% of the bulimic subgroups had a Cluster B (impulsive) disorder. Borderline personality disorder was present in 25% of the bulimic subgroups and was the most common Cluster B condition.

In a study of clinical features, Hatsukami et al. (1984) found that 43.5% of a sample of 108 women with bulimia nervosa had an affective disorder at some time in their lives and 18.5% had a history of alcohol or drug abuse. Although there is a high association of mood disorder with bulimia nervosa, insufficient current evidence is available to support describing bulimia nervosa as a mere forme fruste of mood disorder. Bulimia nervosa theoretically fits well into an addictive model (Szmukler and Tantam 1984).

The percentage of individuals with DSM-III-R bulimia (including anorexic bulimic individuals) who have at least one personality disorder has been reported to be 77% (Powers et al. 1988), 69% (Wonderlich et al. 1990), 62% (Gartner et al. 1989), 61% (Schmidt and Telch 1990), 33% (Ames-Frankel et al. 1992), and 23% (Herzog et al. 1992). All of these studies used established diagnostic interviews, but the findings are not in agreement. This is probably a result of several factors: 1) some of the studies with very small numbers of patients may represent a biased sample; 2) studies used different criteria, ranging from DSM-III to DSM-III-R, for both eating disorders and personality disorders; and 3) some of the Axis II interviewers lacked information about the patients' Axis I diagnosis, which may have led to false-positive personality disorder diagnoses. Nonetheless, substantial evidence indicates that personality disorders are commonly associated with bulimia nervosa.

Treatment

Treatment studies of bulimia nervosa have proliferated in the past 15 years, in contrast to the relatively few treatment studies of anorexia nervosa. This is probably because of the greater prevalence of bulimia nervosa and the fact that this disorder usually can be treated on an outpatient basis. Specific therapy techniques such as behavior therapy, cognitive therapy, psychodynamic therapy, and "psychoeducation therapy" have been conducted in both individual and group therapies. There are no controlled studies in which patients were randomly assigned to individual or group therapy for any of these techniques. Multiple controlled drug treatment studies also have been conducted in the past decade. Often a variety of therapy techniques such as cognitive therapy, behavior therapy, and drug treatment may be used together in either individual or group therapy. Unfortunately, there is no way to predict at present what bulimic patient will respond to what type of therapy or treatment. "The Practice Guideline for the Treatment of Patients With Eating Disorders" (Revision) (American Psychiatric Association 2000b) has a helpful section on developing a treatment plan for the individual patient. Factors that need to be considered are level of care (outpatient, intensive outpatient, partial hospitalization, residential treatment center, or inpatient hospitalization), site of treatment (availability of medical care), and family assessment and treatment.

Psychodynamic Therapy

Lacey (1983) described the use of psychodynamic therapy with cognitive and behavioral techniques in both the individual and the group therapy formats. Common themes that need to be dealt with are poor self-esteem, dependency problems, and a sense of ineffectiveness.

Cognitive-Behavioral Therapy

Fourteen published controlled studies have examined the efficacy of CBT in bulimia nervosa. One of the first and best descriptions of CBT was by Fairburn (1981). All of the subjects in these 14 studies were outpatients, with the exception of one study of the effectiveness of CBT in individual therapy, involving inpatients. Nearly all of the studies used a psychoeducational component that included information on the social-cultural emphasis on thinness; set point theory; the physical effects and medical complications of bingeing, purging, and abuse of laxatives and diuretics; and how dieting and fasting precipitate binge–purge cycles. Self-monitoring was an important part of all of these studies and usually consists of a daily record of the times and durations of meals and a record of binge-eating and purging episodes, as well as descriptions of moods and circumstances surrounding binge–purge episodes. The studies stressed the importance of eating regular meals.

Cognitive restructuring is the basis of all the CBT programs. The first step in cognitive therapy is the assessment of cognition. Patients are asked to write their thoughts on an assessment form so that cognitions can be examined for systematic distortions in the processing and interpretation of events. Two reviews of controlled studies of CBT for bulimia nervosa concluded that CBT benefits most patients (Fairburn et al. 1992a; Gotestam and Agras 1989). CBT was more effective than treatment with antidepressants alone, self-monitoring plus supportive psychotherapy, and behavioral treatment without the cognitive treatment component. One-year follow-up studies with CBT have shown a good maintenance of change, superior to that following treatment with antidepressants.

Behavior therapy is used specifically to stop the binge-eating/purging behaviors. Behavioral approaches include restricting exposure to cues that trigger a binge-purge episode, developing a strategy of alternative behaviors, and delaying the vomiting response to eating. Response prevention is a technique used specifically to prevent vomiting. After eating, a patient is placed in a situation in which it is very difficult for him or her comfortably to vomit. Adding exposure (i.e., requiring the patient to binge) did not seem to enhance the effects of response prevention (Rosen 1982).

The combined effects of CBT and antidepressant medication for bulimia nervosa were examined in three studies. Mitchell et al. (1990) found that group CBT was superior to imipramine therapy for decreasing binge eating and purging, and the combined treatment showed no additive effects for those treated with group CBT alone. Agras et al. (1992) had similar results comparing individual CBT, desipramine therapy, and the combination at 16 weeks. However, at 32 weeks, only the combined treatment given for 24 weeks was superior to medication given for 16

weeks. In a third study, CBT plus medication (desipramine, followed by fluoxetine in nonresponders) was superior to medication alone, but supportive psychotherapy plus medication was not. CBT plus medication was superior to CBT alone.

A study of interpersonal therapy (IPT), which targets interpersonal functioning, showed that IPT was equivalent to CBT in reducing bulimic symptoms and psychopathology; at follow-up, it was actually superior to CBT (Fairburn et al. 1992b). This was the first study to show that bulimia nervosa may be treated successfully without focusing directly on the patient's eating habits and attitudes toward shape and weight. In another study comparing CBT with IPT, bulimic patients had 19 sessions of treatment over a 20-week period and were evaluated for 1 year after treatment in a multisite study. CBT was significantly superior to IPT at the end of treatment for the number of participants recovered (29% vs. 6%). At a 1-year follow-up, no significant difference was found between the two treatments. However, CBT was significantly more rapid in initiating improvement in patients with bulimia nervosa compared with IPT. Therefore, the authors suggested that CBT should be considered the preferred psychotherapeutic treatment for bulimia nervosa (Agras et al. 2000).

Drug Therapy

Studies of antidepressant medications have consistently shown some efficacy in the treatment of bulimia nervosa. These studies were prompted by observations that patients with bulimia nervosa also had significant mood disturbances. Since 1980, more than a dozen double-blind, placebo-controlled trials of various antidepressants were conducted in normal-weight outpatients with bulimia nervosa. (For a review of these studies, see Fairburn et al. 1992a.) All of these trials found a significantly greater reduction in binge eating when antidepressant medication was administered than when placebo was given. Antidepressants improved mood and reduced psychopathological symptoms such as preoccupation with shape and weight. These studies provide evidence for the short-term efficacy of antidepressant medication, but long-term efficacy remains unknown. The average rate of abstinence from bingeing and purging in these studies was 22%, indicating that most patients remain symptomatic at the end of treatment with antidepressants. Both of the systematic studies conducted to evaluate maintenance of change in bulimic symptomatology yielded disappointing results: most subjects did not maintain improvement (Pyle et al. 1990; Walsh et al. 1991). The dosage of antidepressant medication to treat bulimia nervosa was similar to that used in the treatment of depression. The antidepressants used in the controlled treatment studies of bulimia nervosa included desipramine, imipramine, amitriptyline, nortriptyline, phenelzine, and fluoxetine.

The current data suggest that the treatment of choice for bulimia nervosa should be CBT and that a single antidepressant administered in the absence of psychotherapy cannot be considered an adequate treatment.

Obesity

Definition

In contrast to anorexia nervosa and bulimia nervosa, obesity is classified not as a psychiatric disorder but as a medical disorder. Obesity is an excessive accumulation of body fat and operationally is defined as being overweight. The BMI, which is weight (kg) divided by height (m^2), has the highest correlation, 0.8, with body fat measured by other, more precise laboratory methods. *Mildly overweight* is defined as having a BMI of 25–30, or body weight between the upper limit of normal and 20% above that limit on standard height-weight charts. *Obesity* is defined as a BMI greater than 30, or body weight greater than 20% above the upper limit for height (Bray 1978).

Clinical Features

The most obvious clinical features of obesity are physical; these features are discussed in the following section on medical complications. The psychological and behavioral aspects of obesity are best considered grouped in two categories: *eating behavior* and *emotional disturbance*. There is considerable heterogeneity in eating patterns. Most commonly, obese persons complain that they cannot restrain their eating and that they have difficulty achieving satiety. Some obese persons cannot distinguish hunger from other dysphoric states and will eat when they are emotionally upset.

The most methodologically satisfying studies have shown that there is no distinct or excess psychopathology in obesity. In one study of severely obese patients who had gastric bypass surgery, the most prevalent psychiatric diagnosis was major depressive disorder. However, this diagnosis was no more prevalent in the obese patients than in the general population. Self-disparagement of body image is especially present in those who have been obese since childhood. This may be due to the continual bombardment of social prejudice against obese people. The stigmatization and prejudice against obese types is well documented in studies of educational disadvantages and of employment prejudices against obese persons. Many obese individuals develop anxiety and depression when they attempt to diet (Halmi et al. 1980).

Because health risks and mortality vary with degree of adiposity, Bray (1986) proposed a classification into low-risk (BMI = 25–30), moderate-risk (BMI = 31–40), and high-risk (BMI > 40) individuals.

Medical Complications

Obesity affects a great variety of physiological functions. Blood circulation may be overtaxed as body weight increases, and congestive heart failure may occur in grossly obese individuals. Hypertension is strongly associated with obesity, and the prevalence of carbohydrate intolerance in grossly obese individuals is approximately 50%. Increased body fat in the upper region of the body as opposed to the lower region is more likely to be associated with the onset of diabetes mellitus. The impairment of pulmonary function becomes extreme in severe obesity and involves hypoventilation, hypercapnia, hypoxia, and somnolence (i.e., pickwickian syndrome). The latter has a high mortality rate. Obesity may accelerate the development of osteoarthritis and of dermatological problems from stretching of the skin, intertrigo, and acanthosis nigricans. Obese women are an obstetrical risk, because they are susceptible to toxemia and hypertension.

Obesity has been associated with several types of cancer. Obese males have a higher rate of prostate and colorectal cancer, and obese females have increased incidences of gallbladder, breast, cervical, endometrial, uterine, and ovarian cancer. Most studies on the topic suggest that obesity influences the development and progression of both endometrial and breast cancer through influences on estrogen production. Low-density lipoprotein levels are increased in obesity, and levels of high-density lipoproteins (HDL cholesterol) are reduced. The low levels of HDL may be one mechanism by which obesity is associated with an increased risk for cardiovascular disease.

Epidemiology, Course, and Prognosis

If obesity is defined as the state of being 20% above ideal weight, then nearly a quarter of the United States population would be considered obese (VanItallie 1985). Socioeconomic status is highly correlated with obesity: the condition is much more common among women (less so among men) of low status. This relationship is also present in obese children. Increasing age and obesity are associated until age 50. The prevalence of obesity is higher in women compared with men; in individuals older than 50 years, this may be due to the increased mortality rate among obese men with advancing age.

Unfortunately, life expectancy and obesity studies are restricted to life insurance studies and therefore do not represent a random American population. Despite these limitations, studies have shown a progressive increase in "excess mortality" as BMI increased (Society of Actuaries 1992). Another study of grossly obese persons showed that excess mortality was greatly increased in younger men (aged 25–34 years) and gradually declined with age (Stevens et al. 1998).

Etiology and Pathogenesis

It is unlikely that obesity has a single etiology. In the first section of this chapter, the complex neural mechanisms involved in the control of feeding behavior were discussed. Lipid, amino acid, and glucose metabolism all seem to affect, in some way, central neural regulatory mechanisms that influence eating behavior. Obesity is regarded today by most investigators as a disorder of energy balance, a disorder with a strong genetic component that is modulated by cultural and environmental influences.

Obesity has a definite familial aspect. Eighty percent of the offspring of two obese parents are obese, compared with 40% of the offspring of one obese parent and only 10% of the offspring of lean parents. Findings of twin studies and adoption studies suggest that genetic factors play a strong role in the development of obesity.

The cloning and sequencing of the mouse obese (Ob) gene and its human homologue in 1994 (Zhang et al. 1994) provided the basis for further research into the pathways that regulate adiposity and body weight. Leptin, the gene product of the Ob gene, was shown to be a 16-kd protein that is present in both rodent and human plasma (Halaas et al. 1995). Intraperitoneal injections of recombinant leptin decrease food intake and increase energy expenditure in wild-type mice. Leptin reduces body fat in mice, and its absence in mice with the Ob gene leads to a massive increase in body fat. In both humans and rodents, leptin is highly correlated with BMI and amount of body fat (Maffei et al. 1995). Weight loss due to food restriction was associated with a decrease in plasma leptin concentrations in mice and obese humans. These findings suggest that leptin serves an endocrine function, regulating body weight and stores of body fat.

Obese individuals have larger and more numerous fat cells. Cellular proliferation tends to occur early in life but also will occur in adult life when the existing fat cells are greatly enlarged. The regulation of fat cell proliferation and size is not well understood. The relation of physical activity to obesity is complex. It is known that obese individuals are less active than are individuals of normal weight. The increase in caloric expenditure from physical activity is small. Animal studies show that physical activity actually decreases food intake and may even prevent the decline in metabolic rate that usually accompanies dieting.

Treatment

For mild obesity (20%–40% overweight), the most effective treatment to date is behavioral modification in groups, a balanced diet, and exercise. Such treatment programs are usually conducted by both commercial and nonprofit large organizations. For moderate obesity (41%–100% overweight), a medically supervised protein-sparing modified fast (400–700 calories per day) is often necessary. This diet may or may not be combined with behavioral modification techniques. A behavior analysis is necessary to set up a sensible behavioral modification program. Antecedents of eating behavior, the eating behavior itself, the consequences of the behavior, and the acceptable rewards for carrying out various prescribed behaviors are all analyzed. Behavioral treatment programs include self-monitoring, nutrition education, physical activity, and cognitive restructuring.

The use of medication such as phenylpropanolamine or fenfluramine was popular in the past. The problem with these drugs is that on withdrawal, a rebound ballooning up of weight occurs; some patients have concomitant lethargy and depression. In 1997, fenfluramine was removed by the U.S. Food and Drug Administration from the market and for approved use for treatment of obesity because of the adverse effects of pulmonary hypertension and mitral valve impairment.

Only one long-term (5 years) controlled study has documented the safety and efficacy of the fenfluramine-phentermine combination (Weintraub 1992). The National Task Force on the Prevention and Treatment of Obesity (1996) reviewed all English-language reports of studies in which human obesity was treated with medication that was given for at least 24 weeks. The task force found that the net weight loss attributable to medication use was modest, ranging from 2 kg to 10 kg. The weight loss tends to reach a plateau by 6 months. Most adverse effects are mild and self-limited, but rare serious outcomes such as pulmonary hypertension have been reported. The task force's conclusion was that pharmacotherapy for obesity, when combined with appropriate behavioral approaches to change diet and amount of physical activity, helps some obese patients to lose weight and maintain weight loss for at least 1 year (National Task Force on the Prevention and Treatment of Obesity 1996). The task force also stated that until more data are available, pharmacotherapy cannot be recommended for routine use in obese individuals. They did acknowledge that it may be helpful in carefully selected patients.

Severe obesity (greater than 100% over normal weight) is the least common form of obesity and is most effectively treated with surgical procedures that reduce the size of the stomach. These procedures produce a substantial weight loss and show a good record of weight loss maintenance.

Behavioral modification is the treatment of choice for overweight children and should include involvement of the parents and the schools. Psychotherapy is not recommended as a treatment per se for obesity, although some patients may have particular problems that may be effectively treated or helped with psychotherapy. For excellent discussions on the treatment of obesity, see Stunkard (1984), Brownell (1984), and Lasagna (1987).

Conclusions

The eating disorders are complex syndromes in which the interactions among environmental, psychological, and physiological factors both create and maintain the disturbed eating behavior. The more precise an understanding we obtain of the connectedness of basic physiological changes, psychological changes, and eating behavior, the better we will be able to design effective treatment interventions.

Many questions remain to be asked about our current treatment interventions. For example, how long should the bulimic patient be treated with antidepressants? Would periodic follow-up behavioral sessions help prevent relapse in bulimic patients treated with behavior therapy? How can we identify the treatment most likely to be effective for a given patient?

Continued prospective longitudinal studies are necessary for bulimia nervosa because no information is available on what happens to this addictive-like bingeing–purging behavior over the course of a lifetime. Although disturbed eating behavior has been present throughout the history of humankind, it has been systematically studied with scientific methodology only in the past few decades. There is a continued need for further study of eating disorders.

References

Agras WS, Rossiter EM, Arnow B, et al: Pharmacologic and cognitive-behavioral treatment for bulimia nervosa: a controlled comparison. Am J Psychiatry 149:82–87, 1992

Agras WS, Walsh BT, Fairburn CG: A multicenter comparison of cognitive-behavioral therapy and interpersonal psychotherapy for bulimia nervosa. Arch Gen Psychiatry 57:459–466, 2000

Ahima RS, Prabakarn D, Mantzoros C, et al: Role of leptin in the neuroendocrine response to fasting. Nature 382:250–252, 1996

American Psychiatric Association: Diagnostic and Statistical Manual of Mental Disorders, 3rd Edition. Washington, DC, American Psychiatric Association, 1980

American Psychiatric Association: Diagnostic and Statistical Manual of Mental Disorders, 3rd Edition, Revised. Washington, DC, American Psychiatric Association, 1987

American Psychiatric Association: Practice guideline for the treatment of patients with eating disorders (revision). Am J Psychiatry 157 (suppl):1–39, 2000b

Ames-Frankel J, Devlin MJ, Walsh BT, et al: Personality disorders and eating disorders. J Clin Psychiatry 53:90–96, 1992

Barr LC, Goodman WK, Price LH, et al: The serotonin hypothesis of obsessive compulsive disorder: implications of pharmacological challenge studies. Clin Psychiatry 53:17–28, 1992

Bellodi L, Cavallini MC, Bertelli S: Morbidity risk for obsessive-compulsive spectrum disorders in first-degree relatives of patients with eating disorders. Am J Psychiatry 158:563–569, 2001

Ben-Tovin D, Walker K, Gilchrist P: Outcome in patients with eating disorders: a 5 year study. Lancet 357:1254–1257, 2001

Boden G, Chen X, Mazzoli M, et al: Effect of fasting on serum leptin in normal subjects. J Clin Endocrinol Metab 81:3419–3423, 1996

Bohus B, Kovacs GL, de Wied D: Oxytocin, vasopressin and memory: opposite effects on consolidation and retrieval processes. Brain Res 157:414–417, 1978

Booth DA: Food-conditioned eating preferences and aversions with interceptive elements: conditioned appetite and satieties. Ann N Y Acad Sci 443:22–41, 1985

Brambilla F, Bellodi L, Arancio C, et al: Central dopaminergic function in anorexia and bulimia nervosa: a psychoneuroendocrine approach. Psychoneuroendocrinology 26: 393–409, 2001

Braun DL, Sunday SR, Halmi KA: Psychiatric comorbidity in patients with eating disorders. Psychol Med 24:859–867, 1994

Bray GA: Definitions, measurements and classification of the syndromes of obesity. Int J Obesity 2:99–112, 1978

Bray GA: Effects of obesity on health and happiness, in Handbook of Eating Disorders: Physiology, Psychology, and Treatment. Edited by Brownell KD, Foreyt JP. New York, Basic Books, 1986, pp 3–44

Brownell KD: New developments in the treatment of obese children and adolescents, in Eating and Its Disorders. Edited by Stunkard AJ, Stellar E. New York, Raven, 1984, pp 175–184

Bruch H: Perceptual and conceptual disturbance in anorexia nervosa. Psychosom Med 24:187–195, 1962

Charney DS, Wood SW, Krystal JH, et al: Serotonin function and human anxiety disorders. Ann N Y Acad Sci 600:558–573, 1990

Chen H, Charlat O, Tartaglia LA, et al: Evidence that the diabetes gene encodes the leptin receptor: identification of a mutation in the leptin receptor gene in the DB/DB mice. Cell 84:491–495, 1996

Considine RV, Sinha MK, Heiman ML, et al: Serum immunoreactive-leptin concentrations in normal-weight and obese humans. N Engl J Med 334:292–295, 1996

Crisp AH: The possible significance of some behavioral correlates of weight and carbohydrate intake. J Psychosom Res 11:117–123, 1976

Demitrek MA, Kalogeras KT, Altemus M, et al: Plasma and cerebrospinal fluid measures of arginine vasopressin secretion in patients with bulimia nervosa and in healthy subjects. J Clin Endocrinol Metab 74: 1277–1283, 1992

Eagles T, Johnston M, Hunter D, et al: Increasing incidence of anorexia nervosa in the female population of northeast Scotland. Am J Psychiatry 152:1266–1271, 1995

Fairburn C: A cognitive behavioral approach to the treatment of bulimia. Psychol Med 11:707–711, 1981

Fairburn CG, Cooper PJ: The clinical features of bulimia nervosa. Br J Psychiatry 144: 238–246, 1984

Fairburn CG, Agra WS, Wilson GT: The research on the treatment of bulimia nervosa: practical and theoretical implications, in Biology of Feast and Famine: Relevance to Eating Disorders. Edited by Anderson GH, Kennedy SH. New York, Academic Press, 1992a, pp 318–340

Fairburn CG, Jones R, Pevelar RC, et al: Three psychological treatments for bulimia nervosa: a comparative trial. Arch Gen Psychiatry 48:463–469, 1992b

Falk JR, Halmi KA: Amenorrhea in anorexia nervosa: examination of the critical body hypothesis. Biol Psychiatry 17:799–806, 1982

Garfinkel P, Goering L, Spegg C, et al: Bulimia nervosa in a Canadian community sample: prevalence and comparison of subgroups. Am J Psychiatry 52:1052–1058, 1995

Garner DM, Bemis KM: A cognitive-behavioral approach to anorexia nervosa. Cognitive Therapy and Research 6:1223–1250, 1982

Garner DM, Garfinkel PE: Handbook of Psychotherapy for Anorexia Nervosa. New York, Guilford, 1985

Gartner AF, Marcus RN, Halmi KA, et al: DSM-III-R personality disorders in patients with eating disorders. Am J Psychiatry 146:1585–1591, 1989

Gotestam KA, Agras WS: Bulimia nervosa: pharmacologic and psychologic approaches to treatment. Nordisk Psykiatrisk Tidsskrift 43:543–551, 1989

Grahame-Smith DG: Serotonin in affective disorders. Int Clin Psychopharmacol 6 (suppl 4):5–13, 1992

Halaas J, Gajiwala K, Maffei M, et al: Weight-reducing effects of the protein encoded by the obese gene. Science 269:543–546, 1995

Halmi KA: Anorexia nervosa: demographic and clinical features in 94 cases. Psychosom Med 36:18–26, 1974

Halmi KA: Anorexia nervosa and bulimia, in Handbook of Adolescent Psychology. Edited by Hersen M, Van Hasselt T. New York, Pergamon, 1987, pp 265–287

Halmi KA, Falk JR: Common physiological changes in anorexia nervosa. Int J Eat Disord 1:16–27, 1981

Halmi KA, Sunday SR: Temporal patterns of hunger and satiety ratings and related cognitions in anorexia and bulimia. Appetite 16:219–237, 1991

Halmi KA, Stunkard AJ, Mason EE: Emotional responses to weight reduction by three methods: gastric bypass, jejunoileal bypass, diet. Am J Clin Nutr 33:446–451, 1980

Halmi KA, Eckert E, Marchi P, et al: Comorbidity of psychiatric diagnoses in anorexia nervosa. Arch Gen Psychiatry 48:712–718, 1991

Hart K, Ollendick TH: Prevalence of bulimia in working and university women. Am J Psychiatry 142:851–854, 1985

Hatsukami J, Mitchell J, Eckert E, et al: Affective disorder and substance abuse in women with bulimia. Psychol Med 14:704–710, 1984

Herzog DB, Keller MB, Lavori PW, et al: The prevalence of personality disorders in 210 women with eating disorders. J Clin Psychiatry 53:147–152, 1992

Hoek H: The incidence and prevalence of anorexia nervosa and bulimia nervosa in primary care. Psychol Med 21:455–460, 1991

Jimerson DC, Wolfe BE, Metzger ED, et al: Decrease serotonin function in bulimia nervosa. Arch Gen Psychiatry 54:529–534, 1997

Jones D, Fox MM, Babigian HM, et al: Epidemiology of anorexia nervosa in Monroe County, NY, 1960–1976. Psychosom Med 42:551–558, 1980

Kaye WH, Ebert MH, Raleigh M, et al: Abnormalities in CNS monoamine metabolism in anorexia nervosa. Arch Gen Psychiatry 41:350–355, 1984a

Kaye WH, Ebert M, Gwirtsman H, et al: Differences in brain serotonergic metabolism between nonbulimic and bulimic patients with anorexia nervosa. Am J Psychiatry 141:1598–1601, 1984b

Kendler SK, MacLean C, Neale M, et al: The genetic epidemiology of bulimia nervosa. Am J Psychiatry 148:1627–1637, 1991

Kleifield E, Wagner S, Halmi K: Cognitive-behavioral treatment of anorexia nervosa. Psychiatr Clin North Am 19:715–734, 1996

Kurth C, Krahn D, Nairn K, et al: The severity of dieting and bingeing behaviors in college women: interview validation of survey data. J Psychiatry Res 29:211–225, 1995

Lacey JH: An outpatient treatment program for bulimia nervosa. Int J Eat Disord 2:209–241, 1983

Lasagna L: The pharmacotherapy of obesity, in Psychopharmacology: The Third Generation of Progress. Edited by Meltzer HY. New York, Raven, 1987, pp 1281–1284

Levitan RD, Kaplan AS, Joffe RT, et al: Hormonal and subjective responses to intravenous meta-chlorophenylpiperazine in bulimia nervosa. Arch Gen Psychiatry 54: 521–527, 1997

Lilenfeld LR, Kaye WH, Greeno CG, et al: Psychiatric disorders in women with bulimia nervosa and their first degree relatives: effects of comorbid substance dependence. Int J Eat Disord 22:253–264, 1997

Lilenfeld LR, Kaye WH, Greeno CG, et al: A controlled family study of anorexia nervosa and bulimia nervosa: psychiatric disorders in first-degree relatives and effects of proband comorbidity. Arch Gen Psychiatry 55:603–610, 1998

Maffei M, Halaas J, Ravussin E, et al: Leptin levels in human and rodent: measurement of plasma leptin and OB RNA in obese and weight-reduced subjects. Nat Med 1: 1155–1161, 1995

Mantzoros C, Flier JS, Lesem MD, et al: Cerebrospinal fluid leptin in anorexia nervosa: correlation with nutritional status and potential role in resistance to weight gain. J Clin Endocrinol Metab 82:1845–1851, 1997

Mitchell JE, Pyle RL, Eckert ED, et al: A comparison study of antidepressants and structured intensive group therapy in the treatment of bulimia nervosa. Arch Gen Psychiatry 47:149–157, 1990

Morley J, Levine AS: Pharmacology of eating behavior. Annu Rev Pharmacol Toxicol 25: 127–146, 1985

National Task Force on the Prevention and Treatment of Obesity: Long-term pharmacotherapy in the management of obesity. JAMA 276:1907–1915, 1996

Owen WP, Halmi KA, Lasley E, et al: Dopamine regulation in anorexia nervosa. Psychopharmacol Bull 19:578–580, 1983

Pirke KM: Central and peripheral noradrenaline regulation in eating disorders. Psychiatry Res 62:43–49, 1996

Powers PS, Covert DL, Brightwell DR, et al: Other psychiatric disorders among bulimic patients. Compr Psychiatry 29:503–508, 1988

Pyle RL, Mitchell JE, Eckert ED, et al: Maintenance treatment and 6-month outcome for bulimia patients who respond to initial treatment. Am J Psychiatry 147:871–875, 1990

Rosen J: Bulimia nervosa: treatment with exposure and response prevention. Behavior Therapy 13:117–124, 1982

Russell GFM: Metabolic, endocrine and psychiatric aspects of anorexia nervosa. Scientific Basis of Medicine Annual Review 14:236–255, 1969

Russell GFM, Szmukler JI, Dare C, et al: An evaluation of family therapy in anorexia nervosa and bulimia nervosa. Arch Gen Psychiatry 44:1047–1056, 1987

Schmidt ND, Telch MJ: Prevalence of personality disorders among bulimics, non-bulimic binge eaters and normal controls. Journal of Psychopathology and Behavioral Assessment 12:170–185, 1990

Schotte D, Stunkard A: Bulimia vs. bulimic behaviors on a college campus. JAMA 9: 1213–1215, 1987

Society of Actuaries: Life tables for the United States Social Security Area 1900–2080: Actuarial Study No 107, August 1992 (SSA Publ No 11-11536). Washington, DC, U.S. Department of Health and Human Services, 1992

Soubrie P: Reconciling the role of central serotonin neurosis in human and animal behavior. Behav Brain Sci 9:319–363, 1986

Stevens J, Ooi J, Pamuk E, et al: The effect of age on the association between body mass index and mortality. N Engl J Med 338:1–7, 1998

Strober M, Morell W, Burroughs J, et al: A controlled family study of anorexia nervosa. Psychiatry Res 19:329–346, 1985

Strober M, Freeman R, Lampert C, et al: Males with anorexia nervosa: a controlled study of eating disorders in first-degree relatives. Int J Eat Disord 29:263–269, 2001

Stunkard AJ: The current status of treatment for obesity in adults, in Eating and Its Disorders. Edited by Stunkard AJ, Stellar E. New York, Raven, 1984, pp 157–174

Sunday SR, Halmi KA: Taste perceptions and hedonics in eating disorders. Physiol Behav 48:587–594, 1990

Szmukler JI: The epidemiology of anorexia nervosa and bulimia. J Psychiatry Res 19:1243–1253, 1985

Szmukler JI, Tantam D: Anorexia nervosa: starvation dependence. Br J Med Psychol 57:305–310, 1984

Tartaglia LA, Dembski M, Weng X, et al: Identification and expression cloning of a leptin receptor, OB-R. Cell 83:1263–1271, 1995

Theander S: Outcome and prognosis in anorexia nervosa and bulimia, in Anorexia Nervosa and Bulimic Disorders. Edited by Szmukler GI, Slade PD, Harris P, et al: London, Pergamon, 1985, pp 493–508

VanItallie TB: Health implications of overweight and obesity in the United States. Ann Intern Med 103:983–988, 1985

Walsh BT, Hadigan CM, Devlin MJ, et al: Long-term outcome of antidepressant treatment for bulimia nervosa. Am J Psychiatry 148:1206–1212, 1991

Walters EE, Kendler KS: Anorexia nervosa an anorectic-like syndromes in a population-based twin sample. Am J Psychiatry 152:64–71, 1995

Weintraub M: Long-term weight control: the National Heart, Lung and Blood Institute funded multi-modal intervention study. Clin Pharmacol Ther 51:581–585, 1992

Wonderlich SA, Swift WJ, Slotnick HB, et al: DSM-III-R personality disorders and eating disorder subtypes. Int J Eat Disord 9:607–616, 1990

Woodside DB, Garfinkel PE, Lin E, et al: Comparisons of men with full or partial eating disorders, men without eating disorders, and women with eating disorders in the community. Am J Psychiatry 158:570–574, 2001

Zhang Y, Prenca R, Maffei M, et al: Positional cloning of the mouse obese gene and its human homologue. Nature 372:425–432, 1994

CHAPTER 18

Psychopharmacology and Electroconvulsive Therapy

Lauren B. Marangell, M.D.

Jonathan M. Silver, M.D.

Donald C. Goff, M.D.

Stuart C. Yudofsky, M.D.

The skillful practice of psychopharma-cology requires a broad knowledge of psychiatry, pharmacology, and medicine. We begin this chapter with an overview of general principles relevant to the safe and effective use of psychotropic medications. Subsequent sections cover the major classes of psychotropic medications—antidepressants, antipsychotics, anxiolytics, and mood stabilizers—and the disorders for which they are prescribed. The reader should be aware that the psychotropic drug class nomenclature is somewhat arbitrary; for example, many antidepressant medications are also used to treat anxiety disorders.

General Principles

Initial Evaluation

Like all areas of medicine, the art of psychopharmacology rests on proper diagnosis and delineation of medication-responsive target symptoms. Additional considerations include ruling out nonpsychiatric causes, such as endocrine or neurological disorders and substance abuse; noting the presence of other medical problems that will influence drug selection, such as cardiac or hepatic disease; evaluating other medications that the patient is taking that might cause a drug–drug interaction; and evaluating personal and family history of medication responses.

The authors would like to thank Holly Zboyan for her invaluable assistance in the preparation of this chapter.

The "Drug Interactions" subsections contain material developed over many years for other purposes in collaboration with Ann Callahan, M.D., and Terence Ketter, M.D.

Target Symptoms

A key component of a well-considered decision to use a medication is the delineation of target symptoms. The physician should determine and list the specific symptoms that are designated for treatment and should monitor the response of these symptoms to treatment. The goal of treatment is not just to alleviate symptoms but also to restore normal functioning to the greatest extent possible.

Multiple Medications

A frequent and dangerous clinical error is the treatment of specific symptoms of a disorder with multiple drugs, rather than treating, more specifically, the underlying disorder. For example, it is not uncommon for a psychiatrist to receive a referral for a patient who is taking one type of benzodiazepine for anxiety, a different type of benzodiazepine for insomnia, an analgesic for nonspecific somatic complaints, and a subtherapeutic dosage of an antidepressant (e.g., 50 mg/day of imipramine) for feelings of sadness. Often, the somatic complaints, insomnia, and anxiety are components of an underlying depression, which may be aggravated by the polypharmaceutical approach inherent in symptomatic treatment.

However, many patients have psychiatric conditions that require the concomitant use of several psychotropic agents. The carefully considered, rational use of several psychiatric medications must be distinguished from ill-considered polypharmacy. An example of useful combined treatment is augmentation of an antidepressant agent with lithium for patients who have experienced only a partial therapeutic response to an antidepressant alone.

Choice of Drug

Selection of a drug for a given diagnosis or symptom is made on the basis of both patient-specific and drug-specific considerations. Patient-specific factors include comorbid medical and psychiatric disorders, other medications being taken, history of response to medication, family history of medication responses, and life circumstances that will likely be affected by the specific side effects of the chosen agent.

The clinician also must consider the physical, intellectual, and psychological capacities of the patient and of his or her caregivers when selecting a new medication. An elderly patient with mild memory impairment may have difficulty following instructions about increasing the dosage of an antidepressant medication. In general, the more complicated the instructions or the more medications that are prescribed, the more difficulty the patient will have in complying with the therapeutic regimen.

Drug-specific factors include available preparations and cost. In most cases, once-a-day dosing is preferred for patient convenience and compliance. The choice of a particular medication also may depend on whether that drug is available in injectable and liquid forms in addition to tablet, pill, or capsule forms.

Generic Substitution

Generic substitution, when available, may provide a less expensive alternative to the original proprietary (brand-name) formulation; however, some caution is warranted, because generic "equivalents" may not be truly equivalent in all circumstances. After patent expiration, information relevant to producing a medication is in the public domain. At that point, other pharmaceutical companies may produce the medication, provided the drug is formulated according to U.S. Food and Drug Administration (FDA) requirements. The current FDA requirements center around the concept of *bioequivalence;* products are bioequivalent if there is no significant difference in the rate at which or extent to which the active ingredient becomes available to the site of action, given the same dose and conditions (Food and Drug Administration 1992). However, in some cases, even small differences in bioavailability, or other differences in preparations such as type of preservatives or excipients, may become clinically meaningful. For example, a patient may have an allergic reaction to one generic preparation but not another of the same drug because of differences in the dye used to color the pill.

Patient Information and Patient–Physician Communication

A general principle is that the more the patient and his or her family understand about the illness and the reason that medications have been chosen to treat the illness, the more compliant the patient and the more supportive the family will be.

Therapeutic skill and creativity on the part of a clinician are essential for effective treatment with medications. For example, the clinician must expect a patient with major depression associated with significant anxiety and somatic complaints to be concerned about drug side effects. The way in which the clinician discusses such side effects with the patient will ultimately affect the patient's confidence in the treatment plan and his or her compliance with the medication regimen. It is often useful to emphasize that common early side effects, such as nausea, are not dangerous and will likely improve with time. Situations that require immediate intervention to ensure patient safety must

be clearly communicated. For example, it is essential that patients be aware of the signs of lithium toxicity.

Evaluation of Response

The treatment plan should include a predetermined dose and duration that will provide an adequate trial of the medication. Far too frequently, medications are discontinued with the assumption of failure of response without the benefit of an adequate drug trial (e.g., inadequate dosage or duration of treatment). A patient's treatment plan should be revised if the patient has an unusual sensitivity to the medication, if dangerous or disabling side effects emerge, or if the patient does not respond to an adequate drug trial. In such cases, a diagnostic reevaluation of the patient may be indicated, with further tests to detect any underlying nonpsychiatric illness that did not appear during the initial assessment and consideration of alternative treatments.

For patients who do respond, an end point for treatment must be determined. Far too often, medication regimens are continued beyond the point at which therapeutic benefit is derived. A common example is the use of benzodiazepines for the treatment of anxiety in which patients may be maintained for years without the assessment of the therapeutic benefit of the drug by gradual discontinuation.

Antidepressant Drugs

Overview

The modern era of the treatment of depression with medication began in the 1950s when iproniazid, an MAOI used for the treatment of tuberculosis, was noted to elevate mood (Selikoff et al. 1952). Unfortunately, hepatic necrosis was a side effect of iproniazid, and this led to its withdrawal from clinical use. In addition, dangerous hypertensive reactions associated with the MAOIs initially were poorly understood, and most psychiatrists were reluctant to use these drugs. Imipramine, the first of the tricyclic antidepressants (TCAs), was developed as a derivative of chlorpromazine; it was hoped that imipramine would be more effective than chlorpromazine as an antipsychotic agent. Although imipramine did not show antipsychotic efficacy, it was shown to be effective in the treatment of depression (Kuhn 1958). Subsequently, many other antidepressants have been approved for use in the United States. To date, all antidepressants appear to be equally effective for treating major depression, but individual patients may respond preferentially to one agent or another. In addition, these medications are significantly different from one another with regard to side effects, lethality in overdose, pharmacokinetics, and the ability to treat comorbid psychiatric disorders.

Mechanisms of Action

All current antidepressant drugs affect the serotonergic and/or catecholaminergic systems in the central nervous system (CNS), by either presynaptic reuptake inhibition, blocking catabolism, or receptor agonist or antagonist effects (for a review, see Charney 1998; Frazer 1997; W.K. Goodman and Charney 1985). The effects of antidepressants on monoamine availability are immediate, but the clinical response is typically delayed for several weeks. Downregulation of presynaptic autoreceptors, α- and β-noradrenergic receptors, and the serotonin type 1 (5-HT$_1$) receptors more closely parallels the time course of clinical response. This downregulation can be conceptualized as a marker of antidepressant-induced neuronal adaptation. More important, most of the receptors that are immediately affected by antidepressants are linked to G proteins. A defective linkage between the receptor and the G protein may result in abnormal intracellular transduction mechanisms (Bourin and Baker 1996). In actuality, antidepressants most likely act via modulating G proteins, second messenger systems, and gene expression (for a review of molecular mechanisms, see Duman 1998).

Indications

Although the antidepressants have many potential therapeutic uses, the primary approved indication for these drugs is the treatment of major depression, as defined by DSM-IV-TR (American Psychiatric Association 2000). Overall, approximately 70% of patients with depression respond to an adequate trial of antidepressant medication, although far fewer patients achieve full remission of symptoms. In addition, antidepressants are effective for patients with obsessive-compulsive disorder (OCD) (selective serotonin reuptake inhibitors [SSRIs] and clomipramine), panic disorder (TCAs and SSRIs), bulimia (TCAs, SSRIs, and MAOIs), dysthymia (SSRIs), bipolar depression (after treatment with a mood stabilizer), social phobia (MAOIs and SSRIs), posttraumatic stress disorder (PTSD) (SSRIs), irritable bowel syndrome (TCAs), enuresis (TCAs), neuropathic pain (TCAs), migraine headache (TCAs), attention-deficit/hyperactivity disorder (bupropion), smoking cessation (bupropion), and late luteal phase dysphoric disorder (SSRIs); however, the FDA has not evaluated or approved the use of antidepressants to treat many of these conditions.

Clinical Use

Each of the commonly used classes of antidepressants is discussed in the following sections and summarized in Table 18–1.

The antidepressant classes are based on similarity of receptor effects and side effects. All are effective for depression when administered in therapeutic doses. The choice of antidepressant medication is based on the patient's psychiatric symptoms, his or her history of previous treatment response, family members' history of previous response, medication side-effect profile, comorbid psychiatric or medical disorders, and risk of suicide by overdose (Tables 18–2 and 18–3). In general, the SSRIs and the other newer antidepressants are better tolerated and safer than either the TCAs or the MAOIs, although many patients still benefit from these older drugs. In the following sections, clinically relevant information is presented for each of the antidepressant medication classes individually, followed by a discussion of the pharmacological treatment of depression. Principles germane to the use of antidepressants to treat anxiety disorders can be found at the end of the section on anxiety later in this chapter.

Tricyclic and Heterocyclic Antidepressants

Receptor Effects

Most TCAs inhibit the reuptake of norepinephrine, serotonin, and, to a lesser extent, dopamine. These mechanisms are thought to be responsible for the therapeutic action of TCAs. In addition, TCAs block muscarinic cholinergic receptors, H_1 histamine receptors, and α_1-adrenergic receptors. These mechanisms are thought to account for the side effects of the TCAs.

Background

The name *tricyclic* is based on the chemical structure; all tricyclics have a three-ring nucleus. Currently, most clinicians are moving away from use of TCAs as first-line drugs; relative to the newer antidepressants, they tend to have more side

effects, to require gradual titration to achieve an adequate antidepressant dose, and to be lethal in overdose.

Imipramine, amitriptyline, clomipramine, trimipramine, and doxepin are tertiary amines. Desipramine, nortriptyline, and protriptyline are secondary amines. The tertiary amines have more potent serotonin reuptake inhibition, and the secondary amines have more potent noradrenergic reuptake inhibition. The tertiary amines tend to have more side effects than do the secondary amines; in our opinion, the tertiary amines usually do not offer any additional therapeutic benefits. Desipramine and protriptyline tend to be activating. Among the TCAs, nortriptyline is the least likely to produce orthostatic hypotension. Amoxapine has an active metabolite that antagonizes D_2 dopamine receptors and can therefore cause treatment-emergent extrapyramidal side effects (EPS; Coupet et al. 1979; see section on antipsychotic drugs later in this chapter). Maprotiline is characterized as a heterocyclic agent. The receptor effects of maprotiline are most similar to those of protriptyline.

Clinical Use

Before initiation of treatment with TCAs, the physician must obtain a comprehensive cardiovascular history and review of symptoms. Because TCAs often cause orthostasis, other potential risk factors for hypotension should be considered, and patients should be instructed to change from sitting or lying to the standing position slowly. For patients with preexisting heart disease and for all patients older than 40 years, an electrocardiogram (ECG) should be obtained before TCA treatment is initiated. If the initial ECG shows clinically significant abnormalities, another ECG must be obtained after the patient's medication has reached a steady-state level. For patients with bundle branch block,

TABLE 18–1. Commonly used antidepressant drugs

Generic (trade) name	Starting dosage (mg)[a]	Usual daily dosage (mg)	Available oral dosages (mg)	Mean drug [active metabolite] half-life (hours)
Tricyclics and tetracyclics				
Tertiary amine tricyclics				
Amitriptyline (Elavil, Endep)	25–50	100–300	10, 25, 50, 75, 100, 150	15.6 [26.6]
Clomipramine (Anafranil)	25	100–250	25, 50, 75	32 [69]
Doxepin (Sinequan)	25–50	100–300	10, 25, 50, 75, 100, 150	16.8
Imipramine (Tofranil, Tofranil PM)	25–50	100–300	10, 25, 50, 75, 100, 125, 150	7.6 [17.1]
Trimipramine (Surmontil)	25–50	100–300	25, 50, 100	24
Secondary amine tricyclics				
Desipramine (Norpramin)	25–50	100–300	25, 50, 75, 100, 150	17.1
Nortriptyline (Pamelor, Aventyl)	25	50–200	10, 25, 50, 75	26.6
Protriptyline (Vivactil)	10	15–60	5, 10	78.4
Tetracyclics				
Amoxapine (Asendin)	50	100–400	25, 50, 100, 150	8
Maprotiline (Ludiomil)	50	100–225	25, 50, 75	43
Selective serotonin reuptake inhibitors				
Citalopram (Celexa)	20	20–60[b]	20, 40	35
Escitalopram (Lexapro)	10	10–20	10, 20	32
Fluoxetine (Prozac, Sarafem)	50	20–60[b]	10, 20, liq, 90 (weekly)	72 [144]
Fluvoxamine (Luvox)	50	50–300[b]	50, 100	15
Paroxetine (Paxil)	20	20–60[b]	10, 20, 30, 40	20
Paroxetine (Paxil CR)	25[a]	25–75[b]	12.5, 25, 37.5	20
Sertraline (Zoloft)	50	50–200[b]	50, 100	26 [66]
Dopamine-norepinephrine reuptake inhibitors				
Bupropion (Wellbutrin)	150	300	75, 100	14
Bupropion SR (Wellbutrin SR, Zyban)	150	300	100, 150	21
Serotonin-norepinephrine reuptake inhibitors				
Venlafaxine (Effexor)	37.5	75–225	25, 37.5, 50, 75, 100	5 [11]
Venlafaxine (XR) (Effexor XR)	37.5	75–225	37.5, 75, 150	5 [11]
Serotonin modulators				
Nefazodone (Serzone)	50	150–300	100, 150, 200, 250	4
Trazodone (Desyrel)	50	75–300	50, 100, 150, 300	7
Norepinephrine-serotonin modulator				
Mirtazapine (Remeron)	15	15–45	15, 30	20

TABLE 18–1. Commonly used antidepressant drugs *(continued)*

Generic (trade) name	Starting dosage (mg)[a]	Usual daily dosage (mg)	Available oral dosages (mg)	Mean drug [active metabolite] half-life (hours)
Monoamine oxidase inhibitors				
Irreversible, nonselective				
Phenelzine (Nardil)	15	15–90	15	2
Tranylcypromine (Parnate)	10	30–60	10	2
Reversible MAOI-A				
Moclobemide (Aurorix, Manerex)	150	300–600	100, 150	2

[a]Lower starting dosages are recommended for elderly patients and for those with panic disorder, significant anxiety, or hepatic disease.
[b]Dosage varies with diagnosis. See text for specific guidelines.
Source. Dosing information is from American Psychiatric Association 1993. Half-life information is compiled from Amsterdam et al. 1980 and *Physicians' Desk Reference* 2001, 55th Edition. Montvale, NJ, Medical Economics, 2001.

TABLE 18–2. Guidelines for choosing an antidepressant medication

Unipolar depression	All antidepressants are equally effective. Choose on the basis of previous response, side effects, comorbid medical and psychotic disorders.
Depression with melancholic features	TCA[a]
Depression with atypical features	SSRI, MAOI[b]
Depression with psychotic features	Antidepressant plus antipsychotic, or ECT; avoid bupropion
Bipolar depression[c]	Lithium, lamotrigine
Depression + OCD	SSRI, clomipramine
Depression + panic disorder	SSRI, TCA, MAOI[b]
Depression + seizures	Avoid bupropion and TCAs
Depression + Parkinson's disease	Bupropion
Depression + sexual dysfunction	Bupropion, nefazodone, mirtazapine

Note. ECT=electroconvulsive therapy; MAOI=monoamine oxidase inhibitor; OCD=obsessive-compulsive disorder; SSRI=selective serotonin reuptake inhibitor; TCA=tricyclic antidepressant.
[a]Although some data suggest that TCAs are superior in melancholic depression, many clinicians choose the newer agents, even in melancholia, on the basis of improved tolerability and safety.
[b]Although MAOIs are highly effective, they are not used as first-line agents because of their increased risk relative to the newer agents. Other agents may be effective, but there are few data.
[c]Mood stabilizers are first-line treatment for all phases of bipolar disorder (see text section on mood stabilizers).

TCAs should not be used unless all other options have failed.

Dosage guidelines are for healthy adults with minimal anxiety. Patients with significant anxiety, panic, or a tendency to be sensitive to side effects should receive initial dosages that are 50% lower. Similarly, elderly patients and those with cardiovascular or hepatic disease should receive lower initial dosages.

TABLE 18–3. Summary of key features and side effects of antidepressant medications

| Medication | Proposed mechanism/ receptor effects | Dosing | Key features | | | | | Other key side effects |
			Titration required	Sedation	Weight gain	Sexual dysfunction	
TCAs	5-HT + NE reuptake inhibition	Once daily	Yes	Most, yes	Yes	Yes	Anticholinergic,[a] orthostasis, quinidine-like effects on cardiac condition, lethal in overdose
SSRIs	5-HT reuptake inhibition	Once daily	Minimal	Minimal	Rare	Yes	Initial: nausea, loose bowel movements, headache, insomnia
Bupropion SR	DA + NE reuptake inhibition	Multiple, if dose is >200 mg	Some	Rare	Rare	Rare	Initial: nausea, headache, insomnia, anxiety/agitation; seizure risk
Venlafaxine XR	5-HT + NE > DA reuptake inhibition	Once daily	Some	Minimal	Rare	Yes	Similar to SSRIs; dose-dependent hypertension
Nefazodone	$5\text{-}HT_2$ antagonist + weak 5-HT + NE reuptake inhibition	Twice daily	Yes	Yes	Rare	Rare	Initial: nausea, dizziness, confusion, visual changes, sedation
Trazodone	$5\text{-}HT_2$ antagonist + weak $5\text{-}HT_2$ reuptake inhibition	Twice daily	Yes	Yes	Rare	Rare	Initial sedation, priapism, dizziness, orthostasis
Mirtazapine	α_2-Adrenergic + $5\text{-}HT_2$ antagonism	Once daily	Minimal	Yes	Yes	Rare	Anticholinergic,[a] may increase serum lipids; rare: orthostasis, hypertension, peripheral edema, agranulocytosis

TABLE 18–3. Summary of key features and side effects of antidepressant medications (continued)

Medication	Proposed mechanism/ receptor effects	Dosing	Titration required	Key features			Other key side effects
				Sedation	Weight gain	Sexual dysfunction	
MAOIs	Inhibit monoamine oxidase	Two or three times a day	Yes	Rare	Yes	Yes	Orthostatic hypotension, insomnia, peripheral edema; avoid in patients with CHF, avoid phenelzine in patients with hepatic impairment; potentially life-threatening drug interactions; dietary restrictions

Note. CHF = congestive heart failure; DA = dopamine; 5-HT = serotonin; NE = norepinephrine; MAOIs = monoamine oxidase inhibitors; SSRIs = selective serotonin reuptake inhibitors; TCAs = tricyclic antidepressants.

[a]Anticholinergic side effects include dry mouth, blurred vision, constipation, urinary retention, tachycardia, and possible confusion.

Risks, Side Effects, and Their Management

Anticholinergic effects. Anticholinergic side effects result from antagonism of muscarinic receptors. The most common anticholinergic side effects are dry mouth, constipation, urinary retention, blurred vision, and tachycardia. In predisposed patients, such as elderly persons, anticholinergic medications may cause cognitive impairment and confusion. Because the tertiary amines and protriptyline have a particularly high affinity for the muscarinic receptors, these medications are more likely than others to cause anticholinergic side effects.

Cholinergic medications have been reported to relieve some of the anticholinergic side effects (Everett 1976; Yager 1986). Bethanechol chloride may alleviate dry mouth, constipation, urinary hesitancy and retention, and erectile and ejaculatory dysfunction. The addition of a medication to treat side effects should be considered only after dosage reduction and alternative antidepressants with fewer anticholinergic side effects have been attempted.

Sedation. The relative sedating properties of the TCAs appear to parallel their respective histamine receptor binding affinities. Trimipramine, amitriptyline, and doxepin are the most sedating TCAs. Desipramine and protriptyline are less sedating.

Cardiac effects. Many of the TCAs have effects on the cardiovascular system, including orthostatic hypotension and cardiac conduction delays. For many patients, especially those with preexisting heart disease, TCAs have clinically relevant effects on blood pressure, heart rate, cardiac conduction, and cardiac rhythm (Glassman 1984; L. S. Goodman et al. 1986; Roose 1992).

Orthostatic hypotension from TCAs

may not be dose dependent; therefore, lowering the dosage of the antidepressant may not lessen the dizziness or the changes in blood pressure.

Because TCAs at toxic levels (as occur in overdose) can cause life-threatening arrhythmias, many clinicians believe that these drugs can cause dangerous arrhythmias at treatment doses. In fact, TCAs are potent antiarrhythmic agents, possessing quinidine-like properties (Glassman and Bigger 1981). Because prolongation of the P-R and QRS intervals can occur with TCA use, these drugs should not be used in patients with preexisting heart block (especially right bundle branch block and left bundle branch block). In such patients, TCAs often lead to second- or third-degree heart block, both of which are life-threatening conditions (Roose et al. 1987).

Weight gain. Patients treated with TCAs may experience undesirable weight gain. This side effect appears to be unrelated to improvement in the patient's mood (Fernstrom et al. 1986; Kupfer et al. 1979).

Neurological effects. A dose-related risk of seizures has been found with clomipramine, which has led to the recommendation that the daily dosage of this drug should not exceed 250 mg (Clomipramine Collaborative Study Group 1991; see also Anafranil package insert). Overdoses of TCAs, particularly amoxapine and desipramine, are associated with seizures (Wedin et al. 1986). Whether therapeutic dosages of TCAs lower the seizure threshold is controversial (Dailey and Naritoku 1996). Nonetheless, other classes may be safer options for individuals with epilepsy (Rosenstein et al. 1993).

Amoxapine, which has a mild neuroleptic effect, can cause EPS, akathisia, and even tardive dyskinesia (Gammon and

Hansen 1984; Ross et al. 1983; Thornton and Stahl 1984). For this reason, we do not recommend that amoxapine be prescribed as a first-line treatment for depression.

Overdose. The major complications from overdose with TCAs include those that arise from neuropsychiatric impairment, hypotension, cardiac arrhythmias, and seizures. Because the TCAs have significant anticholinergic activity, anticholinergic delirium may occur. This is particularly true for elderly patients and for patients with neuropsychiatric conditions. Other complications of anticholinergic overdose include agitation, supraventricular arrhythmias, hallucinations, severe hypertension, and seizures (Goldfrank et al. 1986). Patients with anticholinergic delirium manifest hot dry skin, dry mucous membranes, dilated pupils, absent bowel sounds, and tachycardia. Anticholinergic delirium constitutes a medical emergency and requires full supportive medical care. Physostigmine, a centrally and peripherally acting reversible anticholinesterase, may be used as a diagnostic agent in cases of suspected anticholinergic toxicity. This agent is administered at a dose of 1–2 mg intramuscularly or intravenously at a slow, controlled rate of no more than 1 mg/minute. Physostigmine should not be used to maintain reversal of the toxicity, however, because a cholinergic crisis may result. A cholinergic crisis is characterized by nausea, vomiting, bradycardia, and seizures. This reaction can be reversed by the administration of a potent anticholinergic drug such as atropine. A more detailed explanation of the treatment of these complications can be found elsewhere (Goldfrank et al. 1986).

Hypotension, which may result from norepinephrine depletion and from other causes related to the peripheral and central effects of TCAs, should be treated with vigorous fluid replacement. Seizures and cardiac complications also may occur with antidepressant overdose (Boehnert and Lovejoy 1985). When the QRS interval is below 0.10, the likelihood of seizures or ventricular arrhythmias decreases (Boehnert and Lovejoy 1985). Ventricular arrhythmias that occur secondary to overdose are typical of the arrhythmias that occur with high doses of quinidine-like agents, and these begin within the first 24 hours after hospital admission (R.J. Goldberg et al. 1985). Ventricular arrhythmias should be treated with lidocaine, propranolol, or phenytoin. Prophylactic treatment with phenytoin and insertion of a temporary pacemaker should be considered in patients with prolonged QRS intervals (i.e., >120 msec; Goldfrank et al. 1986).

Seizures associated with TCA overdose should be managed with standard emergency procedures (i.e., airway maintenance, proper ventilation, and treatment of the seizures with agents such as intravenous diazepam). Because many overdose situations involve combinations of drugs, the clinician should be alert to the possibility that alcohol or benzodiazepines also may have been ingested.

Drug interactions. Because the liver metabolizes the TCAs, drugs that inhibit or induce hepatic microsomal enzymes may alter plasma tricyclic levels. This is particularly true for 2D6 inhibitors. In some individuals, this interaction may cause dangerously high levels of the TCA (Vaughan 1988; see section on drug interactions later in this chapter).

Although several agents affect tricyclic levels, the effect is usually not reciprocal: the TCAs rarely affect the metabolism of other drugs. A notable exception to this general rule is the drug sodium valproate, levels of which may decrease when a TCA is administered concurrently (Preskorn and Burke 1992). By a different mode of action, the TCAs also may interfere with the mechanism of action of two antihypertensive drugs. Both guanethidine and clonidine lose effectiveness if administered concomitantly with drugs, such as TCAs, that block reuptake of catecholamines into adrenergic neurons.

Selective Serotonin Reuptake Inhibitors

Mechanism of Action

SSRIs inhibit the presynaptic serotonin reuptake pump. This reuptake inhibition initially increases serotonin in the synaptic cleft, which then causes presynaptic autoreceptors to downregulate and ultimately increases net serotonin transmission (De Montigny et al. 1981). As discussed earlier in this chapter, the ultimate mechanism of action is likely to be related to secondary effects on signal transduction and gene transcription.

Background

SSRIs were developed in an attempt to formulate reuptake-blocking drugs that lacked the troublesome side effects of the TCAs. SSRIs largely lack four of the five pharmacological properties characteristic of TCAs—blockade of muscarinic receptors, of H_1-histaminergic receptors, and of α_1-adrenergic receptors, and norepinephrine reuptake-blocking properties—leaving only the serotonin reuptake inhibitor property intact. This selectivity has several advantages, including a reduction in dangerous side effects. The SSRIs are much safer in overdose than the TCAs because they do not have life-threatening effects at high plasma concentrations. In addition, SSRIs are unlikely to affect the seizure threshold or cardiac conduction, making these drugs an excellent choice for patients for who have epilepsy or cardiac disease.

Because of the more tolerable side effects and once-a-day dosing, patients are

more likely to comply with SSRI than with TCA treatment. Compliance is particularly important when considering first-line treatment and overall health care costs. In addition, SSRIs have an unusually broad spectrum of action. They are efficacious in the treatment not only of depression but also of many other psychiatric disorders, as listed earlier in this chapter. This broad spectrum of efficacy is advantageous when treating patients who have more than one disorder. For example, only the SSRIs and clomipramine have been shown to be effective for the treatment of OCD in randomized controlled trials.

The SSRIs are started at or near their therapeutic antidepressant doses, without the long titration period required with most TCAs. The most significant disadvantage of these medications is a high incidence of treatment-emergent sexual dysfunction (discussed later), which often persists for as long as the patient continues taking the medication.

All of the SSRIs have a similar spectrum of efficacy and a similar side-effect profile. However, they are structurally and, in some instances, clinically distinct. For example, allergy to one SSRI does not predict allergy to another. Similarly, response or nonresponse to one does not ensure a similar reaction to another medication in the class. The SSRIs also have distinct pharmacokinetic properties, the most important of which are differences in half-life and the propensity to inhibit cytochrome P450 (CYP) enzymes.

Fluvoxamine has an average half-life of 12–15 hours after a single oral dose, but this is prolonged by 30%–50% at steady state (van Harten 1995). Fluvoxamine requires twice-a-day administration at dosages greater than 50 mg/day. Sertraline and paroxetine both have an elimination half-life of approximately 24 hours. Sertraline has an active metabolite, desmethylsertraline, that has a half-life of 62–104 hours. Citalopram has a half-life of 35 hours and no clinically significant metabolites. Escitalopram has a half-life of 27–32 hours. The moderate half-life of these drugs warrants once-daily dosing and allows for washout within about a week. Fluoxetine has a half-life of 2–4 days, and its active metabolite, norfluoxetine, has a half-life of 7–15 days. Although this long half-life results in a longer time to reach steady-state concentrations, the onset of therapeutic effects is not delayed beyond the 2–4 weeks required of all current antidepressant medications. A long half-life may be advantageous for patients who forget to take their medication.

Although drug–drug interactions are significantly less common with SSRIs than with either TCAs or MAOIs, most SSRIs inhibit various hepatic cytochrome P450 enzymes, which may increase levels of other drugs. The individual drugs in the class have different profiles of cytochrome P450 inhibition, as discussed later in this chapter.

Clinical Use

Although all patients with depression should receive a thorough medical evaluation, no specific tests are required before treatment is initiated with an SSRI. The usual starting dosages for the SSRIs are summarized in Table 18–1. These standard dosages should be decreased by 50% for patients with hepatic disease and for elderly persons. In addition, patients with panic disorder or significant anxiety symptoms are often intolerant of the initial stimulating side effects that commonly occur with SSRIs. In these cases, the initial dosage also should be decreased by 50% (or more) and then increased as tolerated to the usual therapeutic dosage. It is often advantageous to apply this approach to patients who generally tend to be sensitive to side effects.

The usual therapeutic dosages for the treatment of depression are citalopram 20 mg, escitalopram 10 mg, fluoxetine 20 mg, paroxetine 20 mg (25 mg for the CR preparation), and sertraline 50–150 mg. Although the manufacturer of fluvoxamine has not pursued FDA approval for the treatment of depression in the United States (fluvoxamine is approved only for the treatment of OCD), this medication is an effective antidepressant at 50–150 mg/day (Claghorn et al. 1996; Walczak et al. 1996). For the treatment of depression, the SSRIs have a flat dose–response curve, meaning that higher dosages tend not to be more effective than standard dosages, although isolated patients respond better to higher dosages. Premature escalation of the SSRI dosage when treating a patient with depression is most likely to add side effects without improved antidepressant efficacy. Therefore, we recommend maintaining the usual therapeutic dosage for 4 weeks. If there is no improvement at that time, a trial of a higher dose may be warranted. If a partial response is evident at 4 weeks, the dosage should remain constant for an additional 2 weeks because improvement to the initial dosage may continue.

The treatment of OCD requires a longer duration and often higher dosages to assess efficacy. A therapeutic trial for OCD is 8–12 weeks. In fixed-dose studies, fluoxetine and sertraline have appeared to be effective at dosages similar to those used to treat depression (Greist et al. 1995a, 1995b; Tollefson et al. 1994). However, some patients clearly benefit from higher doses. To avoid unnecessary side effects, the best course of action often is to treat first with modest dosages of medication and then increase the dosage if needed. The most common reason for nonresponse in patients with OCD is failure to increase the dose adequately.

In the treatment of panic disorder, data indicate that 40–60 mg/day of paroxetine is more efficacious than lower dosages (Ballenger et al. 1998; Oehrberg et al. 1995). However, available data indicate that the other SSRIs are effective for the treatment of panic disorder at their typical antidepressant dosages (Tiller et al. 1999; van Vliet et al. 1996). Use of fluoxetine in panic disorder has been studied only in small, open studies, but the drug appears to show antipanic effects at low dosages (Louie et al. 1993). Fluoxetine should be initiated at 5 mg/day and gradually increased to 20 mg/day, because patients with panic disorder tend to be exquisitely sensitive to side effects (see subsection on the treatment of panic disorder in the section on anxiolytics in this chapter).

Late luteal phase dysphoric disorder appears to respond to dosages similar to those used to treat depression. Interestingly, late luteal phase dysphoric disorder can be successfully treated with medication administered only during the symptomatic period before menses (Gelenberg 1997; Wikander et al. 1998). Fluoxetine is effective in the treatment of bulimia at a dosage of 60 mg/day (Mitchell et al. 1993). Although the other SSRIs also may be effective for the treatment of bulimia, dosing guidelines are not available. The use of SSRIs to attenuate symptoms associated with borderline personality disorder and PTSD may require relatively higher dosages.

Risks, Side Effects, and Their Management

Common side effects.   Mild nausea, loose bowel movements, anxiety, headache, insomnia, and increased sweating are frequent initial side effects of SSRI treatment. They are usually dosage related and may be minimized with low initial dosing and gradual titration. These early adverse effects almost always attenuate after the first few weeks of treatment. Sexual dys-

function, discussed later, is the most common longer-term side effect of the SSRIs.

Neurological effects.   Tension headaches are common early in treatment. These usually can be managed with over-the-counter pain relief preparations. SSRIs may initially worsen migraine headaches, but if the patient can tolerate the first few weeks of treatment with symptomatic relief, SSRIs are often effective in reducing the severity and frequency of migraines (Doughty and Lyle 1995; J.A. Hamilton and Halbreich 1993; Manna et al. 1994). Tremor and akathisia are less common and can be managed with dosage reduction or the addition of a β-blocker.

Stimulation/insomnia.   Some patients complain of jitteriness, restlessness, muscle tension, and disturbed sleep. These side effects typically occur early in treatment, before the antidepressant effect. All patients should be informed of the possibility of these side effects and reassured that if they develop, they tend to be transient. Patients with preexisting anxiety should be started at low dosages with subsequent titration as tolerated. In this way, if overstimulation occurs, it will be less likely to be severe enough to result in a lack of compliance with medication. The short-term use of a benzodiazepine also may help the patient cope with overstimulation in the early stages of treatment, until tolerance to this side effect occurs. Despite these common transient stimulating effects, SSRIs are clearly effective for patients with anxiety or agitated depression. Similarly, insomnia that commonly occurs early in treatment may be tolerable if the patient is reassured that the side effect will be transient. Symptomatic treatment with short-term use of benzodiazepines or low-dose trazodone (e.g., 50–150 mg) at bedtime is reasonable (Jacobsen 1990; Nierenberg and Keck 1989).

Sedation. Despite occasional stimulating effects, SSRIs may induce sedation in some patients. In our experience, patients who experience significant treatment-emergent sedation with these medications often require lower dosages of the medication. Altering the time of administration (e.g., moving the time the medication is taken from morning to evening) often is not successful.

Weight gain or loss. All of the SSRIs have the potential to cause weight gain in some individuals (Bouwer and Harvey 1996; Fisher et al. 1995). In a controlled study, Fava et al. (2000) found that paroxetine was associated with greater weight gain than fluoxetine or sertraline.

Gastrointestinal symptoms. Nausea and diarrhea may occur after treatment with an SSRI. This side effect is dose dependent and often transient.

Sexual dysfunction. Decreased libido, anorgasmia, and delayed ejaculation are common side effects of SSRIs. When possible, the management of sexual side effects should be postponed until the patient has completed an adequate trial of the antidepressant. In some cases, tolerance to sexual side effects develops.

When significant sexual dysfunction persists for more than 1 month despite a positive response to treatment, a reduction in the dosage should be considered. In some cases, this results in a diminution of the symptoms without loss of therapeutic benefit. Unfortunately, in other instances, there is no therapeutic dosage that does not cause the sexual side effect. In such cases, two strategies are available: the antidepressant can be replaced with an alternative, or other drugs may be prescribed to counteract the side effect. The decision to try a different antidepressant

is potentially problematic because an equivalent therapeutic response is not guaranteed. In our experience, switching from one SSRI to another does not tend to decrease sexual side effects. Antidepressants that do not commonly cause sexual dysfunction are bupropion, nefazodone, and mirtazapine.

Several medications have been suggested as antidotes for the sexual side effects associated with antidepressants. Bupropion, 75 or 150 mg/day, has been added to an SSRI regimen with some success for improving libido (Labbate and Pollack 1994). Sildenafil has been used on an as-needed basis prior to sexual activity with some success with improved erectile and ejaculatory function (Ashton and Bennett 1999).

Vivid dreams. Reports of vivid dreams, distinct from nightmares, are common with SSRIs. The mechanism of this side effect is unknown.

Serotonin syndrome. There have been several reports of a medication-induced syndrome that has been attributed to excessive stimulation of the serotonergic system. This condition arises more commonly among patients treated concurrently with two or more serotonergic drugs (e.g., fluoxetine and an MAOI). However, it also may occur in patients receiving SSRI monotherapy. Affected individuals have the constellation of lethargy, restlessness, confusion, flushing, diaphoresis, tremor, and myoclonic jerks. As the condition progresses, hyperthermia, hypertonicity, rhabdomyolysis, renal failure, and death may occur (Metz and Shader 1990). The syndrome must be identified as rapidly as possible because discontinuation of the serotonergic medications is the first step in treatment, followed by emergency medical treatment, as required. Life-threatening serotonin syndrome is fortunately rare and most often occurs with medication combinations that involve MAOIs.

Discontinuation syndromes. Several reports have described a series of symptoms following discontinuation or dose reduction of serotonergic antidepressant medications. The most common symptoms include dizziness, headache, paresthesia, nausea, diarrhea, insomnia, and irritability. Of note, these symptoms are also seen when a patient misses doses. A prospective double-blind, placebo substitution study confirmed that discontinuation symptoms are most common with short-half-life antidepressants, such as paroxetine (Rosenbaum et al. 1998).

Apathy syndromes. We and others have noted an apathy syndrome in some patients after months or years of successful treatment with SSRIs. Patients often confuse this syndrome with a recurrence of depression, but the two conditions are quite distinct. The syndrome is characterized by a loss of motivation, increased passivity, and often feelings of lethargy and "flatness." However, there is no associated sadness, tearfulness, emotional angst, decreased concentration, or thoughts of hopelessness, worthlessness, or suicide. If specifically asked, patients often remark that the symptoms are not experientially similar to their original depressive symptoms. This apathy syndrome has not, to date, been adequately studied, and the pathophysiology is not known. However, there is speculation that subchronic stimulation of central serotonin may attenuate dopamine functioning in several areas of the brain, including the frontal cortex. In this respect, it is notable that the clinical presentation mirrors that of a frontal lobe syndrome.

The syndrome appears to be dose dependent and reversible. Mistakenly inter-preting the apathy and lethargy for a relapse of depression, and hence increasing the dose of medication, will worsen the symptoms. If dosage reduction is not effective, patients may benefit from the addition of a stimulant. Other agents that increase dopamine also may be effective. Other treatments, such as the use of adjunctive olanzapine, are under study based on the ability of this compound to increase frontal lobe dopamine.

Drug interactions. Several deaths have been reported in patients taking a combination of SSRIs and MAOIs, presumably resulting from the serotonin syndrome (Francois et al. 1997; Hodgman et al. 1997; Kolecki 1997). Because of the potential lethality of this interaction, when it is necessary to switch from an SSRI to an MAOI, the patient must remain off the SSRI for a long enough time to ensure that it has been fully eliminated from the body. This time frame is the equivalent of five times the half-life of the SSRI. Therefore, at least 5 weeks are required between the discontinuation of fluoxetine and the institution of an MAOI (Beasley et al. 1993) and about 1 week between other SSRIs and an MAOI. A 2-week waiting period is required when switching from an MAOI to an SSRI to allow resynthesis of the enzyme.

SSRIs vary with regard to inhibition of cytochrome P450 isozymes. Enzyme inhibition may result in increased blood levels of concomitantly administered medications (see section on drug interactions later in this chapter).

Bupropion

Mechanism of Action

Bupropion's mechanism of antidepressant activity remains unclear. Bupropion is metabolized to hydroxybupropion, which appears to be the active entity. Hydroxy-bupropion inhibits the reuptake of norepinephrine and dopamine, hence the designation dopamine-norepinephrine reuptake inhibitor (DNRI).

Background

Bupropion's unique spectrum of putative receptor effects provides a useful addition to the therapeutic armamentarium. The most significant advantage of bupropion is its relative lack of sexual side effects. Indeed, the addition of low doses of bupropion may attenuate the sexual dysfunction caused by other medications. The fact that dopamine is integrally related to the brain's reward mechanisms, which are stimulated by nicotine and other addictive substances, has provided the theoretical underpinning for recent research indicating that bupropion is an effective aid to smoking cessation. Bupropion is being marketed under the name Zyban for smoking cessation.

Overall, bupropion has a favorable side-effect profile with little or no weight gain, few effects on cardiac conduction (Roose et al. 1991), and minimal sexual side effects (Kiev et al. 1994). Disadvantages include an increased risk of medication-induced seizures at higher than recommended dosages and the requirement for twice-daily dosing in most patients.

Clinical Use

We recommend use of the sustained-release preparation rather than the original preparation because of its increased tolerability and decreased seizure risk. The sustained-release preparation is initiated at 150 mg, preferably taken in the morning. After 4 days, the dosage may be increased to 150 mg twice a day. For the short-acting preparation, bupropion is initiated at 75 mg twice a day and increased as tolerated to a total daily dosage of 300 mg. Patients who do not respond after 4 weeks may warrant a trial of 450 mg/day. No single dose should exceed 200 mg. Gradual dose titration helps to minimize initial anxiety and insomnia. The temporary use of anxiolytic or hypnotic agents is reasonable in some patients but generally should be limited to the first few weeks of treatment.

Contraindications

Patients with seizure disorders should not use bupropion. Similarly, consideration of an alternative treatment is advised for patients with a history of significant head trauma, CNS tumor, or an eating disorder.

Risks, Side Effects, and Their Management

The most common side effects of bupropion are initial headache, anxiety, insomnia, increased sweating, and gastrointestinal upset. Tremor and akathisia also may occur. Management of these effects is the same as previously discussed concerning the SSRIs. Bupropion is not associated with anticholinergic side effects, orthostatic hypotension, weight gain, or cardiac conduction changes.

The incidence of seizures is 0.4% with dosages less than 450 mg/day, provided no single dose of the short-acting preparation exceeds 150 mg. The incidence increases to 5% with dosages between 450 and 600 mg/day. The sustained-release preparation has a seizure incidence of 0.1% in dosages less than 300 mg/day and 0.4% in dosages between 300 and 400 mg/day. Higher dosages of the sustained-release preparation have not been evaluated. Patients who have a history of seizures or who are taking concomitant medications that lower the seizure threshold should be given bupropion with caution.

Psychosis.   Reports of delusions, hallucinations, and paranoia are consistent with bupropion-mediated increases in central dopamine. Bupropion should be used with caution in patients with psychotic disorder.

Overdose.   Much more is known about overdose with the immediate-release formulation of bupropion than with the newer, sustained-release formulation. Reported reactions with the immediate-release form include seizures, hallucinations, loss of consciousness, and sinus tachycardia. Treatment of overdose should include induction of vomiting, administration of activated charcoal, and ECG and electroencephalographic (EEG) monitoring. For seizures, an intravenous benzodiazepine preparation is recommended.

Drug interactions.   The combination of bupropion with an MAOI is potentially dangerous, but less so than the combination of serotonergic drugs and MAOIs. Although the practice is not recommended, there are reports of combining MAOIs and bupropion in patients with refractory depression.

In vitro data suggest that bupropion is metabolized by CYP2B6. Bupropion is now known to inhibit CYP2D6. Because of the risk of dose-dependent seizures, caution is warranted when bupropion is combined with other medications that might inhibit its metabolism.

Venlafaxine

Mechanism of Action

Venlafaxine hydrochloride is a potent inhibitor of norepinephrine and serotonin reuptake. At lower dosages, serotonin reuptake inhibition is prominent. At higher dosages, inhibition of norepinephrine reuptake becomes more significant. Inhibition of dopamine reuptake is manifest at the higher end of the dosage range (Ellingrod and Perry 1994).

Background

Venlafaxine is a phenylethylamine antidepressant released in the United States in 1994. Venlafaxine is approved by the FDA for the treatment of both major depression and generalized anxiety disorder. Preliminary data suggest that this agent might also have a role in the treatment of chronic pain conditions and perhaps other disorders for which SSRIs are effective. Venlafaxine is 27% protein bound, a proportion substantially lower than in any of the other antidepressants. This property is advantageous when it is necessary to minimize the likelihood of protein-binding interactions. Venlafaxine is unlikely to inhibit cytochrome P450 enzymes, which further decreases the likelihood of drug interactions. The extended-release formulation of venlafaxine allows for once-a-day dosing. Blood pressure elevation may occur at higher dosages, as discussed in the section on side effects.

Clinical Use

The recommended dosage range of venlafaxine is 75–225 mg/day. The extended-release preparation, which allows for once-daily dosing, is preferred. The usual starting dosage is 37.5–75 mg/day. Doses up to 375 mg/day have been used for patients who are otherwise nonresponsive to treatment. Blood pressure monitoring is recommended because of dose-dependent increases in mean diastolic blood pressure in some patients.

Unlike the SSRIs, venlafaxine demonstrates a positive dose–response relationship; patients with mild depression may respond to lower doses, whereas patients with more severe or recurrent depression may respond better to higher doses. Kelsey (1996) hypothesized that this difference exists because venlafaxine's mechanism of action involves mixed reuptake, with differential effects at higher dosages.

Risks, Side Effects, and Their Management

The side-effect profile of venlafaxine is similar to that of the SSRIs. Like the SSRIs, venlafaxine does not affect cardiac conduction or lower the seizure threshold. For most patients, venlafaxine is not associated with sedation or weight gain. Side effects that differ from those of the SSRIs are hypothesized to be related to the increased noradrenergic activity of this drug at higher doses, specifically dose-dependent anxiety in some patients and hypertension.

Hypertension. Modest dose-dependent increases in blood pressure may occur with venlafaxine treatment. A large meta-analysis found that the magnitude of change in blood pressure with venlafaxine is statistically significant but is unlikely to be of clinical significance at doses of less than 300 mg/day (Thase 1998). For clinically significant treatment-emergent hypertension, dosage reduction or treatment discontinuation should be considered.

Duloxetine

Mechanism of Action

Duloxetine hydrochloride (Cymbalta) binds selectively and with high affinity to both norepinephrine and serotonin transporters. Unlike the case for venlafaxine, the effects of duloxetine on norepinephrine are evident throughout the clinical dosage range.

Background

Duloxetine was recently approved for the treatment of major depression, but at the time of this writing has not been released for use in the United States. Some data suggest that duloxetine may attenuate the painful symptoms that often accompany depression (Detke et al. 2002).

Clinical Use

Although final dosing guidelines for optimal use are not yet established, efficacy has been demonstrated at a dosage of 60 mg bid. At this dose, duloxetine is a moderately potent CYP2D6 inhibitor (Skinner et al. 2003). Caution should be used when CYP2D6 substrates and inhibitors are coadministered with duloxetine.

Risks, Side Effects, and Their Management

Duloxetine appears to be well tolerated; the most common side effects in clinical trials were insomnia, asthenia, nausea, dry mouth, dizziness, and constipation (Detke et al. 2002; Goldstein et al. 2002). Of note, hypertension has not been a problem in clinical trials to date.

Nefazodone

Mechanism of Action

Nefazodone is a 5-HT_2 receptor antagonist and a weak inhibitor of neuronal serotonin and norepinephrine reuptake. Together these properties are believed to enhance 5-HT_{1A}-mediated neuronal transmission.

Background

Nefazodone entered the United States market in 1995. The advantages of nefazodone are a low incidence of sexual dysfunction (R.J. Goldberg 1995) and early attenuation of symptoms of anxiety and insomnia (Armitage et al. 1994; Fawcett et al. 1995). The disadvantages are prominent early sedation, twice-a-day dosing, slow dosage titration, and inhibition of CYP3A3/4.

Clinical Use

The clinically effective dosage range has been determined to be between 300 and 600 mg/day. Because of prominent early side effects, we recommend an initial dosage of 50 mg twice a day or at bedtime, with subsequent increases every 5–7 days, as tolerated, until the total daily dosage reaches 600 mg/day in divided doses or a therapeutic response emerges. The therapeutic range for elderly patients is slightly lower (i.e., between 200 and 400 mg/day in divided doses). As with other antidepressants, an adequate trial of at least 4 weeks is necessary to evaluate efficacy. Patients should be advised to look for signs and symptoms of liver dysfunction (i.e., jaundice), which warrant discontinuation of the medication.

Risks, Side Effects, and Their Management

Common side effects are sedation, nausea, dizziness, confusion, and blurred vision. Nefazodone does not appear to cause weight gain or sexual dysfunction. Although rare, life-threatening hepatic failure has been associated with nefazodone use.

Visual effects. Visual symptoms, such as blurred or abnormal vision, may accompany nefazodone treatment. Nefazodone does not have significant anticholinergic effects, and the mechanism for visual changes is not known. Treatment-emergent visual symptoms are generally mild and transient.

Contraindications and drug interactions. Coadministration of nefazodone with most medications that are metabolized by CYP3A3/4 should be undertaken only with caution, and the dosages of the other medications that are 3A3/4 substrates should be reduced (see the section on drug interactions later in this chapter). The interaction of nefazodone with MAOIs has not yet been evaluated, but it may be as dangerous as the interaction with the SSRIs. Therefore, this combination

should be avoided. Nefazodone use in patients with liver disease should be avoided.

Trazodone

Mechanism of Action

Trazodone, like nefazodone, is a postsynaptic 5-HT$_2$ antagonist and a weak inhibitor of serotonin reuptake.

Background

Trazodone is an older antidepressant associated with significant sedative activity. Currently, trazodone is not recommended as a first-line antidepressant because of an increased risk of orthostatic hypotension, arrhythmias, and priapism. Also, when compared with other available antidepressants, trazodone does not offer an advantage in terms of therapeutic efficacy (Haria et al. 1994). However, trazodone may be useful in patients with insomnia. It is currently common practice to use low dosages of trazodone, such as 50–100 mg, to assist with initial insomnia while starting one of the newer antidepressants to treat the underlying depression. If this strategy is used, we recommend tapering the dosage and discontinuing treatment with trazodone after 4–6 weeks.

Priapism

Trazodone is the only antidepressant that has been associated with priapism (Scher et al. 1983), which may be irreversible and require surgical intervention (Mitchell and Popkin 1983). This risk must always be considered before trazodone is chosen to treat male patients.

Mirtazapine

Mechanism of Action and Receptor Effects

Mirtazapine facilitates central serotonergic and noradrenergic transmission by antagonizing α_2-noradrenergic autoreceptors and heteroreceptors (De Boer 1996). In addition, mirtazapine antagonizes postsynaptic $5-HT_{2A}$, $5-HT_3$, and H_1 receptors. $5-HT_{2A}$ antagonism may be related to the antidepressant properties of this drug and is likely to account for the low occurrence of drug-induced sexual dysfunction. $5-HT_3$ antagonism is thought to prevent nausea. Antagonism of H_1 receptors may account for the side effects of sedation and weight gain. Mirtazapine has moderate activity at α_1 receptors and muscarinic receptors.

Background

Mirtazapine entered the United States market in 1996. It has been shown to reduce anxiety symptoms and sleep disturbances associated with depression as early as 1 week after the start of treatment (Bremmer 1995; Smith et al. 1990). Other advantages are minimal sexual dysfunction, minimal nausea, and once-daily dosing. In addition, mirtazapine is unlikely to be associated with cytochrome P450–mediated drug interactions. The disadvantages of mirtazapine are weight gain and prominent early sedation.

Clinical Use

Mirtazapine treatment is initiated with 15 mg at bedtime. Depending on clinical response and side effects, the dosage can be increased to a maximum of 45 mg at bedtime, although higher dosages are sometimes used in patients with treatment-resistant illness. Elderly patients and those with renal or hepatic disease may require lower dosages.

Monoamine Oxidase Inhibitors

Mechanism of Action

The enzyme monoamine oxidase (MAO) inactivates biogenic amines such as norepinephrine, serotonin, dopamine, and tyramine through oxidative deamination. MAOIs block this inactivation and thereby increase the amount of these transmitters available for synaptic release. There are two types of MAO: A and B. Type A (MAO-A) acts selectively on the substrates norepinephrine and serotonin, whereas type B (MAO-B) preferentially affects phenylethylamine. Both MAO types oxidize dopamine and tyramine. MAO-A inhibition appears to be most relevant to the antidepressant effects of these drugs. Drugs that contain both MAO-A and MAO-B are called *nonselective*. The MAOI antidepressants currently available in the United States are nonselective inhibitors. Because tyramine can be metabolized by either MAO-A or MAO-B, drugs that selectively inhibit either one of these enzymes, but not the other, do not require dietary restrictions. MAO-A–selective drugs, such as moclobemide, are available in other countries for the treatment of depression. MAO-B–selective drugs, such as pargyline and L-deprenyl, are marketed for other indications and do not appear to treat depression in their usual dosages. At higher dosages, both of these drugs become nonselective.

Another important characteristic of MAOIs is the production of reversible versus irreversible enzyme inhibition. An irreversible inhibitor permanently disables the enzyme. This means that MAO must be resynthesized, in the absence of the drug, before the activity of the enzyme can be reestablished. Resynthesis of the enzyme may take up to 2 weeks. For this reason, 10–14 days are required after discontinuation of irreversible inhibitors before instituting other antidepressants or before permitting the use of the drugs or foods that are known to be contraindicated (see the following subsection on clinical use of MAOIs). On the other hand, a reversible inhibitor can move away from the active site of the enzyme, enabling the enzyme to

TABLE 18–4. Summary of monoamine oxidase (MAO) inhibitor reversibility and selectivity

Drug	Reversible inhibition	Enzyme selectivity	Indication
Phenelzine	No	MAO-A + B	Depression
Tranylcypromine	No	MAO-A + B	Depression
L-Deprenyl	No	MAO-B[a]	Parkinson's disease
Pargyline	No	MAO-B[a]	Hypertension
Moclobemide[b]	Yes	MAO-A	Depression

[a]MAO-B is selective at lower doses, nonselective at higher doses.
[b]Not available in the United States.

be available to metabolize other substances. The reversibility and selectivity of the currently available MAOIs are summarized in Table 18–4.

Clinical Use

The MAOIs are not currently used as first-line agents because of the improved tolerability and safety of the newer antidepressants. However, the MAOIs continue to be excellent medications for a subset of patients who do not respond to the newer antidepressants. Patients with a depressive syndrome characterized by mood reactivity (i.e., mood that is responsive acutely to favorable and unfavorable life experiences), oversleeping, overeating, extreme lethargy, and extreme sensitivity to rejection—the so-called atypical subtype—may show a preferential response to MAOI therapy (M.R. Liebowitz et al. 1984; Quitkin et al. 1979; Ravaris et al. 1980; Zisook 1985).

More so than with other medications, it is imperative to review the patient's medical status and current medications before prescribing an MAOI. The importance of following the dietary and medication restrictions, as outlined later, should be discussed with the patient; the discussion should be supplemented with written instructions, as presented in Table 18–5.

Phenelzine is initiated with 15 mg in the morning and increased by 15 mg every

other day until a total daily dosage of 60 mg is reached. If no response occurs within 2 weeks, the dosage may be increased in 15-mg increments to a usual maximum of 90 mg/day. Higher dosages are sometimes used, if tolerated, in patients with severe and refractory depression. Tranylcypromine is initiated at 10 mg and then increased every other day to 30 mg/day. As with phenelzine, higher dosages may be necessary when the condition is refractory to treatment (Amsterdam and Berwish 1989). After tolerance to the hypotensive side effects has developed, usually after 1 or 2 weeks, the patient may take the medication as a single daily dose in the morning. Morning dosing is preferred because these medications tend to be activating, especially tranylcypromine, which is related to amphetamine. Some data suggest that once-daily dosing of the MAOIs may be therapeutically superior to multiple dosing (Weise et al. 1980).

Risks, Side Effects, and Their Management

The following risks and side effects apply to the irreversible, nonselective MAOI antidepressants (phenelzine and tranylcypromine). The most common side effects are orthostatic hypotension, headache, insomnia, weight gain, sexual dysfunction, peripheral edema, and afternoon somnolence. Although the MAOIs do not have

TABLE 18–5. Instructions for patients taking monoamine oxidase inhibitors

While taking this medication

1. Avoid all the foods and drugs indicated on the list (see Table 18–6).
2. In general, all the foods you should avoid are decayed, fermented, or aged in some way. Avoid any spoiled food even if it is not on the list.
3. If you get a cold or flu, you may use aspirin or Tylenol. For a cough, glycerin cough drops or cough syrup without dextromethorphan may be used.
4. All laxatives or stool softeners for constipation may be used.
5. For infections, all antibiotics may be safely prescribed, such as penicillin, tetracycline, or erythromycin.
6. Do not take any other medications without first checking with me. These include any over-the-counter medicines bought without prescription, such as cold tablets, nose drops, cough medicine, and diet pills.
7. Eating one of the restricted foods may cause a sudden elevation of your blood pressure. If this occurs, you will get an explosive headache, particularly in the back of your head and in your temples. Your head and face will feel flushed and full, your heart may pound, and you may perspire heavily and feel nauseated. If this rare reaction occurs, do not lie down because this elevates your blood pressure further. If your blood pressure is high, go to the nearest emergency center for evaluation and treatment. Do not wait for a telephone call from our office.
8. If you need medical or dental care while taking this medication, show these restrictions and instructions to the doctor or dentist. Have the doctor or dentist call my office if he or she has any questions or needs further clarification or information.
9. Side effects such as postural light-headedness, constipation, delay in urination, delay in ejaculation and orgasm, muscle twitching, sedation, fluid retention, insomnia, and excess sweating are quite common. Many of these side effects lessen after the third week.
10. Light-headedness may occur after sudden changes in position. This can be avoided by getting up slowly. If tablets are taken with meals, this and the other side effects are lessened.
11. The medication is rarely effective in less than 3 weeks.
12. Care should be taken while operating any machinery or driving; some patients have episodes of sleepiness in the early phase of treatment.
13. Take the medication precisely as directed. Do not regulate the number of pills without first consulting me.
14. In spite of the side effects and special dietary restrictions, your medication (an MAO inhibitor) is safe and effective when taken as directed.
15. If any special problems arise, call me at my office.

Source.   Adapted from Jenike 1987.

significant affinity for muscarinic receptors, anticholinergic-like side effects are present at the start of treatment. Dry mouth is common but is not as marked as with the TCAs. Fortunately, the more serious risks, such as hypertensive crisis and serotonin syndrome, are not common.

Hypertensive crisis.   The inactivation of intestinal MAO impairs the metabolism of tyramine. Tyramine can function as a false transmitter and displace norepinephrine from presynaptic storage granules. Thus, large amounts of dietary tyramine can result in a hypertensive crisis in patients who are taking MAOIs, because increased amounts of norepinephrine result in profound α-adrenergic activation. This reaction also has been called the "cheese reaction," because tyramine is present in relatively high concentrations in aged cheeses.

Some drugs with sympathomimetic activity, including certain decongestants and cough syrups, should be avoided because of the risk of precipitating a hypertensive crisis (Table 18–6). However, pure antihistamine drugs, such as diphenhydramine, and pure expectorants without dextromethorphan (e.g., guaifenesin) are permissible.

These reactions can range from mild to severe. In the mildest form, the patient may complain of sweating, palpitations, and a mild headache. The most severe form of reaction manifests as a hypertensive crisis, with severe headache, increased blood pressure, and possible intracerebral hemorrhage. If a patient experiences a severely painful or unremitting occipital headache when taking an MAOI, he or she should immediately seek medical assessment and monitoring.

If the blood pressure is severely elevated, pharmacological treatment should be instituted. We often recommend that patients purchase a home blood pressure cuff to help distinguish a true hypertensive crisis from more common, and benign, headaches of other etiologies. Currently, the most common treatment for MAOI-induced hypertension is the calcium channel blocker nifedipine. An oral dose of 10 mg of nifedipine often normalizes blood pressure within 1–5 minutes with little risk of causing overshoot hypotension (Schenk and Remick 1989). If patients are supplied with a prescription for nifedipine in advance, they may administer the medication immediately and then proceed to a hospital for further monitoring and treatment. A drug with α-adrenergic-blocking properties, such as intravenous phentolamine (5 mg) or intramuscular chlorpromazine (25–50 mg), also may be administered. Because treatment with phentolamine may be associated with cardiac arrhythmias or severe hypotension, this approach should be carried out only in

an emergency department setting (Tollefson 1983).

It is advisable to have patients taking MAOIs carry an identification card as notification to emergency medical personnel that they are currently taking an MAOI. Patients should always carry the list of prohibited foods and medications, and they should be told to notify physicians that they are taking an MAOI before accepting any medication or anesthetic (Tables 18–5 and 18–6). When patients have dental procedures performed, local anesthetics without vasoconstrictors (e.g., epinephrine) must be used.

Serotonin syndrome.   The combination of serotonergic drugs, such as the SSRIs, with MAOIs can result in serotonin syndrome, which may be fatal. As the condition progresses, hyperthermia, hypertonicity, myoclonus, and death may occur. The syndrome must be identified as rapidly as possible. Discontinuation of the serotonergic medications is the first step in treatment, followed by emergency medical treatment, as required.

The combination of MAOIs with meperidine, and perhaps with other phenylpiperidine analgesics, also has been implicated in the fatal reactions that were attributed to the serotonin syndrome. Aspirin, nonsteroidal anti-inflammatory drugs, and acetaminophen should be used for mild to moderate pain. Among narcotic agents, codeine and morphine are safe in combination with MAOIs, although doses may need to be lower than usual.

Issues of Treatment

Treatment of Acute Major Depression

The choice of an antidepressant medication is based on factors discussed earlier in this section and outlined in Table 18–2. The initial therapeutic response of the

TABLE 18–6. Dietary and medication restrictions for patients taking monoamine oxidase inhibitors (MAOIs)

Foods that must be avoided while taking an MAOI and for 2 weeks after stopping the medication[a]	Aged cheeses (fresh cheese such as cream cheese, cottage cheese, ricotta cheese, American cheese, and moderate amounts of mozzarella are currently considered safe)
	Aged or fermented meats, such as sausages, salami, and pepperoni (smoked salmon and whitefish are currently considered safe)
	Sauerkraut
	Soy sauce
	Fava beans and broad bean pods
	All food that may be spoiled
	Alcohol may be consumed in moderation, but tap beer should be avoided, including nonalcoholic tap beer
	Yeast or meat extracts such as Marmite and Bovril (yeast and baked goods containing yeast are safe)
	Yogurt, if fresh, is safe
Drugs that must be avoided while taking an MAOI and for 2 weeks after stopping the medication[b]	*All sympathomimetics and stimulant drugs, including*
	Amphetamines — Local anesthetic drugs containing ephedrine or cocaine
	Diet medications — Demerol
	Ephedrine — Levodopa and dopamine
	Isoproterenol — Fenfluramine and dexfenfluramine
	Methylphenidate — Other antidepressant medications
	Phenylpropanolamine — Buspirone
	Phenylephrine

TABLE 18–6. Dietary and medication restrictions for patients taking monoamine oxidase inhibitors (MAOIs) *(continued)*

Drugs that must be avoided while taking an MAOI and for 2 weeks after stopping the medication[b]	*Over-the-counter nasal decongestants and cold, sinus, and allergy medications containing pseudoephedrine, phenylephrine, or phenylpropanolamine*
	Actifed
	Alka-Seltzer Plus
	Allerest
	Contact
	Coricidin D
	CoTylenol
	Dristan
	Neo-Synephrine
	Robitussin PE, DM, CF, Night Relief
	Sine-Aid
	Sine-Off
	Sinex
	Triaminic
	Tylenol
	Vicks Formula 44M, 44D, Nyquil
Safe cold/allergy medications	Tylenol (plain)
	Robitussin (plain)
	Alka-Seltzer (plain)
	Chlor-Trimeton Allergy (without decongestant)
	Steroid inhalers
Other safe medications	Nonsteroidal anti-inflammatory drugs
	Codeine
	Morphine
	Antibiotics
	Laxatives and stool softeners
	Local anesthetics without epinephrine or cocaine

[a]Food restrictions are based on tyramine contact data from Walker et al. 1996.

[b]It is advisable to check the current *Physicians' Desk Reference* for any drug that is not known to be safe before prescribing it in combination with an MAOI.

Source.   Feinburg and Holzer 1997, 2000; Schulman and Walker 1999, 2000; Walker et al. 1997; Wing and Chen 1997.

depressed patient to medications may be detected as early as the first week, but it is often delayed by several weeks. Neurovegetative symptoms usually improve before mood improves. The clinician must inform the patient of this latency in therapeutic response because many patients expect antidepressants to be effective with the first dose. For patients with severe anxiety or insomnia, the concurrent use of a benzodiazepine may be considered. However, we restrict this practice solely to the treatment of depressed patients with marked anxiety, and we discontinue it by tapering the benzodiazepine dosage as the antidepressant begins to exert its therapeutic effect. A patient may experience a return of energy and motivation while still experiencing the subjective symptoms of hopelessness and excessive guilt. For such patients, there may be an increased risk of suicide because a return of energy in an extremely dysphoric individual may provide the impetus and wherewithal for an act of self-destruction. A clinical challenge in the evaluation of side effects of antidepressant drugs is to distinguish symptoms of the illness from complaints that are secondary to side effects.

An adequate trial of antidepressant medication traditionally has been defined as treatment with therapeutic dosages of a drug for a total of 6–8 weeks. On the basis of more recent data, Quitkin et al. (1996) suggested that 4 weeks may be a more clinically meaningful point for reevaluation of treatment. After 4 weeks of antidepressant treatment, the patient can be conceptualized as falling into one of three groups, depending on whether there has been 1) a full response, 2) a partial response, or 3) no response at all. For the fortunate patients who achieve full remission, treatment should continue for a minimum of 4–6 months, or longer when there is a history of a recurrent course (see

the subsection "Maintenance Treatment of Major Depression" later in this chapter). If a partial response has been achieved by 4 weeks, a full response may be evident within an additional 2 weeks without further intervention. If there is no response at all, the dosage should be increased, the medication should be changed to another antidepressant, or the therapy should be augmented with another medication (see the subsection "Treatment-Resistant Depression" later in this chapter). These guidelines are summarized in Figure 18–1.

Treatment of Depression With Psychotic Features

Patients with psychotic depression have been reported to respond to combined treatment with antidepressants and antipsychotics (Nelson and Bowers 1978); they also show a dramatic response to ECT, which is often the treatment of choice in this disorder (Yudofsky 1981). Long-term antipsychotic medications are generally not warranted, but prophylactic antidepressant medication must be continued as in nonpsychotic depression.

Treatment of Bipolar Depression

A history of previous episodes of mania or hypomania should alert the clinician to the diagnosis of bipolar disorder. Because antidepressants can precipitate manic episodes and increase cycling in bipolar patients (Wehr and Goodwin 1979), mood stabilizers (e.g., lithium, valproate) are the appropriate first step in the treatment of bipolar depression (see section "Mood Stabilizers" later in this chapter).

Maintenance Treatment of Major Depression

Antidepressant therapy should not be discontinued before there have been 4–5 symptom-free months (Prien and Kupfer 1986). Most clinicians treat single epi-

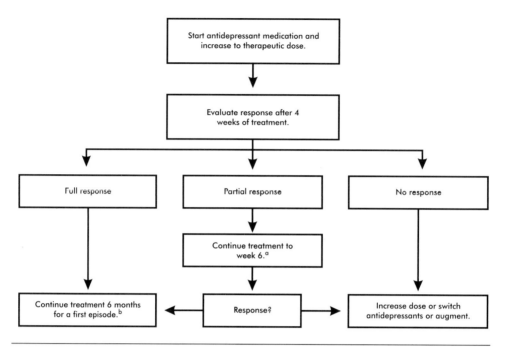

FIGURE 18–1. Algorithm for the acute treatment of major depression.
[a]If no further response is seen at week 5, it is not necessary to wait until week 6.
[b]See text for maintenance treatment guidelines for patients with recurrent depression.

sodes of depression for a minimum of 6 months. Antidepressants should be continued at the same dosage that resulted in remission of the acute episode. Strong evidence indicates that relapse is more likely when the antidepressant dosage is lowered from acute treatment levels (Frank et al. 1990).

Unfortunately, depression is often a recurrent disorder. After one episode of depression, there is a 50% chance that the patient will have a second episode; after three episodes, there is a 90% chance of recurrence (Angst 1990). Therefore, longer periods of antidepressant treatment, often called *maintenance treatment*, are warranted to protect against recurrence (NIMH Consensus Development Conference Statement 1985). In patients with more than three episodes of depression, long-term prophylaxis is strongly recommended. The duration of treatment is individualized on the basis of the severity and effect

of past episodes, and the time between episodes. Some patients may require lifelong antidepressant maintenance treatment. There is no evidence of increased risk associated with long-term use of antidepressants.

Antidepressant Discontinuation

Discontinuation of antidepressant medication should be done in concordance with the guidelines for treatment duration, as outlined earlier. It is advisable to taper the medication while monitoring for signs and symptoms of relapse. Abrupt discontinuation of these medications is also more likely to lead to antidepressant discontinuation symptoms, which are often referred to as *withdrawal* symptoms. The occurrence of these symptoms following medication discontinuation does not imply that antidepressants are "addictive."

Treatment-Resistant Depression

Careful review of the clinical history and response to previous treatment often reveals that patients in whom depression has been resistant to standard antidepressant treatment have had an inadequate therapeutic trial with the antidepressant (Lydiard 1985) or have been noncompliant with the medication. Failure to complete an adequate therapeutic trial with an antidepressant drug does not constitute a depression that is resistant to pharmacotherapy. In another presentation, patients report a history of robust but short-lived responses to several antidepressants. This patient may be manifesting a medication-induced rapid-cycling course. Mild episodes of hypomania during the course of treatment may be overlooked, especially in a high-functioning, productive patient with a premorbid history of hyperthymic personality, which is defined as a chronic state of mild hypomania. Kukopoulos et al. (1983) and Akiskal (1992) claimed that hyperthymia and mild cyclothymia may be predictors of a medication-induced rapid-cycling course and suggested that these patients are at the milder end of a bipolar spectrum. Mixed mood states may ultimately develop if the patient continues taking antidepressants, and the diagnosis of a refractory, agitated depression may be made erroneously. In these cases, treatment with a mood stabilizer (discussed later in this chapter) is indicated.

For patients with true nonresponse and for those who achieve only partial response, treatment options include using an augmentation or combination strategy and switching to another antidepressant. Augmentation involves adding another agent that is not an antidepressant, such as lithium, thyroid hormone, or a psychostimulant. Combination treatment refers to combining two antidepressants with different mechanisms of action to produce synergistic effects. Whether to switch, augment, or combine depends on many factors, including the severity of illness, side effects of the current medication, and the patient's willingness to take more than one medication. For example, if a patient's illness is significantly interfering with daily function, augmentation or combination should be considered if the current antidepressant is well tolerated because this may result in a quicker response. On the other hand, a patient with a milder illness, significant side effects of the current medication, and a general uneasiness about taking medication will probably be better off if the current medication is switched to a different, single antidepressant.

Of the augmentation strategies, lithium augmentation has the best evidence from randomized controlled trials; however, almost all of these data are with the TCAs. Since De Montigny and colleagues first reported successful antidepressant treatment with adjunctive lithium in 1981, there have been many reports of patients who failed to respond to TCA or SSRI treatment alone but whose depressions improved when the antidepressant was combined with lithium (Dinan and Barry 1989; Ontiveros et al. 1991; Thase et al. 1989). Although some of these patients manifested a rapid and dramatic response when lithium was added to their antidepressant regimen, improvement may require several weeks. Patients often respond to dosages of lithium lower than those used for the treatment of bipolar disorder. We typically start with 600 mg at bedtime. If there is no response after 2 weeks, the dosage should be increased as tolerated.

Thyroid supplementation has received a more mixed endorsement in the scientific literature. Goodwin et al. (1982) performed the first double-blind study that found triiodothyronine (T_3) to be a useful adjunct in former nonresponders. However, Gitlin et al. (1987), in a follow-up study, found no benefit to this approach. A study by Joffe (1988) reported that those patients who did respond to the addition of T_3 were less likely to benefit from adjunctive lithium, and vice versa. This double-blind, placebo-controlled trial found a 50% response rate for both lithium and T_3 augmentation. For reasons that are unclear, it appears that T_3 is more effective than thyroxine (T_4) as an augmenting agent in unipolar depression (Joffe and Singer 1990).

Stimulants such as amphetamine and methylphenidate have been used to treat depression for many years. Stimulants should not be used as monotherapy, except perhaps in geriatric patients with prominent apathy, medically ill patients with depression, or patients with post-stroke depression (Lingam et al. 1988). However, psychostimulants are useful for augmentation of antidepressants in the treatment of refractory depression and are generally safe, even for most patients with cardiac disorders. Fawcett et al. (1991) reported the successful use of stimulant-MAOI combinations among a group of patients who were nonresponders to various other treatments, including ECT. Only 1 of their 32 patients could not tolerate the combination because of hypertensive side effects. The nonamphetamine stimulant modafinil has been reported to be useful in a recent uncontrolled report of seven subjects (Menza et al. 2000).

The use of more than one antidepressant for patients with treatment-resistant depression is potentially beneficial. SSRI–TCA combinations have been reported to be effective for patients who do not respond to monotherapy and, perhaps, to cause a more rapid antidepressant effect (Nelson et al. 1991; Weilburg et al. 1989). Some SSRIs can cause tricyclic levels in the blood to rise (Aranow et al. 1989; Downs et al. 1989), but this effect is not

likely to account for the synergism between the two antidepressants. However, because of this pharmacokinetic interaction, augmentation of the TCA dose should be reduced to achieve the same blood levels. Although there are few systematic data, other antidepressant combinations are commonly used in clinical practice to treat refractory depression. The principle of combining two antidepressants is to choose agents that have different mechanisms of action. For example, it makes little sense to combine two different SSRIs. However, the combination of an SSRI with mirtazapine or bupropion may provide mechanistic synergy. When combining antidepressants, it is important first to ensure that the patient has had an adequate trial of a single agent and to be aware of possible drug interactions or additive side effects.

Particular care must be exercised in switching patients from an MAOI to other antidepressant classes. For patients who have completed an MAOI trial without therapeutic response, other antidepressants should not be started until 14 days after the original MAOI has been discontinued. Equal care is required when switching from most other antidepressants to an MAOI. A time period equal to five times the half-life of the drug, including active metabolites, is required between stopping other antidepressant medications and starting an MAOI.

Switching between other antidepressants is less problematic. Current practice is to discontinue the first medication before starting the second one. There is no need for a medication-free period if neither medication is an MAOI. However, some patients report increased side effects and anxiety when switching from fluoxetine to nefazodone. This reaction is most likely because fluoxetine and its active metabolite norfluoxetine inhibit CYP2D6, which metabolizes a metabolite of nefazodone, which is known to be anxiogenic. Therefore, it may be prudent to wait 1–2 weeks between the discontinuation of fluoxetine and the start of nefazodone.

Nonpharmacological options also should be considered in patients who have not adequately responded to treatment. As discussed later in this chapter, ECT is a highly effective treatment. In addition, psychotherapy has an important role in the treatment of depression (as is discussed in various chapters throughout this volume).

Anxiolytics, Sedatives, and Hypnotics

Overview

Anxiety and insomnia are prevalent symptoms with multiple etiologies. Effective treatments are available, but they vary according to diagnosis. In most instances, the best course of action is to treat the underlying disorder rather than reflexively instituting treatment with a nonspecific anxiolytic. For example, a patient who has anxiety symptoms related to paranoid delusions should be given an antipsychotic medication not an anxiolytic. Likewise, patients with panic disorder, OCD, or major depression should receive medications indicated for those disorders. In these cases, anxiety may be a target symptom, one of the group of target symptoms of the underlying disorder.

In some circumstances, anxiolytics can serve a transitional purpose. For example, consider the case of a patient with acute-onset panic disorder, severe anticipatory anxiety, and a family history of depression. An antidepressant medication that also has antipanic effects may be the optimal treatment for this patient, but it will take several weeks for its effects to ap-

pear, during which time there is a risk that the patient's panic disorder will progress to agoraphobia. For this patient, we recommend starting the antidepressant and also targeting acute symptom relief with a benzodiazepine. After 4 weeks, the benzodiazepine should be slowly tapered so that the patient's symptoms are controlled with the antidepressant alone.

In this section, we discuss the pharmacology of medications classified as anxiolytic, sedative, or hypnotic, primarily the benzodiazepines, buspirone, zolpidem, and zaleplon. Subsequently, we present diagnosis-specific treatment guidelines as outlined in Table 18–7. The commonly used anxiolytics and hypnotics, together with their usual dosages, are shown in Table 18–8. In addition, many antidepressant medications are effective in the treatment of anxiety disorders. The pharmacology of the antidepressants was discussed in the previous section; their clinical use in anxiety disorders is included in the diagnosis-specific subsections that follow.

TABLE 18–7. Medications of choice for specific anxiety disorders

Generalized anxiety disorder	Buspirone, benzodiazepines, venlafaxine, SSRIs
Obsessive-compulsive disorder	Clomipramine, SSRIs
Panic disorder	SSRIs, TCAs, MAOIs, benzodiazepines
Performance anxiety	β-Blockers, benzodiazepines
Social phobia	SSRIs, MAOIs, benzodiazepines, buspirone

Note. MAOI = monoamine oxidase inhibitor; SSRI = selective serotonin reuptake inhibitor; TCA = tricyclic antidepressant.

TABLE 18–8.   Commonly used anxiolytic and hypnotic medications

Generic (trade) name	Single dose (mg)	Usual thera- peutic dosage (mg/day)	Approxi- mate dose equivalent (mg)	Methods of administration and supplied form	Approximate elimination half-life, including metabolites[a]
Benzodiazepines					
Alprazolam (Xanax and generics)	0.25–1	1–4	0.5	po: 0.25/0.5 mg	12 hours
Chlordiazepoxide (Librium and generics)	5 25	15 100	10	po: 5/10/25 mg; iv, im[b]	1 4 days
Clonazepam (Klonopin)	0.5–2	1–4	0.25	po: 0.5/2 mg	1–2 days
Clorazepate (Tranx- ene and generics)	3.75–22.5	15–60	7.5	po: 3.75/7.5/30 mg	2–4 days
Diazepam (Valium and generics)	2–10	4–40	5	po: 2/5/10 mg; iv, im[b]	2–4 days
Lorazepam (Ativan and generics)	0.5–2	1–6	1	po, s/l: 0.5/1/2 mg; iv, im[b]	12 hours
Oxazepam (Serax and generics)	10–30	30–120	15	po: 10/15/30 mg	12 hours
Nonbenzodiazepines					
Buspirone (BuSpar)	10–30	30–60	NA	po: 5/10/15 mg	2–3 hours

Note.   NA = not applicable.
[a]The clinical duration of action for the benzodiazepines does not correlate with the elimination half-life. See text for discussion.
[b]Lorazepam im is well absorbed. We do not recommend chlordiazepoxide or diazepam im.
Source.   Adapted from Teboul and Chouinard 1990 and *Physicians' Desk Reference* 2001.

Benzodiazepines

Mechanisms of Action

Benzodiazepines facilitate the inhibitory properties of γ-aminobutyric acid (GABA), the major inhibitory neurotransmitter in the brain (reviewed by Tallman et al. 1980). The benzodiazepine receptor is a subtype of the $GABA_A$ receptor. Activation of the benzodiazepine receptor facilitates the action of endogenous GABA, which results in the opening of chloride ion channels and a decrease in neuronal excitability. Benzodiazepines act rapidly because ion channels can open and close relatively quickly, in contrast to the slower onset of action that occurs when a drug acts via a metabotropic receptor and the resultant cascade of G proteins, second messengers, and subsequent intracellular effects.

Indications and Efficacy

Benzodiazepines are highly effective anxiolytics and sedatives; they also possess muscle relaxant and anticonvulsant properties. Benzodiazepines effectively treat both acute and chronic generalized anxiety (Elie and Lamontagne 1985; Greenblatt et al. 1983; Rickels 1986; Rickels et al. 1983) and panic disorder. The high-potency benzodiazepines alprazolam and clonazepam have received more attention as antipanic agents (Tesar 1990; Tesar et al. 1991), but double-blind studies also have confirmed the efficacy of diazepam (Dunner et al. 1986) and lorazepam (Charney and Woods 1989) in the treatment of panic disorder. Although only a few benzodiazepines have specific, FDA-approved indications for the treatment of insomnia, almost all benzodiazepines may be used for this purpose. Benzodiazepines are most clearly valuable as hypnotics in the general hospital setting, where high levels of sensory stimulation, pain, and acute stress may interfere with sleep. The safe, effective, and time-limited use of benzodiazepine hypnotics may, in fact, prevent chronic sleep difficulties from taking hold (NIMH Consensus Development Conference 1984). Benzodiazepines are also used to treat akathisia and catatonia and as an adjunct in the treatment of acute mania.

Because alcohol and barbiturates also act, in part, via the GABA$_A$ receptor–mediated chloride ion channel, benzodiazepines show cross-tolerance with these substances. As such, benzodiazepines are used frequently for the treatment of alcohol or barbiturate withdrawal and detoxification. Alcohol and barbiturates are more dangerous than benzodiazepines because at high doses they can act directly at the chloride ion channel. In contrast, benzodiazepines have no direct effect on the ion channel; the effects of benzodiazepines are limited by the amount of endogenous GABA.

Choice of Benzodiazepine

The metabolism of benzodiazepines also is important in the choice of the specific therapeutic agent. Lorazepam and oxazepam are not converted to active metabolites by the liver. Therefore, for patients with hepatic dysfunction, lorazepam and oxazepam are clinically indicated for relief of anxiety because their elimination from the body will not be significantly affected (Abernethy et al. 1984).

Risks, Side Effects, and Their Management

Sedation and impairment of performance. Benzodiazepine-induced sedation may be considered either a therapeutic action or a side effect. Residual daytime somnolence is a function of two variables: drug half-life and dosage (Roth and Roehrs 1992). With longer-acting agents, such as flurazepam and quazepam, a morning-after hangover is common, although some tolerance to this effect may develop with time. On the other hand, any benzodiazepine, whether short or long acting, can cause daytime drowsiness if the nighttime dose is too great. In general, it is clinically unclear and theoretically uncertain whether sedation is a desirable component of anxiolytic activity. Many patients both expect and desire some degree of sedation when they are intensely anxious. Anxious patients who have received chronic treatment with benzodiazepines rarely complain about daytime sedation, even when compared with drug-free anxious subjects (Lucki et al. 1986).

Impairment of performance on sensitive psychomotor tests has been well documented after the administration of benzodiazepines. Diazepam, administered at a dosage of 10 mg taken three times a day, was found to cause impaired driving skills in anxious patients during the first weeks of treatment (Linnoila et al. 1983). In contrast, Lucki et al. (1986) found no impairment in performance of a series of cognitive tasks by a group of anxious patients who had been taking benzodiazepines for an average of 5 years. Regardless of whether sedation is a desired effect, patients must be warned that driving, engaging in dangerous physical activities, and using hazardous machinery should be avoided during the acute stages, and possibly during the later stages, of treatment with benzodiazepines.

Dependence, withdrawal, and rebound effects. Concerns about physical and psychological dependence on benzodiazepines are frequently raised by patients and often affect a clinician's choice of treatment. On the basis of the criterion of self-reinforcement, however, most of the benzodiazepines, with the possible exception of diazepam, have low abuse potential when properly prescribed and supervised (American Psychiatric Association 1990; Sellers et al. 1992). Illicit street traffic in potent agents such as alprazolam and triazolam has remained low, possibly because the rapidly developing sedation produced by these drugs interferes with the desired euphoriant effects (Mendelson 1992). Physical dependence often occurs when benzodiazepines are taken in higher than usual dosages or for prolonged periods of time (Busto et al. 1986; Schopf 1983; Tyrer et al. 1983).

If benzodiazepines are discontinued precipitously, withdrawal effects that include hyperpyrexia, seizures, psychosis, and even death may occur. Despite various methodological shortcomings, several studies also suggest that physical dependence may occur even when benzodiazepines are taken in usual clinical doses for prolonged periods beyond several weeks and that the symptoms of withdrawal may arise even when drug discontinuation is not abrupt (Ashton 1991; Noyes et al. 1988). The signs and symptoms of withdrawal may include tachycardia, increased blood pressure, muscle cramps, anxiety, insomnia, panic attacks, impairment of memory and concentration, and perceptual disturbances. In addition, withdrawal-related derealization, hallucinations, and other psychotic symptoms have been reported. These withdrawal symptoms may begin as soon as the day after discontinuation of benzodiazepines and may continue for weeks to months. Evidence indicates that withdrawal reactions peak more rapidly

and more intensely with the benzodiazepines that have a briefer half-life (Busto et al. 1986). These withdrawal effects are rapidly reversed with the readministration of benzodiazepines. Although it is generally believed that there is cross-tolerance for all benzodiazepines, there has been a report of withdrawal symptoms from alprazolam that were not reversed with diazepam (Zipursky et al. 1985).

Memory impairment. Amnesia appears to be mediated through the central benzodiazepine receptor; therefore, this effect may occur with any benzodiazepine (Lister 1985). The degree of anterograde amnesia appears to be related to dosage, and the amnesia may occur in the first several hours after each dose of benzodiazepine is taken, even after repeated use (Lucki et al. 1986).

Disinhibition and dyscontrol. An area of controversy is the allegation that benzodiazepines may, in some instances, cause behavioral disinhibition, leading to acts of aggression (Medawarn and Rassaby 1991). A history of hostility, impulsivity, or borderline or antisocial personality disorder has been implicated as a potential predictor of this reaction.

Overdose. Benzodiazepines are remarkably safe when taken in overdose. Dangerous effects occur when the overdose includes several sedative drugs, especially when alcohol is included, because of synergistic effects at the chloride ion site and resultant membrane hyperpolarization. In an extensive review by Greenblatt et al. (1977), no patient who took an overdose of benzodiazepines alone became seriously ill or had serious complications. When the overdose occurred in combination with other drugs, however, the complications depended on the type and quantity of the nonbenzodiazepines.

Finkle et al. (1979) essentially confirmed these results by finding that in only 2 of 1,239 overdoses with benzodiazepines were the deaths associated with the benzodiazepine alone.

A safe and effective benzodiazepine antagonist, flumazenil, exists that may be used via intravenous injection in an emergency setting to reverse the effects of any potential overdose with a benzodiazepine (Votey et al. 1991). However, medical management of a patient who has had an overdose often still requires physical supportive measures, such as ensuring proper respiratory function.

Drug interactions. Most sedative drugs, including narcotics and alcohol, potentiate the sedative effects of benzodiazepines. In addition, medications that inhibit hepatic CYP3A3/4, as discussed later in this chapter, increase blood levels and hence side effects of clonazepam, alprazolam, midazolam, and triazolam. Lorazepam, oxazepam, and temazepam are not dependent on hepatic enzymes for metabolism and therefore are not affected by hepatic disease or the inhibition of hepatic enzymes.

Use in pregnancy. Anxiolytics, like most medications, should be avoided during pregnancy and breast-feeding when possible. Although there have been concerns that benzodiazepines, when ingested during the first trimester of pregnancy, may increase the risk of the development of cleft palate, this has not been substantiated in controlled studies (Rosenberg et al. 1983; Shiono and Mills 1983).

Buspirone

The azapirones are agonists at the 5-HT$_{1A}$ receptors. Unlike benzodiazepines and barbiturates, they do not interact with the GABA receptor or directly with chloride ion channels. As such, these medications do not produce sedation, interact with alcohol, impair psychomotor performance, or pose a risk of abuse. There is no cross-tolerance between benzodiazepines and azapirones. As such, it is important to bear in mind that these classes of medication are not interchangeable. Like the antidepressants, azapirones have a relatively slow onset of action. Buspirone is the only azapirone currently available in the United States.

Mechanism of Action

The anxiolytic effect of the azapirones is the result of a selective stimulation of the 5-HT$_{1A}$ receptor. Acute administration suppresses neuronal firing in the dorsal raphe through autoreceptor stimulation. Chronic administration desensitizes presynaptic, but not postsynaptic, 5-HT$_{1A}$ receptors (Suranyi-Cadotte et al. 1990).

Indications and Efficacy

Buspirone is effective in the treatment of generalized anxiety. Although it has a longer onset of action, its efficacy is not statistically different from that of the benzodiazepines (Cohn and Wilcox 1986; H.L. Goldberg and Finnerty 1979). Despite its successes in the treatment of generalized anxiety disorder, buspirone does not appear to be effective in the treatment of panic disorder (Sheehan et al. 1990), except perhaps in an auxiliary role for the treatment of anticipatory anxiety (Gastfried and Rosenbaum 1989). Buspirone is also used as an augmenting agent in the treatment of OCD (Harvey and Balon 1995; Laird 1996) and depression (Rickels et al. 1988; Sramek et al. 1996), and some evidence suggests that buspirone may be an effective treatment for social phobia (Munjack et al. 1991; Schneier et al. 1992).

Buspirone is available for oral administration in a variety of dosage forms, including the 15-mg and 30-mg "dividose" tablets. These tablets are scored for division into bisections or trisections. We recommend an initial dosage of 7.5 mg twice a day, increased after 1 week to 15 mg twice a day. The dosage may then be increased as needed to achieve optimal therapeutic response. The usual recommended maximum daily dosage is 60 mg, but many patients safely tolerate and benefit from 90 mg/day. Because buspirone is metabolized by the liver and excreted by the kidneys, it should not be administered to patients with severe hepatic or renal impairment. Buspirone is metabolized by CYP3A3/4. Therefore, the initial dose should be lower in patients who are also taking medications that are known to inhibit this enzyme system, such as nefazodone.

Side Effects

The side effects that are more common with buspirone than with the benzodiazepines are nausea, headache, nervousness, insomnia, dizziness, and light-headedness (Rakel 1990). Restlessness also has been reported, which theoretically may be related to the activity of this drug at the dopamine receptor. Buspirone does not appear to interact with alcohol or other CNS depressants to increase sedation and motor impairment (Moskowitz and Smiley 1982). When administered to subjects who had histories of recreational sedative abuse, buspirone showed no abuse potential (Cole et al. 1982), a finding confirmed by subsequent studies (Sellers et al. 1992). As mentioned previously, buspirone is not sedating and does not impair mechanical performance, such as driving (Moskowitz and Smiley 1982). However, because the side effects in any individual patient cannot be predicted, these activities should be avoided during the initial stages of buspirone therapy.

Drug Interactions

Buspirone should not be administered in combination with an MAOI.

Overdose

No fatal outcomes of buspirone overdose have been reported. However, overdose of buspirone with other drugs may result in more serious outcomes.

Zolpidem and Zaleplon

Zolpidem (Ambien) and Zaleplon (Sonata) are hypnotic medications that act at the omega-1 subtype of the central benzodiazepine receptor. This selectivity is hypothesized to be associated with a lower risk of dependence. Unlike the benzodiazepines, zolpidem and zaleplon do not appear to have significant anxiolytic, muscle relaxant, or anticonvulsant properties. However, amnestic effects may occur.

Indications

Zolpidem is a short-acting hypnotic agent with established efficacy in inducing and maintaining sleep. Because of the short half-life of this medication, most patients report minimal daytime sedation. Zaleplon is an ultra-short-acting hypnotic, which allows this agent to be administered in the middle of the night with minimal residual sedative effects after 4 hours.

Clinical Use

Both zolpidem and zaleplon are available in 5- and 10-mg tablets for oral administration. The maximum recommended dosage for adults is 10 mg/day, administered at night. The initial dosage for elderly individuals should not exceed 5 mg/day. Caution is advised when using these agents in patients with hepatic dysfunction. In general, hypnotics should be limited to short-term use, with subsequent reevaluation for more extended therapy (see discussion of the treatment of insomnia later in this chapter).

TABLE 18–9. Comparison of benzodiazepines, buspirone, and selective serotonin reuptake inhibitors (SSRIs)

Characteristic	Benzodiazepines	Buspirone	SSRIs
Therapeutic effect of single dose	Yes	No	No
Time to full therapeutic action	Days	Weeks	Weeks
Sedation	Yes	No	Unlikely
Dependence liability	Yes	No	No
Impairs performance	Yes	No	No
Suppresses sedative withdrawal symptoms	Yes	No	No
Once-a-day dosing	No	No	Yes
Treats comorbid depression	No	No	Yes
Side effects	Sedation, memory impairment	Dizziness	Gastrointestinal, sexual dysfunction

Risks, Side Effects, and Their Management

In general, the side effects of zolpidem and zaleplon are similar to those of the short-acting benzodiazepines. These agents should not be considered free of abuse potential.

Overdose

Both zolpidem and zaleplon appear to be nonfatal in overdose. However, overdoses in combination with other CNS-depressant agents pose a greater risk. Recommended treatment consists of general symptomatic and supportive measures including gastric lavage. Use of flumazenil may be helpful.

Drug Interactions

Research on drug interactions is limited for these agents, but any drug with CNS-depressant effects could potentially enhance the CNS-depressant effects of zolpidem and zaleplon via pharmacodynamic interactions. In addition, zolpidem is primarily metabolized by cytochrome P450 3A3/4 and zaleplon is partially metabolized by 3A3/4. As such, inhibitors of

this enzyme may increase zolpidem blood levels and toxicity.

Pharmacotherapy for Generalized Anxiety Disorder

Generalized anxiety disorder can be treated with benzodiazepines, buspirone, and certain of the antidepressants (e.g., venlafaxine). Some of these agents are compared in Table 18–9.

Benzodiazepines have the advantage of being rapidly effective and the obvious disadvantages of abuse potential and sedation. Although benzodiazepines are indicated for relatively short-term use only (i.e., 1–2 months), they are, in general, safe and effective for long-term use for the minority of patients who require such medication (Greenblatt et al. 1983; Rickels et al. 1983). Whereas tolerance to sedation often develops, the same is not true of the anxiolytic effects of these agents.

All benzodiazepines indicated for the treatment of anxiety are equally efficacious. The choice of a specific agent usually depends on the pharmacokinetics and pharmacodynamics of the drug. Some patients respond to extremely low dosages, such as 0.125 mg of alprazolam twice a day, although mean dosages are higher. When using benzodiazepines to treat anxiety, we advocate starting with 0.25 mg of alprazolam two or three times a day or an equivalent dosage of another benzodiazepine (Table 18–8) and then titrating according to anxiolysis versus sedation. Benzodiazepines should be avoided in patients with a history of recent and/or significant substance abuse, and all patients should be advised to take their first dose at home in a situation that would not be dangerous in the event of greater than expected sedation.

Buspirone does not cause the sedative or abuse problems of the benzodiazepines, although some clinicians have observed that its anxiolytic properties do not appear to be as potent as those of the benzodiazepines, particularly in patients who have previously received a benzodiazepine (Schweizer et al. 1986). Because buspirone is not sedating (Seidel et al. 1985) and has no psychomotor effects, it has a distinct advantage over the benzodiazepines when optimal alertness and motor performance are necessary. Buspirone has been assessed in individuals with histories of recreational sedative abuse (Cole et al. 1982) and in recently detoxified alcoholic patients (Griffith et al. 1986); in these groups, it showed no abuse potential. Response to buspirone occurs within approximately 2–4 weeks. There is also evidence that the azapirones have modest antidepressant effects, perhaps at high doses (Jenkins et al. 1990; Lucki 1991).

Buspirone does not show cross-tolerance with benzodiazepines and other sedative-hypnotic drugs such as alcohol, barbiturates, and chloral hydrate. Therefore, buspirone does not suppress benzodiazepine withdrawal symptoms (Lader and Olajide 1987). For patients with anxiety who are taking a benzodiazepine and require a switch to buspirone, the benzodiazepine must be tapered gradually to avoid withdrawal symptoms, despite the fact that the patient is receiving buspirone.

Patients with generalized anxiety disorder also respond to antidepressant treatment (Hoehn-Saric et al. 1988; Kahn et al. 1986). In studies comparing benzodiazepines, MAOIs, SSRIs, and TCAs in the treatment of concurrent anxiety and depression, all had some measure of success depending on the degree of depression and the type of anxiety disorder (Keller and Hanks 1995).

The duration of pharmacotherapy for generalized anxiety disorder is controversial. Psychotherapy is recommended for most patients with this disorder, and it may facilitate the tapering of medication. However, generalized anxiety is often a chronic condition, and some patients require long-term pharmacotherapy. As in other anxiety disorders, the need for ongoing treatment should be reassessed every 6–12 months.

Pharmacotherapy for Panic Disorder

Benzodiazepines, TCAs, MAOIs, and SSRIs are all effective in the treatment of panic disorder. Among the benzodiazepines, the higher-potency agents alprazolam and clonazepam are preferred because they are well tolerated in the higher dose ranges often required to treat panic disorder (Spier et al. 1986; Tesar 1990). Clonazepam has the advantage of a longer elimination half-life, which provides more stable plasma drug levels and allows twice-a-day dosing, whereas the shorter half-life of alprazolam is better suited for acute dosage titration. For the treatment of panic disorder, clonazepam is started at 0.5 mg taken twice a day and is increased to a total of 1–2 mg/day in two divided doses. Higher dosage levels may be necessary for complete relief of symptoms. The starting dosage of alprazolam is usually 0.25 or 0.5 mg taken three times a day (Tesar 1990).

Because long-term exposure to high-dose benzodiazepines may place some patients at risk for physical and/or psychological dependence, we recommend the use of antidepressants for the treatment of panic disorder. Many antidepressants have been shown to be effective in this setting, including TCAs (Klein et al. 1987; Zitrin et al. 1983), MAOIs (Sheehan et al. 1980; van Vliet et al. 1993), and SSRIs (den Boer et al. 1995; Oehrberg et al. 1995; Schneier et al. 1990; Westenberg and den Boer 1988). For most patients, the SSRIs should be considered first-line agents. The choice should be based on the same factors discussed in the section on antidepressant drugs. MAOIs usually are reserved for patients who have not responded to SSRIs and TCAs. A major caveat is that patients with panic disorder initially may be highly sensitive to the stimulant effects of small doses of antidepressants. For highly anxious patients with panic disorder, we often initiate treatment with clonazepam or alprazolam and add a low-dose antidepressant, which is then increased slowly. The rapid onset of action of the benzodiazepine is helpful to the patient until the antidepressant becomes effective. When panic symptoms have not been present for several weeks, the benzodiazepine is slowly tapered. In patients with marked residual anticipatory anxiety, longer-term use of a benzodiazepine or buspirone should be considered as an adjunct to the antidepressant. Although some patients respond to lower doses, standard to high-standard antidepressant doses generally are used for the treatment of panic disorder.

For most patients, pharmacotherapy in conjunction with time-limited cognitive-behavioral therapy is highly effective in reducing panic attacks but possibly less

effective in attenuating avoidance behavior. Unfortunately, there are no guidelines for the duration of pharmacotherapy. We recommend attempting to taper medication every 6–12 months if the patient has been relatively symptom-free. However, many patients require longer-term pharmacotherapy.

Pharmacotherapy for Social Phobia

Social phobia responds to a variety of medications, including SSRIs (Black et al. 1992; den Boer et al. 1995; Van Ameringen et al. 1993; Westenberg and den Boer 1993), MAOIs (Liebowitz et al. 1988; Marshall et al. 1994), benzodiazepines (Davidson et al. 1991; Gelernter et al. 1991; Jefferson 1995), and buspirone (Munjack et al. 1991; Schneier et al. 1992). TCAs, although highly effective in the treatment of panic disorder, appear to be ineffective for most patients with social phobia. Similarly, β-blockers, although effective in treating performance anxiety, are not effective in treating generalized social phobia (Jefferson 1995).

The risks and side effects of the SSRIs, MAOIs, and benzodiazepines are discussed extensively elsewhere in the chapter. Dosages for the treatment of social phobia are similar to dosages of these medications for other disorders.

Pharmacotherapy for Performance Anxiety

Several studies have shown the efficacy of β-blockers in the treatment of performance anxiety. Taken within 2 hours of the stressor, propranolol, in doses ranging from 20 to 80 mg, may improve performance on examinations (Drew et al. 1985), in public speaking (Hertley et al. 1983), and in musical performances (Brantigan et al. 1982). A trial dose of 40 mg of propranolol (e.g., during a vacation day) should be administered before the specific performance situation in which the patient anticipates anxiety. This initial dose should not be taken in a high-risk or critical situation in which any unexpected side effect could result in serious consequences. Subsequently, doses of propranolol should be administered approximately 2 hours before the situation in which disabling performance anxiety is expected. The dose may be increased gradually by 20-mg increments during successive performances until adequate relief of performance distress is achieved (Yudofsky and Silver 1987).

Pharmacotherapy for Obsessive-Compulsive Disorder

The discovery of the SSRIs brought about a revolution in the treatment of OCD. Currently, clomipramine and the SSRIs provide the foundation of pharmacological treatment of OCD. In contrast to the experience of patients treated with pharmacotherapy for many other Axis I disorders, most patients with OCD experience only a 35%–60% improvement in symptoms (Jenike 1990). In addition, medication responses may not be apparent until treatment has been given for 10 weeks. Cognitive-behavioral therapy should be combined with pharmacological approaches.

Before initiating clomipramine treatment, the clinician must heed all the precautions associated with the use of any TCA (see discussion of TCAs earlier in this chapter). Initial dosing and titration of clomipramine also must follow the guidelines for TCAs, with the additional caveat that 250 mg is the maximum recommended dosage because there is an increased risk of seizures above this level. Plasma levels are available but are only weakly correlated with therapeutic effect (Mavissakalian et al. 1990). Most patients

with OCD respond to dosages of clomipramine between 150 and 200 mg/day. Because side effects associated with the anticholinergic, antihistaminic, and α_2-adrenergic actions of clomipramine may occur, patients must be monitored for and made aware of the potential for symptoms such as constipation, dry mouth, urinary hesitancy, sedation, and orthostatic hypotension.

As in the treatment of depression, the SSRIs tend to be better tolerated than the TCAs. Fluoxetine has been compared with clomipramine under double-blind conditions and found to have an approximately equivalent antiobsessional effect (Pigott et al. 1990). It has been suggested that an effective antiobsessional dosage of fluoxetine may be higher than its usual antidepressant dosage. Many clinicians seek to establish a daily dose of 60–80 mg in treating OCD. No systematic study of this issue has confirmed this common impression and widely used practice. In fact, a report by Wheadon (1991) found no greater antiobsessional effect of fluoxetine at 40 or 60 mg/day compared with 20 mg/day. Nonetheless, on the basis of the current knowledge of the treatment of OCD, a trial of fluoxetine should not be considered complete until the patient has failed to respond to 80 mg/day after 8 weeks (Jenike 1990).

The other SSRIs are also effective treatments for OCD. Therapeutic dosages of fluvoxamine range from 100 to 300 mg/day in divided doses (Freeman et al. 1994; W.K. Goodman et al. 1990, 1996; Perse et al. 1988). The recommended dosage range for paroxetine in the treatment of OCD is 40–60 mg/day. In a double-blind comparison of three dosages of sertraline (50, 100, and 200 mg/day) and placebo in patients with OCD, all three sertraline groups showed significantly greater improvement than the placebo group after 12 weeks (Greist et al. 1995a).

Several augmentation strategies have been suggested for OCD, none with uniformly positive results in controlled trials but with possible effectiveness in selected patients. OCD augmentation strategies include use of fenfluramine (Hollander et al. 1990), lithium (Feder 1988), antipsychotics (McDougle et al. 1990, 1995), clonazepam (Hewlett et al. 1990), and buspirone (Jenike et al. 1991; Markovitz et al. 1990), typically added to a serotonergic antidepressant.

As in the other anxiety disorders, relatively few data are available to address longer-term treatment of OCD. OCD is often a lifelong disorder with a waxing and waning course, for which many patients require prolonged pharmacotherapy.

Pharmacotherapy for Insomnia

Although the benzodiazepines, zolpidem, and zaleplon are the mainstay of pharmacotherapy for insomnia, other sedating drugs, such as trazodone or chloral hydrate, also may be used. As discussed previously, insomnia should first be addressed diagnostically, and in most cases nonpharmacological interventions should be tried before treatment with a hypnotic is instituted. Hypnotic agents should be administered in the lowest effective dose. Medications commonly prescribed to treat insomnia, their recommended dosages, time of onset, and half-lives are shown in Table 18–10.

Pharmacotherapy for Alcohol Withdrawal

A relatively simple procedure for treating alcohol withdrawal is the benzodiazepine loading dose technique (Sellers et al. 1983). This technique takes advantage of the long half-lives of benzodiazepines such as diazepam and chlordiazepoxide. Doses of 20 mg of diazepam (or 100 mg of chlordiazepoxide) are administered hourly to patients until they have no signs or symptoms of alcohol withdrawal. This state is usually accompanied by mild to moderate sedation. Thereafter, no further doses of benzodiazepine are administered. Because of the long half-life of diazepam and other long-acting benzodiazepines, the therapeutic plasma level of the benzodiazepine is maintained during the period of risk for alcohol withdrawal symptoms. Sullivan and Sellers (1986) recommended that healthy patients receive at least 60 mg of diazepam or 300 mg of chlordiazepoxide in the initial loading dose regimen. This technique has advantages over the method of repeat dosing with benzodiazepines in that the accumulation of benzodiazepines may lead to prolonged sedation and the development of benzodiazepine dependence in a population at high risk for chemical dependence.

Antipsychotic Drugs

Antipsychotic medications, previously referred to as *major tranquilizers* or *neuroleptics*, are effective for the treatment of a variety of psychotic symptoms, such as hallucinations, delusions, and thought disorders, regardless of etiology (other indications are discussed later). The term *major tranquilizer* is a misnomer because sedation is generally a side effect, not the principal treatment effect. Similarly, the term *neuroleptic* is based on the neurological side effects characteristic of the older antipsychotic drugs, such as catalepsy in animals and EPS in humans.

Antipsychotic drugs can be classified in several ways. One classification is based on chemical structure; for example, phenothiazines and butyrophenones constitute two chemical classes. We use the term *conventional* to signify the older antipsychotic drugs, to differentiate them from the newer, *atypical* or "second

TABLE 18–10. Medications commonly prescribed to treat insomnia

Medication (trade name)	Usual adult therapeutic dosage (mg/day)[a]	Time until onset of action (minutes)	Half-life (including metabolites; hours)
Clonazepam (Klonopin)[b]	0.5–2	20–60	19–60
Clorazepate (Tranxene)	3.75–15	30–60	48–96
Estazolam (ProSom)	1–2	15–30	8–24
Lorazepam (Ativan)[b]	1–4	30–60	8–24
Oxazepam (Serax)	15–30	30–60	2.8–5.7
Quazepam (Doral)	7.5–15	20–45	39–120
Temazepam (Restoril)	15–30	45–60	3–25
Triazolam (Halcion)	0.125–0.25	15–30	1.5–5
Chloral hydrate[c]	500–2,000	30–60	4–8
Trazodone (Desyrel)[b,c]	50–150	30–60	5–9
Zaleplon (Sonata)[c]	5–10	30	1.0
Zolpidem (Ambien)[c]	5–10	30	1.5–4.5

[a]Consider lower dosages in the elderly.
[b]Use of this drug as a hypnotic agent is not an indication approved by the Food and Drug Administration.
[c]These drugs are not benzodiazepines.
Source.   Data from Kupfer and Reynolds 1997 and *Physicians' Desk Reference* 2001.

generation" antipsychotics. All conventional antipsychotics are equally effective when given in equivalent doses (Table 18–11). Among the conventional antipsychotics, we commonly distinguish between high- and low-potency agents; as we discuss later, this characteristic predicts side effects. Although the term *atypical antipsychotic* lacks a single consistent definition, it generally implies fewer EPS and superior efficacy, particularly for the negative symptoms of schizophrenia. Atypical antipsychotics are also less likely to produce hyperprolactinemia. Currently, the atypical antipsychotics include clozapine, risperidone, olanzapine, quetiapine, and ziprasidone.

The favorable efficacy and neurological side-effect profiles of atypical antipsychotics have led some authorities to recommend that they be used uniformly as first-line agents, with the exception of clozapine, which is restricted in its use because of the risk of agranulocytosis (Lieberman 1996). The therapeutic advantages of atypical antipsychotics over conventional agents may be greater in first-episode patients than in chronically ill patients, further arguing against second-line status (Sanger et al. 1999). On the other hand, atypical antipsychotics are markedly more expensive and may place some patients at risk for medical morbidity resulting from weight gain (particularly clozapine and olanzapine), hyperprolactinemia (risperidone), and cardiac conduction delay (ziprasidone). Whereas most pharmacoeconomic studies have indicated that increased costs of the atypical antipsychotics are offset by reduced rates of hospitalization, the long-term safety of these drugs remains to be fully characterized. Discussion of the properties common to most of the antipsychotic medications follows, with specific comments on each of the atypical antipsychotics at the end of this section.

Mechanisms of Action

For many years, the prevailing theory regarding the mechanism of action of antipsychotic drugs was based on the observation that all of the available antipsychotics antagonize D_2 dopamine receptors in vitro and that the relative affinities of the typical antipsychotic drugs for striatal D_2 receptors correlate with the dosage required to treat psychotic symptoms (Creese et al. 1976; Seeman et al. 1976). Yet the theory that psychosis results from hyperdopaminergia is overly simplistic. Underactivity of dopamine in mesocortical pathways, specifically those projecting to the frontal lobes, may account for the negative symptoms of schizophrenia (e.g., anergia, apathy, aspontaneity) (K. Davis et al. 1991; Goff and Evins 1998). At the same time, this underactivity in the frontal lobe may serve to disinhibit mesolimbic dopamine activity via a corticolimbic feedback loop (Pycock et al. 1980). An overactivity of mesolimbic dopamine is the result, manifested by the positive symptoms of schizophrenia (e.g., hallucinations, delusions; K. Davis et al. 1991). This revised dopamine hypothesis is concordant with the clinical observation that conventional antipsychotic drugs are more effective in treating positive symptoms than negative symptoms (Breier et al. 1987).

Antagonism of the 5-HT_2 receptor may modify dopamine activity in a regionally specific manner. When combined with conventional antipsychotics, 5-HT_2 blockade preserves firing of nigrostriatal (A9) dopamine neurons (Svensson et al. 1989; Ugedo et al. 1989). Early studies reported that the addition of 5-HT_2 antagonism to conventional antipsychotic agents decreased EPS in rats and improved negative symptoms in patients with schizophrenia (Duinkerke et al. 1993; Gelders 1989). This dual 5-HT_2/D_2 antagonism is believed to account, at

TABLE 18–11. Commonly used antipsychotic drugs

Generic (trade) name	Usual daily dosage (mg)	Methods of administration	Available oral doses (mg)	Approximate oral dose equivalents (mg)[a]
Conventional antipsychotics				
Phenothiazines				
Chlorpromazine (Thorazine)	300–600	po, L, im	10, 25, 50, 100, 200	100
Piperidines				
Thioridazine (Mellaril)	300–600	po, L	10, 15, 25, 50, 100, 150, 200	100
Mesoridazine (Serentil)	150–300	po, im	10, 25, 50, 100	50
Pimozide (Orap)	2–6	po	2	1–2
Piperazines				
Trifluoperazine (Stelazine)	15–30	po, im	1, 2, 5, 10	5
Fluphenazine (Prolixin)	5–15	po, L, im, D	1, 2.5, 5, 10	2
Perphenazine (Trilafon)	32–64	po, L, im	2, 4, 8, 16	10
Thioxanthenes				
Thiothixene (Navane)	15–30	po, L	1, 2, 5, 10	5
Butyrophenones				
Haloperidol (Haldol)	5–15	po, L, im, D	0.5, 1, 2, 5, 10, 20	2
Dibenzoxazepines				
Loxapine (Loxitane)	45–90	po, L	5, 10, 25, 50	15
Molindone (Moban)	30–60	po, L	5, 10, 25, 50, 100	10
Atypical antipsychotics				
Clozapine (Clozaril)	250–500	po	25, 100	50
Risperidone (Risperdal)	4–6	po, L	0.25, 0.5, 1, 2, 3, 4	1
Olanzapine (Zyprexa)	10–20	po	2.5, 5, 7.5, 10, 15, 20	2–3
Quetiapine (Seroquel)	300–600	po	25, 100, 200, 300	100
Ziprasidone (Geodon)	80–160	po, im	20, 40, 60, 80	
Aripiprazole (Abilify)	10–30	po	2, 5, 10, 15, 20, 30	

Note. D = long-acting decanoate preparation; im = short-acting intramuscular; L = liquid; po = oral tablets or capsules.
[a]Equivalent doses from American Psychiatric Association 1997.

least in part, for the superior efficacy and side-effect profile of the atypical antipsychotics (Meltzer et al. 1989), although this model has recently been challenged (Kapur and Seeman 2001). On the basis of this dual antagonism, atypical antipsychotics are often referred to as *serotonin–dopamine antagonists*.

Indications and Efficacy

The most common indications for the use of antipsychotic drugs are the treatment of acute psychosis and the maintenance of a remission of psychotic symptoms in patients with schizophrenia. Although all of the conventional antipsychotic agents have comparable efficacy, their side-effect profiles differ. Clozapine, risperidone, and olanzapine appear to be at least as effective as the older medications for the treatment of positive symptoms and more efficacious for the treatment of negative symptoms of schizophrenia; the other atypical agents are less well studied. Ziprasidone and quetiapine have shown antipsychotic efficacy comparable to that of conventional antipsychotic agents, but their comparative effects on negative symptoms remain to be clarified (Arvanitis and Miller 1997; Goff et al. 1998). Clozapine was effective in approximately 30% of patients who were nonresponsive to several trials of conventional antipsychotics (Kane 1996). Risperidone and olanzapine also may be advantageous for this difficult patient population; however, adequate controlled trials are lacking, and results are not fully consistent (Chakos et al. 2001).

Antipsychotic drugs are also effective in ameliorating psychotic symptoms that result from many diverse etiologies, such as mood disorders with psychotic features, drug toxicities, psychosis secondary to other brain disorders, and delusional disorders. Low dosages of antipsychotics

may be effective in some patients with borderline or schizotypal personality disorders, particularly when used to target psychotic ideation (Gunderson 1986). In the treatment of severe OCD, antipsychotics have been used to augment antiobsessional agents (McDougle et al. 1990). Antipsychotics and other drugs with dopamine receptor–blocking action (e.g., metoclopramide) are also used for their antiemetic effect. Gilles de la Tourette's syndrome may be controlled with antipsychotic agents; haloperidol and pimozide are the most frequently used drugs for this disorder.

The sedative side effect of antipsychotic medications may lead to the misuse of these drugs in several clinical situations. Antipsychotics frequently are improperly prescribed as hypnotic or anxiolytic agents. In addition, antipsychotic drugs are administered to patients who are chronically agitated and violent. Because of the potential long-term risks of these medications (see subsection "Tardive Disorders" later in this section), antipsychotics are not recommended for the treatment of uncomplicated anxiety or insomnia.

Clinical Use

Medication Selection

The choice of antipsychotic medication is often determined, in large part, by the anticipated side effects. When appropriate, involvement of the patient and family members in this process can enhance the treatment alliance and minimize distress when side effects develop. In most circumstances, the atypical antipsychotics (except for clozapine) are best tolerated and are preferred as first-line agents. Head-to-head comparisons of atypical agents have been few, and findings of differential efficacy between agents generally have been inconsistent and contested

(Conley and Mahmoud 2001; Tran et al. 1997). Depot preparations of conventional antipsychotic medications continue to play an important clinical role in the absence of delayed-release formulations of atypical agents. Clozapine is generally reserved for refractory schizophrenia because of the risk of agranulocytosis.

A useful construct for conceptualizing differences in side-effect profiles for the conventional antipsychotics is the concept of "high potency" versus "low potency." Drug potency refers to the milligram equivalence of drugs, not to their relative efficacy. For example, although haloperidol is more potent than chlorpromazine (haloperidol 2 mg = chlorpromazine 100 mg), therapeutically equivalent doses are equally effective (haloperidol 12 mg = chlorpromazine 600 mg). Potency of the antipsychotic drugs has generally been determined in two ways: 1) by ascertaining dosages that are efficacious in clinical trials and clinical practice and 2) by comparing affinities of the drug for the D_2 receptor. Typically, the potency of antipsychotic drugs is rated in comparison with a standard 100-mg dose of chlorpromazine. As a rule, for conventional antipsychotics only, the high-potency antipsychotic drugs have an equivalent dose of less than 5 mg (see Table 18–11). These medications have a high degree of EPS but less sedation, fewer anticholinergic side effects, and less hypotension. Low-potency conventional antipsychotic drugs have an equivalent dose of greater than 40 mg. These drugs have a high level of sedation, anticholinergic side effects, and hypotension but a lower degree of acute EPS. Rates of tardive dyskinesia do not differ between high- and low-potency conventional antipsychotics. Antipsychotic drugs with intermediate potency (i.e., equivalent dose of between 5 and 40 mg) have a side-effect profile that lies between the profiles of these two groups. In most circumstances, high-potency drugs are preferred among the conventional antipsychotics because EPS usually can be minimized by using the lowest effective dosage or by symptomatic treatment, whereas anticholinergic and autonomic side effects are potentially more dangerous and difficult to manage. Intermediate-potency conventional antipsychotic drugs are sometimes useful for those patients who cannot tolerate either high- or low-potency drugs.

The atypical antipsychotics produce fewer EPS than do even the low-potency conventional antipsychotics. Clozapine and quetiapine have the least EPS liability and so are recommended for the treatment of psychosis in patients with Parkinson's disease. Growing evidence suggests that the atypical antipsychotic agents are associated with substantially lower rates of tardive dyskinesia than are the conventional agents. With the notable exception of risperidone, the atypical antipsychotics produce substantially less hyperprolactinemia than do the conventional antipsychotics. Because of associated medical morbidity, as well as the potential effect on self-esteem and compliance, weight gain is also an important side effect associated to varying degrees with all atypical antipsychotic agents except ziprasidone. Concerns about cardiac conduction delay with ziprasidone require careful consideration, as do concerns about cataract formation with quetiapine. Cataracts have been linked to quetiapine in beagle dogs but not in humans or in nonhuman primates. Finally, sedation may be problematic with atypical agents, particularly with clozapine and quetiapine, and the risk of orthostatic hypotension necessitates early dose titration with clozapine, quetiapine, and risperidone.

Optimal Dosages

An optimal dosage or therapeutic range of blood levels has not been identified for most of the antipsychotics. Antipsychotic drugs, with the exception of clozapine, have a high therapeutic index, and they can be administered at dosages substantially above the optimal therapeutic dosage without immediate and obvious adverse events. However, carefully controlled studies have confirmed that more modest dosages of conventional antipsychotic drugs have equal efficacy and are better tolerated. Several reviews of controlled trials of conventional antipsychotics concluded that the optimal dosage for most patients is between 300 and 600 mg/day of chlorpromazine equivalents, with some patients responding to lower dosages and with little benefit at dosages greater than 700 mg/day (Appleton and Davis 1980; Baldessarini et al. 1988; J.M. Davis 1985).

In the initial stages of treatment with antipsychotic medication, sedation may predominate over the specific antipsychotic effects. Many psychiatrists incorrectly believe that if a patient's psychosis does not rapidly resolve with the use of antipsychotic medication, higher dosages are necessary. In fact, as in antidepressant therapy, reversal of psychosis is often gradual and may occur over the course of several weeks to several months. Usual dosages for each of the commonly used antipsychotic medications are summarized in Table 18–11.

Long-Acting Injectable Antipsychotics

For patients with chronic psychotic symptoms who do not comply with a daily medication regimen, clinicians should consider a long-acting depot preparation after stabilization with oral medication. Fluphenazine decanoate and haloperidol decanoate are the only long-acting injectable antipsychotics currently available in the United States.

Conversion to a decanoate preparation is complicated by the highly variable individual pharmacokinetics of the oral and long-term depot agents. Most patients respond to a fluphenazine decanoate dosage of between 10 and 30 mg every 2 weeks (Baldessarini et al. 1988). A loading-dose strategy has been established for haloperidol decanoate, in which patients receive an initial dose that is 20 times the oral maintenance dosage (Ereshefsky et al. 1993). The maximum volume per injection of haloperidol decanoate should not exceed 3 cc, and the maximum dose per injection should not exceed 100 mg. If 20 times the oral dose is greater than 100 mg, the dose is given in divided injections spaced 3–7 days apart. Subsequent medication doses are decreased monthly to about 10 times the oral dose by the third or fourth month. Ten times the oral dose, administered every 4 weeks, is a typical maintenance dose with haloperidol decanoate. For patients who are elderly or debilitated, the initial dose is 10–15 times the previous oral daily dosage. Many clinicians prefer to continue oral medication at approximately half the previous maintenance dose during the first few months of depot neuroleptic administration rather than administer a loading dose of depot medication. This approach allows greater flexibility of initial dose titration. In either approach, breakthrough psychotic symptoms are treated with supplemental oral medication, and the dose of the next scheduled depot injection can be increased accordingly. Steady-state serum concentrations are achieved after approximately 10 weeks (five injection intervals) with fluphenazine decanoate and after approximately 20 weeks with haloperidol decanoate. It should be noted that side effects may take months to subside, and withdrawal dyskinesia may not appear for months after discontinuation of the decanoate formulation.

Risks, Side Effects, and Their Management

Many of the side effects of antipsychotic drugs can be understood on the basis of their receptor-blocking properties. When antipsychotics reduce dopamine activity in the nigrostriatum (via dopamine receptor blockade), extrapyramidal signs and symptoms result, similar to those of Parkinson's disease. Another locus of dopamine receptors resides in the pituitary and hypothalamus (the tuberoinfundibular system), where dopamine is synonymous with prolactin-inhibiting factor. Blockade of dopamine in this system results in hyperprolactinemia. Similarly, antagonism of acetylcholine receptors produces symptoms such as dry mouth, blurred vision, and constipation. Antagonism of α_1-adrenergic receptors results in hypotension, and antagonism of histamine receptors is associated with sedation.

Extrapyramidal Effects

Extrapyramidal symptoms include acute dystonic reactions, parkinsonian syndrome, akathisia, neuroleptic malignant syndrome (NMS), and tardive dyskinesia. Although high-potency antipsychotics are more likely to produce extrapyramidal symptoms, all conventional antipsychotic drugs are equally likely to produce tardive dyskinesia. The atypical antipsychotics produce substantially fewer EPS, although careful titration of risperidone is necessary to avoid neurological side effects. Although use of anticholinergic agents or amantadine may prevent or ameliorate most occurrences of EPS, use of atypical agents is increasingly recommended to avoid these side effects without introducing additional medications. Long-term use of anticholinergics should be minimized because these agents can produce significant side effects, including impairments

of memory and attention. Clozapine appears to be the only agent that does not cause tardive dyskinesia, although preliminary data suggest a reduced risk with olanzapine and risperidone (Jeste et al. 1999; Tollefson et al. 1997); relative tardive dyskinesia rates with quetiapine and ziprasidone have not been reported.

Acute dystonic reactions are among the most disturbing and acutely disabling adverse drug reactions that can occur with the administration of antipsychotic drugs. This reaction most frequently occurs within hours or days of the initiation of a high-potency conventional antipsychotic medication. The uncontrollable tightening of muscles typically involves spasms of the neck, back (opisthotonos), tongue, or muscles that control lateral eye movement (oculogyric crisis). Laryngeal involvement may compromise the airway and result in ventilatory difficulties (stridor). These reactions are often terrifying to the patient and may seriously jeopardize compliance with medications. Intravenous or intramuscular administration of anticholinergic medication is a rapid and effective treatment of acute dystonia. The drugs and dosages used to treat dystonic reactions are listed in Table 18–12. The anticholinergic drug given to reverse the dystonia will wear off after several hours. Because antipsychotic drugs have long half-lives and durations of action, additional oral anticholinergic drugs should be prescribed for several days after an acute dystonic reaction or longer if the antipsychotic drug is continued unchanged. Amantadine should be considered for treatment of EPS in elderly patients who are highly sensitive to anticholinergic activity, particularly if a switch to an atypical agent is not appropriate.

Acute dystonic reactions may be treated prophylactically with anticholinergic medications; for example, benztropine 1–2 mg twice a day may be initi-

TABLE 18–12. Drugs commonly used for the treatment of acute extrapyramidal side effects

Generic (trade) name	Mechanism	Usual dosage	Indications
Benztropine (Cogentin)	Anticholinergic	1–2 mg po bid	D, P
		2 mg iv[a]	Acute dystonia
Diphenhydramine (Benadryl)	Anticholinergic	25–50 mg po tid	D, P
		25 mg im/iv[a]	Acute dystonia
Trihexyphenidyl (Artane)	Anticholinergic	5–10 mg po bid	D, P
Amantadine (Symmetrel)	Dopaminergic	100 mg po bid	P
Propranolol (Inderal)	β-Blocker	20 mg po tid	A
		1 mg iv	

Note. A = akathisia; D = dystonia; im = intramuscularly; iv = intravenously; P = parkinsonian syndrome.
[a]Follow with po medication.

ated at the same time as the antipsychotic agent haloperidol (Goff et al. 1991). Young patients taking high-potency antipsychotic drugs are at particularly high risk for the development of acute dystonia. We suggest that prophylactic treatment be considered for patients for whom the risk of developing extrapyramidal reactions is high, especially patients younger than 40 years starting high-potency conventional agents (Arana et al. 1988). Anticholinergic medication can be tapered and stopped after 10 days.

Parkinsonian syndrome (or pseudoparkinsonism) has many of the features of classic idiopathic Parkinson's disease: diminished range of facial expression (masked facies), cogwheel rigidity, slowed movements (bradykinesia), drooling, small handwriting (micrographia), and pill-rolling tremor. As in Parkinson's disease, the pathophysiology involves disproportionally less dopamine than acetylcholine in the basal ganglia. The onset of this side effect is gradual, and it may not appear for weeks after antipsychotics have been administered. The most common treatments for idiopathic Parkinson's disease restore the dopamine:acetylcholine balance by increasing dopamine. Because dopamine antagonism is putatively involved

in the therapeutic effects of antipsychotics, treatment of parkinsonism most often involves decreasing the level of acetylcholine (although amantadine, a dopaminergic drug, often effectively attenuates parkinsonian side effects without exacerbating the underlying psychotic illness). Drugs used in the treatment of the parkinsonian side effects of antipsychotic agents are listed in Table 18–12.

Tardive Disorders

Tardive dyskinesia is a disorder characterized by involuntary choreoathetoid movements of the face, trunk, or extremities. The syndrome is usually associated with prolonged exposure to dopamine receptor–blocking agents, most frequently, antipsychotic drugs. However, the antidepressant amoxapine and the antiemetic agents metoclopramide and prochlorperazine can also cause tardive dyskinesia. Spontaneous dyskinesias also occur relatively frequently in nonmedicated elderly. The American Psychiatric Association (APA) Task Force on Tardive Dyskinesia estimated a cumulative incidence of 5% per year of exposure among young adults and a prevalence of 30% after 1 year of treatment among elderly patients (American Psychiatric Association 1992). Clozapine seems to carry little or no risk of inducing tardive dyskinesia. The incidence of tardive dyskinesia in association with the other atypical antipsychotics has not yet been adequately determined. Preliminary evidence suggests a level of risk for olanzapine and risperidone between the conventional antipsychotics and clozapine (Jeste et al. 1999; Tollefson et al. 1997).

An evaluation for abnormal movements should be conducted before treatment begins and every 6 or 12 months thereafter. In typical cases, the patient often is not aware of mild involuntary movements. Less common are severe dyskinetic movements, which can be disfiguring or even disabling as a result of involvement of speech or swallowing. Although the most common form of tardive disorder is the dyskinetic variety (nonrhythmic, quick, choreiform movements), other types have been identified. These include tardive akathisia, tardive dystonia, and tardive tics (Fahn 1985).

The most significant and consistently documented risk factor for the development of tardive dyskinesia is increasing age of the patient (Branchey and Branchey 1984; Jeste and Wyatt 1982; Kane and Smith 1982). The duration of exposure to a conventional antipsychotic is also an important factor, as the cumulative incidence has been shown to remain constant at about 5% for the first 8 years in nonelderly patients. Women have been found to be at a greater risk for severe tardive dyskinesia, although the evidence suggests that this finding is limited to geriatric populations (Kennedy et al. 1971; Seide and Muller 1967). Other risk factors may include EPS early in the course of treatment, a history of drug holidays (a greater number of drug-free periods is associated with an increased risk), the presence of brain damage, diabetes mellitus, and a diagnosis of mood disorder.

Because antipsychotic medications are the most effective treatment for most patients with schizophrenia, the situation often arises in which a patient develops tardive dyskinesia but still requires the medication to function. If discontinuation of the antipsychotic drug is clinically possible, gradual improvement in tardive dyskinesia may occur, although involuntary movements often worsen initially with tapering of the antipsychotic, a phenomenon referred to as *withdrawal dyskinesia* (Glazer et al. 1984). Withdrawal dyskinesias also may appear when a patient is switched from a conventional agent to an atypical antipsychotic. Withdrawal dyskinesias typically resolve within 6 weeks; however, suppressed or latent tardive dyskinesia that has been suppressed by D_2 receptor blockade, once it appears, may not resolve. Conversely, movements may be masked temporarily by increasing the dosage of the antipsychotic medication, but the symptoms eventually reemerge, often in a more severe form. Anticholinergic drugs may reversibly worsen dyskinetic movements (Reunanen et al. 1982; Yassa 1985), whereas anticholinergic drugs in high doses may improve tardive dystonia (Burke et al. 1982; Fahn 1985).

No definitive treatment exists for tardive dyskinesia. In several small studies, α-tocopherol (vitamin E) was shown to be of some benefit, most often for patients who had tardive dyskinesia for less than 5 years (Adler et al. 1993; Akhtar et al. 1993; Dabiri et al. 1994; Egan et al. 1992; Elkashef et al. 1990; Lohr and Caligiuri 1996; Lohr et al. 1987), but no benefit was discerned with vitamin E in a recent Department of Veterans Affairs trial (Adler et al. 1998). Vitamin E is a relatively benign antioxidant that may protect neurons from the damaging effects of free radicals, which have been implicated in the etiology of tardive dyskinesia. The typical dosage of vitamin E is 1,600 IU/day. Despite inconsistent evidence for efficacy, prophylaxis with vitamin E has been recommended.

For patients with tardive dyskinesia who cannot discontinue their antipsychotic, a switch to an atypical agent may be prudent. In an open trial, Lieberman et al. (1991) reported a 50% or greater improvement in the severity of tardive dyskinesia among 43% of the patients switched from a conventional antipsychotic to clozapine. Severe tardive dyskinesia, and especially tardive dystonia, was most likely to respond. The efficacy of the other atypical antipsychotics has not been systematically evaluated in this regard, but it is reasonable to attempt to use these agents prior to a clozapine trial.

Neuroleptic Malignant Syndrome

In rare instances, patients taking antipsychotic medications may develop a potentially life-threatening disorder known as *NMS*. Although it occurs most frequently with the use of high-potency conventional antipsychotic drugs, this condition may accompany treatment with any antipsychotic agent, including the atypical antipsychotics. Patients with NMS typically have marked muscle rigidity, although this feature may be absent with the atypical antipsychotics. Other salient features include fever, autonomic instability, elevated white blood cell count (>15,000/mm^3), elevated creatinine phosphokinase (CPK) levels (>300 U/mL), and delirium. The elevated CPK is due to muscle breakdown, which can lead to myoglobinuria and acute renal failure.

In a large prospective study, Rosebush and Stewart (1989) found that NMS was associated most often with the initiation or increase of antipsychotic medication, and in every case the NMS occurred within 1 month of admission to a psychiatric unit. Episodes that occurred in patients taking stable dosages of antipsychotic medications were almost always associated with antecedent dehydration. Lithium use increases the risk appreciably, as does the presence of a mood disorder. Higher dosages, rapid escalation of dosage, and intramuscular injections of antipsychotics are all associated with the development of NMS (Keck et al. 1989). The keys to treatment after recognition of the syndrome are discontinuation of all medications, thorough medical evaluation, intravenous fluids, antipyretic agents, and cooling blankets. Dantrolene and bromocriptine have been reported in uncontrolled trials to improve symptoms of NMS, but their efficacy over supportive care has not been proved and is controversial (Rosebush et al. 1991). Rosebush et al. (1989) reviewed 20 cases of patients who developed NMS while taking conventional agents and found that delaying reinitiation of an antipsychotic by at least 2 weeks after resolution of symptoms was associated with a markedly decreased risk of relapse.

Bromocriptine is a centrally active dopamine agonist that has been used successfully in some cases of NMS (Guze and Baxter 1985). The symptoms of rigidity may respond rapidly, although the temperature elevation, blood pressure instability, and creatinine kinase level may normalize only after several days. This drug should be administered in an initial dosage of 1.25–2.5 mg twice a day, and it may be increased to 10 mg three times a day (Guze and Baxter 1985).

Dantrolene sodium, also used in the treatment of malignant hyperthermia (a rare reaction to anesthetic drugs), is a direct-acting muscle relaxant that may reduce the thermogenesis of NMS caused by the tonic contraction of skeletal muscles (Guze and Baxter 1985). The manufacturer's recommendation for administration of dantrolene for acute malignant hyperthermia is 1 mg/kg by rapid intravenous push. The drug should be continued until the symptoms are reversed or until a maximum dose of 10 mg/kg is given. The oral dosage of dantrolene after a malignant hyperthermic crisis is 4–8 mg/kg/day in four divided doses. This regimen should be continued until all symptoms resolve. The clinician should be aware that dantrolene has a significant potential for hepatotoxicity and thus should not be administered to patients with liver dysfunction.

Anticholinergic Side Effects

Anticholinergic effects include dry mouth, decreased sweating, decreased bronchial secretions, blurred vision (due to inhibition of accommodation), difficulty in urination, constipation, and tachycardia. Bethanechol chloride, a cholinergic drug that does not cross the blood–brain barrier, may effectively treat these side effects at a dosage of 25–50 mg three times a day; it may be required for the duration of therapy with the antipsychotic medication. Central side effects of anticholinergic drugs include impairment in concentration, attention, and memory, and these side effects must be differentiated from symptoms caused by the patient's psychosis.

Adrenergic Side Effects

Antipsychotics also block α-adrenergic receptors, which can result in orthostatic hypotension and dizziness. Orthostatic hypotension is quite commonly associated with low-potency conventional agents, and among the atypical agents, clozapine, risperidone, and ziprasidone require initial dose titration, particularly in the elderly, to avoid orthostatic hypotension. The administration of epinephrine, which stimulates both α- and β-adrenergic receptors, will result in a paradoxical drop in blood pressure as a result of the stimulation of β receptors in the presence of α-receptor blockade. In asthmatic patients who require treatment with antipsychotics as well as episodic treatment with α-adrenergic drugs, specific warnings are necessary regarding the dangers inherent in the use of epinephrine in the treatment of an acute asthmatic attack.

Endocrine and Sexual Side Effects

All the conventional antipsychotic medications and risperidone may produce hyperprolactinemia. Side effects mediated, at least in part, by hyperprolactinemia include gynecomastia, galactorrhea, amenorrhea, and decreased libido.

A combination of anticholinergic effects, α-adrenergic-receptor blockade, and hormonal effects may lead to several types of sexual difficulty. In men, inability to achieve or maintain erections, decreased ability to achieve orgasm, and changes in the pleasurable quality of orgasm have been reported with conventional agents (Ghadirian et al. 1982). Thioridazine may cause painful retrograde ejaculation, in which semen is ejected into the bladder (Shader 1964). Priapism, which necessitates immediate urological consultation, has been reported, especially with thioridazine and chlorpromazine (Mitchell and Popkin 1982), although atypical agents also have been linked to priapism (Deirmenjian et al. 1998; Emes and Millson 1994; Rosen and Hanno 1992). Women may experience changes in the quality of orgasm as well as decreased ability to achieve orgasm with use of antipsychotics.

Weight Gain

Many patients experience weight gain while taking antipsychotic medication. Allison et al. (1999) analyzed results from all published controlled trials of antipsychotic agents and estimated the mean weight change after 10 weeks of treatment for each agent. The effect of conventional antipsychotics ranged from a mean loss of 0.4 kg with molindone to a mean gain of 3.2 kg with thioridazine. Haloperidol produced a mean 1.1-kg weight gain. Among atypical agents, only ziprasidone produced no change in weight; the other atypical agents were associated with the following estimates of weight gain at 10 weeks: risperidone 2.1 kg, olanzapine 4.15 kg, and clozapine 4.45 kg. Insufficient data were available to calculate mean weight gain with quetiapine. Weight gain with atypical agents is quite variable; approximately 20% of the patients treated with olanzapine gain no weight, whereas morbid obesity can occur in about 10% of patients. Weight gain with olanzapine appears to plateau within the first 6 months and is not dose dependent.

Ocular Effects

Antipsychotics may cause pigmentary changes in the lens and retina, especially with long-term treatment. Pigment deposition in the lens of the eye does not affect vision; however, pigmentary retinopathy, which can lead to irreversible blindness, has been associated specifically with the use of thioridazine. Although pigmentary retinopathy has most often been reported with dosages above the recommended ceiling (i.e., 800 mg/day) of thioridazine, this condition also has occurred at usual clinical doses (Ball and Caroff 1986; J.D. Hamilton 1985). The clinician should be aware that drug interactions may increase plasma levels of thioridazine, which may increase the risk of development of this dangerous side effect (Silver et al. 1986).

Quetiapine was associated with cataracts in preclinical safety studies conducted in beagles. Subsequent studies performed in nonhuman primates did not detect an elevated risk of cataracts; postmarketing surveys have not detected an increased risk of cataracts with quetiapine compared with other antipsychotics. However, the incidence of cataracts is elevated in schizophrenia patients in general. Patients starting quetiapine should be informed of the potential risk of cataracts and the recommendation in the package insert that appropriate eye examinations be performed every 6 months. This precaution may be scientifically unsupported at present but remains an issue of liability.

Dermatological Effects

Patients taking antipsychotics, especially the aliphatic phenothiazines (e.g., chlorpromazine), may become more sensitive to sunlight, which can lead to severe sunburn. Especially in the summer months, patients should avoid excessive sun exposure and use ultraviolet-blocking agents such as sunscreens that contain fully protective levels of para-aminobenzoic acid (PABA).

Cardiac Effects

Several reports of sudden death have been attributed to thioridazine or chlorpromazine therapy in young, healthy patients (Aherwadker et al. 1964; Giles and Modlin 1968). Thioridazine slows atrial and ventricular conduction and prolongs refractory periods (Descotes et al. 1979; Hartigan-Go et al. 1996; Yoon et al. 1979). Because the effect is concentration dependent, thioridazine can be quite dangerous if taken in overdose or in combination with quinidine-like drugs (Risch et al. 1981). Chlorpromazine also prolongs QT intervals and atrioventricular conduction, even at relatively low dosages (150 mg/day) (Ban and St. Jean 1964). Pimozide also may produce significant changes in cardiac conduction as a result of its calcium channel blocking properties (Opler and Feinberg 1991). It is recommended that serial ECGs be performed when treatment with pimozide is started, and the drug should be stopped if the QT interval exceeds 520 msec in adults or 470 msec in children (Baldessarini 1985).

Hepatic Effects

Increased levels on liver function tests have been associated with antipsychotic treatment. This reaction appears to be more common with low-potency conventional antipsychotics. Transient elevations in hepatic enzymes have been observed with olanzapine and quetiapine, but these laboratory findings have not been linked to liver injury.

Hematological Effects

Transient leukopenia and, in rare cases, agranulocytosis have been associated with neuroleptic treatment (Balon and Berchou 1986). Although agranulocytosis is strictly defined as a complete absence of all granulocytes in the blood, it also may refer to severe neutropenia, with a neutrophil count of less than 500/mL. This is an idiosyncratic reaction that usually occurs within the first 3–4 weeks after the initiation of treatment with an antipsychotic drug. However, the period of risk for agranulocytosis and leukopenia continues for 2–3 months of treatment. A higher risk for agranulocytosis is associated with low-potency conventional antipsychotic drugs and, most significantly, clozapine (Balon and Berchou 1986). (For discussion of clozapine-induced agranulocytosis, see subsection on the side effects of clozapine later in the chapter.)

Signs and symptoms of this reaction include high fever, stomatitis, severe pharyngitis, lymphadenopathy, and malaise. Treatment of this reaction requires immediate discontinuation of all medications and immediate medical evaluation and treatment. Agranulocytosis usually resolves after discontinuation of the causative agent. There must be vigorous treatment of any infections that develop. Further treatment of psychosis must be with an agent of a completely different chemical class.

Effects on Seizure Threshold

The incidence of seizures with most antipsychotics is quite low (Devinsky et al. 1991). Of all the conventional antipsychotics, molindone and fluphenazine have most consistently been shown to have the lowest potential for this side effect (Itil and Soldatos 1980; Oliver et al. 1982). In a study of patients with epilepsy, the addition of psychotropic medication, including antipsychotics, was generally associated with improved seizure control (Ojemann et al. 1987). Clozapine is an exception among the antipsychotics because it dose-dependently lowers the seizure threshold and has been estimated to produce seizures in as many 10% of the patients receiving the drug for 3.8 years.

Effects on Temperature Regulation

Antipsychotic drugs directly affect the hypothalamus and suppress temperature regulation. In combination with the α-adrenergic receptor– and cholinergic receptor–blocking effects of antipsychotics, this effect becomes particularly serious in hot, humid weather. Severe hyperthermia, rhabdomyolysis, renal failure, and death may result. This potentially life-threatening condition requires immediate medical intervention and supportive treatment. It is mandatory that a cool environment and adequate amounts of fluids be provided for patients taking antipsychotic agents. Also, care must be taken that patients do not overexert themselves in warm weather or hot environments. Special monitoring is also required for acutely agitated or manic patients and for patients in restraints because they are prone to this dangerous condition.

Use in Pregnancy

As a general guideline, antipsychotic drugs should be used in pregnant patients only if absolutely necessary, at the minimal dose required, and for the briefest possible time. Documentation of informed consent from both the mother and the father is necessary. Use of ECT to treat acute psychosis in pregnant mothers should be considered.

Drug Interactions

Antipsychotic drugs have profound effects on multiple CNS receptors, and these effects are compounded when other medications are added. For example, the α-adrenergic-receptor blockade of antipsychotics may interfere with the efficacy of the antihypertensive drug guanethidine. The sedative and anticholinergic effects of antipsychotic drugs are increased with the addition of other sedating or anticholinergic drugs. As mentioned previously, patients taking drugs with potentially serious adverse effects (such as the risk of retinopathy with thioridazine) should be monitored through plasma level determinations when other medications are used concurrently.

Pharmacokinetic interactions with antipsychotic drugs are common and have been reviewed elsewhere (Goff and Baldessarini 1995). Most conventional antipsychotic agents are metabolized by the hepatic CYP2D6 isoenzyme. The activity of this enzyme varies greatly between individuals based on genetic polymorphisms and can be inhibited by certain drugs, such as SSRIs. For example, addition of fluoxetine raised haloperidol serum concentrations by 20% and fluphenazine concentrations by 65% in one study (Goff et al. 1995). Two categories of potential drug-drug interactions are of particular concern. The first includes interactions that can elevate clozapine serum concentra-tions to toxic levels. This has been described with addition of inhibitors of CYP3A4 and CYP1A2 isoenzymes, such as erythromycin and fluvoxamine (L.G. Cohen et al. 1996; Wetzel et al. 1998). The other category of potentially serious interactions includes those that induce metabolism of antipsychotic agents, thereby lowering serum concentrations below a therapeutic threshold. Large reductions in clozapine and haloperidol serum concentrations have been reported with the addition of carbamazepine, phenobarbital, and phenytoin (Arana et al. 1986; Byerly and DeVane 1996). Of note, cigarette smoking can affect antipsychotic metabolism; serum concentrations of clozapine in particular are reduced with smoking and increased after smoking cessation (Byerly and DeVane 1996; Haring et al. 1989).

Atypical Antipsychotic Drugs

Clozapine

Clozapine, a dibenzodiazepine, is the prototypical atypical antipsychotic. Because of the approximately 1% risk of producing a potentially fatal agranulocytosis, the use of clozapine is restricted to patients who have not responded to or cannot tolerate other antipsychotic drugs. Kane et al. (1988) studied patients with chronic schizophrenia who had failed to improve after at least three adequate trials of conventional antipsychotics. Data from this large, multicenter, double-blind prospective study indicated a significant improvement in 30% of the patients taking clozapine, compared with only 4% of those taking chlorpromazine. Clozapine produced significant improvement, compared with chlorpromazine, in positive and negative symptoms, as well as tension and hostility (Kane et al. 1988). Because clozapine appears to be devoid of parkinsonian side effects, it is also useful in low dosages (25 mg/day) for patients with Parkinson's disease and psychosis induced by dopamine agonists (Ostergaard and Dupont 1988). Other indications require higher dosages, as discussed later, and an extended period of titration to achieve therapeutic dosages and clinical response.

Clozapine is a difficult drug for both patient and physician, but when other treatments have failed, there is no doubt that the potential benefits of this remarkable medication are worth the risks for many patients with severe psychotic illnesses.

Mechanism of action. Clozapine shows high in vitro receptor affinities for the D_4, 5-HT$_2$, α_1-adrenergic, muscarinic, and histamine H_1 receptors, and a relatively weak affinity for D_1, D_2, and D_3 receptors (Brunello et al. 1995; Meltzer et al. 1989).

Clinical use. Because of prominent sedation and orthostatic hypotension, clozapine is initiated at a dosage of 12.5 mg/day and quickly increased to 12.5 mg twice a day. The dosage is then increased as tolerated, generally by 25- or 50-mg increments every day or every other day. Clozapine is usually added to the previous antipsychotic agent in a cross-titration in which the previous drug is tapered once a clozapine dosage of approximately 100 mg/day has been achieved. This strategy should be used with caution if the existing medication is a low-potency conventional antipsychotic because of additive α-adrenergic and anticholinergic side effects. Initiation of clozapine in an inpatient setting with monitoring of vital signs can be much more rapid than in an outpatient setting. The typical target dosage is 300–500 mg/day given in divided doses, with a greater amount given in the evening to minimize daytime sedation. Although routine blood level monitoring is not recommended, it should be noted that a serum level of greater than 350 ng/mL is associated with a higher response rate (Perry et al. 1991). Serum levels should be ascertained in nonresponders. The duration of treatment required to assess the medication response is longer than for most medications: typically, 3–6 months (Meltzer 1994). It is important that both the patient and the family understand this time frame before initiating treatment with clozapine. If patients are nonresponsive after 6 months of continuous clozapine treatment, the dosage may be gradually increased to a maximum of 900 mg/day. Not uncommonly, patients may not show a significant reduction in symptoms with clozapine, but review of their course over a 6-month or 1-year period indicates a dramatic reduction in rates of relapse and hospitalization.

Risks, side effects, and their management. *Agranulocytosis.* Agranulocytosis occurs in 0.8% of the patients taking clozapine during the first year of treatment, with a peak incidence at 3 months (Alvir and Lieberman 1994; Alvir et al. 1993). The dispensing of clozapine in the United States is linked to weekly white blood cell monitoring during the first 6 months, then biweekly thereafter. On the basis of the patient's white blood cell and absolute neutrophil count, strict guidelines have been set (Table 18–13). The system of white blood cell monitoring has successfully reduced fatalities from agranulocytosis to extremely low levels (Honigfeld et al. 1998).

If agranulocytosis develops, prompt consultation with a hematologist is indicated. Reverse isolation and prophylactic antibiotics may be used to prevent infection. Granulocyte-stimulating factors may be used to shorten the duration and reduce the morbidity of agranulocytosis (Barnas et al. 1992; Chengappa et al. 1996; Gerson et al. 1992; Nielsen 1993).

TABLE 18–13. Guidelines for hematological monitoring of patients taking clozapine

1. Initial white blood cell (WBC) count must be greater than 3,500/mm^3.
2. A weekly WBC count is required throughout treatment and for 4 weeks after discontinuation of clozapine.[a]
3. If WBC count is 2,000–3,000/mm^3 *or* granulocyte count is 1,000–1,500/mm^3, interrupt therapy and monitor for signs of infection. Check WBC count and differential daily. If there are no symptoms of infection, WBC count returns to greater than 3,000/mm^3, and granulocyte level is greater than 1,500/mm^3, resume clozapine with twice-weekly WBC and differential counts until the total WBC count returns to above 3,500/mm^3.
4. If WBC count is less than 2,000/mm^3 *or* granulocyte count is less than 1,000/mm^3, discontinue clozapine and do not rechallenge. Check WBC count and differential daily. Treat infection with antibiotics. Consider bone marrow aspiration to ascertain granulopoietic status. If granulopoiesis is deficient, consider protective isolation.

[a]Monitoring every 14 days has recently been recommended for patients who have been taking clozapine for 6 months or longer.

Clozapine is contraindicated in patients with myeloproliferative disorders or who are immunocompromised as a result of diseases such as tuberculosis or human immunodeficiency virus (HIV) infection because of their increased risk of developing agranulocytosis. Concomitant medications that are associated with bone marrow suppression, such as carbamazepine, are also contraindicated.

Extrapyramidal effects. EPS are uncommon with clozapine at any dosage, although some patients experience akathisia or hand tremors.

Neuroleptic malignant syndrome. Despite the absence of EPS in clozapine-treated patients, there have been reports of NMS in patients taking clozapine alone (Anderson and Powers 1991; Das Gupta and Young 1991; Miller et al. 1991).

Sedation. Sedation is the most common side effect of clozapine, and it is particularly prominent early in treatment. Sedation generally attenuates with dosage reduction, when tolerance to this side effect develops, or when a disproportionate amount is given at bedtime.

Cardiovascular effects. Hypotension and tachycardia occur in most patients taking clozapine. Rare cases of myocarditis of uncertain etiology also have been reported in patients taking clozapine.

Weight gain. Weight gain occurs in most patients; many patients gain 10% or more of their original body weight (Umbricht et al. 1994).

Hypersalivation. Hypersalivation occurs in one-third of the patients taking clozapine, particularly at night. Although the basis for this side effect is unknown, the symptom is not related to drug-induced parkinsonism. Because clozapine has potent anticholinergic properties, addition of an anticholinergic agent is not recommended for control of drooling.

Fever. For unclear reasons, clozapine treatment is associated with benign, transient temperature elevations, generally within the first 3 weeks of treatment. Patients taking clozapine who develop fevers should be evaluated for infectious etiologies, agranulocytosis, and NMS.

Seizures. Clozapine treatment is associated with a dose-dependent risk of seizures. Although the vast majority of clozapine-induced seizures are tonic-clonic, myoclonic seizures also occur. Dosages of less than 300 mg/day are associated with a 1%–3% seizure risk. Dosages of 300–600 mg/day are associated with a 3%–4% risk, and dosages greater than 600 mg/day are associated with a 5% risk of seizures. Because of this risk, clozapine dosages greater than 600 mg/day are not recommended unless the patient has failed to respond at lower dosages.

Anticholinergic effects.   Anticholinergic effects, such as dry mouth, blurred vision, constipation, and urinary retention, are common early side effects of clozapine treatment.

Obsessive-compulsive symptoms. Treatment with clozapine has been reported to exacerbate symptoms of OCD, probably because of 5-HT$_2$ antagonism (Ghaemi et al. 1995). If this effect occurs, symptoms are usually controlled with the addition of an SSRI.

Drug interactions.   Clozapine should not be combined with any drugs that have the potential to suppress bone marrow function, such as carbamazepine. There have been isolated reports of respiratory arrest in patients who were taking both clozapine and a high-potency benzodiazepine. Because of these reports, benzodiazepines should be avoided, particularly at high doses, in patients who are taking clozapine.

Clozapine is metabolized by hepatic CYP1A2 and, to a lesser degree, CYP3A3/4; therefore, it is subject to changes in serum concentration when combined with medications that inhibit or induce these enzymes (see section on drug interactions later in this chapter). Clozapine serum levels are increased by coadministration of fluvoxamine and erythromycin and decreased by phenobarbital, phenytoin, and

cigarette smoking (Byerly and DeVane 1996). These pharmacokinetic interactions are particularly important because of the dose-dependent risk of seizures.

Risperidone

Risperidone, a novel benzisoxazole derivative, is an atypical antipsychotic medication that combines D$_2$-receptor antagonism with potent 5-HT$_2$ receptor antagonism. Risperidone has a higher affinity for D$_2$ receptors than does clozapine. Risperidone also antagonizes D$_1$, D$_4$, α_1, α_2, and H$_1$ histaminic receptors. Unlike the other atypical agents, risperidone elevates prolactin levels, often higher than levels associated with conventional agents.

Clinical use.   Risperidone is most effective in the 4- to 6-mg range. For initial treatment, we recommend using divided doses, starting at 1 mg twice a day and quickly increasing to 2 mg twice a day. For elderly persons, the initial dosage should be much lower (0.25–0.5 mg/day). After the first week of treatment, the entire dosage can be given at bedtime. This usually helps the patient to sleep and reduces daytime side effects. However, we do not suggest this practice for elderly persons because of an increased risk of falling. In addition, some patients feel an activating effect from risperidone; in these individuals, the medication should be administered in the morning.

Risks, side effects, and their management.   Insomnia, hypotension, agitation, headache, and rhinitis are the most common side effects of risperidone. These tend to lessen with time. Risperidone produces weight gain, which is intermediate in magnitude compared with other atypical agents. Overall, the drug tends to be well tolerated. Risperidone is not associated with significant anticholinergic side effects. Whereas hyperprolactinemia is a common finding with risperidone, the incidence of clinical manifestations is less clear.

Drug interactions. Risperidone is metabolized primarily by the CYP2D6 enzyme (Byerly and DeVane 1996). Medications that inhibit this enzyme, such as many of the SSRIs, cause increased risperidone plasma levels. However, several studies have not found an increase in side effects resulting from such an interaction, possibly because the primary metabolite of risperidone, 9-OH risperidone, is fully active and is excreted unchanged by the kidneys. Inhibition of the 2D6 enzyme may merely alter the balance between parent drug and metabolite without significantly altering total D_2 occupancy. Pharmacodynamic interactions may occur when risperidone is combined with other medications that share a similar physiological effect, such as orthostatic hypotension.

Olanzapine

Olanzapine, a thienobenzodiazepine, represents a modification of the clozapine molecule. Compared with clozapine, olanzapine has greater D_2 and weaker D_4 and α-adrenergic affinity. Despite the structural similarity of these two drugs, olanzapine is not associated with higher than expected rates of agranulocytosis. Although in vitro binding studies have indicated a high affinity for M_1 receptors, anticholinergic side effects are not as prominent as these data would predict.

Olanzapine has dose-dependent therapeutic effects on both positive and negative symptoms and a favorable side-effect profile (Beasley et al. 1996). Acute dystonia is uncommon. Akathisia is more common but is significantly less common than with the conventional antipsychotic medications. In prospective double-blind studies, treatment-emergent tardive dyskinesia was reported to occur in 1% of the olanzapine group compared with 4.6% of the haloperidol group (Tollefson et al. 1997). Olanzapine is associated with modest dose-dependent elevations in serum prolactin levels, but most often these elevations are transient and within the normal reference range (Tollefson et al. 1997).

Clinical use. The recommended starting dosage of olanzapine is 10 mg at bedtime, subsequently titrated on the basis of tolerability and therapeutic effect. The clinically effective range is 7.5–20 mg/day, administered as a single daily dose at bedtime. Higher dosages may be more effective but result in increased side effects. Clinically meaningful improvement may not be evident for the first several weeks after initiating treatment, but improvement usually continues through week 6 and perhaps longer.

Risks, side effects, and their management. *Somnolence.* As one would predict on the basis of the histamine H_1 antagonism, somnolence is a common side effect of olanzapine. Somnolence and psychomotor slowing are dose dependent, and patients often become tolerant to this side effect over time.

Hepatic effects. Increased transaminase levels were reported in 2% of the patients taking olanzapine in premarketing evaluation. In many cases, these levels normalized without medication discontinuation, and all cases to date have been clinically benign. Routine laboratory monitoring is not recommended, but olanzapine should be used with caution in patients with hepatic disease or with additional risk factors for hepatic toxicity. In this group of patients, serum transaminase levels must be monitored.

Weight gain. Treatment-emergent weight gain is common with olanzapine and averages about 7 kg (15 lb). However, approximately 20% of patients may not gain weight. Nutritional education should be provided to patients, along with monitoring of caloric intake by diet diaries, and exercise should be strongly encouraged. Weight reduction groups are often helpful in providing instructional materials and offering support.

Drug interactions. Olanzapine is metabolized by several pathways and is therefore unlikely to be affected by concurrent administration with other medications. Because olanzapine does not appear to inhibit any of the cytochrome P450 enzymes, it should not increase the availability of other medications through this mechanism. Additive pharmacodynamic effects are expected if olanzapine is combined with medications that also have anticholinergic, antihistaminic, or α-adrenergic side effects.

Quetiapine

Quetiapine is a dibenzothiazapine derivative with weak affinity for 5-HT_{1A}, 5-HT_2, D_1, D_2, H_1, α_1, and α_2 receptors. Quetiapine has very "loose" binding to D_2 receptors. Quetiapine's relatively high $5\text{-HT}_2\text{:}D_2$ ratio is consistent with the hypothesized advantageous properties of the atypical antipsychotics, antagonism of H_1 receptors is associated with sedative side effects, and α_1 antagonism is associated with orthostatic hypotension.

Clinical use. Quetiapine is initiated at a dosage of 25 mg twice a day and then increased on day 2 to 50 mg twice a day, on day 3 to 100 mg twice a day, and on day 4 to 100 mg in the morning and 200 mg in the evening. The optimal dosage for most patients appears to range between 400 mg/day and 600 mg/day, although the

drug is safe and efficacious for some patients within a dose range of 150–750 mg. A slower titration and lower daily doses may be warranted for patients with hepatic disease and for elderly patients. Because of its relatively short half-life of 8 hours, quetiapine is usually administered twice daily.

Risks, side effects, and their management. Quetiapine was no different from placebo in doses to 750 mg/day regarding EPS and changes in serum prolactin levels (Arvanitis and Miller 1997).

Somnolence. Somnolence is one of the most common side effects of quetiapine. Somnolence and psychomotor slowing are dose dependent, and patients often become tolerant to this side effect over time.

Ocular changes. The development of cataracts was observed in association with quetiapine treatment in preclinical studies of dogs, but a causal relation has not been established in humans. Postmarketing experience has not detected an increase in incidence of cataracts with quetiapine compared with other antipsychotics; however, cataracts are more common in schizophrenic patients in general compared with the general population.

Cardiovascular effects. As predicted with α_1 antagonism, quetiapine may induce orthostatic hypotension and concomitant symptoms of dizziness, tachycardia, and syncope. The risk of symptomatic hypotension is particularly pronounced during initial dose titration.

Hepatic effects. Increased transaminase levels were reported in 6% of the patients taking quetiapine in premarketing evaluation. These changes usually occur in the first weeks of treatment and to date have been benign. Routine laboratory

Psychopharmacology and Electroconvulsive Therapy

monitoring is not recommended, but quetiapine should be used with caution in patients with hepatic disease or with additional risk factors for hepatic toxicity.

Weight gain. Quetiapine may induce weight gain. In premarketing placebo-controlled studies, a weight gain of 7% or more of body weight was observed in 23% of quetiapine-treated patients, compared with 6% of placebo-control subjects. Early clinical experience suggests that weight gain associated with quetiapine treatment is not generally as marked as has been observed with olanzapine, although insufficient data are available to compare it directly with other agents (Allison et al. 1999).

Drug interactions. Quetiapine is metabolized by the hepatic CYP3A3/4 enzyme. Concurrent administration of cytochrome P450–inducing drugs, such as carbamazepine, decreases quetiapine blood levels. In such circumstances, increased doses of quetiapine are appropriate. Quetiapine does not appreciably affect the pharmacokinetics of other medications. Pharmacodynamic effects are expected if quetiapine is combined with medications that also have antihistaminic or α-adrenergic side effects. Because of its potential for producing hypotension, quetiapine also may enhance the effects of certain antihypertensive agents.

Ziprasidone

Ziprasidone combines a high affinity for $5\text{-}HT_2$ receptors with intermediate affinity for D_2, resulting in a very high $5\text{-}HT_2$:D_2 affinity ratio. Ziprasidone also has substantial agonist activity at $5\text{-}HT_{1a}$ receptors and moderately inhibits reuptake of serotonin and norepinephrine. The FDA delayed approval of ziprasidone until additional safety data could be obtained regarding effects on cardiac conduction.

Ziprasidone delays the QTc interval at maximum therapeutic blood levels by approximately 20 msec, on average, which is a larger effect than with other atypical agents but less than with thioridazine. Although monitoring of ECGs is not routinely required, clinicians should consider the relative risk of cardiac conduction delay compared with the benefits of ziprasidone (which include tolerability and minimal weight gain) when selecting a medication.

Clinical use. Ziprasidone is usually started at a dosage of 20–40 mg twice a day and can be rapidly titrated over 2–4 days to a typical therapeutic dosage of 60–80 mg twice a day in medically healthy, nonelderly patients. In one study, a starting dosage of 60 mg twice a day was well tolerated without significant orthostatic hypotension. Dosing in the elderly and in patients with cardiovascular disease has not been well studied to date. Ziprasidone has a half-life of 5–10 hours and is usually administered twice daily with meals. Food increases absorption by approximately 100%.

Because safety data with ziprasidone are largely derived from studies that excluded subjects with cardiac disease, clinicians should screen patients for cardiac risk factors, preferably with a baseline ECG and serum electrolytes, before initiating ziprasidone. Patients with QTc prolongation at baseline must be monitored very closely; consultation from a cardiologist is recommended. However, ziprasidone may improve cardiovascular risk factors related to obesity and hyperlipidemia.

Risks, side effects, and their management. In the few studies that have been published to date, ziprasidone has been well tolerated. The most common side effects have included headache, dyspepsia, nausea, constipation, abdominal pain, somnolence, and EPS. Ratings of parkinsonism and akathisia with ziprasidone 120 mg/day did not differ from those with placebo. Although dizziness has been reported, rates of orthostatic hypotension have not differed from those with placebo in controlled clinical trials. Ziprasidone produces transient hyperprolactinemia, which returns to predrug baseline levels after 12 hours; prolactin levels are significantly lower with ziprasidone than with haloperidol (Goff et al. 1998).

Cardiovascular side effects. Ziprasidone produced a mean QTc prolongation of 21 msec at maximal blood levels achieved during exposure to typical therapeutic doses. Twenty-one percent of the subjects had QTc prolongation of 60 msec or greater, and 3% developed QTc prolongation of 75 msec or greater. However, in all clinical trials, the rate of QTc intervals greater than 500 msec (considered a threshold for arrhythmia risk) did not differ from that with placebo (<0.1%). Ziprasidone blood levels were increased by about 40% by coadministration of ketoconazole (a metabolic inhibitor) without any change in QTc duration detected. Consistent with the weak relation between drug levels and QTc effect, the 10 published cases of overdose with ziprasidone have been relatively benign.

Weight gain. Ziprasidone produces less weight gain than do other atypical antipsychotic agents. Allison et al. (1999) calculated a mean weight gain of less than 1 kg after 10 weeks of ziprasidone treatment.

Drug interactions. Drugs that inhibit the CYP3A4 isoenzyme reduce metabolism of ziprasidone: concurrent treatment with ketoconazole increased ziprasidone blood levels by approximately 40%. Carbamazepine (and possibly other enzyme inducers) may lower ziprasidone levels by about 35%. Effects of ziprasidone on metabolism of other drugs have not been reported.

Aripiprazole

Aripiprazole (Abilify), the newest addition to the atypical antipsychotic armamentarium, is a D_2 partial agonist, a 5-HT_{1A} partial agonist, and a 5-HT_{2A} antagonist. The D_2 partial agonist feature is distinct from other antipsychotics, which are antagonists at the D_2 receptor.

Clinical use. The recommended starting and target dosage for aripiprazole is 10–15 mg/day administered on a once-a-day schedule.

Risks, side effects, and their management. Aripiprazole is well tolerated, with a low rate of neurological side effects and no significant adverse effects on serum prolactin concentrations, weight, or QTc prolongation.

Neuroleptic malignant syndrome. Two possible cases of NMS occurred during aripiprazole treatment in premarketing clinical trials).

Seizures. Seizures occurred in 0.1% (1 of 926) of aripiprazole-treated patients in short-term, placebo-controlled trials. As with other antipsychotic drugs, aripiprazole should be used cautiously in patients with a history of seizures or with conditions that lower the seizure threshold.

Orthostatic hypotension. Aripiprazole may be associated with orthostatic hypotension, perhaps as a result of its adrenergic receptor antagonism. It should be used with caution in patients with known cardiovascular disease or with conditions that could predispose them to hypotension.

Somnolence. In short-term, placebo-controlled trials, somnolence was reported by 11% of patients on aripiprazole, compared with 8% of patients on placebo. There appears to be a possible dose-response relationship for this side effect, with increased somnolence observed at higher doses (30 mg/day).

Drug interactions. Both CYP3A4 and CYP2D6 are responsible for aripiprazole metabolism. Agents that induce CYP3A4 (e.g., carbamazepine) could cause an increase in aripiprazole clearance and lower blood levels. Inhibitors of CYP3A4 (e.g., ketoconazole) or of CYP2D6 (e.g., quinidine, fluoxetine, paroxetine) can inhibit aripiprazole elimination and cause increased blood levels.

Pharmacological Treatment of Schizophrenia

General Principles

Evidence shows that the long-term outcome for a patient with schizophrenia is better when treatment of the acute episode is initiated rapidly. After a patient's first episode of schizophrenia, the antipsychotic medication should be continued for at least 1 year after a full remission of psychotic symptoms. After that time, a trial period without medication may be considered, except for patients with a history of serious suicide attempts or violent aggressive behavior (American Psychiatric Association 1997). The patient and his or her family should be informed of the early signs and symptoms of relapse, such as suspiciousness, difficulty sleeping, and argumentativeness and should be warned that relapse is highly likely. The patient should be carefully monitored during this period.

For patients with a chronic, relapsing form of schizophrenia, antipsychotic medication should be continued for up to 5 symptom-free years before discontinuation (Johnson 1985) and should probably be continued indefinitely.

Treatment-Resistant Schizophrenia

If the symptoms do not respond to the indicated treatment, minimal side effects (e.g., EPS, hypotension, sedation) occur, and poor compliance is not the cause, the physician can gradually increase the dosage until mild side effects are seen. If no further improvement is seen after an additional 2–4 weeks at this dosage, another antipsychotic drug from another class should be substituted. Atypical antipsychotics should be considered in patients who have not responded to conventional antipsychotic medication. At this time, adequate data do not exist to suggest greater efficacy of one atypical antipsychotic, other than clozapine. A trial of clozapine should be considered for patients who continue to have positive symptoms, frequent relapses, or aggression despite an adequate trial of at least one other antipsychotic medication and for patients with intolerable side effects to at least two different antipsychotic medications from different classes (American Psychiatric Association 1997). At least one of these drugs should be an atypical antipsychotic.

An additional strategy to use with nonresponsive patients is to add another medication to augment the therapeutic effects of the antipsychotic. The most common agents used to augment antipsychotic medications in the treatment of schizophrenia are lithium (Cole et al. 1984; Delva and Letemednia 1982), valproate (Linnoila et al. 1976), and benzodiazepines (Csernansky et al. 1988; Douyon et al. 1989; Nestoros et al. 1982).

Other Uses of Antipsychotic Medications

The use of antipsychotic medications to treat other disorders is addressed elsewhere in this chapter (e.g., in the "Treatment of Mania" section and "Antipsychotic Drugs" subsection in the "Acute Aggression and Agitation" section later in this chapter).

Mood Stabilizers

Overview

In addition to lithium, the anticonvulsant valproate and the atypical antipsychotic olanzapine are approved by the FDA for the treatment of mania. These medications are collectively referred to as *mood stabilizers* because of their ability to stabilize mood oscillations regardless of etiology. In this section, we review the clinical use of lithium and the anticonvulsants that are definite or probable mood stabilizers. The general properties of the antipsychotics, including olanzapine, were reviewed in the preceding section. In this section, we expand on the use of these compounds for the treatment of bipolar disorder (Table 18–14).

Lithium

Mechanism of Action

Lithium is a monovalent cation that is believed to affect intracellular second messenger systems. According to a review by Jope and Williams (1994), lithium inhibits several steps in phosphoinositide metabolism as well as G-protein functioning (Manji et al. 1995). Lithium has been reported to inhibit the stimulation of adenylate cyclase by several different neurotransmitters without suppressing basal adenylate cyclase activity (Belmaker et

al. 1983; Ebstein et al. 1980; Zohar et al. 1982) and to inhibit protein kinase C (PKC) after subchronic administration (Bitran et al. 1995; Lenox et al. 1992; Manji et al. 1993). These effects on signal transduction have broad effects on neuronal function and gene expression (for an excellent review, see Manji et al. 1999).

Indications and Efficacy

Lithium has been proved effective for acute and prophylactic treatment of both manic and depressive episodes in patients with bipolar illness (Consensus Development Panel 1985; Prien et al. 1984) and cyclothymia (Akiskal et al. 1979). However, patients with rapid-cycling bipolar disorder (i.e., four or more mood disorder episodes per year) have been reported to respond less well to lithium treatment (Dunner and Fieve 1974; Prien et al. 1984; Wehr et al. 1988). Lithium is also effective in the prevention of future depressive episodes in patients with recurrent unipolar depressive disorder (Consensus Development Panel 1985) and as an adjunct to antidepressants in depressed patients whose illness is partially refractory to treatment with antidepressants alone. Furthermore, lithium may be useful in the maintenance of remission of depressive disorder after ECT (Coppen et al. 1981; Sackeim et al. 2001). Lithium also has been used effectively in some cases of aggression and behavioral dyscontrol.

Clinical Use

Before they begin treatment with lithium, patients should be told that they might experience nausea, diarrhea, polyuria, increased thirst, and fine hand tremor. These are often transient, but in some patients they persist with therapeutic lithium levels. Because of a narrow range between the therapeutic and toxic doses of lithium and the wide variability of lithium pharmaco-

TABLE 18–14. Characteristics of commonly used mood stabilizers

	Lithium	Valproate	Carbamazepine
Available preparations	Lithium carbonate (Eskalith, Lithonate, Lithotabs, generics; 300-mg tabs, caps) Lithium citrate liquid (8 mEq/5 mL) Extended release (Eskalith CR 450 mg; Lithobid 300 mg)	Divalproex sodium (Depakote 125-, 250-, 500-mg tabs, 125-mg sprinkle caps) Depacon iv Valproic acid (Depakene, generics, 250-mg caps; Depakene 250 mg/5 mL syrup) Divalproex ER 250 mg, 500 mg	Tegretol, generics (200-mg tabs, 100-mg chewable tabs, 100 mg/5 mL suspension) Tegretol-XR sustained release (100-, 200-, 400-mg tabs)
Half-life	24 hours	9–16 hours	24/12 hours[a]
Starting dosage	300 mg bid	250 mg tid or 20 mg/kg	200 mg bid
Blood level	0.8–1.2 mEq/L	45–125 µg/mL	4–12[b] µg/mL
Metabolism	Renal	Hepatic	Hepatic
Contraindications[c]	Unstable renal function	Hepatic dysfunction	Hepatic dysfunction
Pretreatment laboratory evaluation	Chem 20,[d] CBC, thyrotropin, ECG if ≥40 years old or cardiac disease; pregnancy test	Aspartate aminotransferase, alanine aminotransferase, pregnancy test	CBC, aspartate aminotransferase, alanine aminotransferase, pregnancy test

Note. CBC = complete blood count; ECG = electrocardiogram.
[a]24 hours before hepatic autoinduction; 12 hours after autoinduction.
[b]Not correlated with clinical response.
[c]All current mood stabilizers should be avoided in pregnancy. See text for discussion.
[d]Especially blood urea nitrogen, creatinine, sodium, and calcium.

kinetics among different individuals, the optimal dosage for an individual patient cannot be based on the dosage administered. Rather, lithium dosing should be based on the concentration of lithium in the plasma. Lithium carbonate is completely absorbed by the gastrointestinal tract and reaches peak plasma levels in 1–2 hours. The elimination half-life is approximately 24 hours. Steady-state lithium levels are obtained in approximately 5 days.

Therapeutic plasma levels for patients undergoing lithium therapy range from 0.5 to 1.5 mEq/L. Although lower plasma levels are associated with less troubling side effects, most clinicians seek to establish levels of at least 0.8 mEq/L in treating acute manic episodes. Therefore, when intolerable side effects have not intervened, treatment of acute mania with lithium should not be considered a failure until plasma levels of 1.2–1.5 mEq/L have been reached and maintained for 2 weeks. However, when levels this high are necessary for acute treatment, the dosage often may be reduced to the range of 0.8–1.0 mEq/L for maintenance therapy. Although Gelenberg et al. (1989) initially reported that levels in the range of 0.8–1.0 mEq/L provide better prophylaxis against relapse, this finding may be applicable only to patients who require relatively high levels for initial stabilization. Patients who are stabilized with blood levels in the range of 0.4–0.8 mEq/L may do well remaining at these relatively low levels, often with a reduced side effect burden. Therapeutic lithium levels have not been established for other disorders. General guidelines for lithium treatment are listed in Table 18–15.

Contraindications and Pretreatment Medical Evaluation

Lithium should not be administered to patients with fluctuating or unstable renal function. In patients with statically im-

TABLE 18–15. Guidelines for lithium treatment

1. Review medical history and review of systems with particular attention to renal, thyroid, and cardiac status.
2. Order pretreatment pregnancy test and levels of BUN, creatinine, electrolytes, and thyrotropin. If the patient is older than 40 years or has evidence of cardiac disease, order ECG.
3. Inform patient and family of proper use of lithium. Include a discussion of common side effects, the importance of monitoring of lithium levels, early signs and symptoms of toxicity, and potential long-term side effects. If patient is female, include warnings about pregnancy during treatment.
4. Initiate therapy at 300 mg bid, and increase by 300 mg every 3–4 days.
5. Obtain lithium levels (12 hours after last dose) twice a week, until there is a clinical response or the lithium level reaches approximately 1.0 mEq/L.
6. Monitor BUN and creatinine.
7. Monitor thyrotropin every 6–12 months if symptoms of hypothyroidism develop.

Note. BUN = blood urea nitrogen; ECG = electrocardiogram.

paired renal function, another mood stabilizer, such as valproate, is preferred. For patients who are unresponsive to alternative treatments, lithium may be administered if the dosage and dose frequency are suitably reduced to avoid toxic blood levels. Because lithium may affect functioning of the cardiac sinus node, patients with sinus node dysfunction (e.g., sick sinus syndrome) should not receive lithium. Although lithium also has acute and chronic effects on the thyroid, patients with hypothyroidism may receive lithium if the thyroid disease is adequately treated and monitored. Laboratory tests that should be performed before the initiation of lithium or valproate are outlined in Table 18–14.

Although initial uncontrolled reports suggested a markedly increased risk of Ebstein's anomaly of the heart in infants who were exposed to lithium in utero (Nora et al. 1974), subsequent controlled data predicted a 0.1%–0.7% absolute risk (Edmonds and Oakley 1990; Jacobson et al. 1992; Kallen and Tandberg 1983; Zalzstein et al. 1990) compared with 0.01% in the general population. The overall risk of major congenital anomalies in association with lithium exposure is 4%–12%, compared with 2%–4% in comparison groups (L.S. Cohen et al. 1994). The increased risk of malformations must be weighed against the risk for both mother and fetus if lithium discontinuation results in a manic relapse.

Risks, Side Effects, and Their Management

Renal effects. For all patients taking lithium, a measure of serum blood urea nitrogen (BUN) and creatinine should be obtained at baseline and every 3–6 months after lithium therapy has commenced, with more frequent testing if there are specific complaints or signs of renal dysfunction. Most of the effects of lithium on the kidney are reversible after discontinuation of the drug. Although permanent morphological changes in renal structure have been reported, the clinical implications of these changes have yet to be established, and to date there have been no published reports of irreversible renal failure as a result of chronic, nontoxic lithium therapy (Hetmar et al. 1991).

However, lithium inhibits vasopressin with resultant impairment in renal concentrating ability. Termed *nephrogenic diabetes insipidus* (NDI), this condition results in polyuria for up to 60% of patients taking lithium (Lokkegaard et al. 1985).

Proteinuria has been reported as a rare side effect and is thought to be the consequence of either glomerular leakage or the inhibition of tubular resorption (Waller and Edwards 1989; Wood et al. 1989).

Thyroid dysfunction. Reversible hypothyroidism may occur in as many as 20% of the patients treated with lithium (Lindstedt et al. 1977; Myers et al. 1985). Lithium-induced hypothyroidism occurs more frequently in women, in patients with thyroid antibodies, and in patients with an exaggerated thyrotropin response to thyrotropin-releasing hormone (TRH; Calabrese et al. 1985; Myers et al. 1985). Because the development of hypothyroidism in bipolar patients is associated with intractable depression (Yassa et al. 1988) as well as with the development of a rapid-cycling course (Bauer et al. 1990), thyroid function must be monitored every 6–12 months during lithium treatment or if symptoms develop that might be attributable to thyroid dysfunction. If laboratory tests indicate the development of hypothyroidism, the patient should be evaluated clinically for signs and symptoms of hypothyroidism and be referred to an endocrinologist for any further tests. In collaboration with the endocrinologist, the psychiatrist should decide on the appropriate treatment—in most cases, thyroid hormone replacement and continuation of lithium therapy.

Parathyroid dysfunction. The effects of lithium on calcium metabolism may be related to lithium-induced hyperparathyroidism (Anath and Dubin 1983; Mallette and Eichhorn 1986).

Neurotoxicity. Lithium therapy may be associated with several types of neurological dysfunction. Fine resting tremor is a neurological side effect that may be detected in as many as one-half of the patients taking lithium (Vestergaard et al.

1980). β-Adrenergic-blocking drugs, such as propranolol in divided daily doses below 80 mg/day, are effective in treating this tremor (Zubenko et al. 1984). Subjective memory impairment occurs in approximately 28% of the patients taking lithium and is among the most frequent reasons for noncompliance (Goodwin and Jamison 1990).

Cardiac effects. Mitchell and Mackenzie (1982) reported changes in T-wave morphology on the ECG (flattening or inversion) in 20%–30% of patients taking lithium, changes that are most likely benign. Lithium also may suppress the function of the sinus node and result in sinoatrial block. Individuals with sinus disease or conduction defects, therefore, should not be given lithium. Cases have also been reported of aggravation of preexisting ventricular arrhythmias with lithium therapy. An ECG should be checked before treatment with lithium is started in individuals who are older than 40 years or in those with a history or symptoms of cardiac disease.

Weight gain. Weight gain is a frequent side effect of lithium treatment (Peselow et al. 1980; Vendsborg et al. 1976; Vestergaard et al. 1980). Possible mechanisms include influences on carbohydrate metabolism, changes in glucose tolerance, or changes in lipid metabolism. Dieting and exercise should be recommended early in treatment.

Dermatological reactions. Dermatological reactions to lithium include acne, follicular eruptions, and psoriasis (Bakris et al. 1980–1981; Deandrea et al. 1982). Changes in hair, including hair loss, hair thinning, and loss of wave, also have been reported. Except for cases of exacerbation of psoriasis, these reactions are usually benign and may not warrant discontinuation of lithium treatment. Lithium-induced acne responds to topical treatment with steroidal agents, such as tretinoin (Retin-A).

Gastrointestinal side effects. Gastrointestinal difficulties occur frequently with lithium treatment, especially nausea and diarrhea. Although these side effects may be manifestations of toxicity, they also occur at lithium levels within the therapeutic range. Gastrointestinal symptoms may improve with reduction of dosage or ingestion of lithium with meals. Slow-release formulations are more often associated with nausea, whereas sustained-release preparations are more commonly associated with diarrhea.

Hematological side effects. The most frequent hematological change detected in patients taking lithium is leukocytosis (approximately 15,000 white blood cells/mm^3). As reviewed by Brewerton (1986), this change is generally benign; lithium may, in fact, be used to treat several conditions associated with granulocytopenia.

Overdose and toxicity. Because of the narrow range between therapeutic and toxic plasma lithium levels, the physician must devote sufficient time to informing the patient and the family about the signs and symptoms of early lithium toxicity and the circumstances that may increase the chances of toxicity, such as drinking insufficient amounts of fluids, becoming overheated with increased perspiration, or ingesting too much medication. The physician must emphasize the prevention of lithium toxicity through the maintenance of adequate salt and water intake, especially during hot weather and exercise. Toxic lithium levels can produce severe neurotoxic reactions, with symptoms such as dysarthria, ataxia, and intention tremor. The signs and symptoms of lithium toxic-

TABLE 18–16. Signs and symptoms of lithium toxicity

**Mild-to-moderate intoxication
(lithium level = 1.5–2.0 mEq/L)**
  Gastrointestinal
    Vomiting
    Abdominal pain
    Dryness of mouth
  Neurological
    Ataxia
    Dizziness
    Slurred speech
    Nystagmus
    Lethargy or excitement
    Muscle weakness
**Moderate-to-severe intoxication
(lithium level = 2.0–2.5 mEq/L)**
  Gastrointestinal
    Anorexia
    Persistent nausea and vomiting
  Neurological
    Blurred vision
    Muscle fasciculations
    Clonic limb movements
    Hyperactive deep tendon reflexes
    Choreoathetoid movements
    Convulsions
    Delirium
    Syncope
    Electroencephalographic changes
    Stupor
    Coma
    Circulatory failure (lowered blood
      pressure, cardiac arrhythmias, and
      conduction abnormalities)
**Severe lithium intoxication
(lithium level > 2.5 mEq/L)**
  Generalized convulsions
  Oliguria and renal failure
  Death

ity may be divided into those that usually occur at lithium levels between 1.5 and 2.0 mEq/L, those that occur between 2.0 and 2.5 mEq/L, and those that occur above 2.5 mEq/L (Table 18–16), although some patients may become clinically toxic with lithium levels in the standard thera-

TABLE 18–17. Management of lithium toxicity

1. The patient should immediately contact his or her personal physician or go to a hospital emergency department.
2. Lithium should be discontinued and the patient instructed to ingest fluids, if possible.
3. Physical examination should be completed, including vital signs and a neurological examination with complete formal mental status examination.
4. Lithium level, serum electrolytes, renal function tests, and electrocardiogram should be obtained as soon as possible.
5. For significant acute ingestion, residual gastric contents should be removed by induction of emesis, gastric lavage, and absorption with activated charcoal.[a]
6. Vigorous hydration and maintenance of electrolyte balance are essential.
7. For any patient with a serum lithium level greater than 4.0 mEq/L or with serious manifestations of lithium toxicity, hemodialysis should be initiated.[a]
8. Repeat dialysis may be required every 6–10 hours, until the lithium level is within nontoxic range and the patient has no signs or symptoms of lithium toxicity.

[a]Information from Goldfrank et al. 1986.

peutic range. The recommended management of lithium toxicity is reviewed in Table 18–17.

Drug interactions. Because of the narrow therapeutic range of lithium, knowledge of its drug–drug interactions is of paramount importance. Because the kidney excretes lithium, any medication that alters renal function can affect lithium levels. Thiazide diuretics reduce lithium clearance and hence may increase lithium levels. Loop diuretics (e.g., furosemide) do not have this effect. Nonsteroidal anti-inflammatory drugs may also increase lithium levels by decreasing clearance. It is particularly important to inform patients of this effect because these medications are often self-prescribed. Other medications that may increase lithium levels include angiotensin-converting enzyme inhibitors and COX-2 inhibitors (e.g., celecoxib, rofecoxib). Drugs that may decrease lithium levels include theophylline and aminophylline. Lithium may potentiate the effects of succinylocholine-like muscle relaxants. Concerns about increased risk of delirium, NMS, and irreversible brain damage have been raised for the combination of lithium and neuroleptic drugs on the basis of case reports (W.J. Cohen and Cohen 1974). However, a controlled investigation found no difference in side effects or complications between a group of patients with mania treated with antipsychotic medications alone and a group of patients with mania treated with antipsychotic drugs and lithium (Goldney and Spence 1986); this result is concordant with clinical experience. The preponderance of evidence indicates that lithium and antipsychotic medications, including haloperidol, can be safely and effectively combined, with appropriate monitoring.

Valproate

Lambert et al. (1966) were the first to report success in treating bipolar disorder with valproate. Since that time, numerous uncontrolled studies have supported this initial claim. After the early 1980s, several controlled studies established that valproate is effective in acute mania (Gerner and Stanton 1992; Keck et al. 1992; Pope et al. 1991). More recently, a collaborative study by Bowden et al. (1994) directly compared valproate with lithium and placebo in patients with mania. This study found valproate to be as effective as lithium in patients with euphoric mania. It is concordant with previous observations

(Calabrese et al. 1992; McElroy et al. 1992; Post et al. 1987) that valproate was found to be more effective than lithium in patients with rapid-cycling and dysphoric mania. Valproate also has been reported to be especially effective for mania occurring in patients with a history of closed-head trauma (McElroy et al. 1989) and in patients with EEG abnormalities (Pope et al. 1988). Although several open-trial studies have suggested that valproate is also effective for prophylaxis in bipolar disorder, no controlled studies have confirmed this finding to date (Keck et al. 1992). The efficacy of valproate in the treatment of acute bipolar depression has yet to be studied systematically. Divalproex sodium is approved by the FDA for the treatment of mania.

Mechanism of Action

Although many putative mechanisms have been proposed, the basis for the mood-stabilizing effects of valproate is most likely concordant with the mechanism of lithium, specifically by attenuating the activity of PKC and other steps in the signal transduction pathway leading to neuronal adaptation and changes in gene expression (Chen et al. 1994; Manji et al. 1999).

Clinical Use

Before beginning treatment with valproate, patients should be told that they might experience nausea, sedation, and a fine hand tremor. These are often transient, but in some patients they persist. Several valproate preparations are available in the United States, including valproic acid, sodium valproate, divalproex sodium, and an extended-release preparation of divalproex sodium. Divalproex sodium is a dimer of sodium valproate and valproic acid with an enteric coating, and it is much better tolerated than other oral valproate preparations. An intravenous preparation also has become available, but it has not yet been well studied in psychiatric disorders. The half-life of valproate is 10 hours.

Valproate may be initiated gradually with subsequent dosage titration or with a more rapid "loading" strategy. Most commonly, valproate is initiated at a dosage of 250 mg three times a day and subsequently increased by 250 mg every 3 days. Most patients require a dosage of 1,250–2,500 mg/day. Although valproate has a relatively short half-life, moderate doses may be given once a day at bedtime to reduce daytime sedation, often without compromising clinical efficacy. This strategy should not be used when valproate is administered to treat seizure disorders, for which more constant serum levels are required.

In situations for which rapid stabilization is of paramount importance, valproate treatment can be initiated at a dosage of 20 mg per kilogram of body weight (Keck et al. 1993). Some patients require relatively high dosages of valproate, sometimes dosages greater than 4,000 mg/day, to achieve a sufficient plasma level and clinical response, and some patients do not respond until plasma valproate levels are greater than 100 mg/mL. As with all psychotropic medications, the final dosage is more dependent on the balance between clinical response and side effects than on the absolute blood level. However, plasma levels of 45–100 mg/mL are recommended for the treatment of acute mania (Bowden et al. 1996). Patients with less severe symptoms, such as bipolar II disorder or cyclothymia, often respond at lower dosages and blood levels (Jacobsen 1993). Blood levels in other phases of bipolar disorder, such as bipolar depression, or in other indications, such as aggression, have not been established. The extended-release preparation of divalproex sodium has 80%–90% of the bioavailability of the initial divalproex sodium; as a result, dosages may need to be slightly higher when using this preparation.

Contraindications

Valproate is relatively contraindicated for patients with hepatitis or liver disease; it may be pursued as treatment for such patients only as a last resort and with the approval and continuous involvement of a gastroenterologist. Valproate has been linked to spina bifida and other neural tube defects in the offspring of patients exposed to this medication in the first trimester of pregnancy (Lammer et al. 1987; Robert and Guibaud 1982). As such, the risks of continuing valproate during pregnancy must be balanced against the risk of relapse.

Risks, Side Effects, and Their Management

Hepatic toxicity. Although there have been reports of rare, non-dose-related hepatic failure with fatalities—estimated to occur in 1 in 118,000 patients—no cases have occurred in patients older than 10 years who were receiving valproate monotherapy (Dreifuss et al. 1987, 1989). Nonetheless, baseline liver function tests are indicated. If baseline test results are normal, monitoring for clinical signs of hepatotoxicity is more important than routine monitoring of liver enzymes, which has little predictive value and may be less effective than clinical monitoring (Pellock and Willmore 1991).

Transient, mild elevations in the liver enzymes, up to three times the upper limit of normal, do not require the discontinuation of valproate. Although γ-glutamyl transferase (GGT) levels are often checked by clinicians, this test is often elevated without clinical significance in patients receiving valproate and carbamazepine (Dean and Penry 1992). Because increases in transaminase levels are often dose dependent, if there is no suitable alternative treatment, dosage reduction and careful monitoring may be attempted.

Hematological effects.   Valproate has been associated with changes in platelet count, but clinically significant thrombocytopenia has rarely been documented (Dean and Penry 1992).

Gastrointestinal side effects.   Indigestion, heartburn, and nausea are common side effects of valproate therapy. We recommend the divalproex sodium preparation to help mitigate these effects. Patients also may be encouraged to take their doses with food. The symptomatic use of histamine$_2$ blockers or famotidine is sometimes warranted. In most cases, however, dyspepsia is transient and not severe. Pancreatitis has been reported as a rare occurrence among some patients receiving relatively high doses of valproate (M.J. Murphy et al. 1981). If vomiting and severe abdominal pain develop in the context of valproate therapy, a serum amylase level should be obtained immediately.

Weight gain.   Weight gain is a common side effect of valproate treatment. Isojarvi et al. (1996) reported significant weight gain with associated hyperinsulinemia in approximately 50% of a cohort of women taking valproate. This side effect does not appear to be dose dependent. Dieting and exercise should be recommended early in treatment.

Neurological effects.   One of the most common side effects associated with valproate use is benign essential tremor. Although drowsiness is another common side effect of valproate treatment, tolerance often develops once a steady-state level of the drug is reached. In addition, once-a-day bedtime dosing often achieves symptomatic remission with less daytime sedation.

Alopecia.   Both transient and persistent hair loss have been associated with valproate use. When hair loss occurs, it often begins 3 months or longer after the initiation of treatment and is probably not dose related. Patients with valproate-induced alopecia may benefit from zinc supplementation, at a dosage of 22.5 mg/day (Hurd et al. 1984). We routinely recommend supplementation with a multivitamin preparation containing zinc and selenium at the onset of valproate treatment.

Overdose.   Valproate overdose results in increasing sedation, confusion, and ultimately coma. The patient also may manifest hyperreflexia or hyporeflexia, seizures, respiratory suppression, and superventricular tachycardia (Labar 1992). Treatment of valproate overdose should include gastric lavage, ECG monitoring, treatment of emergent seizures, and respiratory support as indicated.

Drug interactions.   Because valproate may inhibit hepatic enzymes, there is the potential for increases in the levels of other medications (Dean and Penry 1992). Valproate is also highly bound to plasma proteins and may displace other highly bound drugs from protein-binding sites. Therefore, coadministered drugs that are either highly protein bound or reliant on hepatic metabolism may require dosage adjustment.

Carbamazepine

Takezaki and Hanaoka (1971) reported that carbamazepine was effective in controlling manic behavior; the first report from the United States of its efficacy for mania was by Ballenger and Post (1980). Subsequently, evidence from controlled studies has indicated that carbamazepine is effective in both the acute and the prophylactic treatment of mania, with overall response rates comparable to those of lithium treatment (Gerner and Stanton 1992; Keck et al. 1992). There is less evidence, however, to support the efficacy of carbamazepine in the acute treatment of depression and in the prophylactic treatment of unipolar depression. In two controlled studies, carbamazepine treatment was found to be effective in a subgroup of patients with refractory depression, with response rates greater among the patients with bipolar depression than among those with unipolar depression (Post et al. 1986; Small 1990). A systematic, controlled study of the antidepressant effects of carbamazepine in a more typical group of patients with depression remains to be conducted.

Clinical Use

Carbamazepine should be initiated at a dosage of 200 mg twice a day with increments of 200 mg/day every 3–5 days. Plasma levels of 8–12 µg/mL are based on clinical use in patients with seizure disorders and do not correlate with clinical response in psychiatric disorders. We recommend dosage titration to clinical response and side effects, rather than targeting of a particular dosage or blood level. During the titration phase, patients may be particularly prone to side effects such as sedation, dizziness, and ataxia, which indicate that a more gradual titration, such as 100 mg twice a day, should be instituted. Although the maximum dosage of carbamazepine recommended by the manufacturer is 1,200 mg/day, higher dosages are frequently required on the basis of plasma level determinations and clinical response (Placidi et al. 1986; Post et al. 1984). Tegretol-XR is a sustained-release preparation that is less likely to cause gastrointestinal side effects. Generic preparations of carbamazepine are often poorly tolerated. Because carbamazepine induces its own metabolism (autoinduction), dosage adjustments may be required for weeks or months after the initiation of treatment to maintain therapeutic plasma levels (Eichelbaum et al. 1985). Some investigators have suggested that the carbamazepine metabolite carbamazepine-10,11-epoxide has a major role in the therapeutic activity of carbamazepine in affective illness, especially in the treatment of depression (Post et al. 1983).

Contraindications

Because of the potential for hematological and hepatic toxicity, carbamazepine should not be administered to patients with liver disease or thrombocytopenia or those who are at risk for agranulocytosis. For this reason, carbamazepine is strictly contraindicated in patients receiving clozapine. Because of reports of teratogenicity, including increased risks of spina bifida (Rosa 1991), microcephaly (Bertollini et al. 1987), and craniofacial defects (Jones et al. 1989), carbamazepine is relatively contraindicated for use in pregnant women. Pretreatment evaluation should include a complete blood count, an aspartate aminotransferase level, and an alanine aminotransferase level.

Risks, Side Effects, and Their Management

Hematological disorders. The most serious toxic hematological side effects of carbamazepine are agranulocytosis and aplastic anemia, either of which can be fatal. Whereas carbamazepine-induced agranulocytosis or aplastic anemia is extremely rare, now estimated to occur at a rate of 1 in 125,000 patients (Pellock 1987), leukopenia (total white blood cell count <3,000 cells/mm^3) is more common, with a prevalence of approximately 10%. Persistent leukopenia with thrombocytopenia occurs in approximately 2% of patients, and mild anemia occurs in fewer than 5% of patients. Although it is important to assess hematological function and risk factors before initiating treatment, there appears to be no benefit to ongoing monitoring in the absence of clinical indicators. When carbamazepine-induced agranulocytosis occurs, the onset is rapid, so that a normal complete blood count one day does not provide reassurance that agranulocytosis will not develop the next day. Therefore, as opposed to routine monitoring, we advise patients to call if they develop fever, sore throat, infection, petechiae, or extreme weakness and pallor. Carbamazepine should be discontinued if the absolute neutrophil count is less than 1,000.

Hepatic toxicity. Carbamazepine occasionally causes hepatic toxicity (Gram and Bentsen 1983), usually a hypersensitivity hepatitis that appears after a latency period of several weeks and is associated with elevations in aspartate aminotransferase, alanine aminotransferase, and lactic dehydrogenase (LDH). Cholestasis is also possible, with increases in bilirubin and alkaline phosphatase. Mild, transient elevations in transaminase levels generally can be monitored without discontinuation of carbamazepine. If aspartate aminotransferase or alanine aminotransferase levels increase above three times the upper limit of normal, carbamazepine should be discontinued.

Dermatological conditions. An exanthematous rash is one of the more common side effects associated with use of carbamazepine, occurring in 3%–17% of patients (Warnock and Knesevich 1988). This reaction typically begins within 2–20

weeks after the start of treatment. Carbamazepine is generally discontinued if a rash develops because of the risk of progression to an exfoliative dermatitis or Stevens-Johnson syndrome, a severe bullous form of erythema multiforme (Patterson 1985). In patients who are nonresponsive to all other mood stabilizers, carbamazepine may be reinstituted along with initial prednisone coverage (J.M. Murphy et al. 1991; Vick 1983).

Endocrinological disorders. SIADH with resultant hyponatremia may be induced by carbamazepine treatment. Alcoholic patients may be at greater risk for developing hyponatremia. If a patient taking carbamazepine develops confusion, the serum sodium level should be checked. When hyponatremia develops, it is often transient; however, even more severe cases of this condition can often be managed by fluid restriction, the addition of lithium, or use of the antibiotic demeclocycline (Brewerton and Jackson 1994).

Weight gain does not appear to be a side effect of carbamazepine therapy (Joffe et al. 1986).

Gastrointestinal disorders. Nausea and occasional vomiting are common side effects of carbamazepine, as they are with other mood stabilizers. Dosage reduction and institution of a slower titration rate help to minimize these effects.

Neurological effects. Patients may develop dizziness, drowsiness, and ataxia. These symptoms often occur at therapeutic plasma levels, especially in the early phases of treatment, and in such cases the dosage should be reduced and a slower titration schedule implemented.

Drug interactions. Carbamazepine induces hepatic cytochrome P450 enzymes, which may reduce the levels of other medications. Through the mechanism of hepatic enzyme induction, carbamazepine has been implicated in oral contraceptive failure (Coulam and Annegers 1979); therefore, women should be advised to consider alternative forms of birth control while taking carbamazepine. Similarly, medications or substances that inhibit CYP3A3/4 (discussed in the section on drug interactions later in this chapter) may result in significant elevations of plasma carbamazepine levels (Brodie and MacPhee 1986; Ketter et al. 1995).

Overdose. Carbamazepine overdose is first manifested by neuromuscular disturbances, such as nystagmus, myoclonus, and hyperreflexia, with later progression to seizures and coma. Cardiac conduction changes are possible at higher dosages. Nausea, vomiting, and urinary retention also may occur. Treatment should include induction of vomiting, gastric lavage, and supportive care. Monitoring of blood pressure and respiratory and kidney functioning should follow for several days after a serious overdose.

Lamotrigine

Lamotrigine is an anticonvulsant medication that decreases sustained high-frequency repetitive firing of the voltage-dependent sodium channel, which may then decrease glutamate release (Leach et al. 1991; MacDonald and Kelly 1995). The efficacy of lamotrigine in treating bipolar depression has been established in a double-blind, placebo-controlled trial (Calabrese et al. 1999). This multicenter study included patients with bipolar I disorder who were experiencing a major depressive episode. Participants received lamotrigine monotherapy (50 or 200 mg) or placebo for 7 weeks. The response rate was 51% in the group that received 200

mg, 41% in the group that received 50 mg, and 26% in the control group. A separate 6-month study in patients with rapid-cycling bipolar disorder reported that lamotrigine monotherapy was more effective in preventing relapse than placebo, especially in bipolar II disorder. Most recently, lamotrigine has demonstrated efficacy in preventing mood episodes in a placebo-controlled 18-month comparison with lithium (Bowden et al. 2003). These data suggest that lamotrigine may become a first-line maintenance treatment in bipolar disorder, especially for the depressive phase of the illness. However, lamotrigine has not been shown to treat acute mania.

Lamotrigine treatment is usually initiated at 25 mg once a day and increased in 25-mg increments every other week. The usual target dosage is 200 mg/day. This dosage should be reduced by half for patients who are also taking valproate and increased for those taking carbamazepine because of hepatic enzyme inhibition and induction, respectively. Lamotrigine requires slow dosage titration to minimize the risk to the patient of developing a skin rash. A maculopapular rash develops in 5% of the patients taking lamotrigine, usually within the first 4 weeks of treatment. Stevens-Johnson syndrome may occur, with an estimated risk of 1 in 1,000 patient years (Richens 1994). Stevens-Johnson syndrome is potentially fatal. It is essential to advise patients of this risk and to emphasize that they should call the office immediately if they develop a rash. Development of a rash with concomitant systemic symptoms is a particularly ominous sign and should be evaluated immediately.

Although lamotrigine is generally well tolerated by most patients, common early side effects include headache, dizziness, gastrointestinal distress, and blurred or double vision.

Treatment of Mania

The first step in treating mania is to initiate treatment with a mood stabilizer. Risperidone, quetiapine, and aripiprazole may soon be approved for use in acute mania. Currently lithium, valproate, and olanzapine are indicated as monotherapy agents for the treatment of mania. Valproate appears to be particularly effective for patients with mixed mania and depression (Swann et al. 1997). The efficacy of atypical antipsychotics in the treatment of mania is independent of the presence or absence of psychotic symptoms.

Other factors to consider in selecting a mood stabilizer include previous response to treatment, family history of response to a particular agent, side effects, concomitant medical problems, and concurrent medications. Lithium and valproate both cause gastrointestinal side effects, weight gain, and tremor. Olanzapine is also associated with weight gain and rarely with impaired glucose metabolism (as discussed earlier in this chapter). Starting dosages and rapidity of titration depend on balancing the clinical need for rapid control of symptoms, which dictates faster titration, with the improved tolerability of slower dose escalations.

Conventional antipsychotics should be avoided because they are associated with a greater degree of EPS and tardive dyskinesia compared with the atypical antipsychotics.

When patients fail to respond to a single agent, the next step is to combine medications. Adding a second agent is preferred to substituting one mood stabilizer for another, unless there was a toxic or allergic reaction to the first drug. If these combinations prove ineffective, preliminary data suggest that clozapine is an effective mood stabilizer, even in nonpsychotic patients (Suppes et al. 1992). ECT is an ef-

fective treatment for acute mania and is especially useful for patients who cannot safely wait until medication becomes effective (Hirschfeld et al. 1994). In addition, myriad other medications are being studied for the treatment of bipolar disorder, most often for the manic phase of the illness. Studies are under way to evaluate other anticonvulsants and atypical antipsychotic medications. To date, there are case reports regarding the use of these other agents but not peer-reviewed controlled clinical trial data. The importance of not assuming that all anticonvulsants are effective is illustrated by two negative controlled trials of gabapentin in the treatment of bipolar disorder (Frye et al. 2000), despite numerous positive case reports.

Bipolar Depression

Treatment

A common mistake is to treat bipolar depression in the same manner as unipolar depression, overlooking the need for a mood stabilizer. In bipolar depression, the first pharmacological intervention should be to start or optimize treatment with a mood stabilizer rather than to start an antidepressant medication.

Unless treatment history or comorbid medical problems dictate otherwise, lithium continues to be a first-line treatment for bipolar depression. The response rate to lithium in bipolar depression is 79% (Zornberg and Pope 1993). The efficacy of lamotrigine in treating bipolar depression has been shown in a double-blind, placebo-controlled trial (Calabrese et al. 1999). Lamotrigine can be combined with lithium, valproate, or carbamazepine. As noted earlier in this chapter, lower doses of lamotrigine are started, and the dose titration is more gradual when this medication is added to valproate.

If treatment with a single mood stabilizer is ineffective, some experts recommend adding a second mood stabilizer, whereas others recommend careful addition of an antidepressant (Sachs et al. 2000). Although the switch rate into mania or induction of rapid cycling by antidepressants is controversial (Peet 1994; Wehr and Goodwin 1987), these agents do appear to present a risk for some patients, often with devastating consequences. Controlled comparative data on the use of specific antidepressant drugs in the treatment of bipolar depression are sparse. Current treatment guidelines extrapolate from these few studies and rely heavily on anecdotal clinical experience. Overall, TCAs should be avoided when other viable treatment options exist. ECT, as discussed later in this chapter, should be considered in severe cases.

Prophylaxis

Patients with bipolar disorder require life-long prophylaxis with a mood stabilizer, both to prevent new illness episodes and to reduce the likelihood that the illness will progress to a more malignant course. Ninety percent of bipolar patients relapse on stopping lithium, most within 6 months (Suppes et al. 1991). In addition to the single episode that may occur, each episode may further kindle the illness, thereby inducing a more malignant course of illness with decreased treatment responsiveness. The more episodes a patient has had, the less likely he or she is to respond to treatment (Gelenberg et al. 1989).

Drug Interactions

Pharmacokinetic Interactions

Cytochrome P450 Enzymes

Clinically significant drug interactions are most commonly caused by changes in drug metabolism. Cytochrome P450 enzymes metabolize all psychotropic drugs, except lithium. These enzymes are a heterogeneous group of mixed-function oxidases found predominantly in the liver and, to varying degrees, in the gut and brain. These enzymes catalyze the oxidative metabolism of a large number of drugs as well as many other endogenous and exogenous substances.

If one of these enzymes is inhibited by another drug, the result is an increase in the plasma level of concurrently administered drugs that rely on the enzyme for metabolism. Table 18–18 provides a list of the better-recognized and clinically important substrates and inhibitors for each of the cytochrome P450 enzymes. In most cases, enzyme inhibitors and substrates can be safely combined, provided the dosage of the substrate is lowered if needed.

In general, enzyme inhibition is competitive and depends on both the relative concentration of the inhibitor and its affinity for the enzyme. The effects of inhibitors are relatively rapid (minutes to hours) and are reversible within a time frame that depends on the half-life of the inhibitor. There is a large amount of inter-individual variation in drug metabolism and the propensity for enzyme inhibition to alter metabolism. Part of this variation is the result of genetic polymorphism (Shimada et al. 1994), which is a heritable alteration in the enzyme.

In addition, the cytochrome P450 enzymes can be induced (Watkins et al. 1985). Cytochrome P450 enzyme induction causes the liver to produce a greater amount of the enzyme, which can increase elimination and reduce plasma levels of a second drug or its metabolites. When clinically relevant, the drug dosage should be increased to achieve the same serum concentration. The effects of inducers tend to be delayed days to weeks because this process involves enzyme synthesis. Barbiturates, carbamazepine, phenytoin, rifampin,

TABLE 18–18. Partial list of clinically relevant cytochrome P450 (CYP) substrates and inhibitors

Enzyme	CYP1A2	CYP2C9/10	CYP2C19	CYP2D6	CYP3A3/4/5
Substrates[a]	Aminophylline Amitriptyline Caffeine Clozapine (in part) Imipramine Methadone Olanzapine Propranolol Tacrine Theophylline Verapamil	Phenytoin Warfarin	Barbiturates Diazepam Divalproex	Most antipsychotics Codeine Donepezil Encainide Flecainide Galantamine Lipophilic β-blockers Mexiletine Oxycodone TCAs[c] Tramadol Trazodone Type IC antiarrhythmics Venlafaxine	Acetaminophen Alprazolam Amiodarone Antiarrhythmics Buspirone Calcium channel blockers Carbamazepine Cyclosporine Donepezil Ethosuximide Galantamine Lamotrigine Lidocaine Midazolam Oral contraceptives Oxcarbazine Pimozide Propafenone Protease inhibitors Quinidine Statins Steroids Tamoxifen Triazolam
Inhibitors[b]	Cimetidine Ciprofloxacin Enoxacin Fluvoxamine Grapefruit juice Ketoconazole Norfloxacin	Cimetidine Fluoxetine Fluvoxamine Modafinil Ritonavir	Fluoxetine Fluvoxamine	Bupropion Cimetidine Duloxetine Fluoxetine Paroxetine Phenothiazines Quinidine Ritonavir Sertraline	Diltiazem Fluvoxamine Grapefruit juice Imidazole antifungal agents (e.g., ketoconazole) Some macrolides antibiotics Nefazodone Protease inhibitors Verapamil

Note. TCA = tricyclic antidepressant.
[a]Medications and substances metabolized by a given enzyme. [b]May increase levels of substrates. [c]The 2D6 enzyme is the final common pathway for the metabolism of TCAs.
Source. Adapted from Callahan et al. 1996.

dexamethasone, smoking, and chronic alcohol use all induce cytochrome P450 enzymes.

Protein Binding

Medications are distributed to their sites of action through the circulatory system. In the bloodstream, all the psychotropic medications except lithium are bound to plasma proteins to varying degrees. A drug is considered highly protein bound if more than 90% is bound to plasma proteins. A reversible equilibrium exists between the bound and unbound drug; the unbound fraction is pharmacologically active, whereas the bound fraction is inactive and therefore cannot be metabolized or excreted. When two drugs exist simultaneously in the plasma, competition for protein-binding sites occurs. This can cause displacement of the previously protein-bound drug, which in the free state becomes pharmacologically active. Interactions that occur by this mechanism are called *protein-binding interactions*. They are transient because, although the plasma concentration of free drug initially increases, the drug then becomes subject to redistribution, metabolism, and excretion, producing a new steady-state concentration. This type of interaction is generally not clinically significant unless the drugs involved are highly protein bound (which results in a large change in plasma concentration of free drug from a small amount of drug displacement) and have a low therapeutic index or narrow therapeutic window (in which case small changes in plasma levels can result in toxicity or loss of efficacy (Callahan et al. 1996).

Absorption and Excretion

Changes in plasma level as a result of alterations in absorption or excretion are less common with psychiatric medications. Drugs with anticholinergic effects, such as TCAs, tend to decrease gastrointestinal motility, which allows for longer periods of absorption of other medications (Greiff and Rowbotham 1994). Prolonged absorption may result in increased plasma levels of concomitantly administered medications. Changes in drug plasma concentration as a result of changes in excretion are those most germane to lithium, which is dependent on renal excretion. Any medication that alters the kidney's excretion of lithium may result in clinically significant changes in the serum lithium level (as reviewed by Goodwin and Jamison 1990). These medications are listed in Table 18–18.

Pharmacodynamic Interactions

Pharmacodynamic interactions involve a change in the pharmacological effect of a drug resulting from the action of a second drug at a common receptor or bioactive site. These interactions can be mediated directly or indirectly. Direct pharmacodynamic interactions involve agonist or antagonist actions of two drugs at a common site, which produces increased (additive) or decreased pharmacological effects. Such interactions generally result from known pharmacological actions of a drug, and for this reason agents with a multiplicity of pharmacological effects are more likely to be involved. For example, low-potency antipsychotics and tertiary amine TCAs have anticholinergic, antihistaminic, α-adrenergic antagonist, and quinidine-like effects. In light of this, it can be predicted that the concurrent administration of chlorpromazine and imipramine will result in additive sedation, constipation, postural hypotension, and depression of cardiac conduction.

Indirect interactions involve changes in physiological functions caused by the combined action of two drugs at a common site. These interactions cannot be predicted on the basis of known pharmacological effects, and their mechanisms are poorly understood. Many indirect pharmacodynamic interactions have clinically significant consequences. For example, the adjunctive use of lithium with various antidepressant agents can potentiate antidepressant effects (synergism). On the other hand, the concurrent administration of a serotonin reuptake inhibitor or meperidine with an MAOI can produce a potentially lethal hypermetabolic reaction.

Antiaggression Drugs

Overview

Aggressive and violent behaviors are frequently encountered in patients with underlying disorders as diverse as traumatic brain injury; brain tumor; hereditary or metabolic brain disease; mental retardation; dementia; seizure disorders; sequelae of CNS infections; sequelae of substance abuse; DSM-IV (American Psychiatric Association 1994) Axis I psychiatric disorders such as schizophrenia, bipolar disorder, and conduct disorder; and Axis II personality disorders such as antisocial and borderline personality disorders (Anderson and Silver 1999; Silver and Yudofsky 1987).

In establishing a treatment plan for patients with agitation or aggression, the overarching principle is that diagnosis comes before treatment. The history of the development of symptoms in a biopsychosocial context is usually the most critical part of the evaluation. It is essential to determine the mental status of the patient before the agitated or aggressive event, the nature of the precipitant, the physical and social environment in which the behavior occurs, the ways in which the event is mitigated, and the primary and secondary gains related to agitation and

aggression (Corrigan et al. 1993; Silver and Yudofsky 1994; Yudofsky et al. 1998).

Although no medication has been approved by the FDA specifically for the treatment of aggression, medications are widely used (and commonly misused) in the management of acute or chronic aggression. We divide the use of pharmacological interventions for aggression into two major categories: 1) the use of the sedating effects of medications, as required in acute or severe situations, so that the patient does not harm himself or herself or others, and 2) the use of nonsedating medications for the treatment of chronic aggression (Corrigan et al. 1993; Silver and Yudofsky 1994; Yudofsky et al. 1998).

Acute Aggression and Agitation

Antipsychotic Drugs

Antipsychotics are the most commonly used medications in the treatment of aggression. Although use of these agents is appropriate and effective when aggression is derivative of active psychosis, the use of antipsychotic agents to treat chronic aggression, especially secondary to organic brain injury, is often ineffective and entails risks that the patient will develop serious complications. Usually, it is the sedative side effects rather than the antipsychotic properties of antipsychotics that are used (i.e., misused) to "treat" (i.e., mask) the aggression. Often, patients will develop tolerance to the sedative effects of the medication and, therefore, will require increasing doses. As a result, especially with the older conventional antipsychotic medications, extrapyramidal and anticholinergic-related side effects occur. Paradoxically (and frequently), because of the development of akathisia, the patient may become more agitated and restless as the dose of neuroleptic is increased, especially when a high-potency antipsychotic such as haloperidol is administered. The akathisia is often mistaken for increased irritability and agitation, and a vicious cycle of increasing neuroleptic doses and worsening akathisia occurs.

In patients with acute aggression, we recommend starting a high-potency antipsychotic such as risperidone at low dosages of 0.5 mg orally with repeated administration every hour until control of aggression is achieved. If intramuscular medication were required, haloperidol would be used. If after several administrations of risperidone the patient's aggressive behavior does not improve, the hourly dose may be increased until the patient is sedated sufficiently that he or she no longer shows agitation or violence. Once the patient is not aggressive for 48 hours, the daily dosage should be decreased gradually (i.e., by 25% each day) to ascertain whether aggressive behavior reemerges. In this case, the clinician must decide whether it is best to increase the dose of risperidone or to initiate treatment with a more specific antiaggressive drug. Chronic use of antipsychotics to treat aggression is only indicated if the aggression is due to a psychotic disorder.

Sedatives and Hypnotics

The literature is inconsistent on the effects of the benzodiazepines in the treatment of aggression. The sedative properties of benzodiazepines are especially helpful in the management of acute agitation and aggression.

For treatment of acute aggression, lorazepam 1–2 mg may be administered every hour by either oral or intramuscular route until sedation is achieved (Silver and Yudofsky 1994). Intramuscular lorazepam has been suggested as an effective medication in the emergency treatment of the violent patient (Bick and Hannah 1986). Intravenous lorazepam is also effective, although the onset of action is similar when administered intramuscularly. Caution must be taken with intravenous administration, and it should be injected in doses less than 1 cc (1 mg) per minute to avoid laryngospasm. As is done with neuroleptics, gradual tapering of lorazepam may be attempted when the patient has been in control for 48 hours. If aggressive behavior recurs, medications for the treatment of chronic aggression may be initiated. Lorazepam in 1- or 2-mg doses, administered either orally or by injection, may be given, if necessary, in combination with an antipsychotic medication (risperidone 1–2 mg). Other sedating medications such as paraldehyde, chloral hydrate, or diphenhydramine may be preferable to sedative antipsychotic agents.

Chronic Aggression

Antianxiety Medications

Serotonin appears to be a key neurotransmitter in the modulation of aggressive behavior. In preliminary reports, buspirone, a 5-HT$_{1A}$ agonist, has been reported to be effective in the management of aggression and agitation for patients with head injury, dementia, and developmental disabilities and autism (Silver and Yudofsky 1994). We usually initiate buspirone at 7.5 mg twice a day for 1 week and then increase the dosage to 15 mg twice a day. Dosages of 45–60 mg/day may be required before there is improvement in aggressive behavior, although we have noted dramatic improvement within 1 week.

Anticonvulsants

Several open studies have indicated that carbamazepine may be effective in decreasing aggressive behavior associated with traumatic brain injury dementia (Chatham-Showalter 1996), developmental disabilities, schizophrenia, and a variety of other organic brain disorders (Silver and Yudofsky 1994; Yudofsky et al. 1998). Carbamazepine can be a highly effective medication to treat aggression in the brain-injured patient.

In our experience and that of others, the anticonvulsant valproic acid also may be helpful to some patients with organically induced aggression (Geracioti 1994; Giakas et al. 1990; Mattes 1992; Wroblewski et al. 1997). For patients with aggression and epilepsy whose seizures are being treated with anticonvulsant drugs such as phenytoin and phenobarbital, switching to carbamazepine or to valproic acid may treat both conditions.

Lithium

Although lithium is known to be effective in controlling aggression related to manic excitement, many studies suggest that it also may have a role in the treatment of aggression in selected, nonbipolar patient populations. Included are patients with traumatic brain injury (Bellus et al. 1996), patients with mental retardation who have self-injurious or aggressive behavior, children and adolescents with behavior disorders, prison inmates, and patients with other organic brain syndromes.

Patients with brain injury have increased sensitivity to the neurotoxic effects of lithium (Hornstein and Seliger 1989; Moskowitz and Altshuler 1991). Because of lithium's potential for neurotoxicity and its relative lack of efficacy in many patients with aggression secondary to brain injury, we limit the use of lithium to those patients whose aggression is related to manic effects or recurrent irritability related to cyclic mood disorders.

Antidepressants

The antidepressants that have been reported to control aggressive behaviors are those that act on serotonin. The dosages used are similar to those used for the treatment of mood lability and depression.

We have evaluated and treated many patients with emotional lability that is characterized by frequent episodes of tearfulness and irritability and the full symptomatic picture of neuroaggressive syndrome (Silver and Yudofsky 1994). These patients, who would be diagnosed according to DSM-IV-TR as having "personality change, labile type, due to traumatic brain injury," have responded well to antidepressants.

Antihypertensive Medications: β-Blockers

Since the first report of the use of β-adrenergic receptor blockers in the treatment of acute aggression in 1977, more than 25 articles have appeared in the neurological and psychiatric literature reporting experience in using β-blockers with more than 200 patients with aggression (Yudofsky et al. 1987). Most of these patients had been unsuccessfully treated with antipsychotics, minor tranquilizers, lithium, and/or anticonvulsants before treatment with β-blockers. The β-blockers that have been investigated in controlled prospective studies include propranolol (a lipid-soluble, nonselective receptor antagonist), nadolol (a water-soluble, nonselective receptor antagonist), and pindolol (a lipid-soluble, nonselective β-receptor antagonist with partial sympathomimetic activity). A growing body of preliminary evidence suggests that β-adrenergic receptor blockers are effective agents for the treatment of aggressive and violent behaviors, particularly those related to organic brain syndrome. The effectiveness of propranolol in reducing agitation has been confirmed during the initial hospitalization after traumatic brain injury (Brooke et al. 1992). When a patient requires the use of a once-a-day medication because of compliance difficulties, long-acting propranolol (i.e., Inderal LA) or nadolol can be used. When patients develop bradycardia that prevents the prescribing of therapeutic dosages of propranolol, pindolol can be substituted, using one-tenth the dosage of propranolol. Pindolol's intrinsic sympathomimetic activity stimulates the β receptor and restricts the development of bradycardia.

The major side effects of β-blockers when used to treat aggression are a lowering of blood pressure and pulse rate. Because peripheral β receptors are fully blocked in doses of 300–400 mg/day, further decreases in these vital signs usually do not occur even when doses are increased to much higher levels. Despite reports of depression with the use of β-blockers, controlled trials and our experience indicate that it is a rare occurrence. Because the use of propranolol is associated with significant increases in plasma levels of thioridazine, which has an absolute dosage ceiling of 800 mg/day, the combination of these two medications should be avoided whenever possible.

Conclusions

Table 18–19 summarizes our recommendations for the use of various classes of medication in the treatment of chronic aggressive disorders associated with traumatic brain injury. Acute aggression may be treated by using the sedative properties of neuroleptics or benzodiazepines. In treating aggression, the clinician, when possible, should diagnose and treat underlying disorders and use, when possible, antiaggressive agents specific to those disorders. When there is partial response after a therapeutic trial with a specific medication, adjunctive treatment with a medication that has a different mechanism of ac-

tion should be instituted. For example, a patient with partial response to β-blockers can have additional improvement with the addition of an anticonvulsant.

Electroconvulsive Therapy

Overview

ECT is the use of electrically induced repetitive firings of the neurons in the CNS (i.e., grand mal seizures) to treat psychiatric illnesses such as depression or mania and psychiatric symptoms such as psychosis or catatonia. Although ECT was first used in the late 1930s, before the era of potent psychopharmacological treatment of major mood disorders, the treatment today remains clinically relevant because of its high degree of efficacy, safety, and usefulness.

Mechanisms of Action

The mechanisms of action of ECT are complex and not completely understood. In studies involving both humans and animals, ECT has been found to affect serotonin, GABA, endogenous opiates and their receptors, and catecholamines (including dopamine, norepinephrine, and epinephrine and their receptors).

Indications

The principal diagnostic indication for ECT is major depression, especially when a rapid response is needed for either medical or psychiatric reasons (American Psychiatric Association 2001).

ECT also may be of benefit in the treatment of mania that is not responsive to medications (Small et al. 1986). Patients with schizophrenia who have affective and catatonic symptoms may have a beneficial response to ECT; however, there is no indication that ECT alters the

TABLE 18–19. Pharmacotherapy for aggression and agitation

	Drug	Primary indication
Acute agitation/ severe aggression	High-potency antipsychotic drugs (haloperidol, risperidone) Benzodiazepines (lorazepam)	
Chronic agitation	Atypical antipsychotics (risperidone, olanzapine, quetiapine, clozapine)	Psychosis
	Valproic acid, carbamazepine, ?gabapentin	Seizure disorder, severe aggression
	Serotonergic antidepressants (SSRIs, trazodone)	Depression, mood lability
	Buspirone	Anxiety
	β-Blockers	Aggression without concomitant neuropsychiatric sequelae

Note. SSRI = selective serotonin reuptake inhibitor.

fundamental psychopathology of schizophrenia (Small et al. 1986).

Contraindications

There are relatively few contraindications to ECT (American Psychiatric Association 2001). First, patients with clinically significant space-occupying cerebral lesions or conditions with increased intracranial pressure must not receive this treatment because of the risk of brain stem herniation (Maltbie et al. 1980). Second, patients with significant cardiovascular problems, such as recent myocardial infarction, severe cardiac ischemia, and moderate to severe hypertension (including pheochromocytoma), are more prone to the transient fluctuations in the cardiovascular system that occur during and shortly after ECT. Such patients may or may not safely be given ECT, and they must be evaluated before treatment by a cardiologist familiar with the potential side effects of ECT. Patients with recent intracerebral hemorrhage are at increased risk, as are those with bleeding or unstable vascular aneurysm or abnormalities, or with retinal detachment.

Technique

Anesthesia and Muscle Relaxation

ECT is used primarily for psychiatric inpatients, and it is common for an anesthetist or anesthesiologist to assist the psychiatrist in administering the treatment. The APA Task Force on Electroconvulsive Therapy (American Psychiatric Association 2001) recommended pretreatment with an anticholinergic drug such as atropine (0.4–1.0 mg iv) or glycopyrrolate (0.2–0.4 mg intravenously) to decrease the morbidity of cardiac bradyarrhythmias and aspiration. General anesthesia is induced only to the degree that a light coma is produced, using a fast-acting anesthetic such as methohexital, which has fewer cardiac side effects than slower-acting barbiturates such as thiopental. A starting dose of approximately 0.75–1.0 mg/kg of intravenous methohexital is recommended, but the amount required to induce safe and brief anesthesia may vary from considerably lower to considerably higher amounts depending on the patient's metabolism of the drug. Once the patient is anesthetized, intravenous succinylcholine is used for muscular relaxation.

In general, approximately 0.5–1 mg/kg of intravenous succinylcholine is administered rapidly, immediately after the onset of general anesthesia. If there are preexisting skeletal problems or other orthopedic problems, a higher dose of succinylcholine may be required, whereas a history or evidence of pseudocholinesterase deficiency would call for a lower dose. Once the succinylcholine is administered, the patient is ventilated with 100% oxygen until muscle fasciculations occur and motoric relaxation of the patient is accomplished. Modern ECT devices allow for simultaneous monitoring of the EEG and ECG before, during, and after the ECT procedure. In addition, there should be frequent monitoring of blood pressure, pulse rate, and blood oxygen saturation (with pulse oximetry).

Parameters

Electrodes may be placed unilaterally on the nondominant hemisphere (i.e., the electrodes over the right hemisphere for a right-handed individual) or bilaterally. Although there have been observations that unilateral electrode placement is related to fewer cognitive side effects compared with bilateral stimulus, studies also have suggested that unilateral placement is less efficacious if comparable stimulus doses are used (Abrams 1986; American Psychiatric Association 1990; Malitz and Sackeim 1986; Sackeim et al. 1993). Recent studies that used higher-dose unilateral ECT reported improved efficacy. Sackeim et al. (2000) randomized 80 depressed patients to right unilateral ECT, with an electrical dosage 50%, 150%, or 500% above the seizure threshold, or bilateral ECT, with an electrical dosage 150% above the threshold. In this study, high-dose right unilateral ECT and bilateral ECT were equally effective (response rate = 65%), and both were approximately twice as effective as low- or moderate-

dose ECT. High-dose right unilateral ECT produced less severe cognitive side effects than did bilateral ECT. A separate study by McCall et al. (2000) produced very similar results; specifically, fixed-dose right unilateral ECT produced a higher antidepressant response rate than lower stimulus parameters. Increased stimulation resulted in an increased response rate (stimulations up to 8–12 times the seizure threshold). Unfortunately, higher electrical dosages also were equated with greater cognitive problems.

Course of Treatment

In the United States, ECT treatments are generally given on an every-other-day basis for 2–3 weeks, usually Monday, Wednesday, and Friday. Twice-weekly treatments may be equally effective with fewer cognitive side effects but with a slower onset of action (Lerer et al. 1995). Duration of seizure for longer than 20 seconds per treatment (as assessed by motor activity, not EEG seizure activity) is considered adequate for therapeutic purposes. The number of treatments administered is generally determined by a patient's clinical response; the therapy is discontinued when successive treatments do not elicit further beneficial effects (Weiner 1979). With depressed patients, a typical course of ECT consists of 6–10 treatments, but sometimes more are required. We do not recommend more than 20 treatments in a single course of ECT.

Risks and Side Effects

In general, ECT is an unusually safe procedure, with morbidity and mortality not significantly greater than that associated with general anesthesia. The mortality rate of patients with ECT is 2 per 100,000 treatments (Fink 1978). The most frequent complaints of patients are memory impairment, headaches, and muscle aches

(Gomez 1975); the most significant risks associated with ECT are cardiovascular and intracerebral (Abrams 1992).

Medical Risks

Ictal and postictal fluctuations in autonomic tone can elicit cardiac arrhythmias of many varieties, including premature ventricular contractions during the immediate postictal period. Increase in vagal tone may result in sinus bradycardia or sinus arrest, whereas increases in sympathetic tone can elicit ventricular ectopy and increases in blood pressure and heart rate (Abrams 1992).

Memory Impairment

The initial confusion and cognitive deficits associated with ECT treatment are usually temporary, lasting approximately 30 minutes. Whereas many patients report no problems with their memory, aside from the time immediately surrounding the ECT treatments, others report that their memory is not as good as it was before receiving ECT (Squire and Slater 1983).

Post-ECT Prophylactic Treatment

Despite the acute efficacy of ECT, appropriate prophylactic treatment must be instituted after ECT to prevent relapse. Most commonly, antidepressant medications are used for this purpose. Unfortunately, many patients who receive ECT have been previously nonresponsive to standard antidepressant medications, and the efficacy of these treatments post-ECT is not clear (Sackeim et al. 1990). In such patients, lithium carbonate may be a useful agent for continuation therapy (Coppen et al. 1981; Perry and Tsuang 1979; Shapira et al. 1995). In a recent controlled study, the combination of nortriptyline and lithium resulted in a 39% relapse rate after 24 weeks, compared with 60% for

nortriptyline alone and 84% for those who received placebo following response to ECT (Sackeim et al. 2001). For patients who fail to respond to other prophylactic therapies, maintenance ECT (i.e., an outpatient treatment every week to every several weeks) may be effective (Schwarz et al. 1995).

Conclusions

After more than 50 years of use, ECT remains a safe, specific, and effective treatment regimen in psychiatry. The treatment is particularly effective in patients with severe depressions, including those that have delusional, suicidal, or psychomotor components. It is important, as it is concerning all somatic interventions in psychiatry, that ECT be recognized as a specific therapeutic tool that is only one component of a larger treatment plan and that includes psychosocial and other biological interventions. Adequate time must be allocated to discuss the risks, benefits, side effects, and overall experience of the procedure with patients and their families and to answer their questions.

References

Abernethy DR, Greenblatt DJ, Ochs HR, et al: Benzodiazepine drug-drug interactions commonly occurring in clinical practice. Curr Med Res Opin 8 (suppl 4):80–93, 1984

Abrams R: Is unilateral electroconvulsive therapy really the treatment of choice in endogenous depression? Ann N Y Acad Sci 462:50–55, 1986

Abrams R: Electroconvulsive Therapy, 2nd Edition. New York, Oxford University Press, 1992

Adler LA, Peselow E, Rotrosen J, et al: Vitamin E in the treatment of tardive dyskinesia. Am J Psychiatry 150:1405–1407, 1993

Adler LA, Edson R, Lavori P, et al: Long-term treatment effects of vitamin E for tardive dyskinesia. Biol Psychiatry 43:868–872, 1998

Aherwadker SJ, Eferdigil MC, Coulshed N: Chlorpromazine therapy and associated acute disturbances of cardiac rhythm. Br Heart J 36:1251–1252, 1964

Akhtar S, Jajor TR, Kumar S: Vitamin E in the treatment of tardive dyskinesia. J Postgrad Med 39:124–126, 1993

Akiskal HS: Depression in cyclothymic and related temperaments: clinical and pharmacologic considerations (monograph). J Clin Psychiatry 10:37–43, 1992

Akiskal HS, Khani MK, Scott-Strauss A: Cyclothymic temperamental disorders. Psychiatr Clin North Am 2:527–554, 1979

Allison DB, Mentore JL, Heo M, et al: Antipsychotic-induced weight gain: a comprehensive research synthesis. Am J Psychiatry 156:1686–1696, 1999

Alvir JMJ, Lieberman JA: Agranulocytosis: incidence and risk factors. J Clin Psychiatry 55 (suppl B):137–138, 1994

Alvir JMJ, Lieberman JA, Safferman AZ: Clozapine-induced agranulocytosis: incidence and risk factors in the United States. N Engl J Med 329:162–167, 1993

American Psychiatric Association: Benzodiazepine Dependence, Toxicity, and Abuse: A Task Force Report of the American Psychiatric Association. Washington, DC, American Psychiatric Association, 1990

American Psychiatric Association: Tardive Dyskinesia: A Task Force Report of the American Psychiatric Association. Washington, DC, American Psychiatric Association, 1992

American Psychiatric Association: Practice Guidelines for Major Depressive Disorder in Adults. Washington, DC, American Psychiatric Association, 1993

American Psychiatric Association: Diagnostic and Statistical Manual of Mental Disorders, 4th Edition. Washington, DC, American Psychiatric Association, 1994

American Psychiatric Association: Practice guideline for the treatment of patients with schizophrenia. Am J Psychiatry 154 (suppl):1–63, 1997

American Psychiatric Association: Diagnostic and Statistical Manual of Mental Disorders, 4th Edition, Text Revision. Washington, DC, American Psychiatric Association, 2000

American Psychiatric Association: The Practice of Electroconvulsive Therapy: Recommendations for Treatment, Training, and Privileging. A Task Force Report of the American Psychiatric Association, 2nd Edition. Edited by Weiner RD. Washington, DC, American Psychiatric Association, 2001

Amsterdam JD, Brunswick DJ, Mendels J: The clinical application of tricyclic antidepressant pharmacokinetics and plasma levels. Am J Psychiatry 137:653–662, 1980

Amsterdam J, Berwish NJ: High dose tranylcypromine therapy for refractory depression. Pharmacopsychiatry 22:21–25, 1989

Anath J, Dubin SE: Lithium and symptomatic hyperparathyroidism. J R Soc Med 96:1026–1029, 1983

Anderson ES, Powers PS: Neuroleptic malignant syndrome associated with clozapine use. J Clin Psychiatry 52:102–104, 1991

Anderson KA, Silver JM: Neurological diseases and medical diseases, in Medical Management of the Violent Patient: Clinical Assessment and Therapy. Edited by Tardiff K. New York, Marcel Dekker, 1999, pp 87–124

Angst J: Natural history and epidemiology of depression, in Results of Community Studies in Prediction and Treatment of Recurrent Depression. Edited by Cobb J, Goeting N. Southampton, England, Duphar Medical Relations, 1990

Appleton WS, Davis JM: Practical Clinical Psychopharmacology, 2nd Edition. Baltimore, MD, Williams & Wilkins, 1980

Arana GW, Goff DC, Friedman H, et al: Does carbamazepine-induced reduction of plasma haloperidol levels worsen psychotic symptoms? Am J Psychiatry 143:650–651, 1986

Arana GW, Goff DC, Baldessarini RJ, et al: Efficacy of anticholinergic prophylaxis for neuroleptic-induced acute dystonia. Am J Psychiatry 145:993–996, 1988

Aranow A, Hudson J, Pope HG Jr, et al: Elevated antidepressant plasma levels after addition of fluoxetine. Am J Psychiatry 148:911–913, 1989

Armitage R, Rush AJ, Trivedi M, et al: The effects of nefazodone on sleep architecture in depression. Neuropsychopharmacology 10:123–127, 1994

Arvanitis LA, Miller BG: Multiple fixed doses of "Seroquel" (quetiapine) in patients with acute exacerbation of schizophrenia: a comparison with haloperidol and placebo. (The Seroquel Trial 13 Study Group.) Biol Psychiatry 42:233–246, 1997

Ashton H: Protracted withdrawal syndromes from benzodiazepines. J Subst Abuse Treat 8:19–28, 1991

Ashton AK, Bennett RG: Sildenafil treatment of serotonin reuptake inhibitor–induced sexual dysfunction. J Clin Psychiatry 60: 194–195, 1999

Baldessarini R: Chemotherapy in Psychiatry: Principles and Practice. Cambridge, MA, Harvard University Press, 1985

Baldessarini RJ, Cohen BM, Teicher MH: Significance of neuroleptic dose and plasma level in the pharmacological treatment of psychoses. Arch Gen Psychiatry 45:79–91, 1988

Bakris GL, Smith DW, Tiwari S: Dermatologic manifestations of lithium: a review. Int J Psychiatry Med 10:327–331, 1980–1981

Ball WA, Caroff SN: Retinopathy, tardive dyskinesia, and low-dose thioridazine (letter). Am J Psychiatry 143:256–257, 1986

Ballenger JC, Post RM: Carbamazepine in manic-depressive illness: a new treatment. Am J Psychiatry 137:782–790, 1980

Ballenger JC, Wheadon DE, Steiner M, et al: Double-blind, fixed-dose, placebo-controlled study of paroxetine in the treatment of panic disorder. Am J Psychiatry 155:36–42, 1998

Balon R, Berchou R: Hematologic side effects of psychotropic drugs. Psychosomatics 27:119–127, 1986

Ban TA, St. Jean A: The effects of phenothiazines on the electrocardiogram. Canadian Medical Association Journal 91:537–540, 1964

Barnas C, Zwierzina H, Hummer M, et al: Granulocyte-macrophage colony-stimulating factor (GM-CSF) treatment of clozapine-induced agranulocytosis: a case report. J Clin Psychiatry 53:245–247, 1992

Bauer MS, Whybrow PC, Winokur A: Rapid cycling bipolar affective disorder, I: association with grade I hypothyroidism. Arch Gen Psychiatry 47:427–432, 1990

Beasley CM Jr, Masica DN, Heiligenstein JH, et al: Possible monoamine oxidase inhibitor-serotonin uptake inhibitor interaction: fluoxetine clinical data and preclinical findings. J Clin Psychopharmacol 13:312–320, 1993

Beasley CM, Tollefson G, Tran P, et al: Olanzapine versus placebo and haloperidol: acute phase results of the Northern American double-blind olanzapine trial. Neuropsychopharmacology 14:111–123, 1996

Bellus SB, Stewart D, Vergo JG, et al: The use of lithium in the treatment of aggressive behaviors with two brain-injured individuals in a state psychiatric hospital. Brain Injury 10:849–860, 1996

Belmaker RH, Lerer B, Klein E, et al: Clinical implications of research on the mechanism of action of lithium. Prog Neuropsychopharmacol Biol Psychiatry 7:287–296, 1983

Bertollini R, Kallen B, Mastroiacovo P, et al: Anticonvulsant drugs in monotherapy: effect on the fetus. Eur J Epidemiol 3:164–171, 1987

Bick PA, Hannah AL: Intramuscular lorazepam to restrain violent patients (letter). Lancet 1:206, 1986

Bitran JA, Manji HK, Potter WZ, et al: Down-regulation of PKC alpha by lithium in vitro. Psychopharmacol Bull 31:449–452, 1995

Black B, Uhde TW, Tancer ME: Fluoxetine for the treatment of social phobia (letter). J Clin Psychopharmacol 12:293–295, 1992

Boehnert MT, Lovejoy FH: Value of the QRS duration versus the serum drug level in predicting seizures and ventricular arrhythmias after an acute overdose of tricyclic antidepressants. N Engl J Med 313:474–479, 1985

Bourin M, Baker GB: The future of antidepressants. Biomed Pharmacother 50:7–12, 1996

Bouwer CD, Harvey BH: Phasic craving for carbohydrate observed with citalopram. Int Clin Psychopharmacol 11:273–278, 1996

Bowden CL, Brugger AM, Swann AC, et al: Efficacy of divalproex vs lithium and placebo in the treatment of mania. The Depakote Mania Study Group. JAMA 271:918–924, 1994

Bowden CL, Janicak PG, Orsulak P, et al: Relation of serum valproate concentration to response in mania. Am J Psychiatry 153:765–770, 1996

Bowden CL, Calabrese JR, Sachs G, et al: A placebo-controlled 18-month trial of lamotrigine and lithium maintenance treatment in recently manic or hypomanic patients with bipolar I disorder. Arch Gen Psychiatry 60:392–400, 2003

Branchey M, Branchey L: Patterns of psychotropic drug use and tardive dyskinesia. J Clin Psychopharmacol 4:41–45, 1984

Brantigan CO, Brantigan TA, Joseph N: Effect of beta blockade and beta stimulation on stage fright. Am J Med 72:88–94, 1982

Breier A, Wolkowitz OM, Doran AR, et al: Neuroleptic responsivity of negative and positive symptoms in schizophrenia. Am J Psychiatry 144:1549–1555, 1987

Bremmer JD: A double blind comparison of mirtazapine, amitriptyline, and placebo in major depression. J Clin Psychiatry 56:519–525, 1995

Brewerton TD: Lithium counteracts carbamazepine-induced leukopenia while increasing its therapeutic effect. Biol Psychiatry 21:677–685, 1986

Brewerton TD, Jackson CW: Prophylaxis of carbamazepine-induced hyponatremia by demeclocycline in six patients. J Clin Psychiatry 55:249–251, 1994

Brodie MJ, MacPhee GJ: Carbamazepine neurotoxicity precipitated by diltiazem. BMJ 292:1170–1171, 1986

Brooke MM, Patterson DR, Questad KA, et al: Agitation and restlessness after closed head injury: a prospective study of 100 consecutive admissions. Arch Phys Med Rehabil 73:917–921, 1992

Brunello N, Masotto C, Steardo L, et al: New insights into the biology of schizophrenia through the mechanism of action of clozapine. Neuropsychopharmacology 13:177–213, 1995

Burke RE, Fahn S, Jankovic J, et al: Tardive dyskinesia: late-onset and persistent dystonia caused by antipsychotic drugs. Neurology 32:1335–1346, 1982

Busto U, Sellers EM, Naranjo CA, et al: Withdrawal reactions after long-term therapeutic use of benzodiazepines. N Engl J Med 315:854–857, 1986

Byerly M, DeVane L: Pharmacokinetics of clozapine and risperidone: a review of the literature. J Clin Psychopharmacol 16:177–187, 1996

Calabrese JR, Gulledge AD, Hahn K, et al: Autoimmune thyroiditis in manic-depressive patients treated with lithium. Am J Psychiatry 142:1318–1321, 1985

Calabrese JR, Markowitz PJ, Kimmel SE, et al: Spectrum of efficacy of valproate in 78 rapid-cycling bipolar patients. J Clin Psychopharmacol 12:53S–56S, 1992

Calabrese JR, Bowden CL, Sach GS, et al: A double-blind placebo-controlled study of lamotrigine monotherapy in outpatients with bipolar I depression. Lamictal 602 Study Group. J Clin Psychiatry 60:79–88, 1999

Callahan AM, Marangell LB, Ketter TA: Evaluating the clinical significance of drug interaction: a systematic approach. Harv Rev Psychiatry 4:153–158, 1996

Chakos M, Lieberman J, Hoffman E, et al: Effectiveness of second-generation antipsychotics in patients with treatment-resistant schizophrenia: a review and meta-analysis of randomized trials. Am J Psychiatry 158:518–526, 2001

Charney DS: Monoamine dysfunction and the pathophysiology and treatment of depression. J Clin Psychiatry 59 (suppl 14):11–14, 1998

Charney DS, Woods SW: Benzodiazepine treatment of panic disorder: a comparison of alprazolam and lorazepam. J Clin Psychiatry 50:418–423, 1989

Chatham-Showalter PE: Carbamazepine for combativeness in acute traumatic brain injury. J Neuropsychiatry Clin Neurosci 8: 96–99, 1996

Chen G, Manji HK, Hawver DB, et al: Chronic sodium valproate selectively decreases protein kinase C alpha and epsilon in vitro. J Neurochem 63:2361–2364, 1994

Chengappa KN, Gopalani A, Haught MK, et al: The treatment of clozapine-associated agranulocytosis with granulocyte colony-stimulating factor (G-CSF). Psychopharmacol Bull 32:111–121, 1996

Claghorn JL, Earl CQ, Walczak DD, et al: Fluvoxamine maleate in the treatment of depression: a single-center, double-blind, placebo-controlled comparison with imipramine in outpatients. J Clin Psychopharmacol 16:113–120, 1996

Clomipramine Collaborative Study Group: Clomipramine in the treatment of patients with obsessive-compulsive disorder. Arch Gen Psychiatry 48:730–738, 1991

Cohen LG, Chessley S, Eugenio L, et al: Erythromycin-induced clozapine toxic reaction. Arch Intern Med 156:675–677, 1996

Cohen LS, Friedman JM, Jefferson MD, et al: A reevaluation of risk of in utero exposure to lithium. JAMA 271:146–150, 1994

Cohen WJ, Cohen NH: Lithium carbonate, haloperidol and irreversible brain damage. JAMA 230:1283–1287, 1974

Cohn J, Wilcox CS: Low-sedation potential of buspirone compared with alprazolam and lorazepam in the treatment of anxious patients: a double-blind study. J Clin Psychiatry 47:409–412, 1986

Cole JO, Orzak MG, Beake B, et al: Assessment of the abuse liability of buspirone in recreational sedative users. J Clin Psychiatry 43:69–74, 1982

Cole JO, Gardos G, Rapkin R, et al: Lithium carbonate in tardive dyskinesia and schizophrenia, in Tardive Dyskinesia and Affective Disorders. Edited by Gardos G, Casey D. Washington, DC, American Psychiatric Press, 1984, pp 50–73

Conley RR, Mahmoud RA: Randomized double-blind study of risperidone and olanzapine in the treatment of schizophrenia or schizoaffective disorder. Am J Psychiatry 158:765–774, 2001

Consensus Development Panel: Mood disorders: pharmacologic prevention of recurrences. Am J Psychiatry 142:469–476, 1985

Coppen A, Abou-Saleb MT, Miller P, et al: Lithium continuation therapy following electroconvulsive therapy. Br J Psychiatry 139:284–287, 1981

Corrigan PW, Yudofsky SC, Silver JM: Pharmacological and behavioral treatments for aggressive psychiatric inpatients. Hosp Community Psychiatry 44:125–133, 1993

Coulam CB, Annegers JF: Do anticonvulsants reduce the efficacy of oral contraceptives? Epilepsia 20:519–525, 1979

Coupet J, Rauh CE, Szues-Myers VA, et al: 2-Chloro-11-(1-piperazinyl) dibenz [b, f] [1, 4] oxazepine (amoxapine), an antidepressant with antipsychotic properties: a possible role for 7-hydroxyamoxapine. Biochem Pharmacol 28:2514–2515, 1979

Creese I, Burt DR, Snyder SH: Dopamine receptor binding predicts clinical and pharmacological potencies of antischizophrenic drugs. Science 192:481–483, 1976

Csernansky JC, Riney SJ, Lombrozo L: Double-blind comparison of alprazolam, diazepam, and placebo for the treatment of negative schizophrenic symptoms. Arch Gen Psychiatry 45:655–659, 1988

Dabiri LM, Pasta D, Darby JK, et al: Effectiveness of vitamin E for the treatment of long-term tardive dyskinesia. Am J Psychiatry 151:925–926, 1994

Dailey JW, Naritoku DK: Antidepressants and seizures: clinical anecdotes overshadow neuroscience. Biochem Pharmacol 52: 1323–1329, 1996

Das Gupta K, Young A: Clozapine-induced neuroleptic malignant syndrome. J Clin Psychiatry 52:105–107, 1991

Davidson JRT, Ford SM, Smith RD, et al: Long-term treatment of social phobia with clonazepam. J Clin Psychiatry 52 (suppl):16–20, 1991

Davis JM: Maintenance therapy and the natural course of schizophrenia. J Clin Psychiatry 46:18–21, 1985

Davis K, Kahn R, Ko G, et al: Dopamine in schizophrenia: a review and reconceptualization. Am J Psychiatry 148:1474–1486, 1991

De Boer T: The pharmacologic profile of mirtazapine. J Clin Psychiatry 57 (suppl 4): 19–25, 1996

De Montigny C, Gunberg S, Mayer A, et al: Lithium induces rapid relief of depression in tricyclic antidepressant nonresponders. Br J Psychiatry 138:252–256, 1981

Dean JC, Penry JK: Valproate, in The Medical Treatment of Epilepsy. Edited by Resor SR, Kutt H. New York, Marcel Dekker, 1992, pp 265–278

Deandrea D, Walker N, Mehlmauer M, et al: Dermatologic reactions to lithium: a critical review of the literature. J Clin Psychopharmacol 2:199–204, 1982

Deirmenjian JM, Erhart SM, Wirshing DA, et al: Olanzapine-induced reversible priapism: a case report. J Clin Psychopharmacol 18:351–353, 1998

den Boer JA, van Vliet IM, Westenberg HG: Recent developments in the psychopharmacology of social phobia. Eur Arch Psychiatry Clin Neurosci 244:309–316, 1995

Delva NJ, Letemednia FJJ: Lithium treatment in schizophrenia and schizoaffective disorders. Br J Psychiatry 141:387–400, 1982

Descotes J, Lievre M, Ollagnier M, et al: Study of thioridazine cardiotoxic effects by means of his bundle activity recording. Acta Pharmacologica Toxicologica 44: 370–376, 1979

Detke MJ, Lu Y, Goldstein DJ, et al: Duloxetine, 60 mg once daily, for major depressive disorder: a randomized double-blind placebo-controlled trial. J Clin Psychiatry 63: 308–315, 2002

Devinsky O, Honigfeld G, Patin J: Clozapine-related seizures. Neurology 41:369–371, 1991

Dinan TG, Barry S: A comparison of electroconvulsive therapy with a combined lithium and tricyclic combination among depressed tricyclic nonresponders. Acta Psychiatr Scand 80:97–100, 1989

Doughty MJ, Lyle WM: Medications used to prevent migraine headaches and their potential ocular adverse effects. Optometry and Vision Science 72:879–891, 1995

Douyon R, Angrist B, Peselow E, et al: Neuroleptic augmentation with alprazolam: clinical effects and pharmacokinetic correlates (comment). Am J Psychiatry 146: 1087–1088, 1989

Downs JM, Downs AD, Rosenthal TL, et al: Increased plasma tricyclic antidepressant concentrations in two patients currently treated with fluoxetine. J Clin Psychiatry 50:226–227, 1989

Dreifuss FE, Santılli N, Langer DH, et al: Valproic acid hepatic fatalities: a retrospective review. Neurology 37:379–385, 1987

Dreifuss FE, Langer DH, Moline KA, et al: Valproic acid hepatic fatalities, II: US experience since 1994. Neurology 39:201–207, 1989

Drew PJ, Barnes JN, Evans SJ: The effect of acute beta-adrenoceptor blockade on examination performance. Br J Clin Pharmacol 19:783–786, 1985

Duinkerke SJ, Botter PA, Jansen AAI, et al: Ritanserin, a selective 5HT2/1c antagonist, and negative symptoms in schizophrenia: a placebo-controlled double blind trial. Br J Psychiatry 163:451–455, 1993

Duman RS: Novel therapeutic approaches beyond the serotonin receptor. Biol Psychiatry 44:324–335, 1998

Dunner DL, Fieve RR: Clinical factors in lithium carbonate prophylaxis failure. Arch Gen Psychiatry 30:229–233, 1974

Dunner DL, Ishiki D, Avery DH, et al: Effect of alprazolam and diazepam on anxiety and panic attacks in panic disorder: a controlled study. J Clin Psychiatry 47:458–460, 1986

Ebstein RP, Hermoni M, Belmaker RH: The effect of lithium on noradrenaline-induced cyclic AMP accumulation in rat brain: inhibition after chronic treatment and absence of supersensitivity. J Pharmacol Exp Ther 213:161–167, 1980

Edmonds LD, Oakley GP: Ebstein's anomaly and maternal lithium exposure during pregnancy. Teratology 41:551–552, 1990

Egan MF, Hyde TM, Albers GW, et al: Treatment of tardive dyskinesia with vitamin E. Am J Psychiatry 149:773–777, 1992

Eichelbaum M, Tomson T, Tybring G, et al: Carbamazepine metabolism in man: induction and pharmacogenetic aspects. Clin Pharmacokinet 10:80–90, 1985

Elie R, Lamontagne Y: Alprazolam and diazepam in the treatment of generalized anxiety. J Clin Psychopharmacol 4:125–129, 1985

Elkashef AM, Ruskin PE, Bacher N, et al: Vitamin E in the treatment of tardive dyskinesia. Am J Psychiatry 147:505–506, 1990

Ellingrod VL, Perry PJ: Venlafaxine: a heterocyclic antidepressant. American Journal of Hospital Pharmacy 51:3033–3046, 1994

Emes CE, Millson RC: Risperidone-induced priapism. Can J Psychiatry 39:315–316, 1994

Ereshefsky L, Toney G, Saklad SR, et al: A loading-dose strategy for converting from oral to depot haloperidol. Hosp Community Psychiatry 44:1155–1161, 1993

Everett HC: The use of bethanechol chloride with tricyclic antidepressants. Am J Psychiatry 132:1202–1204, 1976

Fahn S: A therapeutic approach to tardive dyskinesia. J Clin Psychiatry 46:19–24, 1985

Fava M, Judge R, Hoog SL, et al: Fluoxetine versus sertraline and paroxetine in major depressive disorder: changes in weight with long-term treatment. J Clin Psychiatry 61:863–867, 2000

Fawcett J, Kravitz HM, Zajecka JM, et al: CNS stimulant potentiation of monoamine oxidase inhibitors in treatment-refractory depression. J Clin Psychopharmacol 11:127–132, 1991

Fawcett J, Marcus RN, Anton SF, et al: Response of anxiety and agitation symptoms during nefazodone treatment of major depression. J Clin Psychiatry 56 (suppl 6):37–42, 1995

Feder R: Lithium augmentation of clomipramine (letter). J Clin Psychiatry 49:458, 1988

Feinberg SS, Holzer B: The monoamine oxidase inhibitor (MAOI) diet and kosher pizza (letter, comment). J Clin Psychopharmacol 17:226–227, 1997

Feinberg SS, Holzer B: Clarifying the safety of the MAOI diet and pizza (letter, comment). J Clin Psychiatry 61:145, 2000

Fernstrom MH, Krowinski RL, Kupfer DJ: Chronic imipramine treatment and weight gain. Psychiatry Res 17:269–273, 1986

Fink M: Efficacy and safety of induced seizures (ECT) in man. Compr Psychiatry 19:1–18, 1978

Finkle BS, McCloskey KL, Goodman LS: Diazepam and drug-associated deaths: a survey in the United States and Canada. JAMA 242:429–434, 1979

Fisher S, Kent TA, Bryant SG: Postmarketing surveillance by patient self-monitoring: preliminary data for sertraline versus fluoxetine. J Clin Psychiatry 56:288–296, 1995

Food and Drug Administration: Bioavailability and bioequivalence requirements. Federal Register 57:17997–18001, 1992

Francois B, Marquet P, Roustan J, et al: Serotonin syndrome due to an overdose of moclobemide and clomipramine: a potentially life-threatening association. Intensive Care Med 23:122–124, 1997

Frank E, Kupfer DJ, Perel JM, et al: Three-year outcomes for maintenance therapies in recurrent depression. Arch Gen Psychiatry 47:1093–1099, 1990

Frazer A: Antidepressants. J Clin Psychiatry 58(suppl 6):9–25, 1997

Freeman CP, Trimble MR, Deakin JF, et al: Fluvoxamine versus clomipramine in the treatment of obsessive-compulsive disorder: a multicenter, randomized, double-blind parallel group. J Clin Psychiatry 55:301–305, 1994

Frye MA, Ketter TA, Kimbrell TA, et al: A placebo-controlled study of lamotrigine and gabapentin monotherapy in refractory mood disorders. J Clin Psychopharmacol 20:607–614, 2000

Gammon GD, Hansen C: A case of akinesia induced by amoxapine. Am J Psychiatry 141:283–284, 1984

Gastfried DR, Rosenbaum JF: Adjunctive buspirone in benzodiazepine treatment of four patient with panic disorder. Am J Psychiatry 146:914–916, 1989

Gelders YG: Thymosthenic agents, a novel approach in the treatment of schizophrenia. Br J Psychiatry 155(suppl 5):33–36, 1989

Gelenberg AJ: Treating PMS. Biological Therapies in Psychiatry Newsletter 20:1, 1997

Gelenberg AJ, Kane JM, Keller MB, et al: Comparison of standard and low blood levels of lithium for maintenance treatment of bipolar disorder. N Engl J Med 321:1489–1493, 1989

Gelernter CS, Uhde TW, Cimbolic P, et al: Cognitive-behavioral and pharmacologic treatments for social phobia: a preliminary study. Arch Gen Psychiatry 48:938–945, 1991

Geracioti TD Jr: Valproic acid treatment of episodic explosiveness related to brain injury. J Clin Psychiatry 55:416–417, 1994

Gerner RH, Stanton A: Algorithm for patient management of acute manic states: lithium, valproate, or carbamazepine? J Clin Psychopharmacol 12 (suppl):57S–63S, 1992

Gerson SL, Gullion G, Yeh HS, et al: Granulocyte colony-stimulating factor for clozapine-induced agranulocytosis (letter). Lancet 340:1097, 1992

Ghadirian AM, Chouinard G, Annable L: Sexual dysfunction and plasma prolactin levels in neuroleptic-treated schizophrenic outpatients. J Nerv Ment Dis 170:463–467, 1982

Ghaemi SN, Zarate CA Jr, Popli AP, et al: Is there a relationship between clozapine and obsessive-compulsive disorder? A retrospective chart review. Compr Psychiatry 36:267–270, 1995

Giakas WJ, Seibyl JP, Mazure CM: Valproate in the treatment of temper outbursts (letter). J Clin Psychiatry 51:525, 1990

Giles TO, Modlin RK: Death associated with ventricular arrhythmias and thioridazine hydrochloride. JAMA 205:108–110, 1968

Gitlin MJ, Weiner H, Fairbanks L: Failure of T3 to potentiate tricyclic antidepressant response. J Affect Disord 13:267–272, 1987

Glassman AH: The newer antidepressant drugs and their cardiovascular effects. Psychopharmacol Bull 20:272–279, 1984

Glassman AH, Bigger JT: Cardiovascular effects of therapeutic doses of tricyclic antidepressants: a review. Arch Gen Psychiatry 39:815–820, 1981

Glazer WM, Moore DC, Schooler NR, et al: Tardive dyskinesia: a discontinuation study. Arch Gen Psychiatry 41:623–627, 1984

Goff D, Baldessarini R: Antipsychotics, in Drug Interactions in Psychiatry. Edited by Ciraulo D, Shader R, Greenblatt D, et al. Baltimore, MD, Williams & Wilkins, 1995, pp 129–174

Goff D, Evins A: Negative symptoms in schizophrenia: neurobiological models and treatment response. Harv Rev Psychiatry 6:59–77, 1998

Goff D, Arana G, Greenblatt D, et al: The effect of benztropine on haloperidol-induced dystonia, clinical efficacy and pharmacokinetics: a prospective, double-blind trial. J Clin Psychopharmacol 11:106–112, 1991

Goff D, Midha K, Sarid-Segal O, et al: A placebo-controlled trial of fluoxetine added to neuroleptic in patients with schizophrenia. Psychopharmacology 117:417–423, 1995

Goff D, Posever T, Herz L, et al: An exploratory haloperidol-controlled dose-finding study of ziprasidone in hospitalized patients with schizophrenia or schizoaffective disorder. J Clin Psychopharmacol 18:296–304, 1998

Goldberg HL, Finnerty RJ: The comparative efficacy of buspirone and diazepam in the treatment of anxiety. Am J Psychiatry 136:1184–1187, 1979

Goldberg RJ: Nefazodone and venlafaxine: two new agents for the treatment of depression. J Fam Pract 41:591–594, 1995

Goldberg RJ, Capone RJ, Hunt JD: Cardiac complications following tricyclic antidepressant overdose: issues for monitoring policy. JAMA 254:1772–1775, 1985

Goldfrank LR, Lewin NA, Flomenbaum NE, et al: Antidepressants: tricyclics, tetracyclics, monoamine oxidase inhibitors, and others, in Goldfrank's Toxicologic Emergencies, 3rd Edition. Edited by Goldfrank LR, Flomenbaum ME, Lewis NA, et al. Norwalk, CT, Appleton-Century-Crofts, 1986, pp 351–363

Goldney RD, Spence ND: Safety of the combination of lithium and neuroleptic drugs. Am J Psychiatry 143:882–884, 1986

Goldstein DJ, Mallinckrodt C, Lu Y, et al: Duloxetine in the treatment of major depressive disorder: a double-blind clinical trial. J Clin Psychiatry 63:225–231, 2002

Gomez J: Subjective side effects of ECT. Br J Psychiatry 127:609–611, 1975

Goodman LS, Alexander RD, Laciness DJ: Monoamine oxidase inhibitors and tricyclic antidepressants: comparison of their cardiovascular effects. J Clin Psychiatry 47:225–229, 1986

Goodman WK, Charney DS: Therapeutic applications and mechanisms of action of monoamine oxidase inhibitor and heterocyclic antidepressant drugs. J Clin Psychiatry 46 (suppl 12):6–22, 1985

Goodman WK, Price LH, Delgado PL, et al: Specificity of serotonin reuptake inhibitors in the treatment of obsessive-compulsive disorder: comparison of fluvoxamine and desipramine. Arch Gen Psychiatry 47:577–585, 1990

Goodman WK, Kozak MJ, Liebowitz M, et al: Treatment of obsessive-compulsive disorder with fluvoxamine: a multicentre, double-blind, placebo-controlled trial. Int Clin Psychopharmacol 11:21–29, 1996

Goodwin FK, Jamison R: Manic-Depressive Illness. New York, Oxford University Press, 1990

Goodwin FK, Prange AJ, Post RM, et al: Potentiation of antidepressant effects by L-triiodothyronine in tricyclic nonresponders. Am J Psychiatry 139:34–38, 1982

Gram LM, Bentsen KD: Hepatic toxicity of antiepileptic drugs: a review. Acta Neurol Scand Suppl 97:81–90, 1983

Greenblatt DJ, Allen MD, Noel BJ, et al: Acute overdosage with benzodiazepine derivatives. Clin Pharmacol Ther 21:497–514, 1977

Greenblatt DJ, Shader RI, Abernethy DR: Drug therapy: current status of benzodiazepines. N Engl J Med 309:410–416, 1983

Greiff JM, Rowbotham D: Pharmacokinetic drug interactions with gastrointestinal motility modifying agents. Clin Pharmacokinet 27:447–461, 1994

Greist J, Chouinard G, DuBoff E, et al: Double-blind parallel comparison of three dosages of sertraline and placebo in outpatients with obsessive-compulsive disorder. Arch Gen Psychiatry 52:289–295, 1995a

Greist JH, Jefferson JW, Kobak KA, et al: A 1 year double-blind placebo-controlled fixed dose study of sertraline in the treatment of obsessive-compulsive disorder. Int Clin Psychopharmacol 10:57–65, 1995b

Griffith JD, Jasinski DR, Casten GP, et al: Investigation of the abuse liability of buspirone in alcohol-dependent patients. Am J Med 80(suppl 3B):30–35, 1986

Gunderson JG: Pharmacotherapy for patients with borderline personality disorder. Arch Gen Psychiatry 43:698–700, 1986

Guze BH, Baxter LR: Current concepts: neuroleptic malignant syndrome. N Engl J Med 313:163–166, 1985

Hamilton JA, Halbreich U: Special aspects of neuropsychiatric illness in women: with a focus on depression. Annu Rev Med 44:355–364, 1993

Hamilton JD: Thioridazine retinopathy within the upper dosage limit. Psychosomatics 26:823–824, 1985

Haria M, Fitton A, McTavish D: Trazodone: a review of its pharmacology, therapeutic use in depression and therapeutic potential in other disorders. Drugs Aging 4: 331–355, 1994

Haring C, Barnas C, Saria A, et al: Dose-related plasma levels of clozapine. J Clin Psychopharmacol 9:71–72, 1989

Hartigan-Go K, Bateman N, Nyberg G, et al: Concentration-related pharmacodynamic effects of thioridazine and its metabolites in humans. Clin Pharmacol Ther 60:543–553, 1996

Harvey KV, Balon R: Augmentation with buspirone: a review. Ann Clin Psychiatry 7: 143–147, 1995

Hertley LR, Ungapen S, Davie I, et al: The effect of beta-adrenergic blocking drugs on speakers' performance and memory. Br J Psychiatry 142:512–517, 1983

Hetmar O, Poulsen UJ, Ladefoged J, et al: Lithium: long-term effects on the kidney: a prospective follow-up study ten years after kidney biopsy. Br J Psychiatry 158: 53–58, 1991

Hewlett WA, Vinogradov S, Agras WS: Clonazepam treatment of obsessions and compulsions. J Clin Psychiatry 51:158–161, 1990

Hirschfeld RMA, Clayton P, Cohen I, et al: Practice guideline for the treatment of patients with bipolar disorder. Am J Psychiatry 151:1–36, 1994

Hodgman MJ, Martin TG, Krenzelok EP: Serotonin syndrome due to venlafaxine and maintenance tranylcypromine therapy. Hum Exp Toxicol 16:14–17, 1997

Hoehn-Saric R, McLeod DR, Zimmerli WD: Differential effects of alprazolam and imipramine in generalized anxiety disorder: somatic vs psychic symptoms. J Clin Psychiatry 49:293–301, 1988

Hollander E, DeCaria CM, Schneier FR, et al: Fenfluramine augmentation of serotonin reuptake blockade antiobsessional treatment. J Clin Psychiatry 51:119–123, 1990

Honigfeld G, Arellano F, Sethi J, et al: Reducing clozapine-related morbidity and mortality: 5 years of experience with the Clozaril National Registry. J Clin Psychiatry 59 (suppl 3):3–7, 1998

Hornstein A, Seliger G: Cognitive side effects of lithium in closed head injury (letter). J Neuropsychiatry Clin Neurosci 1:446–447, 1989

Hurd RW, Rinsvelt V, Karas WB, et al: Selenium, zinc, and copper changes with valproic acid: possible relation to drug side effects. Neurology 34:1393–1395, 1984

Isojarvi JI, Laatikainen TJ, Knip M, et al: Obesity and endocrine disorders in women taking valproate for epilepsy. Ann Neurol 39:579–584, 1996

Itil TM, Soldatos CL: Epileptogenic side effects of psychotropic drugs: practical recommendations. JAMA 244:1460–1463, 1980

Jacobsen FM: Low-dose trazodone as a hypnotic in patients treated with MAOIs and other psychotropics: a pilot study. J Clin Psychiatry 51:298–302, 1990

Jacobsen FM: Low-dose valproate: a new treatment for cyclothymia, mild rapid cycling disorders, and premenstrual syndrome. J Clin Psychiatry 54:229–234, 1993

Jacobson SJ, Jones K, Johnson K, et al: Prospective multicentre study of pregnancy outcome after lithium exposure during first trimester. Lancet 339:530–533, 1992

Jefferson JW: Social phobia: a pharmacologic treatment overview. J Clin Psychiatry 56 (suppl):18–24, 1995

Jenike MA: Affective illness in elderly patients, part 2. Psychiatric Times 4:1, 1987

Jenike MA: Approaches to the patient with treatment-refractory obsessive-compulsive disorder. J Clin Psychiatry 51 (suppl): 15–21, 1990

Jenike MA, Baer L, Buttolph L: Buspirone augmentation of fluoxetine in patients with obsessive-compulsive disorder. J Clin Psychopharmacol 12:13–14, 1991

Jenkins SW, Ruegg R, Moeller FG: Gepirone in the treatment of major depression. J Clin Psychopharmacol 10 (suppl):77S–85S, 1990

Jeste DV, Wyatt RJ: Understanding and Treating Tardive Dyskinesia. New York, Guilford, 1982

Jeste DV, Lacro JP, Bailey A, et al: Lower incidence of tardive dyskinesia with risperidone compared to haloperidol in older patients. J Am Geriatr Soc 47:716–719, 1999

Joffe RT: T3 and lithium potentiation of tricyclic antidepressants. Am J Psychiatry 145:1317–1318, 1988

Joffe RT, Singer W: A comparison of triiodothyronine and thyroxine in the potentiation of tricyclic antidepressants. Psychiatry Res 32:241–251, 1990

Joffe RT, Post RM, Uhde TW: Effect of carbamazepine on body weight in affectively ill patients. J Clin Psychiatry 47:313–314, 1986

Johnson DAW: Antipsychotic medication: clinical guidelines for maintenance therapy. J Clin Psychiatry 46:6–15, 1985

Jones KL, Lacro RV, Johnson KA, et al: Pattern of malformations in the children of women treated with carbamazepine during pregnancy. N Engl J Med 320:1661–1666, 1989

Jope RS, Williams MB: Lithium and brain signal transduction systems. Biochem Pharmacol 47:429–441, 1994

Kahn RJ, Menair D, Lipman RS, et al: Imipramine and chlordiazepoxide in depressive and anxiety disorders: efficacy in anxious outpatients. Arch Gen Psychiatry 43:79–85, 1986

Kallen B, Tandberg A: Lithium and pregnancy: a cohort study in manic-depressive women. Acta Psychiatr Scand 68:134–139, 1983

Kane JM: Treatment-resistant schizophrenic patients. J Clin Psychiatry 57:35–40, 1996

Kane JM, Smith JM: Tardive dyskinesia: prevalence and risk factors, 1959 to 1979. Arch Gen Psychiatry 39:473–481, 1982

Kane JM, Honigfeld G, Singer J, et al: Clozapine for the treatment-resistant schizophrenic: a double-blind comparison vs chlorpromazine/benztropine. Arch Gen Psychiatry 45:789–796, 1988

Kapur S, Seeman P: Does fast dissociation from the dopamine D2 receptor explain the action of atypical antipsychotics? A new hypothesis. Am J Psychiatry 158:360–369, 2001

Keck PE Jr, Pope HG Jr, Cohen BM, et al: Risk factor for neuroleptic malignant syndrome. Arch Gen Psychiatry 46:914–918, 1989

Keck PE Jr, McElroy SL, Nemeroff CB: Anticonvulsants in the treatment of bipolar disorder. J Neuropsychiatry Clin Neurosci 4:395–405, 1992

Keck PE Jr, McElroy SL, Tugrul KC, et al: Valproate oral loading in the treatment of acute mania. J Clin Psychiatry 54:305–308, 1993

Keller MB, Hanks DL: Anxiety symptom relief in depression treatment outcomes. J Clin Psychiatry 56 (suppl):22–29, 1995

Kelsey JE: Dose-response relationship with venlafaxine. J Clin Psychopharmacol 16 (suppl 2):21S–28S, 1996

Kennedy PF, Hershon HI, McGuire RJ: Extrapyramidal disorders after prolonged phenothiazine therapy. Br J Psychiatry 118:509–518, 1971

Ketter TA, Flockhart DA, Post RM, et al: The emerging role of cytochrome P450 3A in psychopharmacology. J Clin Psychopharmacol 15:387–398, 1995

Kiev A, Masco HL, Wenger TL, et al: The cardiovascular effects of bupropion and nortriptyline in depressed outpatients. Ann Clin Psychiatry 6:107–115, 1994

Klein DF, Ross DC, Cohen P: Panic and avoidance in agoraphobia; application of path analysis to treatment studies. Arch Gen Psychiatry 44:377–385, 1987

Kolecki P: Venlafaxine induced serotonin syndrome occurring after abstinence from phenelzine for more than two weeks (letter). J Toxicol Clin Toxicol 35:211–212, 1997

Kuhn R: The treatment of depressive states with G 22355 (imipramine hydrochloride). Am J Psychiatry 115:459–464, 1958

Kukopoulos A, Caliari B, Tundo A, et al: Rapid cyclers, temperament, and antidepressants. Compr Psychiatry 24:249–258, 1983

Kupfer DJ, Coble PA, Rubinstein MS: Changes in weight during treatment for depression. Psychosom Med 41:535–544, 1979

Kupfer KJ, Reynolds CF: Management of insomnia. N Engl J Med 336:341–346, 1997

Labar DR: Antiepileptic drug toxic emergencies, in The Medical Treatment of Epilepsy. Edited by Resor SR, Kutt H. New York, Marcel Dekker, 1992, pp 573–588

Labbate LA, Pollack MH: Treatment of fluoxetine-induced sexual dysfunction with bupropion: a case report. Ann Clin Psychiatry 6:13–15, 1994

Lader M, Olajide D: A comparison of buspirone and placebo in relieving benzodiazepine withdrawal symptoms. J Clin Psychopharmacol 7:11–15, 1987

Laird LK: Issues in the monopharmacotherapy and polypharmacotherapy of obsessive-compulsive disorder. Psychopharmacol Bull 32:569–578, 1996

Lambert P-A, Cavaz G, Borselli S, et al: Action neuropsychotrop diun nouvel anti-epileptique: le Depamide. Ann Med Psychol (Paris) 1:707–710, 1966

Lammer EJ, Sever LE, Oakley GP: Teratogen update: valproic acid. Teratology 35:465–473, 1987

Leach MJ, Baxter MG, Critchley MA: Neurochemical and behavioral aspects of lamotrigine. Epilepsia 32:S4–S8, 1991

Lenox RH, Watson DG, Patel J, et al: Chronic lithium administration alters a prominent PKC substrate in rat hippocampus. Brain Res 570:333–340, 1992

Lerer B, Shapira B, Calev A, et al: Antidepressant and cognitive effects of twice- versus three-times-weekly ECT. Am J Psychiatry 152:564–570, 1995

Lieberman JA: Atypical antipsychotic drugs as a first-line treatment of schizophrenia: a rationale and hypothesis. J Clin Psychiatry 57 (suppl 11):68–71, 1996

Lieberman JA, Saltz BL, Johns CA, et al: The effects of clozapine on tardive dyskinesia. Br J Psychiatry 158:503–510, 1991

Liebowitz MA, Gorman JM, Fyer AJ, et al: Pharmacotherapy of social phobia: an interim report of a placebo-controlled comparison of phenelzine and atenolol. J Clin Psychiatry 49:252–257, 1988

Liebowitz MR, Quitkin FM, Stewart JW, et al: Phenelzine vs imipramine in atypical depression: a preliminary report. Arch Gen Psychiatry 41:669–677, 1984

Lindstedt G, Nilsson L, Walinder J, et al: On the prevalence, diagnosis and management of lithium-induced hypothyroidism in psychiatric patients. Br J Psychiatry 130:452–458, 1977

Lingam VR, Lazarus LW, Groves L, et al: Methylphenidate in treating post-stroke depression. J Clin Psychiatry 49:151–153, 1988

Linnoila M, Vinkar M, Hiertala O: Effect of sodium valproate on tardive dyskinesia. Br J Psychiatry 129:114–119, 1976

Linnoila M, Erwin CW, Brendle A, et al: Psychomotor effects of diazepam in anxious patients and healthy volunteers. J Clin Psychopharmacol 3:88–96, 1983

Lister RG: The amnestic action of benzodiazepines in man. Neurosci Biobehav Rev 9: 87–94, 1985

Lohr JB, Caligiuri MP: A double-blind placebo-controlled study of vitamin E treatment of tardive dyskinesia. J Clin Psychiatry 57:167–173, 1996

Lohr JB, Cadet JL, Lohr MA, et al: l-Alpha-tocopherol in tardive dyskinesia. Lancet 1(8538):913–914, 1987

Lokkegaard H, Andersen NF, Henriksen E: Renal function in 153 manic-depressive patients treated with lithium for more than five years. Acta Psychiatr Scand 71:347–355, 1985

Louie AK, Lewis TB, Lannon RA: Use of low-dose fluoxetine in major depression and panic disorder. J Clin Psychiatry 54:435–438, 1993

Lucki I: Behavioral studies of serotonin receptor antagonists as antidepressant drugs. J Clin Psychiatry 52 (suppl):24–31, 1991

Lucki I, Rickels K, Geller AM: Chronic use of benzodiazepines and psychomotor and cognitive test performance. Psychopharmacology (Berl) 88:426–433, 1986

Lydiard RB: Tricyclic-resistant depression: treatment resistance or inadequate treatment? J Clin Psychiatry 46:412–417, 1985

MacDonald RL, Kelly KM: Antiepileptic drug mechanisms of action (review). Epilepsia 36:S2–S12, 1995

Malitz S, Sackeim HA, Decina P, et al: The efficacy of electroconvulsive therapy: dose-response interactions with modality. Ann N Y Acad Sci 462:56–64, 1986

Mallette LE, Eichhorn E: Effects of lithium carbonate on human calcium metabolism. Arch Intern Med 146:770–776, 1986

Maltbie AA, Wingfield MS, Volow MR, et al: Electroconvulsive therapy in the presence of brain tumor: case reports and an evaluation of risk. J Nerv Ment Dis 168:400–405, 1980

Manji HK, Bebchuk JM, Moore GJ, et al: Modulation of CNS signal transduction pathways and gene expression by mood-stabilizing agents: therapeutic implications. J Clin Psychiatry 60 (suppl 2):27–39, 1993

Manji HK, Chen G, Shimon H, et al: Guanine nucleotide-binding proteins in bipolar affective disorder: effects of long-term lithium treatment. Arch Gen Psychiatry 52:135–144, 1995

Manji HK, Chen G, Hsiso JK, et al: Regulation of signal transduction pathways by mood-stabilizing agents: implications for the delayed onset of therapeutic efficacy. J Clin Psychiatry 57:34–46, 1999

Manna V, Bolino F, Di Cicco L: Chronic tension-type headache, mood depression and serotonin: therapeutic effects of fluvoxamine and mianserine. Headache 34:44–49, 1994

Markovitz PJ, Stagro SJ, Calabrese JR: Buspirone augmentation of fluoxetine in obsessive-compulsive disorder. Am J Psychiatry 147:798–800, 1990

Marshall RD, Schneier FR, Fallon BA, et al: Medication therapy for social phobia. J Clin Psychiatry 55:33–37, 1994

Mattes JA: Valproic acid for nonaffective aggression in the mentally retarded. J Nerv Ment Dis 180:601–602, 1992

Mavissakalian MR, Jones B, Olson S, et al: Clomipramine in obsessive-compulsive disorder: clinical response and plasma levels. J Clin Psychopharmacol 10:261–268, 1990

McCall WV, Reboussin DM, Weiner RD, et al: Titrated moderately suprathreshold vs fixed high-dose right unilateral electroconvulsive therapy: acute antidepressant and cognitive effects. Arch Gen Psychiatry 57:438–444, 2000

McDougle CJ, Goodman WK, Price LH, et al: Neuroleptic addition in fluvoxamine-refractory obsessive-compulsive disorder. Am J Psychiatry 147:652–654, 1990

McDougle CJ, Fleischmann RL, Epperson CN, et al: Risperidone addition in fluvoxamine-refractory obsessive-compulsive disorder: three cases. J Clin Psychiatry 56:526–528, 1995

McElroy SL, Keck PE Jr, Pope HG Jr, et al: Valproate in psychiatric disorders: literature review and clinical guidelines. J Clin Psychiatry 50 (suppl):23–29, 1989

McElroy SL, Keck PE Jr, Pope HG Jr, et al: Valproate in the treatment of bipolar disorder: literature review and clinical guidelines. J Clin Psychopharmacol 12 (suppl):42S–52S, 1992

Medawarn C, Rassaby E: Triazolam overdose, alcohol, and manslaughter. Lancet 338:1515–1516, 1991

Meltzer HY: An overview of the mechanism of action of clozapine. J Clin Psychiatry 55 (suppl B):47–52, 1994

Meltzer HY, Matsubara S, Lee J-C: Classification of typical and atypical antipsychotic drugs on the basis of dopamine D1, D2, and serotonin2 pKi values. J Pharmacol Exp Ther 251:238–246, 1989

Mendelson WB: Clinical distinction between long-acting and short-acting benzodiazepines. J Clin Psychiatry 53 (suppl):4–7, 1992

Menza MA, Kaufman KR, Castellanos A: Modafinil augmentation of antidepressant treatment in depression. J Clin Psychiatry 61:378–381, 2000

Metz A, Shader RI: Adverse interactions encountered when using trazodone to treat insomnia associated with fluoxetine. Int Clin Psychopharmacol 5:191–194, 1990

Miller DD, Sharafuddin MJA, Kathol RG: A case of clozapine-induced neuroleptic malignant syndrome. J Clin Psychiatry 52: 99–101, 1991

Mitchell JE, Mackenzie TB: Cardiac effects of lithium therapy in man: a review. J Clin Psychiatry 43:47–51, 1982

Mitchell JE, Popkin MK: Antipsychotic drug therapy and sexual dysfunction in men. Am J Psychiatry 139:633–637, 1982

Mitchell JE, Popkin JE: Antidepressant drug therapy and sexual dysfunction in men: a review. J Clin Psychopharmacol 3:76–79, 1983

Mitchell JE, Raymond N, Specker S: A review of the controlled trials of pharmacotherapy and psychotherapy in the treatment of bulimia nervosa. Int J Eat Disord 14: 229–247, 1993

Moskowitz AS, Altshuler L: Increased sensitivity to lithium-induced neurotoxicity after stroke: a case report. J Clin Psychopharmacol 11:272–273, 1991

Moskowitz H, Smiley A: Effects of chronically administered buspirone and diazepam on driving-related skills and performance. J Clin Psychiatry 43:45–55, 1982

Munjack DJ, Bruns J, Baltazar PL, et al: A pilot study of buspirone in the treatment of social phobia. J Anxiety Disord 5:87–98, 1991

Murphy JM, Mashman J, Miller JD, et al: Suppression of carbamazepine-induced rash with prednisone. Neurology 41:144–145, 1991

Murphy MJ, Lyon IW, Taylor JW, et al: Valproic acid associated with pancreatitis in an adult (letter). Lancet 1(8210):41–42, 1981

Myers DH, Carter RA, Burns BH, et al: A prospective study of the effects of lithium on thyroid function and on the prevalence of antithyroid antibodies. Psychol Med 15: 55–61, 1985

Nelson JC, Bowers MB: Delusional unipolar depression: description and drug response. Arch Gen Psychiatry 35:1321–1328, 1978

Nelson JC, Mazure CM, Bowers MB: A preliminary, open study of the combination of fluoxetine and desipramine. Arch Gen Psychiatry 48:303–307, 1991

Nestoros J, Suranyi B, Spees R, et al: Diazepam in high doses is effective in schizophrenia. Prog Neuropsychopharmacol Biol Psychiatry 6:513–518, 1982

Nielsen H: Recombinant human granulocyte colony-stimulating factor (rhG-CSF; filgrastim) treatment of clozapine-induced agranulocytosis. J Intern Med 34:529–531, 1993

Nierenberg AA, Keck PE Jr: Management of monoamine oxidase inhibitor-associated insomnia with trazodone. J Clin Psychopharmacol 9:42–45, 1989

NIMH Consensus Development Conference: Drugs and insomnia: the use of medication to promote sleep. JAMA 251:2410–2414, 1984

NIMH Consensus Development Conference Statement: Mood disorders: pharmacologic prevention of recurrences. Am J Psychiatry 142:469–476, 1985

Nora JJ, Nora AH, Toews WH: Lithium, Ebstein's anomaly and other congenital heart defects. Lancet 1:594–595, 1974

Noyes R Jr, Garvey MJ, Cook BL, et al: Benzodiazepine withdrawal: a review of evidence. J Clin Psychiatry 49:382–389, 1988

Oehrberg S, Christiansen PE, Behnke K, et al: Paroxetine in the treatment of panic disorder: a randomised, double-blind, placebo-controlled study. Br J Psychiatry 167: 374–379, 1995

Ojemann LM, Baugh-Bookman C, Dudley DL: Effect of psychotropic medications on seizure control in patients with epilepsy. Neurology 37:1525–1527, 1987

Oliver AP, Luchins DJ, Wyatt RJ: Neuroleptic-induced seizures: an in vitro technique for assessing relative risk. Arch Gen Psychiatry 39:206–209, 1982

Ontiveros A, Fontaine R, Elie PL, et al: Refractory depression: the addition of lithium to fluoxetine or desipramine. Acta Psychiatr Scand 83:188–192, 1991

Opler LA, Feinberg SS: The role of pimozide in clinical psychiatry: a review. J Clin Psychiatry 52:221–233, 1991

Ostergaard K, Dupont E: Clozapine treatment of drug-induced psychotic symptoms in late stages of Parkinson's disease (letter). Acta Neurol Scand 78:349–350, 1988

Patterson JF: Stevens-Johnson syndrome associated with carbamazepine therapy. J Clin Psychopharmacol 5:185, 1985

Peet M: Induction of mania with selective serotonin re-uptake inhibitors and tricyclic antidepressants. Br J Psychiatry 164:549–550, 1994

Pellock JM: Carbamazepine side effects in children and adults. Epilepsia 28:S64–S70, 1987

Pellock JM, Willmore LJ: A rational guide to routine blood monitoring in patients receiving antiepileptic drugs. Neurology 41:961–964, 1991

Perry P, Tsuang MT: Treatment of unipolar depression following electroconvulsive therapy: relapse rate comparison between lithium and tricyclic therapies following ECT. J Affect Disord 1:123–129, 1979

Perry PJ, Miller DD, Arndt SV, et al: Clozapine and norclozapine plasma concentrations and clinical response of treatment-refractory schizophrenic patients. Am J Psychiatry 148:231–235, 1991

Perse TL, Greist JH, Jefferson JW, et al: Fluvoxamine treatment of obsessive-compulsive disorder. Am J Psychiatry 144:1543–1548, 1988

Peselow ED, Dunner DL, Fieve RR, et al: Lithium carbonate and weight gain. J Affect Disord 2:303–310, 1980

Physicians' Desk Reference, 51st Edition. Montvale, NJ, Medical Economics, 2001

Pigott TA, Pato MT, Bernstein SE, et al: Controlled comparisons of clomipramine and fluoxetine in the treatment of obsessive-compulsive disorders: behavioral and biological results. Arch Gen Psychiatry 47:926–932, 1990

Placidi GF, Lenzi A, Lazzerini F, et al: The comparative efficacy and safety of carbamazepine versus lithium: a randomized double-blind 3-year trial in 83 patients. J Clin Psychiatry 47:490–494, 1986

Pope HG Jr, McElroy SL, Sathin A, et al: Head injury, bipolar disorder, and response to valproate. Compr Psychiatry 29:34–38, 1988

Pope HG Jr, McElroy SL, Keck PE Jr, et al: Valproate in the treatment of acute mania: a placebo-controlled study. Arch Gen Psychiatry 48:62–68, 1991

Post RM, Uhde TW, Ballenger JC, et al: Carbamazepine and its 10-11-epoxide metabolite in plasma and CSF: relationship to antidepressant response. Arch Gen Psychiatry 40:673–676, 1983

Post RM, Uhde TW, Ballenger JC: Efficacy of carbamazepine in affective disorders: implications for underlying physiological and biochemical substrates, in Anticonvulsants in Affective Disorders. Edited by Emrich HM, Okuma T, Muller AS. Amsterdam, The Netherlands, Elsevier, 1984, pp 93–115

Post RM, Uhde TW, Roy-Byrne PP, et al: Antidepressant effects of carbamazepine. Am J Psychiatry 143:29–34, 1986

Post RM, Uhde TW, Roy-Byrne PP, et al: Correlates of antimanic response to carbamazepine. Psychiatry Res 21:71–83, 1987

Preskorn SH, Burke M: Somatic therapy for major depressive disorder: selection of an antidepressant. J Clin Psychiatry 53 (suppl):5–18, 1992

Prien RF, Kupfer DJ: Continuation drug therapy for major depression episodes: how long should it be maintained? Am J Psychiatry 143:18–23, 1986

Prien RF, Kupfer DJ, Mansky PA, et al: Drug therapy in the prevention of recurrences in unipolar and bipolar affective disorders: report of the NIMH Collaborative Study Group comparing lithium carbonate, imipramine, and a lithium carbonate-imipramine combination. Arch Gen Psychiatry 41:1096–1104, 1984

Pycock CJ, Carter CJ, Kerwin RW: Effect of 6-hydroxydopamine lesions of the medial prefrontal cortex on neurotransmitter systems in subcortical sites in the rat. J Neurochem 34:91–99, 1980

Quitkin F, Rifkin A, Klein DF: Monoamine oxidase inhibitors: a review of antidepressant effectiveness. Arch Gen Psychiatry 35:749–760, 1979

Quitkin FM, McGrath PJ, Stewart JW, et al: Chronological milestones to guide drug change: when should clinicians switch antidepressants? Arch Gen Psychiatry 53: 785–792, 1996

Rakel RE: Long-term buspirone therapy for chronic anxiety: a multicenter international study to determine safety. South Med J 83:194–198, 1990

Ravaris CL, Robinson DS, Ives JO, et al: Phenelzine and amitriptyline in the treatment of depression: a comparison of present and past studies. Arch Gen Psychiatry 37: 1075–1080, 1980

Reunanen M, Kaarnen P, Vaisanen E: The influence of anticholinergic treatment on tardive dyskinesia caused by neuroleptic drugs. Acta Neurol Scand 65 (suppl 90): 278–279, 1982

Richens A: Safety of lamotrigine. Epilepsia 35 (suppl 5):S37–S40, 1994

Rickels K: The clinical use of hypnotics: indications for use and the need for a variety of hypnotics. Acta Psychiatr 332 (suppl): 132–141, 1986

Rickels K, Case WG, Downing RW, et al: Long-term diazepam therapy and clinical outcome. JAMA 250:767–771, 1983

Rickels K, Schweizer E, Csanelosi I, et al: Long-term treatment of anxiety and risk of withdrawal: prospective comparison of clonazepam and buspirone. Arch Gen Psychiatry 45:444–450, 1988

Risch SC, Groom GP, Janowsky DS: Interfaces of psychopharmacology and cardiology—part two. J Clin Psychiatry 42:47–57, 1981

Robert E, Guibaud P: Maternal valproic acid and congenital neural tube defects (letter). Lancet 2(8304):937, 1982

Roose SP: Modern cardiovascular standards for psychotropic drugs. Psychopharmacol Bull 28:35–43, 1992

Roose SP, Glassman AH, Giardina EGV, et al: Tricyclic antidepressants in depressed patients with cardiac conduction disease. Arch Gen Psychiatry 44:273–275, 1987

Roose SP, Dalack GW, Glassman AH, et al: Cardiovascular effects of bupropion in depressed patients with heart disease. Am J Psychiatry 148:512–516, 1991

Rosa FW: Spina bifida in infants of women treated with carbamazepine during pregnancy. N Engl J Med 324:674–677, 1991

Rosebush P, Stewart T: A prospective analysis of 24 episodes of neuroleptic malignant syndrome. Am J Psychiatry 146:717–725, 1989

Rosebush PI, Stewart TD, Gelenberg AJ: Twenty neuroleptic rechallenges after neuroleptic malignant syndrome in 15 patients. J Clin Psychiatry 50:295–298, 1989

Rosebush PI, Stewart T, Mazurek MF: The treatment of neuroleptic malignant syndrome: are dantrolene and bromocriptine useful adjuncts to supportive care? Br J Psychiatry 159:709–712, 1991

Rosen SI, Hanno PM: Clozapine-induced priapism. J Urol 148:876–877, 1992

Rosenbaum JF, Fava M, Hoog SL, et al: Selective serotonin reuptake inhibitor discontinuation syndrome: a randomized clinical trial. Biol Psychiatry 44:75–76, 1998

Rosenberg L, Mitchell AA, Parsells JL, et al: Lack of relation of oral clefts to diazepam use during pregnancy. N Engl J Med 309: 1282–1285, 1983

Rosenstein DL, Nelson JC, Jacobs SC: Seizures associated with antidepressants: a review. J Clin Psychiatry 54:289–299, 1993

Ross DR, Walker JI, Paterson J: Akathisia induced by amoxapine. Am J Psychiatry 140:115–116, 1983

Roth T, Roehrs TA: Issues in the use of benzodiazepine therapy. J Clin Psychiatry 53 (suppl):14–18, 1992

Sachs GS, Printz DJ, Kahn DA, et al: The Expert Consensus Guideline Series: medication treatment of bipolar disorder. Postgrad Med Spec No:1–104, 2000

Sackeim HA, Prudic J, Devanand DP, et al: The impact of medication resistance and continuation pharmacotherapy on relapse following response to electroconvulsive therapy in major depression. J Clin Psychopharmacol 10:96–104, 1990

Sackeim HA, Prudic J, Devanand DP, et al: Effects of stimulus intensity and electrode placement on the efficacy and cognitive effects of electroconvulsive therapy. N Engl J Med 328:839–846, 1993

Sackeim HA, Prudic J, Devanand DP, et al: A prospective, randomized, double-blind comparison of bilateral and right unilateral electroconvulsive therapy at different stimulus intensities. Arch Gen Psychiatry 57:425–434, 2000

Sackeim HA, Haskett RF, Mulsant BH, et al: Continuation pharmacotherapy in the prevention of relapse following electroconvulsive therapy: a randomized controlled trial. JAMA 285:1299–1307, 2001

Sanger T, Lieberman J, Tohen M, et al: Olanzapine versus haloperidol treatment in first-episode psychosis. Am J Psychiatry 156:79–87, 1999

Schenk CH, Remick RA: Sublingual nifedipine in the treatment of hypertensive crisis associated with monoamine oxidase inhibitors (letter). Ann Emerg Med 18:114–115, 1989

Scher M, Krieger JN, Juergens S: Trazodone and priapism. Am J Psychiatry 140:1362–1363, 1983

Schneier FR, Liebowitz MR, Davies SO, et al: Fluoxetine in panic disorder. J Clin Psychopharmacol 10:119–121, 1990

Schneier FR, Saoud JB, Campeas RC, et al: Buspirone in social phobia. J Clin Psychopharmacol 13:251–256, 1992

Schopf J: Withdrawal phenomena after long-term administration of benzodiazepines: a review of recent investigations. Pharmacopsychiatrie Neuro-Psychopharmakologie 16:1–8, 1983

Schulman KI, Walker SE: Refining the MAOI diet: tyramine content of pizzas and soy products. J Clin Psychiatry 60:191–193, 1999

Schulman KI, Walker SE: Clarifying the safety of the MAOI diet and pizza (letter, reply). J Clin Psychiatry 61:145–146, 2000

Schwarz T, Loewenstein J, Isenberg KE: Maintenance ECT: indications and outcome. Convuls Ther 11:14–23, 1995

Schweizer E, Rickels K, Lucki I: Resistance to anti-anxiety effects of buspirone in patients with a history of benzodiazepine use. N Engl J Med 314:719–720, 1986

Seeman P, Lee T, Chau-Wong M, et al: Antipsychotic drug doses and neuroleptic/dopamine receptors. Nature 261:717–719, 1976

Seide H, Muller HR: Choreiform movements as side effects of phenothiazine medication in elderly patients. J Am Geriatr Soc 15:517–522, 1967

Seidel WF, Cohen SA, Bliwise NG, et al: Buspirone: an anxiolytic without sedative effect. Psychopharmacology (Berl) 87:371–373, 1985

Selikoff IJ, Robitzek EH, Ornstein GG: Toxicity of hydrazine derivatives of isonicotinic acid in the chemotherapy of human tuberculosis. Quarterly Bulletin of SeaView Hospital 13:17–26, 1952

Sellers EM, Naranjo CA, Harrison M, et al: Oral diazepam loading: simplified treatment of alcohol withdrawal. Clin Pharmacol Ther 34:822–826, 1983

Sellers EM, Schneiderman JF, Romach MK, et al: Comparative drug effects and abuse liability of lorazepam, buspirone, and secobarbital in nondependent subjects. J Clin Psychopharmacol 12:79–85, 1992

Shader RI: Sexual dysfunction associated with thioridazine hydrochloride. JAMA 188:1007–1009, 1964

Shapira B, Gorfine M, Lerer B: A prospective study of lithium continuation therapy in depressed patients who have responded to electroconvulsive therapy. Convuls Ther 11:80–85, 1995

Sheehan DV, Ballenger J, Jacobsen G: Treatment of endogenous anxiety with phobic, hysterical, and hypochondriacal symptoms. Arch Gen Psychiatry 39:51–59, 1980

Sheehan DV, Raj AB, Sheehan KH, et al: Is buspirone effective for panic disorder? J Clin Psychopharmacol 10:3–11, 1990

Shimada T, Yamazaki H, Mimura M, et al: Interindividual variations in human liver cytochrome P-450 enzymes involved in the oxidation of drugs, carcinogens and toxic chemicals: studies with liver microsomes of 30 Japanese and 30 Caucasians. J Pharmacol Exp Ther 270:414–423, 1994

Shiono PH, Mills JL: Oral clefts and diazepam use during pregnancy (letter). N Engl J Med 311:919–920, 1983

Silver JM, Yudofsky SC: Neuropsychiatric aspects of traumatic brain injury, in Textbook of Neuropsychiatry. Edited by Hales RE, Yudofsky SC. Washington, DC, American Psychiatric Press, 1987, pp 179–190

Silver JM, Yudofsky SC: Aggressive disorders, in Neuropsychiatry of Traumatic Brain Injury. Edited by Silver JM, Yudofsky SC, Hales RE. Washington, DC, American Psychiatric Press, 1994, pp 313–354

Silver JM, Yudofsky SC, Kogan M, et al: Elevation of thioridazine plasma levels by propranolol. Am J Psychiatry 143:1290–1292, 1986

Skinner MH, Kuan HY, Pan A, et al: Duloxetine is both an inhibitor and a substrate of cytochrome P4502D6 in healthy volunteers. Clin Pharmacol Ther 73:170–177, 2003

Small JG: Anticonvulsants in affective disorders. Psychopharmacol Bull 26:25–36, 1990

Small JG, Milstein V, Klapper MH, et al: Electroconvulsive therapy in the treatment of manic episodes. Ann N Y Acad Sci 462:37–49, 1986

Smith WT, Glaudin V, Panagides J, et al: Mirtazapine versus amitriptyline versus placebo in the treatment of major depressive disorder. Psychopharmacol Bull 20:191–196, 1990

Squire LR, Slater PC: Electroconvulsive therapy and complaints of memory dysfunction: a prospective three-year follow-up study. Br J Psychiatry 142:1–8, 1983

Spier SA, Tesar GE, Rosenbaum JF, et al: Treatment of panic disorder and agoraphobia with clonazepam. J Clin Psychiatry 47:238–242, 1986

Sramek JJ, Tansman M, Suri A, et al: Efficacy of buspirone in generalized anxiety disorder with coexisting mild depressive symptoms. J Clin Psychiatry 57:287–291, 1996

Sullivan JT, Sellers EM: Treating alcohol, barbiturate, and benzodiazepine withdrawal. Rational Drug Therapy 20:1–8, 1986

Suppes T, Baldessarini RJ, Faedda GI, et al: Risk of recurrence following discontinuation of lithium treatment in bipolar disorder. Arch Gen Psychiatry 48:1082–1088, 1991

Suppes T, McElroy SL, Gilbert J, et al: Clozapine in the treatment of dysphoric mania. Biol Psychiatry 32:270–280, 1992

Suranyi-Cadotte BE, Bodnoff SR, Welner SA: Antidepressant-anxiolytic interactions: involvement of the benzodiazepine-GABA and serotonin systems. Prog Neuropsychopharmacol Biol Psychiatry 14:633–654, 1990

Svensson TH, Tung CS, Grenhoff J: The 5-HT2 antagonist ritanserin blocks the effect of pre-frontal cortex inactivation on rat A10 dopamine neurons in vivo. Acta Physiol Scand 136:497–498, 1989

Swann AC, Bowden CL, Morris D, et al: Depression during mania: treatment response to lithium or divalproex. Arch Gen Psychiatry 54:37–42, 1997

Takezaki H, Hanaoka M: The use of carbamazepine (Tegretol) in the control of manic-depressive psychosis and other manic-depressive states. J Clin Psychiatry 13:173–183, 1971

Tallman JF, Paul SM, Skolnick P, et al: Receptors for the age of anxiety: pharmacology of the benzodiazepines. Science 207:274–281, 1980

Teboul E, Chouinard G: A guide to benzodiazepine selection, part 1: pharmacological aspects. Can J Psychiatry 35:700–710, 1990

Tesar GE: High-potency benzodiazepines for short-term management of panic disorder: the U.S. evidence. J Clin Psychiatry 15 (suppl):4–10, 1990

Tesar GE, Rosenbaum JF, Pollack MH, et al: Double-blind, placebo-controlled comparison of clonazepam and alprazolam for panic disorder. J Clin Psychiatry 52:69–76, 1991

Thase ME: Effects of venlafaxine on blood pressure: a meta-analysis of original data from 3744 depressed patients. J Clin Psychiatry 59:502–508, 1998

Thase ME, Kupfer DJ, Frank E, et al: Treatment of imipramine-resistant depressant, II: an open clinical trial of lithium augmentation. J Clin Psychiatry 50:413–417, 1989

Thornton JE, Stahl SM: Case report of tardive dyskinesia and parkinsonism associated with amoxapine therapy. Am J Psychiatry 141:704–705, 1984

Tiller JW, Bouwer C, Behnke K: Moclobemide and fluoxetine for panic disorder. International Panic Disorder Study Group. Eur Arch Psychiatry Clin Neurosci 249 (suppl): S7–S10, 1999

Tollefson GD: Monoamine oxidase inhibitors: a review. J Clin Psychiatry 44:280–288, 1983

Tollefson GD, Birkett M, Koran L, et al: Continuation treatment of OCD: double-blind and open-label experience with fluoxetine. J Clin Psychiatry 55 (suppl):69–76, 1994

Tollefson G, Beasley C, Tamura R, et al: Blind, controlled, long-term study of the comparative incidence of treatment-emergent tardive dyskinesia with olanzapine or haloperidol. Am J Psychiatry 154:1248–1254, 1997

Tran P, Hamilton S, Kuntz A, et al: Double-blind comparison of olanzapine versus risperidone in the treatment of schizophrenia and other psychotic disorders. J Clin Psychopharmacol 17:407–418, 1997

Tyrer P, Owen R, Dawling S: Gradual withdrawal of diazepam after long-term therapy. Lancet 1(8339):1402–1406, 1983

Ugedo L, Grenhoff J, Svensson TH: Ritanserin, a 5-HT2 receptor antagonist, activates midbrain dopamine neurons by blocking serotonergic inhibition. Psychopharmacology 98:45–50, 1989

Umbricht D, Pollack S, Kane JM: Clozapine and weight gain. J Clin Psychiatry 55 (suppl B):157–160, 1994

Van Ameringen M, Mancini C, Streiner DL: Fluoxetine efficacy in social phobia. J Clin Psychiatry 54:27–32, 1993

van Harten J: Overview of the pharmacokinetics of fluvoxamine. Clin Pharmacokinet 29(suppl 1):1–9, 1995

van Vliet IM, Westenberg HG, Den Boer JA: MAO inhibitors in panic disorder: clinical effects of treatment with brofaromine: a double blind placebo controlled study. Psychopharmacology 112:483–489, 1993

van Vliet IM, den Boer JA, Westenberg HG, et al: A double-blind comparative study of brofaromine and fluvoxamine in outpatients with panic disorder. J Clin Psychopharmacol 16:299–306, 1996

Vaughan DA: Interaction of fluoxetine with tricyclic antidepressants (letter). Am J Psychiatry 145:1478, 1988

Vendsborg PB, Bech P, Rafaelson OJ: Lithium treatment and weight gain. Acta Psychiatr Scand 53:139–147, 1976

Vestergaard P, Amdisen A, Schou M: Clinically significant side effects of lithium treatment. Acta Psychiatr Scand 62:193–200, 1980

Vick NA: Suppression of carbamazepine-induced skin rash with prednisone. N Engl J Med 309:1193–1194, 1983

Votey SR, Bosse GM, Bayer MJ, et al: Flumazenil: a new benzodiazepine antagonist. Ann Emerg Med 20:181–188, 1991

Walczak DD, Apter JT, Halikas JA, et al: The oral dose-effect relationship for fluvoxamine: a fixed-dose comparison against placebo in depressed outpatients. Ann Clin Psychiatry 8:139–151, 1996

Walker SE, Shulman KI, Tailor SA, et al: Tyramine content of previously restricted foods in monoamine oxidase inhibitor diets. J Clin Psychopharmacol 16:383–388, 1996

Walker SE, Shulman KI, Tailor SA: The monoamine oxidase inhibitor (MAOI) diet and kosher pizza (letter, reply). J Clin Psychopharmacol 17:227–228, 1997

Waller DG, Edwards JG: Lithium and the kidney: an update. Psychol Med 19:825–831, 1989

Warnock JK, Knesevich J: Adverse cutaneous reactions to antidepressants. Am J Psychiatry 145:425–430, 1988

Watkins PB, Wrighton SA, Maurel P, et al: Identification of an inducible form of cytochrome P-450 in human liver. Proc Natl Acad Sci U S A 82:6310–6314, 1985

Wedin GP, Oderda GM, Klein-Schwartz W, et al: Relative toxicity of cyclic antidepressants. Ann Emerg Med 15:797–804, 1986

Wehr TA, Goodwin FK: Rapid cycling in manic-depressives induced by tricyclic antidepressants. Arch Gen Psychiatry 36:555–559, 1979

Wehr TA, Goodwin FK: Do antidepressants cause mania? Psychopharmacol Bull 23:61–65, 1987

Wehr TA, Sack DA, Rosenthal NE, et al: Rapid cycling affective disorder: contributing factors and treatment responses in 51 patients. Am J Psychiatry 145:179–184, 1988

Weilburg JB, Rosenbaum JF, Biederman J, et al: Fluoxetine added to non-MAOI antidepressant converts non-responders to responders: a preliminary report. J Clin Psychiatry 50:447–449, 1989

Weiner RD: The psychiatric use of electrically induced seizures. Am J Psychiatry 136:1507–1516, 1979

Weise CC, Stein MK, Pereira-Ogan J, et al: Amitriptyline once daily versus three times daily in depressed outpatients. Arch Gen Psychiatry 37:555–560, 1980

Westenberg HGM, den Boer JA: Clinical and biochemical effects of selective serotonin-uptake inhibitors in anxiety disorders, in Selective Serotonin Reuptake Inhibitors: Novel or Commonplace Agents? Edited by Gastpar M, Wakelin JS. Basel, Switzerland, S Karger, 1988, pp 84–99

Westenberg HG, den Boer JA: New findings in the treatment of panic disorder. Pharmacopsychiatry 26 (suppl):30–33, 1993

Wetzel H, Anghelescu I, Szegedi A, et al: Pharmacokinetic interactions of clozapine with selective serotonin reuptake inhibitors: differential effects of fluvoxamine and paroxetine in a prospective study. J Clin Psychopharmacol 18:2–9, 1998

Wheadon DE: Placebo controlled multi-center trial of fluoxetine in OCD. Paper presented at the Fifth World Congress of Biological Psychiatry, Florence, Italy, June 1991

Wikander I, Sundblad C, Andersch B, et al: Citalopram in premenstrual dysphoria: is intermittent treatment during luteal phases more effective than continuous medication throughout the menstrual cycle? J Clin Psychopharmacol 18:390–398, 1998

Wing YK, Chen CN: Tyramine content in Chinese food (letter, comment). J Clin Psychopharmacol 17:227, 1997

Wood IK, Parmalee DX, Foreman JW: Lithium-induced nephrotic syndrome. Am J Psychiatry 146:84–87, 1989

Wroblewski BA, Joseph AB, Kupfer J, et al: Effectiveness of valproic acid on destructive and aggressive behaviors in patients with acquired brain injury. Brain Inj 11:37–47, 1997

Yager J: Bethanecol chloride can reverse erectile and ejaculatory dysfunction induced by tricyclic antidepressants and mazindol: case report. J Clin Psychiatry 47:210–211, 1986

Yassa R: Antiparkinsonian medication withdrawal in the treatment of tardive dyskinesia: a report of three cases. Can J Psychiatry 30:440–442, 1985

Yassa R, Saunders A, Nastase C, et al: Lithium-induced thyroid disorders: a prevalence study. J Clin Psychiatry 48:14–16, 1988

Yoon MS, Han J, Dersham GH, et al: Effects of thioridazine (Mellaril) on ventricular electrophysiologic properties. Am J Cardiol 43:1155–1158, 1979

Yudofsky SC: Electroconvulsive therapy in general hospital psychiatry: a focus of new indications and technologies. Gen Hosp Psychiatry 3:292–296, 1981

Yudofsky SC, Silver JM: Beta-blockers in the treatment of performance anxiety. Harvard Mental Health Letter 4:8, 1987

Yudofsky SC, Silver JM, Schneider SE: Pharmacologic treatment of aggression. Psychiatr Ann 17:397–407, 1987

Yudofsky SC, Silver JM, Hales RE: Treatment of agitation and aggression, in The American Psychiatric Press Textbook of Psychopharmacology, 2nd Edition. Edited by Schatzberg AF, Nemeroff CB. Washington, DC, American Psychiatric Press, 1998, pp 881–900

Zalzstein E, Koren G, Einarson T, et al: A case-control study on the association between first trimester exposure to lithium and Ebstein's anomaly. Am J Cardiol 41:551–552, 1990

Zipursky RB, Baker RW, Zimmer B: Alprazolam withdrawal delirium unresponsive to diazepam: case report. J Clin Psychiatry 46:344–345, 1985

Zisook S: A clinical overview of monoamine oxidase inhibitors. Psychosomatics 26:240–246, 1985

Zitrin CM, Klein DF, Woerner MG, et al: Treatment of phobias: comparison of imipramine and placebo. Arch Gen Psychiatry 40:125–138, 1983

Zohar J, Ebstein RP, Belmaker RH: Adenylate cyclase as the therapeutic target site of lithium, in Basic Mechanisms in the Action of Lithium. Edited by Emrich HM, Aldenhoff JB, Lux HD. Amsterdam, The Netherlands, Elsevier, 1982, pp 154–166

Zornberg GL, Pope HGJ: Treatment of depression in bipolar disorder: new directions for research. J Clin Psychopharmacol 13:397–408, 1993

Zubenko GS, Cohen BM, Lipinski JF: Comparison of metoprolol and propranolol in the treatment of lithium tremor. Psychiatry Res 11:163–164, 1984

CHAPTER 19

Psychoanalysis, Psychoanalytic Psychotherapy, and Supportive Psychotherapy

Robert J. Ursano, M.D.

Edward K. Silberman, M.D.

Our health is directly and indirectly affected by our behavior: our thoughts, feelings, fantasies, and actions. Because of this effect, both increased morbidity and mortality can result from psychiatric illness. Frequently, psychopathology limits our ability to see options and exercise choices, leading to feelings, thoughts, fantasies, and actions that may be painful, restricted, and repetitive. Psychotherapy is directed toward changing these learned forms of behavior that affect health and performance. Personality is, in fact, a cluster of probable behaviors that each individual characteristically has in a given context (Ursano et al. 2001). Changing these response patterns can change the risk of disease, illness, and negative health behaviors, as well as interpersonal strategies that may decrease productivity and success.

Originally called the *talking cure*, psychotherapy is the generic term for a large number of treatment techniques that are directed toward changing behavior through verbal interchange. Psychotherapy provides understanding, support, new experiences, and new knowledge that can 1) result in learning, 2) increase the range of behaviors available to the patient, 3) relieve symptoms, and 4) alter maladaptive and unhealthy patterns of behavior. In the process of this reorganization, both perception and behavior change.

The target organ of psychotherapy is the brain. Feelings, thoughts, fantasies, and actions are brain functions. If behavior is to change, brain function and activity must alter at some basic level (Kandell 1979, 1989, 1999, 2000). If neuron A used to fire to neuron B, it must now fire to neuron C. Just as past life experience affects the development and maturation of the brain, and therefore brain activity, so too does present life experience, including the experience of psychotherapy.

Our social connectedness, a major focus of psychotherapeutic work, mediates both morbidity and mortality (House et al. 1988) and serves to regulate bodily function (Hofer 1984). The common observation that a phobic individual will approach the phobic object when accompanied by a supportive other illustrates the profound biological activities that accompany interpersonal relations and of which we know very little. How the "outside" (i.e., life experience) changes what is inside (i.e., our biology) is fundamental to an understanding of brain function and to the effectiveness of all psychotherapies. Our understanding of these processes, the science of behavior change, is now emerging (Kandell 1999, 2000; Ursano and Fullerton 1991). For example, Baxter et al. (1992) showed that after psychotherapy, changes in the brain evident through positron emission tomography are similar to those following treatment with fluoxetine, and preclinical studies are now well focused on the close relationship of brain structure, genes, and experience (Meaney 2001; Sapolsky 2000). Psychotherapy is a life experience that affects brain function. The neuroscience of psychotherapy is in its infancy.

Psychotherapy was defined by Harry Stack Sullivan (1954) as primarily a verbal interchange between two individuals in which one of these individuals is designated an expert and the other a help seeker. These two individuals work together to identify the patient's characteristic problems in living, with the hope of achieving behavioral change (Table 19–1). This definition of psychotherapy excludes a substantial number of activities that are inaccurately considered psychotherapy. First, psychotherapy by this definition is verbal. Certainly more than 90% of the interchange in psychotherapy is verbal. Although nonverbal communication can be important, it is never the primary activity of psychotherapy. Second, the requirement that one person be the help seeker

and the other an expert sets the roles, activities, and boundaries of this interchange. Two friends sharing a drink at a bar or restaurant do not fit this picture. In fact, in the bar or restaurant the social setting and rules are very different. In these settings, the rules of interaction dictate an equal sharing of one's problems. If one person is always the listener, the other begins to feel uncomfortable, because this is not the expected interchange. Rather, at the bar or restaurant, one person talks and then the other often says, "Oh yes, me too," or something similar. Not so in psychotherapy. Here the patient reveals his or her problems, but the physician-therapist provides help, not a reciprocal revelation of problems. The two settings have different rules governing the relationship (Epstein 1995).

TABLE 19–1.   Individual psychotherapy

Consists of an interaction between two persons.

Interaction is primarily verbal.

One person is the help seeker and the other an expert.

Goal of the interaction is to identify the characteristic patterns of behavior of the patient that are causing symptoms and problems in living.

Patient has the expectation of help and change.

All medical treatments, including psychotherapy, also show the effects of nonspecific curative factors in their outcomes (Table 19–2). These factors, also called *placebo effects*, include the presence of a confiding relationship, abreaction (i.e., the expression of intense feelings), the provision of new information, and the provision of a rationale or meaning (i.e., diagnosis) that organizes seemingly unrelated symptoms and events and maximizes the patient's probability of success experiences (J.D. Frank 1971). Clinicians use these principles as part of the art and science of medical treatment to increase their patients' relief of pain and suffering.

TABLE 19–2. Nonspecific curative factors of medical intervention

---

Developing a confiding relationship
Maintaining the expectation of help and
  benefit
Providing opportunities for abreaction
Providing new information
Providing a rationale/organization/meaning
  (diagnosis) to seemingly unrelated
  symptoms and events
Maximizing the probability that the patient
  will experience a success

In addition to these nonspecific factors, most medical treatments also have specific curative factors. Similarly, the psychotherapies identify specific technical interventions and procedures directed toward behavioral change.

As in other medical treatments, there are contraindications to and dangers in the use of psychotherapy (Crown 1983; Hadley and Strupp 1976). It is not sufficient to take the position that "the operation was a success but the patient died"—or that psychotherapy was a success but no change occurred. Although the therapist in individual psychotherapy does not "require" behavioral change and, depending on the type of psychotherapy, may or may not directly use technical procedures focused on behavioral change per se (e.g., practice, desensitization), the final result of the therapist's technical expertise is behavioral change. Such change includes alterations in the patient's well-being, physical health, social supports, and societal productivity, as well as symptomatic relief. What is dealt with in treatment is what the patient is able to bring into fo-

cus, what the patient can tolerate talking about, and what the patient can tolerate the therapist talking about (Coleman 1968).

Psychotherapy is both efficacious and cost-effective (Crits-Christoph 1992; Crits-Christoph and Barben 1991; Perry et al. 1999). The effectiveness of psychotherapy is no longer a matter of debate (Luborsky et al. 1975; Parloff 1982; Parloff et al. 1986; Shapiro and Shapiro 1982; Smith et al. 1980; Spiegel and Lazar 1997). However, the answer to the question of which psychotherapy for which patient and by which therapist is still unclear (Parloff 1982).

Smith and colleagues (Smith and Glass 1977; Smith et al. 1980) showed an effect size of psychotherapy of 0.68, a level equivalent to that found in several clinical trials that were stopped early because it would have been unethical to withhold such a clearly effective treatment from patients. Crits-Christoph (1992; Crits-Christoph and Barben 1991) demonstrated somewhat larger effect sizes in a review of well-designed studies of brief psychodynamic psychotherapy. This review also found that after brief psychodynamic psychotherapy, patients were better off than 79% of those on a waiting list in terms of psychiatric symptom levels and social adjustment.

Psychotherapies can be distinguished by their overall goals, the techniques used, and the diagnostic categories to which the techniques can be applied. In this chapter we review psychoanalytically oriented treatments—psychoanalysis and psychoanalytically oriented (psychodynamic) psychotherapy, interpersonal psychotherapy, (IPT) which has many psychodynamic elements (Markowitz et al. 1998), and finally, supportive psychotherapy. The psychoanalytically oriented and supportive psychotherapies remain the most commonly used psychotherapies. Many of the principles of the psychodynamic/psycho- analytic treatments have been incorpo- rated into other treatment modalities and into the clinical assessment process, med- ication management, and ward milieu work. Understanding the principles and phenomena observed in psychodynamic treatment, therefore, is often critical to success with other treatments and evalua- tion techniques (Gabbard 2000). In addi- tion, skill in the briefer forms of psycho- therapy is related to skill in the longer- term treatments, although these treat- ment approaches are not the same.

The psychoanalytically oriented treat- ments and supportive psychotherapy are applied to a wide array of diagnostic problems. Understanding the techniques and the phases of these therapies can also provide important knowledge and skills for assessment and management of medi- cation, compliance, interpersonal stres- sors, and past and present family prob- lems, all of which can greatly affect outcome, relapse, rehabilitation, and so- cial function.

Psychoanalytically Oriented Psychotherapies

Primary to the psychodynamic (psycho- analytically oriented) treatments is the importance of the patient feeling engaged and involved in the work. Through the ex- ploration of the patient's conflicts evi- denced in symptoms, metaphors, and symbols, both defensive patterns and dis- turbances in present interpersonal rela- tionships can be identified in the treat- ment setting as well as in the patient's life. The therapist's ability to hear what the patient has to say and to understand its meaning is central to all psychoanalyt- ically oriented treatments (Solnit 2000). This facet of treatment demands skill in neutral listening and the ability to identify

with the patient's perspective and world- view while not losing one's own.

The therapist is always listening for the continuity present, but hidden, be- tween sessions (Coleman 1968). The therapist operates on the hypothesis that each session is related to the previous one.

In the initial phase of treatment, the therapeutic alliance (i.e., the working alli- ance) is developed (Greenson 1965; Zet- zel 1956). The therapeutic alliance is the reality-based relationship between the an- alyst (or the therapist) and the patient that forms the basis of working together in a cooperative manner (Sonnenberg et al. 1997). The therapeutic alliance is nur- tured through the identification of the pa- tient's initial anxieties about beginning treatment. Fostering the therapeutic alli- ance is a part of the therapist's establish- ment of the conditions under which the patient can favorably hear and deal with the interpretations that the therapist will give later in the treatment (Ponsi 2000).

Few empirical studies of psychoana- lytic treatment have been done (Bachrach et al. 1985; Galatzer-Levy et al. 2000; Kantrowitz et al. 1986, 1987, 1990; Kern- berg et al. 1972; Sandell et al. 2000; Vaughan et al. 2000; Wallerstein 1992). The brief psychodynamic treatments have a somewhat greater empirical database, but much further research is needed here as well (Crits-Christoph 1992; Gomes- Schwartz et al. 1978; Horowitz et al. 1986; Luborsky et al. 1975, 1988; Malan 1980; Milrod et al. 2000). In general, the studies that have been conducted support the efficacy of psychoanalytically oriented treatment approaches. However, method- ological issues are prominent in most of the research in this area. Moreover, the difficulties of long-term studies are sub- stantial. Handbooks for treatment will go far in improving research in the psychoan- alytically oriented treatments (Luborsky 1984).

Psychoanalysis

Psychoanalysis was developed by Sigmund Freud beginning in the late nineteenth century. Originally, Freud used hypnosis to recover forgotten memories related to traumas of early childhood. Historically, he progressed from hypnosis to the "pressure technique" and finally to the modern approach of using free association. Freud found that it was the subjective experience of events in childhood—that is, the psychic reality of the events—rather than the presence or absence of the actual events, that affected development and conflict formation. This discovery led Freud to identify the role of the unconscious and unremembered experiences of childhood and to develop a mechanism, psychoanalysis, to discover and bring these memories into awareness.

The dangers of neglecting the actuality of traumatic events have been highlighted in recent years and must always be considered by the therapist. In the treatment of children this is particularly important because of the need to intervene to protect the child. Often, a neglect of the reality of trauma results if the therapist does not understand that the patient's recall is a mixture of both subjective factors and objective fact, neither of which can be ignored.

Freud identified dreams, slips of the tongue, and free association as important windows on the influence of childhood and the present conflicts of the patient. From the psychoanalytic view, an understanding of the conflicts experienced in childhood is important to gaining knowledge of and changing present behavior (Brenner 1976). The conflicts of childhood are called the *childhood neurosis.*

Conflicts are patterns of feelings, thoughts, and behavior that were "learned" (i.e., incorporated into brain function and patterning) during childhood. "Neurotic"

conflicts result in the patient's feelings of anxiety and depression; somatic symptoms; work, social, or sexual inhibition; and maladaptive interpersonal relations. Typically, such conflicts are between libidinal (i.e., sexual/bodily) and aggressive wishes. Libidinal wishes can be thought of as longings for sexual and emotional gratification or more generally as positive feelings and affects (Kernberg 2001). Aggressive wishes are destructive desires (or, as they are more often conceptualized today, negative feelings and affects) that either are primary or result from frustration and deprivation.

The concept of sexual wishes is quite broad in psychoanalysis and is not limited to only genital feelings. Sexual wishes include wishes to be held and touched, to control, to eat, and many others.

The goal of psychoanalysis is the elucidation of the childhood neurosis (i.e., conflicts) as it presents in the transference neurosis (Table 19–3). This is a major undertaking that requires a reasonably psychiatrically healthy individual who can sustain the treatment. Psychoanalysis is frequently criticized for being used to treat reasonably psychiatrically healthy people. In fact, however, this is the tradition of medicine. For example, one may ask who receives triple bypass surgery: the individual with a single left main descending artery occlusion or the individual who is having a myocardial infarction and in the end stage of congestive heart failure? Clearly, the answer is the former. This underscores the frequently forgotten point that medical treatments are given to patients rather than to diseases. Psychoanalysis is very demanding of patients. It requires an individual who is able to access his or her fantasy life in an active, experiencing manner and is able to leave it behind at the end of a session.

Psychoanalysis focuses on the recovery of childhood experiences as they appear in

TABLE 19-3.   Psychoanalysis

Goal	Resolution of the childhood neurosis as it presents itself in the transference neurosis
Selection criteria	Experiences conflict that is primarily oedipal
	Experiences conflict as internal
	Is psychologically minded
	Is able to obtain symptom relief through understanding
	Is able to experience and observe strong affects without acting out
	Has supportive relationships available in both the present and the past
Duration	Four to five sessions per week; 3–6 years, average duration
Techniques	Free association
	Therapeutic alliance
	Neutrality
	Abstinence
	Defense analysis
	Interpretation of transference

the relationship with the analyst (Chessick 2000; Coltrera 1980; Freud 1912a/1958; Gill 1982; Greenson 1967). This re-creation in the physician–patient relationship of a conflicted relationship with a childhood figure is the *transference neurosis*. Frequently, the transference is paternal or maternal, but it need not be. Sibling, aunt, uncle, and grandparent transferences are all important parts of psychoanalytic work.

Transference is a ubiquitous phenomenon that is increasingly able to be studied empirically (Fried et al. 1992; Luborsky and Crits-Christoph 1990). Several empirical studies support the importance of addressing the transference for a successful outcome of psychodynamic treatment (Brodaty 1983; Donovan 1984; Frances and Perry 1983; Luborsky and Crits-Christoph 1990; Malan 1975, 1976, 1980; Marziali 1984; Marziali and Sullivan 1980). Transference is the result of our tendency to see the past in the present, to exclude new information, and to see what is familiar to us (Table 19–4). This "looking for the familiar" results in our reacting and responding in ways that are characteristic

of our relationships with significant figures from our past. The analyst's relative abstinence (i.e., avoiding gratifying wishes) and neutrality (i.e., not encouraging one side or another of the patient's conflict—either the wishes or the defenses and prohibitions) help create a setting in which the transference can emerge and, more important, in which it can be observed and understood by the analyst and the patient. It is the contrast between the patient's experience of the analyst in the transference and his or her experience in the therapeutic alliance that facilitates the recognition that the transference thoughts and feelings are self-generated.

The transference is not a total distortion of the physician–patient relationship. Rather, it is often an elaboration (without confirming information) of an observation the patient has made about the analyst or his or her office. The patient's understanding of the transference aids in the recall of the past and the recovery of lost feelings.

Countertransference refers to the analyst's transference response to the patient. At times, *countertransference* is also used

TABLE 19–4. Transference and countertransference

Transference	Seeing the past in the present
	Seeing the familiar
	Excluding new information
Countertransference	
Concordant	Identifying with the patient's feelings (the therapist feels as though he or she were the patient)
Complementary	Reacting to the patient's feelings (the therapist feels as though he or she were the transference figure)

to describe the analyst's specific neurotic responses to the patient's transference (Table 19–4). However, this is not clearly different from the first, more general, definition (Blum 1986). Like transference, countertransference is also ubiquitous, and it is not limited to the psychoanalytic setting. In fact, it can be an important part of any relationship, particularly the physician–patient relationship; when present, it may be intense and enduring. Countertransference is increased by life stress and unresolved conflicts in the analyst. It can appear as either an identification with or a reaction to the patient's conscious and unconscious fantasies, feelings, and behaviors (Racker 1957). Skill in recognizing countertransference and transference is an important part of the psychiatrist's armamentarium in all treatment settings, particularly those involving consultation-liaison psychiatry, in which the physician–patient or nurse–patient relationships can be the major reason a consultation was requested.

The design of the psychoanalytic treatment situation fosters the patient's observing capacity so that the transference neurosis can be analyzed (Stone 1961). Transference is not unique to the psychoanalytic situation. It occurs throughout life in all areas and is a frequent accompaniment to hospitalization of any kind. The ability to recognize transference phenomena as they appear in all physician–patient relationships is very important.

Modern psychoanalysis continues to require frequent meetings of the analyst and analysand—usually, four to five sessions per week. (Freud originally met with his patients six times per week.) This frequency of sessions is continued, on average, for 3–6 years. This intensity of meetings is necessary for the patient to develop sufficient trust to explore his or her inner fantasy life. In addition, given the number of events that occur daily in a human life, the frequent meetings enable the patient to explore fantasies rather than only the reality-based perceptions of life events (Freud 1912b/1958). Individuals who are in crisis and who therefore are very concerned and focused on the real events in their life are not good candidates to enter psychoanalysis. Psychoanalysis focuses on the patient's experience and fantasies of his or her life rather than on the real events. In general, the patient in psychoanalysis is encouraged to use the couch so that the patient's focus on fantasies rather than on reality will be further facilitated. In addition, the analyst usually sits out of view, allowing the patient better to elaborate his or her fantasies about the analyst.

Free association is a major element in the technique of psychoanalysis. Freud described free association through an analogy of a train ride (Freud 1913/1958). He suggested that if the analyst and analysand were riding together on a train and the analyst were blind, the analysand would not forget to describe the beautiful mountains or the ugly coal slags. This analogy is meant to convey the sense of the patient's reporting of all thoughts that come to mind without censorship and without dismissing them as too trivial.

Early in treatment, the analyst establishes a therapeutic alliance with the patient that allows for a reality-based consideration of the demands of the treatment and for a working collaboration between analyst and analysand toward the patient's understanding himself or herself (Greenson 1965; Meissner 1998; Zetzel 1956). The analyst focuses on analyzing the defenses the patient uses to minimize conflict and disturbing affects (Freud 1912b/1958, 1913/1958, 1914/1958) (Table 19–5). Defenses such as intellectualization, reaction formation, denial, repression, and other neurotic cognitive mechanisms are identified and repeatedly interpreted to the patient. Through the analysis of defense, the working alliance strengthens, and the patient's ability to observe internal fantasies and to talk about his or her feelings with the analyst increases.

The analysis of the patient's dreams is an important element of psychoanalytic treatment (Freud 1911/1958; Reiser 2001; Sharpe 1961; Ursano et al. 1998). Dreams, as well as slips of the tongue and symptoms, express the conflicts of the patient in "metaphor," evidencing the out-of-awareness (i.e., unconscious) elements of the conflict.

The analyst uses a number of techniques in his or her interventions, including interpretation and clarification (Bibring 1954; Glover 1968). Classically, an interpretation is the linking together of the patient's experience of an event in the present with the transference experience of the analyst and the childhood-significant figure. Rarely are interpretations actually given in one sentence in one session. More frequently, interpretations occur

TABLE 19–5. Defense mechanisms
Repression
Intellectualization
Reaction formation
Regression
Displacement
Sublimation
Reversal
Splitting
Denial
Projection
Inhibition
Projective identification
Asceticism
Omnipotence
Isolation of affect
Devaluing
Identification with the aggressor
Primitive idealization

over a period during which the past, the present, and the transference experiences are linked together.

Medications are infrequently used in psychoanalysis, although some analysts use medication in the treatment of persons with affective disorders. Psychoanalysis is a highly supportive treatment for the individual who experiences frequent contact, quiet inquiry, and intellectual understanding as a supportive environment (de Jonghe et al. 1992; Wallerstein 1989).

The analyst operates under several guiding principles that facilitate the analysis of the transference. These principles include 1) neutrality, by which the analyst favors neither the patient's wishes (i.e., the id) nor the condemnations of these wishes (i.e., the superego); and 2) abstinence, whereby the analyst does not provide gratification to the patient similar to that of the wished-for object (Freud 1915 [1914]/1958). Abstinence is the avoidance of becoming this figure *in reality* and gratifying these wishes or beliefs. The therapist's abstinence leads to his or her being somewhat silent but not withholding, in order better to observe how the patient organizes his or her psychic world. This stance must be explained and the patient educated about the reason for this stance.

The assessment of a patient for psychoanalysis must include diagnostic considerations as well as an assessment of the patient's ability to make use of the psychoanalytic situation for behavioral change. These considerations include the patient's psychological mindedness; the availability of supports in his or her real environment to sustain the psychoanalysis, which can be felt as quite depriving; and the patient's ability to experience and simultaneously to observe highly charged affective states.

Because of the frequency of the sessions and the duration of the treatment, the cost of psychoanalysis can be prohibitive. Low-fee clinics frequently make available a substantial amount of treatment to some patients who could not otherwise afford it.

Psychoanalysis has been useful in the treatment of obsessional disorders, anxiety disorders, dysthymic disorders, and moderately severe personality disorders. Individuals with substantial preoedipal pathology, usually indicated by chaotic life settings and an inability to establish a supportive dyadic relationship, as is often seen in patients with narcissistic, borderline, schizoid, paranoid, and schizotypal personality disorders, are usually not thought to be candidates for traditional psychoanalysis. Psychoanalysis is more frequently recommended after a course of brief psychotherapy has proved to be either ineffective or insufficient.

Psychoanalytic Psychotherapy

Psychoanalytically oriented psychotherapy—also known as *psychoanalytic psychotherapy, psychodynamic psychother-* *apy,* and *explorative psychotherapy*—is a psychotherapeutic procedure that recognizes the development of transference and resistance in the psychotherapy setting (Bruch 1974; Fromm-Reichmann 1950). Both long-term and brief psychodynamic psychotherapy are possible.

Brief psychotherapy, in particular, requires the therapist to confront his or her own ambitiousness and perfectionism as well as any exaggerated ideal of personality structure and function. The time limits of brief psychotherapy give the therapy its unique characteristics and distinguish it from long-term psychotherapy and psychoanalysis (Ursano and Dressler 1974).

Psychoanalytic psychotherapy is usually more focused than the extensive reworking of personality undertaken in psychoanalysis (Dewald 1978). In addition, psychoanalytic psychotherapy is oriented somewhat more to the here and now and there is less of an attempt to reconstruct the developmental origins of conflicts. Psychoanalytically oriented psychotherapy may take as its entire goal the analysis of a set of defenses that are interfering with the patient's development. The accomplishment of this task may substantially open up the patient's life and development.

Psychoanalytic psychotherapy recognizes and interprets transference when it occurs (Table 19–6). However, the entire treatment is not directed toward the establishment and analysis of the transference in the thorough manner of a psychoanalysis. Long-term psychodynamic psychotherapy includes more transference work than do the brief psychodynamic psychotherapies. Psychoanalytic psychotherapy also makes use of techniques that are not available in psychoanalysis. This allows for its application to a broader range of patients, including those with psychotic regressive potentials such as borderline personality disorder.

TABLE 19–6.   Psychoanalytic psychotherapy

Goal	Defense and transference analysis with limited reconstruction of the past
Selection criteria	When a narrower focus and less comprehensive outcome is acceptable
	The same selection criteria as in psychoanalysis are used, but they can include more seriously disturbed patients who can use understanding to resolve symptoms when supportive elements are available in the treatment
Duration	One to three sessions per week for 1–6 years on average
Techniques	Therapeutic alliance
	Face to face
	Free association
	Defense and transference interpretation
	More use of clarification, suggestion, and learning through experience than in psychoanalysis
	Medication

Usually, patients in long-term psychoanalytic psychotherapy are seen one, two, or three times per week; twice per week is desirable in that this frequency allows for sufficient intensity for the transference to unfold and to be interpreted. Patient and therapist meet in face-to-face encounters and free association is encouraged. Psychoanalytic psychotherapy may extend from several months to several years, at times taking as long as a psychoanalysis. The length of treatment is determined by the number of focal problem areas undertaken in the treatment. Medications are used in psychoanalytic psychotherapy and provide another means of titrating the level of regression a patient may experience. The therapist uses interpretations and clarifications as in psychoanalysis. In addition, however, the therapist may use other interpretative techniques such as practice of new behavior patterns and experiences and confrontation (Bibring 1954). *Practice* in this context refers to learning from experience, such as pointing out that the therapist does not respond in the expected transferential manner. Confrontation is not "fighting"; rather, it consists of pointing out to the patient when something is being denied or avoided.

The same patients who are treated in psychoanalysis can be treated in psychoanalytic psychotherapy. However, the focus of the treatment is much narrower and the expected outcome less comprehensive. The psychosocial problems and internal conflicts of patients who could not be treated in psychoanalysis, such as those with major depression, schizophrenia, and borderline personality disorder, can be addressed in a long-term psychoanalytic psychotherapy. The long-term contributions of psychoanalytic psychotherapy to the treatment of major depression and schizophrenia, for which biological treatments have proved efficacious for some of the major symptoms, require further study. Patients with these diagnoses use psychotherapy to modify illness-onset conditions and facilitate readjustment, recovery, and reintegration into family and community life. In long-term psychoanalytic psychotherapy, the regressive tendencies of such patients can be titrated with greater elements of support, the use of medication as needed, and greater reality feedback through the face-to-face encounter with the therapist.

The opening phase of psychodynamic psychotherapy is often marked by the activation of the magical expectations of the patient and the belief that past pains will now be resolved. During the initial phase, the therapist may make few comments and usually accepts the positive transference of the patient. Important aspects of the current problems, the patient's characteristic defense mechanisms and coping styles, and the developmental roots of the central issue become clearer during this phase. In the middle phase of treatment, resistance is likely to appear, as well as the negative transference. The patient experiences the frustration that not all of the wished-for changes are occurring. Defenses are identified and analyzed, and usually the transference is sufficiently evident to be worked with.

Interpersonal Psychotherapy

IPT is a psychotherapy developed by Klerman and colleagues (Klerman et al. 1984a, 1984b; Markowitz 1998; Rounsaville et al. 1985b). Whether conducted briefly or longer term, IPT focuses on current interpersonal problems in outpatient nonbipolar, nonpsychotic depressed individuals. IPT has been the major psychotherapeutic modality used in combined psychotherapy and pharmacological treatment studies. This psychotherapy has also been used for the treatment of drug abuse. It did not, however, have a notable impact on outcome when patients were already participating in a well-run treatment program that included weekly group psychotherapy (Rounsaville et al. 1983, 1985a). IPT derives from the interpersonal school of psychiatry that originated with Adolf Meyer and Harry Stack Sullivan. The un-

derstanding of social supports and of attachment provides further theoretical underpinning for this form of psychotherapy. IPT focuses on reassurance, clarification of feeling states, improvement in interpersonal communication, testing of perception, and interpersonal skills rather than on personality reconstruction.

TABLE 19–7. Interpersonal psychotherapy

Goal	Improvement in current interpersonal skills
Selection criteria	Outpatient, nonbipolar, nonpsychotic depression
Duration	Short- and long-term
	Usually once-weekly meetings
Techniques	Reassurance
	Clarification of feeling states
	Improvement of interpersonal communication
	Testing perceptions
	Development of interpersonal skills
	Medication

In IPT the therapist focuses on the patient's current social functioning (Table 19–7). A complete inventory of current and past significant interpersonal relationships, including the family of origin, friendships, and relations in the community, is a part of the evaluation phase. Patterns of authority, dominance and submission, dependency and autonomy, intimacy, affection, and activities are observed. Cognitions are generally seen as beliefs and attitudes about norms, expectations and roles, and role performance. Defense mechanisms may be recognized, but they are explored in terms of interpersonal relations. Similarly, dreams may be examined as a reflection of current interpersonal problems. In IPT, the therapist may explore distorted thinking by comparing what the patient says with what he or she does or by identifying the patient's view of an interpersonal relationship (Klerman et al. 1984b).

IPT has been primarily used in the treatment of depressed patients (A.F. Frank et al. 1991; O'Hara et al. 2000). In the opening phase of IPT, a detailed symptom history is taken, usually using a structured interview. The symptoms are reviewed with the patient, and the patient receives explicit information about the natural course of depression as a clinical condition. There is an emphasis on legitimizing the patient in the sick role. A second major task of this phase is the assessment of the patient's interpersonal problem areas. There is an attempt to identify one or more of four problem areas: grief reaction, interpersonal disputes, role transition, and interpersonal deficits. Each of these areas is thought to be related to depression.

The middle phase of treatment is directed toward resolving the problem area or areas. Clarifying positive and negative feeling states, identifying past models for relationships, and guiding and encouraging the patient in examining and choosing alternative courses of action constitute the basic techniques for handling each problem area (Weissman and Markowitz 1994). The focus is kept on current dilemmas and not past interpersonal relationships. Interpersonal events, rather than intrapsychic or cognitive events, are the focus of IPT.

Much of IPT is based on psychodynamic theory (Markowitz et al. 1998). The therapist's attitude is one of exploration, similar to the attitude in other insight-oriented psychotherapies when applied in a medical model. Applying the dictum of working "from the surface to the depths" results in much of the resemblance of IPT to psychodynamic psychotherapy. However, Klerman and colleagues found it useful to highlight the differences between these approaches to standardize a psychotherapeutic technique. Collaborative clinical trials have demonstrated the advantage of maintenance IPT in enhancing social functioning during recovery from depression and in reducing symptoms and improving functioning during the acute phase of a depressive episode. These effects require 6–8 months to become apparent. Depressed patients undergoing combined pharmacotherapy and IPT have the best outcomes. IPT has also been effective in the treatment of postpartum depression, improving depressive symptoms and social adjustment (O'Hara et al. 2000).

Comparison of Psychodynamic, Interpersonal, and Cognitive Psychotherapies

Because interpersonal and cognitive psychotherapies are related to the psychodynamic model, there is a high degree of overlap in the problem areas identified in any given patient in these treatments. The conceptualization of the problem, however, is different. In many ways it is complementary rather than mutually exclusive. The psychoanalytic, interpersonal, and cognitive psychotherapies share explorative and change-oriented goals. Cognitive psychotherapy focuses on the patient's thinking; IPT on the patient's interpersonal relations and social supports; and psychoanalytically oriented treatments on the internal experience of the patient and its relationship to past experience. Cognitive and interpersonal psychotherapies are most frequently used to treat depression rather than to treat an entire range of psychopathology. No studies using well-defined psychodynamic psychotherapies and medication have been performed. In this area, IPT and cognitive psychotherapy have been more closely studied.

IPT, cognitive psychotherapy, and the more traditional psychodynamic psychotherapies can be compared (Table 19–8). All three modalities are complex methods of treatment that must be tailored to the individual patient. All demand a high degree of clinical judgment in the therapist, and the therapist requires a considerable investment of time to acquire competency in administering these treatments (Beck et al. 1979).

Empirical studies comparing well-defined psychodynamic psychotherapy with cognitive and interpersonal psychotherapies have not yet been undertaken. Future research must address which form of psychotherapy may be most helpful for which patient. To develop research strategies, it would be helpful to conceptualize this question as related to the mode or modes through which any particular patient can most effectively learn new behaviors. An individual's available learning path (e.g., through the study of cognitions, interpersonal relations, and/or subjective experience) is influenced by state, trait, and contextual variables.

Supportive Psychotherapy

The term *supportive* is generally used to distinguish a type of psychotherapy that is less ambitious, less intensive, and less anxiety-provoking than those designated psychoanalytic, insight-oriented, exploratory, or expressive. Universally, supportive psychotherapy is ranked as the most important type of psychotherapy to learn during residency training (Langsley and Yager 1988). Despite its centrality, supportive therapy has traditionally been described only vaguely, as a residual category of treatment for patients not suitable for other forms of therapy—a modality de-

fined more by what it is not than by what it is. More recently, there has been a growing interest in supportive therapy as a worthy subject in its own right, and increasing numbers of articles and books have been devoted to describing or studying this modality (Novalis et al. 1997; Werman 1984).

In current thought, supportiveness is seen as an essential element in all forms of psychotherapy, which differ in degree rather than presence of supportive techniques (Ornstein 1986). Supportive psychotherapy may best be viewed as one pole on a continuum of therapies with only relative differences in goals, indications, theoretical bases, strategies, and techniques.

Goals

The goals of supportive psychotherapy (Table 19–9) include amelioration of symptoms, maintenance or restoration of function, improved self-esteem, and improved adaptation to internal and external stresses as the distinctive goals of supportive therapy (Munich 1997). These stand in contrast to the goals of psychoanalysis and psychoanalytic therapy, which center on reversing underlying pathology and restructuring personality.

This dichotomy between supportive and psychoanalytic therapy is clearest in cases in which supportive therapy aims to *maintain* or *restore* function (Table 19–10). It is uncertain whether long-term *improvement* in symptoms, self-esteem, or life functioning can occur without concomitant changes in ego structure—at least in the absence of a continuing relationship with the therapist as an "auxiliary ego."

Indications

In common clinical practice, patients at both ends of the health–sickness contin-

TABLE 19–8. Comparison of psychoanalytic, interpersonal, and cognitive psychotherapies

	Psychoanalytic/ psychodynamic psychotherapy	Interpersonal psychotherapy	Cognitive psychotherapy
Treatment focus	Internal experience	Interpersonal relationships and social supports	Thoughts/cognitions
Primary diagnoses treated	Anxiety	Depression	Depression
	Depression	Anxiety	Anxiety
	Personality disorders		
Skill needed by therapist	++++	++++	++++
Therapeutic alliance	++++	++++	++++
Nonjudgmental stance	++++	++++	++++
Focus			
Cognitive	+++ (defense mechanisms)	+	++++ (cognitive distortions)
Interpersonal	++++ (transference and past relationships)	++++ (interpersonal withdrawal, attachment and models)	+
Technique			
Nondirective	++++	+	+
Directive/behavioral interventions	+	++++	++++

Note. Plus signs indicate degree, from small (+) to great (++++).

TABLE 19–9. Supportive psychotherapy

Goal	Support of reality testing
	Provision of ego support
	Maintenance or reestablishment of usual level of functioning
Selection criteria	Very healthy individual faced with overwhelming crises
	Patient with ego deficits
Duration	Days, months, or years—as needed
Techniques	Predictable availability of therapist
	Use of interpretation to strengthen defenses
	Maintenance of reality-based working relationship grounded in support, concern, and problem solving
	Suggestion, reinforcement, advice, reality testing, cognitive restructuring, reassurance, limit setting, and environmental interventions
	Medication
	Psychodynamic life narrative

TABLE 19–10. Goals

Supportive therapy	Psychoanalytic therapy
Maintenance of function	Reversal of pathology
Restoration of function	Restructuring of personality
Coping with pathology	Resolution of unconscious conflict
Alleviation of symptoms	Understanding of symptoms

uum receive supportive psychotherapy: individuals who are generally very psychiatrically healthy and well adapted but who have become impaired in response to stressful life circumstances and individuals who have severe pathology that cannot be cured (Table 19–11). The healthy individual, when faced with overwhelming stress or crises—particularly those that include traumas or disasters—may seek help and be a candidate for supportive psychotherapy. The relatively psychiatrically healthy candidate for supportive psychotherapy is a well-adapted individual with good social support and interpersonal relations, flexible defenses, and good real-

ity testing who is experiencing an acute crisis but is making use of social supports, is not withdrawing, and is anticipating resolution of the crisis. Although functioning below his or her usual level, this patient remains hopeful about the future and makes use of resources available for problem solving, respite, and growth. This candidate uses supportive psychotherapy to reconstitute more rapidly, to avoid errors in judgment by "thinking out loud," to relieve minor symptomatology, and to grow as an individual by learning about the world.

The more typical candidate for supportive psychotherapy has significant deficits in ego functioning, including the following:

- *Poor reality testing.* These patients show an inability to separate fact from fantasy and to recognize the boundaries between self and others. They may become psychotic under the stress of psychodynamic psychotherapy and may develop psychotic transferences.
- *Poor impulse control.* Such patients need promptly to discharge affects through actions that are often destructive to themselves or others. They are

TABLE 19–11. Characteristics of candidates for supportive psychotherapy

Type I: *Patient impaired by overwhelming crisis, trauma, or disaster and functioning below usual level in response to a crisis.*
  Generally very psychiatrically healthy
  Well adapted
  Good social supports
  Good interpersonal relations
  Flexible defenses
  Good reality testing
  Hopeful about future
  Uses resources

Type II: *Patient has chronic ego deficits and impaired functioning.*
  Impaired reality testing
  Difficulty with impulse control
  Limited ability to sublimate
  Limited interpersonal relations
  Frequently high levels of aggression
  Limited ability to self-soothe/refuel
  Low verbal ability and capacity for
    introspection

not able to contain and examine feelings as is required by more explorative, insight-oriented psychotherapies.

• *Poor interpersonal relations.* Patients who are unable to form and maintain stable relationships that include reasonable levels of trust and intimacy are limited in their capacity to maintain therapeutic relationships as well, especially those that arouse powerful feelings.

• *Poor balance of affects.* This category includes patients who are overwhelmed by anger or anxiety as well as those who experience little or no affect of any sort.

• *Lack of ability to sublimate.* These patients are unable to channel energy into creative and socially useful activities, reflecting their low ability to master affects and impulses pleasurably.

• *Low capacity for introspection.* Because self-observation is a necessary step toward the attainment of insight, these patients do poorly in psychotherapies that require self-reflection and curiosity about themselves and their interpersonal relations.

• *Low verbal ability.* Most clinicians do not include high intelligence as a prerequisite for insight-oriented psychotherapy. However, patients for psychodynamic psychotherapies do need to be able to identify and communicate their thoughts and feelings intelligibly to the therapist and to derive relief from doing so.

Ego strength and the ability to form relationships may be more important than diagnosis in the selection of patients for supportive psychotherapy (Werman 1984). Patients with lower ego strength and lower motivation for therapy have been found to benefit more from supportive techniques than from those specific to exploratory therapy (Horowitz et al. 1984). Delineation of the personal qualities needed to benefit from supportive psychotherapy remains an important task for future research.

Theoretical Basis

Psychoanalytic theory is generally viewed as the basis for supportive therapy. The practice of supportive therapy draws heavily on the work of Kohut and the British Object Relations School (Buckley 1994). Thus, the emphasis is less on conflict resolution, as achieved by analysis of transference, than on establishment of a positive and coherent sense of self, mediated by the relationship between patient and therapist.

From this perspective, the therapist provides a "holding environment" in which patients feel secure, understood, and valued and a relationship through which they can develop a more realistic, less negatively biased view of themselves and others (Winston et al. 1986). Therapeutic gain stems from gradual internalization of aspects of the therapist and the therapeutic relationship. The patient forms a secure attachment to the therapist as a necessary precursor to developing increased autonomy.

Cognitive and behavioral theories, with their emphasis on conscious thought, behavioral change, learning, and problem solving, inform many of the techniques of supportive therapy. In general, supportive therapy derives from a broader theoretical base than does psychoanalytic theory alone.

Strategies

The basic strategy of supportive therapy is to map out the patient's major areas of life difficulty and ameliorate them in whatever way possible, rather than to discover causes.

Central to this strategy is helping the patient to strengthen adaptive defenses, diminish use of maladaptive defenses, and improve the balance of impulse and defense—for example, by avoiding overwhelming stress, reducing excessively harsh self-criticism, or containing overly intense impulses. The attempt is to minimize rather than foster regression, and to help the patient contain rather than mobilize affects.

The relationship between patient and therapist forms the basis of supportive therapy. It provides an object of identification and a source of security and reassurance (Pinsker 1994). In supportive therapy, the transparency and spontaneity of the therapist diminish anxiety.

Improved self-esteem is a goal of supportive therapies. In supportive therapy, self-esteem is enhanced by helping the patient to improve adaptive functioning and minimize emotional discomfort and by

fostering the patient's introjection of the therapist's acceptance and positive regard.

Techniques

Skillful practice of supportive psychotherapy may be more difficult than that of change-oriented psychotherapy because the patient may have less capacity to engage beneficially with a therapist (Wallace 1983). Understanding unconscious motivation, psychic conflict, the patient–therapist relationship, and the patient's use of defense mechanisms is essential to comprehending the patient's strengths and vulnerabilities and to providing support (Bellak and Siegel 1983; Karen Horney Clinic Medical Board 1981).

The basic stance of the therapist is both active and reactive, more readily taking positions, answering questions, giving advice, reassuring, praising, and educating the patient. The therapeutic style tends to be more conversational than that in insight-oriented therapy (Pinsker 1994) (Table 19–12). By his or her activity, judicious sharing of personal factual information, planned use of verbal and nonverbal reinforcement, and willingness to intervene with practical help when necessary, the supportive therapist presents as more of a real person.

Typical frequency of meetings ranges from weekly to monthly, and sessions may be either brief or full-length. More-frequent meetings may be appropriate in times of crisis, and unscheduled telephone calls may be viewed as central to the treatment rather than as deviations.

A particular technical challenge in supportive treatment is the therapist's need to maintain spontaneity without acting impulsively or out of countertransference. For example, the therapist must use reinforcement without becoming coercive, give advice or information without pre-

TABLE 19–12. Techniques

Supportive therapy	Psychoanalytic therapy
Activity; spontaneity	Abstinence
Advice; direction	Neutrality
Reinforcement of defenses	Interpretation of defenses
Clarification of conscious processes	Interpretation of unconscious processes
Acknowledgement of needs	Frustration of wishes
Enhancement of reality testing	Facilitation of fantasy
Benign neglect of process	Attention to process
Reassurance	Confrontation
Therapist as participant ally	Therapist as participant observer
Empathic listening	Empathic listening
Tact	Tact

senting as omnipotent (Nurnberg 1984), and respond flexibly to the patient's needs without becoming anxiously protective or overindulgent.

The therapist who is predictably available and safe (i.e., who accepts the patient and puts aside his or her own needs in the service of the treatment) assumes some of the holding functions of the good parent.

Patients in supportive psychotherapy frequently develop an intensely dependent and ambivalent relationship with the therapist. The therapist's respect for the patient's autonomy and need for "refueling" may be important in strengthening the patient's independence and facilitating return to health. The containment of affect is also an important supportive function (Kernberg 1975, 1984). Patients in need of supportive psychotherapy typically fear the destructive power of their own rage and envy. They may be helped to modulate their emotional reactions by the reliable presence of the therapist and a therapeutic relationship that remains unchanged in the face of emotional onslaughts.

The therapist attempts to strengthen defenses and foster the supportive relationship by refraining from interpreting positive transference feelings and waiting until the intensity of feelings has abated before commenting about negative transference feelings (Buckley 1986). Interpretations of the negative transference are limited to those needed to ensure that the treatment is not disrupted. While maintaining a friendly stance toward the patient, the therapist must respect the patient's need to establish a comfortable degree of distance. There is unanimous agreement among authors on supportive psychotherapy that fostering a good working relationship with the patient is the first priority. Studies indicate that in the case of more severely ill patients, this may take many months, in contrast to work with psychiatrically healthier patients (Docherty 1989; A.F. Frank and Gunderson 1990).

Many of the active interventions of supportive psychotherapy are based on the principle of "substitutive psychotherapy" (Werman 1984), in which the psychotherapy substitutes for capacities that the patient lacks. This is sometimes stated as the therapist acting as an "auxiliary ego" for the patient. Techniques that may support the patients' deficient ego functions include suggestion, reinforcement, clarification, limit setting, environmental interventions, and concurrent use of medication (Werman 1984).

Patients may be encouraged to discuss alternative behaviors, goals, and interpretations of events (Castelnuovo-Tedesco 1986). The therapist tries to reinforce the most adaptive defenses of which the patient is capable while discouraging use of more primitive defenses. This judgment is particularly important when assessing the primitive defenses of patients with schizophrenia (McGlashan 1982) or limited self-mutilation in those with severe personality pathology.

Reassurance takes a variety of forms in supportive psychotherapy, including supporting an adaptive level of denial (such as that employed by a patient in coping with a terminal illness), the patient's experience of the therapist's empathic attitude, or the therapist's reality testing of the patient's negatively biased evaluations (Werman 1984). Reassuring a patient is not easy (Peteet 1982). Reassurance requires a clear understanding of what the patient fears.

Communication of the therapist's knowledge of the patient and his or her circumstances is a pedagogical aspect of supportive psychotherapy (Werman 1981). The therapist uses simple, concrete language that has personal meaning for the patient. The therapist may discuss with the highly inhibited patient the advantages of being more assertive or spontaneous, or may point out to the patient with poorly developed social controls the dangers of impulsive behavior. In this manner, the therapist functions as an "auxiliary superego."

Interpretive comments may be used by the supportive therapist, although the form and content of interpretations usually differ from those in psychoanalytically oriented psychotherapy. Interpretations in supportive psychotherapy are given in a manner consistent with the principle of decreasing (rather than increasing) anxiety and strengthening (rather than loosening) defenses. Thus, they deal with material close to the patient's awareness.

The psychodynamic life narrative can be used as a supportive interpretation (Viederman 1983). The narrative is a formulation of the patient's current difficulties (often a life crisis) as the inevitable

product of previous life experiences. The psychodynamic life narrative uses only facts of which the patient is already aware and explanations that do not threaten the patient's self-esteem. It serves to provide the patient with a sense of control through understanding, to help him or her accept emotional responses as justifiable and inevitable, and to strengthen the alliance with the therapist, who is seen as giving something valuable.

The therapist's expressions of interest, advice giving, and facilitation of ventilation reinforce desired behaviors (P. R. Sullivan 1971). Expressions of interest and solicitude are positively reinforcing. Advice can lead to behavioral change if it is specific and applies to frequently occurring behaviors. Desired behaviors can be rewarded by the therapist's approval and by social reinforcement. Ventilation of emotions may be useful if the therapist can help the patient to safely contain and limit these emotions, thus extinguishing the anxiety response to emotional expression. Cognitive and behavioral psychotherapeutic interventions that strengthen the adaptive and defensive functioning of the ego (e.g., realistic and logical thinking, social skills, containment of affects such as anxiety) can contribute to the supportive aspects of psychotherapy (Novalis et al. 1997).

Except in the case of brief treatment aimed at supporting the patient through a life crisis or traumatic event, termination is not a goal in supportive psychotherapy in the same sense as it is in change-oriented therapies. In the most usual situation, the patient's functional deficits necessitate ongoing, long-term support. In such a case, keeping the patient in treatment might be a more appropriate goal than terminating treatment. Over time the treatment may gradually diminish in intensity or, alternatively, may evolve into a more change-oriented treatment. When the latter occurs, it may be appropriate to reevaluate goals and consider possible criteria for termination.

Supportive psychotherapy with special patient populations may require special techniques. Kates and Rockland (1994) described supportive therapy with schizophrenic patients as involving three phases: stabilization, maintenance, and working through/termination.

With somatizing patients who may habitually express feelings through physical symptoms, the first step may be to get the patient talking about him- or herself, while supplying information and advice relevant to the problem. As the therapeutic alliance develops, the patient is encouraged to express more feelings in recounting his or her life story to the therapist.

Supportive therapy with medically ill patients may entail providing the patient with a safe place to ventilate anger and grief over illness-related loss and disability.

Efficacy

Relatively few studies have assessed the efficacy of supportive therapy. Most data come from studies in which supportive psychotherapy was used as a control in testing the efficacy of other treatments (Conte and Plutchik 1986).

Despite its limitations, the research literature offers some evidence that supportive psychotherapy is an effective treatment. The Menninger Psychotherapy Project assessed long-term (i.e., up to 10 years) explorative and supportive psychotherapy in a group of patients with mixed symptomatic and personality pathology. A major result of the study was that psychoanalytic therapy was less effective, and supportive therapy was more effective, then expected.

More recently, this result was confirmed in a group of patients with Axis II Cluster C disorders who were treated

with either supportive or confrontational dynamic psychotherapy.

A larger body of research exists indicating that supportive psychotherapy is an effective component of treatment for patients with a variety of medical illnesses.

The evidence to date, although preliminary, suggests that supportive psychotherapy can be effective in both psychiatric and medical illnesses and may be more cost-effective than more intense psychotherapies. More research is needed regarding the indications, contraindications, and techniques of supportive psychotherapy.

Education

The importance of individual psychotherapy to the practicing clinician makes mandatory the inclusion of instruction on psychotherapy in psychiatric residency training. The skills learned in psychotherapy—both the ability to intervene and the ability to recognize transference, countertransference, and defense—are important in many other treatment modalities. The clinician who is skilled in recognizing these phenomena is better able to conduct a wide array of interventions, including medication management, family therapy, inpatient psychiatric treatment, and consultation-liaison treatment.

The fundamental skills of establishing the therapeutic alliance, understanding the relationship of transference to anxiety and regression, and providing support are central to psychiatric care. Learning psychodynamic psychotherapy provides the opportunity to work with a specific treatment modality as well as to become skilled in a wide array of areas central to clinical care. Learning long-term psychodynamic psychotherapy is not the equivalent of learning the brief psychotherapies or supportive psychotherapy (Levenson and Strupp 1999; Vaughan et al. 2000); however, it may be true that the long-term psychotherapist is best prepared for using the briefer psychotherapy, in which there are fewer opportunities to make mistakes and to correct them. In this era of managed care, it is even more likely that the psychiatrist will be called on to supervise others conducting psychotherapy. For this reason also, skills in psychotherapy are necessary.

The teaching of supportive psychotherapy requires further development of the knowledge base in supportive psychotherapy and the description of the technical procedures. At present, supportive psychotherapy remains a neglected area of teaching despite its complexity. A clearer delineation of the technical procedures used in psychotherapy and their assessment on a supportive versus change-oriented/explorative continuum should be part of psychotherapy supervision. In addition, such clarification will facilitate comparison among the psychotherapies and foster appropriate research questions, including those concerning the use of supportive psychotherapy as part of medication management.

Conclusions

Individual psychoanalytically oriented and supportive psychotherapies are an effective treatment for a wide range of symptoms and disorders. These treatment modalities require accurate diagnosis, treatment planning, and consistent application of principles and technique.

The psychoanalytic treatments—psychoanalysis and psychoanalytic psychotherapy—now span the range of therapeutic approaches—from brief to long-term and focal to broad based. Interpersonal psychotherapy has primarily been used in research, but highlighted in this form of therapy is the importance of focusing on the social relationships as an aspect of understanding the psychoanalytic components of personality and mind–brain interaction. Supportive psychotherapy, probably the most widely practiced of the psychotherapies, continues to be lacking in specific research. Better delineation of the specific technique in supportive psychotherapy will aid this development.

Clinicians require training in each of the psychotherapy modalities and in their application in stand-alone treatment plans and used intermittently or in combination or sequence with medication.

References

Bachrach HM, Weber JJ, Solomon M: Factors associated with the outcome of psychoanalysis (IV). International Review of Psycho-Analysis 12:379–389, 1985

Baxter C, Schwartz S, Berman K, et al: Caudate glucose metabolic rate changes with both drug and behavior therapy for obsessive-compulsive disorder. Arch Gen Psychiatry 49:681–689, 1992

Beck AT, Rush AJ, Shaw BF, et al: Cognitive Therapy of Depression. New York, Guilford, 1979

Bellak L, Siegel H: Handbook of Intensive, Brief, and Emergency Psychotherapy. Larchmont, NY, CPS, 1983

Bibring E: Psychoanalysis and the dynamic psychotherapies. J Am Psychoanal Assoc 2:745–770, 1954

Blum HP: Countertransference and the theory of technique: discussion. J Am Psychoanal Assoc 34:309–328, 1986

Brenner C: Psychoanalytic Technique and Psychic Conflict. New York, International Universities Press, 1976

Brodaty JH: Techniques in brief psychotherapy. Aust N Z J Psychiatry 17:109–115, 1983

Bruch H: Learning Psychotherapy: Rationale and Ground Rules. Cambridge, MA, Harvard University Press, 1974

Buckley P: [Supportive psychotherapy] A neglected treatment. Psychiatr Ann 16:515–517, 521, 1986

Buckley P: Self psychology, object relations theory and supportive psychotherapy. Am J Psychother 48:519–529, 1994

Castelnuovo-Tedesco P: The Twenty-Minute Hour: A Guide to Brief Psychotherapy for the Physician. Washington, DC, American Psychiatric Press, 1986

Chessick RD: Psychoanalysis: clinical and theoretical. Am J Psychiatry 157:846–848, 2000

Coleman JV: Aims and conduct of psychotherapy. Arch Gen Psychiatry 18:1–6, 1968

Coltrera JT: Truth from genetic illusion: the transference and the fate of the infantile neurosis, in Psychoanalytic Explorations of Technique: Discourse on the Theory of Therapy. Edited by Blum HP. New York, International Universities Press, 1980, pp 284–313

Conte HR, Plutchik R: Controlled research in supportive psychotherapy. Psychiatr Ann 16:530–533, 1986

Crits-Christoph P: The efficacy of brief dynamic psychotherapy: a meta-analysis. Am J Psychiatry 149:151–158, 1992

Crits-Christoph P, Barben JP (eds): Handbook of Short-Term Dynamic Psychotherapy. New York, Basic Books, 1991

Crown S: Contraindications and dangers of psychotherapy. Br J Psychiatry 143:436–441, 1983

de Jonghe F, Rijnierse P, Janssen R: The role of support in psychoanalysis. J Am Psychoanal Assoc 40:475–499, 1992

Dewald P: The process of change in psychoanalytic psychotherapy. Arch Gen Psychiatry 35:535–542, 1978

Docherty JP: The individual psychotherapies: efficacy, syndrome-based treatments, and the therapeutic alliance, in Outpatient Psychiatry: Diagnosis and Treatment, 2nd Edition. Edited by Lazare A. Baltimore, MD, Williams & Wilkins, 1989, pp 624–644

Donovan JM: More on transference interpretations (letter). Am J Psychiatry 141:142, 1984

Epstein RS: Keeping Boundaries: Maintaining Safety and Integrity in the Psychotherapeutic Process. Washington, DC, American Psychiatric Press, 1995

Frances A[J], Perry S: Transference interpretations in focal therapy. Am J Psychiatry 140:405–409, 1983

Frank AF, Gunderson JG: The role of the therapeutic alliance in the treatment of schizophrenia: relationship to course and outcome. Arch Gen Psychiatry 47:228–236, 1990

Frank AF, Kupfer DJ, Wagner EF, et al: Efficacy of interpersonal psychotherapy as a maintenance treatment of recurrent depression. Arch Gen Psychiatry 48:1053–1059, 1991

Frank JD: Therapeutic factors in psychotherapy. Am J Psychother 25:350–361, 1971

Freud S: The handling of dream-interpretation in psycho-analysis (1911), in Standard Edition of the Complete Psychological Works of Sigmund Freud, Vol 12. Translated and edited by Strachey J. London, England, Hogarth Press, 1958, pp 89–96

Freud S: The dynamics of transference (1912a), in Standard Edition of the Complete Psychological Works of Sigmund Freud, Vol 12. Translated and edited by Strachey J. London, England, Hogarth Press, 1958, pp 97–108

Freud S: Recommendations to physicians practising psycho-analysis (1912b), in Standard Edition of the Complete Psychological Works of Sigmund Freud, Vol 12. Translated and edited by Strachey J. London, England, Hogarth Press, 1958, pp 109–120

Freud S: On beginning the treatment (further recommendations on the technique of psycho-analysis I) (1913), in Standard Edition of the Complete Psychological Works of Sigmund Freud, Vol 12. Translated and edited by Strachey J. London, England, Hogarth Press, 1958, pp 121–144

Freud S: Remembering, repeating and working-through (further recommendations on the technique of psycho-analysis II) (1914), in Standard Edition of the Complete Psychological Works of Sigmund Freud, Vol 12. Translated and edited by Strachey J. London, England, Hogarth Press, 1958, pp 145–156

Freud S: Observations on transference-love (further recommendations on the technique of psycho-analysis III) (1915 [1914]), in Standard Edition of the Complete Psychological Works of Sigmund Freud, Vol 12. Translated and edited by Strachey J. London, England, Hogarth Press, 1958, pp 157–173

Fried D, Crits-Christoph P, Luborsky L: The first empirical demonstration of transference in psychotherapy. J Nerv Ment Dis 180:326–331, 1992

Fromm-Reichmann F: Principles of Intensive Psychotherapy. Chicago, IL, University of Chicago Press, 1950

Gabbard GO: Psychodynamic Psychiatry in Clinical Practice, 3rd Edition. Washington, DC, American Psychiatric Press, 2000

Galatzer-Levy RM, Bachrach H, Skolnikoff A, et al: Does Psychoanalysis Work? New Haven, CT, Yale University Press, 2000

Gill M: The Analysis of Transference, I: Theory and Technique. New York, International Universities Press, 1982

Glover E: The Technique of Psychoanalysis. New York, International Universities Press, 1968

Gomes-Schwartz B, Hadley S, Strupp H: Individual psychotherapy and behavior therapy. Annu Rev Psychol 29:435–447, 1978

Greenson RR: The working alliance and the transference neurosis. Psychoanal Q 34: 155–181, 1965

Greenson RR: The Technique and Practice of Psychoanalysis. New York, International Universities Press, 1967

Hadley SW, Strupp HH: Contemporary views of negative effects in psychotherapy: an integrated account. Arch Gen Psychiatry 33:1291–1302, 1976

Hofer MA: Relationships as regulators: a psychobiologic perspective on bereavement. Psychosom Med 46:183–197, 1984

Horowitz MJ, Marmar C, Weiss DS, et al: Brief psychotherapy of bereavement reactions: the relationship of process to outcome. Arch Gen Psychiatry 41:438–448, 1984

Horowitz MJ, Marmar CR, Weiss DS, et al: Comprehensive analysis of change after brief dynamic psychotherapy. Am J Psychiatry 143:582–589, 1986

House JS, Landis KR, Umberson D: Social relationships and health. Science 241:540–545, 1988

Kandell ER: Psychotherapy and the single synapse: the impact of psychiatric thought on neurobiologic research. N Engl J Med 301:1028–1037, 1979

Kandell ER: Genes, nerve cells, and the remembrance of things past. J Neuropsychiatry Clin Neurosci 1:103–125, 1989

Kandell ER: Biology and the future of psychoanalysis: a new intellectual framework for psychiatry revisited. Am J Psychiatry 156: 505–524, 1999

Kandell ER: Comment on "Biology and the future of psychoanalysis: a new intellectual framework for psychiatry revisited." Am J Psychiatry 157:839–840, 2000

Kantrowitz JL, Paolitto F, Sashin J, et al: Affect availability, tolerance, complexity, and modulation in psychoanalysis: follow up of a longitudinal, prospective study. J Am Psychoanal Assoc 34:529–559, 1986

Kantrowitz JL, Katz AL, Paolitto F, et al: Changes in the level and quantity of object relations in psychoanalysis: follow up of a longitudinal, prospective study. J Am Psychoanal Assoc 35:23–46, 1987

Kantrowitz JL, Katz AL, Paolitto F: Followup of psychoanalysis five to ten years after termination, I: stability of change. J Am Psychoanal Assoc 38:471–496, 1990

Karen Horney Clinic Medical Board: Guidelines for identifying therapeutic modalities. Am J Psychoanal 41:195–202, 1981

Kates J, Rockland LH: Supportive psychotherapy of the schizophrenia patient. Am J Psychother 48:543–561, 1994

Kernberg OF: Borderline Conditions and Pathological Narcissism. New York, Jason Aronson, 1975

Kernberg OF: Severe Personality Disorders: Psychotherapeutic Strategies. New Haven, CT, Yale University Press, 1984

Kernberg OF: Affect theory. Paper presented at the annual meeting of the American Psychiatric Association, New Orleans, LA, May 2001

Kernberg OF, Burstein ED, Coyne L, et al: Psychotherapy and psychoanalysis: final report of the Menninger Foundation's Psychotherapy Research Project. Bull Menninger Clin 36:1–275, 1972

Klerman GL, Weissman MM, Rounsaville BJ, et al: Interpersonal psychotherapy for depression, in Psychiatry Update: The American Psychiatric Association Annual Review, Vol 3. Edited by Grinspoon L. Washington, DC, American Psychiatric Press, 1984a, pp 56–67

Klerman GL, Weissman MM, Rounsaville BJ, et al: Interpersonal Psychotherapy of Depression. New York, Basic Books, 1984b

Langsley D, Yager J: The definition of a psychiatrist: eight years later. Am J Psychiatry 145:469–475, 1988

Levenson H, Strupp HH: Recommendations for future of training in brief dynamic psychotherapy. J Clin Psychol 55:385–391, 1999

Luborsky L: Principles of Psychoanalytic Psychotherapy: A Manual for Supportive Expressive Treatment. New York, Basic Books, 1984

Luborsky L, Crits-Christoph P: Understanding Transference. New York, Basic Books, 1990

Luborsky L, Singer B, Luborsky L: Comparative studies of psychotherapies: is it true that "everyone has won and all must have prizes"? Arch Gen Psychiatry 32:995–1008, 1975

Luborsky L, Crits-Christoph P, Mintz J, et al: Who Will Benefit From Psychotherapy? New York, Basic Books, 1988

Malan DH: A Study of Brief Psychotherapy. New York, Plenum, 1975

Malan DH: The Frontier of Brief Psychotherapy. New York, Plenum, 1976

Malan DH: Toward the Validation of Dynamic Psychotherapy. New York, Plenum, 1980

Markowitz J (ed): Interpersonal Psychotherapy. Washington, DC, American Psychiatric Press, 1998

Markowitz JC, Svartberg M, Swartz HA: Is IPT time-limited psychodynamic psychotherapy? J Psychother Pract Res 7:185–195 1998

Marziali EA: Prediction of outcome of brief psychotherapy from therapist interpretive interventions. Arch Gen Psychiatry 41:301–304, 1984

Marziali EA, Sullivan JM: Methodological issues in the content analysis of brief psychotherapy. Br J Med Psychol 53:19–27, 1980

McGlashan TH: DSM-III schizophrenia and individual psychotherapy. J Nerv Ment Dis 170:752–757, 1982

Meany MJ: Nature, nurture, and disunity of knowledge. Ann N Y Acad Sci 935:50–61, 2001

Meissner WW: Neutrality, abstinence and the therapeutic alliance. J Am Psychoanal Assoc 46:1089–1128, 1998

Milrod B, Busch F, Leon AC, et al: Open trial of psychodynamic psychotherapy for panic disorder: a pilot study. Am J Psychiatry 157:1878–1880, 2000

Munich RL: Contemporary treatment of schizophrenia. Bull Menninger Clin 61:189–221, 1997

Novalis PN, Rojceicz SJ Jr, Peele R: Clinical Manual of Supportive Psychotherapy. Washington, DC, American Psychiatric Press, 1997

Nurnberg HG: Survey of psychotherapeutic approaches to narcissistic personality disorder. Hillside Journal of Clinical Psychiatry 6:204–220, 1984

O'Hara MW, Stuart S, Gorman LL, et al: Efficacy of interpersonal psychotherapy for postpartum depression. Arch Gen Psychiatry 57:1039–1045, 2000

Parloff MB: Psychotherapy research evidence and reimbursement decisions: Bambi meets Godzilla. Am J Psychiatry 139:718–727, 1982

Parloff MB, Lond P, Wolfe B: Individual psychotherapy and behavior change. Annu Rev Psychol 37:321–349, 1986

Perry JC, Banon E, Ianni F: Effectiveness of psychotherapy for personality disorders. Am J Psychiatry 156:1312–1321, 1999

Peteet JR: A closer look at the concept of support: some applications to the care of patients with cancer. Gen Hosp Psychiatry 4:19–23, 1982

Pinsker H: The role of theory in teaching supportive psychotherapy. Am J Psychother 48:530–542, 1994

Ponsi M: Therapeutic alliance and collaborative interactions. Int J Psychoanal 81:687–704, 2000

Racker H: Meanings and uses of countertransference. Psychoanal Q 26:303–357, 1957

Reiser MF: The dream in contemporary psychiatry. Am J Psychiatry 158:351–359, 2001

Rounsaville BJ, Glazer W, Wilber CH, et al: Short-term interpersonal psychotherapy in methadone-maintained opiate addicts. Arch Gen Psychiatry 40:629–636, 1983

Rounsaville BJ, Gawin F, Kleber H: Interpersonal psychotherapy adapted for ambulatory cocaine abusers. Am J Drug Alcohol Abuse 11:171–191, 1985a

Rounsaville BJ, Klerman GL, Weissman MM, et al: Short-term interpersonal psychotherapy (IPT) for depression, in Handbook of Depression: Treatment, Assessment and Research. Edited by Beckham EE, Leber WB. Homewood, IL, Dorsey Press, 1985b, pp 125–150

Sandell R, Blomberg J, Lazar A, et al: Varieties of long-term outcome among patients in psychoanalysis and long-term psychotherapy: a review of findings in the Stockholm Outcome of Psychoanalysis and Psychotherapy Project (STOPP). Int J Psychoanal 81:921–942, 2000

Sapolsky RM: Glucocorticoids and hippocampal atrophy in neuropsychiatric disorders, Arch Gen Psychiatry 57:925–935, 2000

Shapiro DA, Shapiro D: Meta-analysis of comparative therapy outcome studies: a replication and refinement. Psychol Bull 92:581–604, 1982

Sharpe EF: Dream Analysis. London, England, Hogarth Press, 1961

Smith ML, Glass GV: Meta-analysis of psychotherapy outcome studies. Am Psychol 32:752–760, 1977

Smith ML, Glass GV, Miller TI: The Benefits of Psychotherapy. Baltimore, MD, Johns Hopkins University Press, 1980

Solnit AJ: Recovery and adaptation. Psychoanal Study Child 55:252–274, 2000

Sonnenberg SM, Sutton L, Ursano RJ: Physician–patient relationship, in Psychiatry. Edited by Tasman A, Kay J, Lieberman JA. Philadelphia, PA, WB Saunders, 1997, pp 40–50

Spiegel D, Lazar SG: The need for psychotherapy in the medically ill. Psychoanalytic Inquiry 17 (suppl):45–50, 1997

Stone L: The Psychoanalytic Situation: An Examination of Its Development and Essential Nature. New York, International Universities Press, 1961

Sullivan HS: The Psychiatric Interview. Edited by Perry HS, Gawel ML. New York, WW Norton, 1954

Sullivan PR: Learning theories and supportive psychotherapy. Am J Psychiatry 128:763–766, 1971

Ursano RJ, Dressler DM: Brief vs long term psychotherapy: a treatment decision. J Nerv Ment Dis 159:164–171, 1974

Ursano RJ, Fullerton CS: Psychotherapy: medical intervention and the concept of normality, in The Diversity of Normal Behavior: Further Contributions to Normatology. Edited by Offer D, Sabshin M. New York, Basic Books, 1991, pp 39–59

Ursano RJ, Sonnenberg SM, Lazar SG: Concise Guide to Psychodynamic Psychotherapy: Principles and Techniques in the Era of Managed Care. Washington, DC, American Psychiatric Press, 1998

Ursano RJ, Epstein RS, Lazar SG: Behavioral responses to illness: personality and personality disorders, in Textbook of Medical Surgical Psychiatry: Psychiatry in the Medically Ill. Edited by Rundell JR, Wise MG. Washington, DC, American Psychiatric Publishing, 2001, pp 125–146

Vaughan SC, Marshall RD, Mackinnon RA, et al: Can we do psychoanalytic outcome research? A feasibility study. Int J Psychoanal 81:513–527, 2000

Viederman M: The psychodynamic life narrative: a psychotherapeutic intervention useful in crisis situations. Psychiatry 46: 236–246, 1983

Wallace ER: Dynamic Psychiatry in Theory and Practice. Philadelphia, PA, Lea & Febiger, 1983

Wallerstein RS: Psychoanalysis and psychotherapy: an historical perspective. Int J Psychoanal 70:563–591, 1989

Wallerstein RS: Follow up in psychoanalysis: what happens to treatment gains. J Am Psychoanal Assoc 40:665–690, 1992

Weissman MM, Markowitz JC: Interpersonal psychotherapy. Arch Gen Psychiatry 51: 599–606, 1994

Werman DS: Technical aspects of supportive psychotherapy. Psychiatric Journal of the University of Ottawa 6:153–160, 1981

Werman DS: The Practice of Supportive Psychotherapy. New York, Brunner/Mazel, 1984

Winston A, Pinsker H, McCullough L: A review of supportive psychotherapy. Hosp Community Psychiatry 37:1105–1114, 1986

Zetzel ER: Current concepts of transference. Int J Psychoanal 37:369–376, 1956

CHAPTER 20

Treatment of Children and Adolescents

Stephen J. Cozza, M.D.

Glen C. Crawford, M.D.

Mina K. Dulcan, M.D.

This chapter provides an overview of and an orientation to the psychiatric treatment of children and adolescents. We focus on what is different or unique in the treatment of children and adolescents.

Techniques used in the treatment of child psychiatric conditions have developed from two different sources: the traditions of understanding and treating children based on developmental uniqueness and treatments that were originally designed for adults and were then applied to children and adolescents. Increasingly, more rigorous evaluation and diagnostic procedures have allowed greater specificity in the application of treatments to our younger patients. In addition, expanding research on the efficacy of specific therapeutic approaches continues to enlarge our armamentarium of empirically tested interventions.

Evaluation

The American Academy of Child and Adolescent Psychiatry (AACAP) has pro-

duced a number of practice parameters as guides to evaluation and treatment of specific disorders. Completed practice parameters are listed in Table 20–1.

Special considerations for children make evaluation different from that for adult patients. Practitioners must have a clear understanding of normal development and the differences that may exist among children at the same or different ages in order to distinguish normal from pathological behaviors. Also, practitioners must be able to apply developmental understanding in the diagnostic interview of the child, using approaches like imaginative play or drawings with younger children or with those who are less skilled in verbal communication.

Information from the school is always useful and is essential when there is concern about learning, behavior, or peer functioning. With parental consent, the clinician talks with the teacher; obtains records of testing, grades, and attendance; and requests completion of a standardized checklist, such as the Teacher Report Form of the Child Behavior Checklist

TABLE 20–1. Practice parameters published by the American Academy of Child and Adolescent Psychiatry

Aggressive Behavior in Child and Adolescent Psychiatric Institutions	2002
Anxiety Disorders	1997
Assessment of Children and Adolescents	1997
Assessment of Infants and Toddlers	1997
Attention-Deficit Hyperactivity Disorder	1997
Autism	1999
Bipolar Disorder	1997
Child Custody Evaluations	1997
Conduct Disorder	1997
Depressive Disorders	1998
Enuresis and Encopresis	2002
Forensic Evaluations of Physical or Sexual Abuse	1997
Language and Learning Disorders	1998
Mental Retardation and Comorbid Mental Disorders	1999
Obsessive-Compulsive Disorder	1998
Posttraumatic Stress Disorder	1998
Schizophrenia	2001
Seclusion and Restraint	2002
Sexually Abusive Youth	1999
Stimulant Medications	2002
Substance Use Disorders	1997
Suicide	2001

(Achenbach 1991). Even better, though less convenient, is a visit to the school to observe the youngster with peers in the classroom and on the playground and to talk with teachers and counselors.

A referral to another provider, such as a pediatrician, pediatric neurologist, child psychologist, or speech and language specialist, may be necessary in order to complete the assessment. Psychological evaluation, including an intelligence test and achievement tests, should be obtained when there is any question about learning or IQ, with additional testing obtained as indicated.

Treatment Planning

The planning of a treatment regimen takes into consideration psychiatric diagnosis, target emotional and behavioral symptoms, and the strengths and weaknesses of the patient and family. Resources and risks in the school, neighborhood, and social support network, and any religious group affiliation, also influence the selection of treatment strategies.

The clinician must decide which treatment is likely to be the most efficient or to have the highest risk–benefit ratio and whether treatments should be administered simultaneously or in sequence. Unfortunately, very few systematic prospective studies have been conducted that have compared well-defined treatments for carefully described groups of child patients.

Parents are best included in the choice of treatment strategies, with the strength of the clinician's recommendation depending on the clarity of the indications. The skilled clinician presents the probable course of the disorder if untreated, as well as the best estimate of benefits and risks of all available treatments for a particular child. The child patient is included in decision making as appropriate. The motivation and ability of the responsible adults to carry out the treatment should be considered because the best treatment has little chance of success without the cooperation of the family.

Treatment planning is an ongoing process, with reevaluations done as interventions are attempted and their results observed and as additional information about the child and family comes to light.

Informed Consent

The implementation of any treatment plan requires carefully obtained informed consent from parents before the plan is initiated. The concept of informed consent is more complicated with children because of legal lack of competency. Although parents provide informed consent for children, clinicians should strive to obtain assent from child patients before initiating any treatment. In obtaining such assent, the clinician should be mindful of the cognitive capacities and developmental level of the patient. The challenge may be even greater when pharmacotherapy is considered (Krener and Mancina 1994). Although not always necessary, parents' written consent may be useful in some situations. Printed materials to supplement discussion with the physician in educating parents and children regarding a variety of treatments are now available (Bastiaens and Bastiaens 1993; Dulcan and Lizarralde 2002). In addition, the Internet is becoming an increasingly important source of information about medications and treatments for health care consumers. Because the quality of information available on the World Wide Web varies, patients and their families may require guidance as to the best sources of information about mental health issues. Clinicians should also be prepared to respond to questions or concerns about treatments that may arise from a patient's or parent's "surfing" of the Internet.

Confidentiality

It is essential that the guidelines for confidentiality and for sharing information between parent and child be clear. Adolescents are usually more sensitive to this issue than younger children. In general, either party should be told when information from one party's session will be relayed to the other. In some situations, parents and children may participate in the decision. When children are engaged

in potentially dangerous activities or have serious thoughts of harming themselves or others, parents must be informed. Carefully planned family sessions in which the therapist coaches and supports a parent or child in sharing information may be more useful than secondhand reports.

Psychopharmacology

Important general principles of pediatric psychopharmacology include minimizing polypharmacy and rarely using medication as the only treatment. Most disorders of children and adolescents that require medication are either chronic (e.g., attention-deficit/hyperactivity disorder [ADHD], autistic disorder, or Tourette's disorder) or likely to have recurrent episodes (e.g., mood disorders), and a long-term relationship with the physician is crucial. It is important to educate the family regarding the disorder, its treatment, and the child's needs at each developmental stage. The physician must consider the meaning of the prescription and administration of a medication to the child, the family, the school, and the child's peer group.

Special Issues for Children and Adolescents

Pharmacokinetics, Pharmacodynamics, and Pharmacogenetics

Pharmacokinetics is the study of the movement of drugs into, around, and out of the body by the processes of absorption, distribution, metabolism, and elimination. Although children share some similarities in the physiological processing of medications with adults, developmental differences are clinically relevant, particularly in regard to drug distribution and metabolism.

Factors that most greatly impact on the developmental differences of distribution of drugs in children are differences in proportion of extracellular water volume and body fat. Extracellular water volume decreases substantially from birth through early adolescence. This decrease results in a larger distribution volume for water-soluble drugs in younger children requiring a relatively higher dose to achieve a comparable plasma concentration (Clein and Riddle 1995).

In general, children have lower proportional body fat than adults, thus reducing the distribution volume for lipid-soluble medications. Although this would result in an expected increase in plasma concentrations of such medications in children compared with adults using weight-adjusted dosages, lower plasma levels in children have been reported. This finding indicates that other pharmacokinetic differences, presumably increased metabolism in children, offset this effect (Clein and Riddle 1995).

From late infancy to early childhood, hepatic metabolic activity is at its peak. This substantially greater metabolic rate is related to the proportionally larger liver size of children compared with adults. Relative to body weight, the liver of a toddler is 40%–50% greater and that of a 6-year-old is 30% greater than the liver of an adult. This greater metabolic rate has been postulated as the principal factor contributing to lower drug plasma concentration levels and shorter drug half-lives in children compared with adults (Clein and Riddle 1995).

An understanding of the cytochrome P450 (CYP) enzyme system is becoming increasingly important for those clinicians who prescribe psychiatric medications to children and adolescents. Many medications are either substrates of, or inhibit or induce one or more of, the CYP isoenzymes. Potentially toxic interactions can result from inappropriate combinations of medications that inhibit CYP enzymes. An excellent source of information on this topic is Flockhart and Oesterheld (2000).

Medication dosage also is determined by pharmacodynamics, or how the biological system responds to the drug. For example, interaction with receptors is determined by receptor number, distribution, structure, function, sensitivity, and mechanism of action. Little is known about the influence of growth and development on these variables.

Ideally, medication doses in children should be derived from studies of children rather than adults, but studies of children often are not possible. Protocols using healthy children are not permitted, and few dosage studies have been done in symptomatic children. Dosage may be determined empirically or by weight or surface area. Generally, children are anticipated to require a higher weight-adjusted dose to achieve the same blood levels and therapeutic effects as adults. However, clinicians should remain alert to the possibility that such practice occasionally results in toxicity.

Side Effects

Side effects are common in children being treated with psychiatric medications. Clinicians must actively look for adverse reactions, as children often will not report them and parents may not notice. Occasionally, children will develop an uncharacteristic or paradoxical response to a particular medication. Such a response may be extremely individual in its manifestation, affecting one child but not another. *Behavioral toxicity* is a term that is used to describe a response to medication in which a child demonstrates behavioral or symptomatic aggravation caused by a particular medication (Van Putten and Marder 1987).

Measurement of Outcome

Effective medication management in children requires the identification of clear target symptoms that are monitored during the course of a medication trial. The physician must obtain emotional, behavioral, and physical baseline and posttreatment data. Therapeutic effects can be assessed by interviews and rating scales, direct observation, collection of data from outside sources (e.g., teachers), or specific tests evaluating attention or learning (Conners 1985).

Developmentally Disabled Patients

Medication effects are even more difficult to assess in children and adolescents with mental retardation or pervasive developmental disorders (PDDs). Their impaired ability to verbalize symptoms is relevant to diagnosis, measurement of efficacy, and detection of side effects. These individuals are prone to physical side effects and are at risk for idiosyncratic behavioral effects or simply less prominent therapeutic effects.

Compliance

Taking medication as directed can be particularly problematic for children because the cooperation of two people, parent and child, and often school personnel as well, is required. In general pediatric practice, high compliance to medication regimens is associated with the degree of parental concern about the seriousness of their child's illness, the severity of the child's symptoms, and prior high compliance to treatment (Lewis 1995). Compliance appears to be inversely related to the complexity of the medication regimen (including the number of medicines used and the frequency of dosing). Although experiences in general pediatrics and adult psychiatry indicate that educational efforts may improve compliance, administration

of psychotropic medications in children is more complex. Bastiaens (1992) found no correlation between knowledge of medications and compliance in a group of inpatient children and adolescents. In a later study, he found that compliance in a group of inpatient adolescents correlated better with attitudes toward than with knowledge of pharmacotherapy, indicating a need to examine and explore a child's feelings about taking medication (Bastiaens 1995).

Stimulants

This category of medications is the most studied and most used in pediatric psychopharmacology and is most often prescribed by non–child psychiatrists such as pediatricians and general practitioners. Traditionally, these medications have included dextroamphetamine, methylphenidate, and magnesium pemoline. More recently, newer mixed-agent medications (Adderall) and medications incorporating innovative delivery systems (Concerta, Metadate-CD) have become increasingly popular as first- and second-line stimulant choices. Magnesium pemoline is no longer a recommended agent even for second- or third-line treatment due to potential life-threatening hepatic toxicity.

Contrary to prevailing mythology, hyperactive boys, healthy boys, and healthy adults have similar cognitive and behavioral responses to comparable doses of stimulants. Although it is clear that stimulants do *not* have a "paradoxical" effect in ADHD, the actual mechanism of action remains unclear. It is likely that stimulant therapeutic effect is related to augmentation of dopaminergic and adrenergic activity in the central nervous system (CNS). Stimulants reduce the performance decrement seen as patients with ADHD perform tasks, perhaps by improving motivation and focusing effort.

Indications and Efficacy

The most established indication for stimulant use is in the treatment of ADHD. In preschool-age children, stimulant efficacy is more variable, and the rate of side effects, especially sadness, irritability, clinginess, insomnia, and anorexia, is higher (S.B. Campbell 1985). Previous practices calling for discontinuation of stimulant treatment in adolescents have been abandoned. Most recently, T. Spencer et al. (1996) reviewed studies of stimulant treatment in adolescents and concluded that, although limited, results indicate that stimulants are equally effective in adolescents as in school-age children.

Stimulants have been found to be effective in treating ADHD symptoms in the mentally retarded population (Aman et al. 1991). Of concern, however, is the fact that this population may be prone to more serious side effects, particularly those children who are more severely impaired (Handen et al. 1991). Handen et al. (1999) reported on a double-blind, placebo-controlled, crossover study of the use of methylphenidate in 11 preschool children with developmental disabilities and ADHD. Although the study found a 73% response rate in the subject children, the authors also reported that 45% of the subjects experienced adverse side effects from the medication. Children with fragile X syndrome also have been shown to benefit significantly from stimulant treatment of ADHD symptoms (Hagerman et al. 1988). Despite previous concern about treating children with PDDs with stimulants, Birmaher et al. (1988) described the effective use of this medication in a group of nine autistic children who did not develop significant side effects or show worsening of stereotypies.

The use of stimulants in patients with tics or Tourette's disorder remains controversial. The greatest concern is precipitating new tics. Often, however, patients with Tourette's disorder are far more disabled by their inattention, impulsivity, low frustration tolerance, and oppositional behavior than by their tics. Data suggest that among children who already have Tourette's disorder, methylphenidate improves behavior without significantly worsening tics (Gadow et al. 1995). Law and Schachar (1999) reported the results of a controlled study in a mixed population of boys and girls in which it was concluded that methylphenidate (0.5 mg/kg twice daily) treatment for ADHD was no more likely than placebo to cause or exacerbate tics. Nevertheless, monitoring for tics during stimulant use is still advised.

The short-term efficacy of stimulants in ADHD is well documented. Global judgments by parents, teachers, and clinicians rate 65%–75% of hyperactive children as improved on stimulants, with placebo response reported between 2% and 39% (Wilens and Biederman 1992). Those 25%–35% who are nonresponders demonstrate no change or worsening of symptoms, or they have intolerable side effects to the medications. A study using a wide range of doses of methylphenidate and dextroamphetamine found that 96% of the sample improved behaviorally in response to one or both drugs, although some children did not continue on medication because of adverse effects (Elia et al. 1991). Stimulant effects on various domains (cognitive, behavioral, social) are highly variable within and among individuals. A dose that produces improvement in one domain may have no effect or may even lead to worsening in another. Higher doses of stimulants, in some studies, have been shown to improve behavior but impair cognitive functioning (Sprague and Sleator 1977). Even more puzzling, the response may differ between measures (e.g., math and reading), even in the same domain.

Stimulants have been demonstrated to have no effect on learning disabilities in the absence of an attention deficit (Gittelman et al. 1983). The use of stimulants in populations with comorbid ADHD and learning disorders appears to have a role in treating the underlying ADHD-related attentional and behavioral symptoms (Gadow 1983).

The long-term therapeutic effect of stimulant medication remains unclear. Most studies to date have been of short duration and many suffer from poor design. The National Institute of Mental Health Collaborative Multisite Multimodal Treatment Study of ADHD (MTA) was designed to address these areas of weakness (Richters et al. 1995). Analysis of the MTA 14-month-treatment database suggests that combined medication and behavioral treatments provide no greater clinical benefit in treating core ADHD symptoms than systematic medication management alone, although behavioral treatment may offer some added benefit in other areas of social skills and academic performance. Behavioral treatments appear to hold added benefit for children suffering from ADHD with comorbid anxiety (Jensen et al. 2001).

Initiation and Maintenance

The decision to medicate a child or adolescent with a stimulant is based on the presence of persistent target symptoms that are sufficiently severe to cause functional impairment at school and usually also at home and with peers. Parents must be willing to monitor medication and to attend appointments. Psychoeducation and school consultation are generally implemented first, unless severe impulsivity and noncompliance create an emergency situation.

Multiple outcome measures, determined by using more than one source, setting, and method of gathering data and including premedication baseline school data on behavior and academic performance, are essential. Education for the child, family, and teacher is helpful before the start of medication (Dulcan and Lizarralde 2002). The physician should explicitly debunk common myths about stimulant treatment—for example, that stimulants have a paradoxical sedative action, that they lead to drug abuse, and that they are not needed or are ineffective after puberty. The physician should work closely with parents on dose adjustments and should obtain annual academic testing and more frequent reports from teachers.

No patient characteristics are helpful in suggesting which stimulant drug is best for a particular child. Twenty-five percent of a sample of boys with ADHD taking both methylphenidate and dextroamphetamine were behaviorally positive responders to one of the drugs but not the other. Of the nonresponders to each drug, the majority responded to the other drug (Elia et al. 1991). Methylphenidate is the most commonly used and best studied.

Several longer-acting stimulant preparations (Ritalin-SR, Dexedrine Spansules, Adderall-XR, Metadate-CD, and Concerta) are now available. These particular medications are useful for children who experience a brief duration of action with the standard formulations (2–3 hours), for those who experience severe rebound, or for circumstances in which administering medication every 4 hours is inconvenient, stigmatizing, or impossible. Parents and children should be warned by clinicians that breaking or chewing most long-acting preparations will destroy the sustained-release packaging and could result in excessively high doses of medication. However, Metadate-CD capsules may be opened and "sprinkled" onto foods such as applesauce. An innovative strategy for difficult-to-manage cases is to combine short-acting and longer-acting medication forms (Fitzpatrick et al. 1992).

Adderall, a racemic mixture of four amphetamine salts (D-amphetamine saccharate, D-amphetamine sulfate, D,L-amphetamine sulfate, and D,L-amphetamine aspartate), has been shown in several randomized double-blind, placebo-controlled studies to be as effective as methylphenidate in treating the behavioral symptoms of ADHD (Pliszka 2000; Swanson et al. 1998a, 1998b). In regard to Adderall's side effects, no significant differences from methylphenidate were noted.

Concerta, a newer long-acting single-daily-dose methylphenidate preparation, uses medication packaging with a slow-release osmotic distribution system. In a recent within-subject double-blind trial (Pelham et al. 2001), Concerta was found to be comparable to three-times-daily dosing of methylphenidate. No additional side effects were noted with Concerta, and many parents preferred its ease of use over methylphenidate's traditional multiple-dosing schedule.

Magnesium pemoline is a longer-acting CNS stimulant that is structurally dissimilar to methylphenidate and dextroamphetamine. In 1996, Abbott Laboratories (manufacturer of the Cylert brand of pemoline) identified 13 cases of acute hepatic failure due to hepatotoxicity that had been reported to the FDA since 1975. As a result of clinician awareness of pemoline hepatotoxicity resulting in death, the United Kingdom and Canada have withdrawn pemoline from their markets. Given the availability of newer and safer long-acting agents, current use of pemoline in children and adolescents appears unsupportable (Safer et al. 2001).

Stimulant medication should be initiated with a low dose and gradually titrated upward within the recommended range every week or two according to response and side effects, with body weight as a rough guide to dosage (Table 20–2). When children reach age 3 years, their absorption, distribution, protein binding, and metabolism of stimulants are similar to those of adults (Coffey et al. 1983), although adults experience more side effects than do children at the same milligrams-per-kilogram dose. Giving medication after meals minimizes anorexia. Preschool-age children or patients with ADHD, predominantly inattentive type; mental retardation; or PDDs may benefit from (and have fewer side effects with) lower doses than those required by patients with ADHD with prominent symptoms of hyperactivity or impulsivity. Starting with only a morning dose may be useful in assessing drug effect by comparing morning and afternoon school performance. The need for an after-school dose or medication on weekends should be individually determined. Results from the MTA study suggest that most children continue to benefit from maintenance medication dosages that are similar to the initial titration dose (Vitiello et al. 2001). However, dosage adjustments were often required in children, indicating the need for ongoing monitoring of treatment response and active medication management (Vitiello et al. 2001).

Behavioral checklists such as the Child Attention Profile (CAP; Edelbrock 1991), the Conners Teacher Rating Scale (CTRS), and the Conners Parent Rating Scale (CPRS; Conners and Barkley 1985) are useful in monitoring the effectiveness of medications in a variety of settings.

If symptoms are not severe outside the school setting, children should have an annual drug-free trial in the summer, at least 2 weeks' duration but longer if possible. If school behavior and academic performance are stable, a carefully monitored trial off medication during the school year (but *not* at the beginning) will provide data on whether medication is still needed.

TABLE 20–2. Clinical use of stimulant medications

	Methylphenidate (Ritalin)	Dextroamphetamine (Dexedrine)	Adderall	Concerta
How supplied (mg)	5, 10, 20 Sustained release 20	5, 10 Elixir (5 mg/5 mL) Spansules 5, 10, 15	5, 10, 20, 30	18, 36
Usual single dose range (mg/kg/dose)	0.3–0.7	0.15–0.50	—	—
Usual daily dosage range (mg/day)	10–60	5–40	5–40	18–54
Usual starting dose (mg)	5–10 qd or bid	2.5 or 5.0 qd or bid	2.5–5.0 qd	18
Maintenance number of doses per day	2–3	2–3	1–2	1

Tolerance is reported anecdotally, but compliance is often irregular and should be the first possibility considered when medication appears ineffective. Children should not be responsible for their medication because youngsters are impulsive and forgetful at best, and most dislike the idea of taking medication, even when they can verbalize its positive effects and cannot identify any side effects. They will often avoid, "forget," or simply refuse medication. Lower potency or absorption of a generic preparation may be another possibility. The apparent decreased drug effect also may be due to a reaction to a change at home or school. Greenhill (1995) uses the term *pseudotolerance* to define circumstances in which increased symptomatology is inaccurately ascribed to decreased medication efficacy (e.g., when symptoms are exacerbated due to changes in a child's life rather than changes in response to medication). True tolerance may be more likely with the long-acting formulations (Birmaher et al. 1989); if it occurs, another of the stimulants may be substituted.

Risks and Side Effects

Most side effects are similar for all stimulants (Table 20–3). Insomnia may be due to drug effect, to rebound, or to a preexisting sleep problem. Stimulants may worsen or improve irritable mood (Gadow 1992). Black male adolescents who take stimulants may be at higher risk for elevated blood pressure (Brown and Sexson 1989).

Although stimulant-induced growth retardation has been a significant concern, decrease in expected weight gain is small and may be clinically insignificant, despite statistical significance. The magnitude of the growth retardation is dose related and appears to be greater with dextroamphetamine than with methylphenidate or pemoline. Effect on height can be minimized with the use of "drug holidays." The mech-

TABLE 20–3. Side effects of stimulant medications

Common initial side effects (try dosage reduction)
  Anorexia
  Weight loss
  Irritability
  Abdominal pain
  Headaches
  Emotional oversensitivity, easy crying

Less common side effects
  Insomnia
  Dysphoria (especially at higher doses)
  Decreased social interest
  Impaired cognitive test performance
    (especially at very high doses)
  Less than expected weight gain
  Rebound overactivity and irritability
    (as dose wears off)
  Anxiety
  Nervous habits (e.g., picking at skin, pulling hair)
  Hypersensitivity rash, conjunctivitis, or hives

Withdrawal effects
  Insomnia
  Rebound ADHD symptoms
  Depression (rare)

Rare but potentially serious side effects
  Motor or vocal tics
  Tourette's disorder
  Depression
  Growth retardation
  Tachycardia
  Hypertension
  Psychosis with hallucinations
  Stereotyped activities or compulsions

Side effects reported with pemoline only
  Choreiform movements
  Dyskinesias
  Night terrors
  Lip licking or biting
  Chemical hepatitis (potentially fatal)

Note. ADHD = attention-deficit/hyperactivity disorder.

anism of this side effect does not appear to be mediated through effects on growth hormone (Greenhill et al. 1981, 1984).

Rebound effects, consisting of increased excitability, activity, talkativeness, irritability, and insomnia, beginning 4–15 hours after a dose, may be seen as the last dose of the day wears off or for up to several days after sudden withdrawal of high daily doses of stimulants. This effect may resemble a worsening of the original symptoms (Zahn et al. 1980).

Although psychosis is a well-known side effect of all stimulant medications, psychotic symptoms have not been rigorously studied within the child and adolescent population being treated for ADHD.

Although there is a commonly held notion that stimulants lower the seizure threshold, there is no evidence that stimulants produce an increase in seizure activity. Addiction has *not* been found to result from the prescription of stimulants for ADHD. Naturalistic longitudinal data suggest that children with ADHD who are effectively treated with stimulants are less likely to abuse substances than are other children with ADHD (Biederman et al. 1999).

α_2-Noradrenergic Agonists

Clonidine and guanfacine are α_2-noradrenergic agonists approved for the treatment of hypertension.

Indications and Efficacy

Attention-deficit/hyperactivity disorder. Clonidine is useful in modulating mood and activity level and in improving cooperation and frustration tolerance in subgroup of children with ADHD, especially those who are highly aroused, hyperactive, impulsive, defiant, and labile (Hunt et al. 1990). Steingard et al. (1993) reported that children with ADHD and comorbid tics may have a more positive response to clonidine than do children with ADHD without tics. In a meta-analysis of the literature from 1980 to 1999,

Connor et al. (1999) demonstrated an effect size of clonidine on symptoms of ADHD that was intermediate between that of stimulant medication response (stronger) and tricyclic antidepressant (TCA) medication response (weaker).

Guanfacine has been shown to be effective in open trials of children with ADHD (Horrigan and Barnhill 1995; Hunt et al. 1995) and children with comorbid ADHD and Tourette's disorder (Chappell et al. 1995). A placebo-controlled study also demonstrated guanfacine's effectiveness in treating children with comorbid ADHD and tic disorders (Scahill et al. 2001).

Initiation and Maintenance

Because clonidine and guanfacine have similar pharmacological profiles, blood pressure and pulse should be measured before treatment and at regular intervals throughout. An electrocardiogram (ECG) and baseline laboratory blood studies (especially fasting glucose) may be considered. Clonidine is initiated at a low dose of 0.05 mg (one-half of the smallest manufactured tablet) at bedtime. This low dose converts the side effect of initial sedation into a benefit. An alternate strategy is to begin with 0.025 mg four times a day. Either way, the dose is then titrated gradually upward over several weeks to 0.15–0.30 mg/day (0.003–0.01 mg/kg/day) in three or four divided doses. Young children (ages 5–7 years) may require lower initial and maintenance doses. The transdermal form (skin patch) may be useful to improve compliance and reduce variability in blood levels. It lasts only 5 days in children (compared with 7 days in adults) (Hunt et al. 1990). Once the daily dose is determined using pills, an equivalent-size patch may be substituted (0.1, 0.2, 0.3 mg/day). Patches should not be cut to adjust the dose, as this may damage the delivery membrane, potentially causing an increase in the delivered dose of clonidine (Broderick-Cantwell 1999). Unfortunately, patches do not adhere well in hot, humid climates.

For guanfacine, dosages range from 0.5 to 4.0 mg/day, and a recommended starting regimen is 0.5 mg once or twice a day in children and 1 mg once or twice a day in adolescents, to be increased every 3 or 4 days until therapeutic effect is noted (Silver 1999). Guanfacine is not currently available in a transdermal preparation.

When clonidine or guanfacine is discontinued, it should be tapered over several days to a week, rather than stopped suddenly, to avoid a withdrawal syndrome consisting of increased motor restlessness, headache, agitation, elevated blood pressure and pulse rate, and (in patients with Tourette's disorder) exacerbation of tics (Leckman et al. 1986).

Risks and Side Effects

Sedation and irritability are troublesome side effects of clonidine therapy, although they tend to decrease after several weeks. Dry mouth, nausea, and photophobia have been reported, with hypotension and dizziness possible at high doses. The clonidine skin patch often causes local pruritic dermatitis; daily rotation of the patch site or use of a steroid cream may minimize this. Depression may occur, often in patients with a history of depressive symptoms in themselves or their families (Hunt et al. 1991). Glucose tolerance may decrease, especially in those patients at risk for diabetes. Although guanfacine is less sedating and less hypotensive than clonidine, it shares many of the side effects of this class of medication.

Recent reports of serious adverse drug reactions (including sudden death) in children treated with clonidine, alone or in combination with methylphenidate, have raised concerns about the safety of this medication in the pediatric population (Cantwell et al. 1997; Popper 1995; Swanson et al. 1995, 1999). In all of these cases, the presence of polypharmacy or of other medical conditions made it difficult to implicate clonidine in the adverse events (Wilens and Spencer 1999). Although Popper (1995) identified no clear evidence that the combination of clonidine and methylphenidate is unsafe, he also warned that there was insufficient scientific evidence available on either the potential benefits or the risks of methylphenidate–clonidine treatment and that clinicians should proceed with caution. Cardiovascular screening and monitoring of children treated with clonidine or guanfacine is recommended, as well as gradual titration and tapering of dose to reduce cardiovascular side effects. These medications should not be used unless a parent can supervise them safely and ensure adherence to the prescribed regimen.

Selective Serotonin Reuptake Inhibitors

Five SSRIs have been approved for use in the United States: citalopram, fluoxetine, fluvoxamine, paroxetine, and sertraline. Of these, only two have FDA-approved indications for use in children: fluvoxamine and sertraline for obsessive-compulsive disorder (OCD). However, all of the SSRIs have been used to treat a wide variety of disorders in children and adolescents.

Indications and Efficacy

Depressive disorders. One rigorous double-blind, placebo-controlled trial in 96 children and adolescents with major depressive episode found that fluoxetine produced significantly greater improvement in depressive symptoms than did placebo, as measured by the Children's Depression Rating Scale and the Clinical Global Impressions scale (Emslie et al. 1997).

Keller et al. (2001) undertook a double-blind, placebo-controlled study of paroxetine in 275 adolescents with major depression, randomizing the patients to paroxetine (20–40 mg/day), imipramine (200–300 mg/day), or placebo. Relative to those taking placebo, patients receiving paroxetine demonstrated significantly greater improvement on several measures of depressive symptomatology. Interestingly, imipramine did not produce statistically significant improvement on any measurement instrument compared with placebo. Open-label studies of sertraline have also shown clinical improvement in symptoms of major depressive disorder in adolescent patients (Ambrosini et al. 1999; McConville et al. 1996).

Obsessive-compulsive disorder. Considerable evidence supports the use of SSRIs in children with OCD. In a recent study, D.A. Geller et al. (2001) found that fluoxetine was significantly more effective than placebo, as measured by CY-BOCS scores, in a randomized, controlled study of 103 children and adolescents. March et al. (1998b) conducted a randomized, double-blind, controlled study of sertraline versus placebo in the treatment of 187 children and adolescents with OCD. Over the 12 weeks of the study, patients treated with sertraline showed a significantly greater improvement on the CY-BOCS than did the placebo group (42% of sertraline group versus 26% of placebo group). In another randomized multicenter trial, Riddle et al. (2001) compared fluvoxamine with placebo in 120 children and adolescents diagnosed with OCD. Fluvoxamine-treated subjects demonstrated significantly improved scores on the CY-BOCS throughout the course of the study. Open trials of paroxetine and citalopram have also shown improvements in CY-BOCS scores in children and adolescents with OCD

treated with these medications (Rosenberg et al. 1999; Thomsen 1997; Thomsen et al. 2001). In all cited studies, medications were described as generally well tolerated by both child and adolescent subjects.

Other disorders. In a multicenter double-blind, placebo-controlled study, Walkup et al. (2001) demonstrated fluvoxamine's superiority to placebo in treating social phobia, separation anxiety disorder, and generalized anxiety disorder in children and adolescents ages 6–17 years. Over the 8 weeks of the study, the patients who received fluvoxamine had significantly greater decreases in their Pediatric Anxiety Rating Scale scores than did those receiving placebo. In addition, the fluvoxamine group showed a greater response to treatment overall, as measured by the Clinical Global Impressions—Improvement scale. Compton et al. (2001), in an open trial of sertraline in children and adolescents with social anxiety disorder, found treatment response, as measured by the Clinical Global Impressions—Improvement scale, in 65% of patients by the end of the 8-week study. Birmaher et al. (1994) reported marked to moderate improvement in children and adolescents with mixed anxiety disorders who were treated with fluoxetine in an open study. In another open study by Fairbanks et al. (1997), children taking fluoxetine for various anxiety disorders were "much improved," with the most robust response seen in separation anxiety disorder and social phobia, and a lesser response seen in generalized anxiety disorder.

Dosage and Administration

Fluoxetine, citalopram, and paroxetine may be started at dosages of 5–10 mg/day, which may be increased as needed to 20 mg/day. Although most children will show an adequate response to 20 mg/day or less of these medications, some children may require dosages in excess of 20 mg/day. All three of these medications are available in a liquid formulation that may facilitate medication administration or dosage titration in small children.

For sertraline and fluvoxamine, doses may be started at 25 mg/day and increased as necessary to a dosage of 100–150 mg/day. Doses may be increased every few days as tolerated. Sertraline is also available in a liquid preparation.

Although children and adolescents usually tolerate this class of medication well, they may experience the same constellation of side effects as seen in adults, such as gastrointestinal complaints or headache. In addition, patients may experience a "withdrawal" phenomenon if the medication is stopped abruptly. Withdrawal symptoms include malaise, myalgias, headache, and anxiety and may occur even if only one dose is missed. This withdrawal phenomenon is not usually noted with fluoxetine because of its active metabolites and long half-life. It is therefore preferable to taper the dosage of medication over several days before cessation rather than discontinuing it abruptly. In a patient who has a recurrence of symptoms after an initial good response, a gentle inquiry about medication compliance should be made before instituting a change in dosage.

Adverse Effects

Several cases of "behavioral activation" and manic symptoms presumed to be caused by treatment with SSRIs have been reported in pediatric patients (Diler and Avci 1999; Grubbs 1997; Guile 1996; Minnery et al. 1995; Oldroyd 1997; Tierney et al. 1995). In many of these cases, the manic symptoms appeared within days to weeks of initiating treatment with an SSRI. Symptoms usually resolved

within a few days of reduction in dosage or cessation of medication. In one case (Oldroyd 1997), treatment with a mood stabilizer was necessary. In many of the cases, there was no premorbid or family history of a cyclical mood disorder.

Movement disorders (acute dystonic reactions, akathisia, and ticlike movements) have also been noted in children taking SSRIs (Bates et al. 1998; Boyle 1999; Jones-Fearing 1996; Lenti 1999). Because SSRI-induced movement disorders are thought to be due to serotonin-mediated inhibition of dopaminergic transmission (Lipinski et al. 1989), movement disorders may potentially occur with any of the SSRIs.

Serotonin syndrome is a potentially fatal reaction to serotonergic agents. It is more likely to occur when serotonergic agents are used in combination. Several signs characterize this syndrome: mental status changes, fever, tremor, diaphoresis, and agitation. Although uncommon, serotonin syndrome has been reported in the pediatric population (Gill et al. 1999; Lee and Lee 1999; Mullins and Horowitz 1999; Pao and Tipnis 1997; Spirko and Wiley 1999). It may arise after only one dose of a serotonergic agent. Clinicians should be alert to the possibility of this syndrome occurring in their pediatric patients and should counsel patients and parents as appropriate.

Tricyclic Antidepressants

Until the introduction of the SSRIs into the U.S. market in the late 1980s, TCAs were a mainstay in the pharmacological treatment of a wide variety of disorders in children and adolescents. However, the paucity of clinical studies demonstrating the efficacy of TCAs in children, an increased awareness of the potential cardiac effects of this class of medication, and the availability of alternative medications has resulted in a shift away from using tricyclic agents as first-line agents (Safer 1997). Although TCAs may no longer be considered first line in the treatment of psychiatric conditions in children and adolescents (B. Geller et al. 1999), their continued use and availability warrants their discussion here.

Indications and Efficacy

Depression. Several double-blind, placebo-controlled studies have examined the efficacy of TCAs in treating depressed children and adolescents. Despite promising anecdotal data and results in open trials, only one study has documented superiority of a TCA over placebo (Preskorn et al. 1987). Hypotheses put forward to explain this poor response include suboptimal dosing, an increase in hormone levels in adolescents, a difference in the maturation of the noradrenergic and serotonergic neurotransmitter systems, and speculation that some of the youths studied may have been in the early phase of bipolar disorder (Ambrosini 2000). Given recent findings of the efficacy of SSRIs in the treatment of adolescent depression (Emslie et al. 1997; Keller et al. 2001) and the consistent lack of data demonstrating the efficacy of TCAs, SSRIs should be considered the treatment of choice for this population.

Attention-deficit/hyperactivity disorder. TCAs may be indicated for patients with ADHD who do not respond to stimulants or who develop significant depression while taking stimulants, or for the treatment of ADHD symptoms in patients with tics or Tourette's disorder. The efficacy of TCAs in improving cognitive symptoms does not appear to be as great as that of stimulants. Because other useful and safe medications are available, TCAs should be a second- or third-line medication for treatment of ADHD in children.

Obsessive-compulsive disorder. Clomipramine, a TCA that inhibits serotonin reuptake, is useful in the treatment of OCD in children (DeVeaugh-Geiss et al. 1992; Leonard et al. 1989). Symptoms are rarely eliminated entirely, but when the medication is effective, the force of obsessions and compulsions is reduced sufficiently to improve quality of life. As in depression, the more favorable side effect and safety profiles of the SSRIs makes clomipramine a second- or third-line treatment of OCD in children.

Autistic disorder. Gordon et al. (1993) reported a double-blind study in which clomipramine was significantly more effective than either placebo or desipramine in improving several autistic symptoms (obsessive-compulsive symptoms, reciprocal social interactions, stereotypies, and self-injury). There was no difference between desipramine and placebo noted. In a recent open study examining the use of clomipramine in treating young children (ages 3.5–8.7 years), Sanchez et al. (1996) reported no therapeutic effect, and significant adverse reactions were noted (urinary retention).

Enuresis. All of the TCAs have been found to be equally effective in the treatment of nocturnal enuresis. In 80% of patients, TCAs reduce the frequency of bed wetting within the first week. Total remission, however, occurs in relatively few cases. Wetting returns when the drug is discontinued. Behavioral treatments that avoid drug side effects and have higher remission and lower relapse rates are the best first choice. Imipramine may be useful on a short-term basis or for special occasions (e.g., overnight camp), although desmopressin is now commonly used for such purposes.

Anxiety disorders. The majority of the literature has examined the use of TCAs for separation anxiety disorder and school absenteeism. Of four double-blind, placebo-controlled studies, only one has demonstrated efficacy of a TCA over placebo in treating separation anxiety disorder and school refusal (Gittelman-Klein and Klein 1971, 1973). Several case studies of the effectiveness of TCAs in treating childhood panic disorder have also been reported (Black and Robbins 1989; Garland and Smith 1990). The efficacy of imipramine in patients with anxiety disorders is controversial (Bernstein et al. 1990; Klein et al. 1992), and other medications are now available.

Initiation and Maintenance

Pharmacokinetics for TCAs is different in children than in adolescents or adults. The smaller fat-to-muscle ratio in children leads to a decreased volume of distribution, and children are not protected from excessive dosage by a large volume of fat in which the drug can be stored. Children have larger livers relative to body size, leading to faster metabolism (Sallee et al. 1986), more rapid absorption, and lower protein binding than in adults (Winsberg et al. 1974). As a result, children are likely to need a higher weight-corrected dose of TCAs than adults. Prepubertal children are prone to rapid dramatic swings in blood levels from toxic to ineffective and should have divided doses to produce more stable levels (Ryan 1992). Parents must be reminded to supervise closely the administration of medication and to keep pills in a safe place, due to the danger of overdose.

The usefulness of plasma levels is limited by the relative rarity of laboratories able to perform them satisfactorily. Medication cannot be safely titrated by plasma level, as there is no known level below which toxicity can be guaranteed not to occur. Plasma levels (drawn 9–11 hours after the last dose) can identify rapid and slow metabolizers. Determination of levels is recommended for patients who fail to respond to usual doses (possibly low levels) or those who have severe side effects at usual doses (possibly very high levels). If the patient's history suggests head trauma or seizures, an electroencephalogram (EEG) is indicated before starting treatment.

Depression. For imipramine, the starting dose is 25 mg/day, which may be increased every 4 days by 1 mg/kg/day to a maximum dose of 5 mg/kg/day. Optimum plasma level of imipramine appears to be 150–250 ng/mL (Preskorn et al. 1987; Ryan 1990).

Nortriptyline may have fewer side effects and a more precise therapeutic window of 75–150 ng/mL, usually attained at 0.5 to 2.0 mg/kg/day (Ryan 1990). It has a longer half-life than imipramine and may be given twice a day in children. Variability in metabolism is greater for nortriptyline than for imipramine (B. Geller et al. 1986).

Attention-deficit/hyperactivity disorder. Imipramine is begun with 10 or 25 mg/day and increased weekly. The maximum dose is 5 mg/kg/day (given in three divided doses). Plasma levels do not predict efficacy. Some patients respond to a daily dose as low as 2 mg/kg. Nortriptyline is given at 25–75 mg/day in two divided doses (Saul 1985).

Obsessive-compulsive disorder. Doses of clomipramine used to treat OCD are generally lower than TCA doses used to treat depression. Response is delayed for 10–14 days, as in the treatment of depression, and is unlike the immediate response seen in the treatment of ADHD or enuresis (Rapoport 1986). Clomipramine is started at 25 mg/day (or every other day) and gradually increased over 2 weeks to a maximum of 100 mg/day or 3 mg/kg/day, whichever is less.

Divided doses are preferable during titration. Chronic treatment (years) is required.

Enuresis. Daily charting of wet and dry nights is used before starting medication to obtain a baseline and subsequently to monitor progress. Much lower doses are needed than for the treatment of depression. Imipramine is started at 10–25 mg at bedtime and increased by 10- to 25-mg increments weekly to 50 mg (75 mg in preadolescents), if necessary. Maximum dose is 2.5 mg/kg/day (Ryan 1990). Tolerance may develop, requiring a dose increase. For some children, TCAs lose their effect entirely. If medication is used chronically, the child or adolescent should have a drug-free trial at least every 6 months because enuresis has a high spontaneous remission rate.

Anxiety disorders. In separation anxiety disorder and school nonattendance, psychological interventions such as family therapy, consultation with school personnel, and cognitive-behavioral techniques should be used before and along with medication. For children with school phobia, the recommended starting dose is 25 mg/day of imipramine. The dose is titrated upward every 3–5 days, as tolerated, to an expected therapeutic range of 3–5 mg/kg/day. A twice-daily dosing regimen is recommended to minimize side effects from a large single dose.

Risks and Side Effects

The quinidine-like effect of the TCAs slows cardiac conduction time and repolarization. At doses of more than 3 mg/kg/day of imipramine, children and adolescents may develop an increased pulse and small but statistically significant ECG changes (intraventricular conduction defects, such as lengthened P-R interval, that

may progress to a first-degree atrioventricular heart block and occasional widening of the QRS complex) (Wilens et al. 1996). Prolongation of the QTc interval may be a sensitive indicator of cardiac effect (Wiles et al. 1991). The tendency of prepubertal children to have wider swings in blood levels may place them at higher risk for serious cardiac conduction changes. A minority of the population has a genetic defect in TCA metabolism, increasing risk for toxicity.

Anticholinergic side effects may occur in children, although less commonly than in adults. Most of these side effects are transient and/or respond to a decrease in dose. Of particular importance for children are dry mouth, which may lead to an increase in dental caries in long-term use (Herskowitz 1987), drying of bronchial secretions (especially problematic for asthmatic children), sedation, anorexia, constipation, nausea, tachycardia, palpitations, and increased diastolic blood pressure.

Other reported side effects include abdominal pain, chest pain, headache, orthostatic hypotension (rare in young patients), syncope, mild tremors of hands and fingers, weight loss, and tics. The seizure threshold may be lowered, with worsening of preexisting EEG abnormalities and rarely a seizure. Seizures appear to be more common with clomipramine. Side effects with a probable allergic mechanism include rash, worsening of eczema, and rarely thrombocytopenia (M. Campbell et al. 1985).

Behavioral toxicity may be manifested by irritability, worsening of psychosis, mania, agitation, anger, aggression, forgetfulness, or confusion. CNS toxicity may be mistaken for exacerbation of the primary condition. A drug blood level is often required to differentiate the two. As depressed children, especially those who are anergic and withdrawn, improve with TCA treatment, crying and verbalizations of sadness and anger may transiently increase.

Sudden cessation of moderate or higher doses results in a flulike anticholinergic withdrawal syndrome, with nausea, cramps, vomiting, headaches, and muscle pains. Other manifestations may include social withdrawal, hyperactivity, depression, agitation, and insomnia (Ryan 1990). TCAs should therefore be tapered over a 2- to 3-week period. The short half-life of TCAs in prepubertal children often produces daily withdrawal symptoms if medication is given only once a day. These symptoms also may indicate that poor compliance is resulting in missed doses. Because of the predictability of TCA-induced ECG changes, a rhythm strip is useful in monitoring compliance.

The physician should be alert to the risk of intentional overdose or accidental poisoning, not only by the patient but by other family members, especially young children.

Cautionary note on the use of desipramine: Six cases of sudden death have been reported in children being treated with desipramine, three of whom died immediately after physical exertion (Riddle et al. 1991, 1993; Varley and McClellan 1997). A causal relationship between the medication and the deaths has not been established. A cardiac etiology has been suspected; however, a recent review of cardiovascular changes in children treated with TCAs (Wilens et al. 1996) concluded that although changes in blood pressure, heart rate, and ECG parameters are identifiable, they are probably of minor significance. In a study of the effects of desipramine on cardiac function during exercise, 9 children and 13 adults were evaluated before and during a course of treatment with desipramine. One 31-year-old subject experienced a brief episode of ventricular tachycardia during exercise while receiving desipramine. The

study concluded that desipramine had only minor effects on the cardiovascular response to exercise, and that these effects did not appear to be age related (Waslick et al. 1999). A further study by Walsh et al. (1999) showed that desipramine reduced parasympathetic input to the heart, as measured by R-R interval variability. Although such a reduction in parasympathetic tone could, theoretically, increase vulnerability to cardiac arrhythmias, the R-R interval variability did not differ with age in the 42 subjects studied (who ranged in age from 7 to 66 years). Nevertheless, given that other safe and effective medications are available, the use of desipramine in prepubertal children is discouraged.

Other Antidepressants

Venlafaxine

Venlafaxine is a serotonin-norepinephrine reuptake inhibitor (SNRI) approved for the treatment of depression. Unlike the SSRIs, the SNRIs have both serotonergic and noradrenergic properties. Although some TCAs also possess dual-neurotransmitter activity, the SNRIs do not have α_1-, cholinergic-, or histaminic-blocking properties. Few studies have examined the use of venlafaxine in children. In one double-blind, placebo-controlled study, Mandoki et al. (1997) compared venlafaxine and cognitive-behavioral therapy with placebo and therapy in the treatment of 33 pediatric patients (ages 8 to 17 years) diagnosed with major depression. Although no significant differences were found between the two groups, the short treatment time and low dose of venlafaxine used may account for this apparent lack of effect. Olvera et al. (1996) conducted an open trial of venlafaxine in 14 children and adolescents (ages 8–17 years) with ADHD and found that venlafaxine reduced impulsivity and hyperactivity as measured by the Conners Rating Scales. Although initial reports of venlafaxine's use in a variety of disorders are promising, further controlled studies are needed to determine the efficacy and safety of venlafaxine in these disorders.

Bupropion

Bupropion is a compound of the aminoketone class and is structurally unrelated to other antidepressants. Conners et al. (1996) reported that bupropion was superior to placebo in the treatment of ADHD in children in a multisite, double-blind, placebo-controlled study. Another study found the efficacy of bupropion in treating ADHD to be not statistically significantly different from that of methylphenidate (Barrickman et al. 1995). Substance-abusing adolescent patients with ADHD may benefit from treatment with bupropion because of its lack of abuse potential. An open study by Riggs et al. (1998) suggested that bupropion could be useful in treating adolescents with comorbid ADHD, conduct disorder, and a substance use disorder. Bupropion has been reported to exacerbate tics in children with comorbid ADHD and Tourette's disorder and thus may not be suitable for use in this population (T. Spencer et al. 1993).

Although bupropion is marketed in the United States as an antidepressant and as an aid in smoking cessation, the literature on its use in treating childhood depression is limited. A small open-label study by Arredondo (1993) showed an improvement in 8 of 10 adolescent inpatients treated with bupropion. More recently, Daviss et al. (2001) used bupropion to treat 24 adolescents with ADHD and a mood disorder (major depressive disorder or dysthymic disorder). Patients were treated with the sustained-release preparation of bupropion over 8 weeks.

Fourteen of the 24 adolescents showed improvement in both depression and ADHD symptoms, 7 showed improvement in depression only, and one showed improvement in ADHD only. Double-blind, placebo-controlled studies of bupropion's efficacy in childhood mood disorders are needed.

Bupropion is administered in two or three daily doses, beginning with a low dose (37.5 or 50 mg twice daily), with gradual upward titration over 2 weeks to a usual maximum of 250 mg/day (300–400 mg/day in adolescents). A long-acting preparation of this medication is also available that allows once- or twice-daily dosing. The most serious side effect of bupropion is a decrease in the seizure threshold, seen most frequently in patients with an eating disorder. Bupropion is contraindicated in this population. Other side effects reported in children include skin rash, perioral edema, nausea, increased appetite, agitation, exacerbation of tics, and mania.

Monoamine Oxidase Inhibitors

Monoamine oxidase inhibitors (MAOIs) have been useful in the treatment of depressed adolescents who do not respond to TCAs (Ryan et al. 1988b), but the availability of safer effective treatments makes MAOIs a distant therapeutic choice. More recently, case reports have described benefit from MAOIs in children with elective mutism (Golwyn and Sevlie 1999) and in adolescents with severe melancholic depression (Strober et al. 1998). MAOIs should be used with extreme caution, if at all, in suicidal or impulsive outpatients because of the risk of severe reactions with dietary indiscretions or drug interactions. Patients taking MAOIs always require instruction on diet restrictions and potential drug interactions with prescription and over-the-counter medications.

Mood-Stabilizing Agents

Lithium has been approved since 1970 in the United States for the treatment of mania in patients 12 years of age and older. The antiepileptic drugs carbamazepine, divalproex sodium, and clonazepam are used for a variety of (non–FDA approved) psychiatric indications, although divalproex sodium has an FDA-approved indication for the treatment of mania in adults. The efficacy of these agents as mood stabilizers may be unrelated to their anticonvulsant effects. Wide variations in the bioavailability and rate of absorption of the available generic mood stabilizers have led to recommendations that the brand name (or at least a single generic) product be prescribed. Data on children and adolescents are far more limited than those from studies of adults, but side effect patterns appear to be similar, and extrapolation may be made from the treatment of children for epilepsy. The anticonvulsants have complex interactions with many other drugs.

Lithium

Indications and efficacy.   Lithium may be considered in the treatment of children and adolescents with bipolar affective disorder, mixed or manic (Strober et al. 1990; Varanka et al. 1988). It is not indicated for prophylaxis of bipolar disorder in children and adolescents unless there is well-documented history of recurrent episodes. Lithium augmentation has been effective in some open trials with adolescents who have tricyclic-refractory depression (Ryan et al. 1988a; Strober et al. 1992). However, fewer adolescents than adults respond to this strategy. Interestingly, in a double-blind, placebo-controlled study of prepubertal children with major depressive disorder without a history of symptoms of mania but with a family history of either bipolar disorder

or multigenerational major depressive episodes, B. Geller et al. (1998) found that lithium was not statistically more effective than placebo in the treatment of depression. It is not yet clear whether lithium is efficacious for the treatment of behavior disorders without an apparent mood disorder in children of bipolar parents or for children and adolescents who have behavior disorders accompanied by mood swings. The combination of lithium and methylphenidate may be more effective in the treatment of combined disruptive behavior disorders (ADHD/conduct disorder) and mood disorders than either medication used alone (Carlson et al. 1992).

In children with severe impulsive aggression, especially when it was accompanied by explosive affect, lithium was equal or superior to haloperidol in reducing aggression, hostility, and tantrums, with fewer side effects (M. Campbell et al. 1984). These positive findings were replicated in subsequent placebo-controlled studies by M. Campbell et al. (1995) and more recently by Malone et al. (2000).

Initiation and maintenance.   Lithium should not be prescribed unless the family is willing and able to comply with regular multiple daily doses and with blood monitoring of lithium levels. In addition to the usual detailed medical history and physical examination, complete blood count (CBC) with differential, liver function tests, electrolytes, serum thyroxine and thyroid-stimulating hormone (TSH), blood urea nitrogen (BUN), creatinine, and ECG should be determined before starting lithium. Some clinicians recommend determining renal concentrating ability (urine specific gravity or osmolality after overnight fluid deprivation) (C. Popper, personal communication, 1992). A patient with a history suggesting increased risk of seizures warrants an EEG. Height, weight, TSH, creatinine, and morning urine specific gravity (or osmolality) should be obtained every 3–6 months.

Lithium levels, drawn 10–12 hours after the last dose, should be obtained twice weekly during initial dose adjustment and monthly thereafter. Three to 4 days are required to reach steady-state levels after a dose change. Therapeutic levels are the same as for adults, 0.6–1.2 mEq/L, which can usually be attained with 900–1,200 mg/day, in divided doses, although daily doses of up to 2,000 mg may be required (M. Campbell et al. 1985). The starting dose is 150–300 mg/day, gradually titrated upward in divided doses according to serum levels and clinical effects. Because lithium excretion occurs primarily through the kidney, and most children have more efficient renal function than adults, children may require higher doses for body weight than do adults (Weller et al. 1986). In prepubertal children, dose may be titrated more rapidly with a regimen based on body weight (Weller et al. 1986) or on a serum level drawn 24 hours after a single 600-mg dose (Fetner and Geller 1992). More steady blood levels may be obtained by using a slow-release formulation. Lithium should be taken with food to minimize gastrointestinal distress. Some difference may be present in pharmacokinetics between lithium carbonate and lithium citrate, and clinicians should not assume equal dosing when shifting between the two forms (Reischer and Pfeffer 1996). Given lithium's teratogenicity, the clinician should address this potential with sexually mature female adolescent patients and should consider contraceptive options as appropriate.

Risks and side effects. The younger the child, the more likely the occurrence of side effects (M. Campbell et al. 1991). Autistic children have more frequent and severe side effects from lithium than do children with conduct disorder, even at lower doses (M. Campbell et al. 1991). Children may experience side effects at serum levels that are lower than those in adults: most commonly, weight gain, vomiting, headache, nausea, tremor, enuresis, stomachache, weight loss, sedation, and anorexia (M. Campbell et al. 1991). Common, early onset side effects, which seem to be related to rapid increase in serum level, include nausea, diarrhea, muscle weakness, thirst, urinary frequency, a dazed feeling, and hand tremor. Polydipsia and polyuria secondary to vasopressin-resistant diabetes insipidus may result in enuresis (M. Campbell et al. 1985). In growing children, the consequences of hypothyroidism (which could resemble retarded depression) are potentially more severe than in adults. The calcium mobilization from bones that has been noted in adults might cause a significant problem in growing children (Herskowitz 1987). Lithium's tendency to aggravate acne may be especially significant for adolescents. Lithium's effects on glucose are controversial, but both hyperglycemia and exercise-induced hypoglycemia are possible. Rarely, lithium may cause extrapyramidal side effects (EPS) in children (Samuel 1993).

Toxicity is closely related to serum levels, and the therapeutic margin is narrow. Symptoms of lithium toxicity include vomiting, drowsiness, hyperreflexia, sluggishness, slurred speech, ataxia, anorexia, convulsions, stupor, coma, and death. Adequate salt and fluid intake is necessary to prevent levels rising into the toxic range. The family should be instructed in the importance of preventing dehydration from heat or exercise and in the need to stop the lithium and contact the physician if the child or adolescent develops an illness with fever, vomiting, diarrhea, and/or decreased fluid intake.

Carbamazepine

Indications and efficacy. Some evidence suggests potential benefit for carbamazepine in the treatment of juvenile bipolar disorder, although no controlled studies have been reported. Kowatch et al. (2000) completed a random-assignment open study that compared the effect sizes of lithium, divalproex sodium and carbamazepine in the treatment of bipolar I and II in children and adolescents. The authors concluded that, similar to lithium and divalproex sodium, carbamazepine had a large effect size and was generally well tolerated.

Initiation and maintenance. Hemoglobin, hematocrit, white blood cell (WBC) count, platelets, liver function, BUN, and creatinine should all be measured before a patient begins taking carbamazepine. The degree of laboratory monitoring necessary is controversial. A conservative recommendation includes CBC and liver function studies weekly for the first 4 weeks, monthly for 4 months, and every 3 months thereafter (Silverstein et al. 1983). A more modest regimen involves CBC (with differential and platelet count), serum iron, BUN, and creatinine after the first month and then every 3–6 months (Trimble 1990). Tests always should be done if a rash, sore throat, fever, malaise, lethargy, weakness, vomiting, increased urinary frequency, anorexia, jaundice, easy bruising, bleeding, or mouth ulcers develop. If the neutrophil count drops below 1,000, or if hepatitis occurs, carbamazepine should be stopped (Silverstein et al. 1983).

The initial dosage of carbamazepine is 100 mg/day taken with food. Children eliminate carbamazepine more rapidly than do adults (Jatlow 1987), and plasma levels (drawn approximately 12 hours after the last dose) are crucial because dosage calculated by weight correlates poorly with plasma concentration. Titration should be gradual (weekly increase of 100 mg/day), guided by plasma levels, to a usual plateau of 8–12 µg/mL. The usual daily dosage range is 10–50 mg/kg, divided into three doses for children and into two doses for older adolescents. Autoinduction of hepatic enzymes may lead to declining plasma concentrations, especially during the first 6 weeks, requiring an increase in dose. Carbamazepine deteriorates if it is stored under humid conditions.

Risks and side effects. The most common adverse effects of carbamazepine are drowsiness, nausea, rash, diplopia, nystagmus, and reversible dose-related leukopenia. Other side effects include vomiting, vertigo, ataxia, tics, muscle cramps, exacerbation of seizures, rare blood dyscrasias, hepatotoxicity, severe skin reactions (e.g., Stevens-Johnson or systemic lupus–like syndromes), and inappropriate secretion of antidiuretic hormone (in rare cases leading to acute renal failure) (Evans et al. 1987; Trimble 1990). Teratogenic effects from carbamazepine have also been demonstrated. Adverse behavioral reactions, such as extreme irritability, agitation, insomnia, obsessive thinking, hallucinations, delirium, psychosis, paranoia, hyperactivity, aggression, and mania, may be seen during the first 1–4 weeks of treatment (Evans et al. 1987; Herskowitz 1987; Pleak et al. 1988).

Divalproex Sodium

Indications and efficacy. Two open-label, uncontrolled trials of divalproex sodium in the treatment of adolescents with mania have been conducted (Papatheodorou et al. 1995; West et al. 1994); both found that divalproex sodium was generally well tolerated and beneficial. As described earlier, Kowatch et al. (2000) conducted an open study in which children and adolescents with bipolar disorder I and II were randomly assigned to treatment with lithium, divalproex sodium, or carbamazepine. Like carbamazepine and lithium, divalproex sodium had a large effect size and was generally well tolerated. Although divalproex sodium may be beneficial in the treatment of mania in bipolar disorder, larger controlled studies are required.

Initiation and maintenance. The initial laboratory workup for divalproex sodium is the same as that for carbamazepine. Liver function tests and CBC may be repeated weekly for the first month, and then every 4–6 months. For children younger than age 10 years, monthly liver function tests are advisable (Trimble 1990). Divalproex sodium may be initiated at 250 mg once or twice daily, depending on the weight of the child. Trough plasma levels should be drawn after reaching a dosage of 15 mg/kg/day dispensed in three divided doses. Dosages should be titrated to achieve a serum level within the therapeutic range (50–120 µg/mL). Clinicians are cautioned that the use of mg/kg loading doses for divalproex sodium may lead to supratherapeutic levels in overweight children (Good et al. 2001).

Risks and side effects. The most frequently experienced adverse effects of divalproex sodium are nausea, vomiting, and gastrointestinal distress (which may be diminished by using enteric-coated divalproex sodium), sedation, weight gain, and tremor (Trimble 1990). Acute hepatic failure is almost always restricted to children younger than age 3 years, especially those with mental retardation or who are on anticonvulsant polytherapy. Other side effects are similar to those seen in adults. Of uncertain significance is a report of menstrual disturbances, polycystic ovaries, and hyperandrogenism in a

series of women treated with divalproex sodium for epilepsy (Isojarvi et al. 1993). These findings have been challenged in a recent review of the literature (Genton et al. 2001).

Antipsychotic Medications

Indications and Efficacy

Antipsychotic medications are more fully discussed in Chapter 18. Their use in children and adolescents has been reviewed by Findling et al. (1998) and Bryden et al. (2001). The recent introduction of "atypical" antipsychotic medications (clozapine, risperidone, olanzapine, quetiapine, and ziprasidone) has added significantly to the child and adolescent psychiatrist's pharmaceutical armamentarium. The use of these agents in children and adolescents is specifically reviewed by Toren et al. (1998) and Remschmidt et al. (2000). Studies examining the efficacy and safety of these atypical medications with children and adolescents, although promising, remain limited, particularly with the newer agents.

Schizophrenia. Few studies examining the efficacy of typical antipsychotic medications in schizophrenic children exist (Findling et al. 1996). Of the two investigations with more stringent diagnostic admission criteria, both controlled studies (Pool et al. 1976; Realmuto et al. 1984) demonstrated moderate effectiveness of antipsychotic medication in adolescent patients with schizophrenia. Medication-induced side effects in both studies were substantial, particularly sedation (in low-potency agents) and EPS (in high-potency agents), supporting the belief that children may be at higher risk than adults for developing side effects with the typical antipsychotic agents. E.K. Spencer et al. (1992) reported preliminary results of the first double-blind, placebo-controlled trial of haloperidol in schizophrenic prepubertal children. Findings similarly support moderate improvement of symptoms in those taking haloperidol rather than placebo.

The more limited effect of typical antipsychotic medications, coupled with higher side-effect profiles (to include tardive dyskinesia), in children has led clinicians to consider the use of atypical antipsychotics in the treatment of pediatric populations. Open trial and double-blind, controlled studies examining the efficacy of clozapine in adolescent patients with treatment-resistant, childhood-onset schizophrenia (Frazier et al. 1994; Kumra et al. 1996; Remschmidt et al. 1994) have demonstrated the superiority of clozapine to standard treatments, specifically haloperidol. Because treatment with clozapine is compounded by the risk of serious side effects (agranulocytosis, seizures, and significant weight gain), its use is reserved for treatment of those select patients who have failed to respond to trials of standard or other atypical antipsychotics.

Information regarding the use of risperidone in the treatment of schizophrenia in the pediatric population is limited to several case reports and open-label studies (Armenteros et al. 1997; Grcevich et al. 1996; Quintana and Keshavan 1995) in which positive and negative symptoms of the disorder appeared to have improved. As an atypical antipsychotic, risperidone may eventually prove to have greater efficacy than current standard treatments; however, controlled investigation is required.

The literature on the use of olanzapine in the treatment of schizophrenia in children and adolescents is sparse (Krishanmoorthy and King 1998; Kumra et al. 1998; Mandoki 1997; Sholevar et al. 2000). Reports are limited to retrospective and open-label studies; no controlled trials have been published. Mandoki (1997) described olanzapine's efficacy in this population as similar to that of clozapine; however, Kumra et al. (1998) suggested that although olanzapine was effective in treating refractory schizophrenia, it may not be as effective as clozapine. Krishanmoorthy and King (1998) reported their open-label use of olanzapine in five preadolescent children with varying diagnoses (including schizophrenia). In all five children, medication was discontinued prematurely due either to lack of clinical response or to the development of adverse side effects. Controlled studies examining olanzapine's efficacy and safety in pediatric populations are still needed.

Pervasive developmental disorders. In some hyper- or normoactive autistic children, haloperidol (in doses of 0.5–4.0 mg/day) has been found to decrease behavioral target symptoms such as hyperactivity, aggressiveness, temper tantrums, withdrawal, and stereotypies (Anderson et al. 1989). Haloperidol's efficacy in enhancing learning is controversial, but such enhancement clearly will not occur in the absence of a highly structured behavioral/ educational program. The majority of hypoactive autistic children do not respond well to haloperidol (M. Campbell et al. 1985) but may do better with pimozide (Ernst et al. 1992).

Atypical antipsychotic agents may eventually prove to be more effective and safer in this population. Six open trials have described the effectiveness of risperidone in the treatment of disruptive behavior in children with severe developmental disorders (Fisman and Steele 1996; Hardan et al. 1996; Horrigan and Barnhill 1997; McDougle et al. 1997; Perry et al. 1997; Zuddas et al. 2000). Masi et al. (2001) reported the benefits of low-dose risperidone (0.5 mg/day) in an open trial studying preschool children with PDDs. Risperidone effectively targeted both the disruptive behaviors and the affective dysregulation and was well tolerated. Although controlled studies are still clearly required, these preliminary data suggest that risperidone may be an effective and safe treatment in children of varying ages with PDDs, particularly in targeting serious aggressive behaviors. In two of these studies (Perry et al. 1997; Zuddas et al. 2000), long-term (greater than 6 months) therapeutic benefit was reported.

Two open-label reports of olanzapine (Malone et al. 2001; Potenza et al. 1999) in the treatment of children and adolescents with autism and PDD not otherwise specified (NOS) suggest that olanzapine may be a safe and effective treatment of core symptoms in this population. However, a similar open-label trial of quetiapine in the treatment of six male children and adolescents with autism (Martin et al. 1999) suggested no therapeutic benefit and reported serious side effects in the treatment group. Clearly, further study of the use of atypical agents in this population is required.

Tourette's disorder. The efficacy of antipsychotic medications is often difficult to evaluate in patients with Tourette's disorder because of the natural waxing and waning of symptoms. Haloperidol in low doses is initially effective for up to 70% of patients (Cohen et al. 1992). Unfortunately, side effects often limit haloperidol's usefulness, and withdrawal of the drug may lead to severe exacerbation of symptoms for up to several months. Pimozide, a high-potency antipsychotic that also blocks calcium channels, has been demonstrated to be effective in the treatment of Tourette's disorder. Although considered an alternative medication to haloperidol and clonidine, one study suggests that pimozide may result in less cog-

nitive impairment than haloperidol when prescribed at effective lower doses (Sallee and Rock 1994).

As has occurred with other disorders, atypical agents may eventually prove to be more effective and safer in this population. Risperidone was reported to be effective in reducing symptoms in two open-label studies of chronic tic/Tourette's disorder (Bruun and Budman 1996; Lombroso et al. 1995). In a double-blind, parallel-group study comparison of risperidone versus pimozide in the treatment of adolescents and adults with Tourette's disorder, Bruggeman et al. (2001) reported a favorable efficacy and tolerability profile for risperidone in this population, suggesting its potential benefit as a first-line agent in the treatment of Tourette's disorder.

A pilot study comparing ziprasidone and placebo in the treatment of children and adolescents with Tourette's disorder reported significant clinical improvement with ziprasidone, which was also well tolerated by the study subjects (Sallee et al. 2000). Additional studies are needed to establish this agent's safety and efficacy.

Conduct disorder and aggression. Studies of hospitalized, severely aggressive children, ages 6–12 years, have demonstrated short-term efficacy of haloperidol (1–6 mg/day or 0.04–0.21 mg/kg/day), thioridazine (mean = 170 mg/day), and molindone (mean = 26.8 mg/day) compared with placebo in reducing, although not eliminating, aggression, hostility, negativism, and explosiveness. Chlorpromazine can lead to unacceptable sedation at relatively low doses (M. Campbell et al. 1985; Greenhill et al. 1985). A more recent double-blind study of risperidone (up to 3 mg/day) in the treatment of 10 youths with conduct disorder reported significant improvement in aggressive symptoms with risperidone in comparison with placebo, with few side effects (Findling et al. 2000). In a double-blind, parallel-group-design study, Buitelaar et al. (2001) similarly found significant efficacy for risperidone (1.5–4.0 mg/day), compared with placebo, in the treatment of aggression in hospitalized adolescents with disruptive behavior disorders and subaverage cognitive abilities. Risperidone was well tolerated in this study group as well.

Initiation and Maintenance

Medication should not be used as the sole treatment in the aforementioned complex disorders. Before medication is initiated, a complete physical examination and baseline laboratory workup, including CBC, differential, liver profile, and urinalysis, should be performed. For those using clozapine, a baseline EEG is recommended, and a weekly WBC count with differential is mandatory. Antipsychotic medication use has been linked to the development of type 2 diabetes mellitus that may or may not be related to weight gain. Patients treated with the atypical agents clozapine and olanzapine should be monitored for changes in weight, as well as changes in fasting glucose levels. Both typical and atypical antipsychotic agents have been shown to increase QT intervals on ECG, potentially leading to dysrhythmias and sudden death. Clinicians should consider the use of ECG monitoring when appropriate.

Doses must be titrated individually, with careful attention to positive and negative effects. Age, weight, and severity of symptoms do not provide clear guidelines. The initial dose should be very low, with gradual increments no more than once or twice a week. Although divided doses are often used during titration, in most cases, once a therapeutic dosage has been reached, a single daily dose (usually at bedtime) can be used. Children metabolize these drugs

more rapidly than do adults but also require lower plasma levels for efficacy (Teicher and Glod 1990). Antipsychotic medications can interact with a wide variety of other drugs (Teicher and Glod 1990).

Schizophrenia.   Older adolescents with schizophrenia may require medication dosages in the adult range. Young adolescents fall in between, and doses must be empirically determined because few data exist. It may require several weeks for full therapeutic effect to be achieved. Although data are sparse, they are suggestive of the benefit and safety of atypical antipsychotics as first-line agents in this population. Because of its potentially lethal side effects, clozapine should be used only in cases refractory to treatment with typical or other atypical agents and should be started at very low dosages—12.5 mg/day or 25 mg/day—and titrated slowly upward (to minimize side effects) to an expected dosage range of 25–500 mg/day. Risperidone should also be initiated at low doses (0.5–1.0 mg) and titrated slowly, to prevent development of EPS, up to an expected dosage range of 2.0–4.0 mg/day. Olanzapine may be started at 5.0 mg/day and titrated upward to an expected range of 10.0–20.0 mg/day.

Pervasive developmental disorders.   It is important to give a trial of sufficient length to determine if the drug is effective, barring serious side effects requiring immediate discontinuation. Typical daily doses are 0.5–4.0 mg of haloperidol. If the drug appears to be helpful, it should be continued for at least several months. At 3- to 6-month intervals, the drug should be discontinued to observe for withdrawal dyskinesias and to determine if the drug continues to be necessary. Some children may have physical withdrawal symptoms or a rebound phenomenon consisting of worsening of behavior for up to 8 weeks after the medication is stopped (M. Campbell et al. 1985). Developmentally disturbed children treated with risperidone may benefit from dosages as low as 0.5–1.0 mg/day (Fisman and Steele 1996; Masi et al. 2001) but may require doses up to 6.0 mg/day (Perry et al. 1997). Therapeutic daily dosages for olanzapine may range from 5.0 to 20.0 mg.

Tourette's disorder. Careful monitoring of patients with Tourette's disorder for several months before starting medication is possible, since this is a chronic disorder and not usually an emergency. This monitoring permits the clinician to establish a baseline of symptoms and to assess the need for psychological and educational interventions. An initial dose of haloperidol is 0.5 mg/day. This may be slowly increased to up to 1–3 mg/day, divided in twice-daily doses (Cohen et al. 1992). Pimozide, which may be given in a single daily dose, is started at 1 mg/day and may be gradually increased to a maximum of 6–10 mg/day (0.2 mg/kg). The usual dose range is 2–6 mg/day (Cohen et al. 1992). Risperidone doses in the range of 1.0–2.5 mg/day appear to be useful (Lombroso et al. 1995). Sallee et al. (2000) initiated ziprasidone at 5 mg/day, titrating as high as 40 mg/day to achieve clinical effect in children with Tourette's disorder.

Risks and Side Effects

Acute EPS, including dystonic reactions, parkinsonian tremor, rigidity and drooling, and akathisia, occur as in adults. Laryngeal dystonia is potentially fatal. Acute dystonia may be treated with oral or intramuscular diphenhydramine, 25 mg or 50 mg, or benztropine mesylate, 0.5–2.0 mg. Adolescent boys seem to be more vulnerable to acute dystonic reactions than are adult patients, so the physician may be more inclined to use prophylactic antiparkinsonian medication. In children, however, reduction of antipsychotic dose is preferable to the use of antiparkinsonian agents (M. Campbell et al. 1985).

For treatment or prevention of parkinsonian symptoms, adolescents may be given the anticholinergic drug benztropine mesylate, 1–2 mg/day, in divided doses. Chronic parkinsonian symptoms are often drastically underrecognized by clinicians (Richardson et al. 1991). The neuromuscular consequences may impair the performance of age-appropriate activities, and the subjective effects may lead to noncompliance with medication. Akathisia may be especially difficult to identify in young patients or those with limited verbal abilities.

Tardive or withdrawal dyskinesias, some transient but others irreversible, seen in 8%–51% of antipsychotic-treated children and adolescents (M. Campbell et al. 1985), mandate caution regarding casual use of these drugs. Tardive dyskinesia has been documented in children and adolescents after as brief a period of treatment as 5 months (Herskowitz 1987) and may appear even during periods of constant medication dose. Cases of tardive dyskinesia have been reported in youths treated with risperidone (Feeney and Klykylo 1996), indicating that atypical antipsychotics may also cause this serious adverse reaction. In children with autism or Tourette's disorder, it may be especially difficult to distinguish medication-induced movements from those characteristic of the disorder. Before patients begin taking an antipsychotic medication, they should be examined carefully for abnormal movements by using a scale such as the Abnormal Involuntary Movement Scale (AIMS 1988) and should be periodically reexamined. Parents and patients (if they are able) should receive regular explanations of the risk of movement disorders.

Potentially fatal neuroleptic malignant syndrome has been reported with antipsychotic agents in children and adolescents (Silva et al. 1999), with a presentation similar to that seen in adults.

Weight gain may be problematic with the long-term use of the low-potency antipsychotics as well as the newer atypical antipsychotic medications. Abnormal laboratory findings seem to be reported less often for children than for adults, but the clinician should be alert to the possibility, especially of agranulocytosis or hepatic dysfunction. If an acute febrile illness or easy bruising occurs, medication should be withheld and CBC with differential and liver enzymes should be determined (M. Campbell et al. 1985).

Another concern is behavioral toxicity, manifested as worsening of preexisting symptoms or development of new symptoms such as hyperactivity or hypoactivity, irritability, apathy, withdrawal, stereotypies, tics, or hallucinations (M. Campbell et al. 1985). Low-potency antipsychotic drugs such as chlorpromazine and thioridazine can produce cognitive dulling and sedation that interfere with the patient's ability to benefit from school (M. Campbell et al. 1985) and are probably best avoided. Children and adolescents are more sensitive than adults to this sedation (Realmuto et al. 1984). Children may be at greater risk of antipsychotic-induced seizures than are adults because of their immature nervous systems and the high prevalence of abnormal EEGs in seriously disturbed children (Teicher and Glod 1990).

Anticholinergic side effects such as hypotension, dry mouth, constipation, nasal congestion, blurred vision, and urinary retention are unusual. Miscellaneous side effects include abdominal pain, enuresis (Realmuto et al. 1984), photosensitivity, and various neuroendocrine effects that may be especially distressing to adolescents.

Kumra et al. (1996) reported a high incidence of serious adverse effects (neutropenia and seizure activity) in children who were treated with clozapine, indicating a need for extremely close monitoring of children treated with this medication.

Side effects are a significant problem of long-term use of haloperidol for Tourette's disorder. Frequent complaints include lethargy, feeling like a "zombie," dysphoria, personality changes, weight gain, parkinsonian symptoms, akathisia, and intellectual dulling (Cohen et al. 1992). Dysphoria and school avoidance also have been reported (Mikkelsen et al. 1981). Pimozide appears to have a similar but less severe side-effect profile.

Antipsychotic medications have been associated with prolongation of the QTc interval, torsades de pointes, and sudden death (Glassman and Bigger 2001). Certain antipsychotics appear to be at greater risk for causing these problems. Recently, the FDA placed a black box warning on the use of thioridazine due to its significantly greater risk for causing QTc prolongation and sudden death. Pimozide and haloperidol have also been associated with torsades de pointes. Ziprasidone has been shown to have a clear effect on cardiac repolarization, resulting in QTc prolongation greater than that caused by most antipsychotic agents but less than that caused by thioridazine. Although no serious cardiac events occurred during the premarketing testing of ziprasidone, its association with sudden death remains unclear at this time (Glassman and Bigger 2001). Clinically, the prudent use of ECG monitoring at baseline and during dosage titration in medications that are of higher risk seems indicated.

Anxiolytics, Sedatives, and Hypnotics

Benzodiazepines

Indications and efficacy. Little research has examined the use of benzodiazepines in the treatment of pediatric psychiatric conditions. Benzodiazepines may be useful in the short-term treatment of children with severe anticipatory anxiety (Pfefferbaum et al. 1987). Although an open trial of alprazolam for children with avoidant and overanxious disorders was promising, a double-blind study did not find superiority of this drug over placebo in the context of an intensive treatment program (Simeon et al. 1992). Efficacy may have been limited by low doses and the short duration of treatment.

Preliminary evidence suggests that clonazepam may be useful in the treatment of panic disorder and antipsychotic-induced akathisia in adolescents (Biederman 1987; Kutcher et al. 1987, 1989, 1992). In a small open trial, clonazepam was found effective in diminishing tics in children with ADHD and comorbid tic disorders when used adjunctively with clonidine (Steingard et al. 1994). In a double-blind, placebo-controlled study, Graae et al. (1994) reported the clinical effectiveness of clonazepam in the treatment of anxiety disorders (predominantly separation anxiety disorder) in children. However, statistical superiority over placebo was not found, and most children evidenced side effects, notably sedation and disinhibition.

Initiation and maintenance. Infants and children absorb diazepam faster and metabolize it more quickly than do adults (Simeon and Ferguson 1985). Usual daily dose ranges for children and adolescents are as follows: lorazepam, 0.25–6.0 mg; diazepam, 1–20 mg; and alprazolam, 0.25–4.0 mg. Clonazepam has been used at a dosage of 0.5–3.0 mg/day. The dosage schedule depends on the patient's age (more frequent dosing in children) and the specific drug (Coffey 1990; Kutcher et al. 1992). When the medication is being discontinued, the dosage needs to

be tapered gradually to avoid withdrawal seizures or rebound anxiety.

Risks and side effects. In addition to the risks of substance abuse and physical or psychological dependence, side effects of benzodiazepines include sedation, cognitive dulling, ataxia, confusion, emotional lability, and worsening of psychosis. Paradoxical or disinhibition reactions may occur, manifested by acute excitation, irritability, increased anxiety, hallucinations, increased aggression and hostility, rage reactions, insomnia, euphoria, and/or incoordination (Coffey 1990; Graae et al. 1994; Reiter and Kutcher 1991; Simeon and Ferguson 1985).

Buspirone

Buspirone is a nonbenzodiazepine anxiolytic that is reported to be less sedating and have less risk of abuse or dependence than do the benzodiazepines. It may also have weak antidepressant efficacy.

Indications and efficacy. All data on buspirone treatment in children are anecdotal. Suggested uses include generalized anxiety disorder (Kutcher et al. 1992), mixed anxiety disorders (Simeon et al. 1994), as a supplementary drug in the treatment of OCD, and for reducing aggression and anxiety in patients with mental retardation (Ratey et al. 1991), PDDs (Buitelaar et al. 1998; Realmuto et al. 1989), or conduct disorder. Pfeffer et al. (1997) conducted an open trial in which buspirone (up to 50 mg/day) was used to treat 25 prepubertal children who were hospitalized with aggressive behavior and anxiety. Seventy-five percent of the children completed the study, and although improvements were demonstrated in overall functioning (as measured by the Global Assessment of Functioning), only 3 of the children were considered to have derived enough benefit from the medication to continue with treatment after the conclusion of the study. Randomized, controlled clinical studies are needed to assess the safety and efficacy of buspirone for pediatric psychiatric conditions.

Initiation and maintenance. Tentative guidelines for children and adolescents suggest a starting dose of 2.5–5.0 mg/day, increasing to three times a day over 2–3 days (Kutcher et al. 1992). The dose may be increased gradually to a maximum of 20 mg/day in children and 60 mg/day in adolescents, in three divided doses. The therapeutic effects may be delayed for 1–2 weeks after reaching the proper dose, with maximal effects not seen for an additional 2 weeks (Coffey 1990).

Risks and side effects. Reported adverse effects include insomnia, dizziness, anxiety, nausea, headache, restlessness, agitation, depression, and confusion (Coffey 1990). Possible psychotic symptoms were reported in two children treated with buspirone (Soni and Weintraub 1992), indicating that clinicians should closely monitor children who are prescribed this medication.

Beta-Blocking Agents
Indications and Efficacy

β-Adrenergic blockers may be useful in patients with otherwise uncontrollable rage reactions and impulsive aggression or self-injurious behavior, especially those with evidence of organicity. Propranolol has been found to be effective in daily doses of 50–960 mg, with a median of 160 mg (Williams et al. 1982). Anecdotal reports suggest that propranolol may be effective in the treatment of agitated, hyperaroused children and adolescents with PTSD (Famularo et al. 1988) and children and adolescents with "hyperventilation attacks" (Joorabchi 1977). In an open trial, a single 40-mg dose of propranolol appeared to be helpful in reducing test anx-

iety and improving performance in high school students (Faigel 1991). Pindolol and nadolol, with fewer side effects and longer half-lives, have been suggested as alternatives. A study by Connor et al. (1997) examined the use of nadolol in the treatment of overt aggression in 12 developmentally delayed youths aged 13–24 years. Seven of the 12 participants received nadolol exclusively. In this open, prospective pilot study, 10 of the 12 patients showed improvement in observer-rated measures of aggression and severity of illness. However, randomized controlled studies are necessary to elucidate the benefit, if any, of this class of medication in pediatric psychiatric populations.

Initiation and Maintenance

Initial workup should include a recent history and physical examination, with particular attention to medical contraindications: asthma, diabetes, bradycardia, heart block, cardiac failure, or hypothyroidism. Fasting blood sugar and glucose tolerance test may be indicated if there is risk of diabetes. An ECG may be considered.

In children and adolescents, the initial dosage of propranolol is 10 mg three times a day, increasing by 10–20 mg every 3–4 days, and pulse and blood pressure should be monitored (minimum pulse 50, blood pressure 80/50). The standard daily dosage range is 10–120 mg for children and 20–300 mg for adolescents, divided into three doses (2–8 mg/kg/day) (Coffey 1990). The short elimination half-life in children (2–3 hours) may necessitate four doses daily. Dose is titrated to clinical effect or side effects. Maximum improvement at a given dose may not be seen for up to 8 weeks. If a β-blocker is to be discontinued, it should be tapered gradually to avoid rebound hypertension and tachycardia. Because β-blockers may alter the blood levels of other medications, caution must be observed when β-blockers (especially propranolol, which is highly protein bound) are used in combination with other agents.

Risks and Side Effects

Side effects of β-blockers are generally the same as in adults. Tiredness, mild hypotension, and bradycardia are the most common. Decreased sexual interest and performance, dysphoria, insomnia, nightmares, or hypoglycemia (in patients with diabetes) may occur.

Naltrexone

Abnormalities of endogenous opioids have been suggested to occur in persons who have autism and in mentally retarded persons who engage in self-injurious behavior. Naltrexone, a potent opiate antagonist, has been found to be effective in the treatment of hyperactivity in autistic children in several double-blind and placebo-controlled studies (M. Campbell et al. 1993; Kolmen et al. 1995, 1997; Willemsen-Swinkels et al. 1995, 1996). Although earlier reports suggested that naltrexone treatment increased social interaction and decreased self-injury in autistic patients, these later controlled studies failed to demonstrate statistical difference from response to placebo in these behaviors. A recent double-blind, placebo-controlled crossover study in autistic children (Feldman et al. 1999) also failed to demonstrate improvement in communication skills with naltrexone in comparison with placebo. However, the study was limited by a short period of assessment per drug (2 weeks). In their randomized, placebo-controlled crossover study of 25 patients with Rett syndrome who received naltrexone, Percy et al. (1994) showed a worsening of motor function and a more rapid progression of the disorder in 40% of the patients receiving naltrexone, compared with none of those receiving placebo.

Two case reports suggest that naltrexone may be of benefit in alcohol dependence in adolescents. Wold and Kaminer (1997) described a decrease in craving and 30 days of abstinence from naltrexone treatment in a 17-year-old youth. Lifrak et al. (1997) reported on two adolescents who experienced decreased craving and either a reduction in drinking days or successful maintenance of abstinence with naltrexone. All of the patients in the above case reports were treated with naltrexone at 50 mg/day. These reports, while anecdotal, suggest that naltrexone may have a place in the treatment of alcohol dependence in adolescents, as it does in adults, although further study is needed.

In doses of 0.5–2.0 mg/kg/day, naltrexone appears to be safe, with only mild side effects noted. No changes in any laboratory measures, ECG, or vital signs have been demonstrated in children or adolescents. Clearly, further controlled trials are needed, but cautious clinical use of naltrexone in patients with severe behavioral symptoms or adolescents with alcohol dependence may be indicated, particularly given its benign side-effect profile in this age group.

Desmopressin

Desmopressin is an analogue of antidiuretic hormone administered as a nasal spray or oral tablet to treat nocturnal enuresis. Desmopressin acts by increasing water absorption in the kidneys, thereby reducing the volume of urine. Onset of action is rapid, and side effects are mild (nasal mucosal dryness or irritation, headache, epistaxis, and nausea) in patients with normal electrolyte regulation. In their review of the literature, Thompson and Rey (1995) concluded that desmopressin is superior to placebo in the treatment of nocturnal enuresis. They further noted that behavioral methods are more effective, and that the relapse rate after cessation of desmopressin is high. Most of the studies cited at the time of their review were of brief duration, usually 2 weeks.

The usual dose is 20–40 μg intranasally at bedtime or 200–400 μg orally. Randomized, double-blind studies have demonstrated that oral desmopressin is just as effective as the intranasal preparation and may be better tolerated (Janknegt et al. 1997; Skoog et al. 1997). Relapse is likely on discontinuation of treatment. Although water intoxication is rare, children should be encouraged to limit fluid intake in the evenings when taking desmopressin.

Electroconvulsive Therapy

Experience in the use of electroconvulsive therapy (ECT) in adolescents is limited, and reports of use in prepubertal children are extremely rare. Rey and Walter (1997) published a review of the literature identifying 60 reports describing 396 patients under 18 years of age who had received ECT. Improvement rates were noted to be 63% for depression, 80% for mania, 42% for schizophrenia, and 80% for catatonia. Although the authors concluded that ECT in adolescents appears to be effective and relatively safe, they noted that many of the published reports were limited by small numbers and lack of consistent diagnostic standardization. No controlled studies were identified.

Psychotherapy

Individual Psychotherapy

All individual therapies have certain common themes (Strupp 1973):

- Relationship with a therapist who is identified as a helping person and who

has some degree of control and influence over the patient
- Instillation of hope and improved morale
- Use of attention, encouragement, and suggestion
- Goals of helping the patient to achieve greater control, competence, mastery, and/or autonomy; to improve coping skills; and to abandon or modify unrealistic expectations of himself or herself, others, and the environment

In the treatment of children, it is essential to consider the patients' environment and family dynamics. In most cases, work with parents and school, and often pediatricians, welfare agencies, courts, or recreation leaders, must accompany individual therapy. The cooperation of parents, and often teachers, is required to maintain the child in treatment and to remove any secondary gain resulting from the symptoms. The therapist must be aware of a patient's level of physical, cognitive, and emotional development in order to understand the symptoms, set appropriate goals, and tailor effective interventions.

Communication With Children and Adolescents

Children are less able to use abstract language than are adults. They use play to express feelings, to narrate past events, to work through trauma, and to express wishes and hopes. It is less threatening and anxiety provoking if the therapist uses the metaphor of the play and bases questions and comments on characters in the play rather than on the child (even if the connection is clear to the therapist). Effective communications are tailored to the child's stage of language, cognitive, and affective development. The therapist must be aware that the vocabulary of some bright and precocious children exceeds their emotional understanding of events and concepts.

Dramatic play with dolls or puppets, drawing, painting, or modeling with clay, as well as questions about dreams, wishes, or favorite stories or television shows, can provide access to children's fantasies, emotions, and concerns. Adolescents may prefer creative writing or more complex expressive art techniques.

The Resistant Child or Adolescent

It is not surprising that many children or adolescents do not cooperate in therapy. Most are brought to treatment by adults. These young patients often do not wish to change themselves or their behaviors and view their parents' and teachers' complaints as unreasonable or unfair. In addition, a child or adolescent may refuse to participate in or may attempt to sabotage therapy for a variety of dynamic reasons (Gardner 1979). Effective interventions are tailored to the cause of the resistance.

A child who is anxious or having difficulty separating from a parent may be helped by initially permitting the parent to remain in the therapy room. When a child or adolescent does not talk, whether from anxiety or opposition, the therapist often addresses this reluctance, either directly or through play. Long silences are not generally helpful and tend to increase anxiety or battles for control. Attractive play materials help to make therapy less threatening and to encourage participation while the therapist builds an alliance. However, the therapist must guard against the danger of sessions becoming mere play or recreation instead of therapy. Gardner (1979) has developed a variety of techniques that incorporate therapeutic activities with storytelling, drama, and game boards. Using behavioral contingencies in therapy also may improve motivation, especially of materially deprived children.

Types of Individual Psychotherapy

Psychodynamic psychotherapies. *Psychodynamically oriented psychotherapy* is grounded in psychoanalytic theory but is more flexible and emphasizes the real relationship with the therapist and the provision of a corrective emotional experience rather than the transference. Frequency is typically once or twice a week, most commonly over a period of 1–2 years, although shorter, time-limited dynamic psychotherapies are also available (Dulcan 1984). Interaction between the parents and the therapist is more active. Goals of therapy include symptom resolution, change in behavior, and return to normal developmental process. Change occurs via transference interpretation and maturation of defenses, catharsis, development of insight, ego strengthening, improved reality testing, and sublimation (Adams 1982). The therapist forms an alliance with the child or adolescent, reassures, promotes controlled regression, identifies feelings, clarifies thoughts and events, makes interpretations, judiciously educates and advises, and acts as an advocate for the patient (Adams 1982).

Supportive therapy. This type of therapy has less ambitious goals than does dynamically oriented psychotherapies and is usually focused on a particular crisis or stressor. The therapist provides support to the patient until a stressor resolves, a developmental crisis has passed, or the patient or environment changes sufficiently so that other adults can take on the supportive role. There is a real relationship with the therapist, who facilitates catharsis and provides understanding and judicious advice.

Time-limited therapy. All of the various models of time-limited therapy have in common a planned, relatively brief duration; a predominant focus on the presenting problem; a high degree of structure and attention to specific, limited goals; and active roles for both therapist and patient. Length of treatment varies among models from several sessions to 6 months. The short duration is used to increase patient motivation, participation, and reliance on resources within the patient's world rather than on the therapist. Theoretical foundations include psychodynamic, crisis, family systems, cognitive, behavioral or social learning and guidance, or educational theories (Dulcan 1984; Dulcan and Piercy 1985).

A model of interpersonal psychotherapy has been modified for depressed adolescents (IPT-A; Mufson et al. 1994). This 12-week treatment focuses on improving interpersonal relationships in the lives of depressed adolescents through role clarification and enhanced communication. This modality has been elaborated in a treatment manual and has demonstrated efficacy in preliminary study. In a 12-week study of adolescents with major depression randomized to either weekly treatment with IPT-A or clinical monitoring, 75% of the patients receiving IPT-A, versus 46% of the patients in the clinical monitoring group, had improved (as evidenced by Hamilton Rating Scale for Depression scores of less than 6) at week 12 compared with the clinical monitoring group (Mufson et al. 1999).

Cognitive-behavioral therapy. The CBT techniques developed for the treatment of depression in adults have been adapted for use in children and adolescents. Studies have demonstrated the benefits of CBT for depression in adolescents (Clarke et al. 1999), for OCD in children and adolescents (March 1995), for posttraumatic stress symptoms in children and adolescents (King et al. 2000; March et al. 1998a), for social phobia in female adolescents (Hayward et al. 2000), and for

school refusal in children and adolescents (King et al. 1998). Caution is needed to ensure that the homework assignments that are an integral part of this therapy are not perceived as aversive when added to homework assigned in school.

Parent Counseling

Parent counseling or guidance is primarily a psychoeducational intervention, conducted in a mental health setting. It may be conducted with a single parent or couple, or in groups. In counseling sessions, parents learn about normal child and adolescent development. Efforts are made to help parents better understand their child and his or her problems and to modify practices that seem to be contributing to the current difficulties (whatever their original cause). The therapist's understanding of the parents' point of view and of the hardships of living with a disturbed child is crucial to the therapist's successful work with the child. For some parents who have serious difficulties of their own, parent counseling may merge into or pave the way for marital therapy or individual treatment of one or more parents.

Behavior Therapy

In behavior therapy, symptoms are viewed as resulting from bad habits, faulty learning, or inappropriate environmental responses to behavior rather than as stemming from unconscious or intrapsychic motivation. Attention is focused on observable behaviors, psychophysiological responses, and self-report statements. Behavioral approaches are characterized by detailed assessment of problematic responses and the environmental conditions that elicit and maintain them, the development of strategies to produce change in the environment and therefore in the patient's behavior, and repeated assessment to evaluate the success of the intervention.

Indications and Efficacy

Behavior therapy is by far the most thoroughly evaluated psychological treatment for children. Maximally effective behavior therapy programs require home and school cooperation, focus on specific target behaviors, and ensure that contingencies follow behavior quickly and consistently.

Behavior therapy is the most effective treatment for simple phobias, for enuresis and encopresis, and for the noncompliant behaviors seen in oppositional defiant disorder and conduct disorder. For youngsters with ADHD, behavior modification can improve both academic achievement and behavior, when specifically targeted. Both punishment (time-out and response cost) and reward components are required. Behavior modification is more effective than medication in improving peer interactions, but skills may need to be taught first. Many youngsters require programs that are consistent, intensive, and prolonged (months to years). A wide variety of other childhood problems, such as motor and vocal tics, trichotillomania, and sleep problems, are treated by behavior modification, either alone or in combination with pharmacotherapy.

Parent Management Training

Effective training packages, based on social learning theory, have been developed for parents of noncompliant, oppositional, and aggressive children (Barkley and Benton 1998; Forehand and McMahon 1981; Patterson 1975; Webster-Stratton 1992, 2000) and delinquent adolescents (Patterson and Forgatch 1987). Such behaviors in children have been found to lead to inappropriately harsh or ineffective parental responses. Through training, parents are taught to give clear instructions, to positively reinforce good behavior, and to use punish-

ment effectively. One frequently used negative contingency is the time-out, so called because it puts the child in a quiet, boring area where there is a time-out from accidental or naturally occurring positive reinforcement. The most powerful parent training programs use a combination of written materials, verbal instruction, and videotapes in social learning principles and contingency management, modeling by the therapist, and behavioral rehearsal of skills to be used.

Classroom Behavior Modification

Techniques for behavior modification in schools include token economies, class rules, and attention to positive behavior, as well as response cost programs in which reinforcers are withdrawn in response to undesirable behavior. Although teachers often resist what they perceive as extra work, an effective program for children with attention and conduct problems required only that teachers observe every 30 minutes whether children were on task and provide verbal feedback (Pelham and Murphy 1986). Reinforcers such as positive recognition or stars on a chart may be dispensed by teachers or more tangible rewards or privileges by parents through the use of daily report cards. Even special education teachers rarely have sophisticated skills in behavior modification, and therapists may need to work closely with teachers and other school staff to develop appropriate programs.

Behavioral Treatment of Specific Symptoms

Behavioral treatments are useful for treating enuresis, encopresis, and certain anxiety disorders in children. Particularly in the case of enuresis or encopresis, an evaluation for other psychiatric disorders and sexual abuse as well as a medical history and physical examination should precede behavioral treatment.

Enuresis. In younger children, especially those who wet only at night, enuresis is largely a consequence of delayed maturation. While waiting for the child to outgrow it, the most useful strategy is to minimize secondary symptoms by discouraging the parents from punishing or ridiculing the child. Older children can be taught to change their own beds, thus reducing expectable negative reactions from parents. A simple monitoring and reward procedure that includes a chart with stars to be exchanged for rewards may be effective for some children who are motivated to stop wetting the bed.

Two additional programs found to be effective in treating nocturnal enuresis are the urine alarm device and dry bed training (DBT). The urine alarm is a conditioning treatment that results in dryness in up to 75% of children (Mikkelsen 2001). The success rate can be increased and relapses minimized by the addition of contingencies for wet and dry nights, diminished gradually once urinary control is achieved (Kaplan et al. 1989). DBT (Azrin et al. 1974) is an equally effective, but somewhat more cumbersome, behavioral program that includes positive practice, contingent response, and the urine alarm in combination.

Children who are secondarily enuretic (having previously been dry) and those who have accompanying psychiatric problems are more difficult to treat. Other interventions may be necessary before they are motivated to participate in or be responsive to behavioral techniques.

Encopresis. The treatment of encopresis is somewhat more complex because encopresis frequently results from chronic constipation and stool withholding, which creates physiological consequences requiring medical treatment. In addition, children with encopresis more commonly have associated psychiatric disorders than do those with enuresis.

Behavioral treatment of encopresis must be integrated into a plan that also includes educational and psychological approaches (Levine 1982). Because encopresis often results in stool retention and impaction, an initial bowel cleanout is sometimes required. This regimen is followed by a bowel "retraining" program using oral mineral oil, a high-roughage diet, ample fluid intake, and a mild suppository. The behavioral program focuses on the development of a regular toileting routine with scheduled positive toilet practicing. Behaviors that progressively approximate the appropriate passing of feces in the toilet are rewarded. Routine pants checks followed by contingent positive or negative response are often included. Administration of enemas by parents is contraindicated, as that alone does not improve bowel function and is toxic to the parent–child relationship.

Anxiety disorders. Desensitization, either in vivo or in fantasy, is the treatment of choice for simple phobias, often supplemented by modeling. The principles and techniques are essentially the same as those used with adults, with modification for developmental level. In vivo desensitization, often combined with contingency management and parent guidance, may be effective in the treatment of school avoidance (school phobia) resulting from separation anxiety disorder.

Behavioral approaches that use exposure plus response prevention (ERP) appear to be effective in the treatment of OCD in children and adolescents. March and colleagues (1994) developed a protocoled, time-limited ERP treatment that has demonstrated therapeutic effect in an open trial with children and adolescents with OCD.

Behavioral Medicine Techniques

Behavioral methods can be used to treat somatic symptoms. These interventions should be carried out in collaboration with the primary physician and any necessary medical specialists. Children are just as sensitive as adults are to implications that their symptoms are not "real," so care must be taken to explain the interaction of psychological processes and physical symptoms and to develop a working alliance.

Family Treatment

Attempts to treat children and adolescents without considering the persons with whom they live and the patients' relationships with other significant persons are doomed to failure. Any change in one family member, whether resulting from a psychiatric disorder, psychiatric treatment, a normal developmental process, or an outside event, is likely to produce change in other family members and in their relationships. Family constellations vary widely from the traditional nuclear family, to single-parent family, a blended or step-family, an adoptive or foster family, or a group home. The term *parents* in this chapter applies to adults filling the parenting role, whatever their actual relationship to the patient.

Evaluation of Families

Data should be gathered on each person living with the patient, as well as on others who may be important or have been so in the past (e.g., noncustodial parents, grandparents, siblings who are no longer living at home). It is often useful to have at least one session that includes all significant family members. For families with young children, techniques such as the use of family drawings or puppet play or the assignment of family tasks to be carried out in the session are often useful. A variety of schemas exist by which to assess a family's structure and dynamic functioning.

The family's developmental stage offers a clue to predictable transitional crises as children are born, become adolescents, and are launched from the nuclear family (Carter and McGoldrick 1980).

Family Therapy

Family therapy addresses primarily the interaction *among* family members rather than the processes *within* an individual. In the most general sense, family therapy is psychological treatment conducted with an identified patient and at least one biological or functional (i.e., by marriage, adoption, and so forth) family member. Related techniques include therapy with an individual patient that takes a family systems perspective or therapy sessions with family members other than the identified patient, based on noncompliance with treatment, severity of illness, or other factors. These days, it is rare for family therapists to insist that all family members attend sessions.

Family therapy may be particularly useful when there are dysfunctional interactions or impaired communication within the family, especially when these appear to be related to the presenting problem. It also may be useful when symptoms seem to have been precipitated by difficulty with a developmental stage for an individual or the family or by a change in the family such as divorce or remarriage. If more than one family member is symptomatic, family therapy may be both more efficient and more effective than multiple individual treatments. Family therapy should be considered when one family member improves with treatment but another, not in treatment, worsens. In any case, the family must have, or be induced to have, sufficient motivation to participate. When the identified patient is relatively unmotivated to participate or to change, family therapy is likely to be more effective than individual therapy. Attention to family systems issues also may be useful when progress is blocked in individual therapy or in behavior therapy.

Family therapy is contraindicated as a sole treatment method in cases of clearly organic physical or mental illness or if the family equilibrium is precarious and one or more family members are at serious risk of decompensation. In these situations, family therapy may be useful in combination with other treatments, such as medication or hospitalization. It is counterproductive to include in family therapy sessions a patient who is acutely psychotic, violent, or delusional regarding the family. Family sessions may not be helpful when a parent has severe, intractable, or minimally relevant psychopathology or when the child strongly prefers individual treatment. Children should not be included in sessions in which parents persist (despite redirection) in criticizing the children or in sharing inappropriate information, when the most critical need is marital therapy, or when parents primarily need specific, concrete help with practical affairs.

A variety of family therapies are considered when treating children and adolescents (Table 20–4).

TABLE 20–4. Models of family therapy

Structural
Behavioral
Multigenerational
Psychoeducational
Strategic
Multiple family group

Group Therapy

Indications

Group therapy is particularly appropriate for children, who are often more willing to reveal their thoughts and feelings to peers than to adults. Establishing rewarding social relationships, a crucial developmental task for children of all ages, is especially difficult for those youths with a psychiatric disorder. Group therapy offers unparalleled opportunities for the clinician to evaluate youths' behavior with peers, to model and facilitate practice of important skills, and to provide youngsters with companionship and mutual support. Interventions by peers may be far more acute and powerful in their effect than those by an adult therapist. An additional benefit is the larger number of patients who can benefit from limited therapist time.

Target symptoms include absent or conflictual peer relationships, aggression, withdrawal, timidity, difficulty with separation, and deficient social interactive or problem-solving skills. These problems often are not apparent or accessible to intervention in individual therapy sessions. Group therapy can be a powerful modality in the treatment of adolescents with eating disorders or substance abuse.

Group psychotherapy is contraindicated for those who are acutely psychotic, paranoid, or actively suicidal. Adolescents who have sociopathic traits or behaviors should not be included in groups with teenagers who might be victimized or intimidated. Severely aggressive or hyperactive children probably should not be included in outpatient groups because of the difficulty in controlling their behavior, the contagion of problem behaviors, and the risk of intimidating less assertive children. Groups should *not* be used as a repository for unmotivated, nonverbal, difficult patients.

Hospital and Residential Treatment

Indications

Because children should be treated in the setting that is least restrictive and disruptive to their lives, hospital or residential treatment is indicated only in emergencies or for youngsters who have not responded to efforts at outpatient treatment because of severity of the disorder, lack of motivation, resistance, or disorganization of patients and/or family. Programs vary widely in their criteria for admission.

Placement in a residential treatment center may be indicated for children and adolescents with chronic behavior problems such as aggression, running away, truancy, substance abuse, school phobia, or self-destructive acts that the family, foster home, and/or community cannot manage or tolerate. Some parents harbor negative attitudes toward their children or adolescents or have severe psychopathology of their own. Children for whom it is not advisable to return home—because of factors in the youngsters, their families, or both—may be referred to a residential treatment center following a hospital stay. Because of the increase in managed care environments, admission criteria have been restricted and lengths of stay have been substantially reduced.

Short-term hospitalization is more often an acute event, stemming from immediate physical danger to self or others, acute psychosis, a crisis in the environment that reduces the ability of the caregiving adults to cope with the child or adolescent, or the need for more intensive, systematic, and detailed evaluation and observation of the patient and family than is possible on an outpatient basis or in a day program. Managed care pressures have forced hospital lengths of stay to decrease significantly, often allowing only clinical stabilization of the patient before his or her discharge from the hospital. Briefer hospitalizations of severely ill child psychiatric patients require a well-coordinated transfer to less intense and restrictive levels of care in the clinical continuum (residential, day, and intensive outpatient treatments) to enhance clinical stability.

Longer-term hospitalization may be indicated for those patients who do not improve sufficiently in a brief period and who continue to require a secure setting and intensive treatment.

Differences in Settings

Residential treatment centers, compared with hospital units, tend to be longer term, tend to be more open to and integrated with the community, and tend not to use the medical model. Usually, residential centers have a lower staff-to-patient ratio and less highly trained personnel. These centers are more likely to be organized based on a family group model and organized by sections or cottages.

Inpatient units for children can be classified according to the usual length of stay on such units. The lengths of stay on brief-stay or crisis intervention units average 3–10 days. These units emphasize rapid evaluation, triage, stabilization, and development of a treatment plan that will be implemented on an outpatient basis or in another facility. Stays on intermediate units last several weeks to months, and more definitive treatment can be conducted. Children may stay on long-term units from several months to longer than 1 year. On these units, care for the most severely impaired youth is provided. Increasing financial pressures have resulted in reduced overall lengths of stay in all types of units.

Treatment Planning

Ideally, hospitalization forms part of a comprehensive continuum of care for children. With ever-shorter lengths of stay, rapid and efficient planning and execution of evaluation and treatment strategies are essential. The goal is not to eliminate all psychopathology but to address the "focal problem" that precipitated hospitalization and then to discharge the patient to home, residential treatment, or foster placement, where he or she can receive outpatient or day treatment (Harper 1989).

Day Treatment

A day program (also called *partial hospitalization*) may be best for the child who requires more intensive intervention than can be provided in outpatient visits but who is able to live at home. Day treatment is less disruptive to the patient and family than hospitalization or residential placement and can offer an opportunity for more intensive work with parents, who may even attend the program on a regular basis. A day program may be used as a transition for a child who has been hospitalized or to avert a hospitalization. It may be implemented in combination with placement in a foster or group home.

Adjunctive Treatments

At times, an intervention that is not a psychiatric treatment may be recommended as part of a treatment plan. These programs may be crucial for the child's well-being and/or the treatment of the psychiatric disorder, or they may be facilitative, speeding progress or improving level of function.

Parent Support Groups

Parents of children with psychiatric disorders, together with mental health professionals and teachers, have established groups that provide education and support for parents, as well as advocacy for services and fundraising for research. National organizations with local chapters include Parents Anonymous, for abusive or potentially abusive parents; the Association for Retarded Citizens; the Autism Society of America; Children and Adults with Attention Deficit/Hyperactivity Disorder (CHADD); and the Learning Disabilities Association of America. The National Alliance for the Mentally Ill (NAMI) established a Child and Adolescent Network (NAMI-CAN) as its concerns broadened to include children and adolescents. Local groups focused on a particular disorder or on more generic issues can provide a powerful adjunct to direct clinical services. The Child and Adolescent Bipolar Foundation is a new addition, offering resources to parents and professionals at its web site (www.bpkids.org).

Special Education

Modified school programs are indicated for those children who cannot perform satisfactorily in regular classrooms or who need special structure or teaching techniques to reach their academic potential. These programs range in intensity from tutoring or resource classrooms several hours a week to special classrooms in mainstream schools to public or private schools that serve only children with special educational needs. Resources differ from community to community, but most communities have programs for mentally retarded youth, for those with learning disabilities (specific developmental disorders), and for those whose emotional and/or behavioral problems require a special setting for learning or for the control of their behavior. Classes are small, with a high teacher-to-student ratio and teachers who are specially trained.

Foster Care

Placement in a foster home may be needed when parents are unwilling or unable to care for a child. Indications are clearest in cases of physical neglect or physical or sexual abuse. Other families may be unable to provide the appropriate emotional or physical environment. Court intervention is required for placement. Although foster placement can be a suitable and effective intervention, children in foster care may have a variety of unmet physical, developmental, and mental health needs, often making foster care less than optimal and clearly unsatisfactory as a long-term solution (Rosenfeld et al. 1997).

References

Abbott Laboratories: Press Release: Focus on Cylert, 1996

Abnormal Involuntary Movement Scale (AIMS). Psychopharmacol Bull 24:781–783, 1988

Achenbach TM: Manual for the Teacher's Report Form and 1991 Profile. Burlington, VT, University of Vermont, Department of Psychiatry, 1991

Adams PL: A Primer of Child Psychotherapy, Second Edition. Boston, MA, Little, Brown, 1982

Aman MG, Marks RE, Turbott SH, et al: Clinical effects of methylphenidate and thioridazine in intellectually subaverage children. J Am Acad Child Adolesc Psychiatry 30:246–256, 1991

Ambrosini PJ: A review of pharmacotherapy of major depression in children and adolescents. Psychiatr Serv 51:627–633, 2000

Ambrosini PJ, Wagner KD, Biederman J, et al: Multicenter open-label sertraline study in adolescent outpatients with major depression. J Am Acad Child Adolesc Psychiatry 38:566–572, 1999

Anderson LT, Campbell M, Adams P, et al: The effects of haloperidol on discrimination learning and behavioral symptoms in autistic children. J Autism Dev Disord 19:227–239, 1989

Armenteros JL, Whitaker AH, Welikson M, et al: Risperidone in adolescents with schizophrenia: an open pilot study. J Am Acad Child Adolesc Psychiatry 36:694–700, 1997

Arredondo DE: Bupropion treatment of adolescent depression. Scientific Proceedings of the 146th Meeting of the American Psychiatric Association, San Francisco, CA, May 1993

Azrin NH, Sneed TJ, Foxx RM: Dry-bed training: rapid elimination of childhood enuresis. Behav Res Ther 12:147–156, 1974

Barkley RA, Benton CM: Your Defiant Child. New York, Guilford, 1998

Barrickman LL, Perry PJ, Allen AJ, et al: Bupropion versus methylphenidate in the treatment of attention-deficit hyperactivity disorder. J Am Acad Child Adolesc Psychiatry 34:649–657, 1995

Bastiaens L: Knowledge, expectations and attitudes of hospitalized children and adolescents in psychopharmacological treatment. J Child Adolesc Psychopharmacol 3:157–171, 1992

Bastiaens L: Compliance with pharmacotherapy in adolescents: effects of patients' and parents' knowledge and attitudes toward treatment. J Child Adolesc Psychopharmacol 5:39–48, 1995

Bastiaens L, Bastiaens DK: A manual of psychiatric medications for teenagers. J Child Adolesc Psychopharmacol 3:M1–M59, 1993

Bates GDL, Khin-Maung-Zaw F: Movement disorder with fluoxetine. J Am Acad Child Adolesc Psychiatry 37:14–15, 1998

Bernstein GA, Garfinkel BD, Borchardt CM: Comparative studies of pharmacotherapy for school refusal. J Am Acad Child Adolesc Psychiatry 29:773–781, 1990

Biederman J: Clonazepam in the treatment of prepubertal children with panic-like symptoms. J Clin Psychiatry 48 (suppl):38–41, 1987

Biederman J, Wilens T, Mick E, et al: Pharmacotherapy of attention-deficit/hyperactivity disorder reduces risk for substance use disorder. Pediatrics 104:E20, 1999

Birmaher B, Quintana H, Greenhill LL: Methylphenidate treatment of hyperactive autistic children. J Am Acad Child Adolesc Psychiatry 27:248–251, 1988

Birmaher B, Greenhill LL, Cooper TB, et al: Sustained release methylphenidate: pharmacokinetic studies in ADHD males. J Am Acad Child Adolesc Psychiatry 28: 768–772, 1989

Birmaher B, Waterman GS, Ryan N, et al: Fluoxetine for childhood anxiety disorders. J Am Acad Child Adolesc Psychiatry 33: 993–999, 1994

Black B, Robbins DR: Case study: panic disorder in children and adolescents. J Am Acad Child Adolesc Psychiatry 29:36–44, 1989

Boyle SF: SSRIs and movement disorders. J Am Acad Child Adolesc Psychiatry 38: 354–355, 1999

Broderick-Cantwell JJ: Case study: accidental clonidine patch overdose in attention-deficit/hyperactivity disorder patients. J Am Acad Child Adolesc Psychiatry 38:95–98, 1999

Brown RT, Sexson SB: Effects of methylphenidate on cardiovascular responses in attention deficit hyperactivity disordered adolescents. Journal of Adolescent Health Care 10:179–183, 1989

Bruggeman R, van der Linden C, Buitelaar JK, et al: Risperidone versus pimozide in Tourette's disorder: a comparative double-blind parallel-group study. J Clin Psychiatry 62:50–56, 2001

Bruun RD, Budman CL: Risperidone as a treatment for Tourette's disorder. J Clin Psychiatry 57:29–31, 1996

Bryden KE, Carrey NJ, Kutcher SP: Update and recommendations for the use of antipsychotics in early onset psychoses. J Child Adolesc Psychopharmacol 11:113–130, 2001

Buitelaar JK, van der Gaag RJ, van der Hoeven J: Buspirone in the management of anxiety and irritability in children with pervasive developmental disorders: results of an open-label study. J Clin Psychiatry 59:56–59, 1998

Buitelaar JK, van der Gaag RJ, Cohen-Kettenis P, et al: A randomized controlled trial of risperidone in the treatment of aggression in hospitalized adolescents with subaverage cognitive abilities. J Clin Psychiatry 62:239–248, 2001

Campbell M, Small AM, Green WH, et al: Behavioral efficacy of haloperidol and lithium carbonate. Arch Gen Psychiatry 41:650–656, 1984

Campbell M, Green WH, Deutsch SI: Child and Adolescent Psychopharmacology. Beverly Hills, CA, Sage, 1985

Campbell M, Silva RR, Kafantaris V, et al: Predictors of side effects associated with lithium administration in children. Psychopharmacol Bull 27:373–380, 1991

Campbell M, Anderson LT, Small AM, et al: Naltrexone in autistic children: behavioral symptoms and attentional learning. J Am Acad Child Adolesc Psychiatry 32:1283–1291, 1993

Campbell M, Adams PB, Small AM, et al: Lithium in hospitalized aggressive children with conduct disorder: a double-blind and placebo-controlled study. J Am Acad Child Adolesc Psychiatry 34:445–453, 1995

Campbell SB: Hyperactivity in preschoolers: correlates and prognostic implications. Clin Psychol Rev 5:405–428, 1985

Cantwell DP, Swanson J, Connor DF: Case study: adverse response to clonidine. J Am Acad Child Adolesc Psychiatry 36:539–544, 1997

Carlson GA, Rapport MD, Kelly KL, et al: The effects of methylphenidate and lithium on attention and activity level. J Am Acad Child Adolesc Psychiatry 31:262–270, 1992

Carter E, McGoldrick M (eds): The Family Life Cycle: A Framework for Family Therapy. New York, Gardner, 1980

Chappell PB, Riddle MA, Scahill L, et al: Guanfacine treatment of comorbid attention-deficit hyperactivity disorder and Tourette's syndrome: preliminary clinical experience. J Am Acad Child Adolesc Psychiatry 34:1140–1146, 1995

Clarke GN, Rohde P, Lewinsohn PM, et al: Cognitive-behavioral treatment of adolescent depression: efficacy of acute group treatment and booster sessions. J Am Acad Child Adolesc Psychiatry 38:272–279, 1999

Clein PD, Riddle MA: Pharmacokinetics in children and adolescents. Child Adolesc Psychiatr Clin N Am 4:59–75, 1995

Coffey BJ: Anxiolytics for children and adolescents: traditional and new drugs. J Child Adolesc Psychopharmacol 1:57–83, 1990

Coffey BJ, Shader RI, Greenblatt DJ: Pharmacokinetics of benzodiazepines and psychostimulants in children. J Clin Psychopharmacol 3:217–225, 1983

Cohen DJ, Riddle MA, Leckman JF: Pharmacotherapy of Tourette's syndrome and associated disorders. Psychiatr Clin North Am 15:109–129, 1992

Compton SN, Grant PJ, Chrisman AK, et al: Sertraline in children and adolescents with social anxiety disorder: an open trial. J Am Acad Child Adolesc Psychiatry 40:564–571, 2001

Conners CK: Methodological and assessment issues in pediatric psychopharmacology, in Diagnosis and Psychopharmacology of Childhood and Adolescent Disorders. Edited by Wiener JM. New York, Wiley, 1985, pp 69–110

Conners CK, Barkley RA: Rating scales and checklists for child psychopharmacology. Psychopharmacol Bull 21:816–832, 1985

Conners CK, Casat CD, Gualtieri CT, et al: Bupropion hydrochloride in attention deficit disorder with hyperactivity. J Am Acad Child Adolesc Psychiatry 35:1314–1321, 1996

Connor DF, Ozbayrak KR, Benjamin S, et al: A pilot study of nadolol for overt aggression in developmentally delayed individuals. J Am Acad Child Adolesc Psychiatry 36:826–834, 1997

Connor DF, Fletcher KE, Swanson JM: A meta-analysis of clonidine for symptoms of attention-deficit hyperactivity disorder. J Am Acad Child Adolesc Psychiatry 38:1551–1559, 1999

Daviss WB, Bentivoglio P, Racusin R, et al: Bupropion sustained release in adolescents with comorbid attention-deficit/hyperactivity disorder and depression. J Am Acad Child Adolesc Psychiatry 40:307–314, 2001

DeVeaugh-Geiss J, Moroz G, Biederman J, et al: Clomipramine hydrochloride in childhood and adolescent obsessive-compulsive disorder: a multicenter trial. J Am Acad Child Adolesc Psychiatry 31:45–49, 1992

Diler RS, Avci A: SSRI-induced mania in obsessive-compulsive disorder. J Am Acad Child Adolesc Psychiatry 38:6–7, 1999

Dulcan MK: Brief psychotherapy with children and their families: the state of the art. J Am Acad Child Adolesc Psychiatry 23:544–551, 1984

Dulcan MK, Lizarralde C (eds): Helping Parents, Youths and Teachers Understand Medications for Emotional and Behavioral Problems: A Resource Book of Medication Information Handouts, 2d Edition. Washington, DC, American Psychiatric Press, 2002

Dulcan MK, Piercy PA: A model for teaching and evaluating brief psychotherapy with children and their families. Professional Psychology: Research and Practice 16:689–700, 1985

Edelbrock CS: Child Attention Profile, in Attention-Deficit Hyperactivity Disorder: A Clinical Workbook. Edited by Barkley RA. New York, Guilford, 1991

Elia J, Borcherding BG, Rapoport JL, et al: Methylphenidate and dextroamphetamine treatments of hyperactivity: are there true nonresponders? Psychiatry Res 36:141–155, 1991

Emslie GJ, Ruch AJ, Weinberg WA, et al: A double-blind, randomized, placebo-controlled trial of fluoxetine in children and adolescents with depression. Arch Gen Psychiatry 54:1031–1037, 1997

Ernst M, Magee HJ, Gonzalez NM, et al: Pimozide in autistic children. Psychopharmacol Bull 28:187–191, 1992

Evans RW, Clay TH, Gualtieri CT: Carbamazepine in pediatric psychiatry. J Am Acad Child Psychiatry 26:2–8, 1987

Faigel HC: The effect of beta blockade on stress-induced cognitive dysfunction in adolescents. Clin Pediatr (Phila) 30:441–445, 1991

Fairbanks JM, Pine DS, Tancer NK, et al: Open fluoxetine treatment of mixed anxiety disorders in children and adolescents. J Child Adolesc Psychopharmacol 7:17–29, 1997

Famularo R, Kinscherff R, Fenton T: Propranolol treatment for childhood posttraumatic stress disorder, acute type. Am J Dis Child 142:1244–1247, 1988

Feeney DJ, Klykylo W: Risperidone and tardive dyskinesia. J Am Acad Child Adolesc Psychiatry 35:1421–1422, 1996

Feldman HM, Kolmen BK, Gonzaga AM: Naltrexone and communication skills in young children with autism. J Am Acad Child Adolesc Psychiatry 38:587–593, 1999

Fetner HH, Geller B: Lithium and tricyclic antidepressants. Psychiatr Clin North Am 15:223–241, 1992

Findling RL, Grcevich SJ, Lopez I, et al: Antipsychotic medications in children and adolescents. J Clin Psychiatry 57 (suppl 9): 19–23, 1996

Findling RL, Schulz SC, Reed MD, et al: The antipsychotics: a pediatric perspective. Pediatr Clin North Am 45:1025–1032, 1998

Findling RL, McNamara NK, Branicky LA, et al: A double-blind pilot study of risperidone in the treatment of conduct disorder. J Am Acad Child Adolesc Psychiatry 39:509–516, 2000

Fisman S, Steele M: Use of risperidone in pervasive developmental disorders: a case series. J Child Adolesc Psychopharmacol 6: 177–190, 1996

Fitzpatrick PA, Klorman F, Brumaghim JT, et al: Effects of sustained-release and standard preparations of methylphenidate on attention deficit disorder. J Am Acad Child Adolesc Psychiatry 31:226–234, 1992

Flockhart DA, Oesterheld JR: Cytochrome P450-mediated drug interactions. Child Adolesc Psychiatr Clin N Am 9:43–76, 2000

Forehand RL, McMahon RJ: Helping the Noncompliant Child: A Clinician's Guide to Parent Training. New York, Guilford, 1981

Frazier JA, Gordon CT, McKenna M, et al: An open trial of clozapine in 11 adolescents with childhood-onset schizophrenia. J Am Acad Child Adolesc Psychiatry 33:658–663, 1994

Gadow KD: Effects of stimulant drugs on academic performance in hyperactive and learning disabled children. Journal of Learning Disabilities 16:290–299, 1983

Gadow KD: Pediatric psychopharmacology: a review of recent research. J Child Psychol Psychiatry 33:153–195, 1992

Gadow KD, Sverd J, Sprafkin J, et al: Efficacy of methylphenidate for attention deficit hyperactivity disorder in children with tic disorder. Arch Gen Psychiatry 52:444–455, 1995

Gardner RA: Helping children cooperate in therapy, in Basic Handbook of Child Psychiatry, Vol 3: Therapeutic Interventions. Edited by Harrison SI. New York, Basic Books, 1979, pp 414–433

Garland EJ, Smith DH: Case study: panic disorder on a child psychiatric consultation service. J Am Acad Child Adolesc Psychiatry 29:785–788, 1990

Geller B, Cooper TB, Chestnut EC, et al: Preliminary data on the relationship between nortriptyline plasma level and response in depressed children. Am J Psychiatry 143: 1283–1286, 1986

Geller B, Cooper TB, Zimerman B, et al: Lithium for prepubertal depressed children with family history predictors of future bipolarity: a double-blind, placebo-controlled study. J Affect Disord 51:165–175, 1998

Geller B, Reising D, Leonard HL, et al: Critical review of tricyclic antidepressant use in children and adolescents. J Am Acad Child Adolesc Psychiatry 38:513–516, 1999

Geller DA, Hoog SL, Heiligenstein JH, et al: Fluoxetine treatment for obsessive compulsive disorder in children and adolescents: a placebo-controlled clinical trial. J Am Acad Child Adolesc Psychiatry 40: 773–779, 2001

Genton P, Bauer J, Duncan S, et al: On the association between valproate and polycystic ovary syndrome. Epilepsia 42:305–310, 2001

Gill M, LoVecchio F, Selden B: Serotonin syndrome in a child after a single dose of fluvoxamine. Ann Emerg Med 33:457–459, 1999

Gittelman R, Klein DF, Feingold I: Children with reading disorders, II: effects of methylphenidate in combination with reading remediation. J Child Psychol Psychiatry 24:193–212, 1983

Gittelman-Klein R, Klein DF: Controlled imipramine treatment of school phobia. Arch Gen Psychiatry 25:204–207, 1971

Gittelman-Klein R, Klein DF: School phobia: diagnostic considerations in the light of imipramine effects. J Nerv Ment Dis 156:199–215, 1973

Glassman AH, Bigger JT: Antipsychotic drugs: prolonged QTc interval, torsade de pointes, and sudden death. Am J Psychiatry 158:1774–1782, 2001

Golwyn DH, Sevlie CP: Phenelzine treatment of selective mutism in four prepubertal children. J Child Adolesc Psychopharmacol 9:109–113, 1999

Good CR, Feaster CS, Krecko VF: Tolerability of oral loading of divalproex sodium in child psychiatry inpatients. J Child Adolesc Psychopharmacol 11:53–57, 2001

Gordon CT, State RC, Nelson JE, et al: A double-blind comparison of clomipramine, desipramine, and placebo in the treatment of autistic disorder. Arch Gen Psychiatry 50:441–447, 1993

Graae F, Milner J, Rizzotto L, et al: Clonazepam in childhood anxiety disorders. J Am Acad Child Adolesc Psychiatry 333:372–376, 1994

Grcevich SJ, Findling RL, Rowane WA, et al: Risperidone in the treatment of children and adolescents with schizophrenia: a retrospective study. J Child Adolesc Psychopharmacol 6:251–257, 1996

Greenhill LL: Attention-deficit hyperactivity disorder. Child Adolesc Psychiatr Clin N Am 4:123–168, 1995

Greenhill LL, Puig-Antich J, Chambers W, et al: Growth hormone, prolactin, and growth responses in hyperkinetic males treated with D-amphetamine. J Am Acad Child Adolesc Psychiatry 20:84–103, 1981

Greenhill LL, Puig-Antich J, Novacenko H, et al: Prolactin, growth hormone and growth responses in boys with attention deficit disorder and hyperactivity treated with methylphenidate. J Am Acad Child Adolesc Psychiatry 23:58–67, 1984

Greenhill LL, Solomon M, Pleak R, et al: Molindone hydrochloride treatment of hospitalized children with conduct disorder. J Clin Psychiatry 46:20–25, 1985

Grubbs JH: SSRI-induced mania. J Am Acad Child Adolesc Psychiatry 36:445, 1997

Guile JM: Sertraline-induced behavioral activation during the treatment of an adolescent with major depression. J Child Adolesc Psychopharmacol 6:281–285, 1996

Hagerman RJ, Murphy MA, Wittenberg MD: A controlled trial of stimulant medication in children with the fragile X syndrome. Am J Med Genet 30:377–392, 1988

Handen BL, Feldman H, Gosling A, et al: Adverse side effects of methylphenidate among mentally retarded children with ADHD. J Am Acad Child Adolesc Psychiatry 30:241–245, 1991

Handen BL, Feldman HM, Jurier A, et al: Efficacy of methylphenidate among preschool children with developmental disabilities and ADHD. J Am Acad Child Adolesc Psychiatry 38:944–951, 1999

Hardan A, Johnson K, Johnson C, et al: Case study: risperidone treatment of children and adolescents with developmental disorders. J Am Acad Child Adolesc Psychiatry 35: 1551–1556, 1996

Harper G: Focal inpatient treatment planning. J Am Acad Child Adolesc Psychiatry 28: 31–37, 1989

Hayward C, Varady S, Albano AM, et al: Cognitive-behavioral group therapy for social phobia in female adolescents: results of a pilot study. J Am Acad Child Adolesc Psychiatry 39:721–726, 2000

Herskowitz J: Developmental neurotoxicology, in Psychiatric Pharmacosciences of Children and Adolescents. Edited by Popper C. Washington, DC, American Psychiatric Press, 1987, pp 81–123

Horrigan JP, Barnhill LJ: Guanfacine for treatment of attention-deficit hyperactivity disorder in boys. J Child Adolesc Psychopharmacol 5:215–223, 1995

Horrigan JP, Barnhill LJ: Risperidone and explosive aggressive autism. J Autism Dev Disord 27:313–323, 1997

Hunt RD, Capper S, O'Connell P: Clonidine in child and adolescent psychiatry. J Child Adolesc Psychopharmacol 1:87–102, 1990

Hunt RD, Lau S, Ryu J: Alternative therapies for ADHD, in Ritalin: Theory and Patient Management. Edited by Greenhill LL, Osman BB. New York, Mary Ann Liebert, 1991, pp 75–95

Hunt RD, Arnsten AF, Asbell MD: An open trial of guanfacine in the treatment of attention-deficit hyperactivity disorder. J Am Acad Child Adolesc Psychiatry 34: 50–54, 1995

Isojarvi JI, Laatikainen TJ, Pakarinen AJ, et al: Polycystic ovaries and hyperandrogenism in women taking valproate for epilepsy. N Engl J Med 329:1383–1388, 1993

Janknegt RA, Zweers HMM, Delaere KPJ, et al: Oral desmopressin as a new treatment modality for primary nocturnal enuresis in adolescents and adults: a double-blind, randomized, multicenter study. J Urol 157:513–517, 1997

Jatlow PI: Psychotropic drug disposition during development, in Psychiatric Pharmacosciences of Children and Adolescents. Edited by Popper C. Washington, DC, American Psychiatric Press, 1987, pp 27–44

Jensen PS, Hinshaw SP, Kraemer HC, et al: ADHD comorbidity findings from the MTA study: comparing comorbid subgroups. J Am Acad Child Adolesc Psychiatry 40:147–158, 2001

Jones-Fearing KB: SSRI and EPS with fluoxetine. J Am Acad Child Adolesc Psychiatry 35:1107–1108, 1996

Joorabchi B: Expressions of the hyperventilation syndrome in childhood. Clin Pediatr (Phila) 16:1110–1115, 1977

Kaplan SL, Breit M, Gauthier B, et al: A comparison of three nocturnal enuresis treatment methods. J Am Acad Child Adolesc Psychiatry 28:282–286, 1989

Keller MB, Ryan ND, Strober M, et al: Efficacy of paroxetine in the treatment of adolescent major depression: a randomized, controlled trial. J Am Acad Child Adolesc Psychiatry 40:762–772, 2001

King NJ, Tonge BJ, Heyne D, et al: Cognitive-behavioral treatment of school-refusing children: a controlled evaluation. J Am Acad Child Adolesc Psychiatry 37:395–403, 1998

King NJ, Tonge BJ, Mullen P, et al: Treating sexually abused children with posttraumatic stress symptoms: a randomized clinical trial. J Am Acad Child Adolesc Psychiatry 39:1347–1355, 2000

Klein RG, Koplewicz HS, Kanner A: Imipramine treatment of children with separation anxiety disorder. J Am Acad Child Adolesc Psychiatry 31:21–28, 1992

Kolmen BK, Feldman HM, Handen BL, et al: Naltrexone in young autistic children: a double-blind, placebo-controlled crossover study. J Am Acad Child Adolesc Psychiatry 34:223–231, 1995

Kolmen BK, Feldman HM, Handen BL, et al: Naltrexone in young autistic children: replication study and learning measures. J Am Acad Child Adolesc Psychiatry 36: 1570–1578, 1997

Kowatch RA, Suppes T, Carmody TJ, et al: Effect size of lithium, divalproex sodium, and carbamazepine in children and adolescents with bipolar disorder. J Am Acad Child Adolesc Psychiatry 39:713–720, 2000

Krener PK, Mancina RA: Informed consent or informed coercion? Decision-making in pediatric psychopharmacology. J Child Adolesc Psychopharmacol 4:183–200, 1994

Krishanmoorthy J, King BH: Open-label olanzapine treatment in five preadolescent children. J Child Adolesc Psychopharmacol 8:107–113, 1998

Kumra S, Frazier JA, Jacobsen LK, et al: Child-onset schizophrenia: a double-blind clozapine-haloperidol comparison. Arch Gen Psychiatry 53:1090–1097, 1996

Kumra S, Jacobsen LK, Lenane M, et al: Childhood-onset schizophrenia: an open-label study of olanzapine in adolescents. J Am Acad Child Adolesc Psychiatry 37:377–385, 1998

Kutcher SP, MacKenzie S, Galarraga W, et al: Clonazepam treatment of adolescents with neuroleptic-induced akathisia. Am J Psychiatry 144:823–824, 1987

Kutcher SP, Williamson P, MacKenzie S, et al: Successful clonazepam treatment of neuroleptic-induced akathisia in older adolescents and young adults: a double-blind, placebo-controlled study. J Clin Psychopharmacol 9:403–406, 1989

Kutcher SP, Reiter S, Gardner DM, et al: The pharmacotherapy of anxiety disorders in children and adolescents. Psychiatr Clin North Am 15:41–67, 1992

Law SF, Schachar RJ: Do typical clinical doses of methylphenidate cause tics in children treated for attention-deficit hyperactivity disorder? J Am Acad Child Adolesc Psychiatry 38:40–47, 1999

Leckman JF, Ort S, Caruso KA, et al: Rebound phenomena in Tourette's syndrome after abrupt withdrawal of clonidine: behavioral, cardiovascular, and neurochemical effects. Arch Gen Psychiatry 43:1168–1176, 1986

Lee DO, Lee CD: Serotonin syndrome in a child associated with erythromycin and sertraline. Pharmacotherapy 19:894–896, 1999

Lenti C: Movement disorders associated with fluvoxamine. J Am Acad Child Adolesc Psychiatry 38:942–943, 1999

Leonard HL, Swedo SE, Rapoport JL, et al: Treatment of obsessive-compulsive disorder with clomipramine and desipramine in children and adolescents: a double-blind crossover comparison. Arch Gen Psychiatry 46:1088–1092, 1989

Levine MD: Encopresis: its potentiation, evaluation and alleviation. Pediatr Clin North Am 29:315–330, 1982

Lewis O: Psychological factors affecting pharmacologic compliance. Child Adolesc Psychiatr Clin North Am 4:15–22, 1995

Lifrak PD, Alterman AI, O'Brien CP, et al: Naltrexone for alcoholic adolescents. Am J Psychiatry 154:439–440, 1997

Lipinski F, Mallya G, Zimmerman P, et al: Fluoxetine-induced akathisia: clinical and theoretical implications. J Clin Psychiatry 50:339–342, 1989

Lombroso PJ, Scahill L, King RA, et al: Risperidone treatment of children and adolescents with chronic tic disorders: a preliminary report. J Am Acad Child Adolesc Psychiatry 34:1147–1152, 1995

Malone RP, Delaney MA, Luebbert JF, et al: A double-blind placebo-controlled study of lithium in hospitalized aggressive children and adolescents with conduct disorder. Arch Gen Psychiatry 57:649–654, 2000

Malone RP, Cataer J, Sheikh RM, et al: Olanzapine versus haloperidol in children with autistic disorder: an open pilot study. J Am Acad Child Adolesc Psychiatry 40:887–894, 2001

Mandoki M: Olanzapine in the treatment of early onset schizophrenia in children and adolescents. Biol Psychiatry 41:22S, 1997

Mandoki MW, Tapia MR, Tapia MA, et al: Venlafaxine in the treatment of children and adolescents with major depression. Psychopharmacol Bull 33:149–154, 1997

March JS: Cognitive-behavioral psychotherapy for children and adolescents with OCD: a review and recommendations for treatment. J Am Acad Child Adolesc Psychiatry 34:7–18, 1995

March JS, Mulle K, Herbel B: Behavioral psychotherapy for children and adolescents with obsessive-compulsive disorder: an open trial of a new protocol-driven treatment package. J Am Acad Child Adolesc Psychiatry 33:333–341, 1994

March JS, Amaya-Jackson L, Murray MC, et al: Cognitive-behavioral psychotherapy for children and adolescents with post-traumatic stress disorder after a single-incident stressor. J Am Acad Child Adolesc Psychiatry 37:585–593, 1998a

March JS, Biederman J, Wolkow R, et al: Sertraline in children and adolescents with obsessive-compulsive disorder: a multicenter randomized controlled trial. JAMA 280:1752–1756, 1998b

Martin A, Koenig K, Scahill L, et al: Open-label quetiapine in the treatment of children and adolescents with autistic disorder. J Child Adolesc Psychopharmacol 9:99–107, 1999

Masi G, Cosenza A, Mucci M: Open trial of risperidone in 24 young children with pervasive developmental disorders. J Am Acad Child Adolesc Psychiatry 40:1206–1214, 2001

McConville BJ, Minnery KL, Sorter, MT, et al: An open study of the effects of sertraline on adolescent major depression. J Child Adolesc Psychopharmacol 6:41–51, 1996

McDougle CJ, Holmes JP, Bronson MR, et al: Risperidone treatment of children and adolescents with pervasive developmental disorders: a prospective open-label study. J Am Acad Child Adolesc Psychiatry 36:685–693, 1997

Mikkelsen EJ: Enuresis and encopresis: ten years of progress. J Am Acad Child Adolesc Psychiatry 40:1146–1158, 2001

Mikkelsen EJ, Detlor J, Cohen DJ: School avoidance and social phobia triggered by haloperidol in patients with Tourette's disorder. Am J Psychiatry 138:1572–1576, 1981

Minnery KL, West SA, McConville BJ, et al: Sertraline-induced mania in an adolescent. J Child Adolesc Psychopharmacol 5:151–153, 1995

Mufson L, Moreau D, Weissman MM, et al: Modification of interpersonal psychotherapy with depressed adolescents (IPT-A): phase I and II studies. J Am Acad Child Adolesc Psychiatry 33:695–705, 1994

Mufson L, Weissman M, Moreau D, et al: Efficacy of interpersonal psychotherapy for depressed adolescents. Arch Gen Psychiatry 56:573–579, 1999

Mullins ME, Horowitz BZ: Serotonin syndrome after a single dose of fluvoxamine (comment). Ann Emerg Med 34:806–807, 1999

Oldroyd J: Paroxetine-induced mania. J Am Acad Child Adolesc Psychiatry 36:721–722, 1997

Olvera RL, Pliszka SR, Luh J, et al: An open trial of venlafaxine in the treatment of attention-deficit/hyperactivity disorder in children and adolescents. J Child Adolesc Psychopharmacol 6:241-250, 1996

Pao M, Tipnis T: Serotonin syndrome after sertraline overdose in a 5-year-old girl. Arch Pediatr Adolesc Med 151:1064–1067, 1997

Papatheodorou G, Kutcher SP, Katic M: The efficacy and safety of divalproex sodium in the treatment of acute mania in adolescents and young adults: an open clinical trial. J Clin Psychopharmacol 15:110–116, 1995

Patterson GR: Families: Applications of Social Learning to Family Life. Champaign, IL, Research Press, 1975

Patterson GR, Forgatch M: Parents and Adolescents Living Together. Eugene, OR, Castalia, 1987

Pelham WE Jr, Murphy HA: Attention deficit and conduct disorders, in Pharmacological and Behavioral Treatment: An Integrative Approach. Edited by Hersen M. New York, Wiley, 1986, pp 108–148

Pelham WE, Gnagy EM, Burrows-Maclean L, et al: Once-a-day Concerta methylphenidate versus three-times-daily methylphenidate in laboratory and natural settings. Pediatrics 107:E105, 2001

Percy AK, Glaze DG, Schultz RJ, et al: Rett syndrome: controlled study of an oral opiate antagonist, naltrexone. Ann Neurol 35:464–470, 1994

Perry R, Pataki C, Monoz-Silva DM, et. Al: Risperidone in children and adolescents with pervasive developmental disorder: pilot trial and follow-up. J Child Adolesc Psychopharmacol 7:167–179, 1997

Pfeffer CR, Jiang H, Domeshek LJ: Buspirone treatment of psychiatrically hospitalized prepubertal children with symptoms of anxiety and moderately severe aggression. J Child Adolesc Psychopharmacol 7:145–155, 1997

Pfefferbaum B, Overall JE, Boron HA, et al: Alprazolam in the treatment of anticipatory and acute situational anxiety in children with cancer. J Am Acad Child Adolesc Psychiatry 26:532–535, 1987

Pleak RR, Birmaher B, Gavrilescu A, et al: Mania and neuropsychiatric excitation following carbamazepine. J Am Acad Child Adolesc Psychiatry 27:500–503, 1988

Pliszka SR: A double-blind, placebo-controlled study of Adderall and methylphenidate in the treatment of attention-deficit/hyperactivity disorder. J Am Acad Child Adolesc Psychiatry 39:619–626, 2000

Pool D, Bloom W, Mielke DH, et al: A controlled evaluation of Loxitane in seventy-five adolescent schizophrenic patients. Curr Ther Res Clin Exp 19:99–104, 1976

Popper CW: Combining methylphenidate and clonidine: pharmacologic questions and news reports about sudden death. J Child Adolesc Psychopharmacol 5:157–166, 1995

Potenza MN, Holmes JP, Kanes SJ, et al: Olanzapine treatment of children, adolescents, and adults with pervasive developmental disorders: an open-label pilot study. J Clin Psychopharmacol 19:37–44, 1999

Preskorn SH, Weller EB, Hughes CW, et al: Depression in prepubertal children: dexamethasone nonsuppression predicts differential response to imipramine versus placebo. Psychopharmacol Bull 23:128–133, 1987

Quintana H, Keshavan M: Case study: risperidone in children and adolescents with schizophrenia. J Am Acad Child Adolesc Psychiatry 34:1292–1296, 1995

Rapoport JL: Antidepressants in childhood attention deficit disorder and obsessive-compulsive disorder. Psychosomatics 27 (suppl):30–36, 1986

Ratey J, Sovner R, Parks A, et al: Buspirone treatment of aggression and anxiety in mentally retarded patients: a multiple-baseline, placebo lead-in study. J Clin Psychiatry 52:159–162, 1991

Realmuto GM, Erickson WD, Yellin AM, et al: Clinical comparison of thiothixene and thioridazine in schizophrenic adolescents. Am J Psychiatry 141:440–442, 1984

Realmuto GM, August GJ, Garfinkel BD: Clinical effect of buspirone in autistic children. J Clin Psychopharmacol 9:122–125, 1989

Reischer H, Pfeffer CR: Lithium pharmacokinetics. J Am Acad Child Adolesc Psychiatry 35:130–131, 1996

Reiter S, Kutcher SP: Disinhibition and anger outbursts in adolescents treated with clonazepam (letter). J Clin Psychopharmacol 11:268, 1991

Remschmidt H, Schultz E, Martin M: An open trial of clozapine in thirty-six adolescents with schizophrenia. J Child Adolesc Psychopharmacol 4:31–41, 1994

Remschmidt H, Hennighausen K, Clement HW, et al: Atypical neuroleptics in child and adolescent psychiatry. Eur Child Adolesc Psychiatry: 9(suppl 1):I9–I19, 2000

Rey JM, Walter G: Half a century of ECT use in young people. Am J Psychiatry 154:595–602, 1997

Richardson MA, Haugland G, Craig TJ: Neuroleptic use, parkinsonian symptoms, tardive dyskinesia, and associated factors in child and adolescent psychiatric patients. Am J Psychiatry 148:1322–1328, 1991

Richters JE, Arnold E, Jensen PS, et al: NIMH Collaborative Multisite Multimodal Treatment Study of Children with ADHD, I: background and rationale. J Am Acad Child Adolesc Psychiatry 34:987–1000, 1995

Riddle MA, Nelson JC, Kleinman CS, et al: Sudden death in children receiving Norpramin: a review of three reported cases and commentary. J Am Acad Child Adolesc Psychiatry 30:104–108, 1991

Riddle MA, Geller B, Ryan N: Another sudden death in a child treated with desipramine. J Am Acad Child Adolesc Psychiatry 32:792–797, 1993

Riddle MA, Reeve, EA, Yaryura-Tobias JA, et al: Fluvoxamine for children and adolescents with obsessive-compulsive disorder: a randomized, controlled, multicenter trial. J Am Acad Child Adolesc Psychiatry 40:222–229, 2001

Riggs PD, Leon SL, Mikulich SK, et al: An open trial of bupropion for ADHD in adolescents with substance use disorders and conduct disorder. J Am Acad Child Adolesc Psychiatry 37:1271–1278, 1998

Rosenberg DR, Stewart CM, Fitzgerald KD, et al: Paroxetine open-label treatment of pediatric outpatients with obsessive-compulsive disorder. J Am Acad Child Adolesc Psychiatry 38:1180–1185, 1999

Rosenfeld AA, Pilowsky DJ, Fine P, et al: Foster care: an update. J Am Acad Child Adolesc Psychiatry 36:448–457, 1997

Ryan ND: Heterocyclic antidepressants in children and adolescents. J Child Adolesc Psychopharmacol 1:21–31, 1990

Ryan ND: The pharmacologic treatment of child and adolescent depression. Psychiatr Clin North Am 15:29–40, 1992

Ryan ND, Meyer V, Dachille S, et al: Lithium antidepressant augmentation in TCA-refractory depression in adolescents. J Am Acad Child Adolesc Psychiatry 27:371–376, 1988a

Ryan ND, Puig-Antich J, Rabinovich H, et al: MAOIs in adolescent major depression unresponsive to tricyclic antidepressants. J Am Acad Child Adolesc Psychiatry 27:755–758, 1988b

Safer DJ: Changing patterns of psychotropic medications prescribed by child psychiatrists in the 1990s. J Child Adolesc Psychopharmacol 7:267–274, 1997

Safer DJ, Zito JM, Gardner JF: Pemoline hepatotoxicity and postmarketing surveillance. J Am Acad Child Adolesc Psychiatry 40:622–629, 2001

Sallee F, Rock CM: Effects of pimozide on cognition in children with Tourette syndrome: interaction with comorbid attention-deficit hyperactivity disorder. Acta Psychiatr Scand 90:4–9, 1994

Sallee F, Stiller R, Perel J, et al: Targeting imipramine dose in children with depression. Clin Pharmacol Ther 40:8–13, 1986

Sallee FR, Kurlan R, Goetz CG, et al: Ziprasidone treatment of children and adolescents with Tourette syndrome: a pilot study. J Am Acad Child Adolesc Psychiatry 39:292–299, 2000

Samuel RZ: EPS with lithium (letter). J Am Acad Child Adolesc Psychiatry 32:1078, 1993

Sanchez LE, Campbell M, Small AM: A pilot study of clomipramine in young autistic children. J Am Acad Child Adolesc Psychiatry 35:537–544, 1996

Saul RC: Nortriptyline in attention deficit disorder. Clin Neuropharmacol 8:382–384, 1985

Scahill L, Chappell PB, Kim YS, et al: A placebo-controlled study of guanfacine in the treatment of children with tic disorders and attention deficit hyperactivity disorder. Am J Psychiatry 158:1067–1074, 2001

Sholevar EH, Baron DA, Hardie TL: Treatment of childhood-onset schizophrenia with olanzapine. J Child Adolesc Psychopharmacol 10:69–78, 2000

Silva RR, Munoz DM, Alpert M, et al: Neuroleptic malignant syndrome in children and adolescents. J Am Acad Child Adolesc Psychiatry 38:187–194, 1999

Silver LB: Alternative (nonstimulant) medications in the treatment of attention-deficit/hyperactivity disorder in children. Pediatr Clin North Am 46:965–975, 1999

Silverstein FS, Boxer L, Johnson MV: Hematological monitoring during therapy with carbamazepine in children. Ann Neurol 13:685–686, 1983

Simeon JG, Ferguson HB: Recent developments in the use of antidepressant and anxiolytic medications. Psychiatr Clin North Am 8:893–907, 1985

Simeon JG, Ferguson HB, Knott V, et al: Clinical, cognitive, and neurophysiological effects of alprazolam in children and adolescents with overanxious and avoidant disorders. J Am Acad Child Adolesc Psychiatry 31:29–33, 1992

Simeon JG, Knott VJ, Dubois C, et al: Buspirone therapy of mixed anxiety disorders in childhood and adolescence: a pilot study. J Child Adolesc Psychopharmacol 4:159–170, 1994

Skoog SJ, Stokes A, Turner K: Oral desmopressin: a randomized double-blind placebo controlled study of effectiveness in children with primary nocturnal enuresis. J Urol 158:1035–1040, 1997

Soni P, Weintraub AL: Case study: buspirone-associated mental status changes. J Am Acad Child Adolesc Psychiatry 31:1098–1099, 1992

Spencer EK, Kafantaris V, Padron-Gayol MV, et al: Haloperidol in schizophrenic children: early findings from a study in progress. Psychopharmacol Bull 28:183–186, 1992

Spencer T, Biederman J, Steingard R, et al: Bupropion exacerbates tics in children with attention-deficit hyperactivity disorder and Tourette's syndrome. J Am Acad Child Adolesc Psychiatry 32:211–214, 1993

Spencer T, Biederman J, Harding M, et al: Growth deficits in ADHD children revisited: evidence for disorder-associated growth delays? J Am Acad Child Adolesc Psychiatry 35:1460–1469, 1996

Spirko BA, Wiley JF 2d: Serotonin syndrome: a new pediatric intoxication. Pediatr Emerg Care 15:440–443, 1999

Sprague RL, Sleator EK: Methylphenidate in hyperkinetic children: differences in dose effects on learning and social behavior. Science 198:1274–1276, 1977

Steingard R, Biederman J, Spencer TJ, et al: Comparison of clonidine response in the treatment of attention-deficit hyperactivity disorder with and without comorbid tic disorders. J Am Acad Child Adolesc Psychiatry 32:350–353, 1993

Steingard R, Goldberg M, Lee D, et al: Adjunctive clonazepam treatment of tic symptoms in children with comorbid tic disorders and ADHD. J Am Acad Child Adolesc Psychiatry 33:394–399, 1994

Strober M, Morrell W, Lampert C, et al: Relapse following discontinuation of lithium maintenance therapy in adolescents with bipolar I illness: a naturalistic study. Am J Psychiatry 147:457–461, 1990

Strober M, Freeman R, Rigali J, et al: The pharmacotherapy of depressive illness in adolescence, II: effects of lithium augmentation in nonresponders to imipramine. J Am Acad Child Adolesc Psychiatry 31:16–20, 1992

Strober M, Pataki C, DeAntonio M: Complete remission of 'treatment resistant' severe melancholia in adolescents with phenelzine: two case reports. J Affect Disord 50:55–58, 1998

Strupp HH: Psychotherapy: Clinical, Research, and Theoretical Issues. New York, Jason Aronson, 1973

Swanson JM, Flockhart D, Udrea D, et al: Clonidine in the treatment of ADHD: questions about safety and efficacy. J Child Adolesc Psychopharmacol 5:301–304, 1995

Swanson JM, Wigal S, Greenhill L, et al: Analog classroom assessment of Adderall in children with ADHD. J Am Acad Child Adolesc Psychiatry 37:519–526. 1998a

Swanson J, Wigal S, Greenhill L, et al: Objective and subjective measures of the pharmacodynamic effects of Adderall in the treatment of children with ADHD in a controlled laboratory classroom setting. Psychopharmacol Bull 34:55–60, 1998b

Swanson JM, Connor DF, Cantwell D: Combining methylphenidate and clonidine. J Am Acad Child Adolesc Psychiatry 38:617–619, 1999

Teicher MH, Glod CA: Neuroleptic drugs: indications and guidelines for their rational use in children and adolescents. J Child Adolesc Psychopharmacol 1:33–56, 1990

Thompson S, Rey JM: Functional enuresis: is desmopressin the answer? J Am Acad Child Adolesc Psychiatry 34:266–271, 1995

Thomsen PH: Child and adolescent obsessive-compulsive disorder treated with citalopram: findings from an open trial of 23 cases. J Child Adolesc Psychopharmacol 7:157–166, 1997

Thomsen PH, Ebbesen C, Persson C: Long-term experience with citalopram in the treatment of adolescent OCD. J Am Acad Child Adolesc Psychiatry 40:895–902, 2001

Tierney E, Joshi PT, Llinas JF, et al: Sertraline for major depression in children and adolescents: preliminary clinical experience. J Child Adolesc Psychopharmacol 5:13–27, 1995

Toren P, Laor N, Weizman A: Use of atypical neuroleptics in child and adolescent psychiatry. J Clin Psychiatry 59:644–656, 1998

Trimble MR: Anticonvulsants in children and adolescents. J Child Adolesc Psychopharmacol 1:33–56, 1990

Van Putten T, Marder SR: Behavioral toxicity of antipsychotic drugs. J Clin Psychiatry 48 (suppl):13–19, 1987

Varanka TM, Weller RA, Weller EB, et al: Lithium treatment of manic episodes with psychotic features in prepubertal children. Am J Psychiatry 145:1557–1559, 1988

Varley C, McClellan J: Case study: two additional sudden deaths with tricyclic antidepressants. J Am Acad Child Adolesc Psychiatry 36:390–394, 1997

Vitiello B, Severe JB, Greenhill LL, et al: Methylphenidate dosage for children with ADHD over time under controlled conditions: lessons from the MTA. J Am Acad Child Adolesc Psychiatry 40:188–196, 2001

Walkup JT, Labellarte MJ, Riddle MA, et al: Fluvoxamine for the treatment of anxiety disorders in children and adolescents. N Engl J Med 344:1279–1285, 2001

Walsh BT, Greenhill LL, Elsa-Grace V, et al: Effects of desipramine on autonomic input to the heart. J Am Acad Child Adolesc Psychiatry 38:1186–1193, 1999

Waslick BD, Walsh BT, Greenhill LL, et al: Cardiovascular effects of desipramine in children and adults during exercise testing. J Am Acad Child Adolesc Psychiatry 38:179–186, 1999

Webster-Stratton C: Incredible Years: A Troubleshooting Guide for Parents of Children Aged 3 to 8. Toronto, ON, Canada, Umbrella Press, 1992

Webster-Stratton C: How to Promote Children's Social and Emotional Competence. London, England, Paul Chapman, 2000

Weller EB, Weller RA, Fristad MA: Lithium dosage guide for prepubertal children: a preliminary report. J Am Acad Child Psychiatry 25:92–95, 1986

West SA, Keck PE, McElroy SL: Open trial of valproate in the treatment of adolescent mania. J Child Adolesc Psychopharmacol 4:263–267, 1994

Wilens TE, Biederman J: The stimulants. Psychiatr Clin North Am 15:191–222, 1992

Wilens TE, Spencer TJ: Combining methylphenidate and clonidine. J Am Acad Child Adolesc Psychiatry 38:614–161, 1999

Wilens TE, Biederman J, Baldessarini RJ, et al: Cardiovascular effects of therapeutic doses of tricyclic antidepressants in children and adolescents. J Am Acad Child Adolesc Psychiatry 35:1491–1501, 1996

Wiles CP, Hardin MT, King RA, et al: Antidepressant-induced prolongation of QTc interval on EKG in two children, in Abstracts of the Annual Meeting of the American Academy of Child and Adolescent Psychiatry. Washington, DC, 1991, p 70

Willemsen-Swinkels SHN, Buitelaar JK, Nijhof GJ, et al: Failure of naltrexone hydrochloride to reduce self-injurious and autistic behavior in mentally retarded adults: double-blind placebo-controlled studies. Arch Gen Psychiatry 52:766–773, 1995

Willemsen-Swinkels SH, Buitelaar JK, van Engeland H: The effects of chronic naltrexone treatment in young autistic children: a double-blind placebo-controlled crossover study. Biol Psychiatry 39:1023–1031, 1996

Williams DT, Mehl R, Yudofsky S, et al: The effect of propranolol on uncontrolled rage outbursts in children and adolescents with organic brain dysfunction. J Am Acad Child Psychiatry 21:129–135, 1982

Winsberg BG, Perel JM, Hurwic MJ, et al: Imipramine protein binding and pharmacokinetics in children, in The Phenothiazines and Structurally Related Drugs. Edited by Forrest IS, Carr CJ, Usdin E. New York, Raven, 1974, pp 425–431

Wold M, Kaminer Y: Naltrexone for alcohol abuse. J Am Acad Child Adolesc Psychiatry 36:6–7, 1997

Zahn TP, Rapoport JL, Thompson CL: Autonomic and behavioral effects of dextroamphetamine and placebo in normal and hyperactive prepubertal boys. J Abnorm Child Psychol 8:145–160, 1980

Zuddas A, Di Martino A, Muglia P, et. Al: Long-term risperidone for pervasive developmental disorder: efficacy, tolerability, and discontinuation. J Child Adolesc Psychopharmacol 10:79–90, 2000

Index

Page numbers printed in **boldface** type refer to figures or tables.